PRINCIPLES OF
MEDICAL
BIOCHEMISTRY

PRINCIPLES OF MEDICAL BIOCHEMISTRY

2ND Edition

Gerhard Meisenberg, PhD

Department of Biochemistry
Ross University School of Medicine
Roseau, Commonwealth of Dominica, West Indies

William H. Simmons, PhD

Division of Biochemistry
Department of Cell Biology, Neurobiology, and Anatomy
Loyola University School of Medicine
Maywood, Illinois

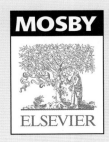

MOSBY

ELSEVIER

1600 John F. Kennedy Blvd.
Ste 1800
Philadelphia, PA 19103-2899

PRINCIPLES OF MEDICAL BIOCHEMISTRY

Notice

Knowledge and best practice in this field are constantly changing. As new research and experience broaden our knowledge, changes in practice, treatment, and drug therapy may become necessary or appropriate. Readers are advised to check the most current information provided (i) on procedures featured or (ii) by the manufacturer of each product to be administered, to verify the recommended dose or formula, the method and duration of administration, and contraindications. It is the responsibility of the practitioner, relying on their own experience and knowledge of the patient, to make diagnoses, to determine dosages and the best treatment for each individual patient, and to take all appropriate safety precautions. To the fullest extent of the law, neither the Publisher nor the Authors assume any liability for any injury and/or damage to persons or property arising out of or related to any use of the material contained in this book.

The Publisher

Library of Congress Cataloging-in-Publication Data
Meisenberg, Gerhard.
    Principles of medical biochemistry / Gerhard Meisenberg, William H. Simmons.—2nd ed.
      p. ; cm.
    Includes bibliographical references and index.
    ISBN-13: 978-0-323-02942-1   ISBN-10: 0-323-02942-6
    1. Biochemistry. 2. Clinical biochemistry. I. Simmons, William H., Ph.D. II. Title.
    [DNLM: 1. Biochemistry. 2. Molecular Biology. QU 34 M515p 2006]
    QP514.2.M45 2006
    612'.015—dc22   2005047921

    ISBN-13: 978-0-323-02942-1
    ISBN-10: 0-323-02942-6

Acquisitions Editor: Alexandra Stibbe
Developmental Editor: Rebecca Gruliow
Publishing Services Manager: Tina K. Rebane
Senior Project Manager: Linda Lewis Grigg
Design Direction: Steven Stave
Cover Designer: Steven Stave
Cover Art: Copyright Photographer/Visuals Unlimited
Cover Images: Lamda repressor and DNA; Plasmids or bacterial DNA, TEM X100,000; Scanning tunneling microscope view of DNA SEM *E. coli*; Bacterial DNA spilling from *E. coli*, TEM X7850; Confocal image of cells at various stages of mitosis.

Printed in China

Last digit is the print number: 9 8 7 6 5 4 3

Preface

It is rumored that among students embarking on a course of study in the medical sciences, biochemistry is the most common cause of pretraumatic stress disorder: the state of mind into which people fall in anticipation of unbearable stress and frustration. No other part of their preclinical curriculum seems as abstract, shapeless, unintelligible, and littered with irrelevant detail as is biochemistry. This prejudice is understandable. Biochemistry is indeed a vast field with an ever-expanding frontier. From embryonic development to carcinogenesis and drug action, biochemistry is becoming the ultimate level of explanation in the medical sciences.

This second edition of *Principles of Medical Biochemistry* is our second attempt at imposing structure and meaning on the blooming, buzzing confusion of this runaway science. We are targeting the same audience as we did with the first edition: first-year medical students, as well as veterinary, dental, and pharmacy students; and students in undergraduate premedical programs.

Despite the ever-increasing importance of biochemistry for the medical sciences, we did not match the increased volume of knowledge in the field by an increased size of the book. Although a biochemistry text must be sufficiently comprehensive to cover all the important topics that are customarily covered in a medical biochemistry course, it can be effective only if it is concise enough for day-to-day use by the students. Therefore we designed the book as a compromise between these two conflicting demands.

This compromise was possible because medical biochemistry is not a random cross-section of the general biochemistry that is taught in undergraduate courses and Ph.D. programs. Biochemistry for the medical professions is "physiological" chemistry: the chemistry needed to understand the structure and functions of the body and their malfunction in disease. Therefore we chose both the topics and their didactic presentation according to their importance for normal and abnormal function of the human body, rather than according to abstract theoretical interest. Thus we paid little attention to details of protein conformation and enzymatic reaction mechanisms, but there are thorough treatments of medically important topics such as lipoprotein metabolism, mutagenesis and genetic diseases, the molecular basis of cancer, nutritional disorders, and the hormonal regulation of metabolic pathways.

In this new edition, we arranged the chapters into only three sections. There is an introductory section (Part One) that deals with the essentials of molecular structure, acid-base relationships, and enzymatic reactions. This is followed by a section (Parts Two, Three, and Four) about molecular biology that includes not only DNA and gene expression, but also chapters about cell and tissue structure, hormones, the cell cycle, and molecular mechanisms of carcinogenesis. The third and last section (Part Five) is about metabolism. Since the time of the first edition, the greatest advances in biochemistry were those related to the human genome. Genomics and proteomics are only now beginning to shed light on the normal workings of the human body and the derangements that we see in diseases. Therefore the most substantial changes in this new edition are in the chapters about molecular genetics. But other fields have seen advances as well, and therefore the whole text has been thoroughly revised and brought up to date.

As in the first edition, there are practice questions at the end of each chapter and case studies at the end of the book. The case study section has been expanded to give a broader and more representative coverage of biochemically interesting diseases. We placed increased emphasis on the case studies because learning medical biochemistry consists of two equally important processes. First, the fundamental principles have to be learned in a systematic way, as extensions of what the students know already; and in parallel with this, the general principles have to be linked to the practice of medicine to become part of the student's clinical reasoning routines. Clinical case studies are essential for this latter purpose.

Contents

PRINCIPLES OF MOLECULAR STRUCTURE AND FUNCTION

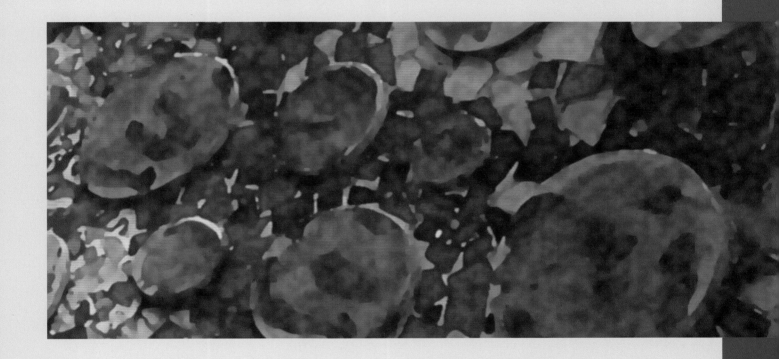

CHAPTER 1

Introduction to Biomolecules

The first question facing the student of biochemistry is this: What is the human body made of? Table 1.1 shows the approximate composition of the proverbial 75-kg textbook adult. Next to water, **proteins** and **triglycerides** are most abundant. The amount of triglycerides is variable, depending on the amount of adipose tissue, and most of it is optional. But proteins are a major component of all tissues and are absolutely essential for cell structure and function. **Carbohydrates** are far less abundant than proteins. Some serve structural functions; others, especially glucose and the storage polysaccharide glycogen, are important sources of metabolic energy. Soluble **inorganic salts** are present in both the intracellular and extracellular fluids, and insoluble salts, most of them related to calcium phosphate, give strength and rigidity to human bones.

This chapter introduces the principles of molecular structure, the types of noncovalent interactions between biomolecules, and the structural features of the major classes of biomolecules.

Water Is the Solvent of Life

Charles Darwin speculated that life originated in a warm little pond. Perhaps it really was a big warm ocean, but one thing is sure: Humans are extremely watery creatures. Almost two thirds of the human body is water (see Table 1.1). The structure of water is simplicity itself, with two hydrogen atoms bonded to an oxygen atom at an angle of 105°:

$$H \overset{O}{\underset{105°}{\diagup\diagdown}} H$$

Water is a lopsided molecule, with its binding electron pairs displaced toward the oxygen atom. This provides the oxygen atom with a high electron density, whereas the hydrogen atoms are electron deficient. The oxygen atom is said to have a partial negative charge (δ^-), and the hydrogen atoms have partial positive charges (δ^+). Therefore, the water molecule forms an electrical **dipole:**

$$\delta^+ \; H \overset{\delta^-}{\underset{}{\diagup O \diagdown}} H \; \delta^+ \qquad \begin{array}{l} \uparrow \text{ negative pole} \\ \downarrow \text{ positive pole} \end{array}$$

Unlike charges attract each other. Therefore, the hydrogen atoms of a water molecule are attracted by the oxygen atoms of other water molecules, forming **hydrogen bonds:**

These hydrogen bonds are weak. No more than 29 kJ, or 7 kcal, are needed to break a hydrogen bond in water, although the breaking of a covalent oxygen-hydrogen bond in the water molecule requires 450 kJ (110 kcal).* Breaking the hydrogen bonds requires no more than heating the water to 100° C. *The hydrogen bonds determine the physical properties of water*, including its boiling point.

The water in the human body always contains inorganic **cations** (positively charged ions), such as

---

*1 kcal = 4.18 kJ.

Table 1.1 Approximate Composition of a 75-kg Adult

Substance	Content (%)
Water	60
Inorganic salt, soluble	0.7
Inorganic salt, insoluble*	5.5
Protein	16
Triglyceride (fat)†	13
Membrane lipids	2.5
Carbohydrates	1.5
Nucleic acids	0.2

* In bones.
† In adipose tissue.

Table 1.2 Typical Ionic Compositions of Extracellular (Interstitial) and Intracellular (Cytoplasmic) Fluids

Ion	Concentration (mmol/liter) in	
	Extracellular Fluid	Cytoplasm
Na^+	137	10
K^+	4.7	141
Ca^{2+}	2.4	10^{-4}*
Mg^{2+}	1.4	31
Cl^-	113	4
$HPO_4^{2-}/H_2PO_4^-$	2	11
HCO_3^-	28†	10†
Organic acids, phosphate esters	1.8	100
pH	7.4	6.5-7.5

* Cytoplasmic concentration. Concentrations in mitochondria and endoplasmic reticulum are much higher.
† The lower HCO_3^- concentration in the intracellular space is caused by the lower intracellular pH, which affects the equilibrium $HCO_3^- + H^+ \rightleftharpoons H_2CO_3 \rightleftharpoons CO_2 + H_2O$.

sodium and potassium, and **anions** (negatively charged ions), such as chloride and phosphate. Table 1.2 shows the typical ionic compositions of intracellular (cytoplasmic) and extracellular (interstitial) fluid. Interestingly, the extracellular fluid has an ionic composition similar to that of seawater. It is a warm little pond that we carry with us so that we can live outside the place of birth.

Predictably, the cations are attracted to the oxygen atom of the water molecule, whereas the anions are attracted to the hydrogen atoms. The **ion-dipole interactions** thus formed are the forces that hold the components of soluble salts in solution, as in the case of sodium chloride (table salt):

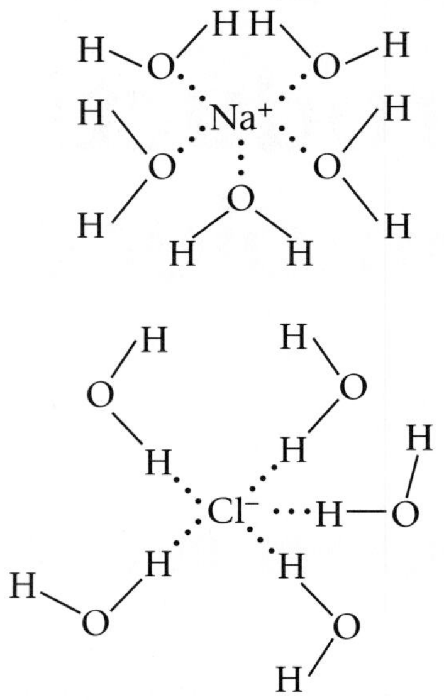

The calcium phosphates in human bones are not soluble because the **electrostatic interactions** (**"salt bonds"**) between the anions and cations in the crystal structure are stronger than their ion-dipole interactions with water.

Water Contains Hydronium Ions and Hydroxyl Ions

Water molecules dissociate reversibly into hydroxyl ions and hydronium ions:

1 $$H_2O + H_2O \rightleftharpoons \underset{\substack{\text{Hydronium} \\ \text{Ion}}}{H_3O^+} + \underset{\substack{\text{Hydroxyl} \\ \text{ion}}}{OH^-}$$

In pure water, only about one in 5 million molecules is in the H_3O^+ or OH^- form:

2 $$[H_3O^+] = [OH^-] = 10^{-7}\,\text{mol}$$

These concentrations are expressed as molar concentrations (mol/liter, mol/L, or M). *One mole of a substance is its molecular weight in grams.* Water has a molecular weight close to 18; therefore 18 g of water are 1 mol. The hydronium ion concentration $[H_3O^+]$ is usually expressed as the **proton concentration**, or the **hydrogen ion concentration** [**H⁺**], regardless of the fact that the proton is actually riding on the free electron pair of a water molecule.

In aqueous solutions, the product of proton (hydronium ion) concentration and hydroxyl ion concentration is a constant:

3 $$[H^+] \times [OH^-] = 10^{-14}\,\text{mol}^2$$

Table 1.3 Relationship Among pH, [H⁺], and [OH⁻]

pH	[H⁺]*	[OH⁻]*
4	10^{-4}	10^{-10}
5	10^{-5}	10^{-9}
6	10^{-6}	10^{-8}
7	10^{-7}	10^{-7}
8	10^{-8}	10^{-6}
9	10^{-9}	10^{-5}
10	10^{-10}	10^{-4}

* [H⁺] and [OH⁻] are measured in mol/liter (M).

The proton concentration [H⁺], otherwise measured in moles per liter, is more commonly expressed as the **pH value;** the negative logarithm of the hydrogen ion concentration:

4
$$pH = -\log[H^+]$$

With equations (3) and (4), the H⁺ and OH⁻ concentrations can be predicted at any given pH value (Table 1.3).

The pH value of an aqueous solution depends on the presence of **acids** and **bases.** According to the **Brønsted definition,** in aqueous solutions *an acid is a substance that releases a proton, and a base is a substance that binds a proton.* The prototypical acidic group is the **carboxyl group,** which is the distinguishing feature of the organic acids:

Carboxylic acid   Carboxylate anion
(protonated form)   (deprotonated form)

The protonation-deprotonation reaction is reversible, and therefore the carboxylate anion fits the definition of a Brønsted base. It is called the **conjugate base** of the acid.

Amino groups are the major basic groups in biomolecules. In this case, the amine is the base and the ammonium salt is the **conjugate acid:**

Amine   Ammonium salt
(deprotonated form)   (protonated form)

Carboxyl groups, phosphate esters, and **phosphodiesters** are the most important acidic groups in biomolecules. They are deprotonated and negatively charged at pH 7. **Sulfhydryl groups** and **phenolic hydroxyl groups** are weakly acidic. They lose their proton only at pH values well above 7. **Aliphatic** (nonaromatic) **amino groups,** including the primary, secondary, and tertiary amines, are basic. They are protonated and positively charged at pH 7. **Aromatic amines** are weakly basic. They become protonated only at pH values well below 7.

Ionizable Groups Are Characterized by Their pK Values

The equilibrium of a protonation/deprotonation reaction is described by the **dissociation constant (K_D).** For the reaction

$$R{-}COOH \rightleftharpoons R{-}COO^- + H^+$$

the dissociation constant K_D is defined as

5
$$K_D = \frac{[R{-}COO^-] \times [H^+]}{[R{-}COOH]}$$

This can be rearranged to

6
$$[H^+] = K_D \times \frac{[R{-}COOH]}{[R{-}COO^-]}$$

The molar concentrations in this equation are the concentrations observed at equilibrium. Because the hydrogen ion concentration [H⁺] is most conveniently expressed as the pH value, it is possible to convert equation (6) into the negative logarithm:

7
$$pH = pK - \log\frac{[R{-}COOH]}{[R{-}COO^-]}$$
$$= pK + \log\frac{[R{-}COO^-]}{[R{-}COOH]}$$

This equation is called the **Henderson-Hasselbalch equation,** and *the pK value is defined as the negative logarithm of the dissociation constant.* The pK value is a property of an ionizable group. If a molecule has more than one ionizable group, then it has more than one pK value.

In the Henderson-Hasselbalch equation, pK is a constant, whereas [R—COOH]/[R—COO⁻] changes with the pH. When, for example, the pH value equals the pK value, log[R—COOH]/[R—COO⁻] must equal zero. Therefore, [R—COOH]/[R—COO⁻] must equal one. Thus, *the pK value corresponds to the*

Table 1.4 Protonation State of a Carboxyl Group and an Amino Group at Different pH Values

	Carboxyl Group		Amino Group	
pH	% of Group Protonated (R—COOH)	% of Group Deprotonated (R—COO⁻)	% of Group Protonated (R—NH₃⁺)	% of Group Deprotonated (R—NH₂)
$pK + 3$	0.1	99.9	0.1	99.9
$pK + 2$	1	99	1	99
$pK + 1$	10	90	10	90
pK	50	50	50	50
$pK - 1$	90	10	90	10
$pK - 2$	99	1	99	1
$pK - 3$	99.9	0.1	99.9	0.1

pH value at which the ionizable group is half-protonated. The pK value is a measure for the "strength" of an acidic or basic group. At pH values below their pK (high [H⁺], high acidity), ionizable groups are mainly protonated; at pH values above their pK (low [H⁺], high alkalinity) they are mainly deprotonated (Table 1.4).

Bonds Are Formed by Reactions between Functional Groups

More than a million chemically different molecules are present in the human body, most of them **macromolecules** ("large" molecules) with molecular weights exceeding 10,000 D. Fortunately, students need not memorize them all. Despite their size and complexity, most biomolecules contain only 3 to 6 different elements out of the 92 that are listed in the periodic table. Carbon (C), hydrogen (H), and oxygen (O) are always present. Nitrogen (N) is present in many biomolecules, and sulfur (S) and phosphorus (P) are present in some. The atoms within a molecule are held together by **covalent bonds.** Covalent bonds are produced by the sharing of electrons between the participating atoms.

Biomolecules contain a limited number of **functional groups,** which determine their physical properties and chemical reactivities. These groups are summarized in Table 1.5. Macromolecules are produced by **condensation reactions** between the functional groups of smaller molecules. In these reactions, two functional groups link up while releasing water. The bonds can be cleaved again by the addition of water. This is called **hydrolysis.** The most important bond types are listed in Table 1.6.

Bond formation is an **endergonic** (energy-requiring) process. This implies that *the construction of large molecules from small ones requires metabolic*

Table 1.5 Functional Groups in Biomolecules

1. Hydrocarbon groups
   —CH₃   Methyl
   —CH₂—CH₃   Ethyl
   —CH₂—   Methylene
   —CH=   Methine
2. Oxygen-containing groups
   R—OH   Hydroxyl (alcoholic)
   ⟩—OH   Hydroxyl (phenolic)
   C=O   Keto ⎤
   —C⟨H   Aldehyde ⎦ Carbonyl
   —C⟨O / OH   Carboxyl
3. Nitrogen-containing groups
   —NH₂   Primary amine
   ⟩NH   Secondary amine
   ⟩N—   Tertiary amine
   —N⁺—   Quaternary ammonium salt
4. Sulfur-containing group
   —SH   Sulfhydryl group

energy. Conversely, bond cleavage by hydrolysis is **exergonic** and releases energy. The digestive enzymes, for example, which catalyze hydrolytic bond cleavages (see Chapter 14), work perfectly well in the lumen of the gastrointestinal tract, where neither adenosine triphosphate (ATP) nor other usable energy sources are available.

Some bonds contain more energy than others. Most ester, ether, acetal, and amide bonds require

Table 1.6 Important Bonds in Biomolecules

Bond	Structure	Formed from	Occurs in
Ether	$R_1\!-\!O\!-\!R_2$	$R_1\!-\!OH + HO\!-\!R_2$	Methyl ethers, some membrane lipids
Carboxylic ester	$R_1\!-\!\overset{\overset{\displaystyle O}{\|\|}}{C}\!-\!O\!-\!R_2$	$R_1\!-\!\overset{\overset{\displaystyle O}{\|\|}}{C}\!-\!OH + HO\!-\!R_2$	Triglycerides, other lipids
Acetal	$R_2\!-\!O$, $O\!-\!R_3$ on C with R_1 and H	$R_2\!-\!O$; $R_1\!-\!\overset{\overset{\displaystyle O}{\|\|}}{C}\!-\!OH + HO\!-\!R_3$ (H)	Disaccharides, oligosaccharides, and polysaccharides (glycosidic bonds)
Mixed anhydride*	$R\!-\!\overset{\overset{\displaystyle O}{\|\|}}{C}\!-\!O\!-\!\overset{\overset{\displaystyle O^-}{\|}}{\underset{\underset{\displaystyle O}{\|\|}}{P}}\!-\!O^-$	$R\!-\!\overset{\overset{\displaystyle O}{\|\|}}{C}\!-\!OH + HO\!-\!\overset{\overset{\displaystyle O^-}{\|}}{\underset{\underset{\displaystyle O}{\|\|}}{P}}\!-\!O^-$	Some metabolic intermediates
Phosphoanhydride*	$R\!-\!O\!-\!\overset{\overset{\displaystyle O^-}{\|}}{\underset{\underset{\displaystyle O}{\|\|}}{P}}\!-\!O\!-\!\overset{\overset{\displaystyle O^-}{\|}}{\underset{\underset{\displaystyle O}{\|\|}}{P}}\!-\!O^-$	$R\!-\!O\!-\!\overset{\overset{\displaystyle O^-}{\|}}{\underset{\underset{\displaystyle O}{\|\|}}{P}}\!-\!OH + HO\!-\!\overset{\overset{\displaystyle O^-}{\|}}{\underset{\underset{\displaystyle O}{\|\|}}{P}}\!-\!O^-$	Nucleotides; most important: ATP
Phosphate ester	$R\!-\!O\!-\!\overset{\overset{\displaystyle O^-}{\|}}{\underset{\underset{\displaystyle O}{\|}}{P}}\!-\!O^-$	$R\!-\!OH + HO\!-\!\overset{\overset{\displaystyle O^-}{\|}}{\underset{\underset{\displaystyle O}{\|}}{P}}\!-\!O^-$	Many metabolic intermediates, phosphoproteins
Phosphodiester	$R_1\!-\!O\!-\!\overset{\overset{\displaystyle O^-}{\|}}{\underset{\underset{\displaystyle O}{\|}}{P}}\!-\!O\!-\!R_2$	$R_1\!-\!OH + HO\!-\!\overset{\overset{\displaystyle O^-}{\|}}{\underset{\underset{\displaystyle O}{\|}}{P}}\!-\!OH + HO\!-\!R_2$	Nucleic acids, phospholipids
Unsubstituted amide	$R\!-\!\overset{\overset{\displaystyle O}{\|\|}}{C}\!-\!NH_2$	$R\!-\!\overset{\overset{\displaystyle O}{\|\|}}{C}\!-\!OH + H\!-\!N\overset{\displaystyle H}{\underset{\displaystyle H}{}}$	Asparagine, glutamine
Substituted amide	$R_1\!-\!\overset{\overset{\displaystyle O}{\|\|}}{C}\!-\!\underset{\underset{\displaystyle H}{\|}}{N}\!-\!R_2$	$R_1\!-\!\overset{\overset{\displaystyle O}{\|\|}}{C}\!-\!OH + H\!-\!\underset{\underset{\displaystyle H}{\|}}{N}\!-\!R_2$	Polypeptides (peptide bond)
Thioester*	$R_1\!-\!\overset{\overset{\displaystyle O}{\|\|}}{C}\!-\!S\!-\!R_2$	$R_1\!-\!\overset{\overset{\displaystyle O}{\|\|}}{C}\!-\!OH + HS\!-\!R_2$	Acetyl-CoA, other "activated" acids
Thioether	$R_1\!-\!S\!-\!R_2$	$R_1\!-\!SH + HO\!-\!R_2$	Methionine

ATP, adenosine triphosphate; CoA, coenzyme A.
* "Energy-rich" bonds.

between 1 and 5 kcal/mol for their formation, and the same amount of energy is released during their hydrolysis. **Anhydride bonds** and **thioester bonds,** however, have free energy contents above 5 kcal/mol. They are classified, rather arbitrarily, as **energy-rich bonds.**

Isomeric Forms Are Common in Biomolecules

What counts in biochemistry is not composition but geometry. **Isomers** are chemically different molecules with identical composition but different geometry. As shown, there are three different types of isomers:

1. **Positional isomers** differ in the positions of functional groups within the molecule. Examples:

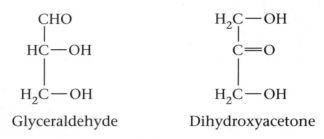

2-Phosphoglycerate   3-Phosphoglycerate

Glyceraldehyde   Dihydroxyacetone

2. **Geometric isomers** differ in the arrangement of substituents at a rigid portion of the molecule. A typical example is *cis-trans* isomers of carbon-carbon double bonds:

cis double bond   *trans* double bond

The two forms are not interconvertible because there is no rotation around the double bond. All substituents (H, R_1, and R_2) are fixed in the same plane. Also, ring systems show geometric isomerism, with substituents sticking out over one or the other surface of the ring. Geometric isomers are called **diastereomers**.

3. **Optical isomers** differ in the orientation of substituents around an **asymmetrical carbon:** a carbon with four *different* substituents. If the molecule has only one asymmetrical carbon, the isomers are mirror images. These mirror-image molecules are called **enantiomers.** They are related to each other in the same way as the left hand and the right hand, and therefore optical isomerism is also called **chirality** (Greek χειρ = "hand").

Unlike positional and geometric isomers, which differ in their melting point, boiling point, solubility and crystal structure, enantiomers have identical physical and chemical properties. They can be distinguished only by the direction in which they turn the plane of polarized light. They do, however, differ in their biological properties.

If more than one asymmetrical carbon is present in the molecule, isomers at a single asymmetrical carbon are not mirror images (enantiomers) but geometric isomers (diastereomers) with different physical and chemical properties.

In the **Fisher projection,** the substituents above and below the asymmetrical carbon face behind the plane of the paper, and those on the left and right face the front. The asymmetrical carbon is in the center of a tetrahedron whose corners are formed by the four substituents. Examples:

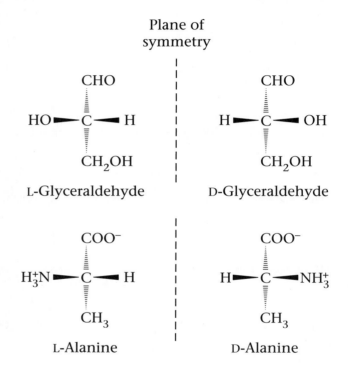

Plane of symmetry

L-Glyceraldehyde   D-Glyceraldehyde

L-Alanine   D-Alanine

The Properties of Biomolecules Are Determined by Their Noncovalent Interactions

The biological properties of a biomolecule depend on its interactions with other molecules. Molecules communicate with one another in the living cell and, being incapable of speech, they have to do it by touch. The surfaces of interacting molecules must be complementary, and noncovalent interactions must be formed between them. These interactions are weak. They break up easily, and therefore *noncovalent binding is always reversible.* There are five types of noncovalent interaction:

1. **Dipole-dipole interactions** usually come in the form of hydrogen bonds: A hydrogen atom is covalently bound to an electronegative atom such as oxygen or nitrogen. This hydrogen attracts another electronegative atom, either in

the same or a different molecule. **Electronegativity** is the tendency of an atom to attract electrons. For the atoms commonly encountered in biomolecules, the rank order of electronegativity is as follows:

$$O > N > S \geq C \geq H$$

Examples:

Hydrogen bond between
ethanol and water

Hydrogen bond between
two peptide bonds

2. **Electrostatic interactions,** or **salt bonds,** are formed between oppositely charged groups:

3. **Ion-dipole interactions** are formed between a charged group and a polarized bond, as in the case of a carboxylate anion and a carboxamide:

4. **Hydrophobic interactions** hold nonpolar molecules and portions of molecules together. There is no strong attractive force between such groups, but *an interface between a nonpolar structure and water is energetically unfavorable.* It limits the ability of the water molecules to form hydrogen bonds with their neighbors. The molecules are forced to reorient themselves in order to maximize their hydrogen bonds with neighboring water molecules, thereby attaining a more ordered and energetically less favorable state. By clustering together, the nonpolar groups minimize their area of contact with water. This allows the water molecules to form more hydrogen bonds and to be more chaotic.

5. **Van der Waals forces** appear whenever two molecules approach each other (Fig. 1.1). A weak attractive force, caused by induced dipoles in the molecules, prevails at moderate distances. On close approximation, however, electrostatic repulsion between the electron shells of the approaching groups overwhelms the attractive force. There is an optimal contact distance at which additional attractive forces are canceled by repulsive forces. Because of van der Waals forces, molecules whose surfaces have complementary shapes tend to bind each other.

Noncovalent interactions determine the biological properties of biomolecules:

- *Water solubility* depends on hydrogen bonds and ion-dipole interactions that the molecules form with water. If a molecule can exist in charged and uncharged states, the charged form is more water soluble.

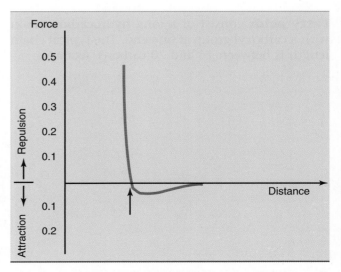

Figure 1.1 Attractive and repulsive van der Waals forces. At the van der Waals contact distance (*arrow*), the opposing forces cancel each other.

- *Higher order structures of macromolecules,* including proteins (see Chapter 2) and nucleic acids (Chapter 6), are formed by noncovalent interactions between portions of the same molecule. Because noncovalent interactions are weak and break easily, many of them are needed to hold a protein or nucleic acid in its proper shape.
- *Binding interactions between molecules* are the essence of life. Structural proteins bind each other, metabolic substrates bind to enzymes, gene regulators bind to DNA, hormones bind to receptors, and foreign substances bind to antibodies.

After this review of functional groups, bonds, and noncovalent interaction, the structures of the major classes of biomolecules—triglycerides, carbohydrates, proteins, and nucleic acids—can now be discussed. More details about these structures are presented in later chapters.

Triglycerides Consist of Fatty Acids and Glycerol

The **triacylglycerols,** better known as **triglycerides** in the medical literature, consist of glycerol and fatty acids. **Glycerol** is a trivalent alcohol:

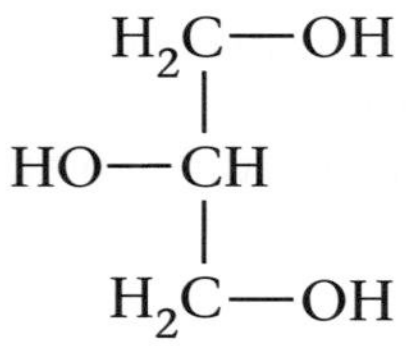

$$H_2C-OH$$
$$HO-CH$$
$$H_2C-OH$$

Glycerol

Fatty acids consist of a long hydrocarbon chain with a carboxyl group at one end. The typical chain length is between 16 and 20 carbons. Example:

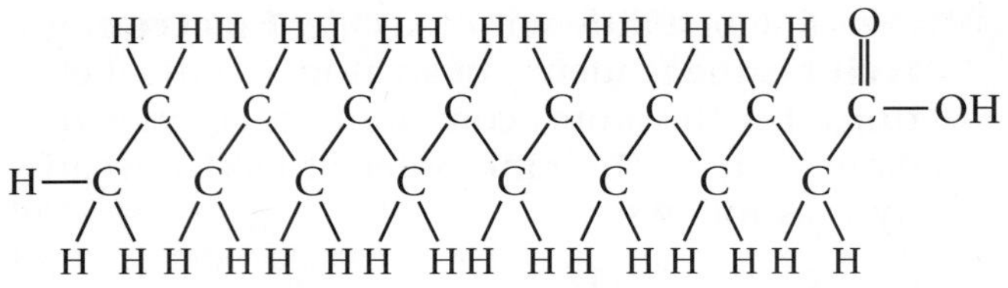

Palmitic acid

Palmitic acid can also be written as

$$H_3C-(CH_2)_{14}-COOH$$

or

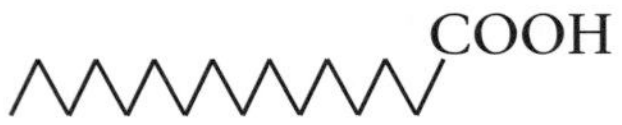

COOH

Fatty acids that have only single bonds between carbons are called **saturated fatty acids.** Those with at least one double bond between carbons are called **unsaturated fatty acids.** Example:

$$H_3C-(CH_2)_5-CH=CH-(CH_2)_7-COOH$$

Palmitoleic acid

Fatty acids have pK values between 4.7 and 5.0, and therefore they are mainly in the deprotonated ($-COO^-$) form at pH 7.

In the triglycerides, all three hydroxyl groups of glycerol are esterified with a fatty acid, as shown in Figure 1.2. The long hydrocarbon chains of the fatty acid residues ensure that *triglycerides are insoluble in water.* In the body, triglycerides minimize contact with water by forming fat droplets.

Collectively, nonpolar biomolecules are called **lipids.** The triglycerides are used only as a storable form of metabolic energy, but other lipids serve more specialized functions: for example, as structural components of membranes (see Chapter 12).

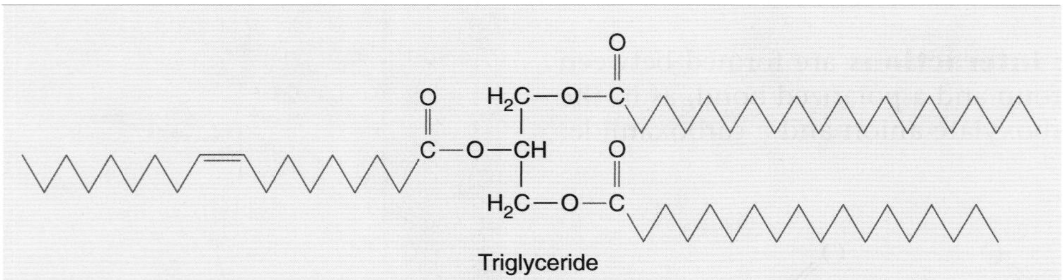

Triglyceride

Figure 1.2 Structure of a triglyceride (fat) molecule. Although the ester bonds can form some hydrogen bonds with water, the long hydrocarbon chains of the fatty acids make fat insoluble.

Monosaccharides Are Polyalcohols with a Keto Group or an Aldehyde Group

Monosaccharides, or "simple" sugars, are the building blocks of all carbohydrates. A monosaccharide is a chain of carbons with a hydroxyl group at each carbon except one. This carbon forms a carbonyl group. **Aldoses** have an aldehyde group, and **ketoses** have a keto group. The length of the carbon chain is variable: for example,

- Triose: 3-carbon sugar
- Tetrose: 4-carbon sugar
- Pentose: 5-carbon sugar
- Hexose : 6-carbon sugar
- Heptose: 7-carbon sugar

D-Glyceraldehyde and dihydroxyacetone are the simplest monosaccharides:

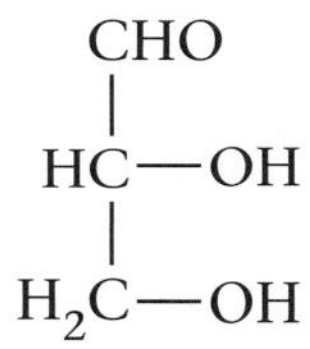

D-Glyceraldehyde (an aldotriose) 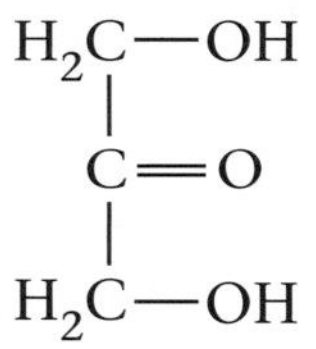   Dihydroxyacetone (a ketotriose)

The most important monosaccharide, however, is the aldohexose **D-glucose:**

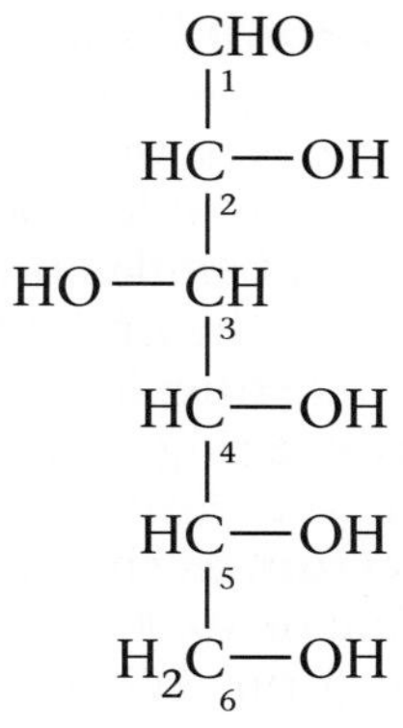

D-Glucose

The carbons are conveniently numbered, starting with the aldehyde carbon or, for ketoses, the terminal carbon closest to the keto carbon. In the structure of D-glucose, carbons 2, 3, 4, and 5 all have four different substituents. These four asymmetrical carbons can form 16 optical isomers. Only one of them is D-glucose. By convention, the "D" in D-glyceraldehyde and D-glucose refers to the orientation of substituents at the asymmetrical carbon farthest removed from the carbonyl carbon (C-2 and C-5, respectively).

Monosaccharides differing in the orientation of substituents around one of their asymmetrical carbons are called **epimers**. In Figure 1.3, for example, D-mannose is a C-2 epimer of glucose, and D-galactose is a C-4 epimer of glucose. *Epimers are not enantiomers but diastereomers.* This means that they have different physical and chemical properties.

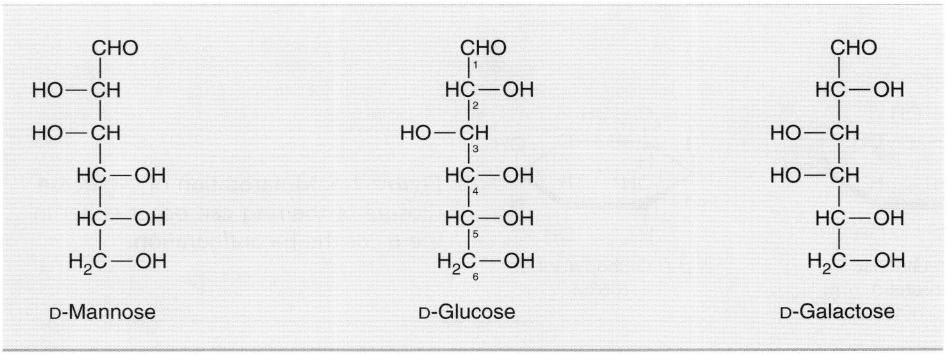

D-Mannose   D-Glucose   D-Galactose

Figure 1.3 D-Mannose and D-galactose are epimers of D-glucose.

Monosaccharides Form Ring Structures

Most monosaccharides spontaneously form ring structures in which the aldehyde (or keto) group forms a hemiacetal (or hemiketal) bond with one of the hydroxyl groups. If the ring contains five atoms, it is called a **furanose** ring; if it contains six atoms, it is called a **pyranose** ring. The ring structures are written in either the Fisher projection or the **Haworth projection,** as shown in Figure 1.4.

In water, only one of 40,000 glucose molecules is in the open-chain form. When the ring structure forms, carbon 1 of glucose becomes asymmetrical. Therefore, two isomers, α-D-glucose and β-D-glucose, can form. These two isomers are called not epimers but **anomers.** In glucose, carbon 1 (the aldehyde carbon) is the **anomeric carbon.** In the ketoses, the keto carbon (usually carbon 2) is anomeric.

Unlike epimers, which are stable under ordinary conditions, *anomers interconvert spontaneously.* This

process of **mutarotation** is caused by the occasional opening and reclosure of the ring, as shown in Figure 1.5. The equilibrium between the α and β anomers is reached within several hours in neutral solutions, but mutarotation is greatly accelerated in the presence of acids or bases.

Complex Carbohydrates Are Formed by Glycosidic Bonds

Monosaccharides combine into larger molecules by forming **glycosidic bonds**: acetal or ketal bonds involving the anomeric carbon of one of the participating monosaccharides. The anomeric carbon forms the bond in either the α or the β configuration. Once the bond is formed, mutarotation is no longer possible, and the bond is locked in its conformation. For example, the structures of maltose and cellobiose in Figure 1.6 differ only in the orientation of their 1,4-glycosidic bond.

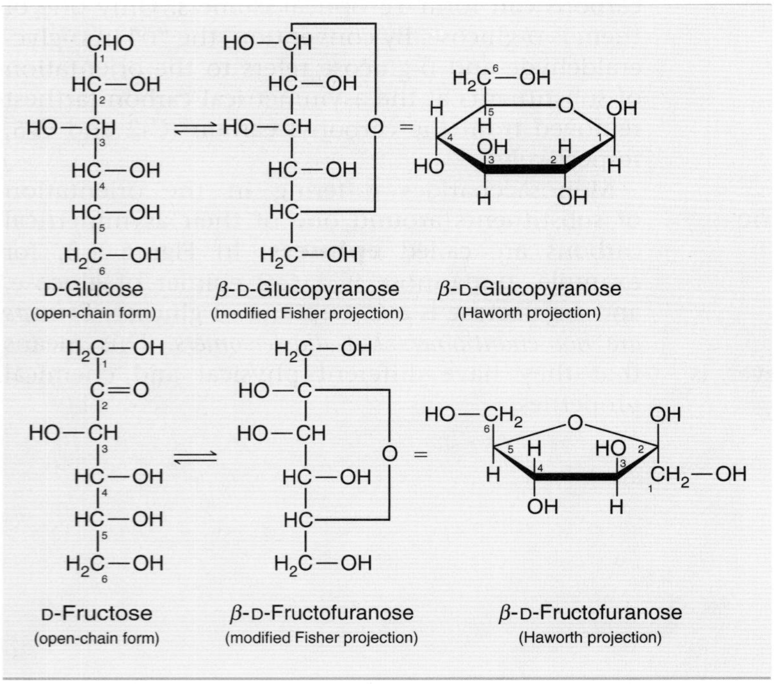

Figure 1.4 The ring structures of the aldohexose D-glucose and the ketohexose D-fructose. The six-member pyranose ring is favored in D-glucose, and the five-member furanose ring in D-fructose.

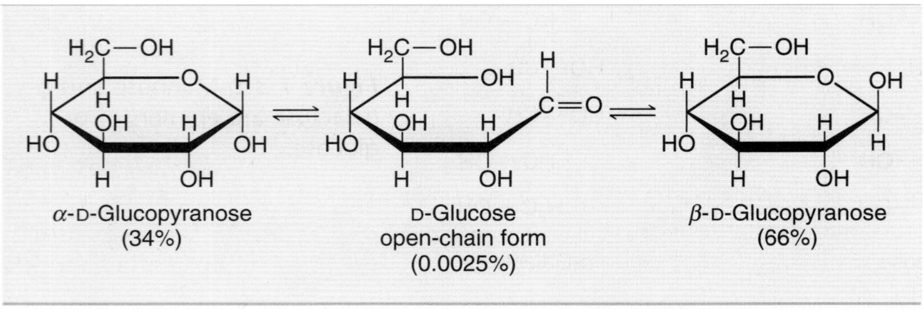

Figure 1.5 Mutarotation of D-glucose. Closure of the ring can occur either in the α- or the β-configuration.

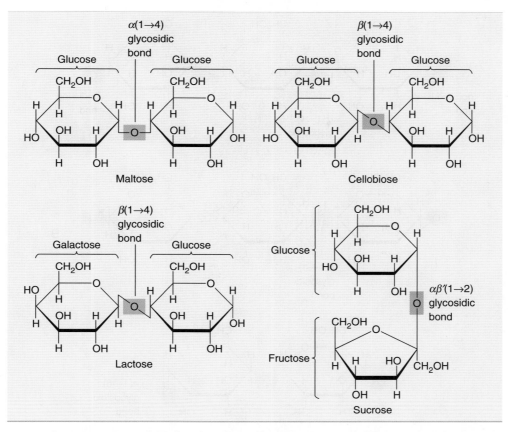

Figure 1.6 Structures of some common disaccharides. Conventionally, the nonreducing end of the disaccharide is written on the left side and the reducing end on the right side.

Structures formed from two monosaccharides are called **disaccharides**. Products with three, four, five, or six monosaccharides are called trisaccharides, tetrasaccharides, pentasaccharides, and hexasaccharides, respectively. **Oligosaccharides** (Greek ολιγοσ = "a few") contain "a few" monosaccharides, and **polysaccharides** (Greek πολυσ = "many") contain "many" monosaccharides (Fig. 1.7).

Sugars can also form glycosidic bonds with noncarbohydrates. In **glycoproteins,** carbohydrate is covalently bound to amino acid side chains, and in **glycolipids,** it is covalently bound to a lipid core. If the sugar binds its partner through an oxygen atom, the bond is called **O-glycosidic;** if the bond is through nitrogen, it is called **N-glycosidic.**

Monosaccharides, disaccharides, and oligosaccharides, commonly known as "sugars," are water soluble because of their high hydrogen bonding potential. Many polysaccharides, however, are insoluble because their large size increases the opportunities for intermolecular interactions. Things become insoluble when the molecules inter-

act more strongly with one another than with the surrounding water.

The carbonyl group of the monosaccharides has reducing properties. *The reducing properties are lost when the carbonyl carbon forms a glycosidic bond.* Of the disaccharides in Figure 1.6, for example, only sucrose is not a reducing sugar, because both anomeric carbons participate in the glycosidic bond. The other disaccharides have a reducing end and a nonreducing end.

Polypeptides Are Formed from Amino Acids

Polypeptides are constructed from 20 different amino acids. All amino acids have a **carboxyl group** and an **amino group,** both bound to the same carbon. This carbon, called the **α-carbon**, also carries a hydrogen atom and a fourth group, the **side chain,** which differs in the 20 amino acids. The general structure of the amino acids can therefore be depicted as shown on the next page,

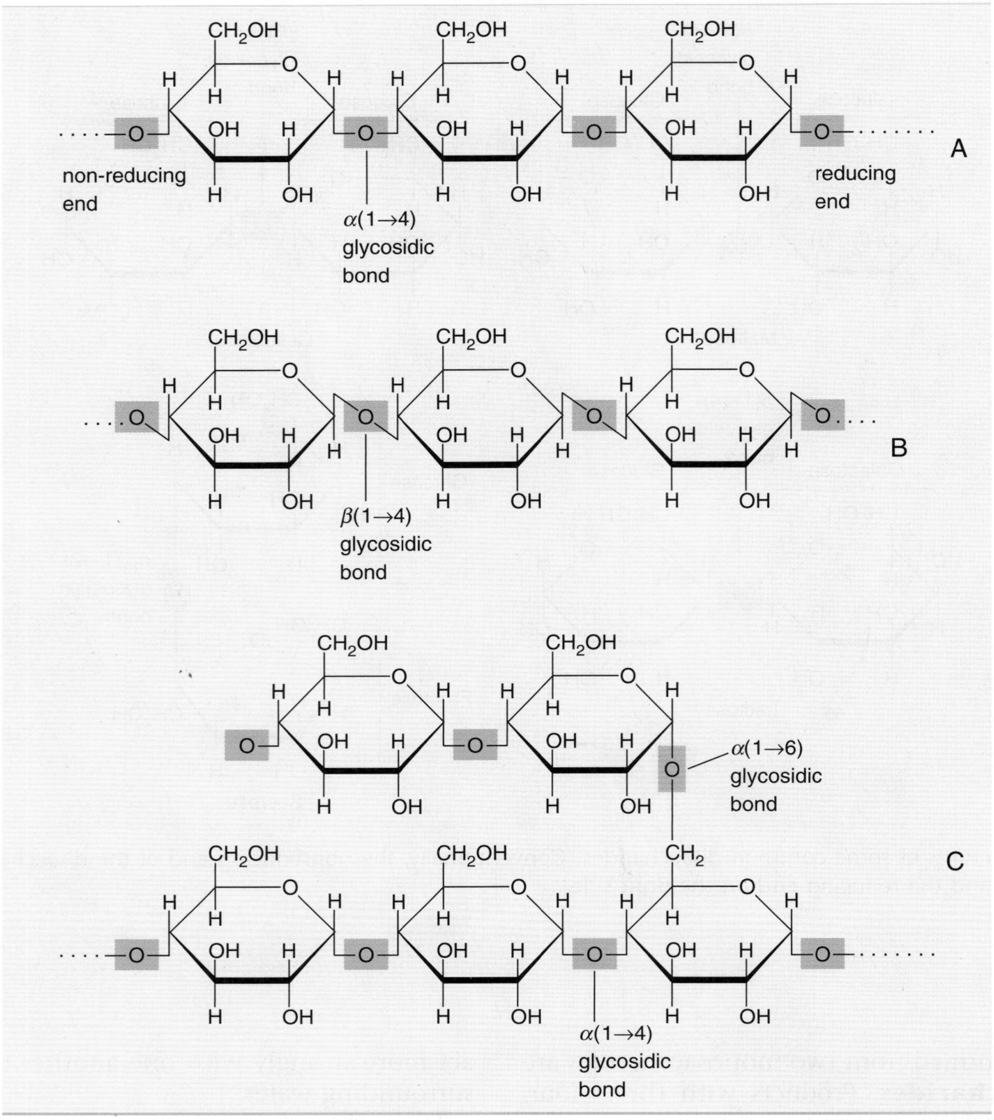

Figure 1.7 Structures of some common polysaccharides. **A,** *Amylose* is an unbranched polymer of glucose residues in α-1,4 glycosidic linkage. Together with amylopectin—a branched glucose polymer with a structure resembling that of glycogen—it forms the starch granules in plants. **B,** Like amylose, *cellulose* is an unbranched polymer of glucose residues. As a major component in the cell walls of plants, it is the most abundant biomolecule on earth. The marked difference in the physical and biological properties between the two polysaccharides is caused by the presence of β-1,4 rather than α-1,4 glycosidic bonds in cellulose. **C,** *Glycogen* is the storage polysaccharide of animals and humans. Like amylose, it contains chains of glucose residues in α-1,4 glycosidic linkage. Unlike amylose, however, the molecule is branched: some glucose residues in the chain form a third glycosidic bond, using their hydroxyl group at carbon 6.

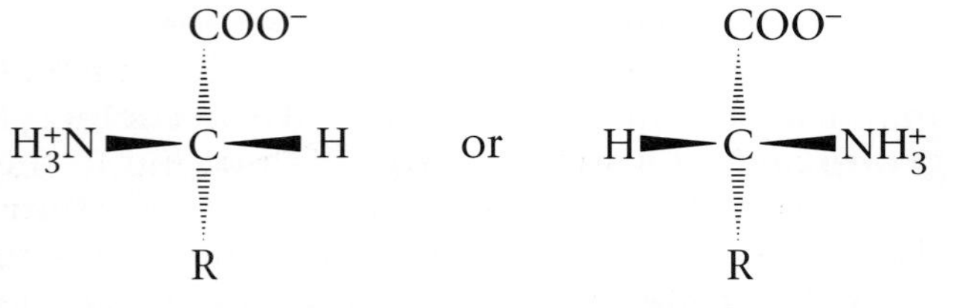

L-Amino acid   D-Amino acid

where R (residue) is the variable side chain. The α-carbon is asymmetrical, but of the two possible isomers, only the L–amino acids occur in polypeptides.

Dipeptides are formed by a reaction between the carboxyl group of one amino acid and the amino group of another amino acid. The substituted amide bond thus formed is called the **peptide bond:**

Dipeptide

Chains of "a few" amino acids are called **oligopeptides,** and chains of "many" amino acids, **polypeptides.**

Nucleic Acids Are Formed from Nucleotides

The nucleic acids consist of three kinds of building blocks:

1. A **pentose sugar,** which is ribose in ribonucleic acid (RNA) and 2-deoxyribose in 2-deoxyribonucleic acid (DNA):

β-D-Ribose β-D-2-deoxyribose

2. **Phosphate,** which is bound to hydroxyl groups of the sugar.
3. The bases **adenine**, **guanine**, **cytosine**, **uracil** (only in RNA), and **thymine** (only in DNA). Chemically, cytosine, thymine, and

uracil are **pyrimidines,** containing a single six-membered ring, whereas adenine and guanine are **purines,** consisting of two condensed rings:

Adenine   Guanine

Cytosine   Uracil   Thymine

A **nucleoside** is obtained when one of the bases forms an *N*-glycosidic bond with C-1 of ribose or 2-deoxyribose (Fig. 1.8). **Nucleotides** have the structure of nucleosides, but with up to three phosphate groups bound to C-5 of the sugar. They are named as phosphate derivatives of the nucleosides. Thus, adenosine monophosphate (AMP), adenosine diphosphate (ADP), and adenosine triphosphate (ATP) contain one, two, and three phosphate residues, respectively.

Nucleic acids are polymers of nucleoside monophosphates. The phosphate group forms a phosphodiester bond between the 5' and 3' hydroxyl groups of adjacent ribose or 2-deoxyribose residues (Fig. 1.9). Most nucleic acids are very large. They can contain thousands and, in the case of deoxyribonucleic acid (DNA), many millions of nucleotides.

Most Biomolecules Are Polymers

The carbohydrates, polypeptides and nucleic acids illustrate how Nature generates molecules of large size and almost infinite diversity by linking simple-structured building blocks into long chains. The macromolecules formed this way are called **polymers** (Greek πολυσ = "many," μεροσ = "part"),

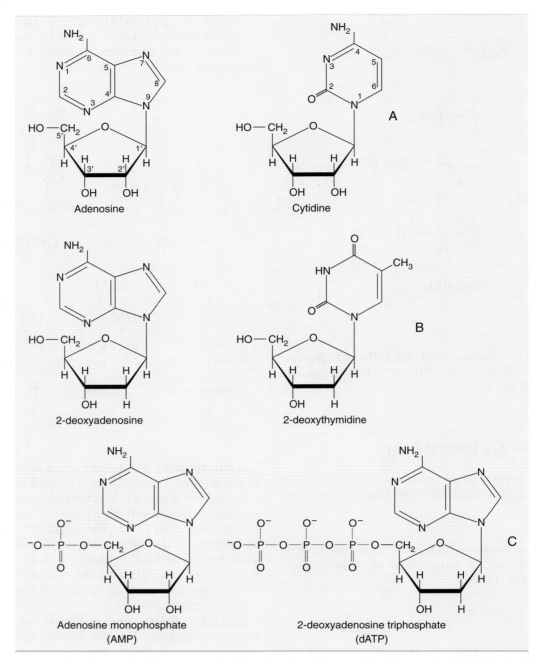

Figure 1.8 Structures of some nucleosides and nucleotides. A prime (') is used for the numbering of the carbons in the sugar, to distinguish it from the numbering of the ring carbons and nitrogen atoms in the bases. **A,** Examples of ribonucleosides. **B,** Examples of deoxyribonucleosides. **C,** Examples of nucleotides.

whereas their building blocks are called **monomers** (Greek μονοσ = "single").

Structural diversity is greatest when more than one kind of monomer is used. Polypeptides, for example, are constructed from 20 different amino acids, and DNA and RNA each contain 4 different bases. Like colored beads in a necklace, these components can be arranged in unique sequences; 20^{100} different sequences are possible for a protein of 100 amino acids, and 4^{100} different sequences are possible for a nucleic acid of 100 nucleotides.

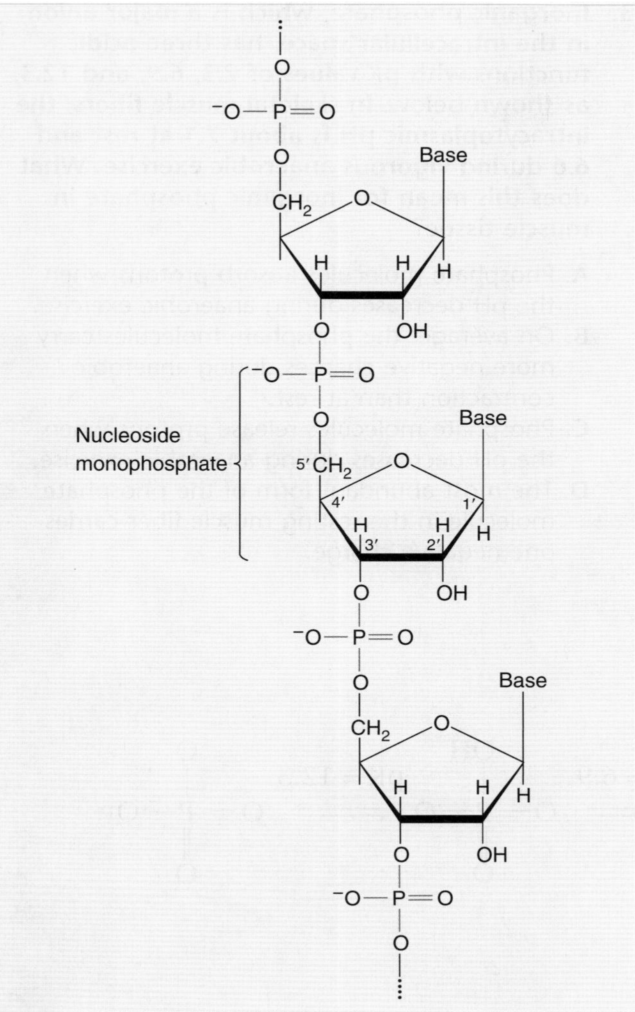

Figure 1.9 Structure of ribonucleic acid (RNA). Deoxyribonucleic acid (DNA) has a similar structure, but it contains 2-deoxyribose instead of ribose. The nucleic acids are polymers of nucleoside monophosphates.

bonds; proteins consist of amino acids linked by peptide bonds; and nucleic acids consist of nucleoside monophosphates linked by phosphodiester bonds. With the exception of the triglycerides, these molecules are hydrophilic. Polysaccharides, polypeptides, and nucleic acids are polymers: long chains of covalently linked building blocks. Forming the bonds in these large molecules requires metabolic energy, whereas cleavage of the bonds releases energy.

Many biomolecules have ionizable groups. Molecules with free carboxyl groups or covalently bound phosphate carry negative charges at neutral pH, and those with aliphatic (nonaromatic) amino groups carry positive charges. These charges make the molecules water soluble, and they permit the formation of salt bonds with inorganic ions and with other biomolecules. The acidity of an ionizable group is its tendency to accept or donate protons (positively charged hydrogen ions). It is described by the pK value. If the pK value is known, it is possible to predict what percentage of an ionizable group is in the protonated or deprotonated state at any given pH.

SUMMARY

All biochemical processes take place in aqueous solutions, and the functions of biomolecules therefore depend in large part on their interactions with water. Water solubility is determined by the ability of a molecule to form hydrogen bonds or ion-dipole interactions with the surrounding water molecules. Hydrophobic interactions, on the other hand, reduce water solubility. These interactions are noncovalent, and they are far weaker than the covalent bonds that hold the atoms within the molecules together.

There are several classes of biomolecules. Triglycerides consist of glycerol and three fatty acids linked by ester bonds; carbohydrates consist of monosaccharides linked by glycosidic

QUESTIONS

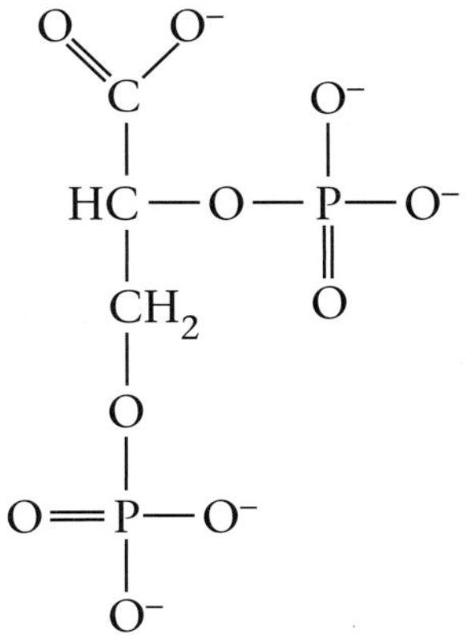

1. The molecule shown here (2,3-bisphosphoglycerate [BPG]) is present in red blood cells, in which it binds noncovalently to hemoglobin. Which functional groups in hemoglobin can make the strongest noncovalent interactions with BPG at a pH value of 7.0?

   A. Sulfhydryl groups.
   B. Alcoholic hydroxyl groups.
   C. Hydrocarbon groups.
   D. Amino groups.
   E. Carboxyl groups.

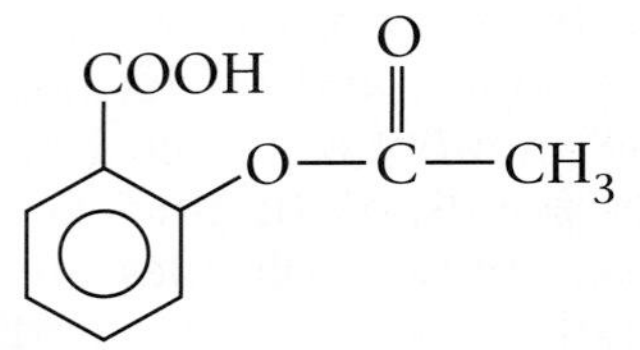

COOH

O
‖
O—C—CH₃

2. **The molecule shown here is acetylsalicylic acid (aspirin). What kind of electrical charge does aspirin carry in the stomach at a pH value of 2 and in the small intestine at a pH value of 7?**

A. Negatively charged in the stomach; positively charged in the intestine.
B. Negatively charged both in the stomach and the intestine.
C. Uncharged in the stomach; negatively charged in the intestine.
D. Uncharged both in the stomach and the intestine.
E. Uncharged in the stomach; positively charged in the intestine.

3. **Inorganic phosphate, which is a major anion in the intracellular space, has three acidic functions with pK values of 2.3, 6.9, and 12.3, as shown below. In skeletal muscle fibers, the intracytoplasmic pH is about 7.1 at rest and 6.6 during vigorous anaerobic exercise. What does this mean for inorganic phosphate in muscle tissue?**

A. Phosphate molecules absorb protons when the pH decreases during anaerobic exercise.
B. On average, the phosphate molecules carry more negative charges during anaerobic contraction than at rest.
C. Phosphate molecules release protons when the pH decreases during anaerobic exercise.
D. The most abundant form of the phosphate molecule in the resting muscle fiber carries one negative charge.

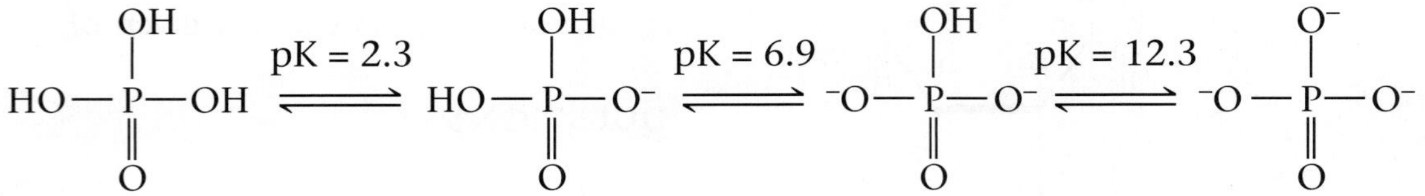

$$HO-\underset{\underset{O}{\|}}{\overset{\overset{OH}{|}}{P}}-OH \;\rightleftharpoons\; \overset{pK = 2.3}{} \; HO-\underset{\underset{O}{\|}}{\overset{\overset{OH}{|}}{P}}-O^- \;\rightleftharpoons\; \overset{pK = 6.9}{} \; {}^-O-\underset{\underset{O}{\|}}{\overset{\overset{OH}{|}}{P}}-O^- \;\rightleftharpoons\; \overset{pK = 12.3}{} \; {}^-O-\underset{\underset{O}{\|}}{\overset{\overset{O^-}{|}}{P}}-O^-$$

CHAPTER 2

Introduction to Protein Structure

Nothing in the cell works without proteins. Membrane proteins join hands with the fibrous proteins of the cytoplasm and the extracellular matrix to keep cells and tissues in shape; enzyme proteins catalyze metabolic reactions; and DNA-binding proteins regulate gene expression.

The simplest proteins consist of a single polypeptide chain: an unbranched polymer of the 20 amino acids, held together by peptide bonds. Some polypeptides are less than 100 amino acids in length, but others have more than 1000. Other proteins consist of two or more polypeptides, held together by noncovalent interactions and sometimes also by covalent bonds. Some proteins even have a nonpolypeptide group attached to them, either covalently or noncovalently. The polypeptide component of these proteins is called the **apoprotein,** and their nonpolypeptide counterpart, the **prosthetic group.**

Prosthetic groups are required because only a limited number of functional groups are available in polypeptides. For example, there are no groups that can easily transfer hydrogen or electrons and none that can bind molecular oxygen, and there are no energy-rich bonds. Whenever such features are needed—for example, for enzymatic catalysis—the protein must employ a prosthetic group.

This chapter is concerned with the structures and properties of the 20 amino acids that occur in proteins, the levels of protein structure, and the physical properties of proteins.

Amino Acids Are Zwitterions

The amino acids have a carboxyl group, an amino group, a hydrogen atom, and a variable side chain R ("residue") bound to the **α-carbon:**

$$
\begin{array}{ccc}
\text{COO}^- & & \text{COO}^- \\
| & & | \\
\text{H}_3^+\text{N} \blacktriangleright \text{C} \blacktriangleleft \text{H} & \text{or} & \text{H} \blacktriangleright \text{C} \blacktriangleleft \text{NH}_3^+ \\
| & & | \\
\text{R} & & \text{R} \\
\text{L-Amino acid} & & \text{D-Amino acid}
\end{array}
$$

Of the two optical isomers, *only the L–amino acids occur in proteins*. D–Amino acids are rare in nature, although they are present in some bacterial products.

The carboxyl and amino groups are called the **α-carboxyl group** and the **α-amino group,** respectively, to distinguish them from similar groups in some of the amino acid side chains. The pK of the α-carbon is always close to 2.0, and the pK of the α-amino group is near 9 or 10. Therefore, the protonation state varies with pH (proton concentration [H⁺]), as illustrated in Figure 2.1.

Below the pK of the carboxyl group, the amino acid is predominantly a cation; above the pK of the amino group, an anion; and between the two pKs, a **zwitterion** (German *Zwitter* = "hermaphrodite"): a molecule carrying both a positive and a negative charge. The **isoelectric point** (**pI**) is defined as *the pH value at which the number of positive charges equals the number of negative charges*. For a simple amino acid such as alanine, the pI is halfway between the pK values of the two ionizable groups. Note that whereas the pK is the property of an individual ionizable group, the pI is a property of the whole molecule.

The pK values of the ionizable groups can be determined by treating an acidic solution of an amino acid with a strong base or by treating an alkaline solution with a strong acid. At pH values close to the pK of an ionizable group, the group releases or absorbs protons as the pH is increased or decreased, respectively. In the **titration curve** of Figure 2.2, each portion of the curve signifies the presence of an ionizable group and its approximate pK value.

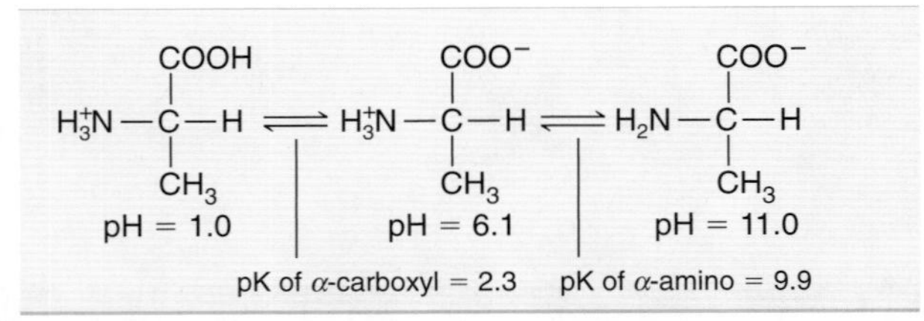

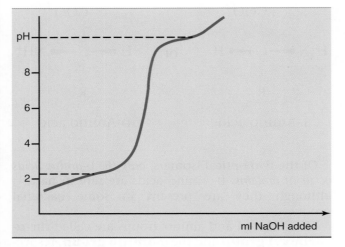

Figure 2.1 The protonation states of the amino acid alanine. The zwitterion is the predominant form in the pH range from 2.3 to 9.9.

Figure 2.2 Titration curve of the amino acid alanine. The two level segments are caused by the buffering capacity of the carboxyl group (at pH 2.3) and the amino group (at pH 9.9).

This implies that ionizable groups stabilize the pH value of the solution against external disturbances. *Any ionizable group buffers the pH of the solution at pH values close to its pK.* The buffering capacity of ionizable groups helps humans maintain a constant pH in body fluids.

Some amino acids have an additional acidic or basic group in the side chain, as illustrated in Figure 2.3. The pI of the acidic amino acids is halfway between the pK values of the two acidic groups, and the pI of the basic amino acids is halfway between the pK values of the two basic groups. The titration curve of these amino acids shows three rather than two buffering areas.

Amino Acid Side Chains Form Many Noncovalent Interactions

The 20 amino acids can be placed in a few major groups, as shown in Figure 2.4. Their functions in proteins are determined by the noncovalent interactions and the covalent bonds that their side chains can form:

1. The **small amino acids** (glycine and alanine) occupy little space. In proteins they are often found in places where two polypeptide chains have to come close together.
2. The **branched-chain amino acids** valine, leucine, and isoleucine have hydrophobic side chains.
3. The **hydroxyl amino acids** serine and threonine form hydrogen bonds with their hydroxyl group. This group also forms covalent bonds with carbohydrate in glycoproteins and with phosphate in phosphoproteins.

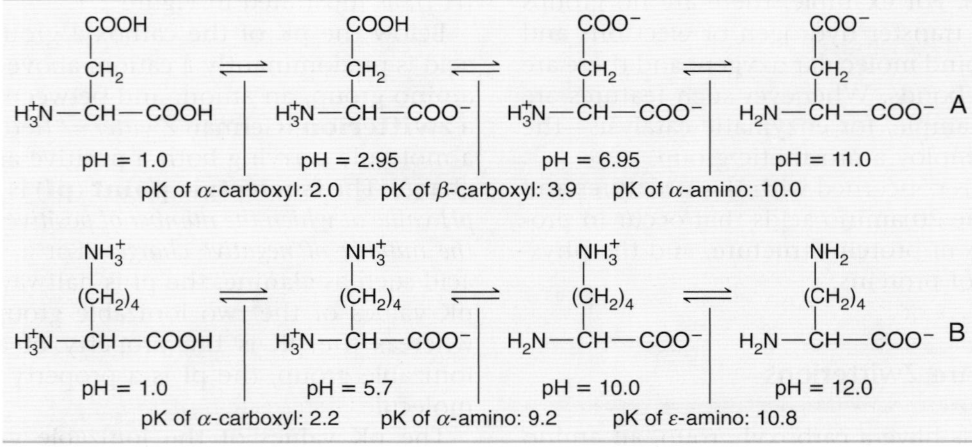

Figure 2.3 Prevailing ionization states of the amino acids aspartate **(A)** and lysine **(B)** at different pH values. The isoelectric points of aspartate and lysine are 2.95 and 10.0, respectively.

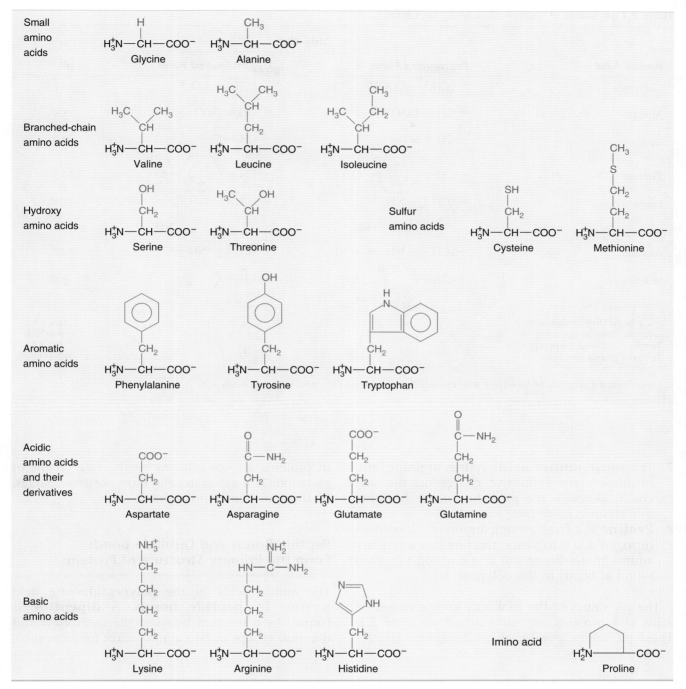

Figure 2.4 Structures of the amino acids in proteins.

4. The **sulfur amino acids** cysteine and methionine are quite hydrophobic, although cysteine also has weak acidic properties. The sulfhydryl (—SH) group of cysteine can form a covalent disulfide bond with another cysteine side chain in the protein.

5. The **aromatic amino acids** phenylalanine, tyrosine, and tryptophan are hydrophobic, although the side chains of tyrosine and tryptophan can also form hydrogen bonds. The hydroxyl group of tyrosine carries a covalently bound phosphate group in some phosphoproteins.

6. The **acidic amino acids** glutamate and aspartate have a carboxyl group in the side chain that is negatively charged at pH 7. The corresponding carboxamide groups in glutamine and asparagine are not acidic but can form strong hydrogen bonds. Asparagine forms an *N*-glycosidic bond with carbohydrate in some glycoproteins.

Table 2.1 pK Values of Some Amino Acid Side Chains*

Amino Acid	Side Chain		pK
	Protonated Form	**Deprotonated Form**	
Glutamate	$-(CH_2)_2-COOH$	$-(CH_2)_2-COO^-$	4.3
Aspartate	$-CH_2-COOH$	$-CH_2-COO^-$	3.9
Cysteine	$-CH_2-SH$	$-CH_2-S^-$	8.3
Tyrosine	$-CH_2-$⬡$-OH$	$-CH_2-$⬡$-O^-$	10.1
Lysine	$-(CH_2)_4-NH_3^+$	$-(CH_2)_4-NH_2$	10.8
Arginine	$-(CH_2)_3-NH-\overset{\overset{\displaystyle NH_2^+}{\|}}{C}-NH_2$	$-(CH_2)_3-NH-\overset{\overset{\displaystyle NH}{\|}}{C}-NH_2$	12.5
Histidine	$-CH_2-$ (imidazole, NH^+)	$-CH_2-$ (imidazole, N)	6.0
α-Carboxyl (free amino acid)			1.8-2.4
α-Amino (free amino acid)			≈9.0-10.0
Terminal carboxyl (peptide)			≈3.0-4.5
Terminal amino (peptide)			≈7.5-9.0

* In proteins, the side chain pK values may differ by more than one pH unit from those in the free amino acids.

7. The **basic amino acids** lysine, arginine, and histidine carry a positive charge on the side chain, although the pK value of the histidine side chain is quite low.
8. **Proline** is a freak among amino acids, with its nitrogen tied into a ring structure as a secondary amino group. Being stiff and angled, it is often found at bends in the polypeptide.

The pK values of the ionizable groups in amino acids and proteins are summarized in Table 2.1. These pK values reveal that most negative charges in proteins are contributed by the side chains of glutamate and aspartate, and most positive charges, by those of lysine and arginine.

Peptide Bonds and Disulfide Bonds Form the Primary Structure of Proteins

The amino acids in the polypeptides are held together by **peptide bonds.** A **dipeptide** is formed by a reaction between the α-carboxyl and α-amino groups of two amino acids; for example:

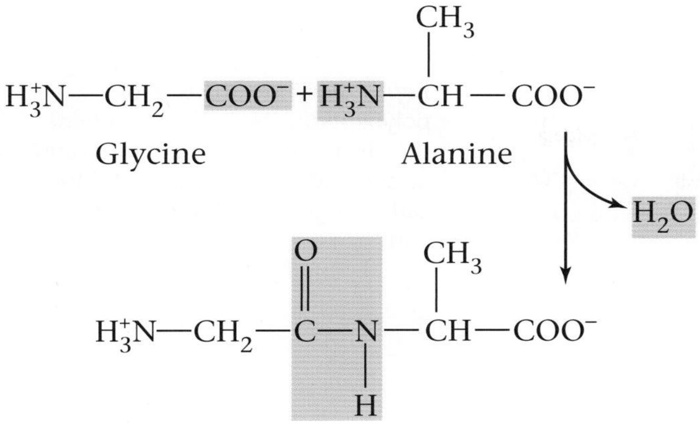

$$H_3^+N-CH_2-COO^- + H_3^+N-CH-COO^-$$

$$\underset{\text{Glycine}}{} \qquad \underset{\text{Alanine}}{\overset{CH_3}{|}}$$

$\rightarrow H_2O$

$$H_3^+N-CH_2-\overset{\overset{\displaystyle O}{\|}}{C}-\underset{\underset{\displaystyle H}{|}}{N}-\overset{\overset{\displaystyle CH_3}{|}}{CH}-COO^-$$

Glycyl-alanine

Adding additional amino acids produces **oligopeptides** and finally **polypeptides,** as shown in Figure 2.5. Each peptide has an **amino terminus**, conventionally written on the left side, and a **carboxyl terminus**, written on the right side. The peptide bond is not ionizable, but it can form hydrogen bonds. Therefore, peptides and proteins tend to be water soluble.

Many proteins contain **disulfide bonds** between the side chains of cysteine residues. They are formed in a reductive reaction in which the two hydrogen atoms of the sulfhydryl groups are transferred to an acceptor molecule:

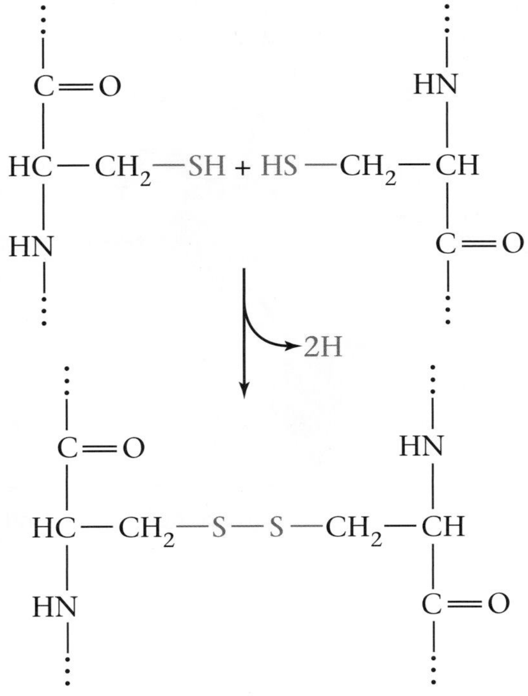

$$\vdots$$
$$C=O \qquad\qquad HN$$
$$HC-CH_2-SH + HS-CH_2-CH$$
$$HN \qquad\qquad C=O$$
$$\vdots \qquad\qquad\qquad \vdots$$

$\rightarrow 2H$

$$\vdots \qquad\qquad\qquad \vdots$$
$$C=O \qquad\qquad HN$$
$$HC-CH_2-S-S-CH_2-CH$$
$$HN \qquad\qquad C=O$$
$$\vdots \qquad\qquad\qquad \vdots$$

The disulfide bond can be formed between two cysteines in the same polypeptide (intrachain) or in different polypeptides (interchain). The reaction takes place in the endoplasmic reticulum, where secreted proteins and membrane proteins are processed. Therefore, *most secreted proteins and membrane proteins have disulfide bonds.* Most cytoplasmic proteins, which do not pass through the endoplasmic reticulum, have no disulfide bonds.

The enzymatic degradation of disulfide-containing proteins yields the amino acid **cystine:**

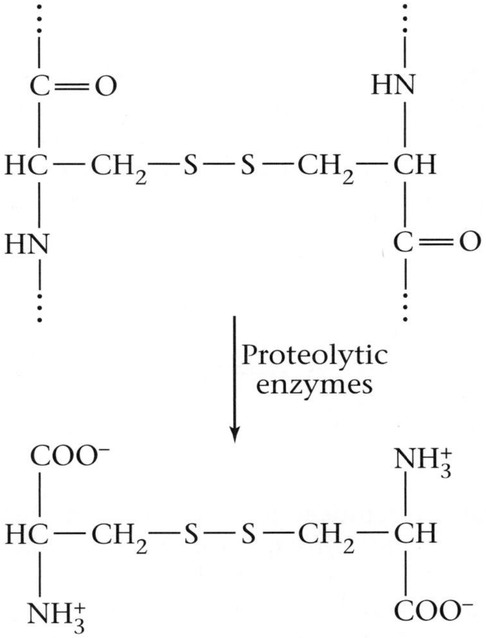

$$\vdots \qquad\qquad\qquad \vdots$$
$$C=O \qquad\qquad HN$$
$$HC-CH_2-S-S-CH_2-CH$$
$$HN \qquad\qquad C=O$$
$$\vdots \qquad\qquad\qquad \vdots$$

$\downarrow$ Proteolytic enzymes

$$COO^- \qquad\qquad NH_3^+$$
$$HC-CH_2-S-S-CH_2-CH$$
$$NH_3^+ \qquad\qquad COO^-$$

The covalent structure of the protein, as described by its amino acid sequence and the positions of disulfide bonds, is called its **primary structure.**

Proteins Can Fold Themselves into Many Different Shapes

The carbon (C) and nitrogen (N) ends of a typical peptide bond have four substituents: a hydrogen, an oxygen, and two α-carbon atoms. The peptide bond is conventionally written as a single bond:

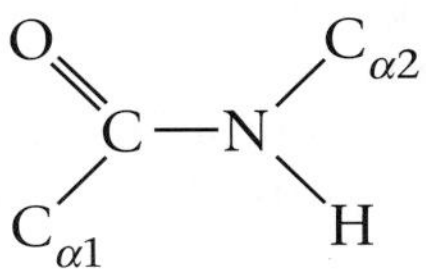

$$\underset{C_{\alpha 1}}{\overset{O}{\|}}C-N\overset{C_{\alpha 2}}{\underset{H}{}}$$

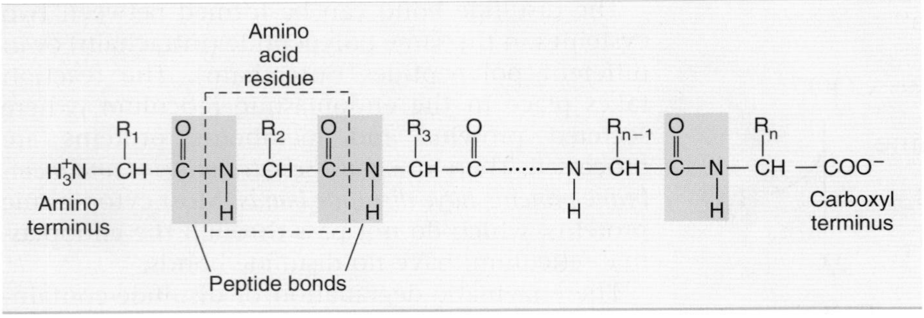

Amino acid residue

$$\underset{\substack{\text{Amino}\\\text{terminus}}}{H_3^+N}-\underset{R_1}{CH}-\underset{O}{C}+\underset{H}{N}-\underset{R_2}{CH}-\underset{O}{C}+\underset{H}{N}-\underset{R_3}{CH}-\underset{O}{C}-\cdots\cdots-\underset{H}{N}-\underset{R_{n-1}}{CH}-\underset{O}{C}-\underset{H}{N}-\underset{R_n}{CH}-\underset{\substack{\text{Carboxyl}\\\text{terminus}}}{COO^-}$$

Peptide bonds

Figure 2.5 The structure of polypeptides. Note the polarity of the chain, with a free amino group at one end of the chain and a free carboxyl group at the opposite end.

A C—N single bond, like a C—C single bond, should show free rotation. In this case, the triangular plane formed by the O=C—$C_{\alpha1}$ portion should be able to rotate out of the plane of the $C_{\alpha2}$—N—H portion. Actually, however, the peptide bond is a resonance hybrid of two structures:

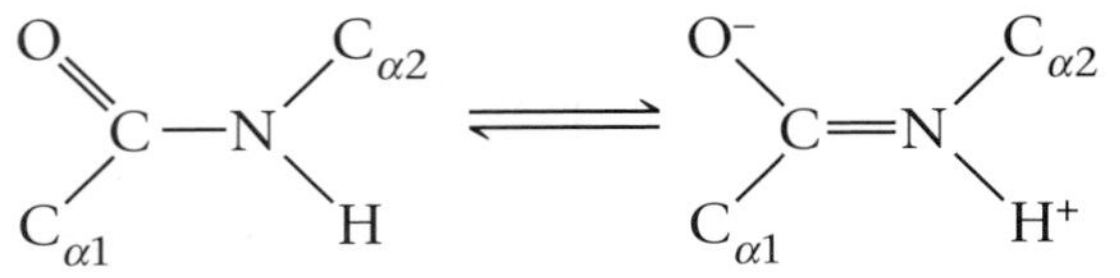

$$\underset{C_{\alpha1}}{\overset{O}{\underset{|}{C}}}-\underset{H}{\overset{C_{\alpha2}}{N}} \rightleftharpoons \underset{C_{\alpha1}}{\overset{O^-}{\underset{|}{C}}}=\underset{H^+}{\overset{C_{\alpha2}}{N}}$$

Its "real" structure is halfway between these two extremes. One consequence is that, like C—C double bonds (see Chapter 12), *the peptide bond does not rotate.* It is rigid, with its four substituents fixed in the same plane. The configuration is *trans,* with the two α-carbons opposite each other.

The other two bonds in the polypeptide backbone, those involving the α-carbon, are "pure" single bonds with the expected rotational freedom. Rotation around the nitrogen—α-carbon bond is measured as the φ (phi) angle, and rotation around the peptide carbon—α-carbon bond, as the ψ (psi) angle (Fig. 2.6). This rotational freedom turns the polypeptide into a contortionist that can bend and twist itself into complex shapes.

Globular proteins have compact shapes. Most are water soluble, but some are incorporated into cellular membranes or into supramolecular aggregates such as the ribosomes. Hemoglobin and myoglobin (Chapter 3), enzymes (Chapter 4), membrane proteins (Chapter 12), and plasma proteins (Chapter 15) are globular proteins. **Fibrous proteins** are long and threadlike, and most serve structural functions. The keratins of hair, skin, and fingernails are fibrous proteins (Chapter 13), as are the collagen and elastin of the extracellular matrix (Chapter 14).

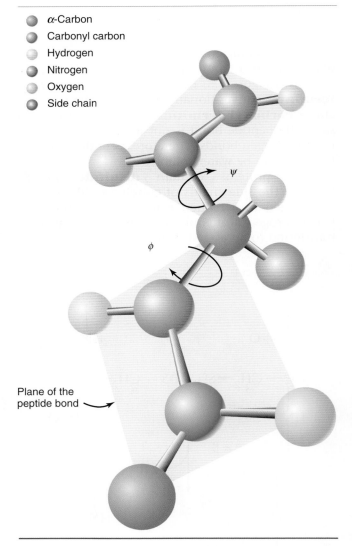

- α-Carbon
- Carbonyl carbon
- Hydrogen
- Nitrogen
- Oxygen
- Side chain

Plane of the peptide bond

Figure 2.6 Geometry of the peptide bond. The φ and ψ angles are variable.

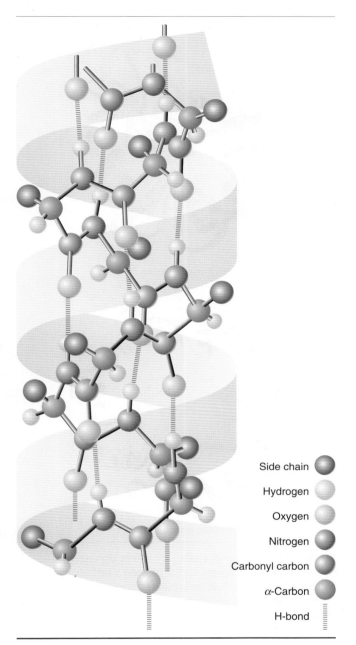

Side chain

Hydrogen

Oxygen

Nitrogen

Carbonyl carbon

α-Carbon

H-bond

Figure 2.7 Structure of the α helix.

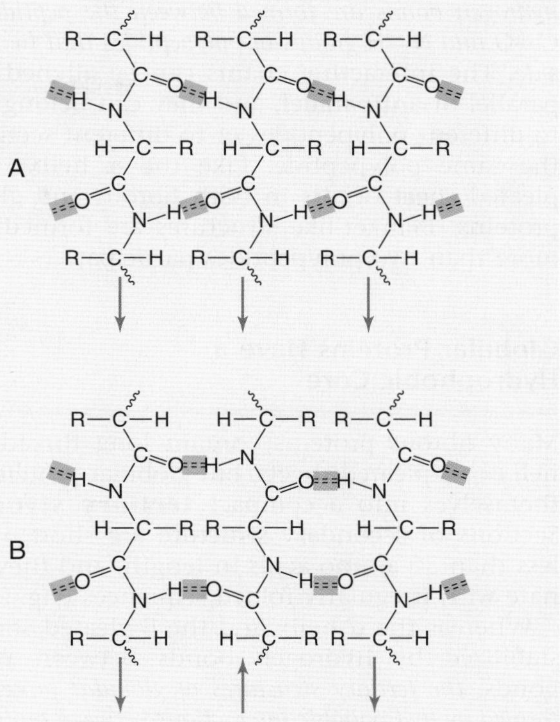

A

B

Figure 2.8 Structure of the parallel and antiparallel β-pleated sheets. **A,** The parallel β-pleated sheet. **B,** The antiparallel β-pleated sheet. The arrows indicate the direction of the polypeptide chain.

axis, the flexed fingers describe the twist of the polypeptide. The threads of screws, nuts, and bolts are right-handed, too. The α helix is very compact. Each full turn has 3.6 amino acid residues, and each amino acid is advanced 1.5 Å along the helix axis ($1\,\text{Å} = 10^{-1}\,\text{nm} = 10^{-4}\,\mu\text{m} = 10^{-7}\,\text{mm}$). Therefore, a complete turn advances by $3.6 \times 1.5 = 5.4$ Å.

The α helix is maintained by hydrogen bonds between the peptide bonds. Each peptide bond C—O is hydrogen-bonded to the peptide bond N—H four amino acid residues ahead of it. Each C—O and each N—H in the main chain are hydrogen bonded. The N, H, and O form a nearly straight line, which is the energetically most favorable alignment for hydrogen bonds.

The amino acid side chains face outward, away from the helix axis. The side chains can stabilize or destabilize the helix, although they are not essential for helix formation. Proline is too rigid to fit into the α helix, and glycine is too flexible. Glycine can assume too many alternative conformations that are energetically more favorable than the α helix.

The α Helix and β-Pleated Sheet Are the Most Common Secondary Structures in Proteins

A **secondary structure** is a regular, repetitive folding pattern that emerges when all the ϕ angles in the polypeptide are the same and all the ψ angles are the same. Only a few secondary structures are energetically possible.

In the **α helix** (Fig. 2.7), the polypeptide backbone forms a right-handed corkscrew. "Right-handed" refers to the direction of the turn: when the thumb of the right hand pushes along the helix

The **β-pleated sheet** (Fig. 2.8) is far more extended than the α helix, with each amino acid advancing by 3.5 Å. In this stretched-out structure, *hydrogen bonds are formed between the peptide bond C—O and N—H groups of polypeptides that lie side by side.* The interacting chains can be aligned either parallel or antiparallel, and they can belong either to different polypeptides or to different sections of the same polypeptide. Like the α helix, the β-pleated sheet occurs in both fibrous and globular proteins. Blanket-like structures are formed when more than two polypeptides participate.

Globular Proteins Have a Hydrophobic Core

Many fibrous proteins contain long threads of α helix or β-pleated sheets, but globular proteins fold themselves into a compact **tertiary structure.** Sections of secondary structure are short, usually less than 30 amino acids in length, and they alternate with irregularly folded sequences (Fig. 2.9).

Whereas the α helix and the β-pleated sheet are stabilized by hydrogen bonds between peptide bonds, *the tertiary structures of globular proteins are formed by hydrophobic interactions between amino acid side chains.* These amino acid side chains form a hydrophobic core.

In some proteins, a single polypeptide folds itself into several compact, globular **domains,** each containing between 100 and 400 amino acid residues. The domains are connected by loose, flexible portions of the polypeptide. Each domain can have a different biological function. There exist, for example, enzyme proteins with multiple domains in which each domain has a different catalytic activity.

Quaternary structures are defined by the interactions between different polypeptides (**subunits**). Therefore, only proteins with more than one polypeptide have a quaternary structure. In some of these proteins, the subunits are held together only by noncovalent interactions, but others are stabilized by interchain disulfide bonds.

The Higher Order Structure Forms While the Polypeptide Is Being Synthesized

Protein structures are formed in a typical sequence:

1. The peptide bonds are formed by the ribosome. The ribosome starts at the amino terminus and then adds one amino acid after another.
2. The growing polypeptide folds itself into a higher order structure. This process begins

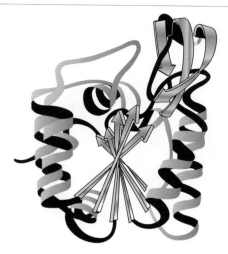

Phosphoglycerate kinase domain 2

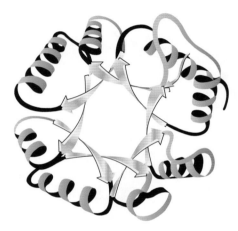

Pyruvate kinase domain 1

Figure 2.9 Structure of globular protein domains containing both α-helical and β-pleated sheet structures. Note that each α-helical or β-pleated sheet structure is formed from only a short section of the polypeptide. These elements of secondary structure are separated by nonhelical portions.

even before the synthesis of the polypeptide has been completed. It usually requires only noncovalent interactions between groups in the polypeptide, although in some cases, correct folding is assisted by helper proteins called **chaperones.**

3. Disulfide bonds are formed between cysteine residues that have been brought in close approximation during the folding process. Thus, the disulfide bridges do not establish the protein's higher order structure. They only stabilize the structure that has been formed already by noncovalent interactions.

4. Other covalent bonds are formed: for example, with phosphate in phosphoproteins and with carbohydrate in glycoproteins, as shown in Figure 2.10.

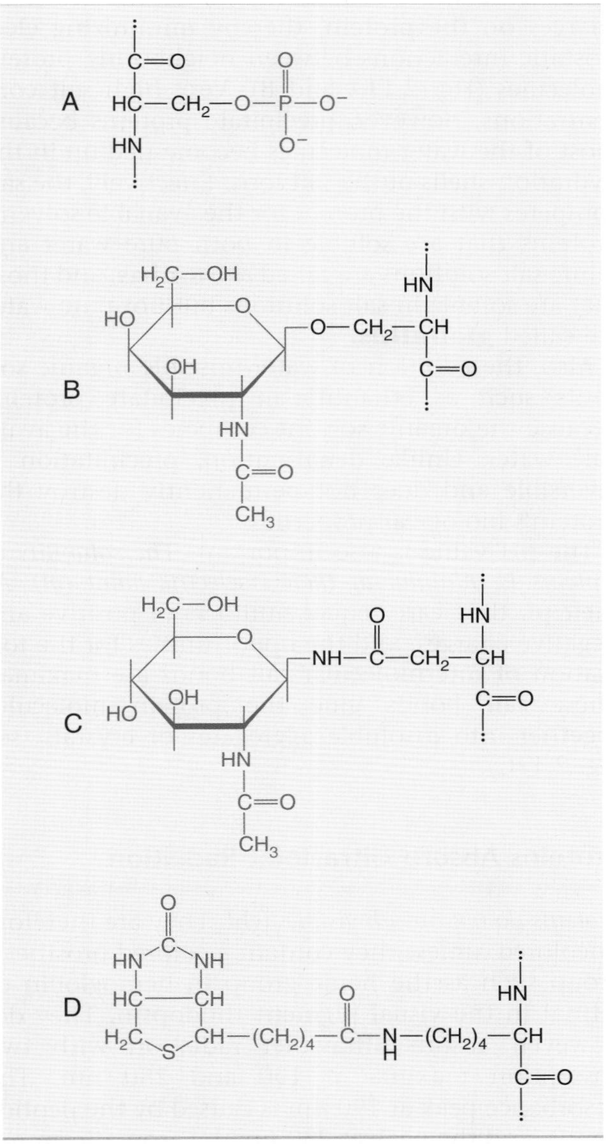

Proteins can also bind noncovalently to other molecules. **Lipoproteins,** for example, are noncovalent aggregates of lipids and proteins held together by hydrophobic interactions (see Chapter 25).

Proteins Lose Their Biological Activities When Their Higher Order Structure Is Destroyed

The covalent bonds in proteins are stable under ordinary conditions. **Peptide bonds** are readily cleaved by proteolytic enzymes such as those in the digestive tract. In the absence of enzymes, however, their hydrolysis requires heating with a strong acid or base. The cleavage of **disulfide bonds** requires reducing or oxidizing agents:

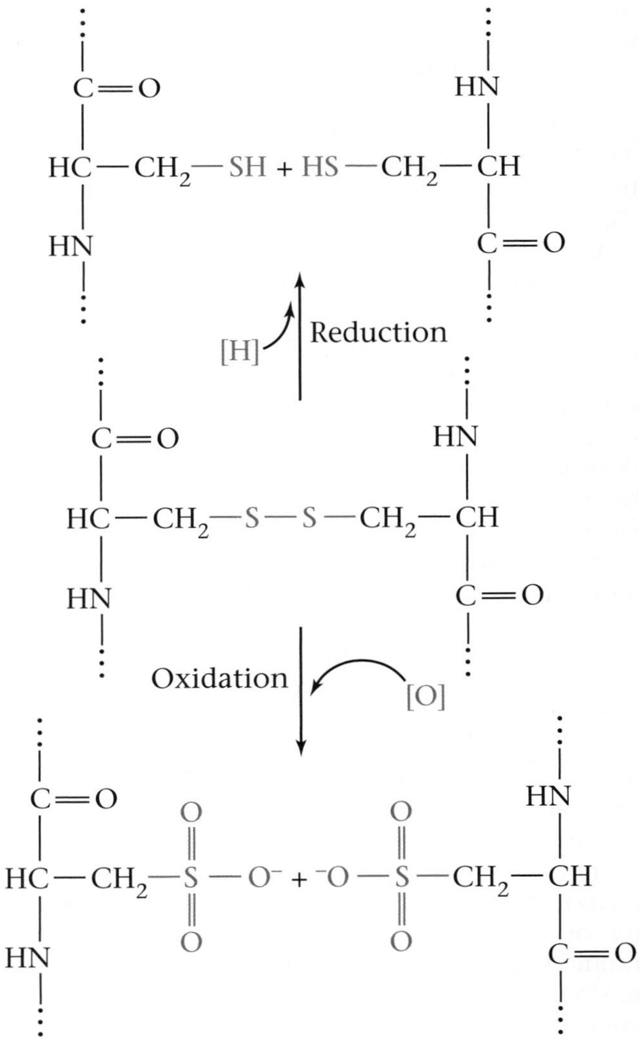

Figure 2.10 Examples of posttranslational modifications in proteins. **A,** A phosphoserine residue. Aside from serine, threonine and tyrosine also can form phosphate bonds in proteins. **B,** An N-acetylgalactosamine residue bound to a serine side chain. Serine and threonine form O-glycosidic bonds in glycoproteins. **C,** An N-acetylglucosamine residue bound to an asparagine side chain by an N-glycosidic bond. These "N-linked" carbohydrates are also common in glycoproteins. **D,** Some enzymes contain covalently bound prosthetic groups. As a coenzyme (see Chapter 5), the prosthetic group participates in the enzymatic reaction. This example shows biotin, which is bound covalently to a lysine side chain.

The noncovalent interactions, however, are so weak that *the higher order structure of proteins can be destroyed by heating.* Within a few minutes of being heated above a certain temperature (usually between 50° and 80° C), the finely crafted higher order structure collapses into a messy tangle work that is known as a **random coil.** This process is called **heat denaturation.**

Denaturation destroys the protein's biological properties. Stated another way, *the biological properties of proteins depend on their higher order structures.* Even the physical properties change dramatically with denaturation. Water solubility, for example, is lost because the denatured polypeptide chains get irrevocably entangled. This happens when an egg is boiled.

The renaturation of a denatured protein is possible only for a few simple-structured proteins under carefully controlled laboratory conditions. Otherwise, *protein denaturation is irreversible.* The boiled egg does not become unboiled when kept in the cold.

Anything that disrupts noncovalent interactions can denature proteins. Many **detergents** and **organic solvents** denature proteins by disrupting hydrophobic interactions. Being nonpolar, they insert themselves between the side chains of hydrophobic amino acids. Strong **acids** and **bases** denature proteins by changing their charge pattern. In a strong acid, the protein loses its negative charges, and in a strong base, it loses its positive charges. This deprives the protein of intramolecular salt bonds. Also, high concentrations of small hydrophilic molecules with high hydrogen bonding potential, such as urea, can denature proteins. They do so by disrupting the hydrogen bonds between water molecules. This limits the extent to which water molecules assume a more "ordered" position at an aqueous/nonpolar interface, and the hydrophobic interactions within the protein are weakened.

Heavy metal ions such as lead, cadmium, and mercury, can denature proteins by binding to carboxylate groups and, in particular, sulfhydryl groups in proteins. This affinity for functional groups in proteins is the reason for their toxicity.

The fragility of life is astonishing. A 6° C rise of the body temperature can be fatal, and the blood pH must never fall below 7.0 or rise above 7.7. These subtle changes in the physical environment do not cleave covalent bonds, but *they disrupt noncovalent interactions.* It is because of the vulnerability of noncovalent higher order structures that humans had to evolve sophisticated regulatory mechanisms for the maintenance of their internal environment.

The Solubility of Proteins Depends on pH and Salt Concentration

Unlike fibrous proteins, most globular proteins are water-soluble. Their solubility is affected by the salt concentration. Raising the salt concentration from zero to one percent or more increases their solubility because the salt ions neutralize the electrical charges on the protein, thereby minimizing electrostatic interactions between neighboring protein molecules (Fig. 2.11A and B). Very high salt concentrations, however, precipitate proteins because most of the water molecules become tied up in the hydration shells of the salt ions. Effectively, the salt competes with the protein for the available solvent. Proteins that are soluble in both pure water and dilute salt solutions are called **albumins,** and those that are soluble in salt solutions but not pure water are called **globulins.**

Also, the addition of water-miscible organic solvents such as ethanol can precipitate proteins because the organic solvent competes for the available water. Unlike denaturation, precipitation is reversible and does not permanently destroy the protein's biological properties.

The pH value is also important. *The solubility of proteins is minimal at their isoelectric point (pI).* At their pI, they carry equal numbers of positive and negative charges, and the opportunities for the formation of intermolecular salt bonds are maximal. These salt bonds glue the protein molecules together into insoluble aggregates or crystals (see Fig. 2.11C).

Proteins Absorb Ultraviolet Radiation

Proteins do not absorb visible light. They are therefore uncolored, unless they contain a colored prosthetic group such as the heme group in hemoglobin or retinal in the visual pigment rhodopsin. They do, however, absorb ultraviolet radiation with two absorption maxima at 190 and 280 nm. The absorbance peak at 190 nm is caused by the peptide bonds, and the peak at 280 nm, by aromatic amino acid side chains. The peak at 280 nm is more useful in laboratory practice because it is relatively specific for proteins. Nucleic acids, however, have an absorbance peak at 260 nm that overlaps the 280 nm peak of proteins (Fig. 2.12).

Proteins Can Be Separated by Their Charge or Their Molecular Weight

Dialysis is used in the laboratory to separate proteins from salts and other small contaminants. The

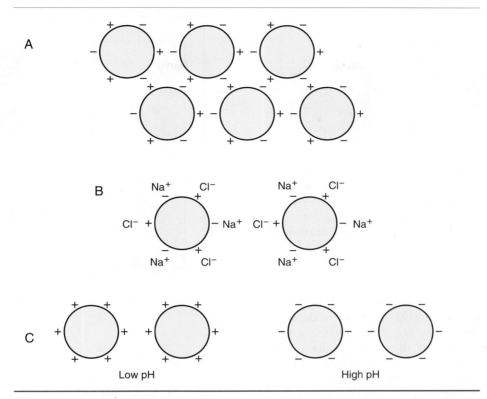

Figure 2.11 Effects of salt and pH on protein solubility. **A,** Protein in distilled water. Salt bonds between protein molecules cause the molecules to aggregate. The protein becomes insoluble. **B,** Protein in 5% sodium chloride (NaCl): Salt ions bind to the surface charges of the protein molecules, thereby preventing intermolecular salt bonds. **C,** The effect of pH on protein solubility: The formation of intermolecular salt bonds is favored at the isoelectric point. At pH values greater or less than the pI, the electrostatic interactions between the molecules are mainly repulsive.

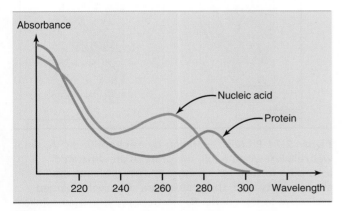

Figure 2.12 Typical ultraviolet absorbance spectra of proteins and nucleic acids. The protein absorbance peak at 280 nm is caused by the aromatic side chains of tyrosine and tryptophan. Nucleic acids absorb at 260 nm because of the aromatic character of their purine and pyrimidine bases.

protein is enclosed in a little bag of porous cellophane as shown in Figure 2.13. The pores allow salts and small molecules to diffuse out, but the large proteins are retained.

The dialysis of kidney patients is based on the same principle. The patient's blood is passed along semipermeable membranes that allow the removal of low-molecular-weight waste products while plasma proteins and blood cells are retained. The blood is dialyzed, not against distilled water (which would lead to a malpractice suit), but against a solution with physiological concentrations of nutrients and inorganic ions.

Electrophoresis is the most common method for protein separation in the clinical laboratory, as illustrated in Figure 2.14. It is based on the movement of charged proteins in an electrical field. At pH values above its pI, the protein carries mainly negative charges and moves to the anode; at pH values below the pI, positive charges prevail and the protein moves to the cathode; and at the pI, the net charge is zero and the protein stays put. Cellulose acetate foil, starch gel, or other carrier materials can be used.

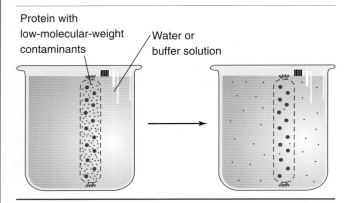

Figure 2.13 The use of dialysis for protein purification. Only small molecules and inorganic ions can pass through the porous membrane.

Electrophoresis is the standard method for the separation of plasma proteins and for the detection of abnormal proteins (see Fig. 2.14). When a structurally abnormal protein differs from its normal counterpart by a single amino acid substitution, *the electrophoretic mobility is changed only if the charge pattern is changed.* When, for example, a glutamate residue is replaced by aspartate, the electrophoretic mobility remains the same because these two amino acids carry the same charge. When, however, glutamate is replaced by an uncharged amino acid such as valine, one negative charge is removed and the two proteins can be separated by electrophoresis.

Electrophoresis can be performed in a crosslinked polyacrylamide or agarose gel that impairs the movement of large molecules. At a pH at which all proteins move to the same pole, they are separated mainly by their molecular weight rather than their charge (see Fig. 2.14B).

SUMMARY

Proteins consist of 20 different amino acids, held together by peptide bonds. The covalent structure of the protein is called its primary structure. It is specified by the amino acid sequence and the positions of additional covalent bonds. Higher order structures are formed by noncovalent interactions that can involve both peptide bonds and amino acid side chains.

Regular, repetitive folding patterns are called secondary structures. The most important secondary structures are the α helix and the β-pleated sheet, both stabilized by hydrogen bonds between the peptide bonds. The tertiary structure, which is prominent in globular proteins, is the overall folding pattern of the polypeptide. It is stabilized mainly by

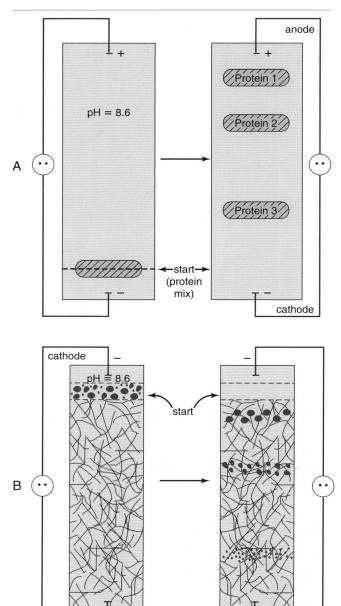

Figure 2.14 Protein separation by electrophoresis. **A,** On a wet cellulose acetate foil, the proteins are separated according to their net change. If, as in this case, an alkaline pH is used, the proteins are negatively charged and move to the anode. **B,** Electrophoresis in a crosslinked polyacrylamide gel. Although small molecules can move in the field, larger ones "get stuck" in the gel. Under suitable pH conditions, this method separates on the basis of molecular weight rather than charge.

hydrophobic interactions between amino acid side chains. Some proteins consist of more than one polypeptide (subunits). Their subunit composition and interactions are referred to as the quaternary structure.

Disulfide bonds, formed between cysteine side chains, are present in many proteins. They are either within the polypeptide (intrachain) or between polypeptides (interchain). Also, non-polypeptide components are common in proteins. These components are called prosthetic groups.

The noncovalent higher order structure of proteins can be destroyed by heating, detergents, nonpolar organic solvents, heavy metals, and extreme pH. This process of denaturation leads to a complete loss of the protein's biological properties. Many laboratory methods are available for the separation of proteins from biological samples.

📖 Further Reading

Blaber ML, Zhang X-J, Matthews BW: Structural basis of amino acid α-helix propensity. Science 260:1637-1640, 1993.

Branden C, Tooze J: Introduction to Protein Structure. New York: Garland Science Publishing, 1998.

Franks F (ed): Characterization of Proteins. Totowa, NJ: Humana Press, 1988.

Kamoun PP: Denaturation of globular proteins by urea: breakdown of hydrogen or hydrophobic bonds? Trends Biochem Sci 13:424-425, 1988.

Thomas PJ, Qu B-H, Pedersen PL: Defective protein folding as a basis of human disease. Trends Biochem Sci 20(11):456-459, 1995.

QUESTIONS

1. **The component of a water-soluble globular protein that is most likely to be present in the center of the molecule rather than on its surface is**

   A. A glutamate side chain.
   B. A histidine side chain.
   C. A phenylalanine side chain.
   D. A phosphate group covalently linked to a serine side chain.
   E. An oligosaccharide covalently linked to an asparagine side chain.

Acetyl-Ala-Glu-His-Ser-Lys-Gly-amide

2. **The above structure is an oligopeptide that is acetylated at its amino end and amidated at its carboxyl end, making the terminal groups nonionizable. This oligopeptide has a pI close to**

   A. 4.3.
   B. 5.1.
   C. 6.0.
   D. 8.4.
   E. 10.8.

3. **Human blood plasma contains about 7% protein. These plasma proteins have pK values close to 4 or 5. In the test tube, these proteins will form an insoluble precipitate after all of the following treatments *except***

   A. Boiling the serum for 5 minutes.
   B. Adding sodium chloride to a concentration of 35%.
   C. Adjusting the pH to 4.5.
   D. Boiling the serum with 6N hydrochloric acid for 10 hours.
   E. Mixing one volume of plasma with two volumes of pure alcohol.

4. **A genetic engineer wants to produce athletes with increased hemoglobin concentration in the erythrocytes, to improve oxygen supply to the muscles. This makes it necessary to increase the water solubility of the hemoglobin molecule. Which of the following amino acid changes on the surface of the hemoglobin molecule is most likely to increase its water solubility?**

   A. Arg → Lys.
   B. Leu → Phe.
   C. Gln → Ser.
   D. Ala → Asn.
   E. Ser → Ala.

CHAPTER 3

Oxygen Transporters: Hemoglobin and Myoglobin

The human body consumes about 500 g of molecular oxygen per day. The transport of this amount from the lungs to the other tissues is no easy feat. At the oxygen partial pressure of 90 torr that prevails in the lung capillaries, only 2.8 ml (4.1 mg) of O_2 can dissolve in 1 liter of plasma. Without oxygen-binding proteins, the 8000 liters of blood that the heart pumps to the tissues every day would be able to supply only about 30 g of oxygen: 6% of the total requirement. Fortunately, human blood contains 150 g of the oxygen binding protein hemoglobin per liter. Thanks to hemoglobin, 1 liter of blood can dissolve 280 mg of oxygen, about 70 times more than hemoglobin-free blood plasma.

Two proteins are specially designed for oxygen binding: **hemoglobin** in red blood cells (RBCs) and **myoglobin** in muscle. The binding of oxygen to these proteins, known technically as **oxygenation,** is reversible:

$$\text{Protein} + O_2 \underset{\text{Deoxygenation}}{\overset{\text{Oxygenation}}{\rightleftharpoons}} \text{Protein } O_2$$

Therefore, oxygen binds to the oxygen-binding proteins when it is plentiful and is released when it is scarce.

The Heme Group Is the Oxygen-Binding Site of Hemoglobin and Myoglobin

None of the functional groups in the common amino acids can bind molecular oxygen. Therefore, the oxygen-binding proteins require **heme** as an oxygen-binding prosthetic group.

Heme consists of a porphyrin, called **protoporphyrin IX,** with a ferrous iron chelated in its center (Fig. 3.1). Protoporphyrin IX contains four five-membered nitrogen-containing rings, known as **pyrrole rings,** held together by methine ($-CH=$) bridges and accompanied by methyl ($-CH_3$), vinyl ($-CH=CH_2$) and propionate ($-CH_2-CH_2-COO^-$) side chains. The porphyrin ring system contains conjugated double bonds (double bonds alternating with single bonds), which absorb visible light. *These double bonds are responsible for the color of human blood.* Oxygenated hemoglobin is red, and deoxyhemoglobin is blue. Therefore, oxygen deficiency, or **hypoxia,** can be recognized as a blue discoloration of the lips and other mucous membranes. This discoloration is called **cyanosis.**

The most important part of the heme group is its iron. Like other heavy metals, ionized iron can form coordinate bonds with the free electron pairs of oxygen and nitrogen atoms. The iron in heme is bound to the nitrogen atoms of the four pyrrole rings. In hemoglobin and myoglobin, the iron forms a fifth bond with a nitrogen atom in a histidine side chain of the apoprotein. This histidine is called the **proximal histidine.** An optional sixth bond can be formed with molecular oxygen:

His

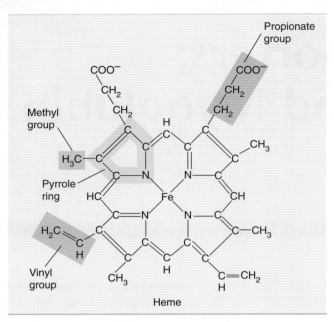

Propionate group

COO⁻

CH₂

CH₂

Methyl group

H₃C

CH₃

Pyrrole ring

HC

Fe

CH

Vinyl group

H₂C

CH₃

CH₃

C=CH₂

Heme

Figure 3.1 Structure of the heme group in hemoglobin and myoglobin. Note that the upper part of the group is hydrophilic because of the charged propionate side chains, whereas the lower part is hydrophobic. The conjugated double bonds in the ring system are responsible for its color. Oxyhemoglobin is red, deoxyhemoglobin blue.

Iron can exist in a ferrous (Fe^{2+}) and a ferric (Fe^{3+}) state. Ferric iron is the more oxidized form because it can be formed from ferrous iron by the removal of an electron:

$$Fe^{2+} \rightleftharpoons Fe^{3+}$$

e^-

e^-

Ferrous iron (reduced form)   **Ferric iron** (oxidized form)

By definition, the removal of an electron qualifies as oxidation. *The heme iron in hemoglobin and myoglobin is always in the ferrous state.* Even during oxygen binding it is not oxidized to the ferric form. It becomes oxygenated but not oxidized.

Myoglobin Is a Tightly Packed Globular Protein

Myoglobin consists of a single polypeptide with 153 amino acids and a tightly bound heme group (molecular weight: 17,000 D, or 17 kDa). Spectroscopic methods such as x-ray diffraction can be used to determine the higher order structure of proteins,

and because of its small size, myoglobin has been a pet subject for structural studies. These studies revealed a globular protein with dimensions of 2.5 × 3.5 × 4.5 nm (Fig. 3.2). *About 75% of the amino acid residues participate in α-helical structures.* Eight α helices with lengths between 7 and 23 amino acids are present, connected by nonhelical segments. Starting from the amino terminus, they are designated by capital letters A through H. The positions of the amino acid residues are specified by the helix letter and their position in the helix. The proximal histidine, for example, which is in position 93 of the polypeptide counting from the amino end, is designated His F8 because it is the eighth amino acid in the F helix.

Many of the α helices are **amphipathic,** with hydrophobic amino acid residues clustered on one edge and hydrophilic residues on the other. The hydrophilic edge contacts the surrounding water, and the hydrophobic edge faces inward to the center of the molecule. Indeed, *the interior of myoglobin is filled with tightly packed nonpolar side chains, and hydrophobic interactions are the major stabilizing force in the tertiary structure.*

The heme group is tucked between the E helix and the F helix, properly positioned by hydrophobic interactions with amino acid side chains and the bond between the iron and the proximal histidine. On the side opposite the proximal histidine, the heme iron faces the **distal histidine** (His E7). There is a cavity between the distal histidine and the heme iron that is just large enough to accommodate an oxygen molecule.

Like most cytoplasmic proteins, *myoglobin contains no disulfide bonds.* Its tertiary structure is maintained only by noncovalent forces.

The Red Blood Cells Are Specialized for Oxygen Transport

Hemoglobin is found only in erythrocytes, or red blood cells (RBCs). Erythrocytes are released from the bone marrow and then circulate for about 120 days before they are scavenged by phagocytic cells in the spleen and other tissues. Unlike all other cells in the body, *erythrocytes have no nucleus* and are therefore no longer able to divide and to synthesize proteins; they are dead. Their hemoglobin is inherited from their nucleated precursors in the bone marrow. They also lack mitochondria and therefore do not consume any of the oxygen they transport. They cover their modest energy needs by the anaerobic metabolism of glucose to lactic acid. In essence, erythrocytes are bags filled with hemoglobin at a concentration of 33%, physically dissolved in the cytoplasm.

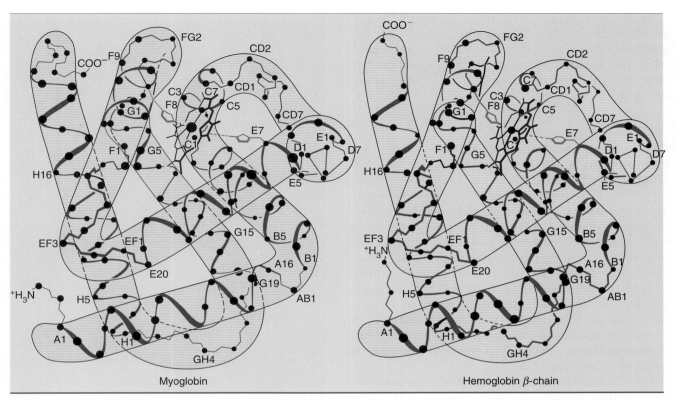

Figure 3.2 Tertiary structures of myoglobin and the β-chain of hemoglobin, as revealed by x-ray diffraction. Only the α-carbons are shown. The amino acid residues are designated by their position in one of the eight helices (A through H, starting from the amino terminus) or nonhelical links. The proximal histidine F8, for example, is the eighth amino acid in the F helix, counting from the amino end.

Table 3.1 The Most Important Human Hemoglobins*

Type	Subunit Structure	Importance
Major adult (HbA)	$\alpha_2\beta_2$	97% of adult hemoglobin
Minor adult (HbA₂)	$\alpha_2\delta_2$	2%-3% of adult hemoglobin
Fetal (HbF)	$\alpha_2\gamma_2$	Major hemoglobin in second and third trimesters of pregnancy

* See also Chapter 10.

The Hemoglobins Are Tetrameric Proteins

Whereas myoglobin consists of a single polypeptide with its heme group, *hemoglobin has four polypeptides, each with its own heme.* Humans have several types of hemoglobin (Table 3.1). **Hemoglobin A (HbA),** consisting of two α chains and two β chains, is the major adult hemoglobin. Also the **minor adult hemoglobin (HbA₂)** and **fetal hemoglobin (HbF)** have two α chains, but instead of the β chains, they have δ chains and γ chains, respectively.

The α chains have 141 amino acids, and the β, γ, and δ chains have 146. *All these chains are structurally related.* The α and β chains are identical in 64 of their amino acids. The β and δ chains differ in 10, and the β and γ chains in 39 of their 146 amino acids.

Although hemoglobin chains are distant relatives of myoglobin, only 28 amino acids are identical in α chains, β chains, and myoglobin. These conserved amino acids include the proximal and distal histidines and some of the other amino acids contacting the heme group. Many of the nonconserved amino acid positions are "conservative" substitutions, and corresponding amino acids have similar physicochemical properties.

Each hemoglobin subunit folds itself into a shape that strikingly resembles the tertiary structure of myoglobin (see Fig. 3.2). Overall, *hemoglobin looks like four myoglobin molecules glued together.* Like myoglobin, each hemoglobin subunit has a hydrophobic core, whereas most of the surface is formed by hydrophilic amino acid residues. There are no disulfide bonds, and the four subunits are held together only by noncovalent interactions.

As in myoglobin, the heme group is tucked between the E and F helices. The immediate environment of the heme iron is the same in each case, with the proximal histidine (His F8) bound on one side and the distal histidine (His E7) on the opposite side.

Oxygenated and Deoxygenated Hemoglobin Have Different Quaternary Structures

The subunits of deoxyhemoglobin are held together by eight salt bonds between the polypeptides, as well as by hydrogen bonds and other noncovalent interactions. Upon oxygenation, the salt bonds break and a new set of hydrogen bonds forms. Overall, the interactions between the subunits are weaker in oxyhemoglobin than in deoxyhemoglobin. Therefore, the conformation of deoxyhemoglobin is called the **T** (tense, or taut) **conformation,** that of oxyhemoglobin the **R** (relaxed) **conformation** (Fig. 3.3).

The conformation of hemoglobin changes with oxygenation because the bond distances between the heme iron and the five nitrogen atoms with which it is complexed shorten when oxygen binds. This distorts the shape of the heme group and exerts a pull on the F helix to which the proximal histidine (F8) belongs. The interactions with the other subunits are destabilized, and the shape of the whole molecule is shifted toward the R conformation.

The most important biological difference between conformations is their oxygen-binding affinity. *The R conformation binds oxygen 150 to 300 times more tightly than the T conformation.*

Proteins that can assume alternative higher order structures are called **allosteric proteins.** *The alternative conformations of an allosteric protein interconvert spontaneously, and their equilibrium is affected by ligand binding.* A **ligand** (Latin *ligare* = "to bind") is any small molecule that binds reversibly to a protein.

Oxygen Binding to Hemoglobin Is Cooperative

The **oxygen binding curve** describes the fractional saturation of the heme groups at varying oxygen partial pressures. The oxygen partial pressure (pO_2) is about 100 torr in the lung alveoli, 90 torr in the lung capillaries, and between 30 and 60 torr in the capillaries of most tissues. In contracting muscles, it can fall to 20 torr.

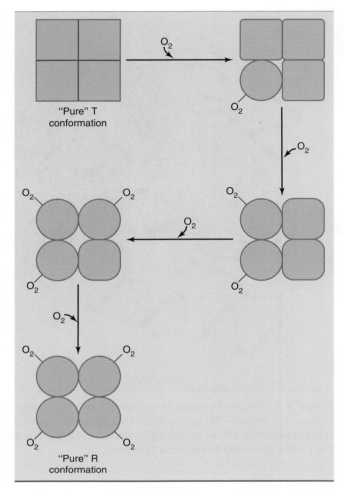

Figure 3.3 Simplified model for the transition from T to R conformation during successive oxygenations of hemoglobin. Partially oxygenated hemoglobin spends most of its time in intermediate conformational states. Actually, different conformations ranging from "pure" T to "pure" R exist in equilibrium in each oxygenation state.

Figure 3.4 shows that *myoglobin binds oxygen far tighter than does hemoglobin.* It is half-saturated with oxygen at 1 torr, whereas hemoglobin requires 26 torr. *This difference in oxygen affinities facilitates the transfer of oxygen from the blood to the tissue.*

The shapes of the oxygen binding curves differ as well. The myoglobin curve is hyperbolic. This has to be expected for a simple equilibrium reaction of the type

$$Mb + O_2 \rightleftharpoons Mb \bullet O_2$$

The binding curve of hemoglobin, however, is sigmoidal. Why? Completely deoxygenated hemoglobin is mainly in the T conformation, which has a very low oxygen affinity. This accounts for the flat part of the curve below about 10 torr. With increasing oxygen partial pressure, however, the first heme

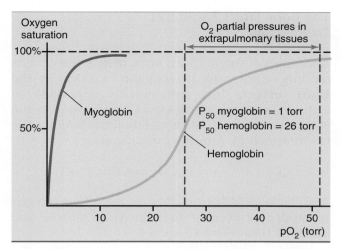

Figure 3.4 Oxygen-binding curves of hemoglobin and myoglobin. The P_{50} is defined as the oxygen partial pressure at which half of the heme groups are oxygenated.

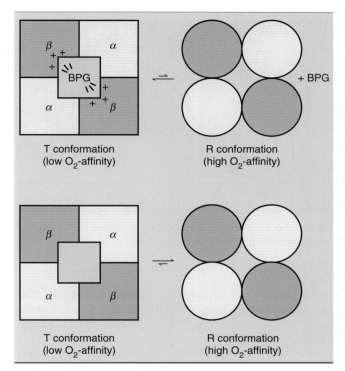

Figure 3.5 Effect of 2,3-bisphosphoglycerate (BPG) on the equilibrium between the T and R conformations of hemoglobin. The salt bonds between BPG and the β-chains stabilize the T conformation.

becomes oxygenated nevertheless. Oxygenation of the first heme destabilizes the T conformation and shifts the structure towards the R conformation. This repeats itself after binding of the second and third oxygen molecules. *Oxygen binding to a heme group in hemoglobin increases the oxygen affinities of the remaining heme groups.* This increase is called **positive cooperativity**.

Cooperativity improves hemoglobin's efficiency as an oxygen transporter. Without cooperativity, an 81-fold increase of the pO_2 would be required to raise the oxygen saturation from 10% to 90%. For hemoglobin, however, a 4.8-fold increase is sufficient to do the same. Thanks to positive co-operativity, hemoglobin is about 96% saturated in the lung capillaries (pO_2 = 90 torr) but only 33% saturated in the capillaries of working muscle (pO_2 = 20 torr). Less oxygen is extracted in other tissues, so that the mixed venous blood is still 60% to 70% oxygenated. Although this oxygen is useless under ordinary conditions, it can keep humans alive for a few minutes after acute respiratory arrest.

2,3-Bisphosphoglycerate Is a Negative Allosteric Effector of Oxygen Binding to Hemoglobin

2,3-Bisphosphoglycerate (BPG) is a small organic molecule that is present in RBCs at a con-centration of about 5 mmol, roughly equimolar with hemoglobin:

$$2,3\text{-BPG}$$

Most of it is noncovalently bound to hemoglobin in a stoichiometry of one molecule of BPG per hemoglobin molecule. Positioned in a central cavity between the subunits, it forms salt bonds with pos-itively charged amino acid residues in the two β chains.

BPG binds to the T conformation but not the R con-formation of hemoglobin. Therefore, the salt bonds that it forms with the β chains stabilize only the T conformation, favoring it over the R conformation (Fig. 3.5). Because the T conformation has the lower oxygen affinity, *BPG decreases the oxygen-binding affinity.*

BPG is a physiologically important regulator of oxygen binding to hemoglobin. The BPG concen-tration in RBCs increases during hypoxic condi-tions, including lung diseases, severe anemia, and adaptation to high altitude. This barely affects

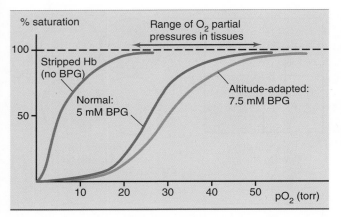

Figure 3.6 Effect of 2,3-bisphosphoglycerate (BPG) on the oxygen-binding affinity of hemoglobin (Hb).

oxygenation in the lung capillaries, but *it enhances the unloading of oxygen in the tissues whose oxygen partial pressures are in the steep part of the oxygen binding curve* (Fig. 3.6).

BPG is characterized as a **negative allosteric effector** with regard to oxygen binding to hemoglobin because it lowers the oxygen affinity. A **positive allosteric effector** would increase the oxygen affinity.

Allosteric interactions between different ligands, such as BPG and O_2, are called **heterotropic effects.** Interactions between identical ligands, as in the cooperativity of oxygen binding, are called **homotropic effects.**

Allosteric proteins are common. Many enzymes, for example, are regulated by positive and negative allosteric effectors that enhance or inhibit enzymatic catalysis, respectively (see Chapter 4). These effectors bind to regulatory sites on the enzyme that are distant from the catalytic sites. *Most allosteric proteins consist of more than one subunit, and the subunit interactions are affected by ligand binding.*

Fetal Hemoglobin Has a Higher Oxygen Binding Affinity than Does Adult Hemoglobin

In HbA, BPG forms salt bonds with the amino termini of the β chains and with the side chains of Lys EF6 and His H21 in the β chains. In the γ chains of HbF, His H21 is replaced by an uncharged serine residue. Therefore, *BPG binds less tightly to HbF than to HbA,* and it reduces the oxygen affinity of HbF less than that of HbA. HbF thereby ends up with the higher oxygen affinity. It is half-saturated at 20 torr, in comparison with 26 torr for HbA. *This facilitates the transfer of oxygen from the maternal blood to the fetal blood in the capillaries of the placenta.*

The Bohr Effect Facilitates Oxygen Delivery

Also, low pH (high acidity) can reduce the oxygen binding affinity of hemoglobin. Known as the **Bohr effect,** this reduction is important in actively metabolizing tissues. Carbon dioxide, the end product of oxidative metabolism, acidifies the environment by forming carbonic acid:

$$CO_2 + H_2O \rightleftharpoons H_2CO_3 \rightleftharpoons HCO_3^- + H^+$$

Also, lactic acid is formed in places where oxygen is needed, especially in exercising muscle and ischemic tissues (see Chapter 21).

Acidity reduces oxygen binding because *oxygenated hemoglobin is more acidic than deoxyhemoglobin.* In other words, oxygen binding releases protons (H^+) from hemoglobin:

$$\text{Hemoglobin} + O_2 \rightleftharpoons \text{Hemoglobin} \cdot O_2 + nH^+$$

An increase in the proton concentration pushes this reaction to the left, favoring the release of oxygen from hemoglobin. About 0.7 protons are released during the binding of each oxygen molecule, most of them as a result of pK changes of those groups that participate in the formation of the intersubunit salt bonds in the T conformation. The equilibrium of the reaction

$$Hb \cdot O_2 + 0.7\ H^+ \rightleftharpoons Hb + O_2$$

is defined by the dissociation constant K_D (see also Chapter 4):

$$K_D = \frac{[Hb] \times [O_2]}{[Hb \cdot O_2] \times [H^+]^{0.7}}$$

This equation can be rearranged to:

$$\frac{[Hb]}{[Hb \cdot O_2]} = K_D \times \frac{[H^+]^{0.7}}{[O_2]}$$

It shows that at a constant oxygen concentration $[O_2]$, an increase of the hydrogen ion concentration $[H^+]$ increases the ratio of deoxyhemoglobin $[Hb]$ over oxyhemoglobin $[Hb \cdot O_2]$.

Also, carbon dioxide (CO_2) decreases the oxygen affinity of hemoglobin. It binds covalently to the terminal amino groups of the α and β chains, forming **carbamino hemoglobin,** as shown on the following page:

$$\text{Hemoglobin}\text{---}NH_2 + CO_2$$

$$\updownarrow$$

$$\text{Hemoglobin}\text{---}NH\text{---}\overset{\overset{\displaystyle O}{\|}}{C}\text{---}O^- + H^+$$

This reversible reaction proceeds spontaneously, without the need for an enzyme. Carbamino hemoglobin has a lower oxygen affinity than does unmodified hemoglobin. Like the pH effect, the CO_2 effect ensures that *oxygen is most easily released in actively metabolizing tissues where it is most needed.*

Most Carbon Dioxide Is Transported as Bicarbonate

Carbon dioxide has higher water solubility than does oxygen, and a significant portion can therefore be transported physically dissolved in the plasma. Also, carbamino hemoglobin, as well as the carbamino derivatives of plasma proteins, transports some CO_2.

About 80% of the CO_2, however, is transported from the peripheral tissues to the lungs as inorganic bicarbonate (Fig. 3.7). CO_2 diffuses into the erythrocyte, where it encounters **carbonic anhydrase,** a highly active enzyme that rapidly establishes equilibrium among CO_2, H_2O, and carbonic acid. Most of the carbonic acid dissociates into a proton and the bicarbonate anion. While the proton binds to hemoglobin as part of the Bohr effect, the bicarbonate leaves the cell in exchange for a chloride ion. This exchange, which requires an anion channel in the membrane, is called the **chloride shift.** The bicarbonate is now transported to the lungs, physically dissolved in the plasma. In the lung capillaries, all these processes run in reverse, and the CO_2 is exhaled.

Anemia Is Commonly Seen in Clinical Practice

Between 38% and 53% of the blood volume consists of RBCs. This percentage can be determined by centrifuging the blood for some minutes. Because of their high protein content, the erythrocytes have a higher density than plasma and settle to the bottom. The percentage of the total volume occupied by this sediment of red cells is called the **hematocrit** (Table 3.2).

Patients whose blood hemoglobin falls below the normal range of 12% to 17% are said to have

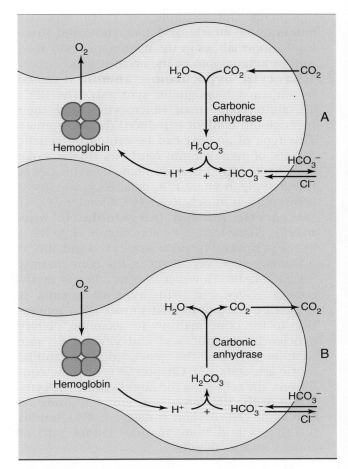

Figure 3.7 The major mechanism of carbon dioxide transport. Note that all processes are reversible. Their direction is determined by the concentrations of the involved substances in the extrapulmonary tissues **(A)** and in the lung capillaries **(B)**.

Table 3.2 Characteristics of Red Blood Cells (RBCs) and Hemoglobin

Diameter of RBCs	$7.3\,\mu m$
Life span of RBCs	120 days
Number of RBCs	4.2-5.4 million/mm³ (female)
	4.6-6.2 million/mm³ (male)
Intracorpuscular hemoglobin concentration	33%
Hematocrit*	38%-46% (female)
	42%-53% (male)
Hemoglobin in whole blood	12%-15% (female)
	14%-17% (male)

* Hematocrit = the percentage of the blood volume occupied by blood cells; measured by centrifugation of whole blood.

anemia. They usually have a reduced hematocrit as well. Chronic anemia can have many causes:

1. **Hemolysis** is the abnormal destruction of erythrocytes. Possible causes include bacterial toxins; enzymes that attack the erythrocyte

membrane (for example, in snake venoms); autoimmune attack; oxidative stress; and structural abnormalities in the membrane, cytoskeleton, or hemoglobin of the erythrocytes.

2. **Microcytic hypochromic anemia** is caused by impaired hemoglobin synthesis. The RBCs are abnormally small (microcytic), and their hemoglobin content is reduced (hypochromia). This type of anemia can be caused by genetic defects of hemoglobin synthesis (thalassemia; see Chapter 10), impaired heme biosynthesis as for example in vitamin B_6 deficiency, and, most commonly, iron deficiency (see Chapter 29).

3. **Macrocytic anemia** (**megaloblastic anemia**) is characterized by abnormally large RBCs in the peripheral blood (macrocytes) and abnormally large RBC precursors in the bone marrow (megaloblasts). However, the number of erythrocytes is reduced. This type of anemia is caused by conditions that impair DNA replication in the bone marrow: for example, dietary deficiencies of folic acid and vitamin B_{12} (see Chapter 29), and the genetic disease familial orotic acidemia (see Chapter 28). In these conditions, the cells grow too large because the cytoplasm of the RBC precursors grows at a normal rate while cell division is delayed. Also, serious blood loss and bone marrow failure can, of course, lead to anemia.

Methemoglobin Is a Nonfunctional Oxidized Form of Hemoglobin

The heme iron in hemoglobin and myoglobin binds molecular oxygen only in the ferrous (Fe^{2+}) state. Its oxidation to the ferric (Fe^{3+}) form produces useless **methemoglobin.** Normally less than 1% of the total hemoglobin is in the form of methemoglobin, but *oxidizing chemicals cause excessive methemoglobin formation.* These chemicals include many aniline dyes, aromatic nitro compounds, and inorganic and organic nitrites. Fortunately, the RBC can defend itself against excessive methemoglobin formation:

1. *Erythrocytes contain reducing substances* such as ascorbic acid (see Chapter 29) and glutathione (see Chapter 22), which destroy many oxidizing agents before they have a chance to react with hemoglobin.

2. *The binding of heme to the apoprotein creates a protective environment for the iron.* When heme is dissociated from the apoprotein, it becomes rapidly oxidized to **hemin** by molecular oxygen. Hemin binds a hydroxyl ion to form **hematin.** Structural abnormalities of the heme binding pocket in the α or β chain can lead to congenital methe-

moglobinemia (congenital means present at birth). The replacement of the proximal histidine by a tyrosine residue, for example, causes methemoglobinemia.

3. *The enzyme **methemoglobin reductase** reduces methemoglobin back to normal hemoglobin,* using the coenzyme NADH as a reductant. Individuals with a genetic deficiency of methemoglobin reductase have congenital methemoglobinemia.

Methemoglobinemia is treated with methylene blue, which reduces the ferric iron to the ferrous state.

Carbon Monoxide Competes with Oxygen for Binding to the Heme Iron

Carbon monoxide (CO) is a product of incomplete combustion, and a small amount is even formed in the human body (see Chapter 27). Like molecular oxygen, *CO binds to the ferrous iron in hemoglobin and myoglobin.* The trouble is that the heme iron binds CO 200 times more tightly than it binds O_2. Therefore, even a low concentration of CO is sufficient to displace O_2 from its binding site on the heme iron. To make matters worse, the binding of CO to one of the heme groups greatly increases the oxygen-binding affinities of the remaining heme groups. This further impairs oxygen transport.

Despite its high affinity, *CO binding is reversible.* In a normally breathing patient with CO poisoning, O_2 gradually displaces the CO from the heme iron. The CO is blown off through the lungs, and the patient recovers slowly in the course of several hours.

The interaction between CO and O_2 at the heme iron is an example of **competitive antagonism:** the two ligands compete for the same site, displacing each other. The outcome depends on the relative affinities and concentrations of the ligands. Because CO has a 200-fold higher binding affinity than does O_2, a CO concentration of only $1/200$ of the O_2 concentration is sufficient to convert half of the oxyhemoglobin to CO hemoglobin. Therefore, *CO poisoning can be overcome by elevated O_2 partial pressure,* and hyperbaric O_2 is the treatment of choice.

Acute CO poisoning is seen after attempted suicide by inhaling car exhaust gas and in people trapped in a burning building. Throbbing headache, confusion, and fainting on exertion occur when 30% to 50% of the heme groups are occupied by CO, and a CO saturation of 80% is rapidly fatal. *Patients with CO poisoning are not cyanotic* because CO hemoglobin has a bright cherry-red color. Smokers have 4% to 8% of their hemoglobin in the CO form. Therefore, smoking is not a good habit for patients who suffer from poor tissue oxygenation, such as those with angina pectoris (myocardial ischemia).

SUMMARY

Humans need oxygen-binding proteins because molecular oxygen is poorly soluble in body fluids. Both hemoglobin in RBCs and myoglobin in the muscles employ heme as a prosthetic group. Myoglobin consists of a single polypeptide with a noncovalently bound heme group. Hemoglobin has four polypeptides, each with its own heme. Adult hemoglobin (HbA) has two α chains and two β chains, and fetal hemoglobin (HbF) has two α chains and two γ chains. Myoglobin has a far higher oxygen-binding affinity than do the hemoglobins, and HbF has a slightly higher affinity than does HbA.

Hemoglobin (but not myoglobin) has allosteric properties. There is positive cooperativity between the heme groups, leading to a sigmoidal oxygen-binding curve. BPG and protons are negative allosteric effectors that decrease the oxygen binding affinity. Hemoglobin deficiency, clinically known as anemia, occurs in many clinical conditions. Hemoglobin can also be poisoned by substances that oxidize the ferrous heme iron to the ferric state and by the competitive antagonist CO that blocks the oxygen-binding site on the heme iron.

QUESTIONS

1. **A pharmaceutical company tries to develop a drug that improves tissue oxygenation by increasing the percentage of oxygen that is released from hemoglobin during its passage through the capillaries of extrapulmonary tissues. This drug, it is hoped, would become a popular doping agent for athletes. The company should try a drug that**

   A. Binds to the heme iron.
   B. Inhibits the degradation of 2,3-BPG, thereby increasing its concentration in erythrocytes.
   C. Binds to ion channels in the RBC membrane, thereby increasing the intracellular pH value.
   D. Binds to the R conformation of hemoglobin but not the T conformation.
   E. Induces the synthesis of hemoglobin γ chains in adults.

2. **A worker in a chemical factory loses consciousness within a few minutes after falling into a vat with the aromatic nitro compound nitrobenzene. This loss of consciousness may be caused by an action of nitrobenzene on hemoglobin, most likely resulting from**

   A. Competitive inhibition of oxygen binding.
   B. Oxidation of the heme iron to the ferric state.
   C. Reductive cleavage of disulfide bonds between the hemoglobin subunits.
   D. Hydrolysis of peptide bonds in hemoglobin α and β chains.
   E. Inhibition of hemoglobin synthesis.

3. **The oxygen-binding curve of hemoglobin is sigmoidal *because***

   A. The binding of oxygen to a heme group increases the oxygen affinities of the other heme groups.
   B. The heme groups of the α chains have a higher oxygen affinity than do the heme groups of the β chains.
   C. The distal histidine allows the hemoglobin molecule to change its conformation in response to an elevated carbon dioxide concentration.
   D. The subunits are held in place by interchain disulfide bonds.
   E. The solubility of the hemoglobin molecule changes with its oxidation state.

CHAPTER 4

Enzymatic Reactions

The living cell presents the student with an exciting array of ever-changing chemical reactions. Hardly any of these reactions would proceed at any noticeable rate if their starting materials, or **substrates,** were simply mixed in a test tube by an overoptimistic chemist. The chemist could possibly force the reactions by increasing the temperature. He or she could also try a nonselective catalyst, such as a strong acid or a strong base. But the human body is not in this lucky position because body temperature and pH must be kept within narrow limits.

Therefore, humans depend on highly selective catalysts called **enzymes.** By definition, *a catalyst is a substance that accelerates a chemical reaction without being consumed in the process.* Because it is regenerated at the end of each catalytic cycle (Fig. 4.1), a single molecule of the catalyst can convert many substrate molecules into product. Therefore, only a tiny amount of the catalyst is needed.

The **thermodynamic properties** of a reaction are those related to energy balance and equilibrium, whereas **kinetic properties** are related to its speed (velocity, or rate of the reaction). Enzymes do not change the equilibrium of a reaction or its energy balance; they only make it go faster. Thus, *enzymes change the kinetic but not the thermodynamic characteristics of the reaction.*

The Equilibrium Constant Describes the Equilibrium of the Reaction

In theory, all chemical reactions are reversible. The reaction equilibrium can be determined experimentally by mixing substrates (or products) with a suitable catalyst and allowing the reaction to proceed to completion. At this point, the concentrations of substrates and products can be measured to determine the **equilibrium constant, K_{equ}.** K_{equ} is *defined as the ratio of product concentration to substrate concentration at equilibrium.* For a simple reaction

$$A \rightleftharpoons B$$

the equilibrium constant is

$$K_{equ} = \frac{[B]}{[A]}$$

[B] and [A] are the molar concentrations of product B and substrate A at equilibrium.

When more than one substrate or product participates, *their concentrations have to be multiplied.* For the reaction

$$A + B \rightleftharpoons C + D$$

the equilibrium constant is

$$K_{equ} = \frac{[C] \times [D]}{[A] \times [B]}$$

The alcohol dehydrogenase (ADH) reaction provides an example. The balance of this reaction is

1
$$H_3C - CH_2OH + NAD^+$$
Ethanol
$$\rightleftharpoons H_3C - CHO + NADH + H^+$$
Acetaldehyde

NAD$^+$ (nicotinamide adenine dinucleotide) is a coenzyme that functions as a hydrogen acceptor in this reaction (see Chapter 5). The equilibrium constant of the reaction is

2
$$K_{equ} = \frac{[Acetaldehyde] \times [NADH] \times [H^+]}{[Ethanol] \times [NAD^+]}$$
$$= 10^{-11} M$$

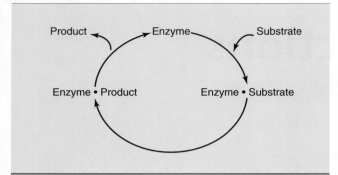

Figure 4.1 The catalytic cycle. The substrate has to bind to the enzyme to form a noncovalent enzyme-substrate complex (enzyme • substrate). The actual reaction takes place while the substrate is bound to the enzyme. Note that the enzyme is regenerated at the end of the catalytic cycle.

What are the relative concentrations of acetaldehyde and ethanol at equilibrium when [NADH] = [NAD⁺] and pH = 7.0? From equation (2) it is possible to obtain

3
$$\frac{[\text{Acetaldehyde}]}{[\text{Ethanol}]} = 10^{-11}\,\text{M} \times \frac{[\text{NAD}^+]}{[\text{NADH}]} \times \frac{1}{[\text{H}^+]}$$
$$= 10^{-11} \times 1 \times 10^{7}$$
$$= 10^{-4}$$

There is 10,000 times more ethanol than acetaldehyde at equilibrium!

Under aerobic conditions, however, NAD⁺ is far more abundant than NADH in the cell. When [NAD⁺] is 1000 times higher than [NADH], equation (3) assumes the numerical values of

$$\frac{[\text{Acetaldehyde}]}{[\text{Ethanol}]} = 10^{-11} \times 1000 \times 10^{7}$$
$$= 10^{-1}$$
$$= \frac{1}{10}$$

The pH is also important. At a pH of 8.0 and an [NAD⁺]/[NADH] ratio of 1000, for example, equation (3) yields

$$\frac{[\text{Acetaldehyde}]}{[\text{Ethanol}]} = 10^{-11} \times 1000 \times 10^{8}$$
$$= 10^{0}$$
$$= 1$$

This example shows that a reaction can be driven toward product formation by raising the concentration of a substrate or lowering the concentration of a product.

To adapt the equilibrium constant to physiological conditions, a "biological equilibrium constant," K'_{equ}, is used. In the definition of K'_{equ}, a value of 1.0 is assigned to the water concentration if water participates in the reaction and a value of 1.0 to a proton concentration of 10^{-7} mol/liter if protons participate in the reaction. The K'_{equ} of the alcohol dehydrogenase reaction, for example, is not 10^{-11} mol/liter but 10^{-4} mol/liter. At a pH of 8.0 in the preceding example, the proton concentration would be given a numerical value of 10^{-1}.

The Free Energy Change Is the Driving Force for Chemical Reactions

During chemical reactions, heat is either released or absorbed. The change in the heat content of the reacting system is characterized as ΔE. It is measured either in kilocalories per mole (kcal/mol) or in kilojoules per mole (kJ/mol, 1 kcal = 4.184 kJ). By convention, *a negative sign of ΔE indicates that heat is released; a positive sign indicates that heat is absorbed.* A more general description of energy changes is the **enthalpy change, ΔH:**

4
$$\Delta H = \Delta E + P \times \Delta V$$

where P is the pressure and ΔV is the volume change. $P \times \Delta V$ is the work done by the system. This can be substantial in a car motor, in which the volume in the cylinder expands against the pressure of the piston, but in the human body, the volume changes (ΔV) are negligible. Therefore, $\Delta H \approx \Delta E$. *The enthalpy change corresponds to the difference in the total chemical bond energies between the substrates and products.*

ΔH is not the only determinant of the reaction equilibrium, and some reactions do occur spontaneously, although they consume heat. The change in **entropy,** designated as ΔS, is important as well. *The entropy is a measure for the randomness or disorderliness of the system.* A cluttered desk is often cited as an example for a system of high entropy. A positive ΔS means that the system becomes more disordered during the reaction. The entropy change and the enthalpy change are combined in the **free energy change, ΔG:**

5
$$\Delta G = \Delta H - T \times \Delta S$$

where T is the absolute temperature measured in Kelvin.

ΔG is the driving force of the reaction. Like ΔE and ΔH in equation (4), it is measured in kilocalories per mole (kcal/mol) or kilojoules per mole (kJ/mol). *A negative sign of ΔG defines an **exergonic reaction.*** It proceeds spontaneously and forms product from substrate. *A positive sign of ΔG signifies an **endergonic reaction.*** It can proceed only in the backward direction. *At equilibrium, ΔG equals zero.*

Equation (5) shows that a reaction can be driven either by a decrease in the chemical bond energies of the reactants (negative ΔH) or an increase in their disorderliness (positive T × ΔS). Low energy content and high randomness are the preferred states. Like most students, Nature tends to slip from energized order into energy-depleted chaos.

Entropy changes are small in most biochemical reactions, but *diffusion is an entropy-driven process* (Fig. 4.2A). There is no making and breaking of chemical bonds during diffusion, and the enthalpy change ΔH is therefore zero. The T × ΔS part of equation (5) remains as the only driving force. Thus, diffusion can produce only a random distribution of the dissolved molecules.

The human body is a very orderly system. To maintain this improbable and therefore thermodynamically disfavored state of affairs, *biochemical reactions must antagonize the spontaneous increase in entropy.* Equation (5) shows that a reaction can reduce entropy (negative T × ΔS) only when it consumes chemical bond energy (negative ΔH). In other words, *humans must consume chemical bond energy to maintain the low-entropy state of the body.*

In the example of Figure 4.2B and C, the cell uses chemical bond energy from adenosine triphosphate (ATP) hydrolysis (ATP → adenosine diphosphate [ADP] + inorganic phosphate [Pᵢ], negative ΔH) to maintain a sodium gradient across the membrane (negative T × ΔS for sodium "pumping"). Without this chemical bond energy, the gradient dissipates, the entropy of the system increases, and the cell dies. That is what death and dying are all about: a sharp rise in the entropy of the body.

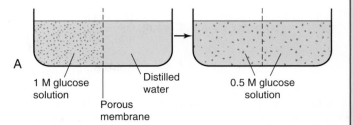

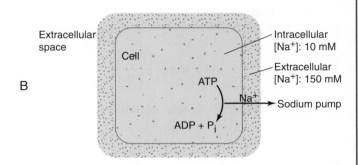

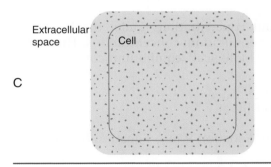

Figure 4.2 Diffusion as an entropy-driven process. **A,** In a hypothetical two-compartment system, molecules diffuse until their concentrations are equal. This is the state of maximal entropy. **B,** The living cell maintains a gradient of sodium ions across its plasma membrane. The cell can maintain this gradient, which represents a low-entropy state, only by "pumping" sodium out of the cell. The pump is fueled by the chemical bond energy in adenosine triphosphate (ATP). ADP, adenosine diphosphate; Pᵢ, inorganic phosphate. **C,** The dead cell lacks ATP: it cannot maintain its sodium gradient. Without the chemical bond energy of ATP, a high-entropy state develops spontaneously, with intracellular [Na⁺] = extracellular [Na⁺].

The Standard Free Energy Change Determines the Equilibrium

The "real" free energy change ΔG is not a property of the reaction as such, but *it is affected by the relative reactant concentrations.* As a measure for the energy balance of the reaction, the **standard free energy change, $\Delta G^{0\prime}$,** must be defined: *$\Delta G^{0\prime}$ is the free energy change under standard conditions.* Standard conditions are defined by a concentration of 1 mol/liter for all reactants (except protons and water) at a pH of 7.0. As in the definition of K'_{equ}, values of 1 are assigned both to the water con-

centration and to the proton concentration at a pH of 7.

For the reaction

$$A + B \rightarrow C + D$$

the standard free energy change $\Delta G^{0\prime}$ is related to the real free energy change ΔG by the following equation:

6
$$\Delta G = \Delta G^{0\prime} + R \times T \times \log_e \frac{[C] \times [D]}{[A] \times [B]}$$

$$= \Delta G^{0\prime} + R \times T \times 2.303 \times \log \frac{[C] \times [D]}{[A] \times [B]}$$

where R is the gas constant, and T is the absolute temperature measured in Kelvin. The numerical value of R is 1.987×10^{-3} kcal $\times$ mol^{-1} $\times$ K^{-1}. At a "standard temperature" of 25° C (298° K), equation (6) assumes the form of

7
$$= \Delta G^{0\prime} + 1.364 \times \log \frac{[C] \times [D]}{[A] \times [B]}$$

At equilibrium, $\Delta G = 0$, and equation (7) therefore yields

8
$$\Delta G^{0\prime} = -1.364 \times \log \frac{[C] \times [D]}{[A] \times [B]}$$

The reactant concentrations under the logarithm are now the equilibrium concentrations. Their ratio defines the "biological" equilibrium constant K'_{equ}:

9
$$\frac{[C] \times [D]}{[A] \times [B]} = K'_{equ}$$

Substituting Equation 9 into Equation 8 yields

10
$$\Delta G^{0\prime} = -1.364 \times \log K'_{equ}$$

There is a negative logarithmic relationship between $\Delta G^{0\prime}$ and the equilibrium constant $K_{equ}{}'$ of the reaction (Table 4.1). When $\Delta G^{0\prime}$ is negative, product concentrations are higher than substrate concentrations at equilibrium, and when it is positive, substrate concentrations are higher.

Table 4.1 Relationship between the Equilibrium Constant K'_{equ} and the Standard Free Energy Change $\Delta G^{0\prime}$

K'_{equ}	$\Delta G^{0\prime}$ [kcal/mol]
10^{-5}	6.82
10^{-4}	5.46
10^{-3}	4.09
10^{-2}	2.73
10^{-1}	1.36
1	0
10	−1.36
10^2	−2.73
10^3	−4.09
10^4	−5.46
10^5	−6.82

Enzymes Are Both Powerful and Selective

There is no compelling reason why only proteins should catalyze reactions, and catalytic RNAs are indeed known to exist. By and large, however, *almost all enzymes are globular proteins.*

Enzymes can accelerate a chemical reaction enormously. Many reactions that proceed within minutes in the presence of an enzyme would require thousands or even millions of years to reach their equilibrium in the absence of a catalyst. The **turnover number** describes the catalytic power of the enzyme. It is defined as *the number of substrate molecules converted to product by one enzyme molecule per second.* Table 4.2 shows the turnover numbers of some enzymes.

Another key property of enzymes is their **substrate specificity.** Typically, each reaction requires its own enzyme. If, for example, an enzyme is inhibited by a drug or deficient because of a genetic defect, only one reaction is blocked.

The Substrate Must Bind to Its Enzyme Before the Reaction Can Proceed

Enzymatic catalysis, like sex, requires intimate physical contact. It starts with the formation of an **enzyme-substrate complex:**

$$E + S \rightleftharpoons E \cdot S$$

where E = free enzyme, S = free substrate, and $E \cdot S$ = enzyme-substrate complex.

In the enzyme-substrate complex, the substrate is bound noncovalently to the **active site** on the

Table 4.2 Approximate Turnover Numbers of Some Enzymes

Enzyme	Turnover Number [sec^{-1}]*
Carbonic anhydrase	600,000
Catalase	80,000
Acetylcholinesterase	25,000
Triose phosphate isomerase	4,400
α-Amylase	300
Lactate dehydrogenase (muscle)	200
Chymotrypsin	100
Aldolase	11
Lysozyme	0.5
Fructose 2,6-bisphosphatase	0.1

* Turnover numbers are measured at saturating substrate concentrations. They depend on the assay conditions, including temperature and pH.

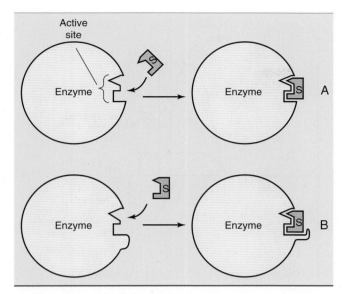

Figure 4.3 The two models of enzyme-substrate binding. **A,** The lock-and-key model. **B,** The induced-fit model. S, substrate.

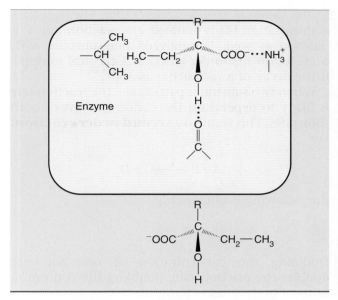

Figure 4.4 A three-point attachment is the minimal requirement for stereoselectivity. In this hypothetical example, the enzyme-substrate complex is formed by a salt bond, a hydrogen bond, and a hydrophobic interaction. The substrate binds, whereas its enantiomer (shown below) is not able to form an enzyme-substrate complex.

surface of the enzyme protein. The active site contains the functional groups for substrate binding and catalysis. If a prosthetic group participates in the reaction as a coenzyme, it is present in the active site.

According to the **lock-and-key model,** substrate and active site bind each other because their surfaces are complementary. In many cases, however, substrate binding induces a conformational change in the active site that leads to further enzyme-substrate interactions and brings catalytically active groups to the substrate. This is called **induced fit** (Fig. 4.3).

The enzyme's substrate specificity is determined by the geometry of enzyme-substrate binding. If the substrate is optically active, generally only one of the isomers is admitted. This has to be expected because the enzyme, being formed from optically active amino acids, is optically active itself. A three-point attachment, as shown schematically in Figure 4.4, is the minimal requirement for stereoselectivity.

Rate Constants Are Useful for Describing Reaction Rates

The rate (velocity) of a chemical reaction can be described by a rate constant k:

$$A \xrightarrow{\ k\ } B$$

In this one-substrate reaction, the reaction rate is defined by:

11 $\quad V = k \times [A]$

The rate constant has the dimension s^{-1} ("per second"), and the velocity V is the change in substrate concentration per second.

For a reversible reaction, the forward and backward reactions must be considered separately:

12 $\quad A \underset{k_{-1}}{\overset{k_1}{\rightleftharpoons}} B$

13 $\quad \begin{aligned} V_{\text{forward}} &= k_1 \times [A] \\ V_{\text{backward}} &= k_{-1} \times [B] \end{aligned}$

At equilibrium, $V_{\text{forward}} = V_{\text{backward}}$. Therefore, the net reaction is zero:

14 $\quad k_1 \times [A] = k_{-1} \times [B]$

15 $\quad \dfrac{[B]}{[A]} = \dfrac{k_1}{k_{-1}} = K_{\text{equ}}$

Equation (15) shows that the equilibrium constant K_{equ}, previously defined as [B]/[A] at equilibrium, is also the ratio of the two rate constants.

In view of only the forward reaction, equation 12 describes a **first-order reaction.** In a first-order reaction, *the reaction rate is directly proportional* *to the substrate concentration.* When the substrate concentration [A] is doubled, the reaction rate V is doubled as well. Uncatalyzed one-substrate reactions follow first-order kinetics. A classical example is the decay of a radioactive isotope.

When two substrates participate, the reaction rate is likely to depend on the concentrations of both substrates. This is called a **second-order reaction:** For

$$A + B \xrightarrow{\quad k \quad} C + D$$

the following is obtained:

16 $\qquad V = k \times [A] \times [B]$

Doubling the concentration of one substrate doubles the reaction rate; doubling the concentrations of both raises it fourfold.

A **zero-order reaction** is independent of the substrate concentration. No matter how many substrate molecules are present in the test tube, only a fixed number is converted to product per second:

17 $\qquad V = k$

Zero-order kinetics are observed only in catalyzed reactions when the substrate concentration is high and the amount and turnover number of the catalyst, rather than the substrate availability, is the limiting factor.

Enzymes Decrease the Free Energy of Activation

Reactions with a negative ΔG can occur. In reality, however, many of these reactions do *not* occur at a perceptible rate. The reason is that in both catalyzed and uncatalyzed reactions, *the substrate must be converted to a* **transition state** *before the product is formed.* The structure of the transition state is intermediate between substrate and product, but its free energy content is higher. Therefore, it is unstable and decomposes almost instantly to form either substrate or product. *The formation of the transition state is the rate-limiting step in the overall reaction.*

The overall reaction in Figure 4.5 is exergonic because the product has lower free energy content than does the substrate, but the formation of the transition state from the substrate is endergonic. *The free energy difference between substrate and transition state is called the* **free energy of activation** *(ΔG_{act}).* It is an energy barrier that must be overcome by the kinetic energy of the reacting molecules as they collide with each other.

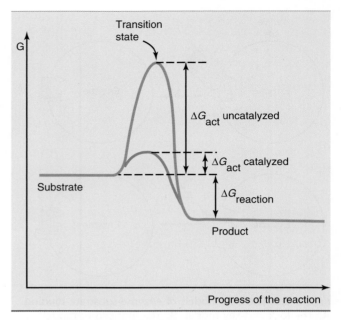

Figure 4.5 Energy profile of a reaction. The enzyme facilitates the reaction by decreasing the free energy content of the transition state. —, Uncatalyzed reaction; —, catalyzed reaction. ΔG_{act}, free energy of activation.

Most chemical systems are **meta-stable:** thermodynamically unstable but kinetically stable. The human body is meta-stable in an oxygen-containing atmosphere. Although CO_2 and H_2O have lower free energy than do molecular oxygen and the organic molecules in the human body, humans do not self-combust spontaneously, because the free energy of activation is too high.

Enzymes stabilize the transition state and decrease its free energy content. As a result, *the enzyme increases the reaction rate by decreasing the free energy of activation.* Forward and backward reactions are accelerated in proportion; therefore, *the equilibrium of the reaction remains unchanged.*

Many Enzymatic Reactions Can Be Described by Michaelis-Menten Kinetics

In Michaelis-Menten kinetics, there are a few simple (or simplistic) assumptions about enzymatic catalysis:

1. *The reaction has only one substrate.*
2. *The molar concentration of the substrate is much higher than that of the enzyme.*
3. *Only the initial reaction rate is considered,* at a time when product is virtually absent and the backward reaction negligible.

4. *The course of the reaction is observed for only a very short time period;* the changes in substrate and product concentrations that take place as the reaction proceeds are neglected.

Enzymatic reactions proceed in three steps:

$$E+S \underset{}{\overset{①}{\rightleftharpoons}} E \cdot S \overset{②}{\rightleftharpoons} E \cdot P \overset{③}{\rightleftharpoons} E+P$$

The conversion of enzyme-bound substrate to enzyme-bound product ($E \cdot S \rightleftharpoons E \cdot P$) requires the formation of the transition state. It is therefore usually the rate-limiting step. At low product concentration, the backward reactions in steps 2 and 3 can be neglected. In addition, steps 2 and 3 can be lumped together to yield

$$E+S \underset{k_{-1}}{\overset{k_1}{\rightleftharpoons}} E \cdot S \overset{k_{cat}}{\longrightarrow} E+P$$

The velocity or rate (*V*) of product formation, which defines the rate of the overall reaction, is

18 $\quad V = k_{cat} \times [E \cdot S]$

where k_{cat} is the **catalytic rate constant.** There is an upper limit to V. This limit is approached when nearly all enzyme molecules are present as enzyme-substrate complex. Therefore, the maximal reaction rate (V_{max}) is

19 $\quad V_{max} = k_{cat} \times [E_T]$

where $[E_T]$ is the concentration of the total enzyme. The k_{cat} corresponds to the turnover number of the enzyme.

The tightness of binding between enzyme and substrate in the enzyme-substrate complex is described by the **"true" dissociation constant:** the equilibrium constant for the reaction $E \cdot S \rightleftharpoons E + S$, or

20 $\quad K_D = \dfrac{[E] \times [S]}{[E \cdot S]} = \dfrac{k_{-1}}{k_1}$

Besides decomposing back to free enzyme and free substrate, the enzyme-substrate complex can undergo catalysis. Under steady-state conditions, the concentration of the enzyme-substrate complex is constant, and its rate of formation equals its rate of decomposition. For

$$E+S \underset{k_{-1}}{\overset{k_1}{\rightleftharpoons}} E \cdot S \overset{k_{cat}}{\longrightarrow} E+P$$

the following is obtained:

21 $\quad \underbrace{k_1 \times [E] \times [S]}_{\substack{\text{Rate of formation} \\ \text{of E}\cdot\text{S}}} = \underbrace{k_{-1} \times [E \cdot S]}_{\substack{\text{Rate of dissociation} \\ \text{of E}\cdot\text{S to E + S}}} + \underbrace{k_{cat} \times [E \cdot S]}_{\substack{\text{Rate of product} \\ \text{formation}}}$

which yields

22 $\quad k_1 \times [E] \times [S] = (k_{-1} + k_{cat}) \times [E \cdot S]$

and

23 $\quad \dfrac{[E] \times [S]}{[E \cdot S]} = \dfrac{k_{-1} + k_{cat}}{k_1} = K_m$

This is the definition of the **Michaelis constant, K_m.** Because k_{cat} is usually far smaller than k_{-1}, K_m is numerically similar to the true dissociation constant of the enzyme-substrate complex (equation 20).

The meaning of K_m becomes clear when equation 23 is remodeled to yield

24 $\quad \dfrac{[E]}{[E \cdot S]} = \dfrac{K_m}{[S]}$

or

25 $\quad [E \cdot S] = [E] \times \dfrac{[S]}{K_m}$

These equations show that when the substrate concentration $[S] = K_m$, the concentration of the enzyme-substrate complex $E \cdot S$ equals that of the free enzyme E: K_m *is the substrate concentration at which the enzyme is half-saturated with its substrate.* Because the reaction rate is proportionate to the concentration of the enzyme-substrate complex (equation 18), K_m *is also the substrate concentration at which the reaction rate is half-maximal.*

The total enzyme (E_T) is present as free enzyme and enzyme-substrate complex:

26 $\quad [E] + [E \cdot S] = [E_T]$

or

27 $\quad [E] = [E_T] - [E \cdot S]$

To obtain the Michaelis-Menten equation, equations (24) and (27) are first combined:

28 $\quad \dfrac{[E_T] - [E \cdot S]}{[E \cdot S]} = \dfrac{K_m}{[S]}$

This becomes

29 $\quad \dfrac{[E_T]}{[E \cdot S]} - 1 = \dfrac{K_m}{[S]}$

and

30 $$\frac{[E_T]}{[E \cdot S]} = \frac{K_m}{[S]} + 1 = \frac{K_m}{[S]} + \frac{[S]}{[S]} = \frac{K_m + [S]}{[S]}$$

Combining equations 18 and 19 yields

31 $$\frac{V_{max}}{V} = \frac{[E_T] \times k_{cat}}{[E \cdot S] \times k_{cat}} = \frac{[E_T]}{[E \cdot S]}$$

Equations 30 and 31 can now be combined to obtain the Michaelis-Menten equation:

32 $$\frac{V_{max}}{V} = \frac{K_m + [S]}{[S]}$$

or

33 $$V = V_{max} \times \frac{[S]}{K_m + [S]}$$

K_m and V_{max} Can Be Determined Graphically

The derivation of K_m and V_{max} is not merely a joyful intellectual exercise for the student. These kinetic properties can actually be used to predict reaction rates at varying substrate concentrations.

In the curve of Figure 4.6, a fixed amount of enzyme has been incubated with varying concentrations of substrate. It shows that *at substrate concentrations far below the K_m, the reaction rate is almost directly proportionate to the substrate concentration,* *and the reaction shows first-order kinetics. Eventually, however, it approaches V_{max}. At substrate concentrations far higher than K_m, the reaction becomes nearly independent of the substrate concentration and shows zero-order kinetics.* Almost all enzyme molecules are present as enzyme-substrate complex, and the reaction is limited no longer by substrate availability but by the amount and turnover number of the enzyme.

K_m can be determined graphically as the point on the x-axis that corresponds to $\frac{1}{2}V_{max}$ on the y-axis.

In a double-reciprocal plot, known as the **Lineweaver-Burk plot** (Fig. 4.7), the relationship between $1/V$ and $1/[S]$ describes a straight line. This line corresponds to the equation

34 $$\frac{1}{V} = \frac{1}{V_{max}} + \frac{K_m}{V_{max}} \times \frac{1}{[S]}$$

which is obtained by turning the Michaelis-Menten equation (equation 33) upside down. The intersection of this line with the y-axis is $1/V_{max}$, and its intersection with the x-axis is $-1/K_m$.

The transition from first-order to zero-order kinetics with increasing substrate concentration can be compared to the ticket sales in a bus terminal. When passengers are scarce, the number of tickets sold per minute depends directly on the number of passengers: tickets are sold with first-order kinetics. However, during rush hour, when a line forms, the rate of ticket sales is no longer limited by passenger availability but by the turnover number of the ticket clerk. No matter how long the line, it progresses at a constant rate, V_{max}. Tickets are now sold with zero-order kinetics.

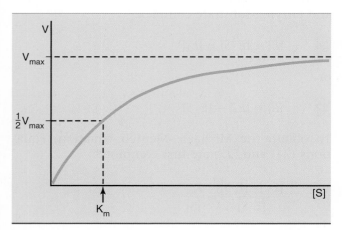

Figure 4.6 Relationship between reaction rate (V) and substrate concentration ($[S]$) in a typical enzymatic reaction. K_m, Michaelis constant; V_{max}, maximal reaction rate.

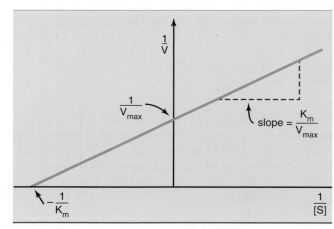

Figure 4.7 A Lineweaver-Burk plot for a typical enzymatic reaction. It is derived from the equation $1/V = 1/V_{max} + K_m/V_{max} \times 1/[S]$. K_m, Michaelis constant; V, reaction rate; V_{max}, maximal reaction rate.

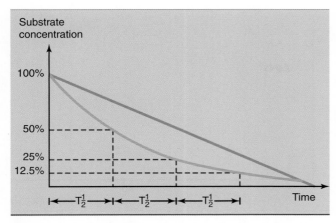

Figure 4.8 The disappearance of the substrate is traced for a zero-order reaction (——) and a first-order reaction (——). The half life (T½), is defined as the time period during which half of the substrate is converted to product in the first-order reaction.

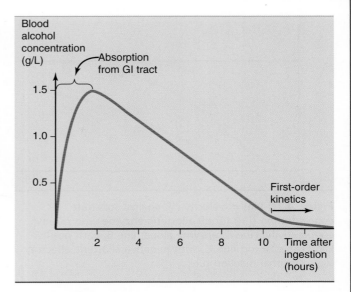

Figure 4.9 Blood alcohol concentration after the ingestion of 120 g of ethanol. The linear decrease of the alcohol level 2 to 10 hours after ingestion shows that a zero-order reaction limits the rate of alcohol metabolism. GI, gastrointestinal.

Substrate Half-Life Can Be Determined for First-Order but Not Zero-Order Reactions

Figure 4.8 shows how the substrate of an irreversible reaction gradually disappears by being converted to product. In a zero-order reaction, the rate of the reaction, corresponding to the slope of the curve, remains constant over time. The first-order reaction, in contrast, slows down as less and less substrate is available.

The **half-life** is the time period during which one half of the substrate is consumed in a first-order reaction. Zero-order reactions do not have a half-life.

Many drugs, for example, are metabolized by enzymes in the liver. The drug concentration is usually so far below the K_m of the metabolizing enzyme that it is metabolized with first-order kinetics. Consequently, the drug's half-life can be determined by measuring its plasma concentrations at different points in time.

Alcohol metabolism is very different. The alcohol level is so high after a few drinks that the metabolizing enzyme, alcohol dehydrogenase, is almost completely saturated. Therefore, a constant amount of about 10 g per hour is metabolized no matter how drunk a person is, and the blood alcohol level declines by about 0.015% every hour (Fig. 4.9).

k_{cat}/K_m Predicts the Enzyme Activity at Low Substrate Concentration

V_{max} is proportionate to the enzyme concentration (equation 19): doubling the enzyme concentration doubles the reaction rate. Therefore, *the amount of*

an enzyme is most conveniently determined by measuring its activity at saturating substrate concentrations. This is done in the clinical laboratory when serum enzymes are determined for diagnostic purposes (see Chapter 15). Enzyme activities can be expressed as **international units (IU)**. One IU is defined as *the amount of enzyme that converts one micromole (μmol) of substrate to product per minute.* Because V_{max} depends on temperature, pH, and other factors, the incubation conditions must be specified.

However, most enzymes in the living cell work with substrate concentrations far below their K_m. *At these low substrate concentrations, the k_{cat}/K_m ratio is the best predictor of the actual reaction rate.* This is apparent when equations 18 and 25 are combined:

35
$$V = \frac{k_{cat}}{K_m} \times [E] \times [S]$$

When the substrate concentration is far below K_m, almost all the enzyme molecules are present as free enzyme rather than enzyme-substrate complex, and

$$[E] \approx [E_T]$$

Therefore, equation 35 yields

36
$$V \approx \frac{k_{cat}}{K_m} \times [E_T] \times [S]$$

It is now evident that at a very low substrate concentration, the reaction rate is directly proportion-

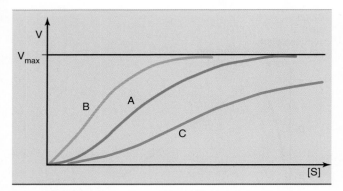

Figure 4.10 Plot of velocity (*V*) against substrate concentration ([*S*]) for an allosteric enzyme with positive cooperativity. Line A, enzyme alone; line B, with positive allosteric effector; line C, with negative allosteric effector; V_{max}, maximal reaction rate.

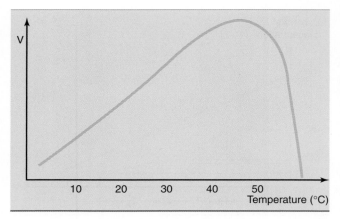

Figure 4.11 Temperature dependence of a typical enzymatic reaction. *V*, reaction rate.

ate to the enzyme concentration [E_T], substrate concentration [S], and k_{cat}/K_m. K_m is a measure for the affinity between enzyme and substrate, with a low K_m signifying high affinity, and k_{cat} is the turnover number of the enzyme.

Allosteric Enzymes Do Not Conform to Michaelis-Menten Kinetics

Not all enzymes show simple Michaelis-Menten kinetics. For example, the sigmoidal relationship between substrate concentration and reaction rate in Figure 4.10 is typical for an allosteric enzyme with more than one active site and positive cooperativity between the active sites. This curve would not yield a straight line in the Lineweaver-Burk plot.

However, the most important feature of allosteric enzymes is their response to **allosteric effectors.** Positive allosteric effectors activate the enzyme, and negative allosteric effectors inhibit it. *These regulatory molecules bind to sites distant from the substrate-binding site.* Their binding is noncovalent and therefore reversible. Allosteric effectors can change both the enzyme's affinity for substrate (K_m) and its turnover number, k_{cat}.

Allosteric enzymes occupy strategic locations in metabolic pathways where they are regulated by substrates or products of the pathway.

Enzyme Activity Depends on Temperature and pH

Chemical reactions are accelerated by increased temperature. The greater the activation energy ΔG_{act} of the reaction, the greater is its temperature dependence. The **Q₁₀ value** is the factor by which the reaction

is accelerated when the temperature rises by 10° C. Most uncatalyzed reactions have Q_{10} values between 2 and 5. Enzymatic reactions have lower activation energies, and their Q_{10} values are therefore most commonly between 1.7 and 2.5. At excessively high temperatures, however, enzymes become irreversibly denatured. This produces the relationship shown in Figure 4.11.

The temperature dependence of enzymatic reactions contributes to the increased metabolic rate during fever. It is, presumably, also responsible for the fact that humans cannot tolerate body temperatures above 42° to 43° C. The most sensitive enzymes may already denature at temperatures above this limit. Protein denaturation is time-dependent, and an enzyme that survives a temperature of 45° C for some minutes may well denature gradually in the course of several hours.

Hypothermia is far better tolerated than hyperthermia, and the temperature of the toes can indeed fall close to 0° C on a cold winter day. This temperature blocks nerve conduction and muscle activity, but it does not kill the cells. However, *the metabolic rate is depressed at low temperatures.* Therefore, a slowdown in the vital functions of brain and heart limits humans' tolerance of hypothermia. Also, a vicious cycle develops when decreased metabolism reduces heat production during hypothermia.

Hypothermia makes cells and tissues more resistant to hypoxia because it decreases their oxygen consumption. This means, for example, that organs used for transplantation are best preserved in the cold.

Enzymes are also affected by the pH as shown in Figure 4.12. The main reason for this effect is that *the protonation state of catalytically active groups in the enzyme depends on the pH.*

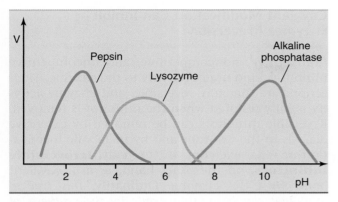

Figure 4.12 The pH dependence of some enzymes. *V*, reaction rate.

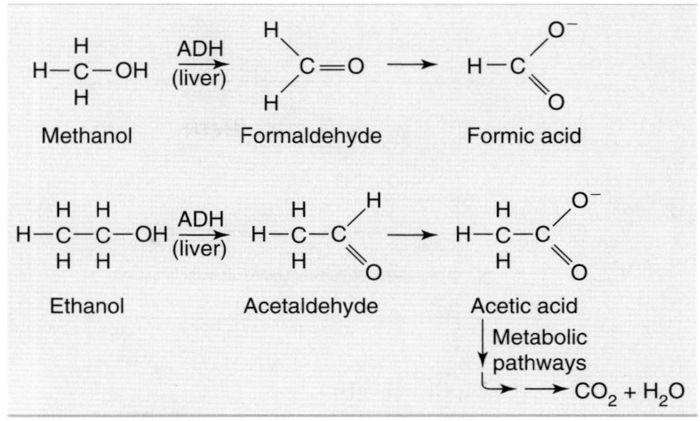

Figure 4.13 Role of alcohol dehydrogenase (ADH) in the metabolism of methanol and ethanol. The two substrates compete for the enzyme. Therefore, ethanol inhibits the formation of toxic formaldehyde and formic acid from methanol.

The pH values of tissues and body fluids are tightly regulated. Deviations of more than 0.5 pH units from the normal blood pH of 7.4 are rapidly fatal. Also, the intracellular compartments have tightly regulated pH values to ensure the proper activity levels of their enzymes. Typical pH values are 6.5 to 7.0 in the cytoplasm, 7.5 to 8.0 in the mitochondrial matrix, and 4.5 to 5.5 in the lysosomes.

Different Types of Reversible Enzyme Inhibition Can Be Distinguished Kinetically

Chapter 3 explained how carbon monoxide (CO) inhibits oxygen transport by competitive binding to the heme iron. Likewise, a **competitive enzyme inhibitor** competes with the substrate by binding to the active site of the enzyme. Competitive inhibitors are structurally related to the normal substrate of the enzyme. The mitochondrial enzyme succinate dehydrogenase (SDH), for example, catalyzes the following reaction:

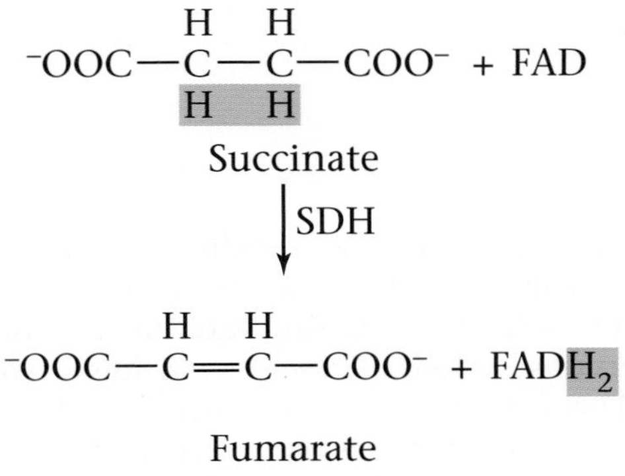

$$^-OOC-\underset{H}{\overset{H}{C}}-\underset{H}{\overset{H}{C}}-COO^- + FAD$$

Succinate

$$\downarrow SDH$$

$$^-OOC-\underset{}{\overset{H}{C}}=\underset{}{\overset{H}{C}}-COO^- + FADH_2$$

Fumarate

This reaction is competitively inhibited by malonate:

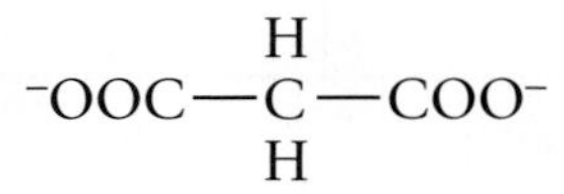

$$^-OOC-\underset{H}{\overset{H}{C}}-COO^-$$

Malonate

Malonate binds to the enzyme by the same electrostatic interactions as the substrate succinate, but it cannot be converted to a product.

In other cases, the inhibitor is converted to a product: *Two alternative substrates can compete for the enzyme.* Methanol, for example, is sometimes swallowed accidentally by people who read "methyl alcohol" on a label and think it is the real stuff. But its ingestion can be fatal because methanol is converted to the toxic metabolites formaldehyde and formic acid in the body (Fig. 4.13).

The methanol-metabolizing enzyme alcohol dehydrogenase can metabolize ethanol as well. Fortunately, the ethanol metabolites are rapidly oxidized to carbon dioxide and water and therefore do not accumulate to toxic levels. When ethanol is administered to a patient with methanol poisoning, the formation of the toxic methanol metabolites is delayed because ethanol competes with methanol for the enzyme. The patient remains drunk but alive.

Competitive inhibitors do not change V_{max} because inhibitor binding is reversible and can be overcome by high concentrations of the substrate. But substrate binding to the enzyme is impaired, and the apparent binding affinity is therefore decreased. Therefore, *competitive inhibitors increase the* K_m (Fig. 4.14).

Some inhibitors bind to the enzyme protein at a site distant from the substrate-binding site. These

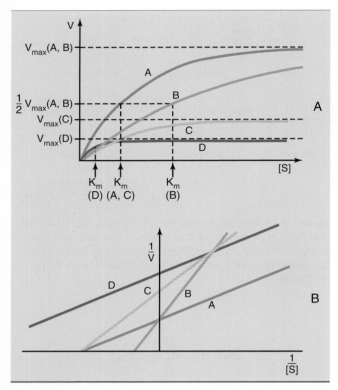

Figure 4.14 The effects of inhibitors on enzymatic reactions. Line A, uninhibited enzyme; line B, competitive inhibitor; line C, noncompetitive inhibitor; line D, uncompetive inhibitor. For noncompetitive inhibition, it is assumed that the inhibitor binds equally well to the free enzyme and the enzyme-substrate complex (see text). The kinetic effects of irreversible inhibitors resemble those shown here for the noncompetitive inhibitor. **A,** Reaction rate (V) plotted against substrate concentration ([S]). **B,** In the Lineweaver-Burk plot, the effects of inhibitors on V_{max} (maximal reaction rate) and K_m (Michaelis constant) are reflected in changes of the intercepts with the y-axis and x-axis, respectively.

Covalent Modification Can Inhibit Enzymes Irreversibly

Competitive, noncompetitive, and uncompetitive inhibitors bind noncovalently to the enzyme. Their actions are therefore reversible, and enzyme activity is fully restored when the inhibitor is removed. Reversible inhibitors can be removed by extensive dialysis in the test tube and by metabolic inactivation or renal excretion in the body. **Irreversible inhibitors,** on the other hand, form a covalent bond with the enzyme. Ordinarily, *this type of inhibition can be overcome only by the synthesis of new enzyme.*

The **organophosphorus compounds,** for example, react with an essential serine residue in acetylcholinesterase, the enzyme that degrades the neurotransmitter acetylcholine (see Chapter 16):

Serine residue
(in acetylcholinesterase)   Sarin

Organophosphates are deadly because acetylcholine accumulates when its degrading enzyme has been destroyed, causing fatal derangements in the nervous system. These agents have two main uses. Those that are most potent on the acetylcholinesterase of insects are used as pesticides by farmers, and those that work best on the human enzyme are used as nerve gases by terrorists and the military.

inhibitors are structurally unrelated to the substrate. Classical **noncompetitive inhibitors** do not prevent substrate binding but do block enzymatic catalysis. *If the noncompetitive inhibitor binds equally well to the free enzyme and the enzyme-substrate complex, it reduces V_{max} without a change in K_m.*

Uncompetitive inhibitors bind only to the enzyme-substrate complex but not the free enzyme. *They thereby reduce both K_m and V_{max}.* Unlike competitive inhibitors, which are most effective at low substrate concentrations, *uncompetitive inhibitors work best when the substrate concentration is high.*

Enzymes Are Classified According to Their Reaction Type

Enzymes are most commonly named after their substrate and their reaction type, with the suffix -*ase* at the end. For example, monoamine oxidase is an enzyme that oxidizes monoamines; and catechol-*O*-methyltransferase transfers a methyl group to an oxygen group in a catechol.

According to their reaction type, enzymes are grouped into six classes, as follows.

OXIDOREDUCTASES

Oxidoreductases catalyze oxidation-reduction reactions: electron transfers, hydrogen transfers, and reactions involving molecular oxygen.

Dehydrogenases transfer hydrogen between a substrate and a coenzyme, most commonly NAD, nicotinamide adenine dinucleotide phosphate (NADP), flavin adenine dinucleotide (FAD), or flavin mononucleotide (FMN). These enzymes are named after the substrate from which the hydrogen is removed. Example:

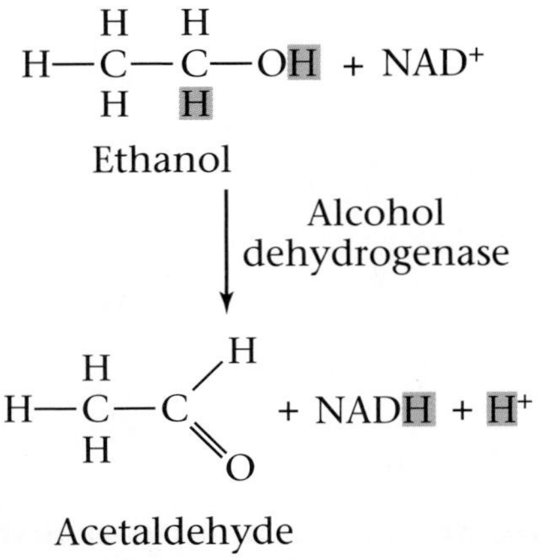

Oxygenases use molecular oxygen as a substrate. **Dioxygenases** incorporate both oxygen atoms of O_2 into their substrate, and **monooxygenases** incorporate only one. Most **hydroxylases** are monooxygenases:

$$Substrate—H + O_2 + NADPH + H^+$$
$$\downarrow$$
$$Substrate—OH + NADP^+ + H_2O$$

where NADPH = the reduced form of nicotinamide adenine dinucleotide phosphate. In this reaction, the second oxygen atom reacts with the reduced coenzyme NADPH to form water.

Peroxidases use hydrogen peroxide or an organic peroxide as one of their substrates. **Catalase** is, technically, a peroxidase. It degrades hydrogen peroxide to molecular oxygen and water:

$$H_2O_2 \rightarrow H_2O + \frac{1}{2}O_2$$

TRANSFERASES

Transferases transfer a group from one molecule to another.

Kinases transfer phosphate from ATP to a second substrate. They are named according to the substrate to which the phosphate is transferred. Example:

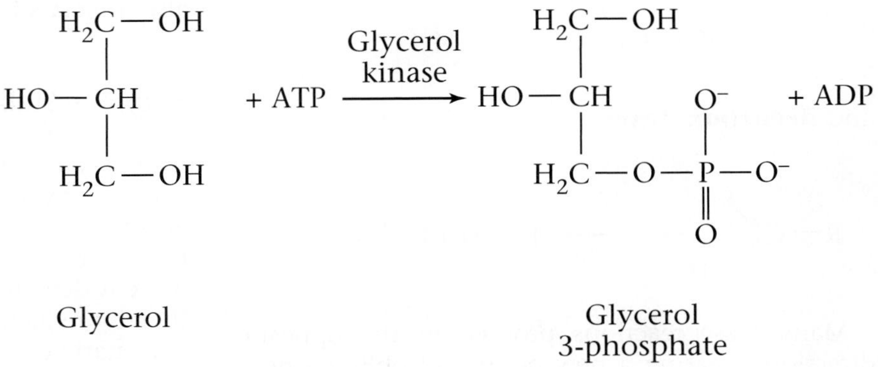

Other examples of transferases include **phosphorylases,** which cleave bonds by the addition of inorganic phosphate; **glycosyl transferases,** which transfer an "activated" monosaccharide to an acceptor molecule; the **transaminases** (see Chapter 26); and the **peptidyl transferase** of the ribosome (see Chapter 6).

HYDROLASES

Hydrolases cleave bonds by the addition of water. Their names indicate the substrates or bonds on which they act: peptidases (proteases), esterases, lipases, phospholipases, glycosidases, phosphatases, and so forth. Digestive enzymes and lysosomal enzymes are hydrolases.

The cleavage specificities of hydrolytic enzymes acting on polymeric substrates are specified by the prefixes *endo-* (from Greek, meaning "inside") and *exo-* (from Greek, meaning "outside"). An exopeptidase, for example, cleaves amino acids from the end of a polypeptide, and an endopeptidase cleaves internal peptide bonds.

LYASES

Lyases remove a group nonhydrolytically, forming a double bond. Examples are the **dehydratases:**

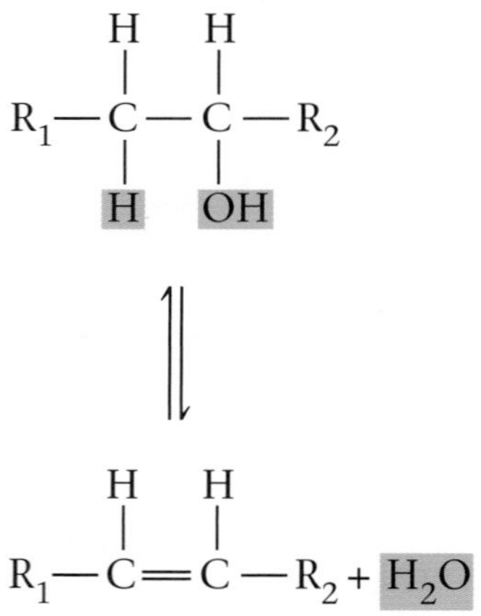

and **decarboxylases:**

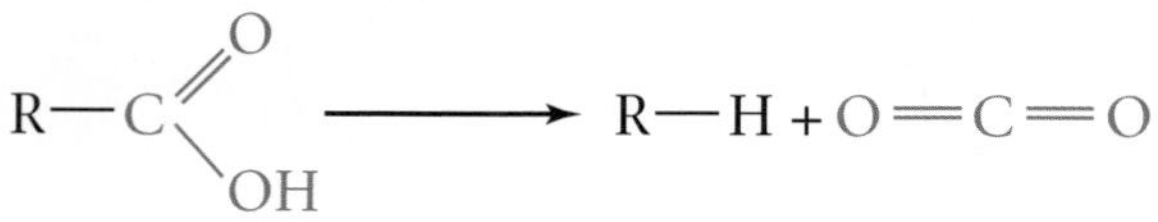

Many lyase reactions proceed in the opposite direction, creating a new bond and obliterating a double bond in one of the substrates. These enzymes are called **synthases**.

ISOMERASES

Isomerases interconvert positional, geometric, or optical isomers.

LIGASES

Ligases couple the hydrolysis of a phosphoanhydride bond to the formation of a bond. These enzymes are often called **synthetases.** Glutamine synthetase, for example, couples ATP hydrolysis to the formation of the amide bond in glutamine:

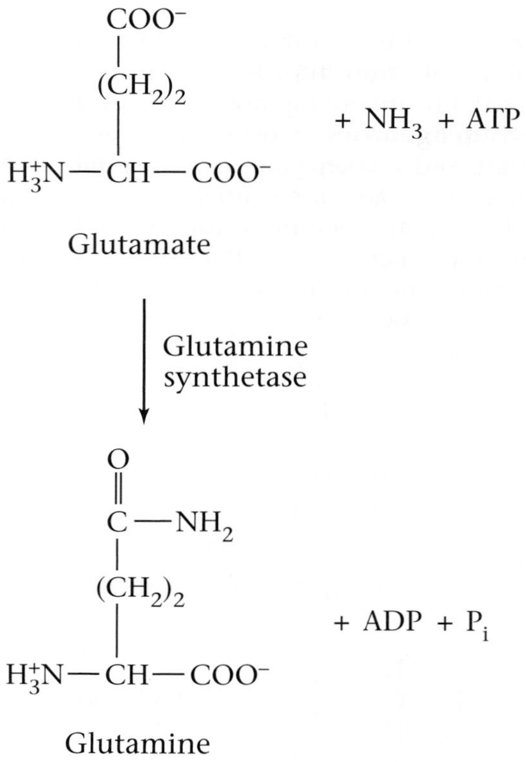

DNA ligase and **aminoacyl–transfer RNA synthetases** (see Chapter 6) are further examples. The biotin-dependent carboxylases (see Chapter 21) also are classified as ligases.

Enzymes Stabilize the Transition State

Enzymes can stabilize the transition state of the reaction by making its formation a more likely event, thereby increasing the entropy of the transition state, or by forming energetically favorable noncovalent interactions with the transition state, thereby reducing its enthalpy. Four mechanisms of enzymatic catalysis are often distinguished:

1. *The **entropy effect** is achieved by the approximation of substrates in a two-substrate reaction. The*

transition state can form only when the substrates collide in the correct geometric orientation and with sufficient energy to bring them to the transition state. The enzyme increases the likelihood of such an event by binding the two substrates to its active site in close proximity and in the correct geometric orientation.

2. ***Steric stabilization of the transition state*** *occurs when the enzyme interacts more strongly with the conformation of the transition state than with that of the substrate.* This decreases the free energy content of the transition state in relation to the substrate, and ΔG_{act} is reduced. This effect is also called "substrate strain" because the enzyme bends the substrate into the shape of the transition state.

3. ***General acid-base catalysis*** *exploits ionizable groups on the enzyme as proton donors or proton acceptors.* Enzymes can also provide electron pair donors and acceptors, which are known as Lewis bases and Lewis acids, respectively. In some cases the enzyme donates a proton to the substrate or removes one from it to form the transition state; in other cases, it stabilizes the transition state through electrostatic interactions. *General acid-base catalysis is the most important reason for the pH dependence of enzymatic reactions.* The ionizable groups that participate in this type of catalysis must be in the correct protonation state. If, for example, the reaction requires a deprotonated glutamate side chain with a pK of 4.0 as a general base and a protonated histidine side chain with a pK of 6.0 as a general acid, only pH values between 4.0 and 6.0 will allow high reaction rates.

4. In ***covalent catalysis,*** *the enzyme forms a transient covalent bond with the substrate.* The serine proteases described in the following paragraph are the most prominent example.

Chymotrypsin Forms a Transient Covalent Bond during Catalysis

The pancreatic enzyme **chymotrypsin** is a prototypical **serine protease.** When the enzyme-substrate complex forms, the targeted peptide bond of the polypeptide substrate is placed right on the hydroxyl group of the catalytic serine residue in the active site, Ser-195. The substrate binds to the active site by hydrogen bonds between peptide bonds in the substrate and the enzyme. In addition, the side chain of the amino acid whose carboxyl group contributes to the targeted bond binds to a hydrophobic pocket on the enzyme. Therefore, chymotrypsin prefers peptide bonds that are formed by the car-

boxyl group of large hydrophobic amino acids (Figure 4.15).

In addition to Ser-195, catalysis requires a deprotonated histidine residue, His-57, and a deprotonated aspartate residue, Asp-102. Although widely separated in the amino acid sequence of the protein, these three amino acids are hydrogen-bonded to each other in the active site of the enzyme.

Catalysis by chymotrypsin is actually a sequence of two reactions. In the first reaction, the peptide bond in the substrate is cleaved, and one of the fragments binds covalently to the serine side chain to form an **acyl-enzyme intermediate.** In the second reaction, this intermediate is cleaved hydrolytically. The acyl-enzyme intermediate does not qualify as a transition state because it occupies a valley in the free energy graph, rather than a peak (Fig. 4.16).

The transition states in both reactions are negatively charged **tetrahedral intermediates.** These intermediates are stabilized by hydrogen bonds with two N-H groups in the main chain of the enzyme.

To form the negatively charged transition state, *a proton must be transferred from the hydroxyl group of Ser-195 to His-57.* Asp-102 remains negatively charged throughout the catalytic cycle. It forms a salt bond with the protonated but not the deprotonated form of His-57, thereby stabilizing the protonated form and increasing the proton affinity of the histidine.

The serine proteases are a large family of enzymes that includes digestive enzymes, such as trypsin, chymotrypsin, and elastase, and blood clotting factors, such as thrombin. They all use the same catalytic mechanism but have different substrate specificities. Trypsin, for example, contains a negatively charged aspartate residue in its substrate-binding pocket and therefore prefers peptide bonds formed by positively charged amino acids; thrombin is extremely selective for a small number of plasma proteins, including fibrinogen.

SUMMARY

All chemical reactions proceed to an equilibrium state that can be described by the equilibrium constant. The position of the equilibrium can be predicted from the standard free energy change of the reaction: the difference in the free energy contents of substrates and products. Enzymes cannot change the equilibrium of the reaction. They can only increase the reaction rate.

Enzymatic catalysis starts with the formation of a noncovalent enzyme-substrate complex. The binding affinity between enzyme and sub-

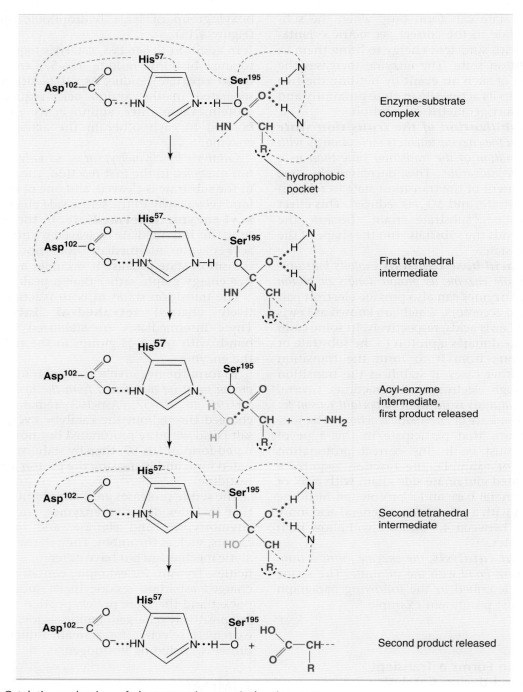

Figure 4.15 Catalytic mechanism of chymotrypsin, a typical serine protease.

strate is the major determinant of the Michaelis constant, K_m. K_m indicates at what substrate concentration the reaction is half-maximal.

All chemical reactions, both catalyzed and uncatalyzed, proceed through an energetically unstable transition state. The formation of the transition state is the rate-limiting step for the overall reaction. Enzymes stabilize the transition state. They reduce its free energy content, thereby lowering the energy barrier for the reaction.

At very low substrate concentrations, the reaction rate increases almost linearly with increasing substrate concentration. The reaction shows first-order kinetics. At very high substrate concentrations, however, the reaction rate cannot be increased by further increases of the substrate concentration because most of the enzyme is already present as enzyme-substrate complex. The reaction shows zero-order kinetics.

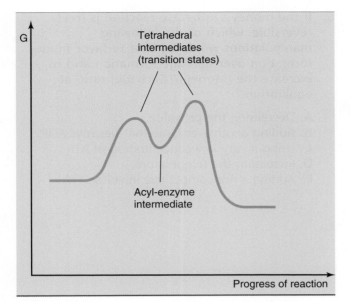

Figure 4.16 Energy profile for the reaction of a serine protease. G, free energy.

The rate of enzymatic reactions increases with increasing temperature, typically with a doubling of the reaction rate for a temperature increase of about 10° C. The pH is also important because most enzymes use ionizable groups for catalysis. These groups must be in the proper protonation state.

Many drugs and toxins act as specific enzyme inhibitors. Some bind to the enzyme reversibly, through noncovalent interactions. Others form a covalent bond with the enzyme, thereby destroying its catalytic activity permanently.

QUESTIONS

1. During a drug screening program, you find a chemical that decreases the activity of the enzyme monoamine oxidase. A fixed dose of the chemical reduces the catalytic activity of the enzyme by the same percentage at all substrate concentrations, with a decrease in V_{max}. K_m is unaffected. This inhibitor is

   A. Definitely a competitive inhibitor.
   B. Definitely a noncompetitive inhibitor.
   C. Definitely an irreversible inhibitor.
   D. Either a competitive or irreversible inhibitor.
   E. Either a noncompetitive or irreversible inhibitor.

2. The irreversible enzymatic reaction

   Oxaloacetate + Acetyl–Coenzyme A (CoA) →
      Citrate + CoA—SH

   is inhibited by high concentrations of its own product citrate. This product inhibition can be overcome, and a normal V_{max} can be restored, when the oxaloacetate concentration is raised but not when the acetyl-CoA concentration is raised. This observation suggests that citrate is

   A. An irreversible inhibitor reacting with the oxaloacetate binding site of the enzyme.
   B. A competitive inhibitor binding to the acetyl-CoA binding site of the enzyme.
   C. A competitive inhibitor binding to the oxaloacetate binding site of the enzyme.
   D. A noncompetitive inhibitor binding to the acetyl-CoA binding site of the enzyme.
   E. A noncompetitive inhibitor binding to the oxaloacetate binding site of the enzyme.

3. An enzymatic reaction works best at pH values between 6 and 8. This is compatible with the assumption that the reaction mechanism requires two ionizable amino acid side chains in the active site of the enzyme, possibly

   A. Protonated glutamate and deprotonated aspartate.
   B. Protonated histidine and deprotonated lysine.
   C. Protonated glutamate and deprotonated histidine.
   D. Protonated arginine and deprotonated lysine.
   E. Protonated cysteine and deprotonated histidine.

4. A biotechnology company has cloned four different forms of the enzyme money synthetase, which catalyzes the reaction

   Garbage + ATP → Money + ADP
      + Phosphate + H$^+$

   The K_m values of these enzymes for garbage and the V_{max} values are as follows:

   - Enzyme 1: K_m = 0.1 mmol,
     V_{max} = 5.0 mmol/min
   - Enzyme 2: K_m = 0.3 mmol,
     V_{max} = 2.0 mmol/min
   - Enzyme 3: K_m = 1.0 mmol,
     V_{max} = 5.0 mmol/min
   - Enzyme 4: K_m = 3.0 mmol,
     V_{max} = 20 mmol/min

   Which of the four enzymes is fastest at a saturating ATP concentration and a garbage concentration of 0.01 mmol/liter?

A. Enzyme 1.
B. Enzyme 2.
C. Enzyme 3.
D. Enzyme 4.

5. **Which of the four forms of money synthetase is fastest at a saturating ATP concentration and a garbage concentration of 10 mmol/liter?**

   A. Enzyme 1.
   B. Enzyme 2.
   C. Enzyme 3.
   D. Enzyme 4.

6. **If the money synthetase reaction is freely reversible, which of the following manipulations would be best to favor money formation over garbage formation and to increase the [Money]/[Garbage] ratio at equilibrium?**

   A. Decreasing the pH value.
   B. Adding another enzyme that destroys ADP.
   C. Using a very low concentration of ATP.
   D. Increasing the temperature.
   E. Adding a noncompetitive inhibitor.

CHAPTER 5

Coenzymes

The time-honored name of coenzyme is applied to two different types of cofactor. A **cosubstrate** is promiscuous, associating with the enzyme only for the purpose of the reaction. It becomes chemically modified in the reaction and then diffuses away for a next liaison with another enzyme. A true **prosthetic group,** in contrast, is monogamous. It is permanently bonded to the active site of the enzyme, either covalently or noncovalently, and stays with the enzyme after completion of the reaction.

Some coenzymes can be synthesized in the body de novo ("from scratch"), but others contain a vitamin or are vitamins themselves. Reactions that depend on such a coenzyme are blocked when the vitamin is deficient in the diet.

Each coenzyme is concerned with a specific reaction type such as hydrogen transfer, methylation, or carboxylation. Thus, test-savvy students can predict the coenzyme of a reaction from the reaction type.

ATP Has Two Energy-Rich Bonds

Metabolic energy is generated by the oxidation of carbohydrate, fat, protein, and alcohol. This energy must be harnessed to drive endergonic chemical reactions, membrane transport, and muscle contraction. Nature has solved this task with a simple trick: *Exergonic reactions are used for the synthesis of the energy-rich compound **adenosine triphosphate (ATP)**, and the chemical bond energy of ATP drives the endergonic processes.* In this sense, ATP serves as the energetic currency of the cell (Fig. 5.1).

ATP is a ribonucleotide, one of the precursors for RNA synthesis. It does not contain a vitamin, and the whole molecule can be synthesized from simple precursors (see Chapter 28). Its most important part

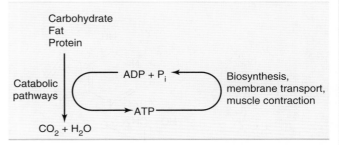

Figure 5.1 The function of adenosine triphosphate (ATP) as the "energetic currency" of the cell. ADP, adenosine diphosphate; P_i, inorganic phosphate.

is a string of three phosphate residues, bound to carbon 5 of ribose and complexed with a magnesium ion (Figs. 5.2 and 5.3).

The first phosphate is linked to ribose by a phosphate ester bond, but *the two bonds between the phosphates are energy-rich phosphoanhydride bonds.* The free energy changes in Figure 5.2 apply to standard conditions. The actual free energy change for the hydrolysis of ATP to adenosine diphosphate (ADP) + inorganic phosphate (P_i) depends on pH; ionic strength; and the concentrations of ATP, ADP, phosphate, and magnesium. It is close to −11 or −12 kcal/mol under "real-cell" conditions. ATP can be hydrolyzed either to ADP and phosphate:

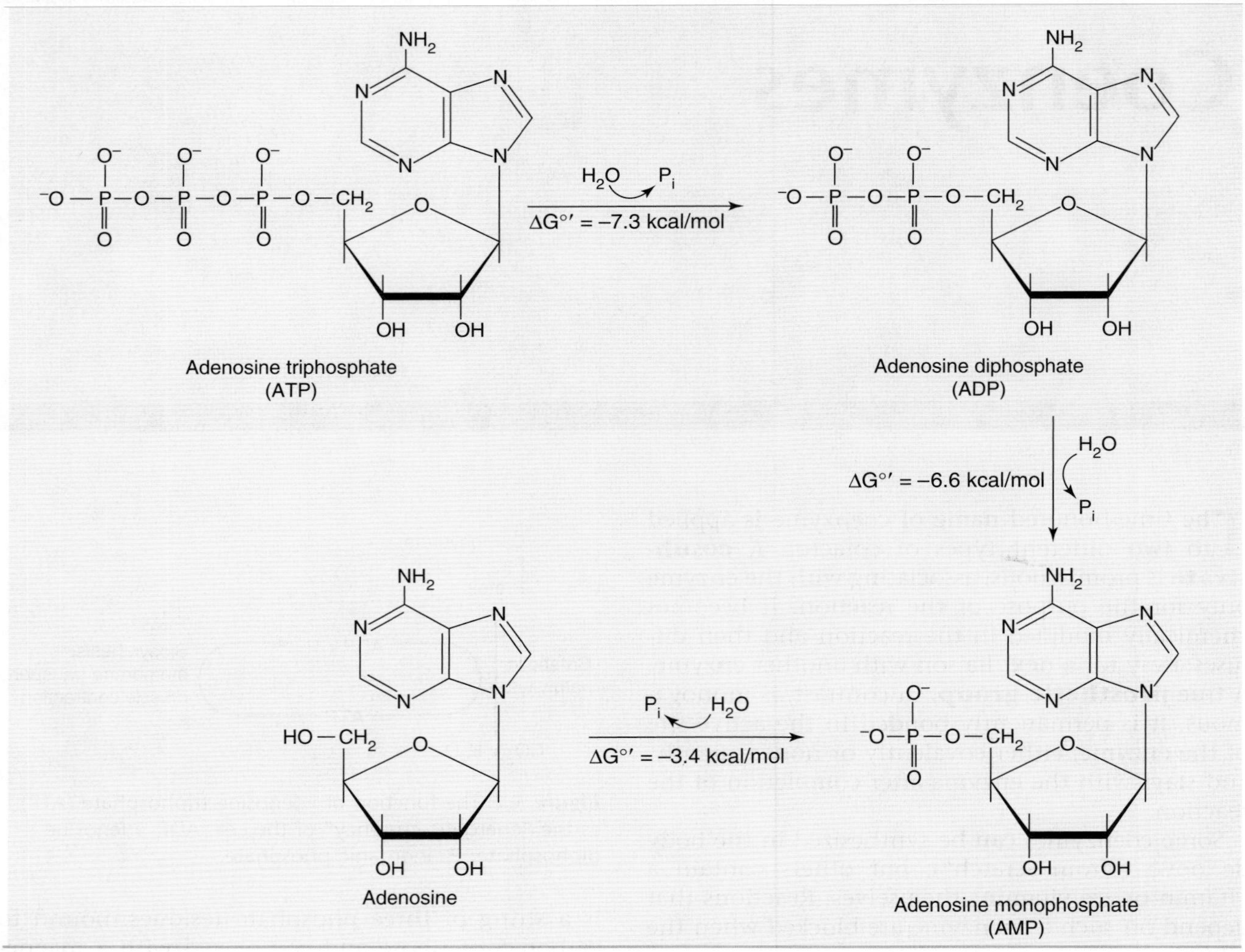

Figure 5.2 Sequential hydrolysis of ATP. $\Delta G^{0\prime}$, standard free energy change; P_i, inorganic phosphate.

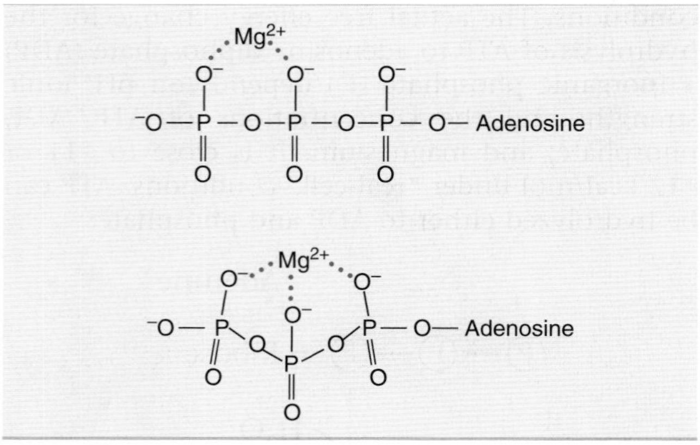

Figure 5.3 Magnesium complexes formed by adenosine triphosphate (ATP). Complexes are the actual substrates of ATP-dependent enzymes.

or to adenosine monophosphate (AMP) and inorganic pyrophosphate (PP_i):

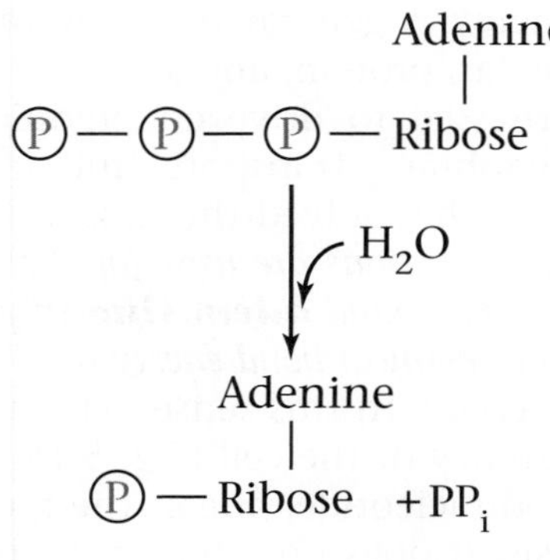

Table 5.1 Uses of Adenosine Triphosphate (ATP)

Process	Function
RNA synthesis	Precursor
Phosphorylation	Phosphate donor
Coupling to endergonic reactions	Energy source
Active membrane transport	Energy source
Muscle contraction	Energy source
Ciliary motion	Energy source

The PP_i formed in the second reaction still contains an energy-rich phosphoanhydride bond:

$$\begin{array}{ccc} O^- & & O^- \\ | & & | \\ {}^-O-P-O-P-O^- \\ \| & & \| \\ O & & O \end{array}$$

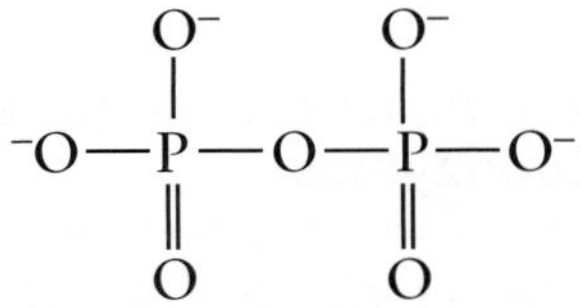

PP_i is rapidly hydrolyzed by pyrophosphatases in the cell. Because this removes PP_i from the reaction equilibrium, the cleavage of ATP to AMP + PP_i releases far more energy than the cleavage to ADP + phosphate.

ATP Is the Phosphate Donor in Phosphorylation Reactions

Table 5.1 lists the most important uses of ATP. Only phosphorylation reactions and the coupling to endergonic reactions are considered here.

Phosphorylation is the covalent attachment of a phosphate group to a substrate, most commonly by the formation of a phosphate ester bond. Assume that the cell is to convert glucose to glucose-6-phosphate, a simple phosphate ester:

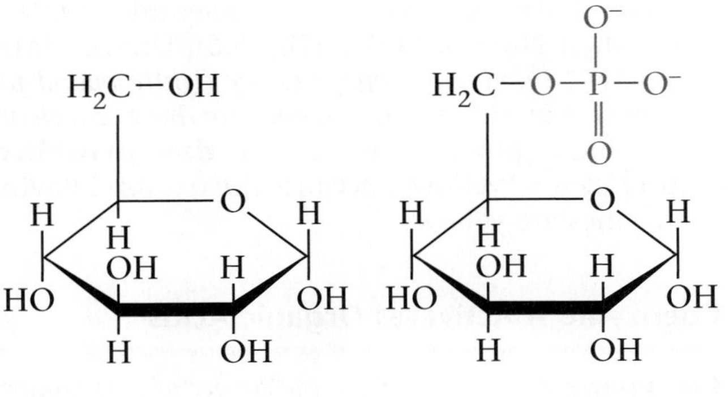

Glucose   Glucose-6-phosphate

An investigator can try to synthesize glucose-6-phosphate by reacting free glucose with P_i:

$$\text{Glucose} + P_i \xrightarrow{\text{Glucose 6-phosphatase}} \text{Glucose-6-phosphate} + H_2O$$

The enzyme glucose-6-phosphatase really exists, but the $\Delta G^{0\prime}$ of the reaction is +3.3 kcal/mol. This translates into an equilibrium constant (K_{equ}) of about 4×10^{-3} L/mol. At an intracellular phosphate concentration of 10 mmol/L, there would be 25,000 molecules of glucose for each molecule of glucose-6-phosphate!

Things look better when ATP supplies the phosphate group:

$$\text{Glucose} + ATP \xrightarrow{\text{Hexokinase}} \text{Glucose-6-phosphate} + ADP$$

The $\Delta G^{0\prime}$ of this reaction is –4.0 kcal/mol. The difference in the $\Delta G^{0\prime}$ values of the hexokinase and glucose-6-phosphatase reactions (7.3 kcal/mol) corresponds to the free energy content of the phosphoanhydride bond in ATP. Now the equilibrium constant is about 10^3. When the cellular ATP concentration is 10 times higher than the ADP concentration, there are 10,000 molecules of glucose-6-phosphate for each molecule of glucose at equilibrium!

ATP Hydrolysis Drives Endergonic Reactions

Phosphorylation reactions are not the only ones driven in the desired direction by ATP. For example, the following reaction takes place in the mitochondria:

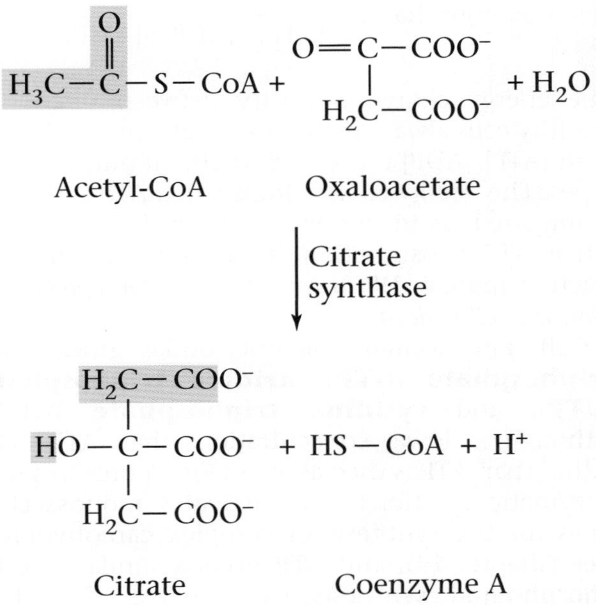

Acetyl-CoA   Oxaloacetate

Citrate   Coenzyme A

The $\Delta G^{0'}$ of this reaction is -8.5 kcal/mol. Therefore it is essentially irreversible in the direction of citrate formation. The cytoplasmic enzyme ATP-citrate lyase, however, couples this reaction to ATP synthesis:

$$\text{Acetyl-CoA} + \text{Oxaloacetate} + \text{ADP} + \text{P}_i \rightarrow$$
$$\text{Citrate} + \text{Coenzyme A} + \text{ATP}$$

The $\Delta G^{0'}$ of this reaction is -1.2 kcal/mol: the sum of the free energy changes for citrate formation (-8.5 kcal/mol) and ATP synthesis ($+7.3$ kcal/mol). The reaction is now reversible and can, under suitable conditions, make oxaloacetate from citrate.

Cells Always Try to Maintain a High Energy Charge

ATP can reach a cellular concentration of 5 mmol/L (2.5 g/liter, or 0.25%) in some tissues, but the life expectancy of an ATP molecule is only about 2 minutes. Although the total body content of ATP is only about 100 g, *60 to 70 kg are produced and consumed every day.*

In the cell, the enzyme adenylate kinase (adenylate = AMP) maintains the three adenine nucleotides in equilibrium:

$$\text{ATP} + \text{AMP} \xrightleftharpoons[]{\text{Adenylate kinase}} 2\,\text{ADP}$$

The energy status of the cell can be described either as the [ATP]/[ADP] ratio or as the **energy charge:**

$$\text{Energy charge} = \frac{[\text{ATP}] + \frac{1}{2}[\text{ADP}]}{[\text{ATP}] + [\text{ADP}] + [\text{AMP}]}$$

The energy charge can vary between 0 and 1. Healthy cells always maintain a high energy charge, with [ATP]/[ADP] ratios of 5 to 200 in different cell types. The energy charge drops when ATP synthesis is impaired, as in hypoxia (oxygen deficiency), or when ATP consumption is increased, as in contracting muscle. *When the energy charge approaches zero, the cell is dead.*

Cells also contain the nucleotides **guanosine triphosphate (GTP)**, **uridine triphosphate (UTP)**, and **cytidine triphosphate (CTP)**, although at lower concentrations than ATP. GTP rather than ATP is used as an energy source in some enzymatic reactions. UTP activates monosaccharides for the synthesis of complex carbohydrates (see Chapter 14), and CTP plays a similar role in phospholipid synthesis (see Chapter 24). The monophosphate, diphosphate, and triphosphate forms are in equilibrium through kinase reactions:

$$\left.\begin{array}{c}\text{GMP}\\\text{UMP}\\\text{CMP}\end{array}\right\} + \text{ATP} \xrightleftharpoons[\text{kinases}]{\substack{\text{Nucleoside}\\\text{monophosphate}}} \left.\begin{array}{c}\text{GDP}\\\text{UDP}\\\text{CDP}\end{array}\right\} + \text{ADP}$$

and

$$\left.\begin{array}{c}\text{GDP}\\\text{UDP}\\\text{CDP}\end{array}\right\} + \text{ATP} \xrightleftharpoons[\text{kinase}]{\substack{\text{Nucleoside}\\\text{diphosphate}}} \left.\begin{array}{c}\text{GTP}\\\text{UTP}\\\text{CTP}\end{array}\right\} + \text{ADP}$$

Dehydrogenase Reactions Require Specialized Coenzymes

In **redox reactions,** electrons are transferred from one substrate to another, either alone or along with protons.

*The cosubstrates **NAD** and **NADP** accept and donate hydrogen (electron + proton) in dehydrogenase reactions.* Nicotinamide is the hydrogen-carrying part of these coenzymes (Fig. 5.4). The additional phosphate in NADP does not affect the hydrogen transfer potential, but it is a recognition site for enzymes. *Most dehydrogenases use either NAD alone or NADP alone.*

NAD$^+$ acquires two electrons and a proton during catabolic reactions and feeds them into the respiratory chain of the mitochondria, where they reduce molecular oxygen to water (see Chapter 21). Also, NADP$^+$ accepts electrons in catabolic pathways, but *it feeds them into biosynthetic pathways.* This enables the cell to make reduced products such as fatty acids and cholesterol from more oxidized precursors (Fig. 5.5).

Some dehydrogenases use flavin adenine dinucleotide (FAD) or flavin mononucleotide (FMN), rather than NAD or NADP (Fig. 5.6). Unlike NAD and NADP, *the flavin coenzymes are tightly bound to the apoprotein either noncovalently or by a covalent bond.* These proteins are called **flavoproteins** (Latin *flavus* = "yellow") because the oxidized flavin coenzymes are yellow.

Coenzyme A Activates Organic Acids

***Coenzyme A (CoA)** is a soluble carrier of acyl groups* (Fig. 5.7). The business end of the molecule is a sulfhydryl group, and its structure can therefore be abbreviated as CoA-SH. The sulfhydryl group forms energy-rich thioester bonds with many organic acids: for example, acetic acid:

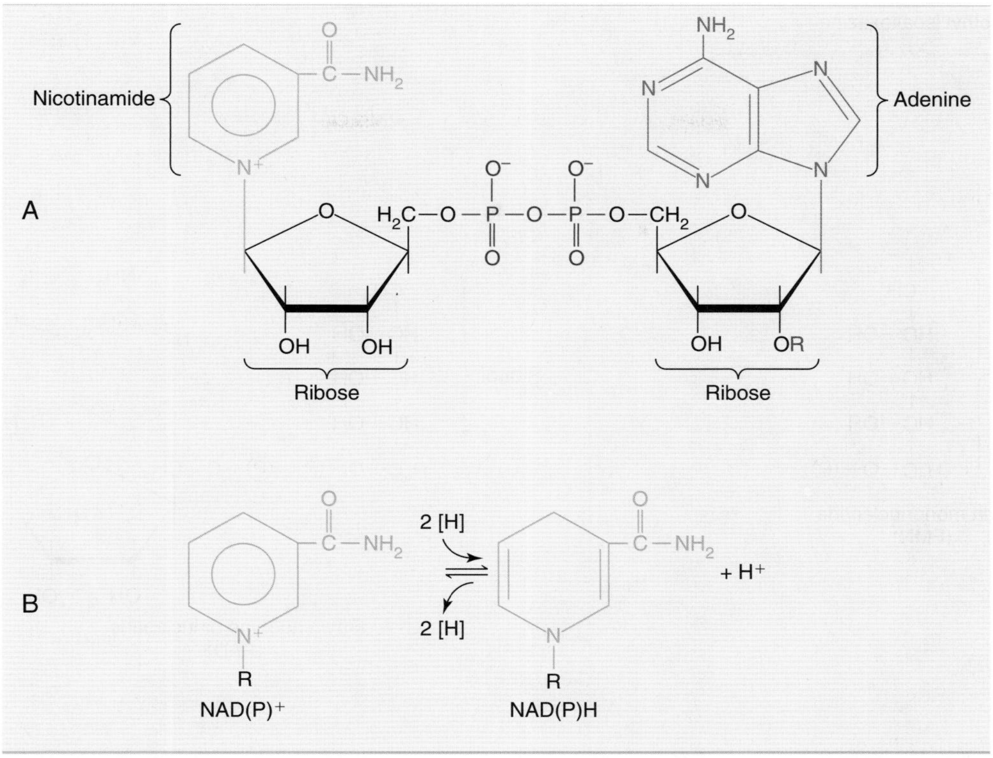

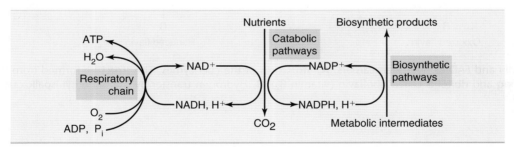

Figure 5.4 Structures of nicotinamide adenine dinucleotide (NAD⁺) and nicotinamide adenine dinucleotide phosphate (NADP⁺). **A,** Structures of the coenzymes. For NAD⁺, R = –H; for NADP⁺, R = –PO₃²⁻. **B,** The reversible hydrogenation of the nicotinamide portion in NAD⁺/NADH (reduced form of nicotinamide adenine dinucleotide) and NADP⁺/NADH.

Figure 5.5 Metabolic functions of nicotinamide adenine dinucleotide (NAD) and nicotinamide adenine dinucleotide phosphate (NADP). ADP, adenosine diphosphate; ATP, adenosine triphosphate; NADH, reduced form of nicotinamide adenine dinucleotide; NADPH, reduced form of nicotinamide adenine dinucleotide phosphate.

$$CoA-S-\overset{\overset{\displaystyle O}{\|}}{C}-CH_3$$

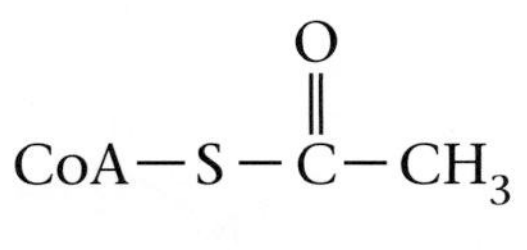

Acetyl-CoA

and fatty acids:

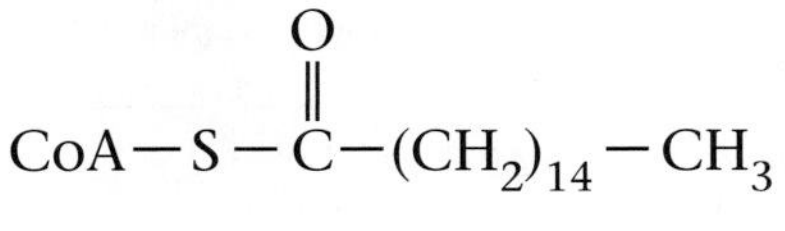

$$CoA-S-\overset{\overset{\displaystyle O}{\|}}{C}-(CH_2)_{14}-CH_3$$

Palmitoyl-CoA

The thioester bonds have a free energy content between 7 and 8 kcal/mol. *In biosynthetic reactions, the acid is transferred from CoA to an acceptor molecule.* This happens, for example, during acetylation reactions (the "A" in "coenzyme A" stands for "acetylation") and in the synthesis of triglycerides (see Chapter 23).

S-Adenosyl Methionine Donates Methyl Groups

Methylation reactions transfer a methyl group (—CH₃) to an acceptor molecule. The donor of the

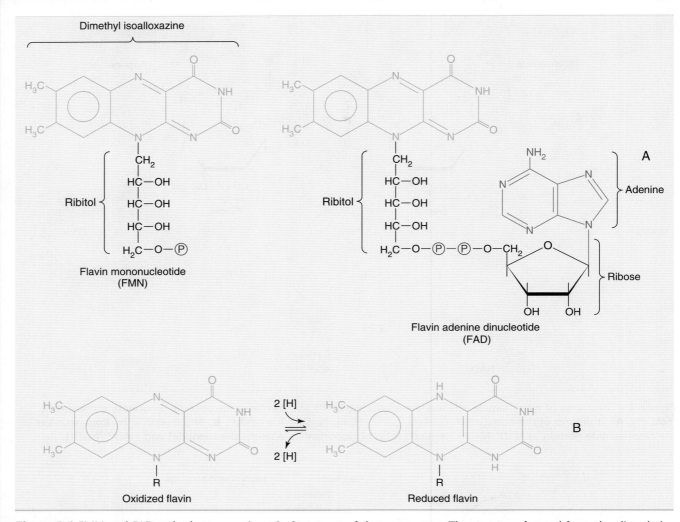

Figure 5.6 FMN and FAD as hydrogen carriers. **A,** Structures of the coenzymes. The structure formed from the dimethyl isoalloxazine ring and ribitol is called riboflavin (vitamin B$_2$). **B,** Hydrogen transfer by the dimethyl isoalloxazine ring of FMN and FAD.

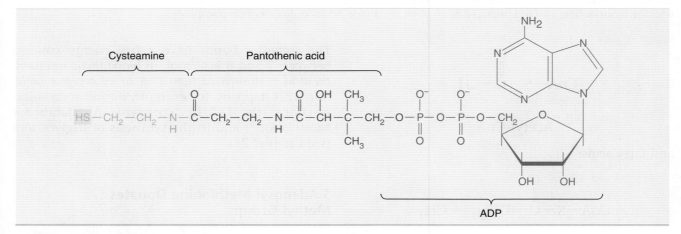

Figure 5.7 The structure of coenzyme A. ADP, adenosine diphosphate.

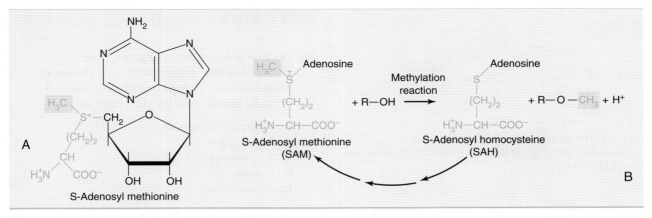

Figure 5.8 *S*-Adenosyl methionine (SAM) as a methyl group donor. **A,** Structure of the coenzyme. **B,** Formation of a methoxyl group in a SAM-dependent methylation.

Table 5.2 Summary of the Most Important Coenzymes

Coenzyme	Present as	Functions in	Vitamin*
Adenosine triphosphate (ATP)	Cosubstrate	Energy-dependent reactions	—
Guanosine triphosphate (GTP)	Cosubstrate	Energy-dependent reactions	—
Uridine triphosphate (UTP)	Cosubstrate	Activation of monosaccharides	—
Cytidine triphosphate (CTP)	Cosubstrate	Phospholipid synthesis	—
NAD and NADP	Cosubstrate	Hydrogen transfers	Niacin
Flavin adenine dinucleotide (FAD) and flavin mononucleotide (FMN)	Prosthetic group	Hydrogen transfers	Riboflavin
Coenzyme A	Cosubstrate	Acylation reactions	Pantothenic acid
S-Adenosyl methionine (SAM)	Cosubstrate	Methylation reactions	—
Heme	Prosthetic group	Electron transfers	—
Biotin	Prosthetic group	Carboxylation reactions	Biotin
Tetrahydrofolate (THF)	Cosubstrate	One-carbon transfers	Folic acid
Pyridoxal phosphate (PLP)	Prosthetic group	Amino acid metabolism	B_6
Thiamine pyrophosphate (TPP)	Prosthetic group	Carbonyl transfers	Thiamine (B_1)
Lipoic acid	Prosthetic group	Oxidative decarboxylations	—

* The vitamins are discussed in Chapter 24.
NAD, nicotinamide adenine dinucleotide; NADP, nicotinamide adenine dinucleotide phosphate.

methyl group is in most cases **S-adenosyl methionine (SAM)** (Fig. 5.8). The methylation reaction converts SAM to *S*-adenosyl homocysteine (SAH), which can be converted back to SAM in a different reaction (see Chapter 26). Like CoA, SAM is a cosubstrate rather than a prosthetic group.

Several other coenzymes participate in enzymatic reactions. These coenzymes, summarized in Table 5.2, will be discussed in the context of the metabolic reactions in which they participate.

Many Enzymes Require a Metal Ion

Many enzymes require alkali metals such as Na^+ and K^+ to maintain their active conformation. Transition metals such as iron, zinc, copper, and manganese, on the other hand, are often found in the active site, where they participate in catalysis. They are suitable for electron transfer reactions because they can easily switch between different oxidation states:

$$Fe^{3+} \underset{e^-}{\overset{e^-}{\rightleftharpoons}} Fe^{2+}$$

$$Cu^{2+} \underset{e^-}{\overset{e^-}{\rightleftharpoons}} Cu^+$$

In other cases, the metal acts as a Lewis acid, or electron pair acceptor. This happens in many oxygenase reactions, when ferrous iron (Fe^{2+}) or monovalent copper (Cu^+) binds molecular oxygen.

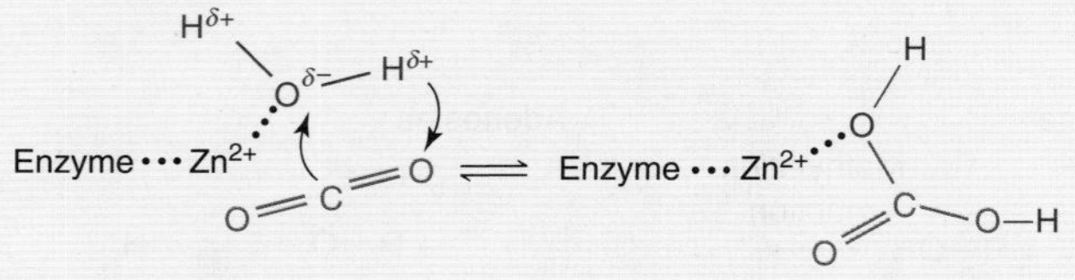

Figure 5.9 The catalytic mechanism of carbonic anhydrase. This enzyme catalyzes the reversible reaction $CO_2 + H_2O \rightleftharpoons H_2CO_3$.

Another example is the carbonic anhydrase reaction shown in Figure 5.9. In this case, the electron density on the oxygen of a water molecule is increased by binding to a zinc ion. This makes the water more reactive for a nucleophilic attack on the carbon of CO_2.

SUMMARY

Some coenzymes are tightly bound to the enzyme as prosthetic groups, whereas others are soluble cosubstrates. They are required because they offer structural features and chemical re-activities that are not present in simple polypeptides. The cosubstrate ATP, for example, contains two energy-rich phosphoanhydride bonds. Breakage of these bonds supplies energy to drive endergonic reactions. NAD, NADP, FMN, and FAD are hydrogen carriers in many dehydrogenase reactions. NAD and NADP are soluble cosubstrates, whereas FMN and FAD are tightly bound prosthetic groups. SAM is a methyl group donor, and CoA activates organic acids for biosynthetic reactions. Many enzymes contain a metal ion in their active site that participates in catalysis.

QUESTIONS

1. **Protein kinases are enzymes that phosphorylate amino acid side chains of proteins in ATP-dependent reactions. A protein kinase can be classified as**

   A. An oxidoreductase.
   B. A hydrolase.
   C. An isomerase.
   D. A lyase.
   E. A transferase.

2. **Cyanide is a potent inhibitor of cell respiration that prevents the oxidation of all nutrients. Cyanide will therefore definitely reduce the cellular concentration of:**

   A. Heme groups.
   B. $FADH_2$.
   C. CoA.
   D. ATP.
   E. SAM.

3. **The reaction**

   Succinyl-CoA + GDP + P$_i$
   $\rightarrow$ Succinate + CoA-SH + GTP

   has a standard free energy change $\Delta G^{0\prime}$ of −0.8 kcal/mol. If the free energy content of a phosphoanhydride bond in GTP is 7.3 kcal/mol, what would be the standard free energy change of the reaction

   Succinyl-CoA + H$_2$O $\rightarrow$ Succinate + CoA-SH?

   A. −8.1 kcal/mol.
   B. +6.5 kcal/mol.
   C. +8.1 kcal/mol.
   D. −6.5 kcal/mol.
   E. +0.8 kcal/mol.

PART TWO

GENETIC INFORMATION: DNA, RNA, AND PROTEIN SYNTHESIS

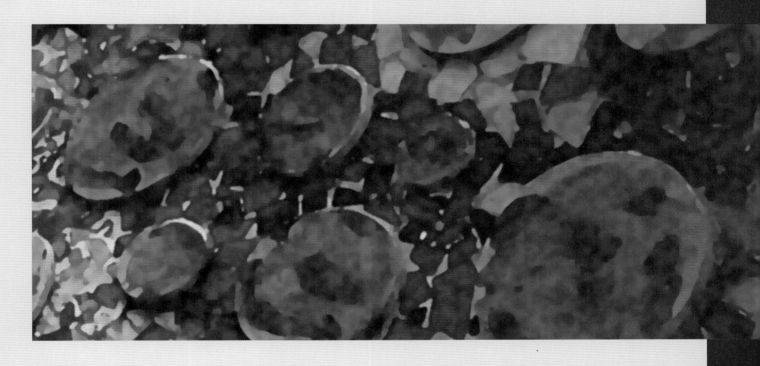

CHAPTER 6

DNA, RNA, and Protein Synthesis

A typical human cell contains about 10,000 different proteins. Their polypeptide chains are synthesized by ribosomes in the cytoplasm, according to instructions from the DNA in the chromosomes. These instructions are mailed from the chromosome to the ribosome in the form of **messenger RNA** (**mRNA**). Therefore, gene expression requires two steps (Fig. 6.1):

1. **Transcription** is the synthesis of an mRNA molecule in the nucleus. The mRNA is the carbon copy of a DNA strand.
2. **Translation** is the synthesis of the polypeptide by the ribosome, guided by instructions in the mRNA.

The functional unit of the genetic databank is the **gene.** *A gene is a length of DNA that directs the synthesis of a polypeptide.* It consists of a transcribed sequence and regulatory sites. The **chromosome** is a much larger structure, consisting of a very long DNA molecule with hundreds or even thousands of genes.

As it is expressed, the genetic message is amplified. A single gene can be transcribed into thousands of mRNA molecules, and each mRNA can be translated into thousands of polypeptides. A red blood cell, for example, contains 5×10^8 copies of the hemoglobin β chain, but the nucleated RBC precursors that make the hemoglobin have only two copies of the β chain gene.

All Living Organisms Use DNA as Their Genetic Databank

Living things are grouped into two major branches on the basis of their cell structure: The **prokaryotes,** which include bacteria, actinomycetes, and blue-green algae, and the **eukaryotes,** which include protozoa, plants, and animals. *Only eukaryotic cells are compartmentalized into organelles by intracellular membranes.* In addition to the nucleus, which is surrounded by a twofold membrane, eukaryotes possess the following structures:

1. **Mitochondria,** which have a twofold membrane and are the largest organelles besides the nucleus. As the powerhouses of the cell, they turn food and oxygen into ATP.
2. The **endoplasmic reticulum,** which is bounded by a single membrane and processes membrane proteins, membrane lipids, and secreted proteins.
3. The **Golgi apparatus,** which is a sorting station that sends secreted proteins, lysosomal enzymes, and membrane components to their proper destinations.
4. **Lysosomes,** which are membrane vesicles filled with hydrolytic enzymes. They degrade many cellular macromolecules, as well as substances that the cell engulfs by endocytosis.
5. **Peroxisomes,** which contain many of those enzymes that generate and destroy toxic hydrogen peroxide.
6. **Cytoskeletal fibers,** which give structural support to the cell. They are also required for cell motility and intracellular transport.

Differences between prokaryotes and eukaryotes are summarized in Figure 6.2 and Table 6.1. Despite these differences, all living cells have three features in common:

1. *All cells are surrounded by a plasma membrane:* a flimsy, fluid, flexible structure that forms a diffusion barrier between the cell and its environment.

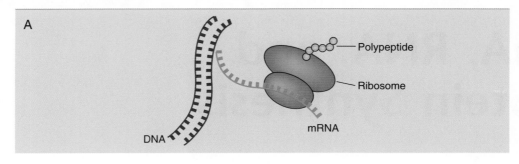

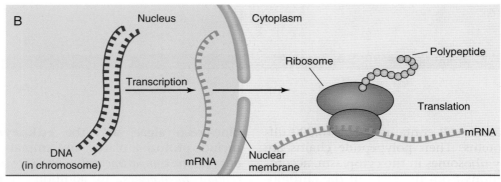

Figure 6.1 Expression of genetic information. In all organisms, the DNA of the gene is first copied into a single-stranded molecule of messenger RNA (mRNA). This process is called transcription. During ribosomal protein synthesis, the base sequence of the mRNA is used to specify the amino acid sequence of a polypeptide. This is called translation. **A,** In prokaryotic cells, translation follows immediately on transcription. **B,** Eukaryotic cells have a nuclear membrane. Therefore, transcription and translation take place in different compartments: transcription in the nucleus and translation in the cytoplasm.

Table 6.1 Typical Differences between Prokaryotic and Eukaryotic Cells

Property	Prokaryotes	Eukaryotes
Typical size	0.4-4 µm	5-50 µm
Nucleus	−	+
Membrane-bounded organelles	−	+
Cytoskeleton	−	+
Endocytosis and exocytosis	−	+
Cell wall	+ (some −)	+ (plants) − (animals)
No. of chromosomes	1 (+plasmids)	>1
Ploidy	Haploid	Haploid or diploid
Histones	−	+
Introns	−	+
Ribosomes	70S	80S

2. *All cells display metabolic activity,* with energy-generating and energy-consuming processes.
3. *All cells store genetic information in the form of DNA,* using it to reproduce themselves and to direct the synthesis of their RNA and protein.

This chapter describes DNA replication and protein synthesis in prokaryotes. The corresponding processes in eukaryotes, described in Chapter 8, are similar but are often more complex.

DNA Contains Four Bases

DNA is a polymer of nucleoside monophosphates (Fig. 6.3B). Its structural backbone is a chain of alternating phosphate and 2-deoxyribose residues that are held together by phosphodiester bonds. Carbons 3 and 5 of 2-deoxyribose participate in these bonds, whereas carbon 1 forms a β-*N*-glycosidic bond with a nitrogen in a purine or pyrimidine base (Fig. 6.4).

One end of the DNA strand has a free hydroxyl group at C-5 of the last 2-deoxyribose, and the other end has a free hydroxyl group at C-3. The carbons of 2-deoxyribose are numbered by a prime (′) to distinguish them from the carbon and nitrogen atoms of the bases, and therefore investigators speak of the 5′ end and the 3′ end. By convention, the 5′ terminus of a DNA (or RNA) strand is written at the left end, and the 3′ terminus at the right end. Thus, the

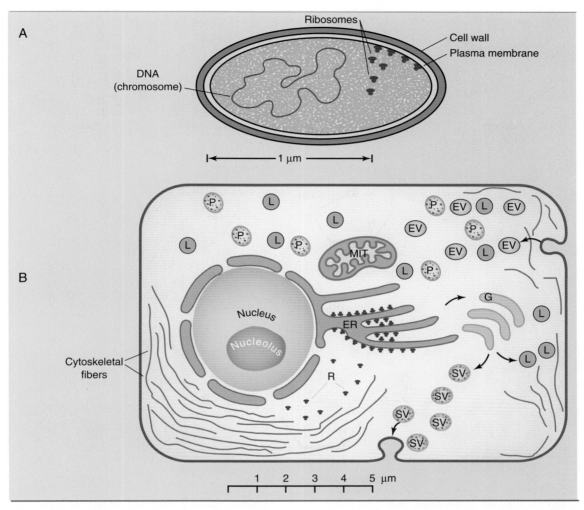

Figure 6.2 Typical elements of prokaryotic and eukaryotic cell structure. **A,** Typical bacterial (prokaryotic) cell. **B,** Typical human (eukaryotic) cell. R, Ribosomes; ER, endoplasmic reticulum; L, lysosome; P, peroxisome; EV, endocytotic vesicle; SV, secretory vesicle; G, Golgi apparatus; MIT, mitochondrion.

tetranucleotide in Figure 6.4 can be written as ACTG but not GTCA.

The variability of DNA structure is produced by its base sequence. With four different bases, there are 4^2 (or 16) different dinucleotides and 4^3 (or 64) different trinucleotides, and 4^{100} possibilities exist for a sequence of 100 nucleotides.

DNA Forms a Double Helix

Cellular DNA is always double-stranded. The vast majority of it is present as a **double helix,** as first described by James Watson and Francis Crick in 1953. The most prominent features of the Watson-

Crick double helix (Figs. 6.5, 6.6, and 6.7) are as follows:

1. *The two strands of the double helix have opposite polarity.* Base-pairing is always antiparallel, not only in the DNA double helix but also in other base-paired structures formed by DNA or RNA.
2. *The 2-deoxyribose/phosphate backbones of the two strands form two ridges on the surface of the molecule.* The phosphate groups are negatively charged.
3. *The bases face inward to the helix axis, but their edges are exposed.* They form the lining of two grooves that are framed by the ridges of the sugar-phosphate backbone. Because the *N*-glycosidic bonds are not exactly opposite each

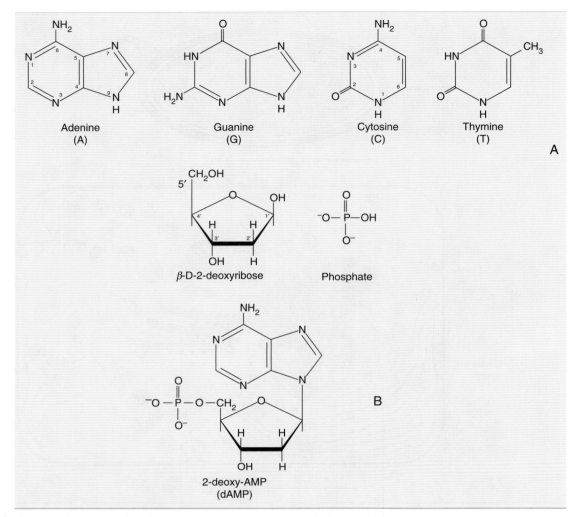

Figure 6.3 The building blocks of DNA. **A,** Structures of the four bases, 2-deoxyribose, and phosphate. A and G are purines; C and T are pyrimidines. **B,** Structure of 2-deoxy-adenosine monophosphate (dAMP), one of the four 2-deoxyribonucleoside monophosphates in the repeat structure of DNA. Note that a nitrogen atom of the base is bound by a β-*N*-glycosidic bond to C-1 of 2-deoxyribose, whereas C-5 forms a phosphate ester bond.

other (see Fig. 6.7), the two grooves are of unequal size. They are called the **major groove** and the **minor groove.**

4. *In each of the two strands, successive bases lie flat, one on top of the other,* like a stack of pancakes. The flat surfaces of the bases are hydrophobic, and successive bases in a strand form numerous van der Waals interactions. This **base stacking** is the strongest noncovalent force in the double helix.

5. *Bases in opposite strands interact by hydrogen bonds.* Adenine (A) always pairs with thymine (T) in the opposite strand, and guanine (G) with cytosine (C). Therefore, the molar amount of adenine in the double-stranded DNA always equals that of thymine, and the amount of guanine equals that of cytosine. Most important, *the base sequence of one strand predicts exactly the base sequence of the opposite strand.* This is essential for DNA replication and DNA repair.

6. *The double strand is wound into a right-handed helix* with about 10.4 base pairs per turn. Each full turn of the helix advances about 3.4 nm along the helix axis. The double helix is usually a stiff, extended shape, but it can also be bent and twisted by DNA-binding proteins.

DNA Can Be Denatured

Like other noncovalent structures, *the Watson-Crick double helix disintegrates at high temperatures.* This is

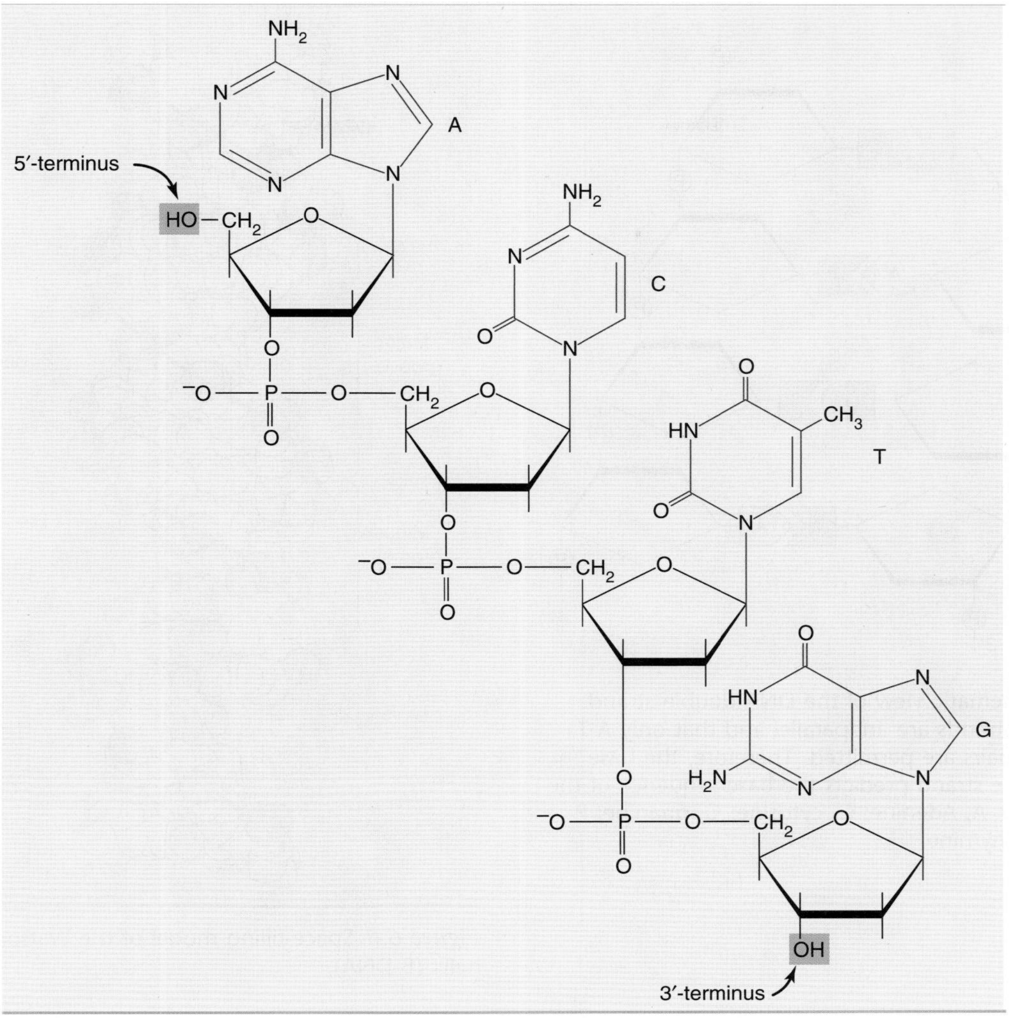

Figure 6.4 Structure of the (2-deoxy-) tetranucleotide ACTG. The DNA strands in chromosomes are far larger, with lengths of many million nucleotide units. A, Adenine; C, cytosine; G, guanine; T, thymine.

called **melting** of the DNA. Because A-T base pairs are held together by two hydrogen bonds and G-C base pairs by three, *A-T–rich sections of the DNA unravel more easily than G-C–rich regions* when the temperature is raised. Eventually, however, the whole molecule is converted to a single-stranded **random coil** (Figs. 6.8 and 6.9). At physiological pH and ionic strength, this typically happens between 85° C and 95° C.

Heat denaturation changes the physical properties of the DNA. It decreases the viscosity of DNA solutions because the single strands are more flexible than the stiff, resilient double helix; and it increases the ultraviolet light absorbance at 260 nm, which is caused by the bases, because base stacking is disrupted.

DNA can also be denatured by a decrease of the salt concentration, by extreme pH values, and by chemicals that disrupt hydrogen bonding or base stacking.

When cooled slowly, denatured DNA molecules "renature" spontaneously. This process is called **annealing.** Although small DNA molecules anneal almost instantaneously, seconds to minutes are required for large molecules.

DNA Is Supercoiled

Many naturally occurring DNA molecules are circular. When a linear duplex is partially unwound by one or several turns before it is linked into a circle, the number of base pairs per turn of the helix is greater than the usual 10.4. The torsional strain in this molecule can be relieved either by partial strand separation or by supercoiling of the duplex around

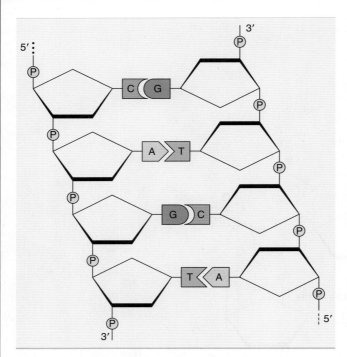

Figure 6.5 Schematic view of the DNA double strand. Note that the strands are antiparallel and that only A-T and G-C base pairs are permitted. Therefore, the base sequence of one strand predicts the base sequence of the opposite strand. A, Adenine; C, cytosine; G, guanine; P, phosphate; T, thymine.

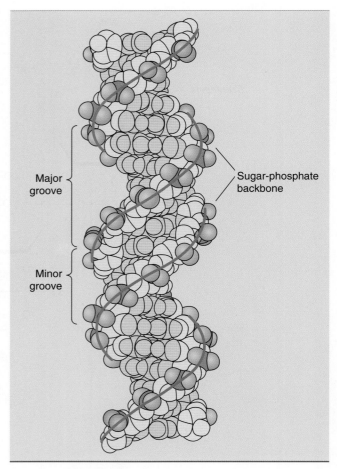

Figure 6.6 Space-filling model of the Watson-Crick double helix (B-DNA).

its own axis, much as a telephone cord twists around itself. This is called a **negative supertwist.** The opposite situation, in which the helix is overwound, is called a **positive supertwist.**

Most cellular DNAs are negatively supertwisted, with 5% to 7% fewer right-handed turns than expected from the number of their base pairs. *This underwound condition favors the unwinding of the double helix during DNA replication and transcription.*

The supertwisting of DNA is regulated by **topoisomerases.** These enzymes cleave a phosphodiester bond either in one strand or in both strands. Then they rotate the DNA around its axis before resealing the molecule (Fig. 6.10). Some topoisomerases only relax positive or negative supertwists, without consuming metabolic energy. Others, however, hydrolyze ATP to pump positive or negative supertwists into the DNA.

DNA Replication Is Semiconservative

DNA is the only molecule in the body that can be used to make identical copies of itself. These copies

are transmitted to the daughter cells during mitosis and even to the next generation through the gametes. In this sense, it is the only immortal molecule in the body. The organism is best understood as an artificial environment, created by genes for the benefit of their own continued existence.

The replication of double-stranded DNA to produce two identical daughter molecules proceeds in two steps (Fig. 6.11):

1. The *double helix unwinds to produce two single strands.* This requires ATP-dependent enzymes to break the hydrogen bonds between bases.
2. *A new complementary strand is synthesized for each of the two old strands.* This is possible because the base sequence of each strand predicts the base sequence of the complementary strand.

The unwinding of the parental double helix creates the **replication fork.** This is the place where the new DNA is synthesized. DNA replication is called **semiconservative** because one strand in

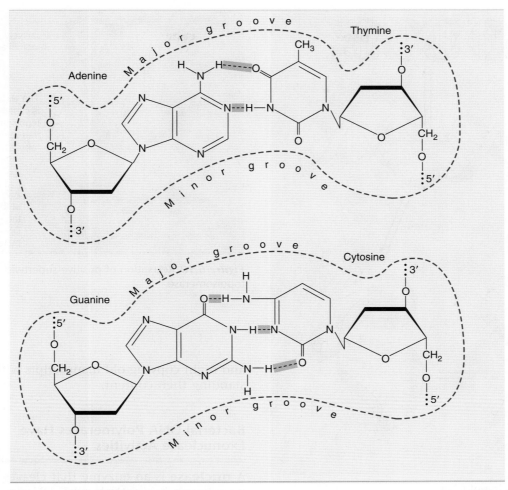

Figure 6.7 Cross sections through an adenine-thymine (A-T) and a guanine-cytosine (G-C) base pair in the DNA duplex. The A-T base pair is held together by two hydrogen bonds (– – –); the G-C base pair, by three.

the daughter molecule is always old and the other strand is newly synthesized.

DNA Is Synthesized by DNA Polymerases

The steps in DNA replication are best known in *Escherichia coli,* an intestinal bacterium that has enjoyed the unfaltering affection of generations of molecular biologists.

The key enzymes of DNA replication in *E. coli,* as in all other cells, are the **DNA polymerases.** *DNA polymerases synthesize the new DNA strand stepwise, nucleotide by nucleotide, in the 5′→3′ direction.* The precursors are the deoxyribonucleoside triphosphates: deoxy-adenosine triphosphate (dATP), deoxy-guanosine triphosphate (dGTP), deoxy-cytosine triphosphate (dCTP), and deoxy-thymidine triphosphate (dTTP). DNA polymerase

elongates DNA strands by linking the proximal phosphate of an incoming nucleotide to the 3′-hydroxyl group at the end of the growing strand, as shown in Fig. 6.12. The pyrophosphate formed in this reaction is rapidly cleaved to inorganic phosphate by cellular pyrophosphatases.

*The DNA polymerases require a single-stranded DNA as a **template.*** Therefore, the parental DNA double helix has to be unwound before the synthesis of new DNA can begin. While synthesizing the new strand in the 5′→3′ direction, the enzyme moves along the template strand in the 3′→5′ direction.

DNA polymerases are "literate" enzymes that can "read" the base sequence of their template, and they incorporate in the new strand only the bases that pair correctly with the base in the template strand. Therefore, *the new strand is exactly complementary to the template strand.* Thus, the DNA polymerases are lacking in creative spirit. They are like the scribe monks in medieval monasteries, who worked day

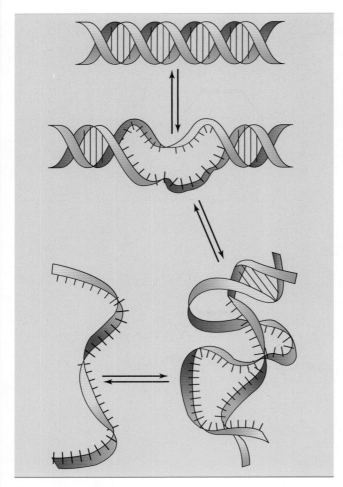

Figure 6.8 Melting of DNA.

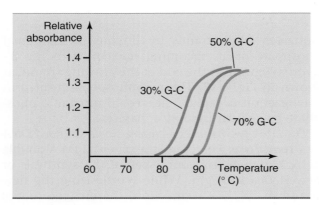

Figure 6.9 Melting of DNA, monitored by the increase of ultraviolet light absorbance at 260 nm. The melting temperature increases with increased guanine-cytosine (G-C) content of the DNA. It is also affected by ionic strength and pH. The melting temperature is the temperature at which the increase in ultraviolet light absorbance is half-maximal.

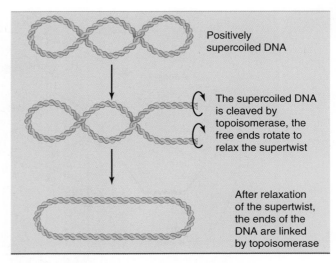

Figure 6.10 Relaxation of positive supertwists in DNA by a topoisomerase.

and night copying old manuscripts without understanding their content.

Bacterial DNA Polymerases Have Exonuclease Activities

A **nuclease** is an enzyme that cleaves phosphodiester bonds in a nucleic acid. DNases cleave DNA, and RNases cleave RNA. Nucleases that cleave internal phosphodiester bonds are called **endonucleases,** and those that cleave bonds at the 5′ end or the 3′ end are called **exonucleases.**

Nobody is perfect, and even DNA polymerase sometimes incorporates a wrong nucleotide in the new strand. The **mutation** created by such an error can be deadly when it leads to the synthesis of a faulty protein. To minimize such mishaps, all bacterial DNA polymerases are equipped with a **3′-exonuclease activity** that they use for proofreading. The exonuclease removes from the 3′ end of the new strand only the nucleotides that are not properly base-paired to the template, leaving well-paired nucleotides in place (Fig. 6.13). *This proofreading mechanism reduces the error rate from 1 in 10^4 or 1 in 10^5 to approximately 1 in 10^7.*

Most bacterial DNA polymerases also have a **5′-exonuclease activity** (see Fig. 6.13). This activity is not used for proofreading, but it removes damaged DNA during DNA repair and erases the RNA primer during DNA replication.

E. coli has three DNA polymerases. They differ in their affinity for the DNA template and consequently in their **processivity,** the number of

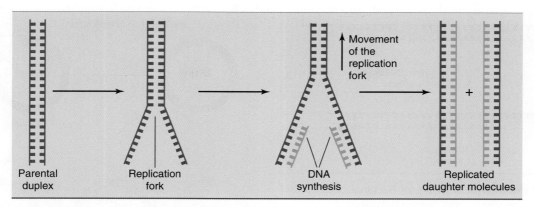

Figure 6.11 The semiconservative mechanism of DNA replication.

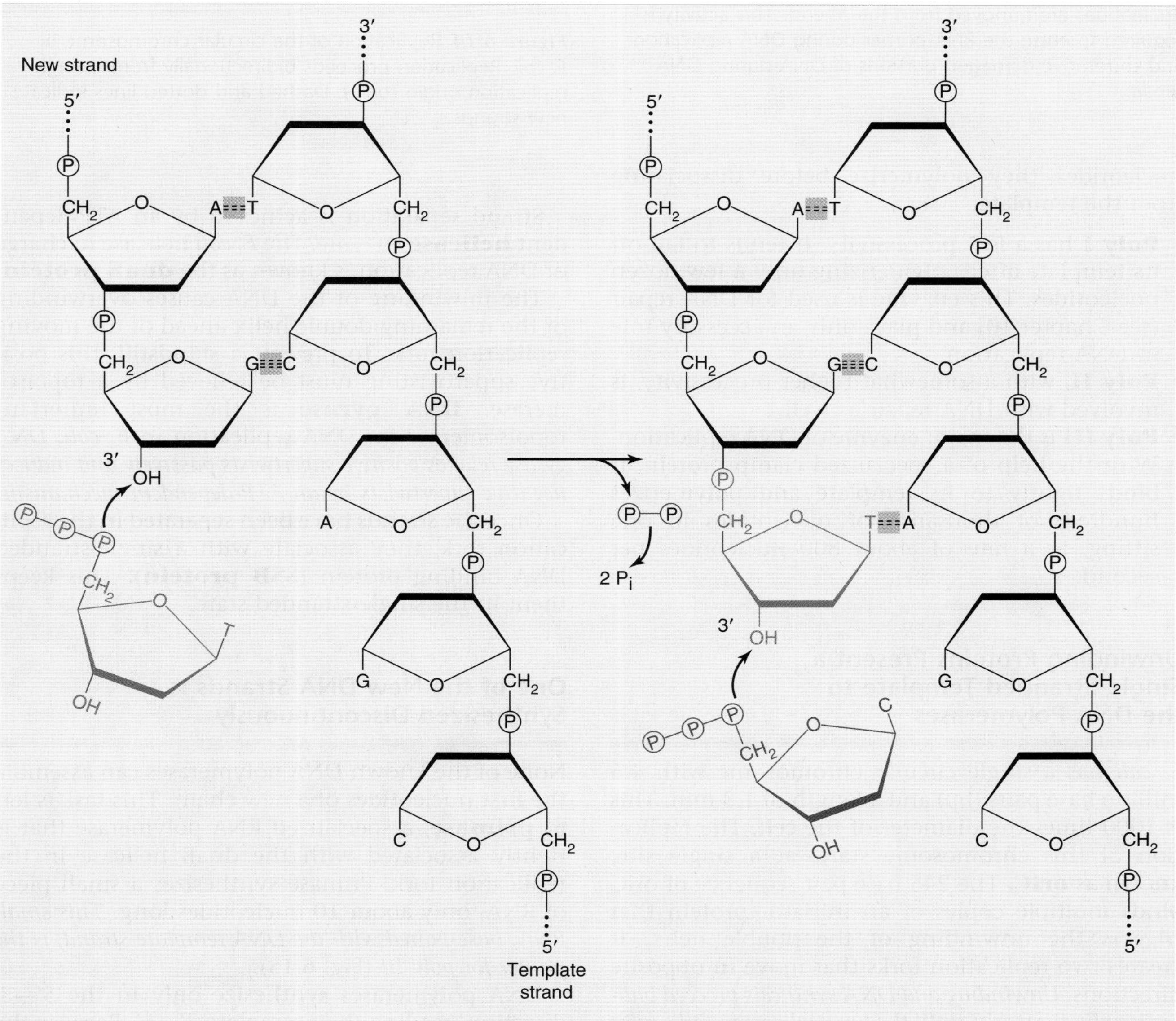

Figure 6.12 Template-directed synthesis of DNA by DNA polymerases. A, Adenine; C, cytosine; G, guanine; P, phosphate; T, thymine.

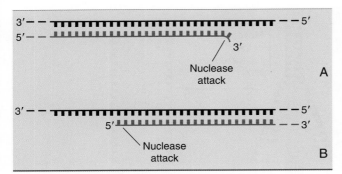

Figure 6.13 Exonuclease activities of bacterial DNA polymerases. The products of these cleavages are nucleoside 5'-monophosphates. **A,** 3'-Exonuclease activity: Only mismatched bases are removed from the 3' end of the newly synthesized DNA strand. This activity is required for proofreading. **B,** 5'-Exonuclease activity: Base-paired nucleotides are removed from the 5' end. This activity is required to erase the RNA primer during DNA replication and to remove damaged portions of DNA during DNA repair.

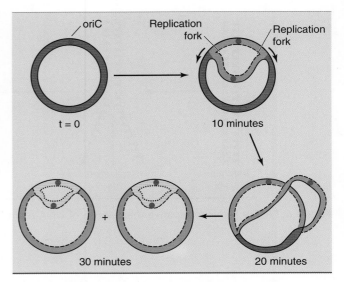

Figure 6.14 Replication of the circular chromosome of *E. coli*. Replication proceeds bidirectionally from a single replication origin (oriC). Dashed and dotted lines indicate new strands.

nucleotides they polymerize before dissociating from the template:

- **Poly I** has a low processivity. It tends to fall off its template after polymerizing only a few dozen nucleotides. This enzyme is used for DNA repair (see Chapter 10) and plays only an accessory role in DNA replication.
- **Poly II,** with a somewhat higher processivity, is involved with DNA repair as well.
- **Poly III** is the major enzyme of DNA replication. With the help of a specialized clamp protein, it binds tightly to its template and polymerizes hundreds of thousands of nucleotides in one sitting, at a rate of about 800 nucleotides per second.

Unwinding Proteins Present a Single-Stranded Template to the DNA Polymerases

E. coli has a single circular chromosome with 4.6 million base pairs (bp) and a length of 1.3 mm. This is 1000 times the diameter of the cell. The replication of this chromosome starts at a single site, known as **oriC.** The 245 base pair sequence of oriC binds multiple copies of an initiator protein that triggers the unwinding of the double helix. It creates two replication forks that move in opposite directions. *Unwinding and DNA synthesis proceed bidirectionally from oriC until the two replication forks meet at the opposite side of the chromosome* (Fig. 6.14). The replication of the whole chromosome takes 30 to 40 minutes.

Strand separation is achieved by an ATP-dependent **helicase** enzyme. The *E. coli* helicase in charge of DNA replication is known as the **dnaB protein.**

The unwinding of the DNA causes overwinding of the remaining double helix ahead of the moving replication fork. To prevent a standstill, this positive supertwisting must be relieved by a topoisomerase. **DNA gyrase** is the most important topoisomerase for DNA replication in *E. coli*. *DNA gyrase relaxes positive supertwists passively and induces negative supertwists by an ATP-dependent mechanism.*

Once the strands have been separated in the replication fork, they associate with a single-stranded DNA binding protein (**SSB protein**). This keeps them in the single-stranded state.

One of the New DNA Strands Is Synthesized Discontinuously

None of the known DNA polymerases can assemble the first nucleotides of a new chain. This task is left to **primase,** a specialized RNA polymerase that is tightly associated with the dnaB helicase in the replication fork. Primase synthesizes a small piece of RNA, only about 10 nucleotides long. *This small RNA, base-paired with the DNA template strand, is the primer for poly III* (Fig. 6.15).

DNA polymerases synthesize only in the 5'→3' direction, reading their template 3'→5'. Because the parental double strand is antiparallel, only one of the new DNA chains, the **leading strand,** can be synthesized by a poly III molecule that simply

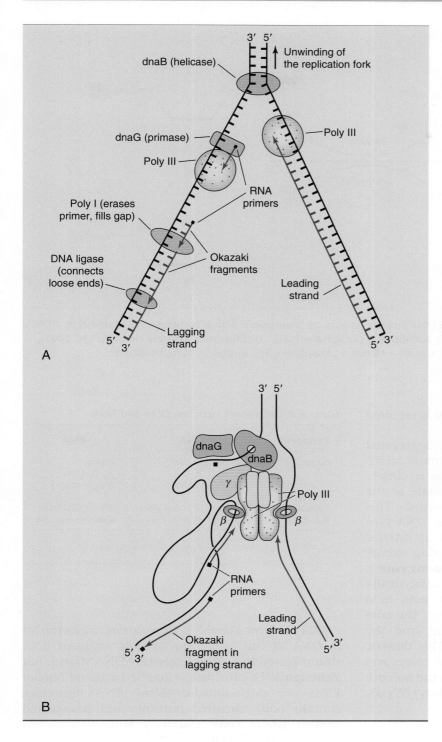

Figure 6.15 The replication fork of *Escherichia coli.* **A,** Because new DNA can be synthesized only in the 5'→3' direction, one of the two new strands (the "lagging strand") is synthesized piecemeal. The primer has to be removed from the lagging strand by DNA polymerase I (Poly I), and the Okazaki fragments have to be connected by DNA ligase. **B,** A model for the actual assembly of proteins in the bacterial replication fork. Note that the DNA template for the lagging strand has to spool through the β clamp backward to account for the direction of DNA synthesis. dnaB, helicase; dnaG, primase; β, clamp protein; γ, clamp loader; Poly III, DNA polymerase III.

travels with the replication fork. The other strand, called the **lagging strand,** has to be synthesized piecemeal.

This requires the repeated action of the primase, followed by poly III. Together they produce DNA strands of about 1000 nucleotides, each with a tiny piece of RNA at the 5' end. The pieces are called **Okazaki fragments.** The RNA primer is soon removed by the 5'-exonuclease activity of poly I, and the gaps are filled by its polymerase activity.

Poly I cannot connect the loose ends of two Okazaki fragments. This task is performed by a **DNA ligase** that links the phosphorylated 5'-terminus of one fragment with the free 3'-terminus of another. The hydrolysis of a phosphoanhydride bond in the reduced form of nicotinamide adenine dinucleotide

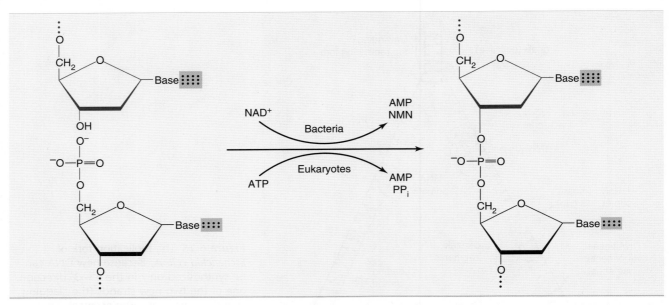

Figure 6.16 Reaction of DNA ligase. The two DNA strands have to be base-paired with a complementary strand in a DNA duplex. AMP, adenosine monophosphate; ATP, adenosine triphosphate; NAD$^+$, nicotinamide adenine dinucleotide; NMN, nicotinamide mononucleotide (contains nicotinamide + ribose + phosphate); PP$_i$, inorganic pyrophosphate.

(NADH) (in bacteria) or ATP (in humans) is required for this reaction (Fig. 6.16).

The enzymes of DNA replication are aggregated in large complexes with multiple enzymatic activities (see Fig. 6.15). The dnaB helicase is closely linked to the primase, to keep the primase in the replication fork where its work is needed. This complex is known as the **primosome.** DNA synthesis itself requires two copies of poly III: one for the leading strand and one for the lagging strand. Indeed, the **DNA polymerase III holoenzyme** is a large complex with two copies of the catalytically active core enzyme (subunit structure $\alpha\varepsilon\theta$) held together by two τ subunits. One copy of the core enzyme synthesizes the leading strand, and the other synthesizes the lagging strand. This dimeric core enzyme associates with other polypeptides and finally with the clamp protein β to form the holoenzyme with a subunit structure of $(\alpha\varepsilon\theta)_2\tau_2\gamma_2\delta\delta'\chi\psi\beta_2$ and a molecular weight of 900,000.

RNA Plays Key Roles in Gene Expression

There are only two strictly chemical differences between DNA and RNA: RNA contains ribose instead of 2-deoxyribose, and uracil instead of thymine. Thymine and uracil are distinguished only by a methyl group. This methyl group does not participate in base-pairing, and thus *both uracil and thymine pair with adenine* (Table 6.2).

Table 6.2 Differences between DNA and RNA

Property	DNA	RNA
Sugar	2-Deoxyribose	Ribose
Bases	A, G, C, T	A, G, C, U
Strandedness in vivo	Double strand	Single strand
Typical size	Often >10^6 base pairs	60-20,000 bases
Function	Genetic information	Gene expression

A, adenine; C, cytosine; G, guanine; T, thymine; U, uracil.

RNA can form a double helix with dimensions similar to DNA. It can also form hybrids, with an RNA strand paired to a complementary DNA strand. But although RNA can form a double helix, *all cellular RNAs are single-stranded.* Most RNA molecules contain both unpaired portions and base-paired regions where complementary sequences within the same strand form a short double helix.

All cellular RNAs are copied from a DNA template in the process of **transcription,** but only **messenger RNA (mRNA)** is translated into protein. **Ribosomal RNA (rRNA)** is a major constituent of the ribosome; and the **transfer RNAs (tRNAs)** are small cytoplasmic RNAs that bind amino acids covalently and deliver them to the ribosome for protein synthesis (Table 6.3). More than 80% of all RNA in *E. coli* is rRNA and only 3% is mRNA, although about one third of the RNA synthesized

Table 6.3 Properties of ribosomal RNA (rRNA), transfer RNA (tRNA), and messenger RNA (mRNA)

Property	rRNA	tRNA	mRNA
Relative abundance	Most abundant	Less abundant	Least abundant
Molecular weight (in *Escherichia coli*)	1.2×10^6	$2\text{-}3 \times 10^4$	Heterogeneous
	0.55×10^6		
	3.6×10^4		
Location (in eukaryotes)	Ribosomes, nucleolus	Cytoplasm	Nucleus, cytoplasm
Function	Structure of ribosomal subunits, peptidyl transferase activity	Brings amino acids to the ribosome	Transmits information for protein synthesis

Table 6.4 Comparison of the Bacterial DNA Polymerases and RNA Polymerase

Property	DNA Polymerase I	DNA Polymerase III	RNA Polymerase
Subunit structure	Single polypeptide	8 Subunits	$\alpha_2\,\beta\beta'\sigma$
Molecular weight	$\approx$103,000	$\approx$170,000*	$\approx$450,000
Substrates	dATP, dGTP, dCTP, dTTP	dATP, dGTP, dCTP, dTTP	ATP, GTP, CTP, UTP
Direction of synthesis	$5'\rightarrow3'$	$5'\rightarrow3'$	$5'\rightarrow3'$
Template required	DNA	DNA	DNA
Primer required	Yes	Yes	No
Speed (bases/sec)	10-20	600-1000	$\approx$50
3'-Exonuclease activity	Yes	Yes	No
5'-Exonuclease activity	Yes	No	No

*Core enzyme ($\alpha + \varepsilon + \theta$ subunits) only. Several other polypeptides are associated with this core enzyme in vivo.

in this organism is mRNA. This is because bacterial mRNA has an average lifespan of only 3 minutes. Most human mRNAs, on the other hand, live for between 1 and 10 hours before they succumb to cellular nucleases.

The σ Subunit Recognizes Promoters

RNA polymerase is the enzyme of RNA synthesis (Table 6.4). Bacterial RNA polymerase has the subunit structure $\alpha_2\beta\beta'\sigma$, but the σ (sigma) subunit is only loosely bound to the other subunits. The **RNA polymerase core enzyme** ($\alpha_2\beta\beta'$) polymerizes nucleotides into RNA, and *the σ subunit is needed to recognize transcriptional start sites.*

RNA polymerase has to bind to a **promoter** before it can initiate transcription. The promoter extends over about 60 base pairs and includes the first 10 to 12 bases of the transcribed sequence. To find the promoter, the RNA polymerase binds nonselectively and with moderately high affinity to double-stranded DNA and slides along the double helix. When its σ subunit encounters a promoter, it binds to it and positions the core enzyme over the transcriptional start site.

The RNA polymerase then separates the DNA double helix on a length of about 18 base pairs, starting at a conserved A-T–rich sequence about 10 base pairs upstream of the transcriptional start site. Strand separation is essential because *transcription, like DNA replication, requires a single-stranded template.*

The σ subunit dissociates away from the core enzyme after the formation of the first 5 to 15 phosphodiester bonds. This marks the transition from the initiation to the elongation phase of transcription. Without the σ subunit, the core enzyme no longer has a specific affinity for the promoter. It is now free to vacate the promoter and travel along the base sequence of the gene.

Although all promoters are recognized by the same σ subunit, they look different in different genes. Only two short segments, which are located about 10 base pairs and 35 base pairs upstream of the transcriptional start site, are similar in all promoters. Even these sequences are somewhat variable, but it is possible to deduce a **consensus sequence** of the most commonly encountered bases (Fig. 6.17).

This diversity is required because genes must be transcribed at different rates. Some are transcribed up to 10 times per minute, whereas others are transcribed only once every 10 or 20 minutes. The rate of transcriptional initiation depends on the base sequence of the promoter. In general, *the more the promoter resembles the consensus sequence, the higher is the rate of transcription.*

P$_R$	CGGCATGATATTGACTTATTGAATAAAATTGGG	TAAATTTGACTCAACG
T7AI	AAAAGAGTTGACTTAAAGTCTAACCTATAG	GATACTTACAGCCAT
lac	ACCCCAGGCTTTACACTTTATGCTTCCGGCTCGTATGTTGTGTGGAATT	
araC	GCCGTGATTATAGACACTTTTGTTACGCGTTTT	TGTCATGGCTTTGGTC
trp	AAATGAGCTGTTGACAATTAATCATCGAACTAG	TTAACTAGTACGCAAG
bioB	CATAATCGACTTGTAAACCAAATTGAAAAGATT	TAGGTTTACAAGTCTA
tRNA$_{tyr}$	CAACGTAACACTTTACAGCGGCGCGTCATTTGA	TATGATGCGCCCCGCT
Str	TGTATATTTCTTGACACCTTTTCGGCATCGCCC	TAAAATTCGGCGTCCT
Tet	ATTCTCATGTTTGACAGCTTATCATCGATAAGC	TTTAATGCGGTAGTTT
Consensus sequence	TTGACA	TATAAT

Figure 6.17 Consensus sequence for promoters in *Escherichia coli*. All of these promoters are recognized by the major σ subunit of *E. coli*. Some belong to *E. coli* genes; others, to bacteriophages infecting *E. coli*. Only the base sequence of the coding strand (nontemplate strand) is shown. Colored bases to the right of the TATAAT consensus indicate start of transcription.

DNA Is Faithfully Copied into RNA

RNA synthesis resembles DNA synthesis in most respects (Fig. 6.18). The RNA polymerase uses ATP, GTP, CTP, and UTP as precursors, synthesizing the RNA 5'→3' while reading the template strand 3'→5' (Fig. 6.19). But unlike the DNA polymerases, RNA polymerase can do without a primer. It starts a new chain simply by placing a ribonucleoside triphosphate in the first position.

Only one strand of the DNA is used as the **template strand.** This strand is complementary to the RNA. The opposite DNA strand, which has the same base sequence as the RNA transcript (T replacing U), is called the **coding strand** (see Fig. 6.19). Transcription by bacterial RNA polymerase proceeds at a rate of 50 nucleotides per second, taking almost 20 times longer than DNA replication.

RNA polymerase has no proofreading nuclease activity, and thus *it has an error rate of about 1 per 10,000,* which is 1000 times higher than the error rate of poly III. This can be tolerated because the damage caused by a single faulty RNA molecule is not nearly as great as the damage caused by a faulty DNA.

The most important principle discussed so far is that *all nucleic acid synthesis requires a DNA template.* DNA is the sovereign master of the organism because it alone controls the synthesis of DNA, RNA, and proteins.

Transcription Is Terminated When the RNA Forms a Hairpin Loop

Transcription continues until the RNA polymerase runs into a **terminator** sequence at the end of the gene. Terminators look different in different genes,

but most of them contain a **palindrome:** a type of symmetrical sequence in which the base sequence of one DNA strand traced in one direction from the symmetry axis is the same as the sequence of the opposite strand traced in the opposite direction. A palindrome is a word or sentence that reads the same in both directions, as in "Madam, I'm Adam."

When a palindrome is transcribed, the RNA transcript forms a **hairpin loop** by internal base-pairing (Fig. 6.20). This hairpin loop causes the RNA polymerase to dissociate from the DNA template and release the RNA.

Transcription Can Be Inhibited by Drugs

Chemotherapeutic agents are, in a sense, weapons of mass destruction that doctors use to exterminate undesirable life forms such as bacteria, fungi, parasites, and cancer cells. To be used effectively in the patient, they must perform their mission without collateral damage to normal cells. As a rule, bacteria are more easily killed in the human body than are fungi and parasites because they are more different from human cells than are the eukaryotic pathogens, and cancer cells are most difficult to eradicate because they are too similar to the normal cells from which they evolved.

Rifampicin inhibits transcription by tight binding to the β subunit of bacterial RNA polymerase. This does not kill the bacteria, but it prevents their growth. Eukaryotic RNA polymerases are not affected; therefore, rifampicin can be used for the treatment of bacterial infections including tuberculosis.

Sometimes this works, but sometimes it does not, because a point mutation that changes the

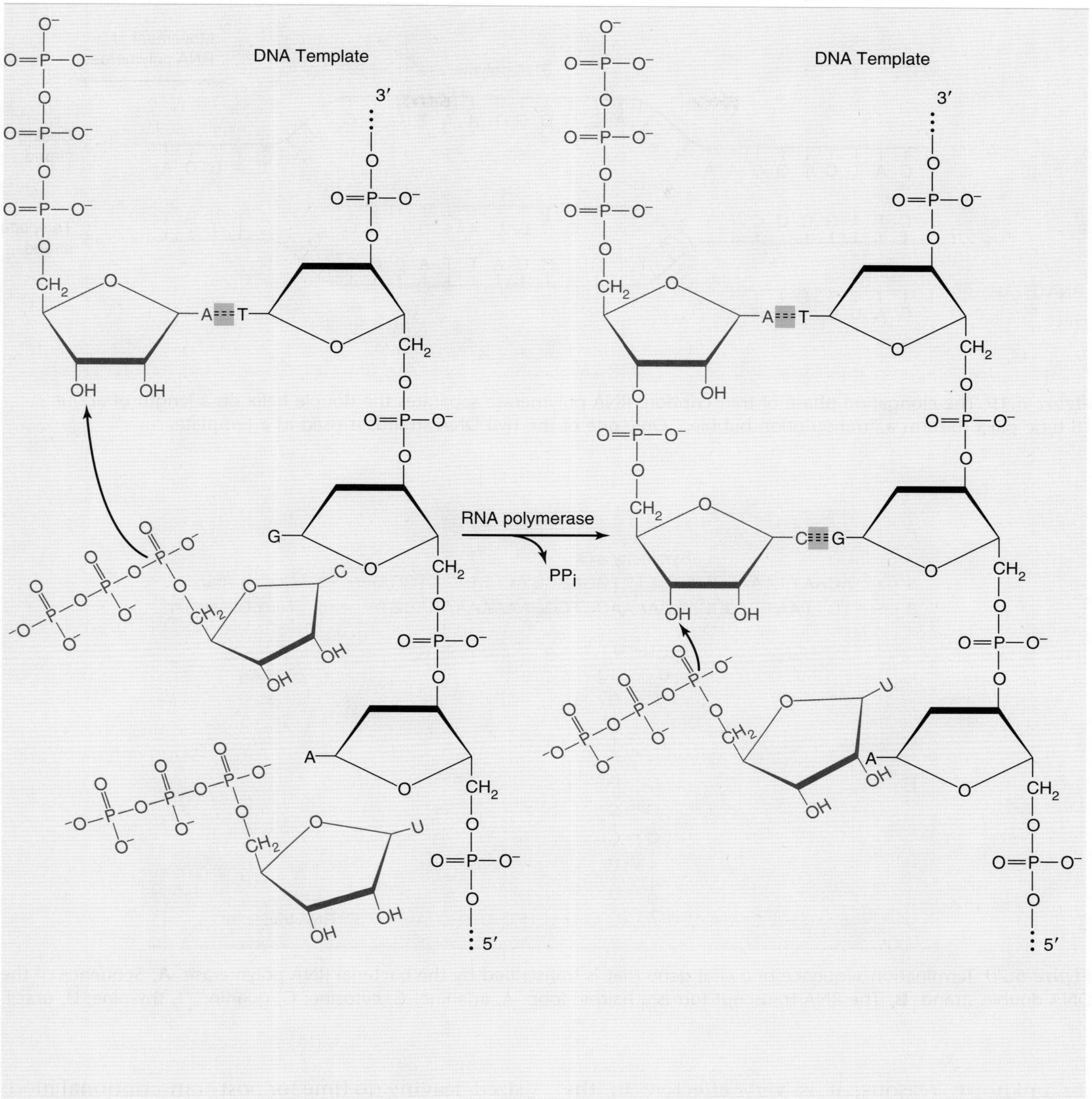

Figure 6.18 Formation of the first phosphodiester bond during transcription. The nucleotide at the 5′ terminus of the RNA remains in the 5′-triphosphate form. Compare this with the mechanism of DNA synthesis shown in Fig. 6.12. A, adenine; C, cytosine; G, guanine; PPi, inorganic pyrophosphate; T, thymine.

rifampicin binding site on the β subunit can make the bacteria resistant to rifampicin. With continued treatment, any resistant mutants in the bacterial population rapidly take over the ecosystem, and the drug becomes ineffective.

Actinomycin D (Fig. 6.21) inhibits transcription by a different mechanism. A planar phenoxazone ring in the molecule becomes intercalated (sandwiched) between two G-C base pairs in double-stranded DNA, and two oligopeptide tails in the molecule clamp the drug to the minor groove of the double helix. RNA polymerase cannot transcribe past the bound drug.

Actinomycin D binds to the DNA of eukaryotes as well as prokaryotes; therefore, it cannot be used for the treatment of bacterial infections. However,

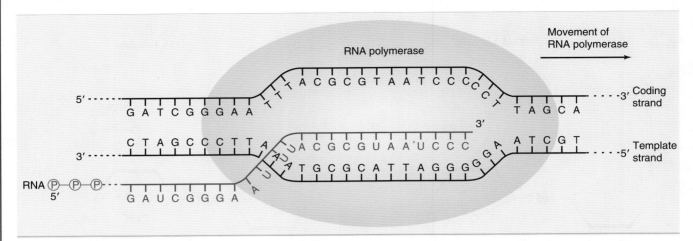

Figure 6.19 The elongation phase of transcription. RNA polymerase separates the double helix on a length of about 18 base pairs to form a "transcription bubble." Only one of the two DNA strands is used as a template.

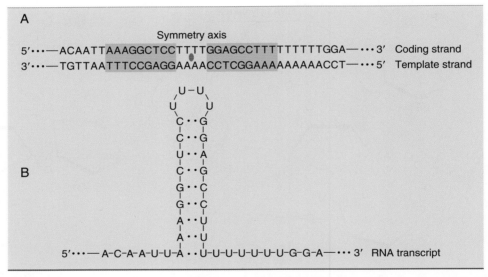

Figure 6.20 Termination sequence of a viral gene that is transcribed by the bacterial RNA polymerase. **A,** Sequence of the DNA double strand. **B,** The RNA transcript forms a hairpin loop. A, adenine; C, cytosine; G, guanine; T, thymine; U, uracil.

for unknown reasons, it is very effective in the treatment of Wilms tumor (nephroblastoma), a rare childhood cancer.

Some RNAs Are Chemically Modified after Transcription

The chemical modification of RNA after its synthesis by RNA polymerase is called **post-transcriptional processing.** Of the three major RNA types, **mRNA** is processed extensively in eukaryotes (see Chapter 8) but not in prokaryotes.

One reason for this difference is that bacterial mRNAs are translated as soon as they are synthe-sized, leaving no time for post-transcriptional modi-fications. In fact, *ribosomes attach to the 5′ end of the mRNA and start translation long before the synthesis of the mRNA has been completed.* In eukaryotes, in contrast, the mRNA has to move from the nucleus to the cytoplasm before it can be translated. This leaves ample time for post-transcriptional processing.

rRNA is modified post-transcriptionally in both prokaryotes and eukaryotes. Each bacterial ribo-some contains three molecules of rRNA: 5S, 16S, and 23S RNA. The "S" refers to the behavior of a molecule in the ultracentrifuge, and its numerical value is roughly related to its size.

These ribosomal RNAs are transcribed from a single gene as one large precursor molecule. This transcript is cleaved into the three rRNAs by specific endonucleases. The ribosome contains a single copy of each rRNA, and this mechanism of synthesis guarantees that the three rRNAs are produced in equimolar amounts. *E. coli* has seven copies of the rRNA gene to synthesize the large quantities of rRNA that are needed by the growing cell. Some copies of this gene contain the sequences of one or several tRNAs as well. Eukaryotes use a similar strategy for the synthesis of their rRNA (Fig. 6.22).

Bacterial rRNA contains some methylated bases, whereas eukaryotic rRNA contains methylated ribose residues. There is also a rather large amount of pseudouridine in eukaryotic rRNA (Fig. 6.23). The methylation of bases and ribose residues requires *S*-adenosyl methionine (SAM) as a methyl group donor.

Most tRNA genes of *E. coli* are integrated into larger transcription units with other tRNA genes and sometimes with rRNA or protein-coding genes. The tRNA is modeled from the transcript by the concerted action of endonucleases and exonucleases. tRNA also contains many unusual or chemically modified bases, both in prokaryotes and in eukaryotes (see Fig. 6.23).

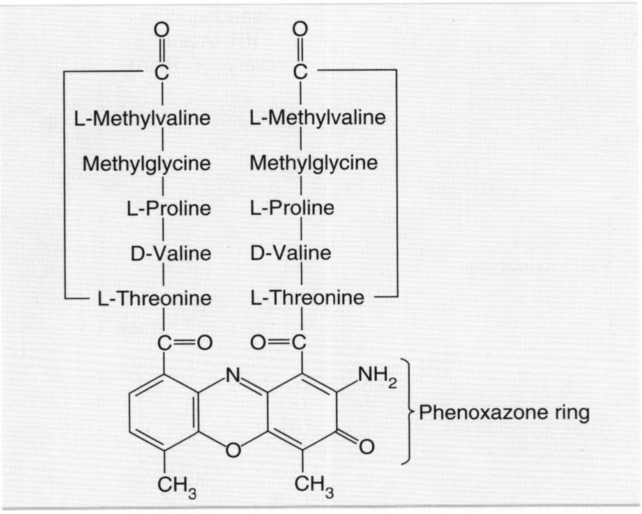

Figure 6.21 Structure of actinomycin D.

The Genetic Code Defines the Relationship between the Base Sequence of the Messenger RNA and the Amino Acid Sequence of the Polypeptide

A single base in the mRNA cannot specify an amino acid in a polypeptide because mRNA has only 4 bases, whereas polypeptides contain 20 amino acids. A sequence of two bases can specify 4^2 (16) amino acids, and a sequence of three bases, 4^3 (64) amino acids.

In fact, *a sequence of three bases on the mRNA codes for an amino acid.* The ribosome reads these base triplets, or **codons,** in the 5'→3' direction. This is the same direction in which the mRNA is itself synthesized by RNA polymerase. *As the ribosome moves*

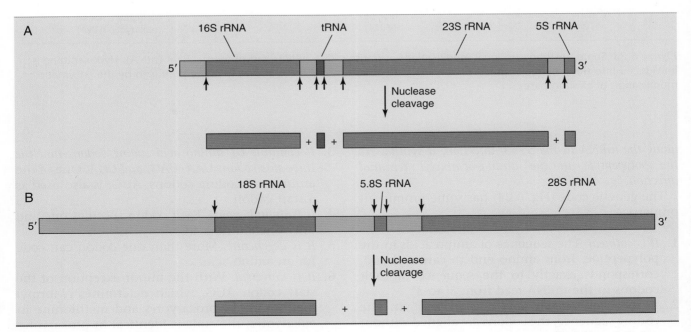

Figure 6.22 Processing of ribosomal RNA (rRNA) precursors in prokaryotes and eukaryotes. **A,** In *Escherichia coli.* **B,** In *Homo sapiens.* tRNA, transfer RNA.

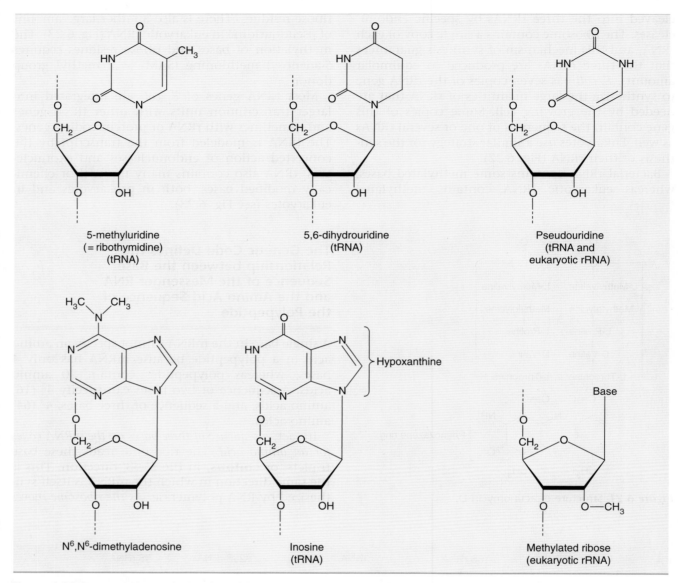

Figure 6.23 Some posttranscriptional modifications in transfer RNA (tRNA) and ribosomal RNA (rRNA). Hypoxanthine is introduced into tRNA by replacement of adenine. The other unusual bases shown here are produced by the enzymatic modification of existing bases.

along the mRNA in the 5′→3′ direction, it synthesizes the polypeptide in the amino→carboxyl terminal direction.

The genetic code (Fig. 6.24) has some prominent properties:

1. *It is colinear.* The sequence of amino acids in the polypeptide, from amino end to carboxyl end, corresponds exactly to the sequence of their codons in the mRNA read from 5′ to 3′.
2. *It is nonoverlapping and "commaless."* In the coding sequence, the codons are aligned without overlap and without empty spaces in between. Each base belongs to one and only one codon.
3. *It contains 61 amino acid coding codons and the three stop codons UAA, UAG, and UGA.* One of the amino acid coding codons, AUG, is also used as a start codon.
4. *It is unambiguous.* Each codon specifies one and only one amino acid.
5. *It is degenerate.* More than one codon can code for an amino acid.
6. *It is universal.* With the minor exception of the start codon AUG, which determines *N*-formyl methionine in prokaryotes and methionine in eukaryotes, the code is identical in prokaryotes and eukaryotes. Other minor variations occur only in the small genomes of mitochondria

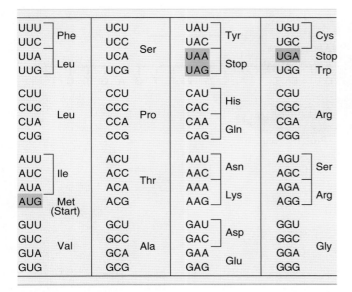

UUU ⎤ Phe UUC ⎦ UUA ⎤ Leu UUG ⎦	UCU ⎤ UCC ⎥ Ser UCA ⎥ UCG ⎦	UAU ⎤ Tyr UAC ⎦ UAA ⎤ Stop UAG ⎦	UGU ⎤ Cys UGC ⎦ UGA Stop UGG Trp
CUU ⎤ CUC ⎥ Leu CUA ⎥ CUG ⎦	CCU ⎤ CCC ⎥ Pro CCA ⎥ CCG ⎦	CAU ⎤ His CAC ⎦ CAA ⎤ Gln CAG ⎦	CGU ⎤ CGC ⎥ Arg CGA ⎥ CGG ⎦
AUU ⎤ AUC ⎥ Ile AUA ⎦ AUG Met (Start)	ACU ⎤ ACC ⎥ Thr ACA ⎥ ACG ⎦	AAU ⎤ Asn AAC ⎦ AAA ⎤ Lys AAG ⎦	AGU ⎤ Ser AGC ⎦ AGA ⎤ Arg AGG ⎦
GUU ⎤ GUC ⎥ Val GUA ⎥ GUG ⎦	GCU ⎤ GCC ⎥ Ala GCA ⎥ GCG ⎦	GAU ⎤ Asp GAC ⎦ GAA ⎤ Glu GAG ⎦	GGU ⎤ GGC ⎥ Gly GGA ⎥ GGG ⎦

Figure 6.24 The genetic code. A, adenine; Ala, alanine; Arg, arginine; Asn, asparagine; Asp, aspartate; C, cytosine; G, guanine; Cys, cysteine; Gln, glutamine; Glu, glutamate; Gly, glycine; His, histidine; Ile, isoleucine; Leu, leucine; Lys, lysine; Met, methionine; Phe, phenylalanine; Pro, proline; Ser, serine; Thr, threonine; Trp, tryptophan; Tyr, tyrosine; U, uracil; Val, valine.

and chloroplasts and in some single-celled eukaryotes.

The near-universality of the genetic code shows that *all surviving life on earth is descended from a common ancestor.* There is no way that a complex and arbitrary system such as the genetic code could have evolved independently in two lineages. Aliens from other planets would also need replicating genetic molecules because inheritance is an essential attribute of life, but there is no reason to expect that they would use the terrestrial genetic code. It is even doubtful that they would use DNA.

The universality of the code is also interesting for genetic engineers. It implies, for example, that *coding sequences of eukaryotic genes that are artificially introduced into prokaryotic cells can be expressed correctly.*

One final problem is that there are three possible **reading frames** for a colinear, nonoverlapping, and commaless triplet code. The ribosome decides among these three possibilities by searching the 5′-terminal region of the mRNA for the initiation codon AUG. Starting with AUG, it then reads successive base triplets as codons until it reaches a stop codon that signals the end of the polypeptide. This implies that *the 5′ and 3′ ends of the mRNA are not translated* (Fig. 6.25).

Transfer RNA Is the Adapter Molecule in Protein Synthesis

The tRNAs are small RNAs, about 80 nucleotides long, that present amino acids to the ribosome for protein synthesis. Their base sequences are quite variable, but all tRNAs share some common structural and functional features (Fig. 6.26):

1. *The molecule is folded into a cloverleaf structure,* with three stem portions whose bases are paired and three loops whose bases are unpaired.
2. *The 3′-terminus is the attachment site for an amino acid.* The tRNA ends with the sequence CCA, and the amino acid is bound to the ribose of the last nucleotide.
3. *One of the three loops of the cloverleaf contains the* **anticodon.** The three bases of the anticodon pair with the codon on the mRNA during protein synthesis.

The other two leaflets of the cloverleaf are called the **dihydrouridine loop** and the **TψC loop** (TψC = thymine–pseudouracil–cytosine). They are named after conserved bases in their structures. A variable loop is also present in most tRNAs. This structure participates in recognition by the aminoacyl-tRNA synthetase and in binding to the ribosome.

The unique feature of tRNA is that it possesses both an anticodon to recognize the codon on the mRNA and a covalently bound amino acid. Thus, *it can match the amino acid to the appropriate codon on the mRNA.*

Amino Acids Are Activated by an Ester Bond with the 3′-Terminus of the Transfer RNA

A cytoplasmic **aminoacyl-tRNA synthetase** attaches an amino acid to the 3′ end of the tRNA, thereby converting it into an **aminoacyl-tRNA** (Fig. 6.27). The balance of the reaction is

$$Amino\ acid + tRNA + ATP$$

$$\downarrow$$

$$Aminoacyl\text{-}tRNA + AMP + PP_i$$

where AMP = adenosine monophosphate and PPi = inorganic pyrophosphate. The ester bond between amino acid and tRNA is almost as energy-rich as a phosphoanhydride bond in ATP, but the reaction is nevertheless irreversible because the pyrophosphate is quickly hydrolyzed in the cell.

There are only 20 different aminoacyl-tRNA synthetases in bacterial cells, each of them specific for

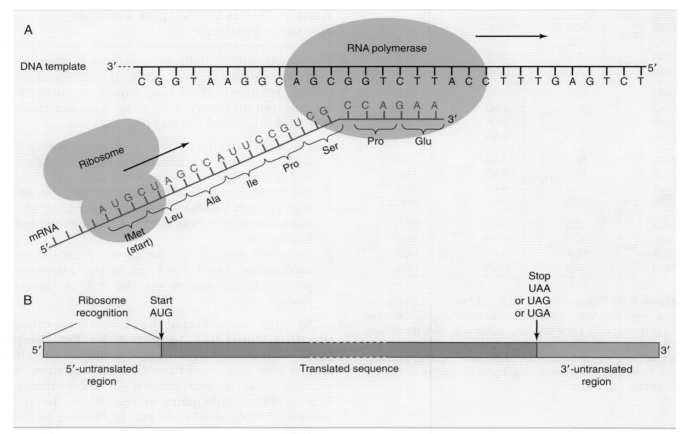

Figure 6.25 The reading frame of messenger RNA (mRNA) and the importance of the start and stop codons. **A,** The determination of the reading frame. The ribosome identifies the start codon AUG, then reads successive base triplets as codons. The cotranscriptional initiation of translation depicted here is specific for prokaryotes. **B,** The overall structure of mRNA. mRNAs have a 5′-untranslated sequence upstream of the start codon and a 3′-untranslated sequence downstream of the stop codon. The 5′-untranslated region is required for the initial binding of the mRNA to the ribosome during the initiation of translation.

one of the 20 amino acids. The number of different tRNAs in the cell is considerably greater than 20; therefore, most amino acids can be loaded on more than one tRNA. In these cases, the aminoacyl-tRNA synthetase can recognize several tRNAs, although it is highly selective for the amino acid. In fact, aminoacyl-tRNA synthetases make only about one mistake in every 40,000 couplings.

This selectivity is needed for the fidelity of the genetic code. When the enzyme attaches the wrong amino acid to the tRNA, the wrong amino acid will be incorporated into the polypeptide in place of the correct one, and when a mutation alters the specificity of an aminoacyl-tRNA synthetase, causing it to attach the wrong amino acid to its tRNAs, the result will be a change in the genetic code. A mutation in the anticodon of a tRNA also changes the genetic code. Such mutations would be fatal.

Many Transfer RNAs Recognize More than One Codon

During protein synthesis, *the codon of the mRNA base-pairs with the anticodon of the tRNA in an antiparallel orientation.* With strict Watson-Crick base-pairing, at least 61 different tRNAs would be needed for the 61 amino acid coding codons. However, most bacteria have fewer than 61 different tRNAs, and human mitochondria have only 22.

This is possible because the rules of base-pairing are relaxed for the third codon base. Uracil at the 5′ end of the anticodon can pair not only with adenine (A) but also with guanine (G) at the 3′ end of the codon, and a G in this position can pair with cytosine (C) or uracil (U). Also, several tRNAs have hypoxanthine as their first anticodon base (the corresponding nucleoside is called inosine). Hypoxan-

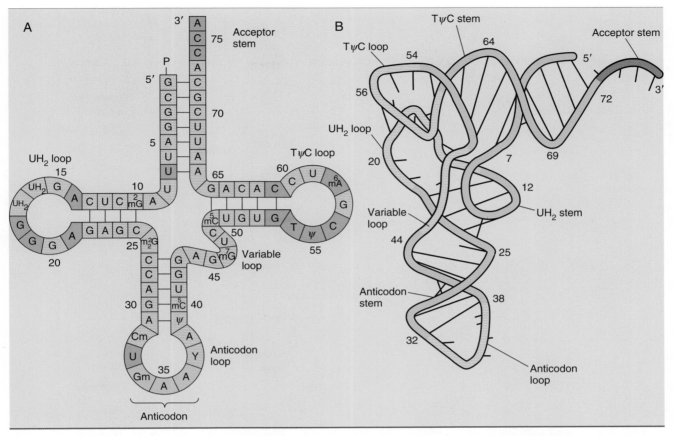

Figure 6.26 Structure of a typical transfer RNA (tRNA), yeast tRNA^Phe. Note the wide separation between the amino acid binding site ("acceptor stem") and the anticodon. **A,** The "cloverleaf" structure. Conserved bases are indicated by dark color. **B,** The tertiary structure. The three stem-loop structures of the cloverleaf are shown in orange. A, adenine; C, cytosine; G, guanine; T, thymine; U, uracil. Modified nucleosides: ψ2, pseudouridine; Cm, 2'-O-methyl cytidine; Gm, 2'-O-methylguanosine; m²G, 2-methylguanosine; m₂²G, 2,2-dimethylguanosine; m⁵C, 5-methylcytidine; m⁶A, 6-methyladenosine; m⁷G, 7-methylguanosine; UH₂, dihydrouridine; Y, "hypermodified" purine.

thine can pair with A, U, or C. This freedom of base-pairing is called **wobble.**

Wobble contributes to the degeneracy of the genetic code. As seen in Figure 6.24, codons specifying the same amino acid usually differ in the third codon base. This is the "wobble position," and in many cases the alternative codons are indeed read by the same tRNA.

Ribosomes Are the Workbenches for Protein Synthesis

Although they enjoy the prestigious status of organelles, ribosomes are not surrounded by a membrane and do not form a separate cellular compartment. They are simply large, catalytically active ribonucleoprotein particles. In bacteria, they are either free floating in the cytoplasm or attached to the plasma membrane, and in eukaryotes they are either free floating in the cytoplasm or bound to the membrane of the endoplasmic reticulum. *E. coli* contains about 16,000 ribosomes, but a typical eukaryotic cell has more than 1 million.

Ribosomes consist of a large and a small subunit. According to their sedimentation rate in the ultracentrifuge, bacterial ribosomes are characterized as 70S ribosomes, with 30S and 50S subunits. The ribosomes in the cytoplasm and on the ER of eukaryotes are a bit larger: 80S, with 40S and 60S subunits. Inactive ribosomes exist as loose subunits that aggregate into complete 70S or 80S particles only when they get ready for protein synthesis.

The composition of bacterial and eukaryotic ribosomes is summarized in Table 6.5. Each ribosomal RNA molecule and, with one exception, each ribosomal protein is present in only one copy per ribosome. The components are held together noncovalently,

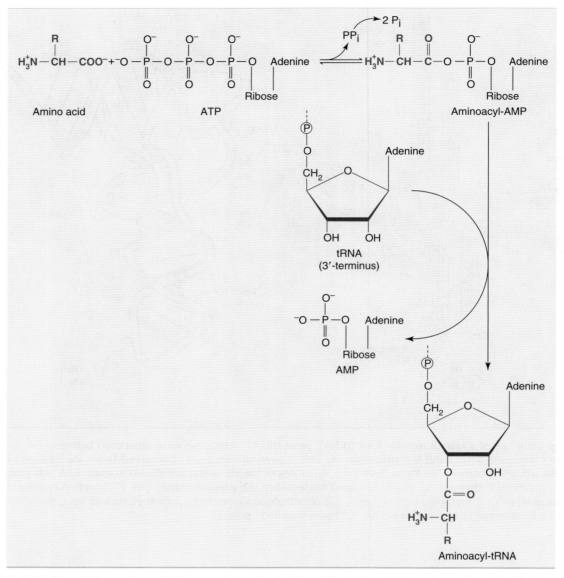

Figure 6.27 Activation of the amino acid for protein synthesis. The activation reactions are catalyzed by highly selective aminoacyl–transfer RNA (tRNA) synthetases in the cytoplasm. The aminoacyl-tRNA is the immediate substrate for ribosomal protein synthesis. AMP, adenosine monophosphate; ATP, adenosine triphosphate; P_i, inorganic phosphate; PP_i, inorganic pyrophosphate.

and ribosomal subunits can be assembled in the test tube from ribosomal proteins and RNAs. Living cells assemble their ribosomes in the cytoplasm (prokaryotes) or the nucleolus (eukaryotes).

Some features of ribosomal protein synthesis are as follows:

1. To start protein synthesis, the ribosome binds to a site near the 5' terminus of the mRNA.
2. mRNA is read in the 5'→3' direction, whereas the polypeptide is synthesized in the amino→carboxyl terminal direction.
3. The ribosome has a binding site for the tRNA that carries the growing polypeptide chain, and another binding site for the incoming aminoacyl-tRNA.
4. The ribosome forms the peptide bond while peptidyl-tRNA and aminoacyl-tRNA are bound to these sites.
5. Energy-dependent steps in ribosomal protein synthesis require GTP rather than ATP.
6. Some steps in protein synthesis require the help of soluble cytoplasmic proteins that are known as **initiation factors, elongation factors,** and **termination factors.**
7. Each ribosome synthesizes only one polypeptide at a time, but an mRNA molecule is read simultaneously by many ribosomes.

Table 6.5 Features of Prokaryotic and Eukaryotic Ribosomes

Property	Escherichia coli	Homo sapiens (Cytoplasmic)*
Diameter (nm)	20	25
Mass (kD)	2700	4200
Sedimentation coefficient†		
Complete ribosome	70S	80S
Small subunit	30S	40S
Large subunit	50S	60S
RNA content	65%	50%
Protein content	35%	50%
rRNA, small subunit	16S	18S
rRNAs, large subunit	5S, 23S	5S, 5.8S, 28S
No. of proteins		
Small subunit	21	34
Large subunit	34	50

* For mitochondrial ribosomes, Chapter 8.
† S, Svedberg unit, which describes the behavior of particles in the ultracentrifuge. Higher S values are associated with heavier particles, but they are not additive.
rRNA, ribosomal RNA.

The Initiation Complex Brings Ribosome, Messenger RNA, and Initiator–Transfer RNA Together

To initiate protein synthesis, *the ribosome has to associate with mRNA and the initiator tRNA.* The initiator tRNA carries the modified amino acid N-formylmethionine (fMet), and its anticodon binds to the AUG start codon on the mRNA. *Bacterial proteins are always synthesized with fMet at their amino terminus.*

The 5′-untranslated region of the mRNA contains the conserved **Shine-Dalgarno sequence** (consensus: AGGAGGU) about 10 nucleotides upstream of the AUG start codon. To form the **30S initiation complex,** the Shine-Dalgarno sequence base-pairs with a complementary sequence on the 16S RNA in the small ribosomal subunit. At the same time, the initiator-tRNA binds to the small ribosomal subunit while pairing its anticodon with the AUG start codon of the mRNA (Fig. 6.28).

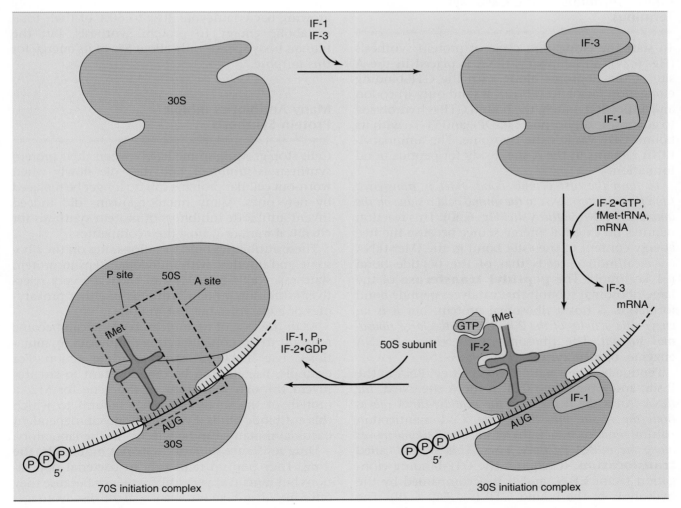

Figure 6.28 Formation of the 70S initiation complex in prokaryotes. AUG, adenine-uracil-guanine; fMet, N-formylmethionine; GDP, guanosine diphosphate; GTP, guanosine triphosphate; IF-1, IF-2, and IF-3, initiation factors 1, 2, and 3; mRNA, messenger RNA; P_i, inorganic phosphate; tRNA, transfer RNA.

The initiation complex also contains three initiation factors: **IF-1, IF-2,** and **IF-3.** IF-1 and IF-3 prevent the ribosomal subunits from associating into a complete 70S ribosome. IF-2, containing a bound GTP molecule, is required for the binding of the fMet-tRNA to the 30S initiation complex.

The **70S initiation complex** is formed when the 50S ribosomal subunit binds to the 30S initiation complex. The initiation factors are released while the bound GTP is hydrolyzed to GDP and inorganic phosphate.

The binding site for the initiator tRNA on the ribosome is called the **P site** because it is occupied by a **p**eptidyl-tRNA during the elongation phase. A second tRNA binding site, the **A site** (A = **a**minoacyl-tRNA, or **a**cceptor) is still empty. It receives incoming aminoacyl-tRNA molecules during the elongation phase.

Polypeptides Grow Stepwise from the Amino Terminus to the Carboxyl Terminus

To start the elongation cycle of protein synthesis (Fig. 6.29), an aminoacyl-tRNA is placed in the A site of the ribosome along with the GTP-binding elongation factor Tu (EF-Tu). If (and only if) codon and anticodon match, the bound GTP is hydrolyzed to guanosine diphosphate (GDP), and EF-Tu with its bound GDP vacates the ribosome. The aminoacyl-tRNA remains in the A site, ready for peptide bond formation.

To form the first peptide bond, fMet is transferred from the initiator-tRNA to the amino acid residue on the aminoacyl-tRNA in the A site (Fig. 6.30). This reaction requires no external energy source because the free energy content of the ester bond in the fMet-tRNA (≈7 kcal/mol) exceeds that of the peptide bond (≈1 kcal/mol). The **peptidyl transferase** of the large ribosomal subunit that catalyzes peptide bond formation is not a ribosomal protein, but *it is an enzymatic activity of the 23S RNA in the large ribosomal subunit.* The ribosome is therefore an RNA enzyme, or **ribozyme.**

Peptide bond formation leaves a free tRNA in the P site and a peptidyl-tRNA in the A site. Next, *the tRNA leaves the P site, and the peptidyl-tRNA moves from the A site into the P site.* Codon-anticodon pairing remains intact; therefore, *the ribosome moves along the mRNA by three bases.* This step is called **translocation.** It requires the GTP-binding elongation factor **EF-G,** and it is accompanied by the hydrolysis of the bound GTP (see Fig. 6.29). The speed of ribosomal protein synthesis is about 20 amino acids per second, and the error rate is about 1 for every 10,000 amino acids.

The stop codons UAA, UAG, and UGA do not have matching tRNAs but are recognized by proteins called **release factors.** After binding to the stop codon, the release factors induce the cleavage of the bond between polypeptide and tRNA. The polypeptide leaves the ribosome, the mRNA is released, and the ribosome dissociates into large and small subunits.

Protein Synthesis Is Energetically Expensive

The hydrolysis of GTP during the formation of the initiation complex is a one-time expense, but each elongation cycle requires the recurrent expense of two GTP bonds for placement and translocation. In addition, two high-energy phosphate bonds in ATP are needed for the formation of the aminoacyl-tRNA.

Therefore, *at least four high-energy bonds are consumed for the synthesis of each peptide bond.* Rapidly growing bacteria devote 30% to 50% of their total metabolic energy to protein synthesis, but the human body spends only about 5% of its energy for this purpose.

Many Antibiotics Inhibit Protein Synthesis

Cells stop growing immediately when their protein synthesis is inhibited, and they die slowly when worn-out cellular proteins can no longer be replaced by new ones. Many microorganisms did indeed invent antibiotic inhibitors of protein synthesis for chemical warfare against their competitors.

These antibiotics bind to various sites on the ribosome and interfere with individual steps in protein synthesis (Table 6.6). Most of them are very selective, inhibiting protein synthesis in either prokaryotes or eukaryotes but not in both.

As in the case of rifampicin, bacteria can become resistant to ribosomally acting antibiotics by mutations that affect the target of drug action. For example, bacteria can become resistant to streptomycin through mutations in the gene for S12, a protein of the small ribosomal subunit to which this antibiotic binds. Even streptomycin-dependent bacterial mutants can be selected in the laboratory.

Drug resistance mutations are not induced by the drug. They pop up randomly in bacterial populations but remain at very low frequency because they offer no advantage (or even a slight disadvantage) in the absence of the drug. However, when the bacteria are exposed to the drug, the susceptible cells die off, and the few surviving drug-resistant

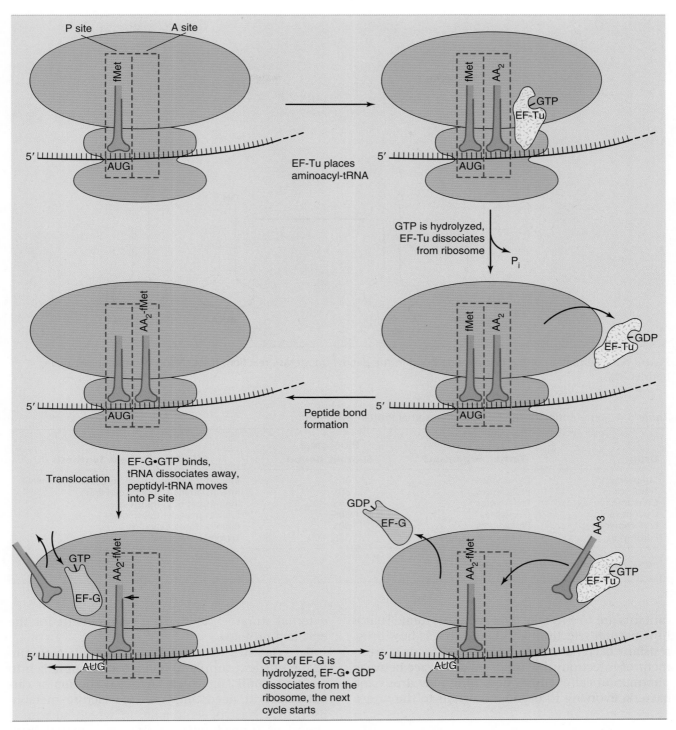

Figure 6.29 The first elongation cycle of ribosomal protein synthesis, which introduces the second amino acid (AA$_2$). EF-G, elongation factor G; EF-Tu, elongation factor Tu; fMet, *N*-formylmethionine; tRNA, transfer RNA.

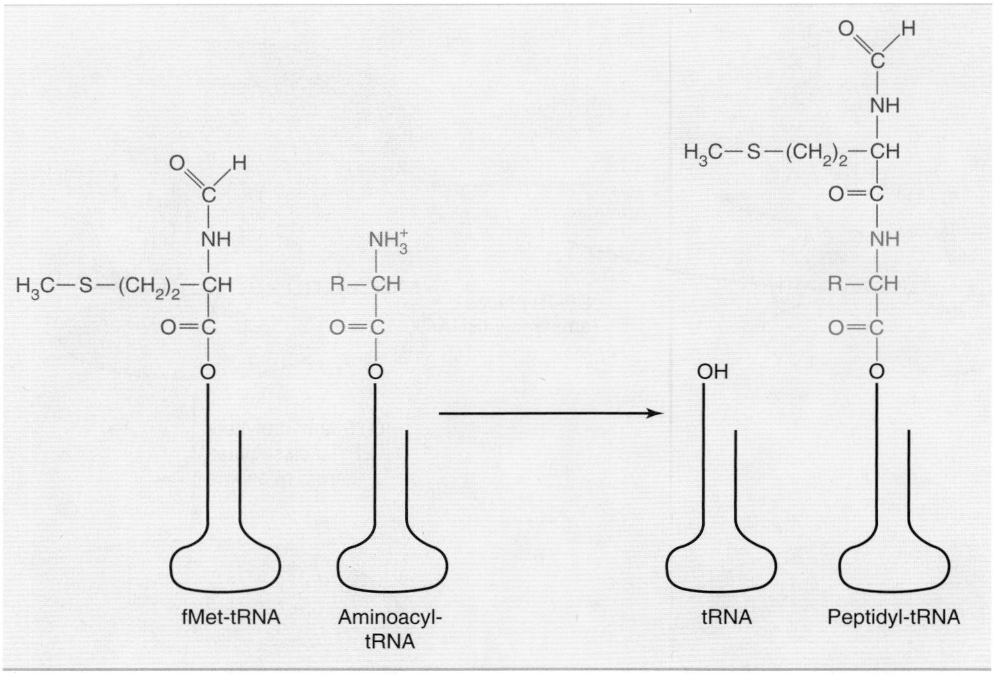

Figure 6.30 Formation of the first peptide bond in the petidyl transferase reaction. fMet, *N*-formylmethionine; tRNA, transfer RNA.

Table 6.6 Some Antibiotic Inhibitors of Ribosomal Protein Synthesis

Drug	Target Organisms	Ribosomal Subunit Bound	Effect on Protein Synthesis
Streptomycin	Prokaryotes	30S	Inhibits initiation, causes misreading of mRNA
Tetracycline	Prokaryotes	30S	Inhibits aminoacyl-tRNA binding
Chloramphenicol	Prokaryotes	50S	Inhibits peptidyl transferase
Cycloheximide	Eukaryotes	60S	Inhibits peptidyl transferase
Erythromycin	Prokaryotes	50S	Inhibits translocation
Puromycin	Prokaryotes, eukaryotes	50S, 60S	Terminates elongation

mRNA, messenger RNA; tRNA, transfer RNA.

mutants are free to take over the ecosystem. That is how natural selection works, and that is how drug-resistant bacteria breed in patients. The drug treatment of infectious diseases is an arms race between pharmaceutical chemists designing new drugs and bacteria evolving to become resistant to the drugs.

Gene Expression Is Tightly Regulated

Some proteins are needed at all times, and the genes that encode them are therefore transcribed at a fairly constant rate at all times. These proteins are called **constitutive proteins,** and their genes are called **housekeeping genes** because they have to work continuously. **Inducible proteins,** in contrast, are synthesized only when they are needed. The transcription of their genes is responsive to

external stimuli that signal a requirement for the encoded protein.

Bacteria have to adjust their metabolic activities to the nutrient supply. When a bacterium falls into a glass of milk, in which lactose is the major carbohydrate, it needs enzymes for lactose metabolism; in a glass of lemonade, in which sucrose is abundant, it needs enzymes of sucrose metabolism; and in a glass of beer, it needs enzymes for alcohol oxidation. In short, having the enzymes for a catabolic, energy-generating pathway makes sense only when the substrate of the pathway is available.

The enzymes of a biosynthetic pathway, on the other hand, are required only when the end product is not available from external sources. The enzymes of tryptophan synthesis, for example, are required only when the cell has to grow on a tryptophan-free medium.

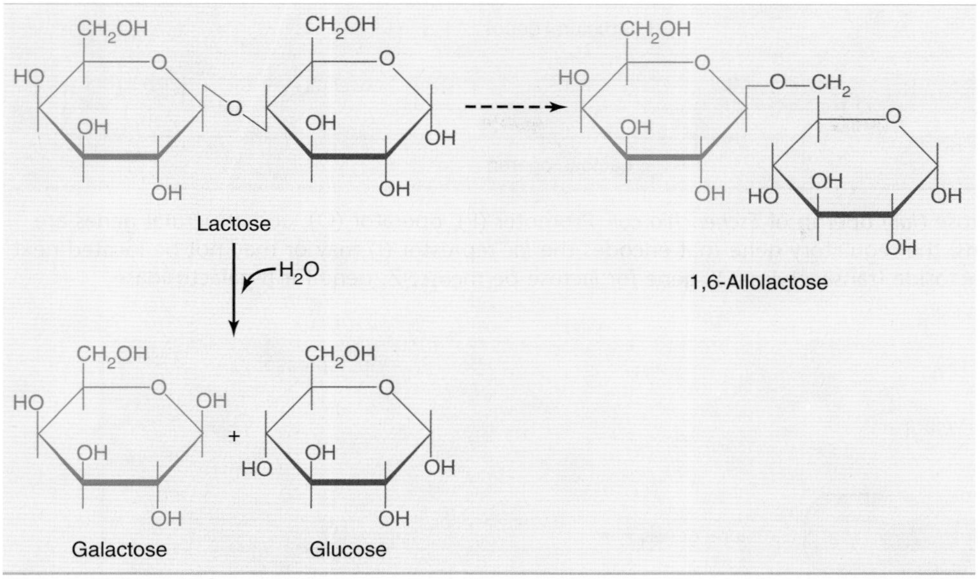

Figure 6.31 The β-galactosidase reaction. A small percentage of the substrate is not hydrolyzed but rather is isomerized to 1,6-allolactose in a minor side reaction.

Also, humans have to adjust their metabolic activity to the supply of nutrients and the need for biosynthetic products. But humans also need regulated gene expression for the formation of specialized cell types. *All cells of the body have the same genes, but different cells make different proteins.* Hemoglobin, for example, is synthesized by erythroid precursor cells in the bone marrow but not by neurons in the cerebral cortex. *Such differences are the result of cell-specific gene expression.*

A Repressor Protein Regulates the Transcription of the *lac* Operon in *Escherichia coli*

E. coli can use the disaccharide lactose (milk sugar) as a source of metabolic energy. Lactose is first transported across the plasma membrane by the membrane carrier **lactose permease,** and then it is cleaved to free glucose and galactose by the enzyme **β-galactosidase** (Fig. 6.31). A third protein, **β-galactoside transacetylase,** is not required for lactose catabolism, but it acetylates several other β-galactosides. It is probably concerned with the removal of nonmetabolizable β-galactosides from the cell.

Being an intestinal bacterium, *E. coli* needs these three proteins only when its host drinks milk. In the absence of lactose, the cell contains only about 10 molecules of β-galactosidase, but several thousand molecules are present when lactose is the only carbon source; the levels of the permease and the transacetylase parallel exactly those of β-galactosidase.

The genes for these three proteins are lined up head-to-tail in the bacterial chromosome. They are regulated in concert because *they are transcribed from a single promoter.* The product of transcription is a **polycistronic mRNA** ("cistron" = gene). The ribosome can synthesize three different polypeptides from this large mRNA because the stop codons of the first two genes are followed by a Shine-Dalgarno sequence and a start codon at which the synthesis of the next polypeptide is initiated.

The array of protein-coding genes, their shared promoter sites, and their associated regulatory sites is called an **operon,** and the protein-coding genes of the operon are called **structural genes.**

Wedged between the three structural genes and their shared promoter is an **operator** (Fig. 6.32), a short regulatory DNA sequence that binds the **lac repressor.** The repressor binding site (operator) overlaps with the binding site for RNA polymerase (promoter). Therefore, *the RNA polymerase cannot bind to the promoter when the* lac *repressor is bound to the operator.*

The *lac* repressor is a tetrameric (Greek τετρα = "four", μεροσ = "part") protein with four identical subunits, encoded by a regulatory gene that is constitutively transcribed at a low rate. This gene is located immediately upstream of the *lac* operon.

In the absence of lactose, the *lac* repressor binds tightly to the operator and prevents the transcription of the structural genes. In the presence of lactose, however, a small amount of 1,6-allolactose is formed. This minor side product of the β-galactosidase reaction (see Fig. 6.31) binds tightly to the *lac* repressor, changing its conformation by an allosteric mechanism. The repressor-allolactose

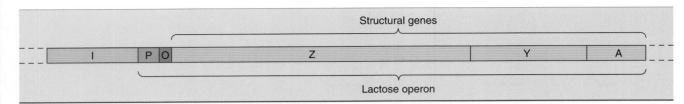

Figure 6.32 Structure of the lactose (*lac*) operon of *Escherichia coli*. Promoter (P), operator (O), and structural genes are contiguous in all bacterial operons; the regulatory gene that encodes the *lac* repressor (I) may or may not be located next to the operon. A, gene for β-galactoside transacetylase; Y, gene for lactose permease; Z, gene for β-galactosidase.

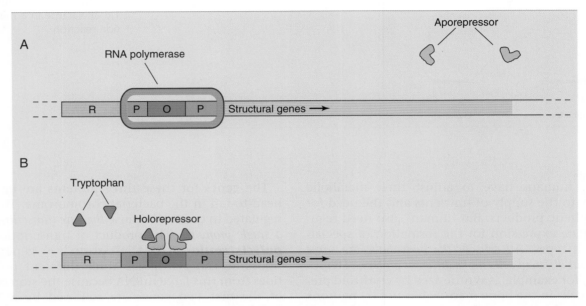

Figure 6.33 Regulation of the tryptophan (*trp*) operon of *Escherichia coli*. **A,** Tryptophan is absent: the aporepressor does not bind to the operator, and the structural genes are transcribed. **B,** Tryptophan is abundant: the "holorepressor" (aporepressor + tryptophan) binds to the operator. The binding of RNA polymerase is prevented, and the structural genes are not transcribed. P, Promoter; O, operator; R, regulatory gene.

complex no longer binds to the operator, and the structural genes can be transcribed. Thus 1,6-allolactose functions as an **inducer** of the *lac* operon.

Anabolic Operons Are Repressed by the End Product of the Pathway

The tryptophan (*trp*) operon of *E. coli* codes for a set of five enzymes that are required for the synthesis of tryptophan. Thus, the bacteria can synthesize their own tryptophan, but *this energetically expensive biosynthetic pathway is required only when external tryptophan is not available.*

The repressor of the *trp* operon is a dimeric protein that binds to an operator site in the middle of the promoter, about 20 to 30 nucleotides upstream of the transcriptional start site. It thereby prevents the binding of RNA polymerase (Fig. 6.33).

Unlike the *lac* repressor, the *trp* repressor cannot bind its operator without outside help. *It is an allosteric protein that becomes an active repressor only when it binds tryptophan.* Therefore, the *trp* operon

is repressed when tryptophan is abundant. In this system, the repressor protein is called an **aporepressor,** and tryptophan is called a **corepressor.** This regulatory strategy is typical for biosynthetic operons.

Glucose Regulates the Transcription of Many Catabolic Operons

When given the choice between glucose and lactose, *E. coli* metabolizes glucose first. The levels of β-galactosidase and the other products of the *lac* operon are very low as long as both sugars are present in the medium, and *the enzymes of lactose metabolism are induced only when glucose is depleted* (Fig. 6.34).

Glucose is the favored tasty treat of bacteria because it is more easily metabolized than is lactose. The thrifty (or lazy) bacterium saves the expense for the synthesis of lactose-metabolizing enzymes by metabolizing glucose first. Not only the *lac* operon but also many other catabolic operons are repressed in the presence of glucose. This is called **catabolite repression.**

Catabolite repression is mediated by **cyclic AMP** (**cAMP**). This small molecule serves as a second messenger of hormone action in humans (see Chapter 17), but in bacteria it is regulated by glucose. *The intracellular cAMP level is low when glucose is plentiful and high when it is scarce.*

When glucose is depleted and cAMP abundant, cAMP binds to the dimeric **catabolite activator protein** (**CAP**). CAP alone does not bind to regulatory DNA sites, but *the CAP-cAMP complex binds at the promoters of many catabolic operons,* including the *lac* operon (Figs. 6.35 and 6.36A). The DNA-bound CAP-cAMP complex provides additional sites of interaction for RNA polymerase, thereby facilitating its binding to the promoter and the initiation of transcription.

Transcriptional Regulation Depends on DNA-Binding Proteins

The *lac* operon and the *trp* operon illustrate the important features of transcriptional regulation:

1. *Gene expression is most commonly regulated at the level of transcription.* Regulation of mRNA processing and translation also occur, especially in eukaryotes, but transcriptional regulation is of prime importance.

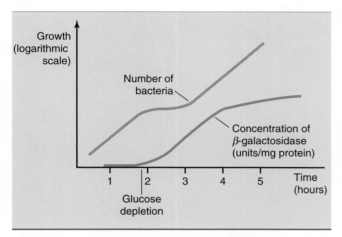

Figure 6.34 Growth of *Escherichia coli* bacteria on a mixture of glucose and lactose.

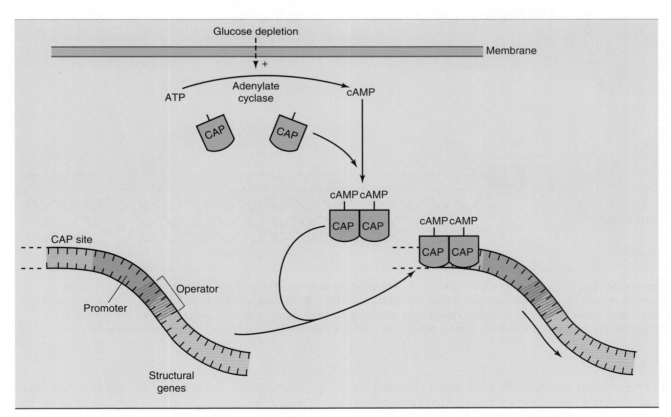

Figure 6.35 The mechanism of catabolite repression. The promoter of the *lac* operon is intrinsically weak and permits a high rate of transcription only when the complex of catabolite activator protein (CAP) and cyclic AMP (cAMP) is bound to the DNA of the promoter. The cAMP level is low in the presence of glucose but rises in the absence of glucose when the cAMP-forming enzyme adenylate cyclase is activated. The CAP binds the promoter only when it is complexed with cAMP. ATP, adenosine triphosphate.

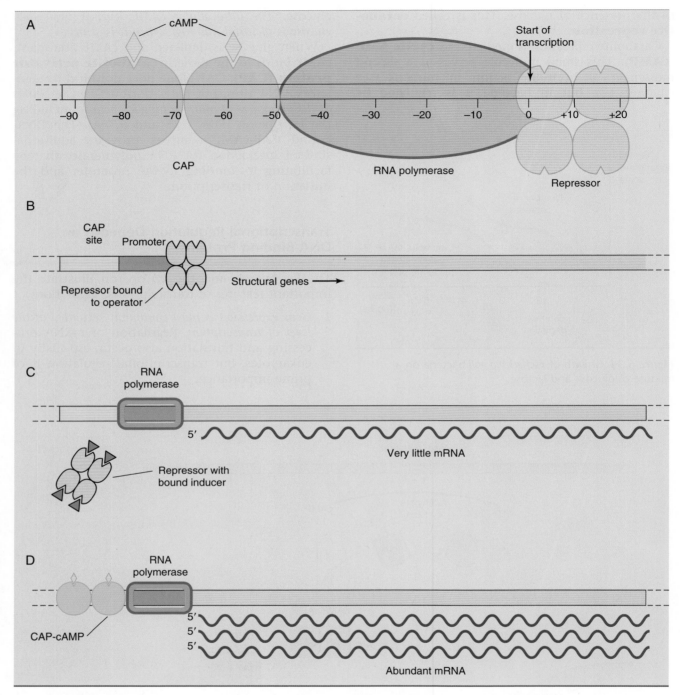

Figure 6.36 Regulation of the lactose operon. **A,** The binding sites for RNA polymerase, repressor, and catabolite activator protein (CAP)–cyclic adenosine monophosphate (cAMP). **B,** Lactose absent, glucose present: RNA polymerase cannot start transcription. **C,** Lactose present, glucose present: weak binding of RNA polymerase to the promoter. **D,** Lactose present, glucose absent: strong binding of RNA polymerase to the promoter; high rate of transcription.

2. *Prokaryotes coordinate the transcription of functionally related genes by arranging them in operons.* Eukaryotes, however, do not use this strategy. They work with monocistronic mRNAs, and functionally related genes need not be close together in the genome.

3. *Transcription is controlled by proteins that bind to regulatory DNA sequences in the vicinity of the transcriptional start site.* The proteins can recognize these sites because the edges of the DNA bases are exposed in the major and minor grooves of the double helix.

4. *Many transcriptional activators and repressors are allosterically controlled by small molecules such as 1,6-allolactose, cAMP, or tryptophan.* However, other control mechanisms are possible. These include interactions with other regulatory proteins and covalent modification by protein phosphorylation.

5. *DNA-binding gene regulator proteins act either as activators or repressors.* This action is called **positive control** or **negative control** of transcription, respectively. The stimulation of transcription by CAP-cAMP is an example of positive control, and the actions of the *lac* repressor and the *trp* repressor are examples of negative control.

6. *Many transcriptional regulators are either dimers (CAP,* trp *repressor) or larger oligomers (*lac *repressor) with identical or slightly different subunits.* Their structures are therefore symmetrical. The symmetry of the proteins is reflected in the DNA sequences to which they bind, which are in many cases palindromic (Fig. 6.37). The oligomeric nature of the gene regulators facilitates allosteric changes in their conformation, and their responses to effector molecules can be accentuated by positive cooperativity.

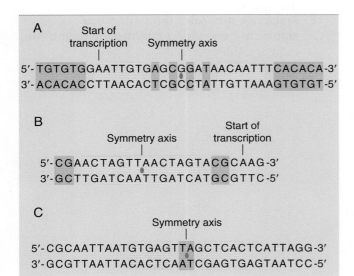

Figure 6.37 Incomplete palindromic sequences in the binding sites of transcriptional regulator proteins. Most transcriptional regulators bind their cognate DNA sites in a dimeric form, each subunit interacting with one leg of the palindrome left and right of the symmetry axis. **A,** The *lac* operator. **B,** The *trp* operator. **C,** The CAP-cAMP binding site of the *lac* operon. A, adenine; C, cytosine; G, guanine; T, thymine.

SUMMARY

DNA as it occurs in cells is a large double-stranded molecule with a length of several million nucleotides. It contains the four bases adenine (A), guanine (G), cytosine (C), and thymine (T), bound to a backbone of 2-deoxyribose and phosphate. Bases in opposite strands interact, forming A-T base pairs and G-C base pairs. Therefore, the base sequence of one strand predicts the base sequence of the opposite strand.

For replication, the parental DNA double helix is unwound and new complementary strands are synthesized; one of the old strands is always used as a template. The new strands are synthesized by DNA polymerases, with deoxyribonucleoside triphosphates as precursors.

For gene expression, DNA is copied into RNA by RNA polymerase. This process is called transcription. The gene is defined as the length of DNA that codes for a polypeptide or for a functional RNA in cases in which the RNA is not translated into protein (e.g., rRNA and tRNA). The RNA transcript of a protein-coding gene is called a messenger RNA (mRNA).

The correspondence between the base sequence of the mRNA and the amino acid sequence of the encoded polypeptide is called the genetic code. The amino acids are specified by base triplets called codons. There are 61 amino acid coding codons and three stop codons. The amino acid coding codons are recognized by tRNAs during protein synthesis, and each tRNA presents the appropriate amino acid to the ribosome. During protein synthesis, the ribosome moves along the mRNA in the 5'→3' direction while polymerizing the polypeptide in the amino→carboxyl terminal direction.

Genes contain regulatory DNA sequences near the transcriptional start site that bind regulatory proteins. The enhancement of transcription by a DNA-binding protein is called positive control, and the inhibition of transcription is called negative control.

📖 Further Reading

Benkovic SJ, Valentine AM, Salinas F: Replisome-mediated DNA replication. Annu Rev Biochem 70:181-208, 2001.

QUESTIONS

1. The base triplet 5′-GAT-3′ on the template strand of DNA is transcribed into mRNA. The anticodon that recognizes this sequence during translation is

   A. 5′-GAT-3′.
   B. 5′-GAU-3′.
   C. 5′-UAG-3′.
   D. 5′-AUC-3′.
   E. 5′-ATC-3′.

2. The high fidelity of DNA replication in *E. coli* would not be possible without

   A. The high processivity of DNA polymerase III.
   B. The s subunit of DNA polymerase I.
   C. The 5′-exonuclease activity of DNA polymerase I.
   D. The 3′-exonuclease activity of DNA polymerase III.
   E. The extremely high accuracy of the aminoacyl-tRNA synthetases.

3. Stop codons are present on

   A. The coding strand of DNA, where they signal the end of transcription.
   B. The template strand of DNA, where they signal the end of transcription.
   C. The mRNA, where they signal the end of translation.
   D. The tRNA, where they signal the end of translation.
   E. Termination factors, where they signal the end of translation.

4. As a result of a mutation, an *E. coli* cell produces an aberrant aminoacyl-tRNA synthetase that attaches not leucine but isoleucine to one of the leucine-tRNAs. This kind of mutation would lead to

   A. A disruption of codon-anticodon pairing during protein synthesis.
   B. Premature chain termination during ribosomal protein synthesis.
   C. Impaired initiation of ribosomal protein synthesis.
   D. Inability of the aminoacyl-tRNA to bind to the ribosome.
   E. A change in the genetic code.

5. Like lactose, the pentose sugar arabinose can be used as a source of metabolic energy by *E. coli*. The most reasonable prediction for the regulation of the arabinose-catabolizing enzymes would be that

   A. Enzymes of arabinose catabolism are induced when glucose is plentiful.
   B. A repressor protein prevents the synthesis of arabinose-catabolizing enzymes in the absence of arabinose.
   C. The catabolite activator protein prevents the synthesis of arabinose-catabolizing enzymes in the absence of arabinose.
   D. Arabinose acts as a corepressor that is required for the binding of the repressor to the operator.
   E. Arabinose stimulates the synthesis of arabinose-catabolizing enzymes by raising the cellular cAMP level.

CHAPTER 7

Viruses

There are three essential attributes of life: a membrane that physically separates the living cell from its environment; the generation and utilization of metabolic energy; and reproduction.

Viruses have dispensed with cell structure and metabolism, but they reproduce, and they use a nucleic acid as their genetic databank. However, being unable to hold the proteins and substrates for its replication together in a cellular structure, and unable to generate metabolic energy, the viral nucleic acid depends on a host cell for its replication. Thus, viruses are villains not by choice but by necessity.

All viruses are obligatory intracellular parasites. They do nothing useful for the organism that harbors them, and the physician encounters them only as the causes of viral diseases. Because they are very simple and depend heavily on normal host cell functions for their replication, they offer few targets for the development of chemotherapeutic drugs. This chapter introduces the life cycles of the major types of viruses.

Viruses Can Replicate Only in a Host Cell

Outside its host cell, the virus exists as an inert particle, the **virion:** a package of nucleic acid wrapped in a protective protein coat. *The viral genome can be formed from any kind of nucleic acid:* double-stranded DNA, single-stranded DNA, single-stranded RNA, or double-stranded RNA. Viruses are genetic paupers, with anywhere between 3 and 250 genes, in comparison with 4300 genes in *Escherichia coli* and 25,000 to 30,000 in humans.

The viral nucleic acid is wrapped into a protective protein coat, or **capsid.** The virus can encode only a small number of structural proteins, and therefore capsids are formed from a few proteins that poly-merize into a regular, crystalline structure. The protein coat protects the nucleic acid from physical insults and enzymatic attack, and it is required to recognize and invade the host cell.

Many animal viruses are enclosed by an **envelope:** a piece of host cell membrane appropriated by the virus while budding out of its host cell. The envelope is studded with viral proteins, the **spike proteins** (Fig. 7.1).

The viral nucleic acid can be replicated only in the host cell, and host cell ribosomes are required for the synthesis of the viral proteins. Some of these proteins are enzymes for viral replication, whereas others form the capsid or appear as spike proteins in the viral envelope.

Bacteriophage T$_4$ Destroys Its Host Cell

Viruses that infect bacteria are called **bacterio-phages** ("bacteria-eaters"), and bacteriophage T$_4$ is a classical example.

T$_4$ is one of the most complex viruses known (Fig. 7.2). Its DNA genome with about 150 genes is tightly packed into the head portion of the virus particle. Attached to the head is a short neck followed by a cylindrical tail with two coaxial hollow tubes, a base plate, and six spidery tail fibers. These structures are built from about 40 virus-encoded polypeptides, each present in many copies.

T$_4$ is constructed like a syringe that injects its DNA into the host cell. First, the tail fibers bind to a **virus receptor** on the surface of a prospective victim. The virus receptor is a normal component of the bacterial cell wall, and only the bacterial strains that carry it can be infected. Next, the sheath of the tail contracts, its inner core penetrates the cell wall, and the viral DNA is injected into the cell. Only the DNA enters the host cell, and the protein coat remains outside (Fig. 7.3).

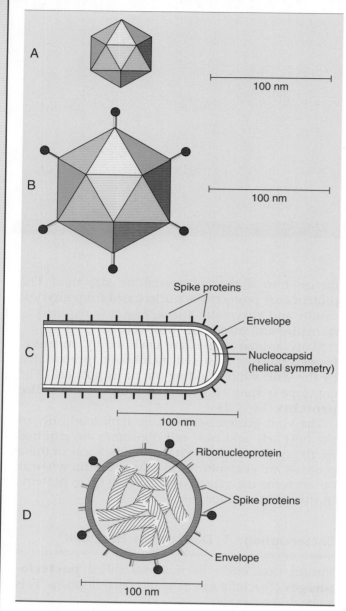

Figure 7.1 Sizes and structures of some typical viruses. **A,** Papilloma (wart) virus: a nonenveloped DNA virus of icosahedral shape (spherical symmetry). **B,** Adenovirus: another nonenveloped DNA virus. **C,** Rabies virus: an enveloped RNA virus. **D,** Influenza virus: an enveloped RNA virus containing eight segments of ribonucleoprotein with helical symmetry.

Some viral genes are transcribed immediately by the bacterial RNA polymerase. One of these "immediate-early" genes encodes a DNase that degrades the host cell chromosome. The viral DNA is not attacked by this DNase because it contains hydroxymethyl cytosine instead of cytosine.

During the later stages of the infection, viral proteins substitute for the σ subunit of bacterial RNA polymerase and direct the transcription of the

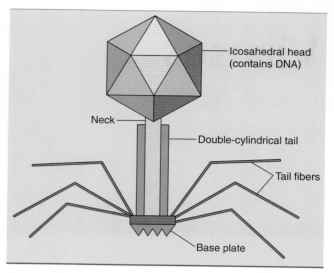

Figure 7.2 Structure of bacteriophage T_4, one of the most complex DNA viruses known. Its capsid consists of approximately 40 different proteins.

"delayed-early" and "late" viral genes. The promoters of these genes are not recognized by the bacterial σ subunit.

The early viral proteins include enzymes for nucleotide synthesis, DNA replication, and DNA modification. The late proteins include the viral coat proteins. At this time, *new virus particles are assembled from the replicated viral DNA and the newly synthesized coat proteins.* Finally, at the end of the infectious cycle, virus-encoded phospholipase and lysozyme destroy the bacterial plasma membrane and cell wall.

This mode of virus replication is called the **lytic pathway** because it ends with the lysis (destruction) of the host cell. It takes approximately 20 minutes, and about 200 progeny viruses are released from the lysed host cell.

DNA Viruses Substitute Their Own DNA for the Host Cell DNA

Some but not all features of lytic infection by bacteriophage T_4 are typical for viral infections in general:

1. *Infection is initiated by specific binding of the virus to the surface of its host cell.* A viral protein in the capsid or the envelope has to bind selectively to a cellular surface component on the host cell that serves as a "virus receptor." Only cells that possess the virus receptor can be infected. The human body can combat viral infections with antibodies that coat the viral surface proteins.

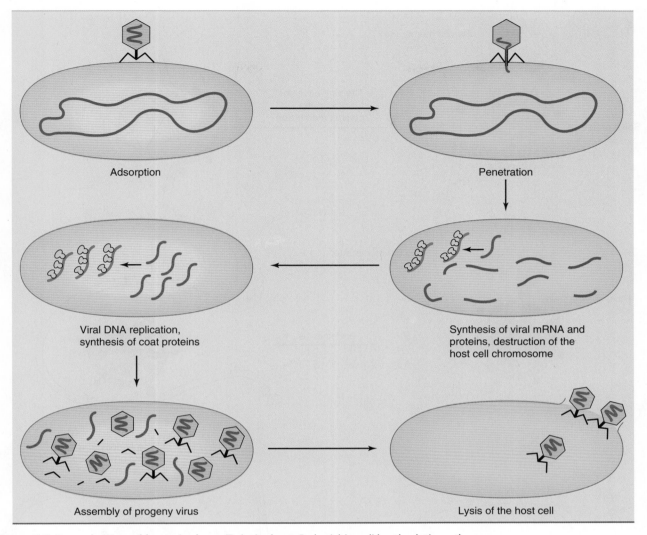

Figure 7.3 Reproduction of bacteriophage T$_4$ in its host *Escherichia coli* by the lytic pathway.

2. *Many bacteriophages inject their nucleic acid into the host cell.* Animal and human viruses use different strategies. Some enveloped viruses fuse their envelope with the plasma membrane of the host cell, whereas others trigger their own endocytosis (Fig. 7.4).

3. *All viruses abuse the host cell ribosomes for the synthesis of their proteins.* DNA replication and transcription of the smaller viruses depend heavily on host cell enzymes but larger viruses, including T$_4$, synthesize many of the required enzymes themselves.

4. *The viruses of eukaryotes replicate either in the nucleus or the cytoplasm.* Most DNA viruses replicate in the nucleus, where they can take advantage of the host's DNA and RNA polymerases, but most RNA viruses replicate in the cytoplasm.

5. *Many viruses inhibit vital processes of the host cell,* but T$_4$'s barbaric practice of cutting the host's

DNA to pieces is not common among animal viruses.

6. *Bacteriophages kill their victims, but virus-infected human cells often survive.* In most viral infections of animal or human cells, virus particles are shed continuously by the infected cell.

λ Phage Can Integrate Its DNA into the Host Cell Chromosome

Like T$_4$ phage, λ phage is constructed as a syringe that injects its DNA into the host cell. Its genome, with about 50 genes, is a linear double-stranded DNA molecule (48,502 base pairs) with single-stranded ends of 12 nucleotides each. These single-stranded overhangs have complementary base sequences (Fig. 7.5). After entering the host cell, the

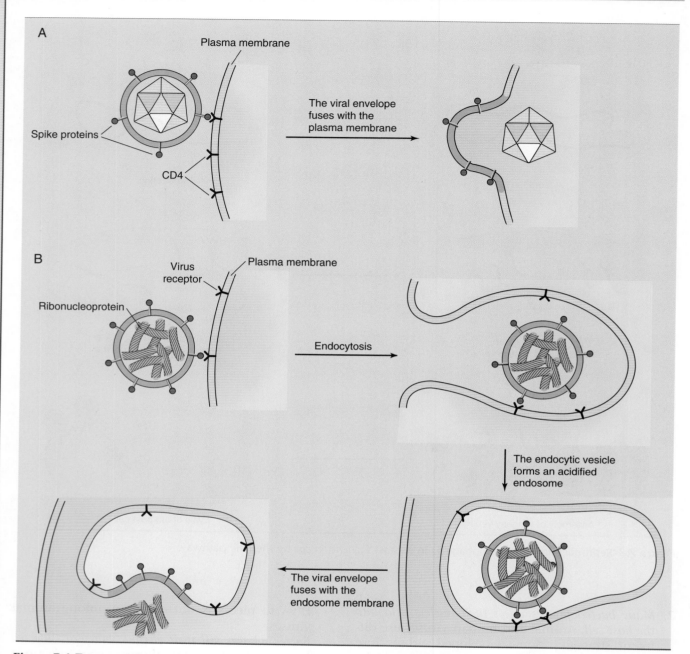

Figure 7.4 Two strategies for the uptake of an enveloped virus into its host cell. An initial noncovalent binding between a viral spike protein and the host cell membrane is essential in both cases. **A,** Uptake of human immunodeficiency virus (a retrovirus) is triggered by binding to the membrane glycoprotein CD4. The uptake of the nucleocapsid into the cytoplasm does not depend on endocytosis but is effected by direct fusion of the viral envelope with the plasma membrane. Only CD4-positive cells can be infected by this virus. **B,** Uptake of influenza virus, an enveloped RNA virus. Endocytosis is triggered by binding of the virus to the cell surface. The fusion of the viral envelope with the membrane of the endosome is facilitated by the low pH (<5.0) of this organelle.

single-stranded ends anneal (base-pair), and the viral DNA is linked into a circle by a bacterial DNA ligase. Lytic infection can now proceed as described previously for T_4 phage.

Unlike T_4, however, λ phage can also pursue an alternative lifestyle: Rather than destroying its host cell by brute force, it can integrate itself into a specific site of the host cell chromosome, between the galactose and biotin operons. *The viral DNA is now part of the host cell chromosome,* and it is replicated during each cycle of cell division. This mode of virus replication is called the **lysogenic pathway** (Fig. 7.6). The integrated virus DNA is called a **prophage,** and the bacterium is characterized as **lysogenic.**

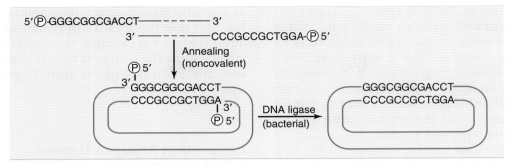

Figure 7.5 Circularization of λ phage DNA. This event takes place immediately after the entry of the viral DNA into the host cell and does not require virally encoded proteins. The circular DNA is then either replicated in the lytic pathway or integrated into the bacterial chromosome.

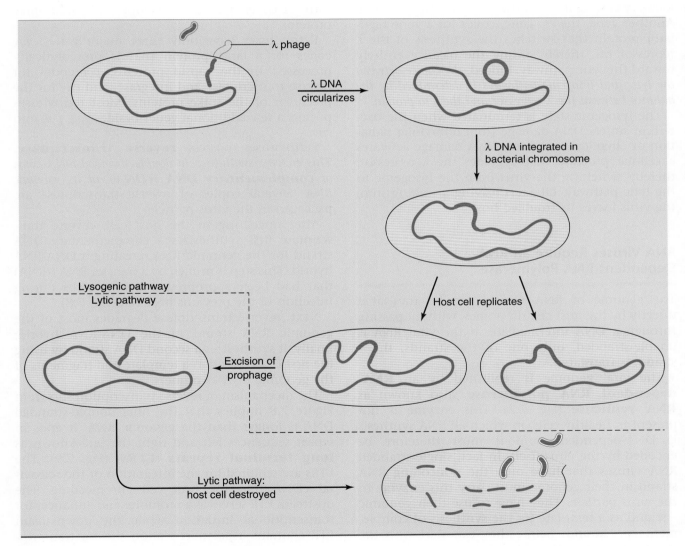

Figure 7.6 The lysogenic pathway of λ phage.

The integration of the viral DNA requires a virus-encoded **integrase.** Another viral gene, which becomes activated under the same conditions as the integrase gene, codes for the λ **repressor.** *The λ repressor maintains the lysogenic state by preventing the transcription of all phage genes except its own.* It even makes the lysogenic bacterium resistant to reinfection by λ phage because the genes of any incoming λ phage become repressed as well.

The lysogenic state can be maintained for hundreds or thousands of cell generations, but the viral genes, although dormant in the prophage, can be reactivated. *Whenever the concentration of the λ repressor falls below a critical limit, the genes of the lytic pathway become derepressed.*

One of the derepressed genes, the *xis* gene, codes for an excisionase. This enzyme turns the prophage loose by cutting it out of the bacterial chromosome. Another gene, the *cro* gene, codes for a gene regulator protein that switches the synthesis of the λ repressor off, thereby tilting the balance entirely toward the lytic pathway. Indeed, *the choice between the lytic and lysogenic pathways is determined by the balance between the λ repressor and the Cro protein.*

The lysogenic state is terminated when the bacterium suffers DNA damage from ultraviolet radiation or chemical mutagens. DNA damage activates a cellular protease that degrades the λ repressor, thereby switching the virus from the lysogenic to the lytic pathway. Like rats leaving a sinking ship, the virus leaves its troubled host.

RNA Viruses Require an RNA-Dependent RNA Polymerase

The genome of RNA viruses can be translated directly by the host cell ribosomes, without passing through a DNA intermediate. If the viral RNA is double-stranded, only one of the strands, the + strand, is translated.

The viral genome is replicated by an **RNA-dependent RNA polymerase,** also known as **RNA replicase** (Fig. 7.7). This enzyme is not present in healthy cells, in which all RNA synthesis is DNA-dependent, and it must therefore be encoded by the virus itself. In fact, single-stranded RNA viruses that have only the noncoding RNA strand in their genome must carry this enzyme in the virus particle. They have to use their genomic – strand as a template for the synthesis of complementary + strands before they can start with the synthesis of the viral proteins.

The viral RNA replicases have no proofreading 3′-exonuclease activity, and their error rate is about one in every 10,000 nucleotides. Therefore, *RNA viruses have high mutation rates,* and they can elude the host defenses by inventing new antigenic variants very fast. For example, the development of vaccines against the common cold is hampered by the high mutation rate of the rhinoviruses that cause this illness.

Retroviruses Replicate through a DNA Intermediate

The retroviruses are a rather uniform group of viruses infecting eukaryotic hosts. Their genome consists of two identical copies of a positive RNA strand, about 10,000 nucleotides long, which is enclosed by an icosahedral capsid. The capsid, in turn, is covered by an envelope with viral spike proteins.

Retroviruses have only three major genes: *gag* codes for a large protein that is proteolytically processed to the capsid proteins, *pol* codes for reverse transcriptase and integrase, and *env* for the precursor of the spike proteins. Most retroviruses possess a few additional genes besides *gag*, *pol*, and *env*.

Retroviruses possess **reverse transcriptase.** *This enzyme synthesizes a double-stranded DNA copy, or* **complementary DNA (cDNA),** *of its genomic RNA.* Several copies of reverse transcriptase are packaged in the virus particle.

After uncoating in the host cell, reverse transcriptase first synthesizes a complementary DNA strand for the genomic RNA, creating a DNA-RNA hybrid. This step is primed by a transfer RNA (tRNA) that had been appropriated by the virus during infection of the previous host cell (Fig. 7.8).

Next, reverse transcriptase degrades most of the genomic RNA strand in the DNA-RNA hybrid; finally, it synthesizes a second DNA strand by using the first DNA strand as a template and fragments of the genomic RNA as primers.

The mechanism of reverse transcription shown in Figure 7.8 implies that the final double-stranded DNA is longer than the genomic RNA. It ends in repeat sequences left and right that are known as **long terminal repeats** (**LTRs**) (Fig. 7.9). The LTRs are required for the integration of the retroviral cDNA into the host cell chromosome. The upstream LTR serves as a promoter and enhancer for transcriptional initiation while the downstream LTR contains a polyadenylation site for transcriptional termination (see Chapter 8).

Like the RNA replicases, reverse transcriptases do not proofread their product. Thus, *retroviruses have high mutation rates.* This makes them fast-moving

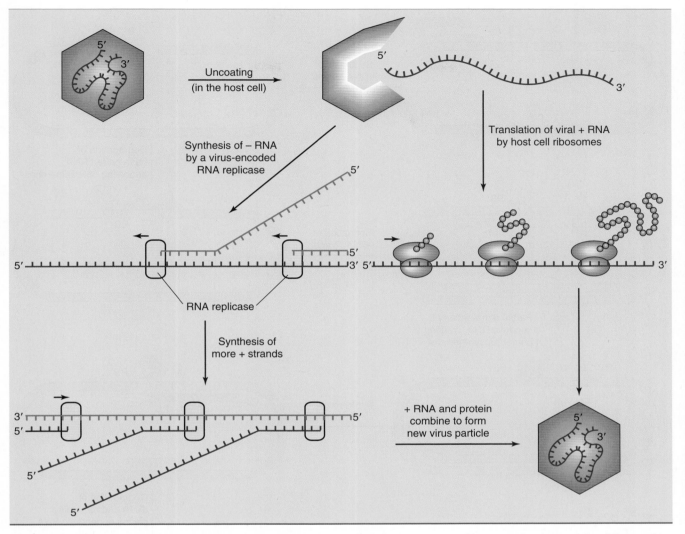

Figure 7.7 The replicative cycle of a positive (+)–stranded animal RNA virus. ⌐⌐, positive strand; ⌐⌐, negative (–) strand.

targets for the immune system and also for scientists who try to develop vaccines for retroviral diseases such as acquired immunodeficiency syndrome (AIDS). An AIDS vaccine is still not in sight because of the high mutation rate of the retroviral *env* gene. The human AIDS virus evolved from a related chimpanzee virus very recently, sometime during the 20th century. This "instant evolution" was possible because of the short generation time of the virus, its high mutation rate, and changed selection pressures in the new host species.

With the help of a virus-encoded **integrase,** *the cDNA produced by the reverse transcriptase becomes integrated into the host cell DNA as a* **DNA provirus.** The integrase makes staggered cuts in the chromosomal DNA. As a result, four to six base pairs of chromosomal DNA become duplicated and form short **direct repeats** that flank the retroviral insertion site.

The viral genes are transcribed by a host cell RNA polymerase only after their integration into the host cell genome. The RNA transcript is translated by the host cell ribosomes. It can also be packaged into virus particles to form the genomic virus RNA of the next generation (Fig. 7.10).

In most retroviral infections the cell survives but produces virus particles for the rest of its lifetime. Only the AIDS retrovirus kills its host. The body's main defense against retroviruses, as against other viral infections, is the destruction of the infected cells by T lymphocytes. The immune system can recognize virus-infected cells because they display viral spike proteins on their surface (see Fig. 7.10).

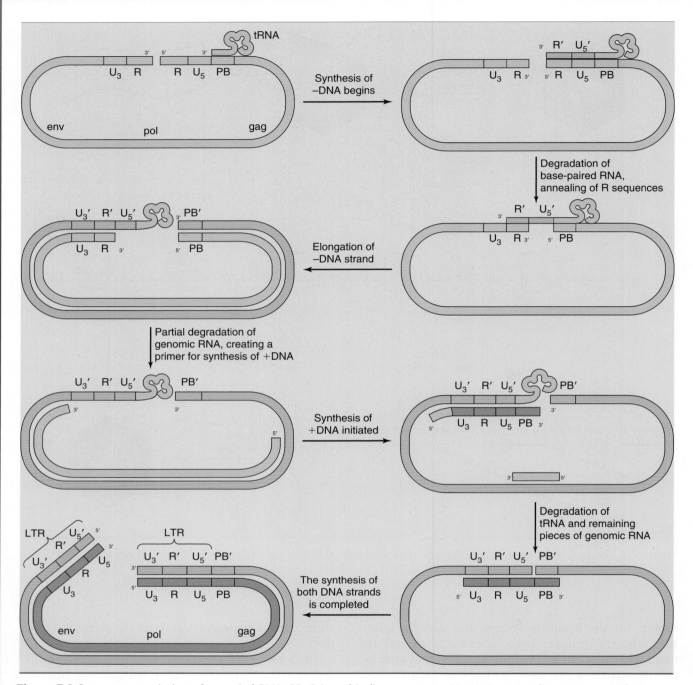

Figure 7.8 Reverse transcription of retroviral RNA. PB, Primer-binding sequence; U₃, U, R, noncoding sequences that become the long terminal repeats (LTR). ◻, RNA; ◼, negative (−) DNA strand; ◼, positive (+) DNA strand.

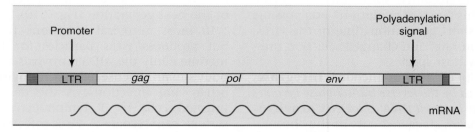

Figure 7.9 The structure of integrated retroviral complementary DNA (cDNA). After integration into the host cell genome, all three genes are transcribed into a single mRNA. *gag, pol,* and *env* are the structural genes of the virus. LTR, long terminal repeat; ◼, direct repeats (target site duplications).

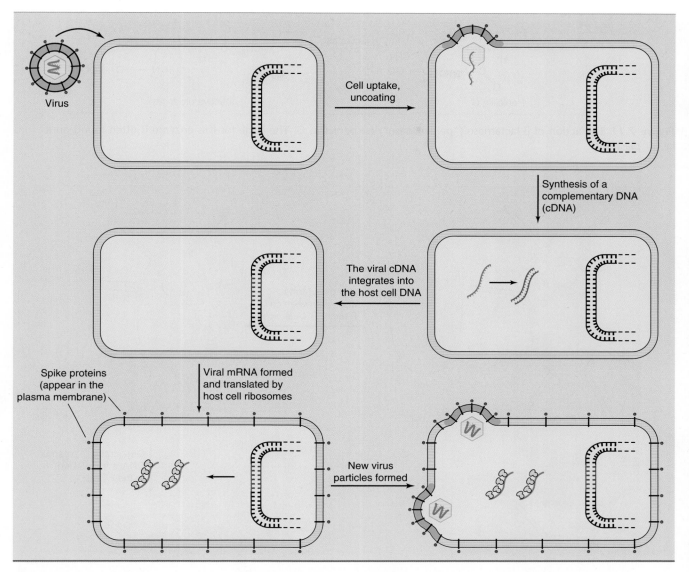

Figure 7.10 The life cycle of a retrovirus. The viral reverse transcriptase converts the viral RNA *(green)* into a double-stranded DNA *(red)*, which becomes integrated into the host cell genome. mRNA, messenger RNA.

Plasmids Are Small "Accessory Chromosomes" or "Symbiotic Viruses" of Bacteria

Plasmids are small circles of double-stranded DNA with between 2000 and 200,000 base pairs, found in prokaryotes and some lower eukaryotes. Their replication is controlled by plasmid genes that maintain an adequate copy number of the plasmid throughout the cell generations.

Most plasmids carry additional genes, but in contrast to the chromosomal genes, *the plasmid genes are dispensable in most situations.* Toxin production, antibiotic resistance, the ability to degrade unusual metabolic substrates, and genetic recombination are some typical abilities conferred by plasmids.

R factor plasmids (R = resistance) are especially important because they carry genes for antibiotic resistance. Most of the resistance genes encode drug-inactivating enzymes. Penicillin, for example, is degraded by a plasmid-encoded **β-lactamase,** also known as **penicillinase** (Fig. 7.11). R factor containing bacteria have been selected by the widespread use of antibiotics and are now a major problem for the treatment of many bacterial infections.

Some Plasmids Are Transmissible

Some of the larger plasmids are infectious. A classical example is the **F factor** (F = fertility) of *E. coli,*

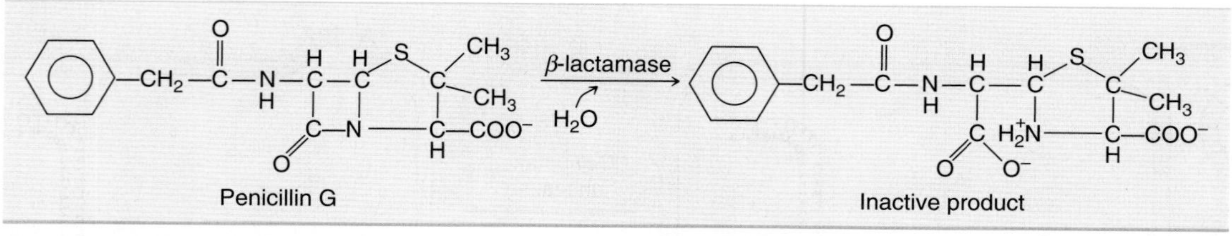

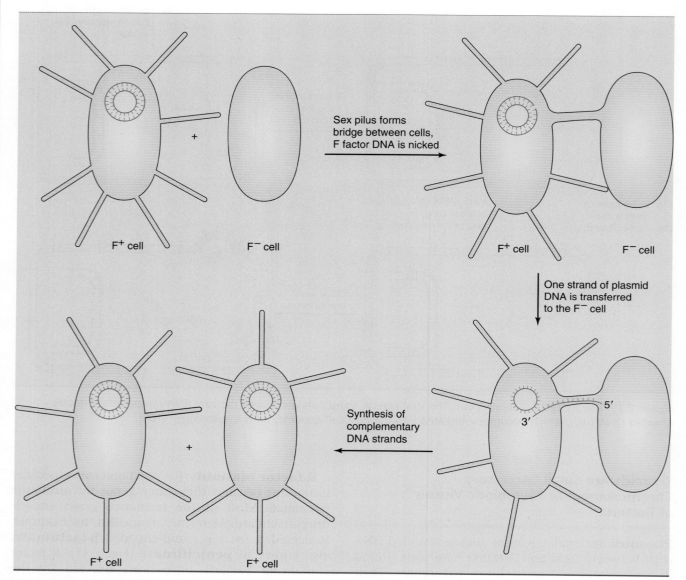

Figure 7.11 The action of β-lactamase ("penicillinase") on penicillin G. The gene for this enzyme is often found on R factor plasmids.

Figure 7.12 Cell-to-cell transfer of the F factor during conjugation in *Escherichia coli*.

a large plasmid with 94,500 base pairs. The F factor carries a set of about a dozen genes that control the formation of sex pili, hairlike processes protruding from the cell surface in all directions.

Once an F factor–bearing cell (F⁺ cell) encounters a cell without F factor (F⁻ cell), a delicate bridge is formed between the cells by one of the sex pili. At this point, one strand of the plasmid DNA is nicked, the double helix unravels, and one of the strands worms its way into the F⁻ cell (Fig. 7.12). This is followed by the synthesis of a new complementary DNA strand both in the F⁺ cell and

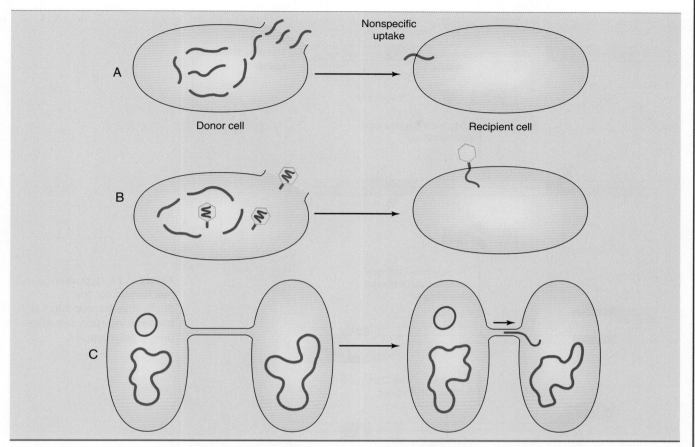

Figure 7.13 Transfer of DNA between bacterial cells. The three mechanisms of DNA transfer shown here are collectively known as "parasexual" processes. **A**, Transformation. **B**, Transduction. **C**, Conjugation.

the ex–F⁻ cell. This type of DNA transfer is called **conjugation.**

The F factor behaves as an infectious agent that can spread in the bacterial population. It is of no immediate benefit for the host cell, but sometimes it carries bacterial genes from cell to cell. On occasion, the F factor acquires genes from the bacterial chromosome and transfers them into the F⁻ cell along with its own genes. In rare cases, it becomes integrated into the bacterial chromosome and pulls a complete copy of the chromosome into the F⁻ cell during conjugation.

Also, some R factor plasmids are self-transmissible. Therefore, *drug resistance is often transmissible* within a bacterial species and sometimes even between different species.

Bacteria Can Exchange Genes by Transformation and Transduction

Bacteria can acquire new DNA in ways other than by conjugation (Fig. 7.13). In **transformation,** a piece of foreign DNA is taken up by the bacterium and becomes integrated into the chromosome by homologous recombination (see "Genetic Recombination Requires the Cutting and Joining of DNA" covered later in this chapter). Some bacteria have specialized systems for the uptake of foreign DNA. For most, however, including *E. coli,* transformation is an exceedingly rare event in nature. Special treatments are necessary to achieve transformation of these bacteria in the laboratory.

In **transduction,** a bacteriophage carries a fragment of host cell DNA from cell to cell. The host cell DNA is erroneously packaged into a virus particle, and the virus injects bacterial DNA instead of (or in addition to) viral DNA into the next host cell.

Jumping Genes Can Change Their Position in the Genome

Most genes occupy a fixed position on the genomic map, but *some genes can move from one place to*

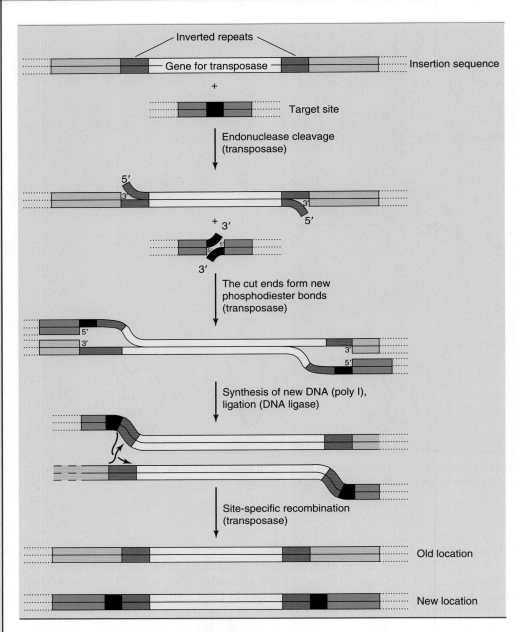

Figure 7.14 Hypothetical mechanism for the duplicative transposition of a bacterial insertion sequence. poly I, polymerase I.

another. The mobile genes of prokaryotes include insertion sequences and transposons.

An **insertion sequence** is a small mobile element, about 1000 base pairs long, that is framed by **inverted repeats** of between 9 and 41 base pairs. Most insertion sequences are present in 5 to 30 copies that are identical or nearly identical, including the inverted repeats at their ends. The inverted repeats are flanked by short (4 to 12 base pairs) direct repeats that differ in different copies of the insertion sequence.

Insertion sequences contain a solitary gene for **transposase,** an enzyme required for transposi-

tion. There are two forms of transposition. In **conservative transposition,** the insertion sequence vacates its old position to settle in a new place. In **duplicative transposition,** in contrast, the insertion sequence replicates. One copy stays in the old location, and the other moves to a new site. A hypothetical mechanism is shown in Figure 7.14.

The transposase recognizes the inverted repeats of its own insertion sequence. It cannot transpose unrelated insertion sequences with different inverted repeats. The direct repeats are target site duplications that arise because the transposase, like the retroviral integrase, makes staggered cuts in the DNA of the

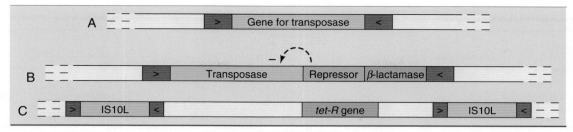

Figure 7.15 Examples of mobile elements in bacteria. **A,** An insertion sequence: a gene for transposase that is flanked by inverted terminal repeat sequences (▪). **B,** Transposon Tn3. Besides the transposase gene, this transposon contains both a gene for a repressor that regulates the expression of the transposase gene and a gene for the penicillin-degrading enzyme β-lactamase. Bacteria carrying this transposon are resistant to penicillin. **C,** Transposon Tn10. This transposon contains a gene for tetracycline resistance (*tet-R* gene). Unlike Tn3, it is not framed by simple inverted repeats but rather by two identical insertion sequences (IS10L), each of them containing a transposase gene.

target site. Transposition is a rare event, occurring perhaps once every 100,000 cell generations.

Insertion sequences are of no obvious advantage to the cell, and they can cause crippling mutations when they jump into an important gene. Therefore, they are often considered **selfish DNA:** molecular parasites that promote only their own survival.

Like insertion sequences, **transposons** are flanked by inverted repeats and contain a gene for transposase. Unlike insertion sequences, however, *transposons also contain useful genes* such as antibiotic resistance genes. In **composite transposons,** the useful genes are flanked not by simple inverted repeats but by insertion sequences (Fig. 7.15). Indeed, *any gene that becomes framed by two insertion sequences becomes transposable.*

Transposons can jump back and forth among the bacterial chromosome, plasmids, and bacteriophages. Self-transmissible plasmids can spread them from cell to cell by conjugation, and bacteriophages can spread them by transduction. Transposons are more than "selfish DNA": They offer the services of useful genes to their host cell.

Genetic Recombination Requires the Cutting and Joining of DNA

Nature is a savvy genetic engineer, cutting and joining DNA molecules to create new gene combinations. This is achieved with two types of genetic recombination.

Site-specific recombination depends on specific sequences on one or on both DNA molecules. For example, the integrase of λ phage recognizes both the phage DNA and the target site on the bacterial chromosome; the retroviral integrase is specific for the long terminal repeats of the retroviral

cDNA; and transposase recognizes the inverted terminal repeats of its transposon.

General recombination, also known as **homologous recombination,** requires no specific DNA sequence, but *it depends on sequence identity or similarity between the recombining molecules.* Therefore, foreign DNA that is acquired by transformation, transduction, or conjugation can be integrated into the bacterial chromosome, but only if it is similar to the chromosomal DNA. *Eukaryotes use homologous recombination during prophase of meiosis I to exchange DNA between homologous chromosomes.* Thus, the chromosomes in human gametes are patchworks of maternally derived genes and paternally derived genes.

The molecular mechanism of homologous recombination is best known for *E. coli* (Fig. 7.16). In this system, a complex of the recB, recC, and recD proteins acts as an endonuclease and helicase to generate single-stranded DNA. The single-stranded DNA then invades a DNA duplex, catalyzed by the recA protein. This occurs only when the base sequence of the invaded double strand is similar or identical to the base sequence of the invading single strand.

After a second strand break and the crosswise joining of the loose ends by DNA ligase, a cross-shaped intermediate called the **Holliday intermediate** (named after Robin Holliday, who proposed this structure in 1964) is formed. This intermediate is resolved by the successive action of an endonuclease (ruvC in *E. coli*) and DNA ligase.

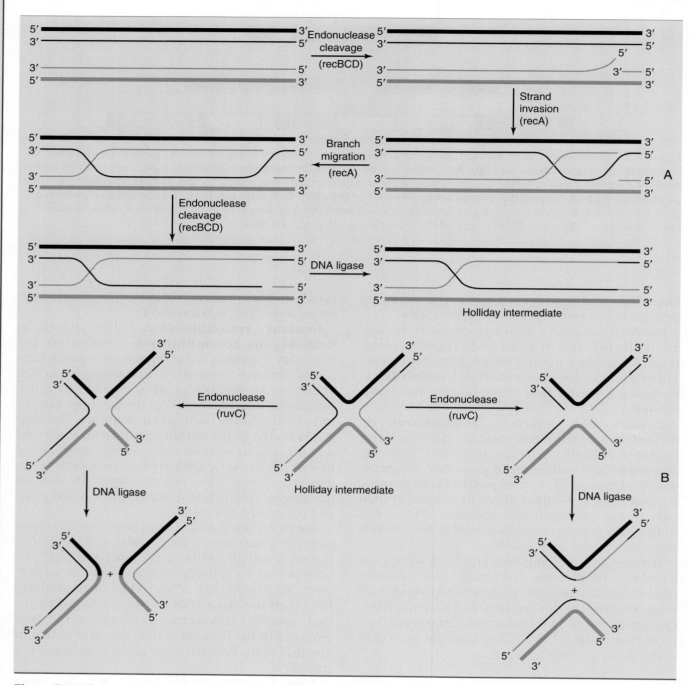

Figure 7.16 The hypothetical mechanism of homologous recombination. This type of recombination results in a reciprocal exchange between two duplex DNA molecules. The proteins required for recombination (recBCD, recA, ruvC) have been described in *E. coli.* Proteins with equivalent functions are thought to exist in other organisms as well, both prokaryotes and eukaryotes. **A,** Formation of the Holliday intermediate. The Holliday intermediate itself can undergo further branch migration (not shown). **B,** Resolution of the Holliday intermediate.

SUMMARY

Viruses are infectious particles made of nucleic acid and protein. Although they have no cellular structure and no metabolism, they can replicate within a host cell by exploiting the host's enzymes, ribosomes, and metabolic energy.

DNA viruses substitute their own genomic DNA for the host cell DNA, directing the synthesis of viral messenger RNA (mRNA) and viral proteins. RNA viruses substitute their own RNA for the host's mRNA, directing the synthesis of viral proteins without the need for transcription. Retroviruses synthesize a DNA copy of their genomic RNA and integrate it into the host cell genome.

Prokaryotic cells contain many semi-autonomous genetic elements. Plasmids are small circular DNA duplexes that function as accessory chromosomes. Some plasmids are infectious, transmitting themselves from cell to cell by conjugation. Insertion sequences and transposons are "jumping genes" on the bacterial chromosome and on plasmids. Some viruses, plasmids, and mobile elements mediate the exchange of genetic information between cells. This information transfer requires genetic recombination: the joining of two DNA molecules from different sources into a single molecule.

QUESTIONS

1. **In order to infect a new host cell, a virus has to bind specifically to a "virus receptor" on the surface of the host cell. In the case of the AIDS virus (a retrovirus), this initial interaction involves the viral**

   A. Spike proteins.
   B. Reverse transcriptase.
   C. Capsid proteins.
   D. RNA.
   E. Integrase.

2. **The Holliday intermediate is a cruciform structure that appears as an intermediate in**

   A. The integration of phage into the bacterial chromosome.
   B. The integration of a retroviral cDNA into the host cell genome.
   C. Homologous recombination.
   D. The replication of bacteriophage T_4.
   E. The duplicative transposition of a bacterial insertion sequence.

3. **An inhibitor of reverse transcriptase would be useful to**

   A. Prevent λ phage from integrating into the host cell chromosome.
   B. Prevent lytic infection by T_4 bacteriophage.
   C. Inhibit homologous recombination between two DNAs.
   D. Cure rabies, a disease caused by an RNA virus.
   E. Cure AIDS, a disease caused by a retrovirus.

CHAPTER 8

The Human Genome

The principles of DNA replication and gene expression that were described in Chapter 6 apply to all living things on Earth. All cells have genes of double-stranded DNA, replicate their DNA, and express genetic information through an RNA intermediate.

Although the clockwork of life is similar in prokaryotes and eukaryotes, eukaryotes are more complex. Prokaryotes must be mean and lean to ensure fast reproduction. Therefore, they keep their genomes as small as possible and gene expression as simple as possible. These pressures are somewhat relaxed in slow-reproducing eukaryotes.

Humans, for example, have 700 times more DNA than *Escherichia coli,* although they have only seven times more genes (Table 8.1). This disparity comes from the fact that 90% of *E. coli* DNA, but only 1.2% of human DNA, codes for proteins.

Eukaryotes owe their evolutionary success to their great complexity, but complexity comes at a steep price. It requires a larger number of genes and more sophisticated systems for the regulation of gene expression. Metazoan animals have the same genes in every cell of the body, but different genes are expressed in different cell types and at different stages during the development of the organism. This requires control mechanisms of mind-boggling complexity.

Chromatin Consists of DNA and Histones

Prokaryotic DNA is a naked double helix, circular and with a length of about 1 mm. Eukaryotic DNA is linear, has a length of several centimeters, and is tightly packaged with a set of small proteins that are known as histones.

The histones are basic proteins, with numerous positive charges on the side chains of lysine and arginine residues. These positive charges can bind to the negatively charged phosphate groups of the DNA. This means that *the binding of histones to DNA does not depend on the base sequence of the DNA.*

There are only five types of histones in eukaryotic cells (Table 8.2). With the exception of histone H1, whose structure varies in different species and even in different tissues of the same organism, the histones are well conserved throughout the phylogenetic tree. For example, histones H3 and H4 from pea seedlings and calf thymus differ in only four and two amino acid positions, respectively. Presumably, the histones were invented by the very first eukaryotes, perhaps as early as 2 billion years ago, and have served the same essential functions ever since.

Chromatin consists of about 50% DNA and 50% histones. It is conspicuous in histological preparations for its affinity for basic dyes such as hematoxylin and fuchsin. **Euchromatin** has a loose structure, whereas **heterochromatin** is more tightly condensed and deeper staining. *Genes are actively transcribed in euchromatin but are repressed in heterochromatin.*

The Nucleosome Is the Structural Unit of Chromatin

Under the electron microscope, chromatin looks like beads on a string. The "string" is the DNA double helix, and the "beads" are **nucleosomes:** little disks formed from two copies each of histones H2A, H2B, H3, and H4. One hundred forty-six base pairs of DNA are wound around this histone core in a left-handed orientation. The DNA between the nucleosomes, typically 50 to 60 base pairs in length, is associated with a solitary molecule of histone H1 (Fig. 8.1). Histone H1 participates in the formation of higher-order chromatin structures.

Table 8.1 Genomes of Various Organisms

		Genome Size	
Species	Type of Organism	Mega–Base Pairs	Gene Number
Prokaryotes			
Escherichia coli	Intestinal bacterium	4.639	4289
Mycoplasma genitalium	Genitourinary pathogen	0.58	468
Mycobacterium tuberculosis	Tubercle bacillus	4.447	4402
Rickettsia prowazekii	Typhus bacillus	1.111	834
Treponema pallidum	Syphilis spirochete	1.138	1041
Helicobacter pylori	Stomach ulcer bacterium	1.667	1590
Eukaryotes			
Saccharomyces cerevisiae	Baker's yeast	12.069	6300
Caenorhabditis elegans	Roundworm	97	19000
Drosophila melanogaster	Fruit fly	137	14000
Homo sapiens	Pride of creation	3000	30000

Table 8.2 The Five Types of Histones

Type	Size (Amino Acids)	Location
H1	215	Linker
H2A	129	Nucleosome core
H2B	125	Nucleosome core
H3	135	Nucleosome core
H4	102	Nucleosome core

The packaging of DNA into nucleosomes is only the first step in the condensation of genomic DNA. The diameter of a nucleosome is about 11 nm, but most chromatin is coiled up into fibers with a diameter of about 30 nm. These two packaging operations compress the length of the genomic DNA by a factor of 40. This may be sufficient for dispersed euchromatin in the interphase nucleus, but fully condensed metaphase chromosomes are 200-fold more compact than the 30-nm fiber. This further compaction is achieved with the help of **scaffold proteins** to which long loops of DNA are attached.

Chromatin Structure Is Regulated by Covalent Modifications of Histones and DNA

Both nucleosomes and the higher order chromatin structures are inimical to transcription. Both the 30-nm fiber and the interaction between DNA and the histone core must be destabilized for efficient transcription. The condensation of chromatin is regulated by multiple mechanisms:

1. *The acetylation of lysine side chains in histones destabilizes chromatin structures and favors transcription.*

Acetylation weakens the binding of the histone to DNA by eliminating the positive change on the lysine side chain.

2. *The methylation of some lysine side chains in histones favors the formation of tightly condensed heterochromatin and reduces transcription, whereas methylations on other lysine and arginine side chains have the opposite effect.* These effects are probably mediated by nonhistone proteins that are recruited by the methylated histone.

3. *The methylation of cytosine to 5-methylcytosine in the DNA causes chromatin condensation and gene silencing.* This effect is mediated by chromosome-condensing nonhistone proteins that are attracted by the methylated cytosine bases. About 3% of the cytosine bases in human DNA are methylated.

4. *The phosphorylation of serine side chains in histones is characteristic of mitosis and meiosis.* The role of histone phosphorylation in the formation of condensed mitotic chromosomes is still enigmatic.

5. *ATP–dependent chromatin remodeling complexes can loosen the nucleosome structure temporarily to facilitate transcription.* Again, little is known about the constituents, regulation, and biological functions of these complexes.

All Eukaryotic Chromosomes Have a Centromere, Telomeres, and Replication Origins

Chromosomes need specialized structures to ensure their structural integrity, their replication, and their transmission during mitosis (Fig. 8.2).

*Eukaryotic chromosomes have multiple **replication origins**,* spaced about 100,000 base pairs apart. Multiple origins are needed because eukaryotic

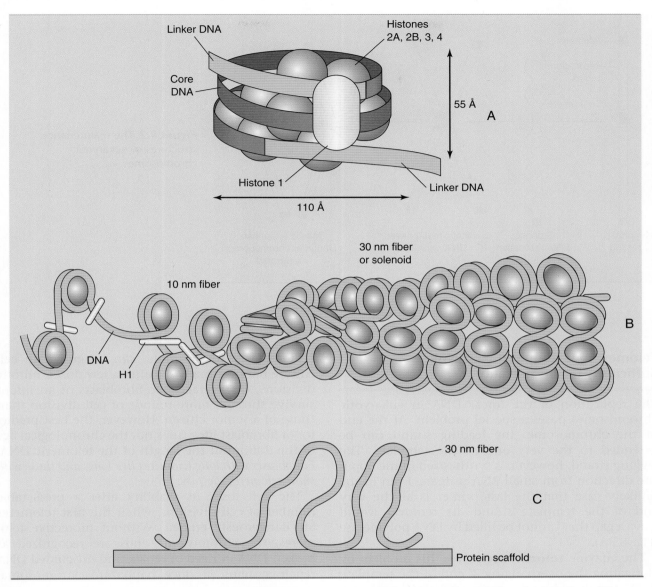

Figure 8.1 Structure of chromatin. **A,** The nucleosome. **B,** Formation of the 30-nm fiber. **C,** Attachment of the 30-nm fiber to the central protein scaffold of the chromosome. Each loop of 30-nm fiber from one scaffold attachment to the next measures approximately 0.4 to 0.8 µm and contains 45,000 to 90,000 base pairs.

chromosomes are 10 to 100 times longer than bacterial chromosomes and because eukaryotic replication forks move at a rate of only 50 nucleotides per second, which is only 6% of the speed of bacterial replication forks. With a single replication origin, the replication of the largest human chromosome would take at least one month.

The **centromere** *is the point where the chromosome attaches to the mitotic spindle.* It consists of several hundred thousand base pairs of highly repetitive DNA, present as tightly condensed heterochromatin. Several dozen proteins attach to the centromeric heterochromatin to form a **kinetochore.** The kinetochore is the immediate attachment point for the spindle fibers during mitosis and meiosis.

Telomeres *are repetitive sequences that cap the ends of the chromosomes.* They consist of the repeat sequence TTAGGG repeated in tandem between 500 and 5000 times. The telomeric repeats bind proteins to cap the chromosome end and protect it from enzymatic attack.

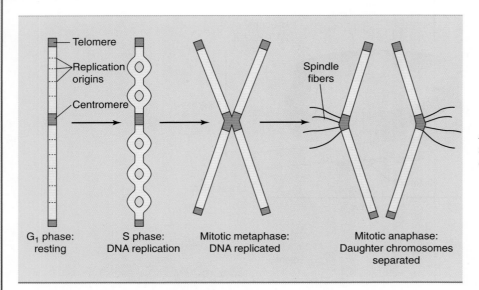

Figure 8.2 The maintenance structures of eukaryotic chromosomes.

The figure labels, left to right:

G₁ phase: resting — Telomere, Replication origins, Centromere

S phase: DNA replication

Mitotic metaphase: DNA replicated

Mitotic anaphase: Daughter chromosomes separated — Spindle fibers

Telomerase Is Required (but Not Sufficient) for Immortality

The replication of the linear DNA in eukaryotic chromosomes poses a special problem. At the end of the chromosome, the leading strand can be extended to the very end of the template. The lagging strand, however, is synthesized in the opposite direction from small RNA primers. Even in the unlikely case that the last primer is at the very end of the template strand, its removal would leave a gap that cannot be filled by DNA polymerase (Fig. 8.3A).

The enzyme **telomerase** solves this problem by elongating the overhanging 3′ end of the template DNA strand, adding the correct TTAGGG sequence of the telomere repeat. There is no DNA template available for this reaction, and therefore *telomerase itself contains the template,* in the form of a 150-nucleotide RNA. One section of this RNA is complementary to the telomeric repeat sequence. It is used as a template to extend the overhanging 3′-terminus. This extended 3′ end is in turn used as a template for the extension of the opposite strand (see Fig. 8.3B and C).

Telomerase is required for immortality. The Olympic gods were considered immortal, and so they presumably expressed telomerase in all their cells, but in the human body, only the cells of the germline are immortal. They have telomerase, and therefore egg and sperm have long telomeres. The expression of telomerase tapers off during embryonic development, and from that time on, the cells lose 50 to 100 base pairs of DNA from the telomeres with every round of DNA replication.

Fibroblasts, for example, can be grown in cell culture but eventually die after a few dozen mitotic divisions. On average, the fibroblasts of an infant survive through more rounds of cell division than those of a senior citizen. However, the best predictor of fibroblast lifespan is not the chronological age of the donor but the length of the telomeric DNA. *Fibroblasts with long telomeres live long, and those with short telomeres die fast.*

The cell loses its viability after a predictable number of cell divisions, when the first telomeres are dangerously eroded. Without protective telomeres, the chromosome ends are recognized as broken DNA in need of repair, and misguided DNA repair systems produce haphazard chromosomal rearrangements. More commonly, however, aged cells respond to undersized telomeres with growth arrest and programmed cell death long before the telomeres have disappeared altogether.

Cancer cells express telomerase and are immortal. This suggests that the lack of telomerase in somatic cells is not only a curse that seals humans' earthly fate but also a protective mechanism to reduce the cancer risk. In order to become malignant, a somatic cell not only has to escape the controls that normally limit its growth but also has to find ways to derepress its telomerase.

Knockout mice that are lacking telomerase altogether are healthy for a few generations, although they do eventually develop defects in replicative tissues. And, counterintuitively, they have an increased rather than reduced cancer risk. The reason is not known.

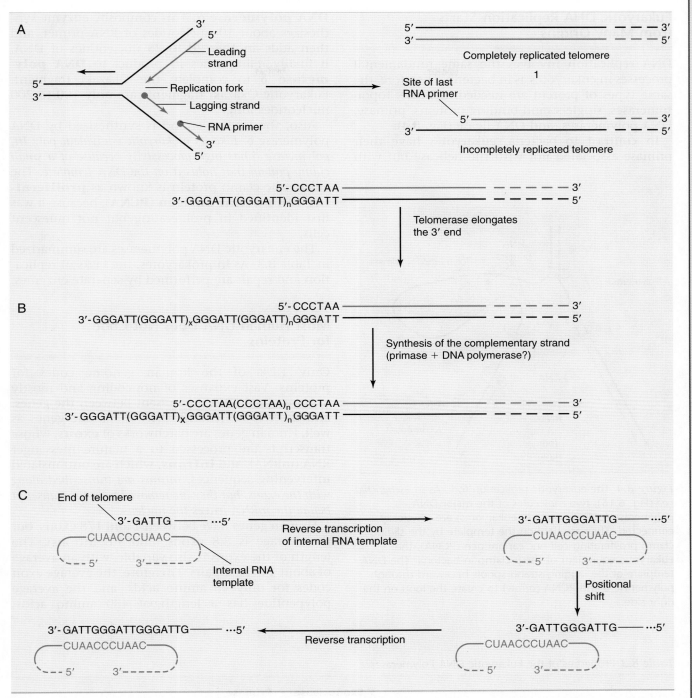

Figure 8.3 The terminal replication problem of telomeric DNA in eukaryotic chromosomes. **A,** The problem: One of the daughter chromosomes is incompletely replicated because DNA replication proceeds only in the 5′ → 3′ direction. direction, and the replication of the lagging strand ends at the site of the last RNA primer. **B,** The solution: Telomerase elongates the overhanging 3′ end of the incompletely replicated telomere. This is followed by the synthesis of the complementary strand. Although the mechanism of complementary strand synthesis is not firmly established, it is probably affected by the regular mechanism of DNA replication, with the combination of primase and DNA polymerase activities. **C,** The hypothetical mechanism of telomere extension by telomerase.

Eukaryotic DNA Replication Starts from Many Origins

DNA replication involves the same fundamental processes in eukaryotes as in bacteria. Therefore, the same types of protein are needed: helicase, topoisomerases, single-strand binding proteins, primase, DNA polymerases, and DNA ligase (Fig. 8.4).

In contrast to bacteria, eukaryotes have their primase associated not with the helicase but with

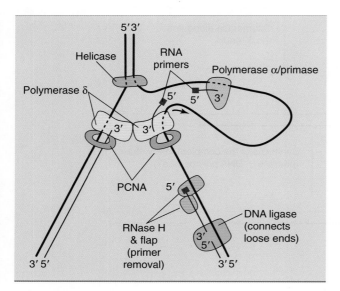

Figure 8.4 The eukaryotic replication fork. As in *Escherichia coli* (Fig. 6.15), two molecules of the major DNA polymerase (polymerase δ in eukaryotes) are physically connected. They are held on the template by the sliding clamp proliferating cell nuclear antigen (PCNA), the eukaryotic equivalent of the β-clamp in bacteria. The DNA template of the lagging strand spools backward through polymerase δ and PCNA (*arrow*) to create the loop on the right side.

DNA polymerase α. This composite enzyme synthesizes about 10 nucleotides of RNA primer, and then adds another 20 to 25 nucleotides of DNA. It finally relinquishes its product to **DNA polymerase δ** to complete the Okazaki fragment. Eukaryotic Okazaki fragments are only 100 to 200 nucleotides long.

Also, the leading strand is synthesized by DNA polymerase δ. *Like its prokaryotic equivalent poly III, polymerase δ has high processivity because of a small clamp protein that holds it on the DNA template.* The eukaryotic clamp protein is known as **proliferating cell nuclear antigen** (**PCNA**), because it was first identified in proliferating but not quiescent cells.

The eukaryotic DNA polymerases are summarized in Table 8.3. As in prokaryotes, the tasks of replication and repair are performed by separate enzymes.

Most Human DNA Does Not Code for Proteins

Only 1.2% of the human genome codes for proteins. Vast expanses of noncoding and mostly untranscribed DNA are present between the genes, and there is noncoding DNA *within* the genes as well. Human genes are patchworks of **exons,** whose transcripts are processed to a mature messenger RNA (mRNA), and **introns,** which are untranslated intervening sequences. *Introns are transcribed along with the exons, but they are removed from the transcript before the mRNA leaves the nucleus.*

Human genes have between 1 and 178 exons, but the average is 8.8 exons (and 7.8 introns). The length of the exons is also variable, with an average of about 145 base pairs. Therefore, the average exon codes for only 48 amino acids, and the average polypeptide has a length of 430 amino acids.

Table 8.3 Properties of the Eukaryotic DNA Polymerases

Polymerase	Location	MW (D)	3'-Exonuclease Activity	Primase Activity	Processivity	Function
α	Nucleus	335,000*	−	+	Low	Initiates DNA replication
δ	Nucleus	170,000†	+	−	High	Major enzyme of DNA replication
ε	Nucleus	256,000‡	+	−	High	Repair
β	Nucleus	37,000	−	−	Low	Repair
γ	Mitochondria	160,000–300,000§	+	−		

*With catalytic subunit of MW 165,000 D.
†With catalytic core of MW 125,000 D.
‡With catalytic core of MW 215,000 D.
§With catalytic subunit of MW 125,000 D.
MW, molecular weight.

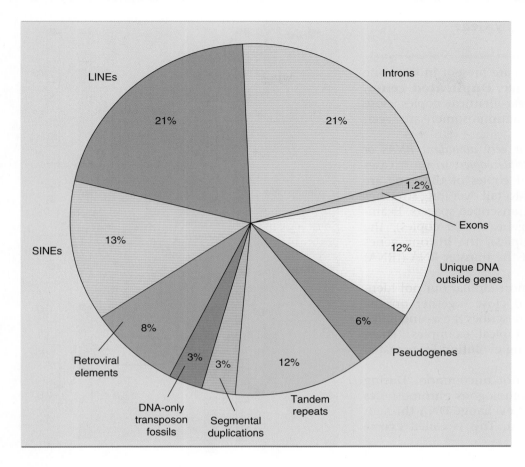

Figure 8.5 The approximate composition of the human genome. LINEs, long interspersed elements; SINEs, short interspersed elements.

Introns are generally far longer than exons, and more than 90% of the DNA within genes belongs to introns (see Figure 8.11 for an example).

It is not known why human genes have introns, why they have so many of them, and why the introns are so long. In some genes, regulatory DNA sequences in introns participate in the regulation of gene expression. Otherwise, introns appear to be useless junk DNA.

However, the intron-exon structure of human genes is important for evolution. *Different structural and functional domains of a polypeptide are often encoded by separate exons.* The immunoglobulin chains, for example, consist of several globular domains with similar amino acid sequence and tertiary structure. Each of these domains is encoded by its own exon (see Chapter 15). This suggests that the immunoglobulin genes arose by **exon duplication** from a single-exon gene.

In other cases, exons from different genes appear to have combined to form a new functional gene. This is called **exon shuffling.** *The exons are the building blocks from which the multitude of eukaryotic genes has been assembled in the course of evolution.*

In addition to introns, exons, and unique DNA between the genes, the genome is cluttered with miscellaneous repetitive sequences. These sequences are repetitive because they are mobile or have been mobile in the past. Like the insertion sequences and transposons described in Chapter 7, they can or could clone themselves into new locations.

Figure 8.5 gives an overview of the composition of the human genome. One commentator wrote about the human genome: "In some ways it may resemble your garage/bedroom/refrigerator/life: highly individualistic, but unkempt; little evidence of organization; much accumulated clutter (referred to by the uninitiated as 'junk'); virtually nothing ever discarded; and the few patently valuable items indiscriminately, apparently carelessly, scattered throughout."

Gene Families Originate by Gene Duplication

Most protein-coding genes are present in only one copy in the haploid genome. **Duplicated genes,** with two identical or near-identical copies close together on the same chromosome, are seen occasionally.

Some genes that code for very abundant RNAs or proteins are present in multiple copies. In most cases identical or near-identical copies of the gene are arranged in tandem, head-to-tail over long stretches of DNA, separated by untranscribed spacers. Examples include the rRNA genes (≈200 copies), the 5S rRNA gene (≈2000 copies), the histone genes (≈20 copies), and most of the transfer RNA (tRNA) genes.

In other cases, two or more similar but not identical genes are positioned close together on the chromosome. Chapter 10 describes the α- and β-like globin gene clusters as typical examples. These **gene families** arise during evolution by repeated gene duplications.

Gene duplications are not uncommon. During prophase of meiosis I, homologous chromosomes align in parallel, and they exchange DNA through homologous recombination. This is called **crossing over** (Fig. 8.6A).

Normal crossing over is a strictly reciprocal process in which neither chromosome gains or loses genes. But *if the chromosomes are mispaired during crossing over, one chromosome acquires a deletion and the other a duplication.* The duplicated genes are bound to change by occasional mutations, and eventually they can acquire distinctive new biological functions.

In many cases, however, one of the duplication products acquires crippling mutations that prevent its transcription or translation. The result is called a **pseudogene.** Pseudogenes still have the intron-exon structure of the functional gene from which they were derived, and they are located close to their functional counterpart on the chromosome.

The Genome Contains Many Tandem Repeats

Tandem repeats, also known as **simple-sequence DNA,** consist of a short DNA sequence of between two and a few dozen base pairs that is repeated head-to-tail many times. In the telomeres, for example, the sequence TTAGGG is repeated hundreds to thousands of times. *The centromeres have even more simple-sequence DNA than the do telomeres, but the repeat sequences differ in different chromosomes.*

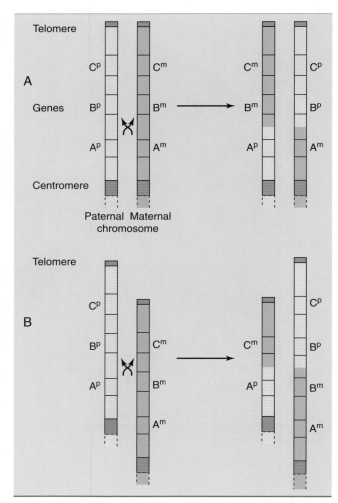

Figure 8.6 Gene duplication by crossing over between mispaired chromosomes in meiosis. **A,** Normal meiotic recombination. This is an example of homologous recombination. It creates new combinations of the paternally derived and maternally derived genes. **B,** Recombination between mispaired chromosomes. This is a rare event because, ordinarily, homologous recombination occurs only between DNA molecules of related base sequence. Note that one chromosome acquires a gene deletion and the other a gene duplication. Repeated gene duplications followed by divergent evolution of the duplicated genes create gene families.

After partial endonuclease digestion, the centromeric and telomeric DNA can be separated from bulk genomic DNA by density gradient centrifugation. The repetitive DNA thus isolated is called **satellite DNA.**

Most of the simple-sequence DNA outside the centromeres and telomeres occurs in the form of simple repeats with two to five base pairs in the repeat unit. These units are repeated from a few times to more than 50 times in any one location, and the same repeat can be present at many differ-

Table 8.4 Diseases That Are Caused by the Expansion of a Trinucleotide Repeat Sequence in a Gene

| Disease | Type of Disease | Inheritance | Amplified Repeat* | Repeat Number | | Location in Gene |
				Normal	Disease	
Huntington disease	Neural degeneration	AD	CAG	6–34	36–120	Coding sequence (Gln)
Myotonic dystrophy	Muscle loss, cardiac arrhythmia	AD	CTG	5–37	100–5000	3'-Untranslated region
Fragile X	Mental retardation	XR	CGG	6–52	200–3000	5'-Untranslated region
Friedreich ataxia	Loss of motor coordination	AR	GAA	7–22	200–1000	Intron

*A, adenine; C, cytosine; G, guanine; T, thymine.
AD, autosomal dominant; AR, autosomal recessive; Gln, glutamine; XR, X-linked recessive.

ent sites all over the genome. Dinucleotide repeats are most abundant, but repeats of three, four, or five bases are common as well. Most of them are scattered in the junk DNA, and their functions, if any, are not known. These repeat sequences are known as **microsatellites.** Tandem repeats with longer repeat units are called **minisatellites.**

Microsatellite Expansions Can Cause Disease

The length of tandem repeats is prone to change through mutation. The resulting length variations are innocuous and are therefore not removed by natural selection. They can survive in the population as part of the normal genetic variation. A variable repeat is referred to as a **variable number of tandem repeats** (**VNTR**). Chapter 11 describes how VNTRs are used for DNA fingerprinting and paternity testing.

The few tandem repeats that are located in genes tend to be mutational hot spots. **Huntington disease,** for example, is caused by the expansion of the trinucleotide repeat CAG in the coding sequence of a brain-expressed gene. In the normal gene, the CAG is repeated 6 to 34 times, coding for a polyglutamine tract in the protein huntingtin.

In Huntington disease, the CAG sequence of the gene (and the glutamine sequence in the encoded protein) is expanded to a copy number in excess of 36. This glutamine-expanded huntingtin protein forms abnormal complexes with other proteins, leading to progressive cell death in the basal ganglia of the brain and in the cerebral cortex. This autosomal dominant disease first manifests with personality changes and a motor disorder in adults and gradually progresses to severe dementia.

The greater the trinucleotide expansion, the earlier is the onset of the disease. During transmission from the father to the children, the repeat tends to expand even further and *the disease tends to become more severe in successive generations.* Some other diseases that are caused by trinucleotide expansions are listed in Table 8.4.

Some DNA Sequences Are Copies of Functional RNAs

In addition to pseudogenes, which are the degenerate offspring of functional duplicated genes, the human genome also contains **processed pseudogenes.** Although pseudogenes still have the intron-exon structure of the gene from which they were derived, *a processed pseudogene consists only of exon sequences, with an oligo-A tract of 10 to 50 nucleotides at the 3' end.* This structure is framed by direct repeats of between 9 and 14 base pairs (Fig. 8.7). Unlike pseudogenes, processed pseudogenes are not located near their functional counterparts.

Processed pseudogenes arise during evolution by the reverse transcription of a cellular RNA. Fully processed eukaryotic mRNAs no longer have introns, but they possess a poly-A tail at the 3' end. Therefore, reverse transcriptase produces a complementary DNA (cDNA) without introns but with part of the poly-A tail included. This cDNA becomes integrated in the genome. The direct repeats are target site duplications that arise when an integrase enzyme inserts the cDNA into the chromosome. Chapter 7 showed that target site duplications are also produced when a DNA transposon or a retrovirus integrates itself into the genome.

Having lost their promoter during retrotransposition, processed pseudogenes are rarely if ever transcribed. The existence of processed pseudogenes in the human genome shows that *reverse transcriptase and integrase are (or at least were) present in "normal" human cells.* These enzymes are encoded by integrated retroviruses and other parasitic elements.

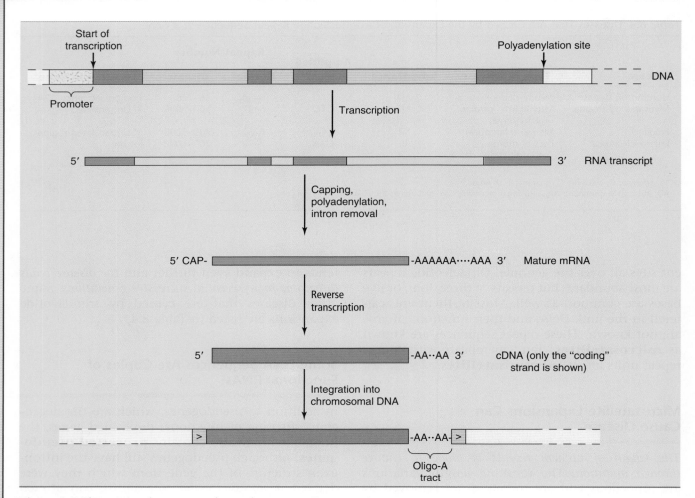

Figure 8.7 The origin of a processed pseudogene. ■, Exons; □, introns.

Table 8.5 Mobile Elements in the Human Genome

Class	Length	Number in Genome	Encoded Proteins	Mode of Movement	Current Activity
DNA-only transposons	Variable, 220 average	400,000	Transposase (defunct)	Direct transposition	Fossils only
Retrovirus-like retrotransposons	Up to 10,000 bp, but 350 bp average	700,000	Reverse transcriptase (usually defunct)	Retrotransposition	Few are still active
LINE-1 elements	Up to 6000 bp, but most are truncated	900,000	Reverse transcriptase, RNA-binding protein	Retrotransposition	Still active
Alu sequences	Up to 300, many are truncated	1,300,000	None	Retrotransposition	Still active

bp, base pairs.

Some Repetitive DNA Sequences Are Mobile

The human genome is inhabited by a vast population of repetitive sequences. These sequences have lengths of up to a few thousand base pairs. They are not aligned in tandem but are scattered all over the genome as **interspersed elements.**

These elements are repetitive because they can insert copies of themselves into new genomic locations. The human genome contains several types, as summarized in Table 8.5.

Insertion sequences and transposons are called **DNA transposons,** to distinguish them from mobile elements that move through an RNA intermediate. DNA transposons were at one time active in the human or prehuman genome, but they mutated into irrelevance approximately 30 million years ago. Only their molecular fossils can still be inspected by genome sequencers.

Retroviral retrotransposons are more abundant than DNA transposons. They contain remnants of retroviral *gag, pol,* and *env* genes and long terminal repeats. They are no longer infectious because they are mutationally degraded and unable to form a complete set of viral proteins. A few can still make their own reverse transcriptase and integrase and can use them to move around in the genome, although they can no longer make infectious virus particles.

Apparently only one family of retroviral retrotransposons has been active in the human genome during the past 6 million years, since human ancestors differentiated from the ancestors of chimpanzees. However, *most retroviral retrotransposons are the dead bodies of retroviruses, left to rot in the genomic soil.*

L1 Elements Encode a Reverse Transcriptase

The **L1 elements** are the most abundant type of **long interspersed elements** (LINEs). A full-length L1 element has nearly 6000 base pairs and ends in a poly-A tract. There are no long terminal repeats but only short direct repeats that originated during retrotransposition.

In all, there are 900,000 L1 elements in the human genome, but most of them are badly truncated at the 5′ end. Truncation seems to be a common accident during retrotransposition. Only about 5000 are full-length. Two randomly selected L1 elements from different parts of the genome are about 95% identical in sequence.

Full-length L1 elements contain two genes, but these genes are intact in only 60 to 100 of the 5000 full-length L1 elements. One of the two genes codes for an RNA-binding protein and the other for a protein with reverse transcriptase and nuclease (and possibly integrase) activities.

With the help of these two proteins, L1 elements can move into new genomic locations. The L1 element is first transcribed into RNA by a cellular RNA polymerase. The L1-encoded proteins then copy this RNA into a cDNA and insert the cDNA into the genome.

Alu Sequences Spread with the Help of Reverse Transcriptase from Other Mobile Elements

The L1 reverse transcriptase acts preferentially on the transcript of the L1 element. On occasion, however, it produces a processed pseudogene by reverse-transcribing and integrating a cellular mRNA. It also spreads other long and short interspersed elements.

The most populous tribe of **short interspersed elements** (SINEs) are the **Alu sequences,** with 1.3 million copies in the haploid genome. A full-length Alu sequence measures 282 base pairs, contains an adenine-rich tract of between 7 and 50 base pairs at the 3′ end, and is flanked by direct repeats of 7 to 21 base pairs.

When two Alu sequences from different parts of the genome are compared, they differ on average in about 20% of their bases. Many Alu sequences can be transcribed by RNA polymerase III, but they do not encode any proteins. Most of the transcripts are rapidly degraded in the nucleus.

On occasion, however, the RNA transcript of an Alu sequence is copied into a cDNA by reverse transcriptase from an L1 element or a retrovirus-like element, followed by integration into the genome (Fig. 8.8). By abusing their reverse transcriptase and integrase, Alu sequences are the parasites of other parasitic elements.

Whereas L1 sequences might be the descendants of a virus, *the Alu sequences are clearly of cellular origin.* The Alu consensus sequence is more than 80% identical to the sequence of **7SL RNA,** a small cytoplasmic RNA that participates in the targeting of proteins to the endoplasmic reticulum (see Chapter 9). Inasmuch as the 7SL RNA is present in all eukaryotes but Alu sequences are abundant only in vertebrates, the Alu sequences probably originated by the reverse transcription of 7SL RNA after the divergence of the earliest vertebrates 550 million years ago.

Retrotranspositions of L1 and Alu sequences still occur in the human genome. Alu sequences have in a few instances been observed to cause mutations by jumping into an important gene. They also cause chromosome misalignment during meiosis when nonhomologous copies of a repetitive element pair up. This can lead to large duplications and deletions, by the mechanism shown schematically in Figure 8.6B.

Thus, the human genome is a graveyard that harbors the rotting relics of an estimated 4.3 million copies of parasitic DNA. Mobile, "parasitic" DNA elements are more common in sexually reproducing organisms than in those with asexual reproduction, and *the mobile elements that gave rise to*

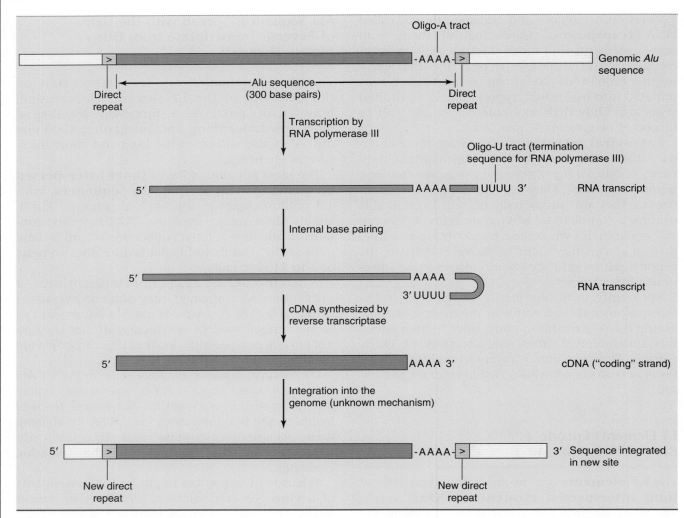

Figure 8.8 Hypothetical mechanism for the retroposition of Alu sequences. Transcription by RNA polymerase III typically starts at the first base of the Alu sequence and ends at a T-rich sequence downstream of the Alu sequence. Note that the direct repeats flanking the sequence arise as target site duplications during integration. Therefore they differ in different copies of the Alu sequence. L1 sequences are thought to move by the same mechanism. cDNA, complementary DNA.

nearly half of the human genome are best understood as sexually transmitted parasites.

Humans Have Approximately 30,000 Genes

The precise number of genes in the human genome is unknown, but most estimates are between 25,000 and 35,000. Genes have telltale sequences, including promoter elements, a start codon followed by a substantial string of amino acid coding codons, intron-exon junctions, and a polyadenylation signal at the end of the gene. However, these sequences are so variable that the computer programs that have been designed for gene hunting

cannot agree among themselves about the exact number.

Another approach is to extract fully processed mRNA from the cytoplasm of cells, copy it into a cDNA with the help of reverse transcriptase, and clone the cDNA in bacteria. The sequences identified with this method are called **expressed sequence tags.** Because they are transcribed, processed, and transported into the cytoplasm, they presumably represent protein-coding genes.

Molecular geneticists can also use the comparative method. Random mutations in the junk DNA cause no damage and can therefore survive. However, mutations in important coding and regulatory sequences are likely to disrupt gene function. They are therefore removed by natural selection.

Table 8.6 The Eukaryotic RNA Polymerases

Type	Location	Transcripts	Inhibition by α-Amanitin
I	Nucleolus	Pre-rRNA	–
II	Nucleus	Pre-mRNA	+++
III	Nucleus	tRNA, 5S rRNA	+
Mitochondrial	Mitochondria	Mitochondrial RNAs	–

mRNA, messenger RNA; rRNA, ribosomal RNA; tRNA, transfer RNA.

As a result, *the important coding and regulatory sequences of genes show little variation among species, and the junk DNA shows much variation.* For example, the DNA of humans and chimpanzees differs in 1.5% of the nucleotide positions overall, but the difference is far less than this in the coding and regulatory sequences of the genes.

Eukaryotes Have Three Nuclear RNA Polymerases

E. coli has a single RNA polymerase for the synthesis of all its cellular RNA, but eukaryotes employ separate enzymes for the synthesis of ribosomal RNA (rRNA), mRNA, and tRNA (Table 8.6).

RNA polymerase I synthesizes the common precursor of the 5.8S, 18S, and 28S rRNA. *This enzyme is active in the nucleolus,* where the ribosomal RNA is synthesized and ribosomal subunits are assembled from rRNA and proteins. Ribosomal proteins are synthesized in the cytoplasm. They are then transported into the nucleolus, where the ribosomal subunits are assembled, and the assembled ribosomal subunits are finally exported to the cytoplasm.

RNA polymerase II is present in the nucleoplasm where it synthesizes the mRNA precursors, and **RNA polymerase III,** also in the nucleoplasm, synthesizes the tRNAs, the small 5S rRNA, and other small RNAs.

RNA polymerase II and, at higher concentrations, RNA polymerase III are inhibited by **α-amanitin,** a poison from the toadstool *Amanita phalloides.* This toxin is the most common cause of fatal mushroom poisoning worldwide.

Transcriptional Initiation Requires General Transcription Factors

Eukaryotic promoters are as variable as their prokaryotic counterparts. The most consistent promoter element in protein-coding genes is the **TATA box,** located 25 to 30 base pairs upstream of the transcriptional start site. There are also poorly defined initiator (Inr) elements at the transcriptional start site.

These elements are required for the correct positioning of RNA polymerase II. Therefore, they must be present in the correct 5′→3′ orientation, and they must be on the correct strand of the double helix.

Whereas promoter recognition in bacteria requires only the σ subunit, eukaryotes employ a whole set of **general transcription factors** for this purpose. They are called "general" because they are required for the transcription of all genes that are transcribed by a particular RNA polymerase. They are named by the acronym TF, followed by the number of the RNA polymerase they work with and an identifying letter. *The RNA polymerase must bind to the promoter-associated transcription factors before it can start transcription.*

The formation of the initiation complex for RNA polymerase II starts with the binding of the TATA-binding protein **TBP** to the TATA box. This induces a sharp bend in the DNA double helix. TBP is only one of about 11 subunits of transcription factor IID (**TFIID**). The other subunits are also known as TBP-associated factors (**TAFs**). They assemble on TBP as soon as TBP is bound to the TATA box.

Figure 8.9 shows a hypothetical sequence of events. After TFIID, the transcription factors **TFIIB, TFIIF, TFIIE,** and **TFIIH** are added along with RNA polymerase II. *TFIIH is the only transcription factor with enzymatic activities.* As an ATP-dependent helicase, it unwinds a short stretch of the DNA to provide a single-stranded template for RNA polymerase II. It also has protein kinase activity.

Transcriptional Activator and Repressor Proteins Are Essential for Regulated Gene Expression

Chapter 6 described transcriptional repressors, such as the *lac* repressor, and transcriptional activators, such as the catabolite activator protein (CAP).

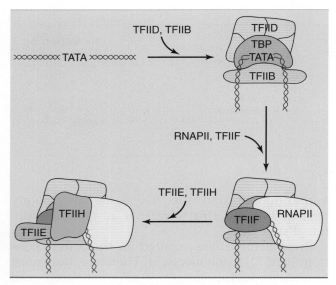

Figure 8.9 The formation of the transcriptional initiation complex by the assembly of general transcription factors and RNA polymerase II (RNAPII). Transcription factor IID (TFIID) contains multiple subunits. One subunit, the TATA-binding protein (TBP), binds the TATA box. TFIIB, TFIIE, TFIIF, and TFIIH, transcription factors IIB, IIE, IIF, and IIH.

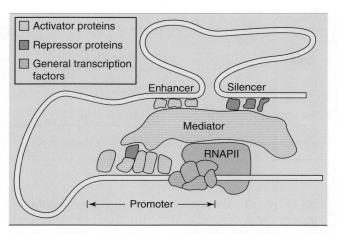

Figure 8.10 The mediator is a large protein complex that mediates the effects of activator and repressor proteins on transcriptional initiation. RNAP II, RNA polymerase II.

Repressors tend to be more common than activators in bacteria.

In eukaryotes, however, the nonselective repression of transcription by histones has to be overcome by the competitive binding of sequence-specific activator proteins to the DNA. Therefore, transcriptional activators tend to be more common than repressors in eukaryotes. Transcriptional activators and general transcription factors are loosely referred to as "transcription factors."

Ultimately, DNA-bound activator proteins stabilize the transcriptional initiation complex, whereas transcriptional repressors destabilize it. *Promoters have multiple binding sites for regulatory proteins upstream from the transcriptional start site.* These sites are different in different genes.

In most cases, the effects of the activator and repressor proteins that bind to these sites are relayed to the transcriptional initiation complex through a large protein complex called **mediator** (Fig. 8.10).

Mediator does not bind to DNA, but it binds to RNA polymerase II and it activates the protein kinase activity of TFIIH. It also binds to activator and repressor proteins that are associated with the promoter upstream of the general transcription factors. Thus, *mediator is the link between the regulatory DNA-binding proteins and the transcriptional initiation complex.*

Regulatory Sites on the DNA Can Be at a Great Distance from the Transcriptional Start Site

The promoters of most eukaryotic genes stretch over about 300 base pairs, with binding sites for the general transcription factors near the transcriptional start site and binding sites for specific activators and repressors a bit upstream.

Enhancers and **silencers** are regulatory DNA sequences that can be thousands or even tens of thousands of base pairs away from the transcriptional start site, either upstream in the junk DNA between the genes or downstream in an intron. They bind activator and repressor proteins, respectively. Through bending and looping of the DNA, these bound proteins can affect transcription by interacting with the mediator.

In recombinant DNA experiments, enhancers and silencers influence transcription even when they are on the "wrong" strand of the double helix or in the "wrong" 5'→3' orientation.

Typical enhancers look as if an overenthusiastic sorcerer's apprentice had stuffed as many binding sites for regulatory proteins as possible into as small a space as possible. Figure 8.11 shows an example. Most binding sites are only 15 to 20 base pairs long. Many activator and repressor proteins respond to hormones, second messengers, or nutrients. Their binding sites are therefore called **response elements.**

There often are multiple binding sites for an activator or repressor protein crowded together. This may be necessary to overcome the inhibitory effects of the histones. When one binding site is

Table 8.7 The Major Types of DNA-Binding Proteins in Eukaryotes

Structural Motif	Structural Features	Examples
Helix-turn-helix proteins	Two α helices separated by a β turn; "recognition helix" fitting in major groove of DNA	"Homeodomain" proteins (proteins regulating embryonic development); also, most prokaryotic repressors
Zinc finger proteins	Contain zinc bound to Cys and His side chains	Receptors for steroid and thyroid hormones
Leucine zipper proteins	Two α helices, one with basic residues for DNA binding, one with regularly spaced Leu for dimerization	C/EBP (gene activator in liver); c-Myc, c-Fos, c-Jun (growth regulators, proto-oncogene products)
Helix-loop-helix proteins	DNA-binding α helix and two dimerization helices separated by a nonhelical loop	Myo D-1, myogenin (proteins that induce muscle differentiation)

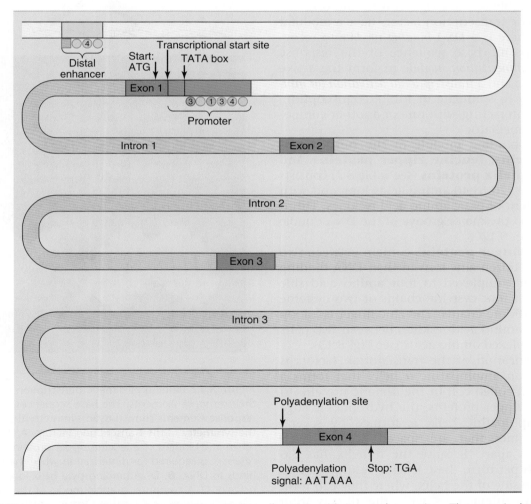

Figure 8.11 The gene for the liver protein transthyretin (prealbumin), with its regulatory sites. The gene is drawn to scale to show its intron-exon structure and the multiple upstream binding sites for regulatory proteins. Note that in this gene, as in most others, the introns are far longer than the exons. Sites for the binding of regulatory proteins are clustered in the promoter and a distal enhancer. With the exception of AP1, which is present in all nucleated cells, the regulatory proteins are present in hepatocytes but not in most other cell types. ■, AP1; ○, C/EBP; (1), (3) and (4), hepatocyte nuclear factors 1, 3, and 4.

covered by histones, a neighboring site may still be accessible.

Gene Expression Is Regulated by DNA-Binding Proteins

Most activator and repressor proteins bind their response elements in a dimeric form, either as homodimers of two identical subunits or as heterodimers of two slightly different subunits. The symmetry of the dimeric transcription factors is matched by their response elements, which tend to possess an incomplete dyad symmetry (see also Fig. 6.37). Some recurrent structural motifs have been described in regulatory DNA-binding proteins. These are summarized in Table 8.7 and Figures 8.12 and 8.13.

The dimeric transcription factors have a modular structure. There is a *DNA-binding module* to recognize the specific base sequence of the response element; a *dimerization module* to form the active dimeric state; and a *transcriptional activation (or inhibition) region* to stimulate or inhibit transcription, usually by interacting with one or another component of the mediator.

The DNA-binding module of the **helix-turn-helix proteins, leucine zipper proteins,** and **helix-loop-helix proteins** (see Table 8.7) consists of an α helix, 20 to 40 amino acids long and with a high content of basic amino acid residues. This α helix fits into the major groove of the DNA double helix (see Fig. 8.12C).

The **zinc finger proteins** contain between two and about a dozen zinc ions in their DNA-binding region, each complexed to four amino acid side chains: either four cysteine chains or two cysteine and two histidine chains. The zinc finger is a loop of about 12 amino acid residues between two pairs of zinc-complexed amino acids (see Fig. 8.13).

The dimerization of the transcription factors is effected by an amphipathic α helix that forms a two-stranded coiled coil in the dimeric protein. In the leucine zipper proteins, the hydrophobic edge of this amphipathic helix is formed by several leucine residues that are spaced exactly seven amino acids apart. Because the α helix has 3.6 amino acids per turn, these leucine residues are all on the same side of the helix, where they can form hydrophobic interactions with the dimerization partner.

The activator and repressor proteins are regulated in several ways:

1. *Their synthesis is regulated by other activator and repressor proteins.* This regulation can be cell type–specific. For example, some activator and repressor proteins are present mainly in liver and

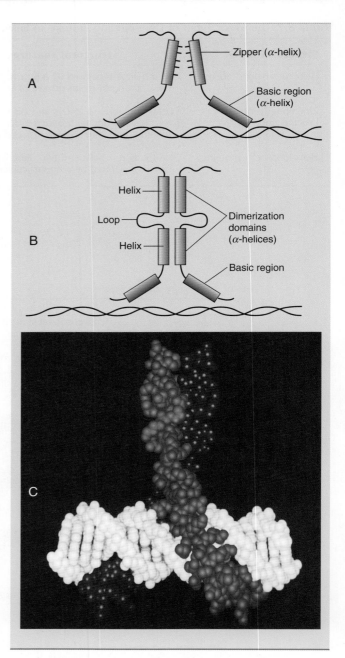

Figure 8.12 Binding of dimeric transcription factors to their response elements. The base sequences of the response elements show a dyad symmetry that matches the symmetry of the transcription factors. **A,** The schematic binding of a leucine zipper protein. The "zipper" is required for dimerization while the basic region binds to DNA. **B,** DNA binding by a helix-loop-helix protein. **C,** A computer graphic model of the binding of the carboxyl-terminal portion ("basic region") of the leucine zipper protein C/EBF to its cognate binding site.

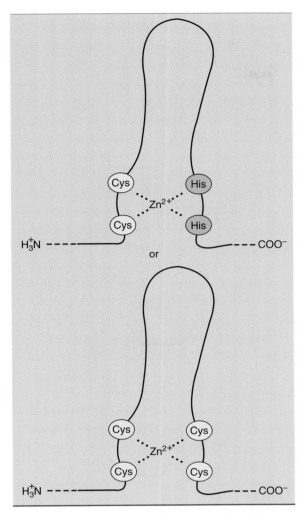

Figure 8.13 The zinc finger. This structural motif occurs in 2 to 12 copies in the DNA-binding region of the zinc finger proteins. The amino acid residues on each side of the zinc are separated by approximately 3 or 4 amino acid residues, and the intervening loop contains approximately 12 residues. Cys, cysteine; His, histidine.

kidney, whereas others are expressed only in muscles.

2. *Some are regulated by the noncovalent binding of a hormone or another small molecule.* The most prominent examples are the receptors for steroid and thyroid hormones.

3. *Many are regulated by covalent phosphorylation and dephosphorylation.* The protein kinases and protein phosphatases acting on these gene regulators are themselves responsive to stimuli such as growth factors, hormones, nutrients, and metabolic products.

4. *Protein-protein interactions are important.* For example, the effects of some transcriptional activators can be blocked by other nuclear proteins that bind to the transcriptional activator domain.

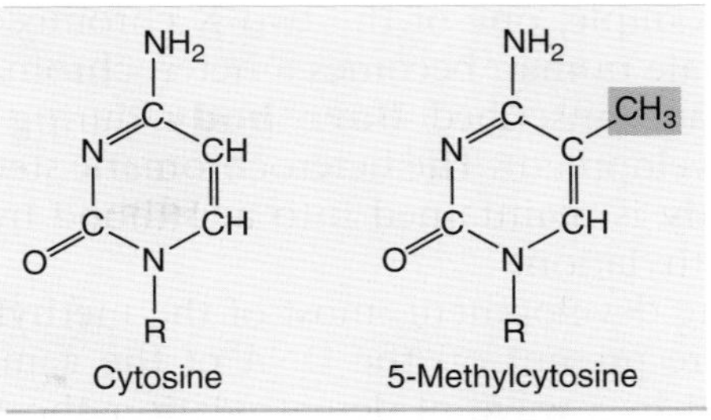

Figure 8.14 Structure of 5-methylcytosine in DNA. The methyl group does not interfere with the normal base pairing of cytosine.

One fundamental task of transcriptional regulation in multicellular organisms is the establishment and maintenance of cell differentiation. Figure 8.11 shows the gene for transthyretin, a plasma protein that is formed only in the liver and the choroid plexuses of the brain. This gene is regulated by at least five different proteins that bind to 10 binding sites. With the exception of AP1, which is abundant in all nucleated cells, these transcription factors are more abundant in hepatocytes than in other cells.

Another important task for transcriptional regulation is the response to external signals. Some lipid-soluble hormones, including the steroid and thyroid hormones, manipulate gene expression by binding to activator or repressor proteins. Water-soluble hormones and growth factors, however, act indirectly by activating protein kinases. The hormone-regulated protein kinases enter the nucleus, where they phosphorylate gene regulator proteins.

Genes Can Be Silenced by Methylation

The methylation of cytosine residues to **5-methylcytosine** (Fig. 8.14) is a mechanism for the long-term regulation of gene expression. The methylcytosine is present in the sequence 5'-CG-3', and about 60% of human genes have **CG islands** in their vicinity.

The CG sequence is a palindrome, and usually the cytosines on both strands are methylated. This is because after DNA replication of a methylated (but not unmethylated) CG sequence, a **maintenance methyltransferase** methylates the CG sequence in the new strand. Thus, *the methylation pattern of the DNA is heritable.*

Methylcytosine attracts a set of DNA-binding proteins, which in turn attract histone deacetylases. The removal of acetyl groups from histones leads to tighter packing of the chromatin. Therefore, *genes that have methylated CG islands nearby are not transcribed.*

For example, one of the two X chromosomes in the female human becomes a heterochromatic and largely untranscribed **Barr body** during embryonic development. The heterochromatic state of the Barr body is maintained into adulthood by extensive methylation.

During development, most of the methyl groups that were present on the DNA of the gametes are removed in a wave of demethylation shortly after fertilization. Tissue-specific methylation then takes place in the developing embryo, when the embryonic cells differentiate into specialized cell types. An understanding of DNA methylation in different cell types is important for understanding human reproductive cloning.

Some genes, however, maintain the methylation pattern that they had acquired in the germline. These methylation patterns differ in the male and female germlines. Therefore, *some genes are expressed only when they come from the father, and some are expressed only when they come from the mother.* This is called **imprinting.** Only a small number of genes are imprinted in the human genome.

Eukaryotic Messenger RNA Is Extensively Processed by Nuclear Enzyme Systems

The introns in human genes are transcribed along with the exons but are spliced out of the transcript in the nucleus. *Only fully processed, mature mRNA translocates to the cytoplasm, where it is translated.* mRNA processing includes not only the removal of the introns but also the modification of the two ends:

1. *The 5′ end of the mRNA receives a cap.* The cap is a methylguanosine residue that is linked to the first nucleotide of the RNA through an unusual 5′-5′-triphosphate linkage (Fig. 8.15). The cap binds a set of proteins that protect the 5′-end of the mRNA from 5′-exonucleases; it helps guiding the mRNA through the nuclear pore complex into the cytosol, and it helps in the initial interaction between the mRNA and the ribosome.
2. *The 3′ end of the mRNA receives a poly-A tail of about 200 nucleotides.* Multiple copies of a **poly-A binding protein** (**PABP**) bind to the poly-A tail. This helps in nuclear export and retards the action of 3′-exonucleases. Only the histone mRNAs have no poly-A tails, and their half-lives are only a few minutes. Histones are synthesized only during the S phase of the cell cycle when the DNA is replicated, and their synthesis must be switched off quickly once the DNA is completely replicated.

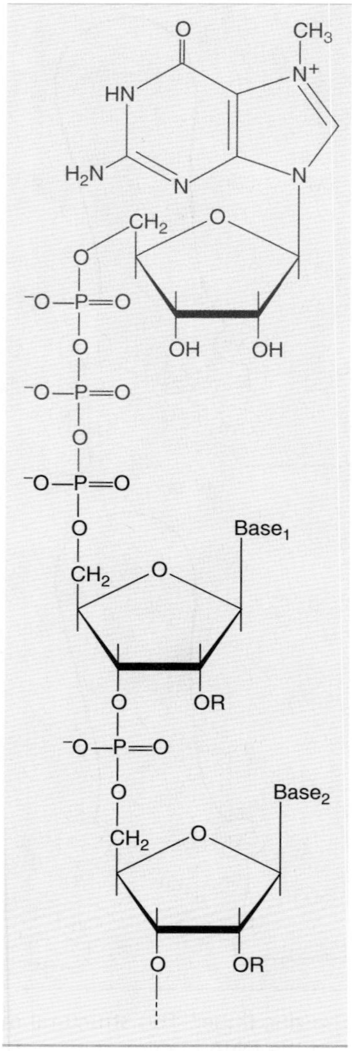

Figure 8.15 Structure of the cap at the 5′ end of eukaryotic messenger RNAs. Transfer and ribosomal RNAs do not have caps. R = H or CH_3.

The Pre–Messenger RNA Is Processed during Transcription

The "post-transcriptional" processing of mRNA is actually cotranscriptional. It occurs while RNA polymerase II is synthesizing the mRNA, and it is guided by proteins that interact directly with the RNA polymerase (Fig. 8.16).

The RNA is synthesized in the 5′→3′ direction, and *5′ capping is the first modification of the pre-mRNA.* It is done when about 25 nucleotides of the RNA have been polymerized.

Next, *the introns are removed by nuclear enzyme complexes called spliceosomes.* The spliceosome contains five small RNAs (U1, U2, U4, U5, and U6), each between 106 and 185 nucleotides long. These are associated with proteins to form **small nuclear ribonucleoprotein particles (snRNPs**

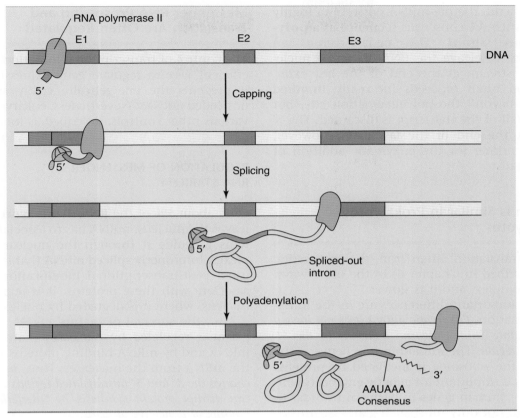

Figure 8.16 The "post-transcriptional" processing of messenger RNA (mRNA) actually takes place while RNA polymerase II is synthesizing the mRNA. E1, E2, and E3, exons; P, promoter.

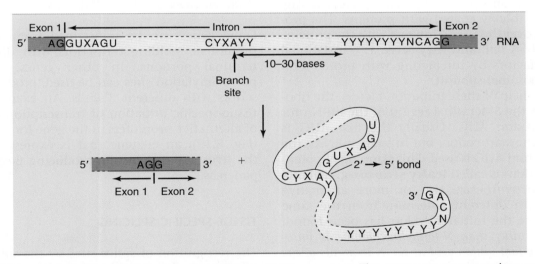

Figure 8.17 The splicing of introns from messenger RNA (mRNA) precursors. The consensus sequences base-pair with RNA components of the spliceosomes. A, adenine; C, cytosine; G, guanine; N = any base; U, uracil; X, purine; Y, pyrimidine.

["**snurps**"]). Overall, about 50 proteins are involved in splicing.

The intron-exon junctions of protein-coding nuclear genes are marked by more or less conserved consensus sequences. There is also a conserved "branch site" within the intron, about 30 nucleotides from the 3' end (Fig. 8.17). Splicing releases the intron as a cyclic lariat structure, with the 5' end forming a bond with the 2' hydroxyl group at the branch site.

Near its 3' end, the pre-mRNA possesses a highly conserved AAUAAA consensus sequence as a **polyadenylation signal.** This signal recruits an endonuclease to cleave the RNA about 20 nucleotides downstream, at the end of the last exon. Transcription often proceeds for many hundred nucleotides beyond the polyadenylation site, but the cut-off tail of the transcript is discarded. The 3' terminus at the end of the last exon, however, serves as a primer for the enzymatic addition of the poly-A tail.

Translation Is Similar in Prokaryotes and Eukaryotes

Eukaryotic translation differs from the prokaryotic system (described in Chapter 6) in the usual ways: It is more complex, and it is slower.

The most important differences are in the initiation of translation. *Eukaryotic mRNA does not have a ribosome-binding Shine-Dalgarno sequence in the 5'-untranslated region.* The initial binding between the mRNA and the ribosome is mediated by proteins instead. This is important for genetic engineers who try to express human genes in bacteria. In order to be translated, not only must such genes be intronless and coupled to a bacterial promoter but also a Shine-Dalgarno sequence must be engineered into the gene construct.

Figure 8.18 shows that the ends of eukaryotic mRNAs are thickly coated with proteins. The proteins that cover the 5'-end interact with the proteins on the poly-A tail, and they serve as translational initiation factors by interacting with proteins on the 40S ribosomal subunit.

With the help of these initiation factors, the ribosome scans the 5'-terminal region of the mRNA for the start codon AUG. Usually the first AUG is chosen as the start codon, but in some mRNAs, the second or third AUG is used. This skipping of potential start codons is called **leaky scanning.** It allows the cell to synthesize two or more alternative proteins with different N-termini from the same mRNA. Once the initiator codon has been found, *methionine rather than N-formylmethionine is introduced as the first amino acid at the N-terminus of the polypeptide.*

The steps in the elongation cycle are analogous to those in bacterial protein synthesis, and the elongation factors are functionally equivalent (Table 8.8). However, *eukaryotes add only two amino acids per second to the growing polypeptide chain, in comparison with 20 per second in bacteria.*

Messenger RNA Processing and Translation Are Often Regulated

The control of transcriptional initiation is the most efficient way to regulate gene expression because it prevents the energetically costly synthesis of unneeded mRNAs. Nevertheless, eukaryotes also use various other controls, described as follows.

REGULATION OF MESSENGER RNA STABILITY

Only about 5% of the RNA that is synthesized ever leaves the nucleus. mRNA has to associate with proteins to guide it through the nuclear pore complexes. Improperly spliced mRNA that is lacking the usual post-transcriptional modifications does not associate with these proteins. It is retained in the nucleus, where it is degraded by nucleases.

Also, the survival of mature mRNA in the cytoplasm is regulated by nucleases that degrade the mRNA and by mRNA-binding proteins that protect the mRNA from the nucleases. Thus, *mutations that change the 3' and 5' untranslated regions of the mRNA can disrupt protein synthesis by interfering with the binding of protective proteins.*

TISSUE-SPECIFIC INITIATION AND TERMINATION OF TRANSCRIPTION

Some genes can be transcribed from alternative promoters, yielding transcripts with different 5'-terminal portions. In other genes, alternative polyadenylation sites can be used, producing transcripts with different 3'-ends. An example of the tissue-specific initiation of transcription is the use of alternative promoters in the gene for glucokinase (Fig. 8.19), an enzyme that is expressed only in the liver and the insulin-producing β-cells of the pancreas.

TISSUE-SPECIFIC SPLICING

The recognition of splice sites by the spliceosomal system can be variable. Thus, an exon that is included in the mature mRNA in one cell type can be skipped in another. Alternative splicing is common in multicellular eukaryotes. About 60% of the genes in the human genome are thought to be subject to alternative splicing. This means that although humans have only about 30,000 genes, alternative splicing enables them to make far more than 30,000 different polypeptides. Figure 8.20

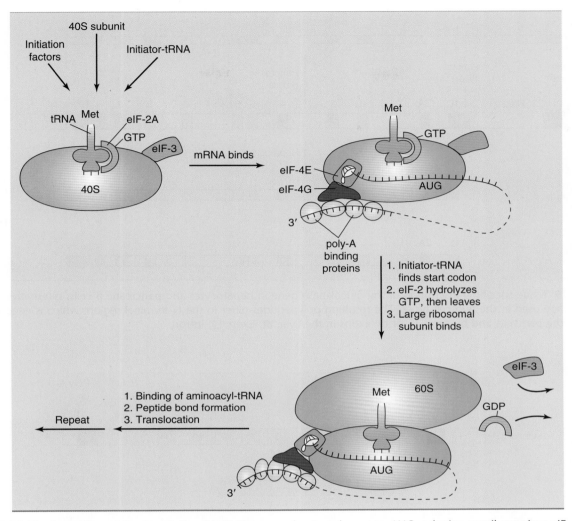

Figure 8.18 The formation of the translational initiation complex in eukaryotes. AUG, adenine-uracil-guanine; eIF, eukaryotic initiation factor.

Table 8.8 Initiation Factors and Elongation Factors of Eukaryotic Protein Synthesis

Eukaryotic Protein	Equivalent Prokaryotic	GTP Hydrolysis	Function
Initiation Factors			
eIF-2A	IF-2	+	Places the initiator-tRNA on the 40S subunit
eIF-2B	—	–	Regenerates the GTP-form of eIF-2A
eIF-3	IF-3	–	Binds 40S subunit, prevents aggregation with 60S subunit
eIF-6	—	–	Binds 60S subunit, prevents aggregation with 40S subunit
eIF-4E	—	–	Cap-binding protein
eIF-4G	—	–	Binds eIF-4A and poly-A binding protein
Elongation Factors			
EF-1α	EF-Tu	+	Places aminoacyl-tRNA in the A site of the ribosome
EF-1βγ	EF-Ts	–	Regenerates the GTP-bound form of EF-1α
EF-2	EF-G	+	Translocation

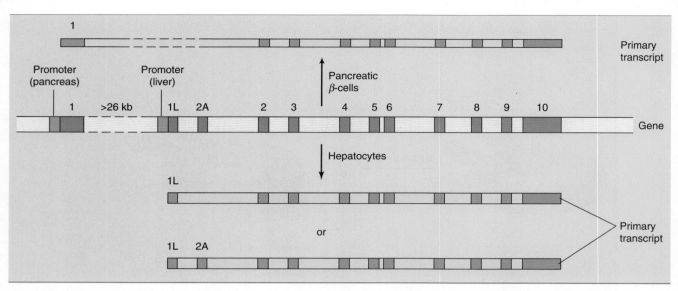

Figure 8.19 Tissue-specific transcription of the glucokinase gene in hepatocytes and pancreatic β cells. Alternative promoters are used in the two cell types. The resulting polypeptides differ in the N-terminal region, which is encoded by exon 1 in the pancreas and by exon 1L or by exons in the liver. ■, Exon; □, intron.

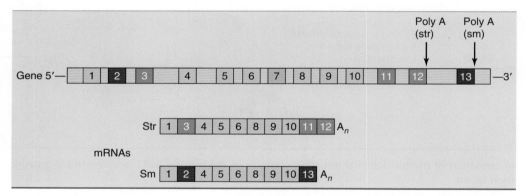

Figure 8.20 The tropomyosin gene is a good example of tissue-specific splicing. Only 10 of the 13 exons are used in striated muscle, and 9 are used in smooth muscle. In this case, alternative polyadenylation signals are used in striated muscle and smooth muscle: Poly A (str) and Poly A (sm).

shows as an example the tissue-specific splicing of the muscle protein tropomyosin.

TRANSLATIONAL REPRESSORS

Ribosomal protein synthesis can be regulated by mRNA-binding proteins. For example, the mRNA of the PABP has an oligo-A tract in its 5′-untranslated region. When PABP is abundant, it binds to this oligo-A tract to prevent its own continued synthesis.

MESSENGER RNA EDITING

In mRNA editing, a base in the mRNA is altered enzymatically. If this creates or obliterates a stop codon, the length of the encoded polypeptide is altered. mRNA editing is rare in mammals, but when it occurs, it can lead to the production of alternative polypeptides from the same gene in different cell types.

Diphtheria Toxin Inhibits Protein Synthesis

Diphtheria is a bacterial infection of the upper respiratory tract that leads to necrosis (death) of mucosal cells and airway obstruction. The offending bacterium, *Corynebacterium diphtheriae*, causes this disease by secreting a toxic protein. This toxin binds to a surface receptor on the mucosal cells

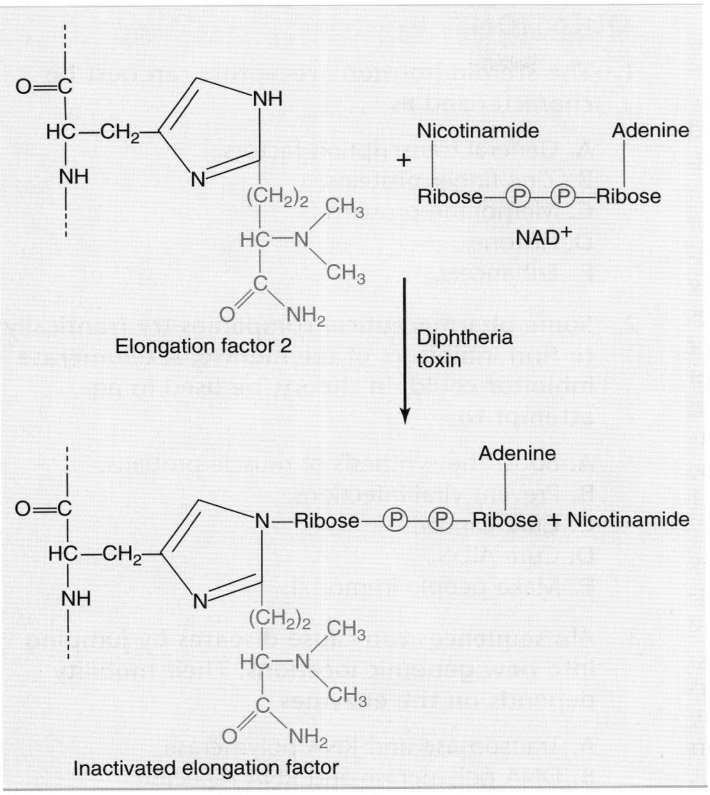

Figure 8.21 Covalent modification of the eukaryotic elongation factor 2 ("translocase") by diphtheria toxin. The amino acid side chain in the elongation factor is diphthamide, a post-translationally modified histidine. NAD+, nicotinamide dinucleotide.

and is then cleaved by a protease, and one of the proteolytic fragments then enters the cell. *This active fragment is an enzyme that inactivates the elongation factor EF-2* (Fig. 8.21). Because the toxin inactivates the elongation factor irreversibly, a single toxin molecule is sufficient to inactivate thousands of EF-2 molecules.

Interestingly, the gene for diphtheria toxin is not a regular denizen of the bacterial chromosome but belongs to a temperate phage that is carried as a prophage in the bacterial genome. Only lysogenic strains of *C. diphtheriae* are pathogenic. Nonlysogenic strains are peaceful members of the normal bacterial flora on human skin and mucous membranes.

Mitochondria Have Their Own DNA

Human mitochondria contain a small circular chromosome with 16,569 base pairs of DNA. Four to ten copies of this chromosome are present in each mitochondrion. It codes for a total of 13 polypeptides, 22 tRNAs, and 2 rRNAs (12S and 16S). The genes are transcribed by a mitochondrial RNA polymerase, and the mRNA is translated by small mitochondrial ribosomes that are more similar to bacterial ribosomes than to human cytoplasmic ribosomes.

The mitochondria have their own protein-synthesizing system because *they are the descendants of symbiotic bacteria*. Once upon a time, more than 1.5 billion years ago, their already aerobic ancestors invaded a eukaryotic cell that had not yet learned the use of oxygen for ATP synthesis. What may have started as an attempt at parasitism soon turned into a peaceful coexistence, and in time the bacteria evolved (or degenerated) into the present-day mitochondria.

One after another most of the original bacterial genes relocated into the nucleus, and for good reason. Oxidative metabolism pollutes the environment with DNA-damaging side products such as superoxide and hydroxyl radicals. Therefore, the nucleus is a safer place for genes than is the mitochondrion. In addition, in the nucleus the genes could profit from the genetic recombination that comes with sexual reproduction. This means that the *human nuclear genome is of hybrid origin, being descended in part from a primordial eukaryote and in part from a symbiotic prokaryote.*

SUMMARY

Eukaryotes have far larger genomes than do prokaryotes, and their DNA is packaged into chromosomes with the help of basic proteins called histones. Both histones and DNA can be modified covalently to regulate gene expression.

Only 1.2% of human nuclear DNA codes for proteins. Human genes are interrupted by noncoding introns that are far longer than the coding exons and are separated from neighboring genes by variable expanses of junk DNA. About 45% of the human genome is formed by the remnants of mobile DNA sequences that are best understood as "molecular parasites." These mobile elements move by retrotransposition, using a reverse transcriptase that is encoded either by L1 elements or by retrovirus-like elements.

Transcription is meticulously regulated by proteins that bind to promoters and other regulatory sites in and around the genes. The mRNA transcripts must be modified by capping, polyadenylation, and the removal of introns before the mature mRNA is allowed to leave the nucleus for translation. Translational initiation is also a complex process, and protein synthesis can be regulated at the level of translation as well as transcription.

📖 Further Reading

Alberts et al: Molecular Biology of the Cell, 4th ed. New York: Garland Science Publishing, 2002, p 203.

Holmberg CI, Tran SEF, Eriksson JE, Sistonen L: Multisite phosphorylation provides sophisticated regulation of transcription factors. Trends Biochem Sci 27:619-627, 2002.

Kazazian HH Jr, Goodier JL: LINE drive: retrotransposition and genome instability. Cell 110:277-280, 2002.

Kraus WL, Wong J: Nuclear receptor-dependent transcription with chromatin. Is it all about enzymes? Eur J Biochem 269:2275-2283, 2002.

Orphanides G, Reinberg D: A unified theory of gene expression. Cell 108:439-451, 2002.

Schmid CW: Alu: a parasite's parasite? Nature Genet 35:15-16, 2003.

Venter JC, Adams MD, Myers EW, et al: The sequence of the human genome. Science 291:1304-1351, 2001.

Woychik NA, Hampsey M: The RNA polymerase II machinery: structure illuminates function. Cell 108:453-463, 2002.

QUESTIONS

1. **The steroid hormone receptors can best be characterized as**

   A. General transcription factors.
   B. Zinc finger proteins.
   C. Membrane proteins.
   D. Histones.
   E. Enhancers.

2. **Some pharmaceutical companies try frantically to find inhibitors of telomerase. A telomerase inhibitor could, in theory, be used in an attempt to**

   A. Boost the synthesis of muscle proteins.
   B. Prevent viral infections.
   C. Cure cancer.
   D. Cure AIDS.
   E. Make people immortal.

3. **Alu sequences can cause diseases by jumping into new genomic locations. Their mobility depends on the enzymes**

   A. Transposase and RNA polymerase.
   B. DNA polymerase and RNA replicase.
   C. Peptidyl transferase and transposase.
   D. Primase and integrase.
   E. RNA polymerase and reverse transcriptase.

4. **Eukaryotic enhancers are**

   A. Regulatory DNA sequences within the coding sequences of genes that affect the rate of transcriptional elongation.
   B. Binding sites for general transcription factors in the promoter.
   C. Proteins that bind to regulatory base sequences in DNA.
   D. DNA sequences outside the promoter region that contain multiple binding sites for regulatory proteins.
   E. Proteins that enhance the rate of translational initiation by binding either to the ribosome or to the mRNA.

5. **In the year 2045, the Surgeon General determines that reverse transcriptase is hazardous to your health because it leads to insertional mutations. In order to eliminate reverse transcriptase from the human body, genetic engineers would have to excise all full-length, intact copies of**

   A. DNA transposons and Alu sequences.
   B. Retroviral retrotransposons and Alu sequences.
   C. L1 elements and Alu sequences.
   D. Pseudogenes and retroviral retrotransposons.
   E. L1 elements and retroviral retrotransposons.

CHAPTER 9

Protein Targeting

The first task of a newborn protein is the formation of its higher order structure. *Most polypeptides fold spontaneously into their proper conformation during translation.* Protein folding is driven by noncovalent interactions between groups in the polypeptide. In some instances, however, helper proteins called **chaperones** assist in the folding process.

The formation of the higher order structure is not always successful. According to one estimate, one third of all newly synthesized proteins fail to fold properly. These misfolded proteins are rapidly degraded.

Next, *covalent modifications are introduced.* Disulfide bridges are formed, and carbohydrate groups and phosphate groups are attached to amino acid side chains. These reactions are collectively called **post-translational processing.**

During or after post-translational processing, *the protein is transported to its proper destination.* At the end of its life cycle, it is degraded by proteases. This chapter traces the fate of eukaryotic proteins from the cradle to the grave.

A Signal Sequence Directs Polypeptides to the Endoplasmic Reticulum

Ribosomes can be found both free-floating in the cytoplasm and attached to the membrane of the rough endoplasmic reticulum (ER), depending on the proteins they make. *Free cytoplasmic ribosomes synthesize the proteins of the cytoplasm, nucleus, and mitochondria. The ER-bound ribosomes synthesize secreted proteins; plasma membrane proteins; and the proteins of the ER, Golgi apparatus, and lysosomes.*

The site of protein synthesis is determined by a **signal sequence:** a highly variable sequence of about 20 to 25 mainly hydrophobic amino acid residues at the amino end of the polypeptide. *If the polypeptide has a signal sequence, it goes to the ER; if not, it remains in the cytosol.*

As soon as it emerges from the ribosome, the signal sequence binds to a cytoplasmic **signal recognition particle (SRP)**. This soluble complex is formed from a small RNA molecule of about 300 nucleotides (the **7SL RNA**) and six protein subunits. *Binding of the SRP halts translation* until the SRP–signal sequence–ribosome complex binds to an **SRP receptor** on the ER membrane (Fig. 9.1).

The SRP receptor brings the ribosome in contact with a **protein translocator,** a donut-shaped protein in the membrane of the rough ER. The tunnel on the large ribosomal subunit from which the growing polypeptide emerges is placed on the central hollow of the protein translocator while the SRP detaches. A pore opens in the translocator, through which the polypeptide is pushed into the lumen of the rough ER.

The signal sequence is no longer required beyond this stage. Before translation is completed, it is cleaved off by a **signal peptidase** on the inner surface of the ER membrane.

Soluble secreted proteins pass through the rough ER and the smooth ER and are then ferried to the Golgi apparatus in transfer vesicles, as shown in Figure 9.2. *The Golgi apparatus is a sorting station in which secreted proteins are packaged into secretory vesicles.* These vesicles are destined to fuse with the plasma membrane and release their contents by **exocytosis.** This system of organelles forms the **secretory pathway.** It is used by all protein-secreting cells in the body (Table 9.1).

While soluble proteins move through the lumen of the organelles, membrane proteins are inserted into the ER membrane and then travel as

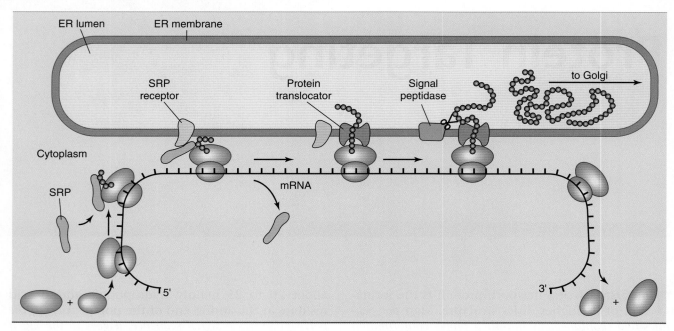

Figure 9.1 The synthesis of a secreted protein by ribosomes on the rough endoplasmic reticulum (ER). The ribosome forms a tight seal on the translocator during translocation, to prevent other molecules from diffusing in and out of the ER while the polypeptide is threaded through the pore. mRNA, messenger RNA; SRP, signal recognition particle.

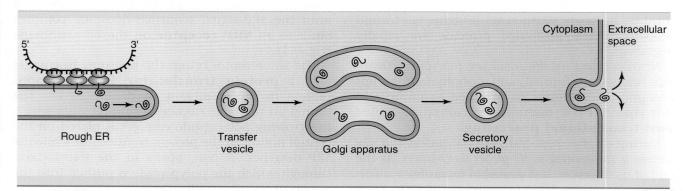

Figure 9.2 The secretory pathway. The proteins are transported to the cell periphery through ER, transfer vesicles, Golgi apparatus, and secretory vesicles. The release from the cell is by exocytosis (fusion of the secretory vesicle membrane with the plasma membrane).

Table 9.1 Use of the Secretory Pathway by Different Cell Types

Cell	Secreted Products	Reference Chapter
Pancreatic acinar cells	Zymogens	Chapter 19
Pancreatic β cells	Insulin, C-peptide	Chapter 16
Fibroblasts	Collagen, elastin, glycoproteins, proteoglycans	Chapter 14
Goblet cells	Glycoproteins ("mucins"), proteoglycans	Chapter 14
Intestinal mucosal cells	Chylomicrons	Chapter 23
Hepatocytes	Serum albumin, other plasma proteins, VLDL	Chapter 15

VLDL, very-low-density lipoprotein.

constituents of the organelle membranes. Proteins of the plasma membrane travel all the way through the secretory pathway, whereas proteins of the ER membrane and the Golgi membrane are retained in their respective organelles.

Table 9.2 Post-translational Processing in the Secretory Pathway

Type of Processing	Examples
Removal of signal sequence	All proteins of the secretory pathway
Disulfide bond formation	Most proteins of the secretory pathway
Glycosylation	Collagen, other glycoproteins, proteoglycans
Amino acid modifications	Collagen, elastin
Partial proteolytic cleavage	Insulin, other peptide and protein hormones

Glycoproteins Are Processed in the Secretory Pathway

This road to the periphery is also an assembly line on which the proteins are modified covalently. The most important types of covalent modification in the secretory pathway are listed in Table 9.2.

Most secreted proteins and membrane proteins are glycoproteins, with oligosaccharides covalently bound to serine, threonine, or asparagine side chains. *The oligosaccharides are synthesized from nucleotide-activated monosaccharide precursors.*

The enzymes that catalyze these reactions are called **glycosyl transferases,** because they transfer the sugar from the nucleotide to the amino acid side chain or the growing oligosaccharide (Figs. 9.3 and 9.4; Table 9.3). The synthesis of the activated sugars is discussed in Chapter 22.

O-linked oligosaccharides are bound to the oxygen in the side chains of serine and threonine.

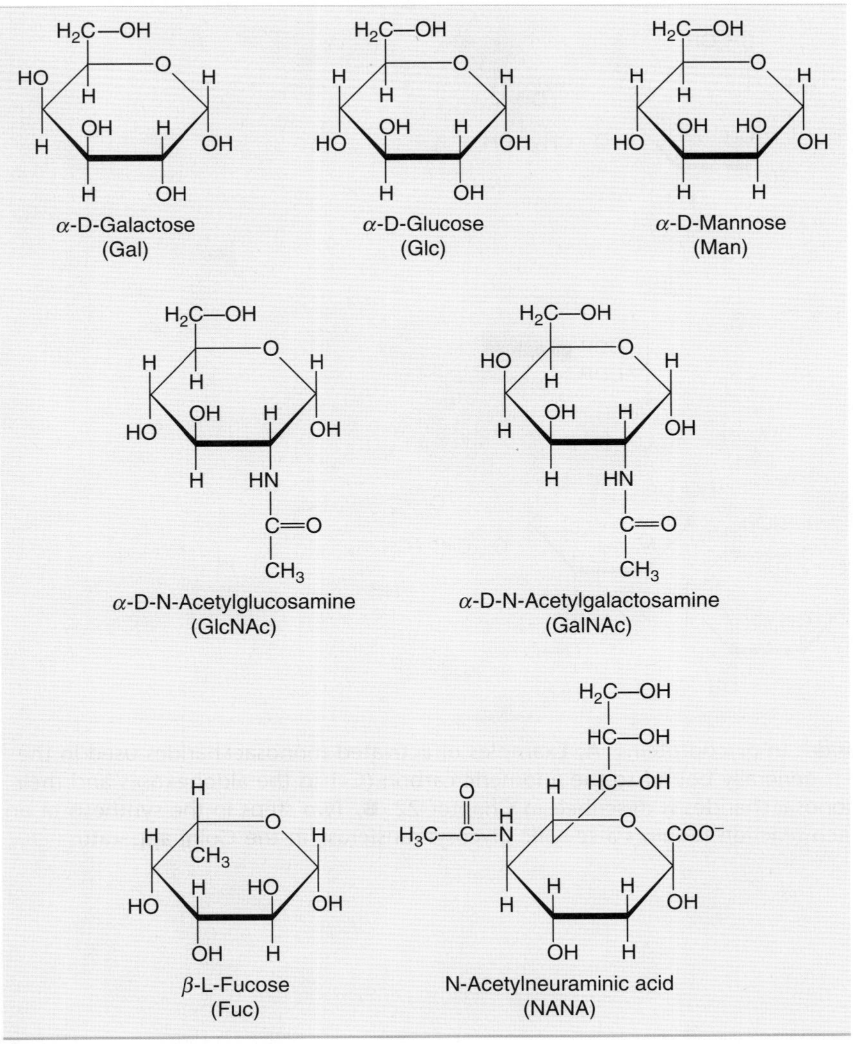

Figure 9.3 The structures of some monosaccharides in glycoproteins.

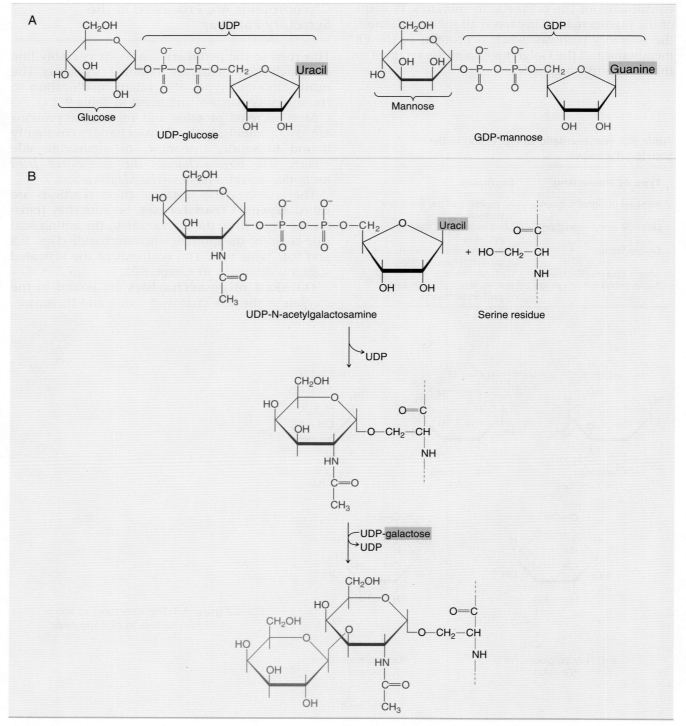

Figure 9.4 Synthesis of *O*-linked oligosaccharides in glycoproteins. **A,** Examples of activated monosaccharides used in the synthesis of oligosaccharides. The nucleotide is generally bound to the anomeric carbon (C-1 in the aldohexoses and their derivatives). The synthesis of the activated monosaccharides is described in Chapter 22. **B,** Two steps in the synthesis of an *O*-linked oligosaccharide in a glycoprotein. Each reaction requires a specific glycosyltransferase in the Golgi apparatus.

Table 9.3 Monosaccharides Commonly Found in Glycoproteins

Monosaccharide	Type	Activated Form	Comments
Galactose (Gal)	Aldohexose	UDP-Gal	Common
Glucose (Glc)	Aldohexose	UDP-Glc	Rare in mature glycoproteins
Mannose (Man)	Aldohexose	GDP-Man	Very common in *N*-linked oligosaccharides
Fucose (Fuc)	6-Deoxyhexose	GDP-Fuc	Both in *O*- and *N*-linked oligosaccharides
N-Acetylglucosamine (GlcNAc)	Amino sugar	UDP-GlcNAc	Linked to asparagine in *N*-linked oligosaccharides
N-Acetylgalactosamine (GalNAc)	Amino sugar	UDP-GalNAc	Common
N-Acetylneuraminic acid (NANA)	A sialic acid (acidic sugar derivative)	CMP-NANA	Often in terminal positions of both *O*- and *N*-linked oligosaccharides

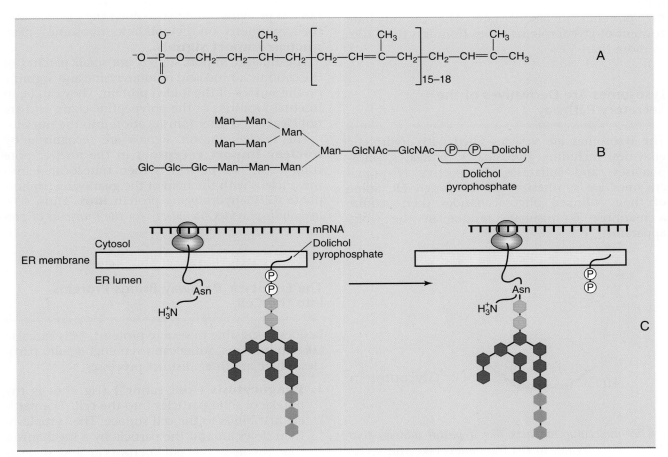

Figure 9.5 Synthesis of *N*-linked oligosaccharides in glycoproteins. **A,** Structure of dolichol phosphate. This lipid is present in the endoplasmic reticulum (ER) membrane, in which it is used as a carrier of the core oligosaccharide. **B,** Structure of the dolichol-bound precursor oligosaccharide in *N*-linked glycosylation. This oligosaccharide is synthesized by the stepwise addition of the monosaccharides from activated precursors. The second phosphate residue in dolichol pyrophosphate is introduced by UDP–α-D-*N*-acetylglucosamine (GlcNAc) during the synthesis of the oligosaccharide. Glc, α-D-glucose; Man, α-D-mannose; P, phosphate. **C,** Transfer of the precursor oligosaccharide to an asparagine side chain of the polypeptide. This transfer reaction is cotranslational. Asn, asparagine; mRNA, messenger RNA.

They are synthesized in the Golgi apparatus by the stepwise addition of monosaccharides.

N-linked oligosaccharides are bound to the nitrogen in the side chain of asparagine. N-*linked glycosylation starts with the construction of a mannose-rich oligosaccharide on* **dolichol phosphate,** a lipid in the membrane of the rough ER. The whole oligosaccharide is then transferred to an asparagine side chain of a newly synthesized polypeptide (Fig. 9.5).

In the ER and Golgi apparatus, the glucose residues and one or more of the mannose residues are removed by exoglycosidases. The remaining core structure is again extended by glycosyl transferases in the Golgi apparatus.

The oligosaccharides of glycoproteins range in size from two sugar residues in the simplest O-linked oligosaccharides to more than 15 in some of the more complex N-linked oligosaccharides. Most are branched, and in many cases the terminal positions are occupied by the acidic amino sugar **N-acetylneuraminic acid** (**NANA**) (see Fig. 9.3).

The oligosaccharides of glycoproteins are important for their biological functions, including the maintenance of their higher order structure, water solubility, and antigenicity and the regulation of the protein's metabolic fate. The carbohydrate content of glycoproteins varies from less than 10% to more than 50%.

Lysosomes Are Derivatives of the Secretory Pathway

The lysosomes are vesicles filled with hydrolytic enzymes, including glycosidases, proteases, phosphatases, and sulfatases. Prospective lysosomal enzymes are synthesized at the rough ER. Some of their N-linked oligosaccharides then acquire a mannose 6-phosphate residue in the Golgi apparatus:

This molecular tag acts like a postal address that directs the enzymes to the lysosomes. Like the secretory vesicles, lysosomes are formed by budding from the Golgi apparatus.

In a rare, recessively inherited condition known as **I cell disease,** one of the enzymes for the attachment of mannose 6-phosphate is deficient. As a result, *the enzymes are not sorted into the lysosomes but secreted.* High levels of lysosomal enzymes circulate in the blood, and undegraded lipids and polysaccharides accumulate in the cells. The accumulation of these products leads to mental deterioration, skeletal deformities, and death between 5 and 8 years of age.

I cell disease is a form of **lysosomal storage disease.** In this group of diseases, nonmetaboliz-

able products accumulate because of an inherited deficiency in one or more lysosomal enzymes.

Nuclear Proteins Possess Their Own Targeting Sequences

The nuclear envelope is riddled with 3000 to 4000 **nuclear pore complexes.** They are freely permeable for small molecules, but large proteins and nucleic acids need permission to pass. RNAs and ribosomal subunits that are exported from the nucleus need **nuclear export signals,** and the nuclear proteins that have to enter the nucleus after their synthesis on cytoplasmic ribosomes need **nuclear import signals.**

The nuclear import signals are small patches of the cationic amino acid residues lysine and arginine on the surface of the folded protein. They can be in internal locations of the polypeptide chain and are not cleaved off after translocation into the nucleus.

The nuclear import signals are recognized by **nuclear import receptors** in the nuclear pore complexes. The protein is then translocated into the nucleus with the help of the guanosine triphosphate (GTP)–hydrolyzing protein **Ran.** Thus, *GTP hydrolysis provides the energy for the transport of proteins into the nucleus.*

The Endocytic Pathway Brings Proteins into the Cell

Besides being able to secrete proteins, cells can also take up proteins. Some can even engulf solid particles. There are three distinct processes:

1. **Phagocytosis** ("cell eating") (Fig. 9.6) is the uptake of solid particles into the cell. The particle first binds to the cell surface. The cytoplasm then flows around the particle by a mechanism that involves the polymerization and depolymerization of actin microfilaments. The phagocytic vacuole thus formed fuses with lysosomes or other intracellular vesicles, and its contents are digested within the cell. Unicellular eukaryotes use phagocytosis for their own nutrition. In the human body, however, the process is limited to professional phagocytes: macrophages, neutrophils, and dendritic cells. These cells protect humans from aberrant cells and microbial invaders. They also engulf inanimate objects, such as dust particles in the lungs and urate crystals in the joints of patients with gout.

2. **Pinocytosis** ("cell drinking") is the nonselective uptake of fluid droplets into the cell.

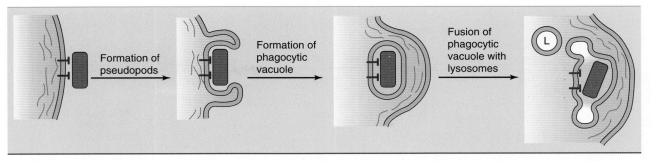

Figure 9.6 Phagocytosis is triggered by the binding of a solid particle to a protein in the plasma membrane that functions as a receptor (T). It requires the reversible depolymerization and repolymerization of actin microfilaments (∽) under the plasma membrane. Pseudopods are formed that flow round the particle. The phagocytic vacuole fuses with lysosomes (L), and the particle is digested by lysosomal enzymes.

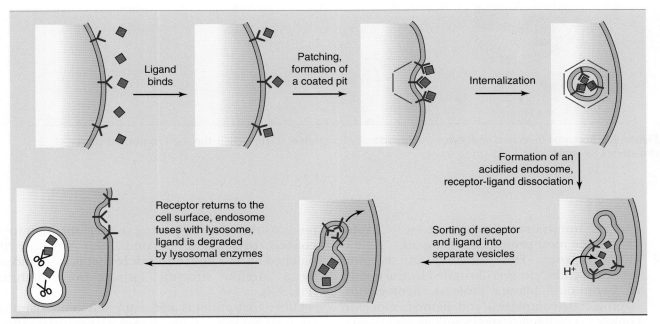

Figure 9.7 Receptor-mediated endocytosis is triggered by the binding of a ligand to a receptor in the plasma membrane. Fusion of the endocytic vesicle with intracellular vesicles creates an acidified endosome.

Pinocytic vesicles contain dissolved substances according to their concentrations in the extracellular medium. Secretory cells use pinocytosis to retrieve the membrane material that is added to the plasma membrane during exocytosis.

3. **Receptor-mediated endocytosis** (Fig. 9.7) is a mechanism for the selective uptake of soluble proteins and other high-molecular-weight materials. *Unlike pinocytosis, it requires a cell surface receptor to which the endocytosed product binds selectively.* Binding is followed by the clustering of receptor-ligand complexes on the cell surface and, finally, by the formation of an endocytic vesicle.

Endocytic vesicles tend to fuse with each other and with intracellular vesicles to form larger structures called **endosomes,** which rapidly become acidified to a pH of about 5.0. Materials can be transferred from the endosome to the Golgi apparatus. More commonly, however, the endosome fuses with a lysosome to form a **secondary lysosome** in which the endocytosed material is digested by lysosomal enzymes. In most but not all cases, the receptor is recycled to the cell surface.

The most important uses of receptor-mediated endocytosis are as follows:

1. *The uptake of nutritive substances.* The uptake of low-density lipoprotein (LDL) (see Chapter 25)

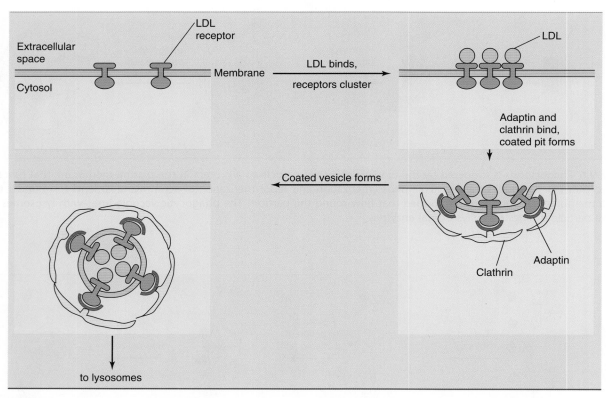

Figure 9.8 Receptor-mediated endocytosis of low-density lipoprotein (LDL). LDL is the most important source of cholesterol for most cells.

and the iron-transferrin complex (see Chapter 29) are the most prominent examples.

2. *Waste disposal.* This function of receptor-mediated endocytosis is illustrated by the uptake of "worn-out" plasma proteins, hemoglobin-haptoglobin complexes, and heme-hemopexin complexes by hepatocytes or reticuloendothelial cells (see Chapter 15). The endocytosed products are digested by lysosomal enzymes.

3. *Mucosal transfer.* Single-layered epithelia can endocytose a protein on one side and exocytose it on the opposite side. This process is called **transcytosis.** The secretion of immuno-globulin A (IgA) across mucosal surfaces (see Chapter 15) is an example.

Endocytosis Is Regulated by Cytoplasmic Proteins

Pinocytosis and receptor-mediated endocytosis are regulated by proteins on the cytoplasmic surface of the vesicle. Receptor-mediated endocytosis is initiated when the cytoplasmic protein **adaptin** is recruited to the plasma membrane by the ligand-bound receptor. The structural protein clathrin then binds to the adaptin, pulling the membrane into a **coated pit.** Within seconds, this structure is pinched off as a **coated vesicle** that is surrounded by a cagelike structure formed from clathrin (Fig. 9.8).

Other coat proteins and many different adaptins are used for other types of vesicular transfer. They regulate the complex trafficking of vesicles and their contents in the intersecting secretory and endocytic pathways.

The Secretory and Endocytic Organelles Are Derived from the Plasma Membrane

Bacteria also secrete proteins. They have no lyso-somes and are therefore unable to digest macro-molecular nutrients inside the cell. They have to secrete their digestive enzymes into the environ-ment and absorb the breakdown products.

Being incapable of phagocytosis, bacteria cannot eat one another. They can only poison each other with secreted toxins and digest each other with secreted enzymes. Pathogenic bacteria secrete enzymes to eat their way through the host tissues,

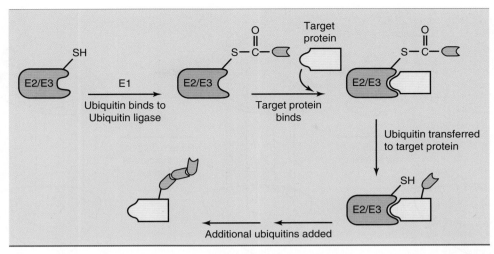

Figure 9.9 The ubiquitination of proteins. The multiubiquitin chain attached by ubiquitin ligase (E2/E3 complex) directs the target protein to the proteasome. There are about 300 distinct E2/E3 complexes in the cell.

regulatory proteins to manipulate host responses, and toxins to poison the cells of the immune system.

The secreted proteins and membrane proteins of bacteria are synthesized by ribosomes that are attached to the plasma membrane. Indeed, bacterial signal sequences can direct nascent polypeptides to the ER membrane in eukaryotic cells. *The organelles of the secretory pathways probably evolved from an infolding of the plasma membrane, and endocytosis, phagocytosis, and lysosomes were added as further refinements.*

ubiquitin ligases recognize the presence of oxidized amino acids in the protein, others recognize the presence of abnormal hydrophobic patches on the surface of partially denatured proteins, and still others recognize sequence motifs that are normally buried in the center of the protein but become exposed in misfolded proteins.

Some ubiquitin ligases recognize intact proteins that are naturally short-lived in the cell, and some even respond to regulatory signals. This means that *the cell can regulate the life spans of distinct classes of proteins.*

Ubiquitin Marks Cellular Proteins for Destruction

Most proteins that are taken into the cell by phagocytosis, pinocytosis, or receptor-mediated endocytosis are degraded by lysosomal enzymes. More selective mechanisms are needed for the degradation of cellular proteins. Specifically, the cell must remove damaged proteins selectively: those that are partially unfolded and those that have been chemically altered.

These worn-out proteins are marked for destruction by **ubiquitin,** a small protein with 76 amino acids. Figure 9.9 shows that ubiquitin is first bound to a **ubiquitin ligase (E2-E3 complex)** by a **ubiquitin-conjugating enzyme (E1).**

There are about 300 distinct ubiquitin ligase complexes present in the cell. *Each ubiquitin ligase targets a different kind of structurally aberrant protein.* Some

The Proteasome Degrades Ubiquitinated Proteins

Whereas the ubiquitin ligases are the judges that condemn a protein to death, the **proteasome** is the executioner. It consists of a hollow cylinder whose inner surface is lined with proteases and that has a large cap on both sides (Fig. 9.10). The cap scavenges ubiquitinated proteins, denatures them with the help of ATP hydrolysis, and feeds them into the hollow cylinder for degradation.

Proteasomes are abundant in the cell. They are found both in the cytoplasm and the nucleus, and they constitute about 1% of the total cellular protein. The ER contains no proteasomes, but misfolded and damaged proteins can be retrotranslocated from the ER lumen to the cytoplasm, where they are degraded by the ubiquitin-proteasome system.

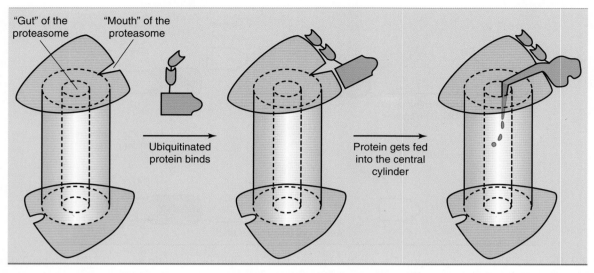

Figure 9.10 The proteasome. The cover on the hollow cylinder recognizes ubiquitinated proteins, denatures them, and feeds them into the central cavity, in which they are degraded by proteases.

SUMMARY

The formation of the peptide bonds by the ribosome is only a first step in protein synthesis. The newly synthesized proteins have to fold themselves into their proper higher order structure during translation, and this is followed by post-translational modifications such as disulfide bond formation, glycosylation, and phosphorylation.

Secreted proteins and proteins of the ER, Golgi apparatus, plasma membrane, and lysosomes have a signal sequence at their amino end that directs them to the rough ER. Their post-translational processing takes place mainly in the ER and Golgi apparatus.

Cellular proteins are marked for destruction by the attachment of the small protein ubiquitin. The ubiquitinated proteins are then fed into the proteasome. This mechanism preferentially removes abnormal proteins and those that are naturally short-lived in the cell.

QUESTIONS

1. **A signal sequence has to be expected in the precursors of all the following proteins *except***

    A. Ribosomal proteins.
    B. The sodium-potassium ATPase in the plasma membrane.
    C. Collagen in the extracellular matrix of connective tissues.
    D. Signal peptidase.
    E. Acid maltase, a lysosomal hydrolase.

2. **The deficiency of a ubiquitin ligase can potentially result in**

    A. The abnormal accumulation of ubiquitin in the cell.
    B. Failure to direct lysosomal proteins to the lysosomes.
    C. The excessive breakdown of some classes of proteins.
    D. The buildup of abnormal proteins in the cells.
    E. An increased mutation rate.

CHAPTER 10

Introduction to Genetic Diseases

The human body is a clone of cells that are descended from the fertilized ovum, or the zygote. Because the zygote is formed from egg and sperm, each with a complete set of genes, human genes are present in two copies. Human bodies are **diploid,** whereas human gametes are **haploid.** In all, human somatic cells have 22 pair of **auto-somes** (non–sex chromosomes) and one pair of **sex chromosomes:** XX in females and XY in males.

Thus, in theory, one half of human genes *should* be identical to genes in the father and the other half *should* be identical to genes in the mother, and the genes *should* be identical in all cells of the body. In reality, however, they are not. Maintaining a bloated genome of 3 billion base pairs is such a formidable task that errors are unavoidable. These errors are called **mutations,** and they are a major cause of disease and disability.

Somatic mutations can produce cells with reduced viability or impaired function. *They accumulate with age and contribute to normal aging.* The most dangerous somatic mutations, however, are those that cause the cell to grow out of control. *Mutations of this type cause cancer* (which is responsible for 20% of all deaths in the modern world). This implies that *all mutagenic agents are carcinogenic.*

Germline mutations arise in the gametes or their diploid ancestors in the gonads. They are transmitted to the offspring and can cause genetic diseases.

This chapter introduces the various types of mutation and the DNA repair systems that the body employs to protect itself against mutations, and it presents the hemoglobinopathies as examples of genetic diseases with well-understood pathogeneses.

Mutations Are an Important Cause of Poor Health

According to one estimate, at least one new muta-tion can be expected to occur in each round of cell division, even in cells with unimpaired DNA repair and in the absence of external mutagens.

As a result, *every child is born with an estimated 100 to 200 new mutations that were not present in the parents.* Most of these mutations change only one or a few base pairs, and a large majority is in the junk DNA, in which they cause no damage. They only create DNA diversity that can be used for DNA fingerprinting, paternity testing, and phylogenetic studies.

However, *an estimated one or two new mutations are "mildly detrimental."* This means they are not bad enough to cause a disease on their own, but they can impair physiological functions to some extent, and they can contribute to multifactorial diseases. Finally, *about 1 per 50 infants is born with a diagnos-able genetic condition that can be attributed to a single major mutation.*

Children are, on average, a little sicker than their parents because they have new mutations on top of those inherited from the parents. This **mutational load** is kept in check by **natural selection.** In most traditional societies, almost half of all children used to die before they had a chance to reproduce. Investigators can only guess that those who died had, on average, more "mildly detrimental" muta-tions than those who survived.

There Are Four Types of Genetic Disease

According to the type of mutation and its clinical expression, four types of genetic disease can be distinguished:

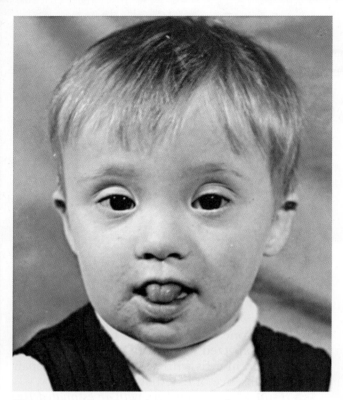

Figure 10.1 The physical appearance of a patient with Down syndrome. This disorder is characterized by moderately severe mental deficiency combined with physical stigmata.

1. **Aneuploidy** is an aberration in chromosome number, caused by the faulty segregation of chromosomes either during meiosis or during mitosis in the germline. About 1 in 400 infants is born aneuploid. In **trisomy 21,** for example (**Down syndrome**) (Fig. 10.1), one of the smallest autosomes is present in three rather than the usual two copies. Presumably the proteins that are encoded by the 225 genes on chromosome 21 are 50% overproduced in these patients.

2. **Chromosomal rearrangements** are caused by chromosome breakage, sometimes followed by a failed attempt at repair. They can also be caused by recombination between mispaired chromosomes during meiosis. For example, in large **deletions,** part of a chromosome is lost, and in **translocations,** part of a chromosome has been transferred to another chromosome. *Those chromosomal rearrangements that change the copy number of genes usually cause disease, whereas those that do not are usually asymptomatic.* About 1 per 1000 infants is born with a symptomatic chromosomal rearrangement.

3. **Single-gene disorders,** also known as **mendelian disorders** because of their predictable inheritance pattern, are caused by small

mutations that affect only a single gene. Therefore, the signs and symptoms of the disease can be attributed to a single faulty protein. **Dominant diseases** are expressed in heterozygotes, who carry a single copy of the mutation, and **recessive diseases** are expressed only in homozygotes, who have the mutation in both copies of the gene. Severe dominant diseases are often caused by a new mutation, whereas recessive mutations can be passed through many generations of unaffected carriers before they cause disease in a homozygote.

4. **Multifactorial disorders** are caused not by a single major mutation but by a constellation of environmental and genetic risk factors. *Most of the common diseases that the general practitioner sees, from allergies to diabetes, are multifactorial.* Even the susceptibility to infectious diseases, from herpes simplex to tuberculosis and polio, is known to be influenced by the patient's genetic constitution.

Both mutational load and common genetic polymorphisms can contribute to the risk of a multifactorial disorder. **Polymorphisms** are "normal" genetic variants that are fairly common in the population. For example, the susceptibility to autoimmune diseases is influenced by normal polymorphisms that regulate immune defenses. Presumably the variants that favor specific kinds of autoimmune disease are common in the population because they also protect people from specific kinds of infectious disease.

Many genetic diseases are not inherited, but arise through new mutations. The risk for these diseases increases with parental age. The children of older fathers have an increased risk of small mutations that cause single-gene disorders and multifactorial disease. These mutations arise as replication errors in the spermatogonia. The children of older mothers have an increased risk for aneuploidy.

A Change in the Base Sequence of DNA Can Change the Amino Acid Sequence of the Encoded Polypeptide

A **point mutation** is a change in a single base pair of the DNA. It is called **transition** if a purine is replaced by another purine or a pyrimidine by another pyrimidine, and **transversion** if a purine is replaced by a pyrimidine or a pyrimidine by a purine.

If it occurs in the coding sequence of a gene, *the most common consequence of a point mutation is a single amino acid substitution in the polypeptide.* Some amino acid substitutions leave the biological functions of the protein intact, but others destroy them either partially or completely. For example:

```
-ACA-TTA-CGC-        -ACA-TCA-CGC-
-Thr-Leu -Arg-   →   -Thr -Ser  -Arg-
```

Because of the degeneracy of the genetic code, some point mutations produce a codon that still codes for the same amino acid. **Silent mutations** of this kind are asymptomatic and can be identified only by DNA sequencing. For example:

```
-ACA-TTA-CGC-        -ACA-CTA-CGC-
-Thr -Leu -Arg-      -Thr -Leu -Arg-
```

A **nonsense mutation** generates a stop codon. *It causes the premature termination of translation,* usually with the complete loss of function in the truncated protein. For example:

```
-ACA-TTA-CGC-        -ACA-TAA-CGC-
-Thr -Leu -Arg-      -Thr -Stop . . . . .
```

Small **deletions** and **insertions** of one or two base pairs in the coding sequence of a gene amounts to a **frameshift mutation.** Beyond the site of the mutation the mRNA is translated in the wrong reading frame, which produces a garbled amino acid sequence. The protein product is most likely nonfunctional. For example:

```
-CTC-ATC-GGA-CTT-        -CTC-TCG-GAC-TT-
-Leu -Ile -Gly -Leu-     -Leu -Ser  -Asp- . . .
```

However, the insertion or deletion of three base pairs, or any multiple of three, does not result in a frameshift.

Splice-site mutations change an intron-exon junction or the branch site within the intron. They cause abnormal splicing and the synthesis of an abnormal protein.

Promoter mutations, as well as mutations in other regulatory sites, leave the structure of the polypeptide intact but change its rate of synthesis.

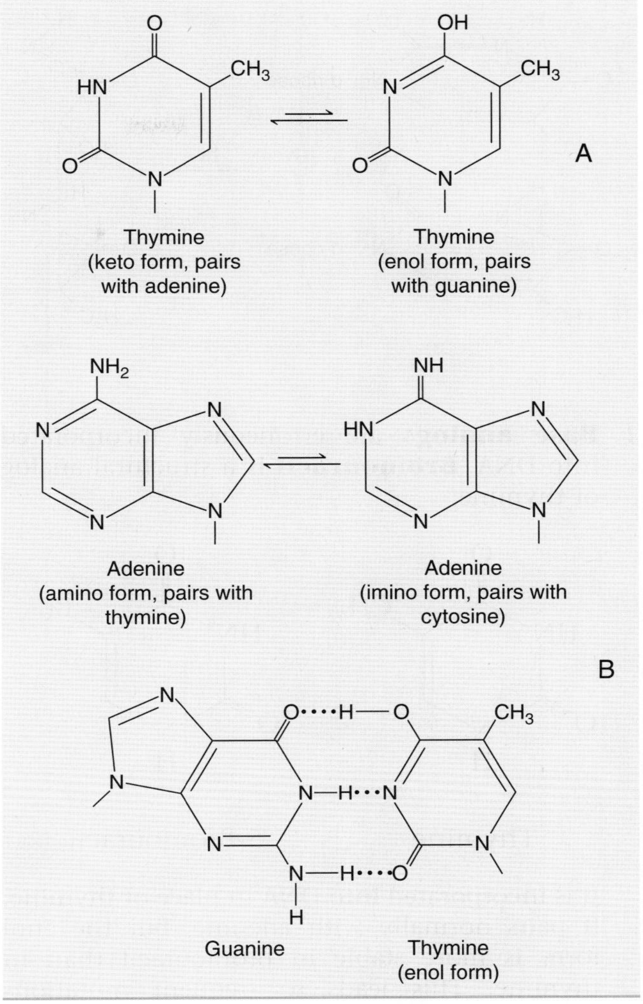

Mutations Can Be Induced by Radiation and Chemicals

The **basal mutation rate,** which is observed in the absence of environmental mutagens, is caused mainly by errors during DNA replication. Spontaneous **tautomeric shifts** in the bases contribute to these errors. Thymine, for example, normally is present in the keto form and pairs with adenine. Very rarely, however, it shifts spontaneously to the enol form, which pairs with guanine. If a thymine in the template strand happens to be in the rare enol form at the moment of DNA replication, G instead of A is incorporated in the new strand.

Similarly, adenine has a rare imino form that pairs with cytosine rather than thymine (Fig. 10.2). Fortunately, these bases spend very little time in their less stable forms; thus, mutations caused by tautomeric shifts are rare.

Figure 10.2 Spontaneous tautomeric shifts of DNA bases as a cause of point mutations. **A,** Alternative structures of thymine and adenine. **B,** A base pair between guanine and the enol form of thymine.

Radiation is an important environmental cause of mutations. **Ionizing radiation,** including **x-rays** and **radioactive radiation,** is sufficiently energy rich to displace electrons from their orbits, creating unstable intermediates that react with the DNA. **DNA double-strand breaks** are the most important type of damage caused by ionizing radiation. *Ionizing radiation penetrates the whole body and can therefore cause both somatic and germline mutations.*

Ultraviolet radiation is a normal component of sunlight. It cannot penetrate beyond the outer layers of the skin, but it can nevertheless form **pyrimidine dimers** from adjacent pyrimidine bases (Fig. 10.3). Therefore, *sunlight is mutagenic,* causing both sunburn and skin cancer.

Many chemicals are also mutagenic:

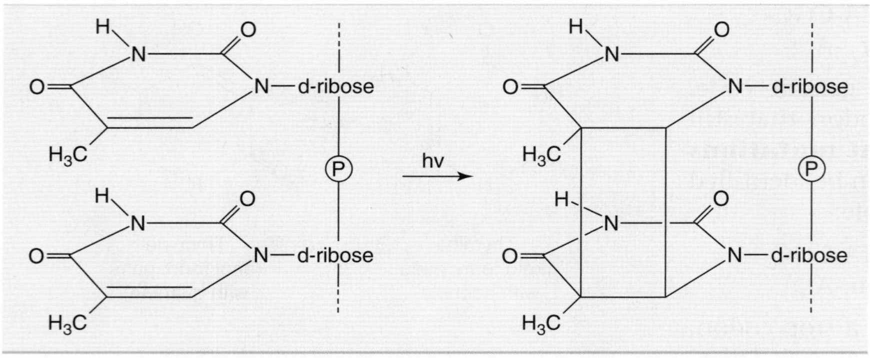

Figure 10.3 Formation of a thymine dimer by ultraviolet radiation. Note that the two thymine residues are in the same strand of the double helix.

1. **Base analogs** are erroneously incorporated into DNA. **Bromouracil** is a structural analog of thymine:

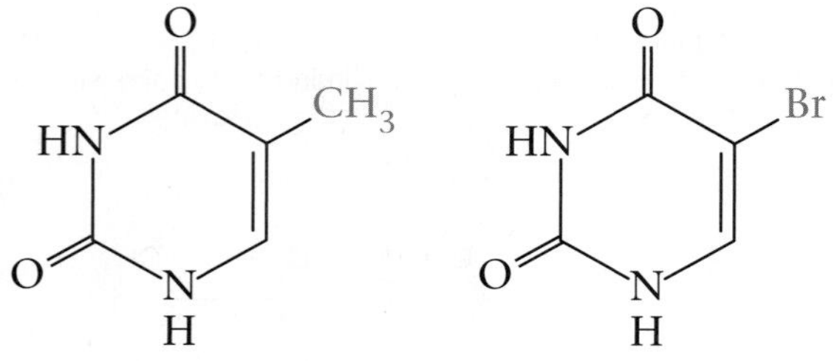

Thymine   5-Bromouracil

It is incorporated into DNA in place of thymine. It pairs normally with adenine, but the enol form is more stable in bromouracil than in thymine. This leads to frequent mutations through spontaneous tautomeric shifts.

2. **Alkylating agents** attach alkyl groups to nitrogen or oxygen atoms in the bases. Examples:

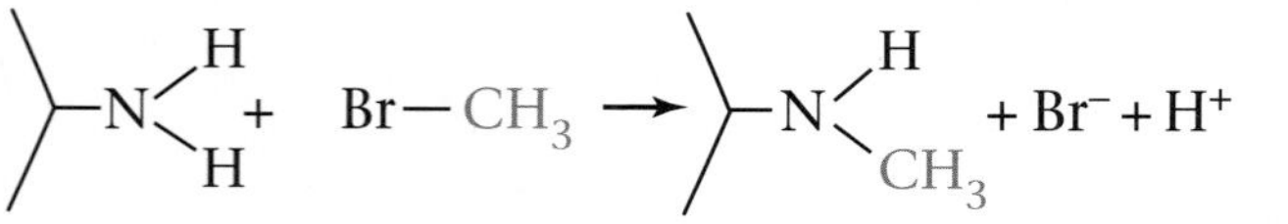

Methyl bromide

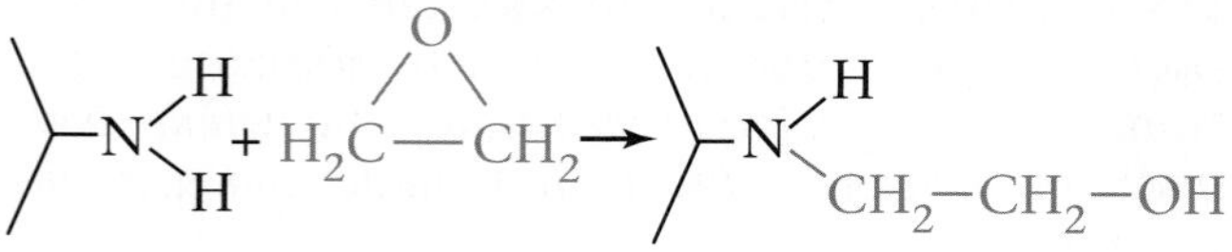

Ethylene oxide

Methyl bromide was used as a grain fumigant before it was banned for this use because of its carcinogenic properties; ethylene oxide is used for the sterilization of surgical instruments.

3. **Deaminating agents** turn the bases adenine, guanine, and cytosine into hypoxanthine, xanthine, and uracil, respectively. These bases make aberrant base pairing and lead to errors during DNA replication (Fig. 10.4).

4. **Intercalating agents** are planar fused-ring structures that insert themselves between the stacked DNA bases, causing frameshift mutations during DNA replication (Fig. 10.5).

DNA damage must be repaired before the S phase in order to prevent fixation of an irreversible mutation when the DNA is replicated. Therefore, *mutagens are most mutagenic during the S phase of the cell cycle.*

The use of radiation for cancer treatment is based on this principle. Because the cancer cells are the most rapidly dividing cells in the irradiated area, they are most likely to be in S phase when the mutagenic radiation is applied.

Mismatch Repair Is Coupled to DNA Replication

Base substitutions are the most common errors during DNA replication, and small insertions and deletions are important as well. To repair such damage, the repair enzymes have to proceed like a plumber who replaces a damaged piece of pipe: *identify the damage, remove the damaged part, and replace it with a good part.*

The biggest problem in the repair of replication errors is the distinction between the old template strand and the newly synthesized strand. The mismatch-recognizing component of the system is located at the replication fork, where it scans the newly synthesized DNA for mismatches. The new strand is distinguished from the old by the presence of frequent nicks. In the lagging strand, the nicks are present from the beginning, until the Okazaki fragments are sealed by DNA ligase, but even the leading strand is known to have occasional nicks.

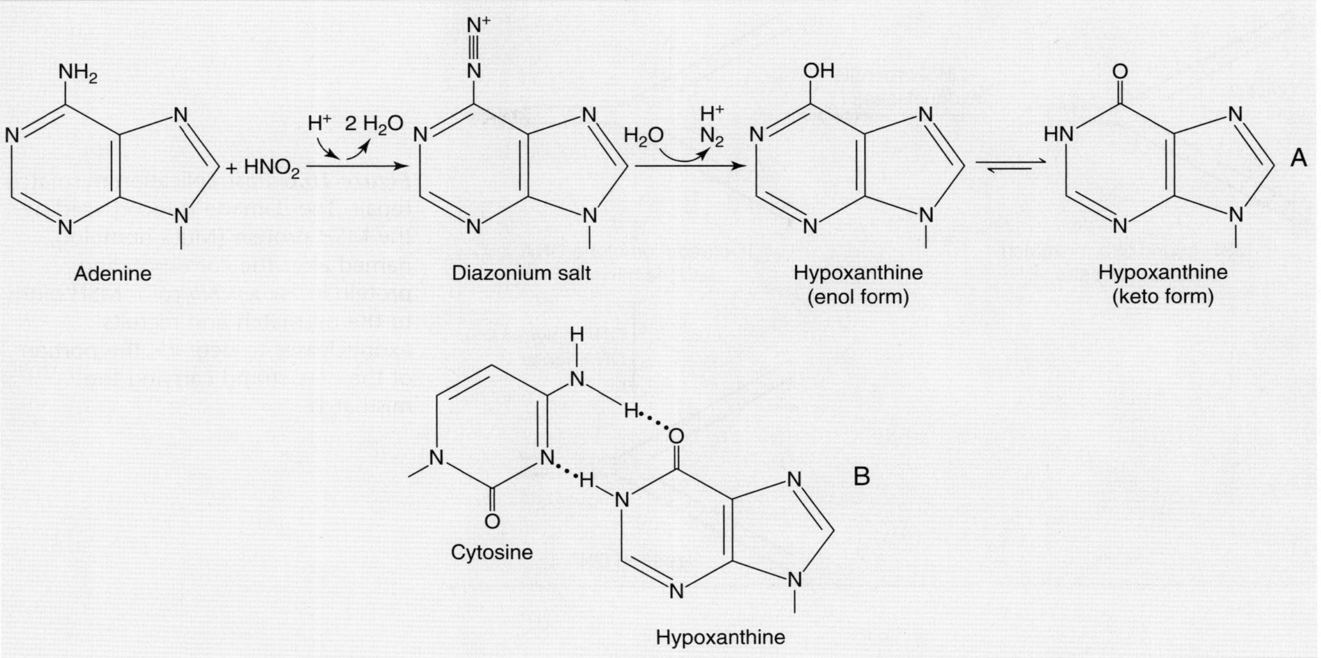

Figure 10.4 The action of a deaminating agent. HNO$_2$ can be formed from dietary nitrates in the intestine. **A,** The reaction of nitrous acid with adenine. **B,** Hypoxanthine pairs with cytosine instead of thymine.

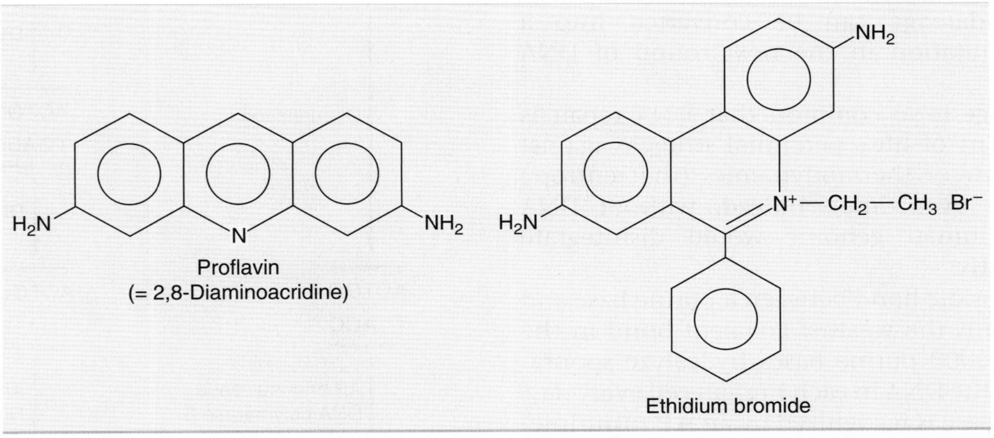

Figure 10.5 Structures of intercalating agents. These planar ring systems cause frameshift mutations by inserting themselves between the DNA bases.

The mismatch repair system recruits exonucleases to the nicks that are closest to the damage. The exonucleases remove the damaged piece, and this sets the stage for DNA polymerase and DNA ligase to fill the gap and connect the loose ends (Fig. 10.6). **Hereditary nonpolyposis colon cancer (HNPCC)** is a dominantly inherited cancer susceptibility syndrome that accounts for 2% to 3% of all colon cancers. Affected individuals have an 80% chance of developing colon cancer by the age of 65, and they are also at increased risk for tumors of the endometrium, ovary, stomach, and small intestine. *These patients are born with a heterozygous deficiency in one or another component of the mismatch repair system.* Their cells can still repair mismatches because they have an intact backup copy of the gene. On occasion, however, a somatic cell loses this backup copy through a random mutation and becomes unable to perform mismatch repair.

This does not matter for nondividing cells such as neurons, but *any dividing cell with a homozygous inactivation of postreplication mismatch repair develops a mutator phenotype.* The mutation rate is increased about 100-fold. Most of these cells gradually mutate to their death, but on occasion, one of them mutates into a cancer cell. Mismatch repair defects lead mainly to cancer in the colon mucosa because of the high mitotic rate of this tissue.

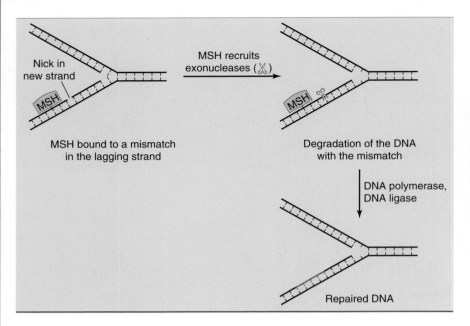

Figure 10.6 Postreplication mismatch repair. The damage is recognized by the MSH protein (MutS homolog, named after the corresponding protein in *Escherichia coli*). MSH binds to the mismatch and recruits exonucleases to degrade the portion of the new strand carrying the mismatch.

Damaged DNA Can Be Repaired

Replication errors arise only in dividing cells, but even resting cells suffer chemical damage to their DNA. Such damage can be converted into a permanent mutation in the next round of DNA replication.

DNA damage is so common that DNA repair is required as part of life's perennial struggle against the second law of thermodynamics (that entropy tends to rise over time). Indeed, without DNA repair, the human genome would disintegrate almost instantly.

The *N*-glycosidic bond between a purine base and 2-deoxyribose is the weakest covalent bond in the DNA. About 5000 purine bases hydrolyze spontaneously from the DNA in each human cell every day. This loss of a base is recognized by an **AP (ap**urinic) **endonuclease** that cleaves the phosphodiester bond on one side of the baseless nucleotide. The other phosphodiester bond is cleaved by DNA polymerase β, which also fills the resulting gap. This is followed by DNA ligase (Fig. 10.7).

Base Excision Repair Removes Abnormal Bases

Base excision repair is designed for the removal of abnormal bases. The key enzymes are **DNA glycosylases,** which recognize the abnormal base and cleave its bond with 2-deoxyribose. There are many different DNA glycosylases for deaminated, alkylated, and oxidized bases and for bases with opened rings or other kinds of damage.

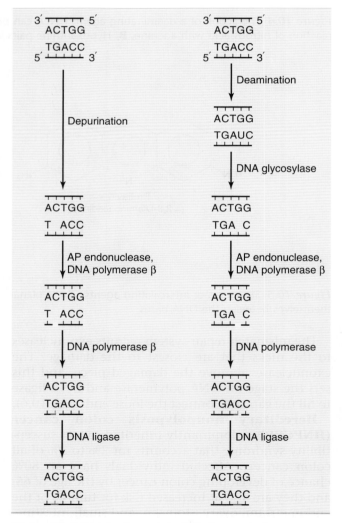

Figure 10.7 Repair of apurinic (AP) sites and of deaminated cytosine (uracil).

For example, in each cell, about 100 cytosine residues in the DNA are deaminated to uracil every day. Being recognized as an abnormal base, uracil is removed by a DNA glycosylase. The baseless site created by this enzyme is then recognized by AP endonuclease, and the remaining steps are identical to the repair of apurinic sites (see Fig. 10.7).

The advantage of having thymine rather than uracil in DNA is evident. If DNA contained uracil, the deamination of cytosine could not be recognized by the repair enzymes, and the mutation rate would be unpleasantly high.

The mutation rate is indeed unpleasantly high for 5-methylcytosine residues. Chapter 8 showed that the methylation of the cytosine in a CG sequence is an important mechanism for gene silencing. The deamination of methylcytosine produces thymine, which is a normal DNA base and therefore not removed by base excision repair:

5-Methylcytosine   Thymine

For this reason, CG sequences in and around genes are important **mutational hot spots.**

Nucleotide Excision Repair Removes Bulky Lesions

Nucleotide excision repair is designed for lesions that are bulky enough to distort the geometry of the DNA double helix: pyrimidine dimers and other photoproducts, adducts formed by the covalent binding of large foreign molecules to DNA, and some alkylated bases.

The components of the nucleotide excision repair system form a "repair crew" that scans the DNA, recognizes the lesion, and removes a piece of about 25 nucleotides from the damaged strand. The resulting gap is filled by a DNA polymerase and DNA ligase (Fig. 10.8).

Defects in one or another component of this system lead to **xeroderma pigmentosum (XP)**. Patients with this recessively inherited condition cannot repair sunlight-induced DNA damage in the skin. They present at an early age with numerous freckles and ulcerative lesions on sun-exposed skin. Skin cancer develops at multiple sites early in life, and the only effective treatment for this otherwise fatal disease is the complete avoidance of sunlight.

Seven subtypes of XP have been identified in different patients, each caused by the deficiency of a different polypeptide in the repair system.

One variant of nucleotide excision repair is recruited to the DNA by the transcriptional machinery, and therefore it repairs only transcribed genes. This type of repair is important in terminally differentiated cells such as neurons. Unlike the cells in the germinal layer of the epidermis that are ravaged by XP, neurons are not destined to replicate and differentiate into other cell types.

Recessively inherited defects in this type of nucleotide excision repair lead to **Cockayne syndrome (CS)**. There is not much photosensitivity and no increased cancer risk in this condition, but the patients present with growth retardation, neurological degeneration, a wizened appearance, and early senility. CS comes in two types that are caused by deficiencies of two different gene products.

The neurological degeneration and early senility in CS show that *the preferential repair of transcribed genes is important for the maintenance of nondividing end-stage cells that cannot be replaced once they are fatally injured by a mutation in an important gene.*

The Repair of DNA Double-Strand Breaks Is Difficult

DNA double-strand breaks are dangerous because they can lead to major chromosomal rearrangements. *Human cells can repair double-strand breaks by homologous recombination,* as shown in Figure 10.9. The problem with this mechanism is that the repair enzymes have to find the corresponding sequence on the homologous chromosome, which is not an easy task in a nucleus with a diploid genome of 6 billion base pairs.

Therefore, *many double-strand breaks are repaired by nonhomologous mechanisms instead.* These repair systems can avert the disaster of a major chromosomal rearrangement, but they are likely to create a "scar" by inserting or deleting a few bases where the ends of the broken DNA are joined. Thus, they are mutagenic. The repair systems for DNA double-strand breaks and related types of DNA damage are still incompletely known, and in many cases the only clues come from patients with clinically defined chromosome breakage syndromes (Table 10.1).

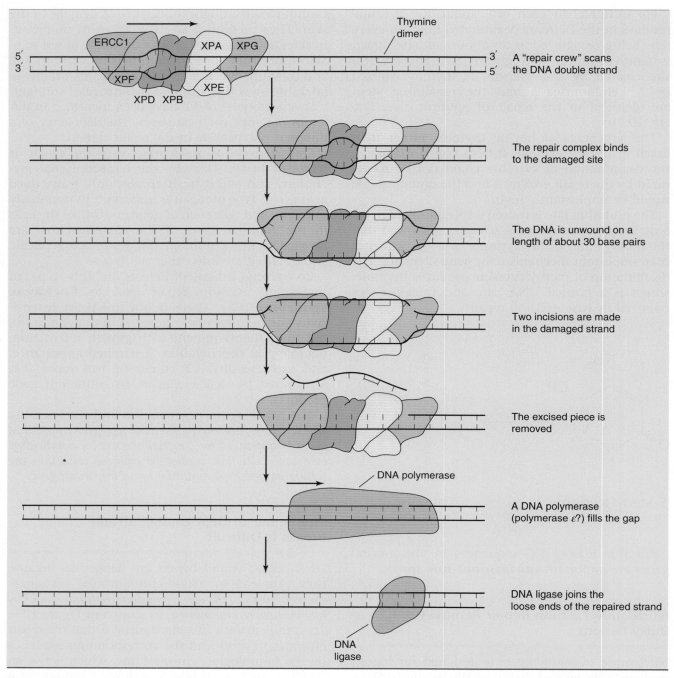

Figure 10.8 The hypothetical sequence of events during the excision repair of a thymine dimer in humans. The repair complex may contain more than a dozen different polypeptides. Some of them *(XPB, XPD)* have helicase activity; others recognize the damage *(XPA, XPE)* or act as endonucleases *(XPG, ERCC1/XPF)*. The "XP" in the names of many of the repair proteins stands for "xeroderma pigmentosum," a disease that is caused by defects of excision repair proteins. Each XP protein is related to a different subtype ("complementation group") of this disease.

Many Genes Are Not Essential for Life

Scientists do not know the functions of every one of the 30,000 human genes, but the mere fact that a gene exists is bona fide evidence that it is good for something. If a gene were good for nothing, it would have mutated out of existence long ago.

The importance of a gene can be determined with **knockout mice.** These genetically modified animals are lacking one or both copies of a gene, and their abnormalities allow conclusions about the normal functions of the gene. One surprising finding is that in more than half the cases that have been examined, mice with a homozygous deletion

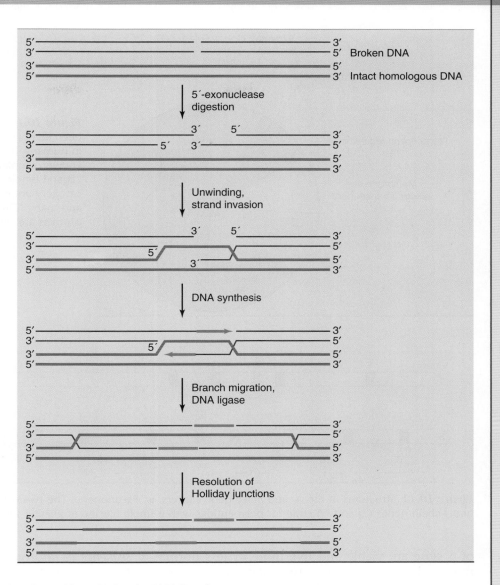

Figure 10.9 A hypothetical mechanism for the repair of DNA double-strand breaks by homologous recombination. This mechanism is similar to the one described in Figure 7.16.

Table 10.1 Inherited Diseases That Are Caused by a Defect in DNA Repair.

Disease	Clinical Manifestation	Type of Protein Affected	Affected Function
Xeroderma pigmentosum	Cutaneous photosensitivity	Proteins of nucleotide excision repair	Genome-wide nucleotide excision repair
Cockayne syndrome	Poor growth, neurological degeneration, early senility	Proteins of nucleotide excision repair	Transcription-coupled nucleotide excision repair
Hereditary nonpolyposis colon cancer	Cancer susceptibility	Proteins of mismatch repair	Postreplication mismatch repair
Ataxia-telangiectasia	Motor incoordination, immune deficiency, chromosome breaks, lymphomas	Protein kinase activated by DNA double-strand breaks	Cell cycle arrest after DNA breakage
Bloom syndrome	Poor growth, butterfly rash, immunodeficiency, cancer susceptibility, chromosome breaks	DNA helicase	Recombinational repair?
Werner syndrome	Early senility	DNA helicase and exonuclease	Unknown
Fanconi anemia	Anemia, leukemia, skeletal deformities, chromosome breakage	Heterogeneous, at least 8 different proteins	Repair of DNA crosslinks?
Breast cancer susceptibility	Breast and ovarian cancer	BRCA1, interacts with repair enzymes	Recombinational repair, transcription-coupled repair of oxidative damage
Spinocerebellar ataxia	Motor incoordination	Heterogeneous	Repair of DNA single-strand break

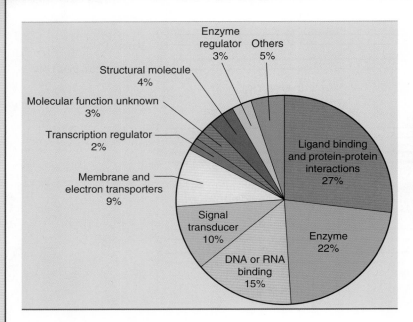

Figure 10.10 The functions of proteins that have been identified as targets of single-gene disorders in humans. In many cases, the functions are not known completely. Thus, many proteins in the "ligand binding and protein-protein interactions" category are in all likelihood signal transducers, and many "DNA and nucleic acid binding" proteins are probably transcriptional regulators.

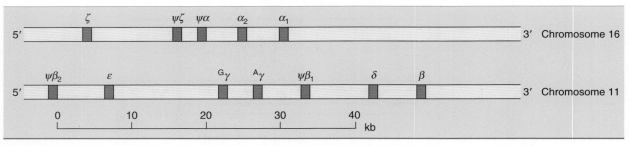

Figure 10.11 Structures of the α- and β-like gene clusters. ψ, Pseudogene. The two α-chain genes are identical, and the two γ-chain genes (Gγ and Aγ) code for polypeptides with a single glycine or alanine substitution, respectively.

of a gene are viable and live more or less normal murine lives. This means that *most genes are not essential for life,* and in many cases the defects that arise from a complete lack of the gene are too subtle to be recognized by simple inspection.

Knockout humans have not been created intentionally so far, but Nature creates knockout humans all the time, in the form of patients with genetic diseases. As in knockout mice, the phenotypes range all the way from minimal impairment to a failure of early embryonic development.

Figure 10.10 gives an overview over the types of protein that have been identified as mutated in genetic diseases. The overall composition is quite similar to the composition of the human proteome. The **proteome** is the sum total of the proteins produced by the organism, in the same sense that the genome is the sum total of its DNA. The large proportion of known or suspected regulatory proteins and signal transducers is a typical feature of all multicellular eukaryotes.

Not all deviations from the "normal" state cause disease. It has been estimated that *the coding sequence of an average protein-coding gene has about four single-nucleotide polymorphisms* with a population frequency of more than 1% for the less common allele. Most of these variations do not lead to disease. If they did, they would be removed by natural selection and would not occur at such high frequencies in the population.

Hemoglobin Genes Are Present in Two Gene Clusters

Abnormalities in the structure or synthesis of hemoglobin, known collectively as **hemoglobinopathies,** are among the most common genetic diseases worldwide. Figure 10.11 shows that hemoglobin genes are found in two clusters: α-like genes on chromosome 16, and β-like genes on chromosome 11. Besides the α, β, γ, and δ chain genes already described in Chapter 3, these clusters also contain genes for embryonic hemoglobins: the α-like ζ chain and the β-like ε chain. Both gene clusters also contain pseudogenes.

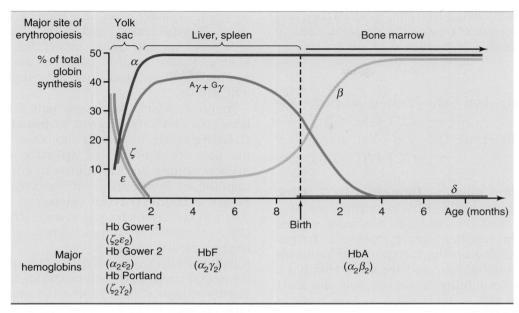

Figure 10.12 Synthesis of globin chains during different stages of development. Hb, hemoglobin; HbA, adult hemoglobin; HbF, fetal hemoglobin.

Interestingly, *humans have two identical α-chain genes, both of which contribute to similar extents to the overall production of α chains.* There are also two very similar γ chain genes: the ^{A}γ gene and the ^{G}γ gene, whose products differ only by the presence of either alanine or glycine in one of the amino acid positions.

Figure 10.12 shows the expression of the hemoglobin genes during prenatal and postnatal development. Whereas ε and ζ chains are limited to the early embryonic stage, α and γ chains prevail in the fetus. *The newborn has about 75% fetal hemoglobin (HbF) ($α_2γ_2$) and 25% adult hemoglobin (HbA) ($α_2β_2$), but HbF becomes almost completely replaced by HbA within the first 4 months after birth.*

Many Point Mutations in Hemoglobin Genes Are Known

About 800 structural variants of hemoglobin have been described in humans so far. The majority are single amino acid substitutions that can be traced to a single base substitution in the gene, and most of them are harmless. Some, however, cause disease:

1. *Mutations that affect the heme-binding pocket cause methemoglobinemia.* Replacement of the proximal histidine by tyrosine, for example, makes the heme group inaccessible to methemoglobin reductase. Heterozygotes with this condition are cyanotic but otherwise in good health.

2. *Unstable hemoglobins cause hemolytic anemia.* Mutations that lead to spontaneous denaturation of hemoglobin cause the formation of insoluble protein aggregates in the erythrocytes that are known as **Heinz bodies.** The abnormal cells are removed by macrophages in the spleen, which results in anemia.

3. *Mutations that affect the interface between the subunits produce hemoglobins with abnormal oxygen-binding affinity.* An increased O_2 affinity leads to poor tissue oxygenation and a compensatory increase in erythropoiesis with polycythemia (increased number of red blood cells [RBCs]); and reduced O_2 affinity causes cyanosis (blue lips).

4. *Mutations that lead to abnormal processing of mRNA, premature degradation of mRNA, or increased proteolytic degradation of the α or β chain cause anemia.* Affected patients present with thalassemia.

5. *Hemoglobins with reduced water solubility cause sickling disorders.* In these diseases, crystalline precipitates of the insoluble hemoglobin distort the shape of the cell, damage the membrane, and cause premature destruction of the cell.

Sickle Cell Disease Is Caused by a Point Mutation in the β-Chain Gene

Sickle cell disease is a severe hemolytic disease that is common among people of African origin but also occurs in persons living in India, Saudi Arabia, and the Mediterranean. *It is caused by the replacement of a glutamate residue in position 6 of the β chain by valine:*

$$H_3^+N-Val-His-Leu-Thr-Pro-Glu-Glu-\cdots\cdots$$
$$\cdots\cdots-CCT\ GAG\ GAG-\cdots\cdots$$
$$H_3^+N-Val-His-Leu-Thr-Pro-Val-Glu-\cdots\cdots$$
$$\cdots\cdots-CCT\ GTG\ GAG-\cdots\cdots$$

This mutation produces **hemoglobin S (HbS,** subunit structure $\alpha_2\beta^S_2$). HbS is synthesized at a normal rate, is stable, and has a normal oxygen affinity. The mutation, however, replaces a charged amino acid residue on the surface of the molecule with a hydrophobic one, and therefore HbS has a reduced water solubility. However, *only the deoxy form of HbS is sufficiently insoluble to form a fibrous precipitate in the erythrocyte.*

Because the mutation changes the charge pattern of the molecule, *HbS can be separated from HbA by electrophoresis* (Fig. 10.13).

Only homozygotes (genotype SS) have sickle cell disease. Therefore, the mode of inheritance is characterized as autosomal recessive. First signs of the disease do not appear until about 6 months after birth, when the fetal hemoglobin has been replaced by adult hemoglobin.

After this age, the erythrocytes are prone to assume bizarre, sickle-like shapes in oxygen-depleted capillaries and veins, and the sickled cells are liable to rupture in the blood vessels or be eaten by splenic macrophages. This leads to anemia with hemoglobin levels in the range of 6 to 11 g/dL.

The most ominous aspect of sickle cell disease is not the anemia but the tendency of the sickled cells

to block capillary beds and thereby cause infarctions. Painful bone and joint infarctions are common; multiple renal infarctions can lead to kidney failure; many patients develop poorly healing leg ulcers, and some are crippled by recurrent strokes.

Frequent attacks of severe pain in the joints, bones, or abdomen, known as **painful crisis** or **sickling crisis,** impair the subjective well-being of the patients. Episodes of **aplastic crisis** (bone marrow failure) are less common, and the sudden trapping of erythrocytes in the enlarged spleen, known as **sequestration crisis,** can cause sudden death in children with the disease. There is a high rate of mortality from infections, renal failure, and cerebrovascular accidents.

Patients with sickle cell disease should avoid anything that could lead to hypoxia: vigorous exercise, staying at high altitude, and drugs that depress respiration, such as heroin. Also, dehydration should be avoided because it leads to a temporary increase in the hemoglobin concentration. Indeed, *intravenous fluids are the standard treatment for sickling crisis.*

Anything that reduces the concentration of deoxygenated HbS is beneficial. **Cyanate** increases the oxygen affinity of hemoglobin by covalent modification of the amino termini of the α and β chains:

$$Polypeptide-NH_2 + O=C=NH$$
$$cyanate$$
$$\downarrow$$
$$Polypeptide-NH-\overset{\overset{\displaystyle O}{\|}}{C}-NH_2$$

Carbamoyl hemoglobin
(high O_2-affinity)

This reaction competes with the formation of carbamino hemoglobin, which has a reduced oxygen affinity (see also Chapter 3):

$$Polypeptide-NH_2 + CO_2$$
$$\downarrow$$
$$Polypeptide-NH-\overset{\overset{\displaystyle O}{\|}}{C}-O^- + H^+$$

Carbamino hemoglobin
(low O_2-affinity)

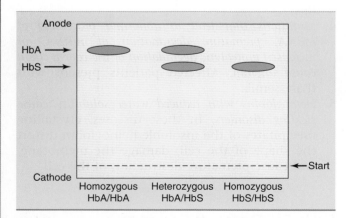

Figure 10.13 Electrophoresis of hemoglobin A and hemoglobin S at a pH of 8.6. Electrophoretic separation is possible because the sickle cell mutation removes a negative charge from the β chain. HbA, adult hemoglobin; HbS, hemoglobin S (sickle cell).

Unfortunately, cyanate reacts not only with hemoglobin but also with the terminal amino groups of other proteins. Therefore, it is too toxic for general use. Even the inhalation of low concentrations of carbon monoxide (CO) can help. This counterintuitive measure reduces sickling by converting some of the deoxy HbS to the nonsickling CO HbS.

affected homozygotes are likely to die before they have a chance to reproduce.

The connection between hemoglobin S and malaria is not altogether surprising. The malaria parasite, *Plasmodium falciparum*, spends part of its life cycle in erythrocytes, in which it is protected from immune attack, and the presence of HbS appears to create a less hospitable environment for the parasite.

SA Heterozygotes Are Protected from Tropical Malaria

Sickle cell heterozygotes (genotype SA) have about 70% HbA and 30% HbS. Their RBCs do not sickle under ordinary conditions, and therefore *SA heterozygotes are healthy.*

The heterozygous carrier state, also known as **sickle cell trait,** can be detected in the laboratory by exposing hemolyzed RBCs to anoxic conditions in vitro. If HbS is present, the solution becomes turbid because HbS becomes insoluble.

Figure 10.14 shows the distribution of the sickle cell trait in the native populations of the Old World. The HbS allele is common in many tropical areas because *sickle cell heterozygotes have improved malaria resistance.* Therefore, natural selection favors the sickle cell gene in the heterozygous state, although

The Thalassemias Are Caused by Reduced α or β Chain Production

In thalassemia, the structure of hemoglobin is normal, but its rate of synthesis is reduced. *All thalassemias are characterized by anemia.* They can be classified as follows:

- **α-Thalassemia:** deficiency of α chains.
- **β-Thalassemia:** deficiency of β chains.
- **Thalassemia minor:** heterozygous thalassemia; borderline anemia.
- **Thalassemia major:** homozygous thalassemia; severe anemia.

The thalassemias are common in the Mediterranean, Africa, the Middle East, India, and Southeast Asia. The heterozygous conditions are thought to provide some protection against malaria.

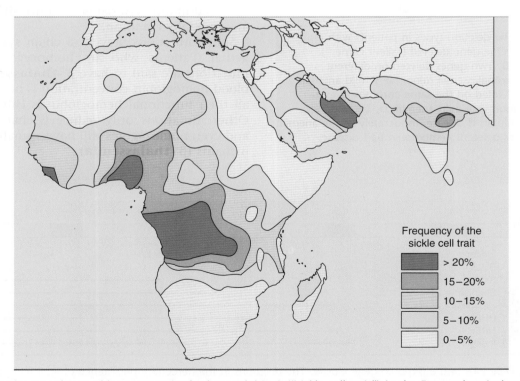

Frequency of the sickle cell trait

- > 20%
- 15–20%
- 10–15%
- 5–10%
- 0–5%

Figure 10.14 The prevalence of heterozygosity for hemoglobin S ("sickle cell trait") in the Eastern hemisphere. In the United States, 8% of African Americans have the sickle cell trait, and approximately 1 per 600 has the disease.

α-Thalassemia Is Most Often Caused by Large Deletions

Large deletions that remove one or both of the α-chain genes on the chromosome are the most common cause of α-thalassemia. Because "normal" people have four α chain genes in their somatic cells, diseases are of graded severity, depending on the number of genes that are lost (Fig. 10.15).

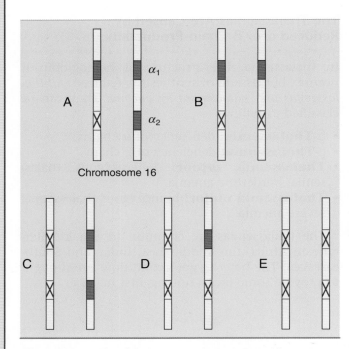

Figure 10.15 The deletion types in patients with α-thalassemia. **A,** One gene deleted ("silent carrier"): asymptomatic. **B,** Two genes deleted on different chromosomes: α-thalassemia minor, very mild anemia. **C,** Two genes deleted on the same chromosome: α-thalassemia minor, very mild anemia. **D,** Three genes deleted: hemoglobin H disease, moderately severe anemia. **E,** All four genes deleted: hemoglobin Bart disease, hydrops fetalis.

Because α chains are present in fetal as well as adult hemoglobin, *a complete lack of α chains is fatal before or at birth.* Under these conditions, an abnormal hemoglobin of subunit structure γ_4 (**hemoglobin Bart**) is formed; this hemoglobin has a 10-fold higher oxygen affinity than does hemoglobin A and cannot function as an effective oxygen carrier. An unstable β_4 tetramer (**hemoglobin H**) is the predominant hemoglobin in patients with deletions of three α-chain genes.

In most areas of the "thalassemia belt," only the smaller deletions are prevalent. About 2% of African Americans, for example, have the thalassemia minor genotype of Figure 10.15B. In parts of India and Melanesia, a majority of individuals are either "silent carriers" or have α-thalassemia minor. The large deletions are most common in Southeast Asia, where the severe homozygous deletion type is a frequent cause of stillbirth.

Many Different Mutations Can Cause β-Thalassemia

Some cases of β-thalassemia (and δβ thalassemia [Fig. 10.16]) are caused by large deletions, but most patients have single-base substitutions. In all, more than 170 β-thalassemia mutations have been identified. Promoter mutations, splice-site mutations, nonsense and frameshift mutations, and a mutation in the polyadenylation signal all have been observed in different patients. Splice-site mutations are especially common.

Some mutations prevent β chain synthesis altogether. Patients who are homozygous for such mutations are said to have β^0-**thalassemia.** Their blood hemoglobin concentration is below 4%, and all their functional hemoglobin is HbF and HbA$_2$. Other mutations only reduce β chain synthesis, and even homozygotes still have a small amount of β chains (β^+-**thalassemia**).

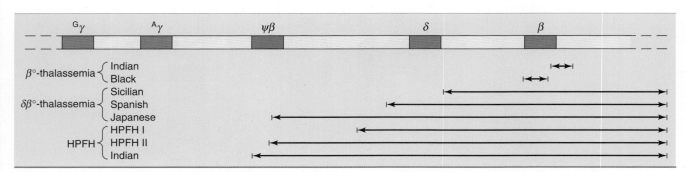

Figure 10.16 Deletions in the β-globin gene cluster. The deletions in the hereditary persistence of fetal hemoglobin (HPFH) group suggest that DNA sequences between the $^A\gamma$ and δ genes are important for the developmental switch-off of γ-chain synthesis.

Because of the large number of mutations, most β-thalassemia "homozygotes" are actually **compound heterozygotes** who have two different mutations in their two β-chain genes. These patients show a wide range of residual β chain production and clinical severity. The milder forms, with clinical expression intermediate between the classical minor and major forms, are called **thalassemia intermedia.** The patients are normal at birth because of the abundance of fetal hemoglobin, but *anemia develops during the first 6 months after birth, when the fetal hemoglobin is phased out.*

Unlike the β chains and γ chains, the excess α chains that are produced in β-thalassemia cannot form a soluble tetramer. They form an insoluble precipitate instead. Cells with this precipitate are recognized as deviant by the macrophages in bone marrow and spleen. This leads to **abortive erythropoiesis** through the destruction of RBC precursors in the bone marrow, and the premature destruction of circulating RBCs in the spleen. These processes aggravate the anemia.

The bone marrow responds to the anemia by working overtime, and a massive expansion of the red bone marrow leads to facial deformities ("chipmunk facies") and radiological abnormalities. Eventually, extramedullary erythropoiesis develops in the liver and spleen.

Untreated patients with homozygous β⁰-thalassemia are likely to die of severe anemia and intercurrent infections in infancy or childhood. Regular blood transfusions alone can keep them alive to an age of about 20 years, when they succumb to iron overload. *Severe anemia by itself increases intestinal iron absorption, and repeated blood transfusions introduce additional iron that cannot be excreted.*

Iron overload can be prevented with **desferrioxamine,** an iron chelator that is administered continuously through a subcutaneous infusion pump. Desferrioxamine forms a soluble iron complex that can be excreted by the kidneys.

High Levels of Fetal Hemoglobin Protect from the Effects of β-Thalassemia and Sickle Cell Disease

Patients with β⁰-thalassemia can survive (although with difficulty) because they still possess small amounts of HbA_2 and HbF. HbF accounts for less than 2% of the hemoglobin in normal adults and occurs only in a fraction of the RBCs, but in homozygous β⁰-thalassemia, it is the major hemoglobin. *In these patients, the severity of the disease is inversely related to the HbF level.*

In some patients, including some of the deletion types (see Fig. 10.16), the symptoms of β-thalassemia remain mild because of high levels of HbF expression. These conditions are called **hereditary persistence of fetal hemoglobin (HPFH).** Elevated levels of HbF are also seen in some nonthalassemic persons with near-normal levels of HbA. In some cases of nondeletion HPFH, the condition could be traced to a point mutation in the promoter region of one of the γ chain genes.

A high level of HbF in adults is protective in all β-chain abnormalities, including β-thalassemia and sickle cell disease. Some drugs can induce γ chain expression in adults. These include hydroxyurea, several derivatives of butyric acid, and the antitumor drug azacytidine. Unfortunately, these agents have many undesirable side effects. Azacytidine induces at least part of its effect by preventing the methylation of newly synthesized DNA in regulatory regions of the γ chain genes.

SUMMARY

Mutations are changes in DNA structure that arise as spontaneous replication errors or in response to DNA damage. Somatic mutations contribute to aging and are the principal cause of cancer, whereas germline mutations cause genetic diseases. Mutations can prevent the normal expression of a gene or cause the synthesis of a defective protein with impaired or abnormal biological properties.

Cells use a variety of DNA repair systems to keep the mutation rate at a tolerable level. Inherited defects of DNA repair can increase cancer risk and cause premature aging.

The hemoglobinopathies are classical examples of genetic diseases. In sickle cell disease, a point mutation leads to a Glu→Val substitution in the hemoglobin β chain. The erythrocytes of affected homozygotes sickle because deoxy HbS has an abnormally low solubility, and the patients develop a hemolytic anemia and multiple tissue infarctions.

In the thalassemias, hemoglobin α chains or β chains are underproduced. The hemoglobinopathies are the most common genetic diseases in many parts of the world because heterozygous carriers of the offending mutations have improved malaria resistance.

📖 Further Reading

Byrne M, Agerbo E, Ewald H, et al: Parental age and risk of schizophrenia. A case-control study. Arch Gen Psychiat 60:673-678, 2003.

Crow JF: The origins, patterns and implications of human spontaneous mutation. Nature Rev Genet 1:40-47, 2000.

Maki H: Origin of spontaneous mutations: specificity and directionality of base-substitution, frameshift, and sequence-substitution mutageneses. Annu Rev Genet 36:279-303, 2002.

Moses RE: DNA damage processing defects and disease. Annu Rev Genomics Hum Genet 2:41-68, 2001.

Steward RE, MacArthur MW, Laskowski RA, Thornton JM: Molecular basis of inherited diseases: a structural perspective. Trends Genet 19:505-513, 2003.

Van den Bosch M, Lohman PHM, Pastink A: DNA double-strand break repair by homologous recombination. Biol Chem 383:873-892, 2002.

QUESTIONS

1. You examine a 10-month-old infant who has numerous scaly and ulcerative skin lesions, premalignant changes, and areas of hyperpigmentation. These lesions are present only on sun-exposed skin. This is most likely caused by a defect in

   A. Post-replication mismatch repair.
   B. The repair of double-strand DNA breaks.
   C. Removal of deaminated bases.
   D. Base excision repair.
   E. Nucleotide excision repair.

2. The most important type of DNA damage in the child described in question 1 is

   A. Double-strand DNA breaks.
   B. Pyrimidine dimers.
   C. Replication errors.
   D. Insertions and deletions.
   E. Base methylations.

3. An 18-month-old girl of Middle Eastern ancestry, who was initially treated for recurrent lung infections, is found to have a blood hemoglobin concentration of 4.6%. The erythrocytes are smaller than normal and of somewhat irregular shape, and the mean intracorpuscular hemoglobin content is only 55% of normal. HbF and HbA_2 are elevated. This is most likely a case of

   A. Sickle cell disease.
   B. A DNA repair defect.
   C. α-Thalassemia major.
   D. β-Thalassemia major.
   E. β-Thalassemia minor.

4. Some patients with sickle cell disease have relatively mild symptoms because they also have

   A. Bone marrow depression.
   B. Elevated β-chain synthesis.
   C. Reduced α-chain synthesis.
   D. Reduced γ-chain synthesis.
   E. Iron overload.

5. Schizophrenia affects about 1% of the population in every generation. Genetic factors are known to be important, and it is also known that schizophrenic persons have, on average, fewer children than do unaffected individuals. On average, schizophrenic persons have somewhat older fathers than do unaffected individuals. This effect is especially pronounced in those without a family history of the disease. This suggests that many cases of schizophrenia are caused by

   A. Common polymorphisms.
   B. New point mutations.
   C. Nondisjunction.
   D. Chromosomal rearrangements.
   E. Somatic mutations.

CHAPTER 11

DNA Technology

Converting scientists' knowledge of the human genome into better ways to diagnose and treat diseases requires a sophisticated tool kit. There are several operations that occur in many applications: cutting DNA into handy fragments; separating DNA fragments by size; identifying DNA with a specific, known sequence; amplifying minute amounts of DNA to get enough material for analysis; sequencing DNA; and bringing therapeutic DNAs into the patient's cells. This chapter introduces the basic tools and procedures of genetic diagnosis and recombinant DNA technology.

Restriction Endonucleases Cut Large DNA Molecules into Smaller Fragments

A typical human DNA molecule has a length of about 100 million base pairs. For isolation, sequencing, or genetic manipulations, it is mandatory to break these unwieldy molecules into smaller fragments.

This can be done with **restriction endonucleases.** *These enzymes cleave double-stranded DNA very selectively at palindromic sequences of four to eight nucleotides.* The size of the resulting **restriction fragments** depends on the cleavage specificity of the enzyme. If the enzyme recognizes a specific sequence of four bases, then the restriction fragments that it produces will be, on average, 256 base pairs in length; that is, this sequence would appear by chance only once in every 256 bases (4^4). In the case of an enzyme that recognizes an eight-base sequence, the average length of the restriction fragments would be 65,536 base pairs (4^8). Several hundred restriction endonucleases that recognize different palindromic sequences are available commercially.

Most restriction enzymes cut not in the center of their recognition sequence but one or two base pairs away from the symmetry axis in both strands. Therefore, *they produce a double-stranded DNA with short single-stranded ends* (Fig. 11.1 and Table 11.1).

Because the single-stranded overhangs are complementary to one another, *every restriction fragment can anneal (base-pair) with any other restriction fragment produced by the same restriction enzyme.* Once annealed, the restriction fragments can be linked covalently by DNA ligase. This property of restriction enzymes makes them ideal tools for **recombinant DNA technology:** the cutting and joining of DNA in the test tube.

Restriction endonucleases are bacterial enzymes that the bacteria use as a defense against DNA viruses. Susceptible sites in the bacterial genome are protected by methylation, but the unmethylated DNA of a viral intruder is cleaved. This system is not absolutely reliable. If the viral DNA encounters the methyltransferase first, it gets methylated and can no longer be cleaved by the restriction enzyme.

DNA Is Sequenced by Controlled Chain Termination

Genome sequencing is performed with pieces of genomic DNA that have been propagated in bacteria. These snippets of cloned DNA are cut out of the bacterial DNA by restriction endonucleases and denatured by alkali treatment before being used for sequencing.

In the **dideoxy method** of DNA sequencing, single-stranded target DNA is used as a template for the synthesis of a complementary strand in vitro. DNA synthesis is started with a short oligonucleotide primer and allowed to proceed until several hundred nucleotides have been polymerized.

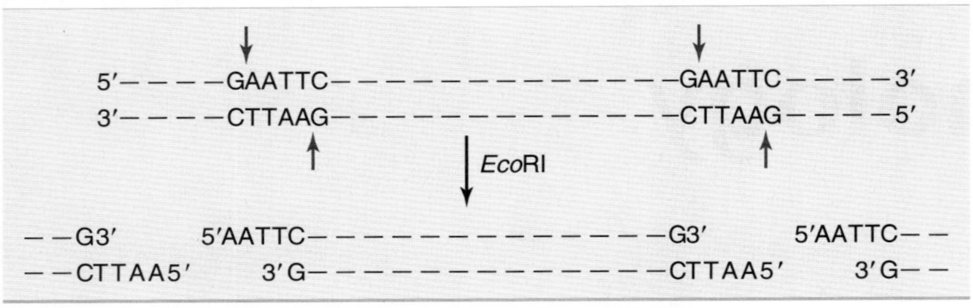

Figure 11.1 Generation of restriction fragments by the restriction endonuclease *Eco*RI. Both strands are cut. Note that the double-stranded DNA fragments have single-stranded ends.

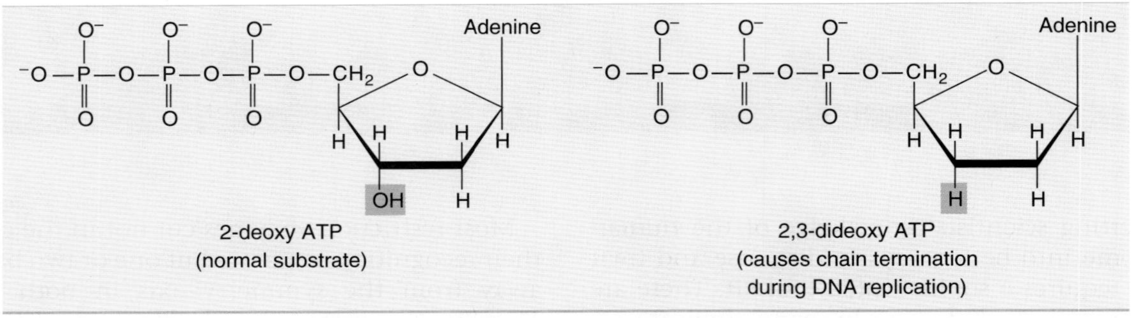

Figure 11.2 Structure of a dideoxynucleoside triphosphate. DNA polymerases can incorporate a dideoxynucleotide into a new DNA strand, but further chain growth is prevented by lack of a free 3′-hydroxyl group. ATP, adenosine triphosphate.

Table 11.1 Examples of Restriction Endonucleases*.

Enzyme	Source	Cleavage Specificity	No. of Cleavage Sites on λ Phage DNA[†]
*Eco*RI	*Escherichia coli* RY 13	5′ G↓A A T T C 3′ 3′ C T T A A↑G 5′	5
*Eco*RII	*E. coli* R 245	5′↓C C T G G 3′ 3′ G G A C C↑5′	>35
*Hin*dIII	*Haemophilus influenzae* R$_d$	5′ A↓A G C T T 3′ 3′ T T C G A↑A 5′	6
*Hae*III	*Haemophilus aegypticus*	5′ G G↓C C 3′ 3′ C C↑G G 5′	>50
*Bam*HI	*Bacillus amyloliquefaciens*	5′ G↓G A T C C 3′ 3′ C C T A G↑G 5′	5

* The first three letters in the name of each enzyme indicates the bacterium from which it is derived. Enzymes with a short recognition sequence, such as *Hae*III, cleave at many sites in natural DNA molecules and generate restriction fragments of small average size; those with a long recognition sequence cleave fewer sites and generate longer fragments.
[†] The λ phage DNA (see Chapter 7) consists of 48,513 base pairs.

However, included in the incubation mixture are not only the deoxyribonucleoside triphosphates but also small quantities of the corresponding dideoxyribonucleoside triphosphates (Fig. 11.2). The DNA polymerase can incorporate these analogs into the DNA, but *DNA synthesis cannot continue in the absence of a 3′-hydroxyl group.*

Each of the four dideoxyribonucleotides is added only in small quantities, so that chain termination occurs with a probability of less than 1% in each step. Each is labeled with a different fluorescent group, so that they can be distinguished from one another. Polyacrylamide gel electrophoresis produces a string of closely spaced fluorescent bands according to the chain length of the products. The fluorescence is scanned automatically by a laser beam and read by a computer (Fig. 11.3). Most modern automated sequencing machines use a different technique called capillary electrophoresis to separate the mixture of different-sized fluorescent DNA chains.

Complementary DNA Probes Are Used for In Situ Hybridization

The direct identification of mutations is becoming increasingly important for the diagnosis of genetic

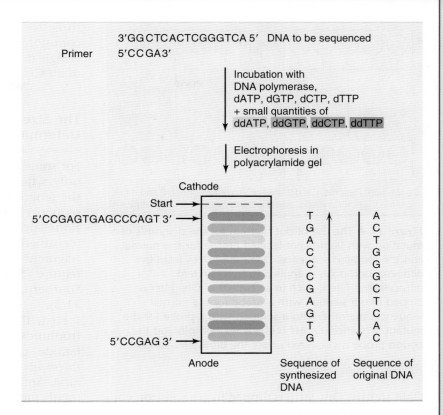

Figure 11.3 DNA sequencing with the dideoxy method. Each of the four dideoxynucleotides (ddATP, ddCTP, ddGTP, and ddTTP) is labeled with a different fluorescent tag. They are added with a large excess of the deoxynucleotides dATP, dCTP, dGTP, and dTTP.

diseases. It is best done with a **molecular probe.** *A probe is a single-stranded DNA or RNA that is complementary to the target DNA.* To be detectable, the probe must be labeled either with a radioactive isotope or with a fluorescent group.

A messenger RNA (mRNA), for example, can be used as a probe. In a denatured restriction digest, *the mRNA probe binds to all restriction fragments that contain exon sequences of its gene.* The same can be done with a **complementary DNA (cDNA) probe** that is made from the mRNA with the help of reverse transcriptase.

A cDNA with a strong fluorescent label can be used for **in situ hybridization.** This procedure can be used to test for gene deletions. A chromosome spread is prepared from a metaphase cell, the chromosomal DNA is denatured, and the probe is applied. *If the gene is present, the probe binds; if it is deleted, it does not bind.*

In situ hybridization can also be used to test for aneuploidy in interphase cells. *If a probe for a specific gene or chromosomal region binds to two spots in the amorphous chromatin, the chromosome is present in two copies; if it binds to three spots, the chromosome is present in three copies.*

Dot Blotting Is Used for Genetic Screening

The diagnosis of small mutations requires a synthetic **oligonucleotide probe.** *The probe must be at least 17 or 18 nucleotides long* because shorter probes are likely to hybridize with multiple sites in the genome. Oligonucleotides of this size can be synthesized by chemical methods.

Oligonucleotide probes that discriminate between two genetic variants (alleles) are called **allele-specific oligonucleotides.** Most applications involve a pair of oligonucleotide probes with identical lengths, one complementary to the normal sequence and the other complementary to the mutation.

These probes are applied under conditions of high **stringency.** These are conditions of high temperature and/or low ionic strength that destabilize base-pairing and permit annealing only if the sequences match precisely. Under conditions of low stringency, the probes would bind irrespective of the mismatch, and discrimination would be impossible.

Dot blotting (Fig. 11.4) is a rapid screening test for the detection of small mutations. The extracted DNA is denatured and applied to two strips of nitrocellulose paper. This material binds single-stranded

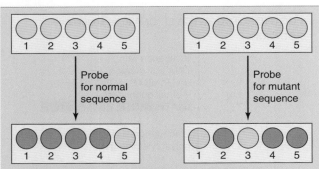

Conclusion: Patients 1 and 3 are homozygous normal, 2 and 4 are heterozygous, and 5 is homozygous for the mutation.

Figure 11.4 The use of dot blotting for the diagnosis of a mutation with fluorescent-labeled probes for the normal and the mutated sequence. Denatured DNA from five different individuals is applied to two different nitrocellulose filters, each in a single dot. One filter is dipped into a solution with a probe for the normal sequence, the other into a solution with a probe for the mutant sequence. Excess probe is washed off, and the bound probe is visualized under the ultraviolet lamp.

DNA tightly. One strip is dipped into a solution containing an oligonucleotide probe for the normal sequence, and the other is dipped into a solution with a probe for the mutation. *If only the probe for the normal sequence binds, the patient is homozygous normal; if only the probe for the mutation binds, the patient is homozygous for the mutation; and if both probes bind, the patient is heterozygous.*

Dot blotting is simple, rapid, and inexpensive. Thus, it can be used to test large numbers of people for polymorphisms and recessive mutations.

Cystic fibrosis (CF), for example, is a severe recessively inherited disease that affects one in 2500 newborns of European descent. About 4% of the population are heterozygous carriers of a CF mutation, and the risk for two carrier parents of having an affected child is 25%.

CF is easy to prevent. All that is needed is to screen the whole population for CF mutations, identify all couples at risk, and persuade them to refrain from producing affected children. Other than a child-free lifestyle, the options for these couples include donor gametes, intrauterine or postnatal adoption, prenatal diagnosis with selective termination of affected pregnancies, and preimplantation genetic diagnosis with selective implantation of unaffected embryos.

More than 100 CF mutations are known, but a 3–base pair deletion (ΔPhe^{508} mutation) accounts for 50% to 70% of all CF mutations in the white population. For genetic screening, the DNA of large numbers of people is subjected to dot blotting with three to more than a dozen probes for the most common CF mutations in the local population. This design misses the rare mutations, but 80% to 90% of all CF carriers are identified.

The Size of Restriction Fragments Is Determined by Southern Blotting

For some applications, scientists want to know not only whether a base sequence is present but also the length of the restriction fragment carrying the sequence. For example, small insertions and deletions such as the ΔPhe^{508} mutation in CF can be identified by measuring the length of the restriction fragment carrying the mutation. Such applications require **Southern blotting,** named after Ed Southern, who developed the method in 1975 (Fig. 11.5).

First, the restriction digest is separated by electrophoresis in a crosslinked agarose or polyacrylamide gel. *This method separates the restriction fragments by their size rather than their charge/mass ratio.* Small fragments move fast, and large fragments move slowly because they are retarded by the gel. Even restriction fragments differing in length by only one or a few base pairs can be separated.

The restriction fragments are not tightly bound to the gel slab in which they were separated and are therefore leached out easily. In Southern blotting, the DNA is denatured by dipping the gel into a dilute sodium hydroxide solution and then transferred ("blotted") to nitrocellulose paper. In effect, *a replica of the gel with its separated restriction fragments is made on the nitrocellulose.*

The desired fragment is identified simply by dipping the nitrocellulose paper in a neutral solution of the probe and washing off the excess unbound probe.

To make a probe for Southern blotting, the base sequence must be known. In organisms whose genome sequence has not yet been identified, however, sometimes only the sequence of the encoded protein is known. The exact base sequence of the gene cannot be predicted because the genetic code is degenerate. All amino acids except methionine and tryptophan have more than one codon. To make a probe, it is necessary to choose a sequence rich in methionine and/or tryptophan and synthesize all possible complementary oligonucleotides (Fig. 11.6).

Whereas Southern blotting identifies DNA fragments, **Northern blotting** is similarly used for RNA. **Western blotting** is a method for the separation of polypeptides that are then analyzed by a monoclonal antibody.

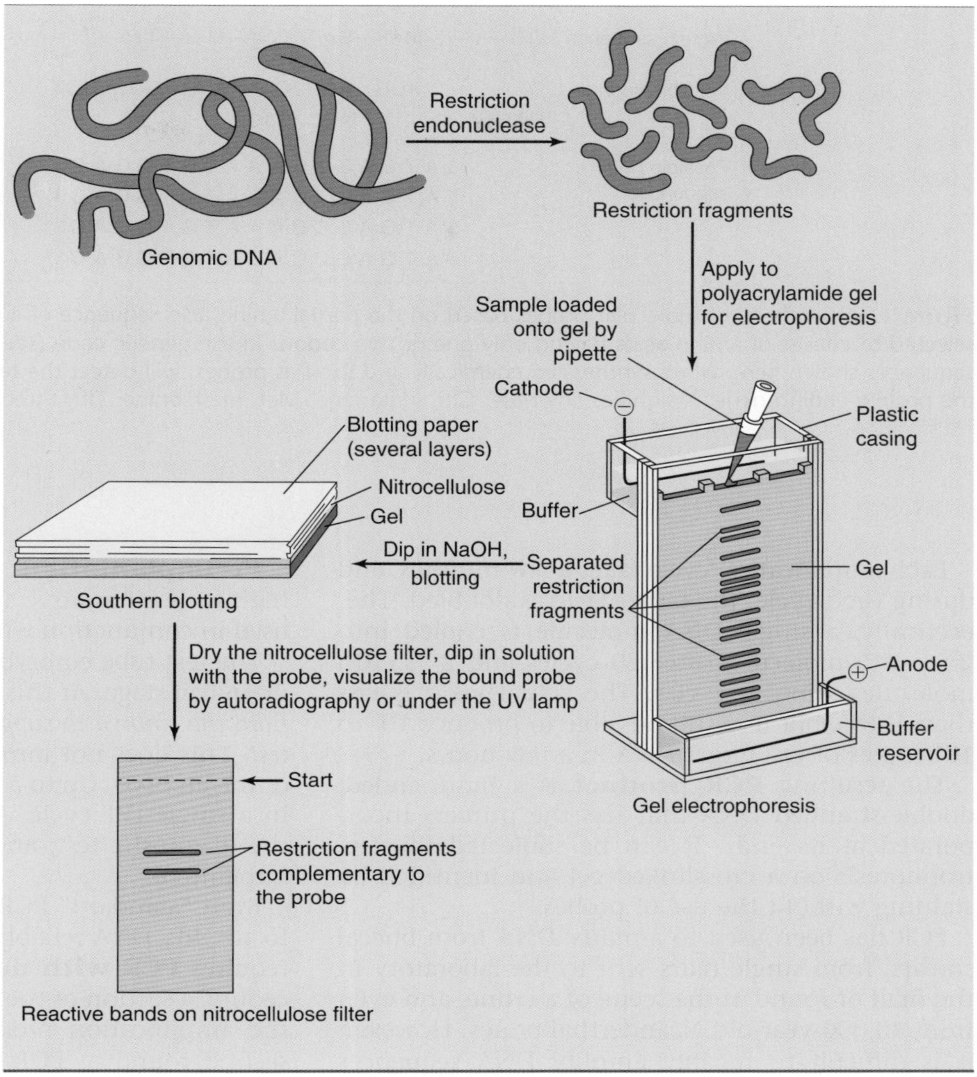

Figure 11.5 Identification of restriction fragments by Southern blotting. Only the restriction fragments with sequence complementarity to the probe are seen in the last step. This method provides two important pieces of information: It shows whether DNA sequences with complementarity to the probe are present in the genomic DNA, and it shows the approximate length of the restriction fragment carrying these sequences. UV, ultraviolet.

DNA Can Be Amplified with the Polymerase Chain Reaction

Southern blotting requires about 10 μg of DNA. This amount can be obtained from 1 mL of blood or from 10 mg of chorionic villus biopsy material. When less than this amount is available for analysis, the DNA has to be amplified with the **polymerase chain reaction (PCR).**

The procedure, described in Figure 11.7, employs a heat-stable DNA polymerase such as **Taq polymerase.** This enzyme is derived from *Thermus aquaticus,* a thermophilic bacterium that was originally isolated from a hot spring in Yellowstone National Park. It functions best at temperatures close to 60° C and can survive repeated heating to 90° C.

PCR is used to amplify only the DNA of interest. This specificity is achieved by the choice of primers. *Two oligonucleotide primers that are complementary to sequences on the two strands of the target DNA are required.*

The primers are added to the DNA in very large (>10^8-fold) molar excess, along with Taq polymerase and the required nucleotides dATP, dGTP, dCTP, and dTTP. *This mix is repeatedly heated to 90° C in order to denature the target DNA, and cooled to 60° C for annealing of the primers and polymerization.*

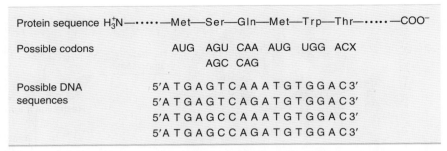

Figure 11.6 Synthesis of molecular probes based on the partial amino acid sequence of a protein. The sequence is selected to consist of amino acids having only one or two codons in the genetic code (see Fig. 6.25). The possible DNA sequences shown here, when synthesized chemically and used as probes, will detect the template (noncoding) strand in the protein-coding gene. X signifies any base. Gln, glutamine; Met, methionine; Thr, threonine; Trp, tryptophan.

Each amplification cycle takes a few minutes, and during each cycle, the target DNA is doubled. Theoretically, a single DNA molecule is copied into 2^{20} ($>10^{6}$) molecules after 20 cycles and 2^{30} ($>10^{9}$) molecules after 30 cycles. The actual yield is less than 100%, but it is still possible to produce 10^{6} to 10^{8} copies of the target DNA in a few hours.

The resulting **PCR product** is a blunt-ended, double-stranded DNA that has the primers incorporated at its ends. It can be subjected to electrophoresis on a crosslinked gel and identified by staining without the use of probes.

PCR has been used to amplify DNA from buccal smears, from single hairs sent to the laboratory in the mail or found at the scene of a crime, and even from 40,000-year-old Neanderthal bones. However, it is difficult to reliably amplify DNA sequences longer than three kilobases. Individual exons can be amplified easily, but most genes are too large to be amplified in one piece.

Also, the Taq polymerase has no proofreading 3'-exonuclease activity. Therefore, it misincorporates bases at a rate of about one every 5000 or 10,000 base pairs.

Polymerase Chain Reaction with Nested Primers Is Used for Preimplantation Genetic Diagnosis

Prenatal diagnosis *(antenatal diagnosis) is used to detect severe genetic defects early in pregnancy and is often followed by the termination of affected pregnancies.* Fetal cells are obtained either by chorionic villus sampling at about 10 weeks of gestation or by amniocentesis at about 16 weeks. The cells can be propagated in cell culture to obtain enough DNA for diagnostic tests, but this is often not necessary when PCR is employed.

Preimplantation genetic diagnosis is a high-tech alternative to prenatal diagnosis and is used in conjunction with in vitro fertilization (IVF).

The test-tube embryo is allowed to grow to the 8- or 16-cell stage. At this point, *a single cell is removed from the embryo to supply the DNA for the diagnostic test.* This does not impair the further development of the embryo. Up to a dozen embryos are obtained in a single IVF cycle. All of them are subjected to the diagnostic test, and only the healthy ones are implanted.

Even "standard" PCR is not sufficiently powerful to amplify DNA reliably from a single cell. This feat requires **PCR with nested primers.** In this procedure, a section of the target DNA is amplified, and the amplification product is then subjected to a second round of PCR with a more closely spaced primer pair.

Figure 11.8 describes the use of PCR with nested primers for the preimplantation diagnosis of the ΔPhe^{508} mutation. This three–base pair deletion is readily identified by PCR because *the mutated sequence yields a PCR product three base pairs shorter than normal.* This difference is sufficient for separation by polyacrylamide gel electrophoresis.

This method can be employed for all small insertions and deletions. It is especially useful for conditions that are caused by a microsatellite expansion, such as Huntington disease and fragile X mental retardation (see Chapter 8). In these cases, the exact size of the expanded repeat sequence can be determined by electrophoresis of the PCR products.

Base-substitution mutations yield PCR products of the same length as the normal sequence. Therefore, the PCR products cannot be separated by electrophoresis, and the distinction between normal and abnormal requires an allele-specific oligonucleotide probe.

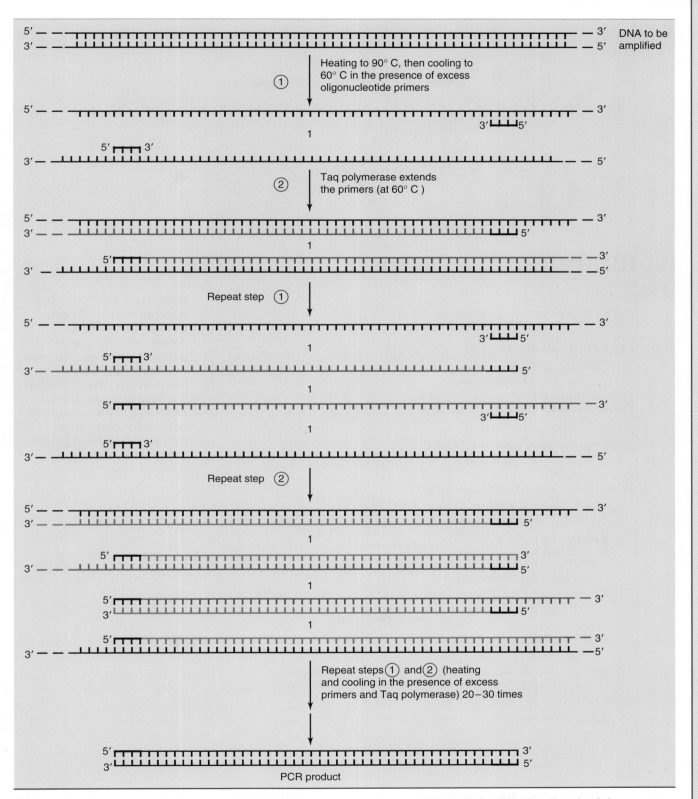

Figure 11.7 The polymerase chain reaction (PCR). The sequence to be amplified is defined by the 5′ ends of the oligonucleotide primers. The primers base-pair with the heat-denatured DNA strands by Watson-Crick base pairing. The Taq polymerase catalyzes DNA polymerization at 60° C and survives a temperature of 90° C during heat denaturation of the DNA. Neither primer nor Taq polymerase has to be added during repeated amplification cycles. Note that the amount of DNA between the primers increases geometrically: it doubles during each cycle of heating and cooling. ⊔⊔⊔, Oligonucleotide primer.

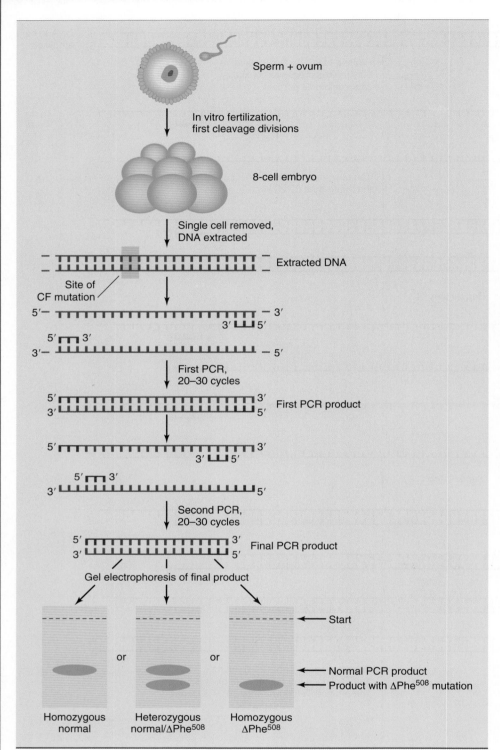

Figure 11.8 Preimplantation diagnosis of cystic fibrosis, through the use of the polymerase chain reaction (PCR) with nested primers. The most common cystic fibrosis mutation, the ΔPhe^{508} mutation, is a three-base-pair deletion that results in a PCR product three nucleotides shorter than normal. The two PCR products can be separated by gel electrophoresis.

Labels in figure:
- Sperm + ovum
- In vitro fertilization, first cleavage divisions
- 8-cell embryo
- Single cell removed, DNA extracted
- Extracted DNA
- Site of CF mutation
- First PCR, 20–30 cycles
- First PCR product
- Second PCR, 20–30 cycles
- Final PCR product
- Gel electrophoresis of final product
- Start
- Normal PCR product
- Product with ΔPhe^{508} mutation
- Homozygous normal
- Heterozygous normal/ΔPhe^{508}
- Homozygous ΔPhe^{508}

Polymerase Chain Reaction Can Be Used for Deletion Scanning

PCR can also detect large deletions that remove a whole exon or even a whole gene. **Duchenne muscular dystrophy (DMD)** is a severe X-linked recessive muscle disease that is caused by mutations in the gene for the muscle protein dystrophin. The gene is enormous, with 79 exons scattered over more than 2 million base pairs of DNA. Two thirds of affected patients have large deletions in which one or several exons have been removed from the gene.

Deletions can be identified by the PCR amplification of deletion-prone exons, as outlined in Figure

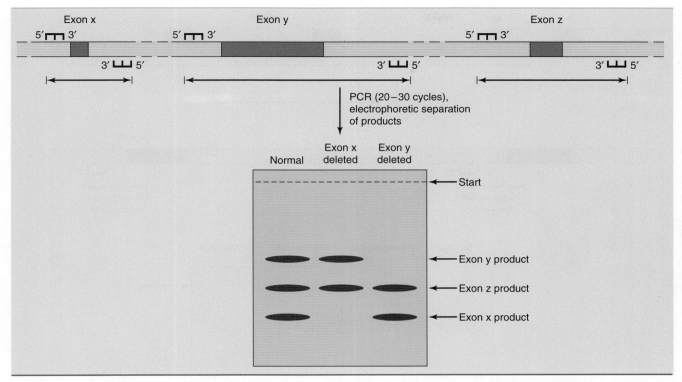

Figure 11.9 The principle of deletion scanning with the polymerase chain reaction (PCR). Note that the primer pairs are designed to generate PCR products of different lengths that can be separated from each other by polyacrylamide gel electrophoresis. This method has been employed to amplify deletion-prone exons in patients with Duchenne muscular dystrophy. ■, Exons; ⊔⊔, primer.

11.9. *If one of the target exons is deleted, its PCR product is absent.*

A more complex application of PCR has been described for the diagnosis of α-thalassemia deletions in Southeast Asia and China (Fig. 11.10). The homozygous deletions can readily be identified through PCR, but the heterozygous carrier state is more easily diagnosed with restriction endonuclease digestion and Southern blotting, as shown in Figure 11.11.

Allele-Specific Polymerase Chain Reaction Can Detect Point Mutations

A synthetic oligonucleotide can prime DNA synthesis only if its 3′ end is properly base-paired to the target DNA.

Single-base substitutions can be identified through PCR, with the use of primers whose 3′ ends pair with the alternative bases. *A primer whose 3′ end pairs with the normal base amplifies only the normal sequence, and a corresponding primer whose 3′ end pairs with the mutated base amplifies only the mutation.* These allele-specific primers are used in conjunction with a second primer that recognizes a nearby unmutated sequence, as shown in Figure 11.12.

Allelic Heterogeneity Is the Greatest Challenge for Molecular Genetic Diagnosis

All patients with sickle cell disease have the same mutation. Thus, a single pair of allele-specific oligonucleotide probes or allele-specific primers is sufficient for molecular diagnosis. In CF, any mutation that prevents the synthesis of a functional gene product leads to the same disease, but only a few mutations are common in the population. Therefore, most carriers can be identified with a small assortment of oligonucleotide probes, one for each common mutation.

In the worst cases, all mutations for the disease are rare. In the X-linked clotting disorder hemophilia B, for example, more than 2000 different mutations in the gene for clotting factor IX have been observed in different patients. This degree of **allelic heterogeneity** prevents the use of allele-specific oligonucleotide probes. There are three ways to obviate this problem:

1. *Scanning the gene for a mismatch.* This is done by amplifying the exons of the gene and hybridizing the PCR products from the patient with the corresponding products from the normal gene.

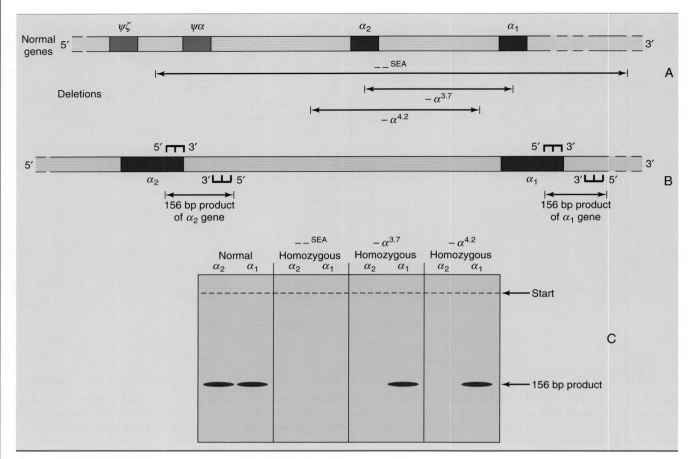

Figure 11.10 The use of the polymerase chain reaction (PCR) for the diagnosis of α-thalassemia deletions. **A,** The three most common α-thalassemia deletions in Southeast Asia and China. **B,** The use of two primer pairs for the amplification of two 156–base pair segments at the 3′ ends of the $α_1$ and $α_2$ genes. The 5′ primers of the two amplifications are identical. They are complementary to a shared sequence near the 3′ ends of the two α-chain genes. The 3′ primers are different. They are complementary to sequences immediately 3′ of the two genes. The amplifications of the two segments are performed in different test tubes. The sizes of the primers and amplification products are not to scale. **C,** Identification of the PCR products from the $α_2$ and $α_1$ genes by polyacrylamide gel electrophoresis. This method can identify the lethal hydrops fetalis genotype during prenatal diagnosis. It also can distinguish between heterozygosity for the $--^{SEA}$ deletion and homozygosity for one of the two smaller deletions in patients with clinical signs of α-thalassemia minor. ⊔⊔, Primer. bp, base pair.

The mismatch can be detected either by chemical reagents that cleave selectively at the site of the mismatch or by electrophoresis under partially denaturing conditions.

2. *Sequencing of the whole gene.* This brute-force approach is becoming increasingly popular because affordable DNA sequencers are now widely available.

3. *Tracking the mutation by linkage with a genetic marker.* In this case, no attempt is made to identify the mutation, but a known genetic marker that is located next to the mutated gene is analyzed instead. The mutated gene is inherited along with the marker simply because both are located on the same DNA molecule, and recombination between the gene and the marker is very rare.

Single-Nucleotide Polymorphisms, Restriction-Site Polymorphisms, and Variable Number of Tandem Repeats Are Used as Genetic Markers

In theory, any DNA polymorphism can be used as a genetic marker for gene tracking. According to one definition, a polymorphism is any variable site in the DNA for which the frequency of the less common allele is above 1% in the population. *There*

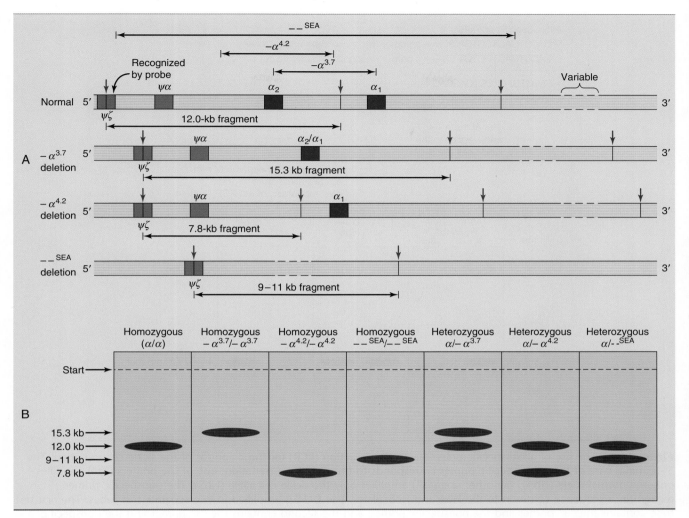

Figure 11.11 The use of Southern blotting for the diagnosis of the most common α-thalassemia deletions (compare Fig. 11.10). The genomic DNA, extracted from leukocytes, cultured fibroblasts, or cultured amniotic cells, is cleaved with the restriction endonuclease *Bg*/II (↓). The probe that is used to detect the fragments hybridizes to a sequence in the 3′ portion of the zeta pseudogene (ψζ). **A,** Fragments generated in three different deletion types. **B,** The appearance of restriction fragments after Southern blotting. kb, kilobase.

are several million polymorphisms in the human genome, most of them **single-nucleotide polymorphisms (SNPs)**.

Some SNPs obliterate or create a cleavage site for a restriction endonuclease. This subset of SNPs produces **restriction-site polymorphisms (RSPs)**. They are convenient genetic markers because they give rise to restriction fragments of different sizes that can be separated by gel electrophoresis. This method is more accurate and foolproof than the identification of "ordinary" SNPs with allele-specific probes.

However, *polymorphic microsatellites are the most useful genetic markers*. These microsatellites are tandemly repeated sequences with two to more than a dozen nucleotides in the repeat unit (Fig. 11.13B). The repeat number and, therefore, the length of these microsatellites vary among people. Most people are heterozygous, carrying two different-length variants on the two copies of the chromosome. These polymorphisms are called **variable number of tandem repeats (VNTRs).** *Whereas RSPs have only two alleles, VNTRs come in multiple alleles.*

Most SNPs, RSPs, and VNTRs do not cause disease. But when a disease-causing mutation arises on a chromosome next to a polymorphic site, mutation and polymorphism travel together through the generations until they are divorced by a crossing-over in meiosis. Therefore, *the inheritance of the defective gene can be traced by tracing the inheritance of the polymorphic marker with which it is associated.*

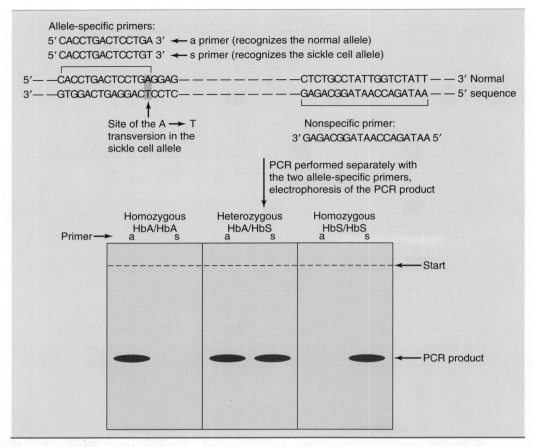

Figure 11.12 The use of allele-specific polymerase chain reaction (PCR) for the diagnosis of the sickle cell mutation. The 3'-terminal base of the allele-specific primer corresponds to the site of the mutation: one of the primers ("a") amplifies only the normal allele (HbA); the other one ("s") amplifies only the sickle cell allele (HbS). The nonspecific primer recognizes a sequence common to the HbA and HbS alleles. The DNA is amplified in two separate test tubes. The first test tube contains the "a" primer and the nonspecific primer, and the second contains the "s" primer and the nonspecific primer.

The linkage pattern is likely to be different in different families. For example, a disease gene may be inherited along with a shorter fragment of a VNTR in some families but with a longer fragment in others. Therefore, linkage cannot be used for population screening; it can be used only for studies of families in which the genotypes of one or more affected individuals are known.

Tandem Repeats Are Used for DNA Fingerprinting

Polymorphic DNA sequences can also be used to identify criminals—and, as has happened in many cases, for exonerating prisoners who had been wrongly convicted. This application is called **DNA fingerprinting.**

Any polymorphism can be used, but *VNTRs are by far the most useful polymorphisms for DNA finger-printing.* **Microsatellites** are short VNTRs, usually with 2 to 4 nucleotides in the repeat unit and a total length well below 1000, whereas **minisatellites** have longer repeat units and a total length of more than 1000 nucleotides.

DNA fingerprinting can be performed with Southern blotting or PCR (Fig. 11.14). Southern blotting requires a large amount of DNA: for example, that from a drop of seminal fluid from a sex offender. PCR is used when only a small amount of DNA is available: for example, that from a single hair of the murderer stuck under the victim's fingernail. However, because of its high sensitivity, PCR is more vulnerable to contamination by extraneous DNA. This could put the laboratory technician at risk of being wrongly convicted!

VNTRs are also used for paternity testing. DNA typing is replacing the time-honored immunological methods of blood group typing and human leukocyte antigen (HLA) typing for this purpose

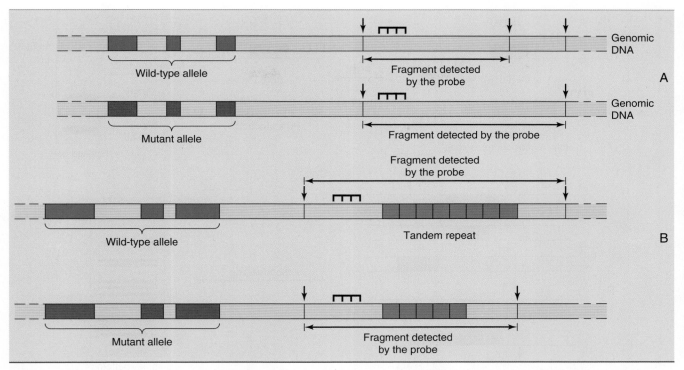

Figure 11.13 Restriction-site polymorphisms and variable numbers of tandem repeats (VNTRs) used for linkage analysis. **A,** A restriction-site polymorphism, caused by a base substitution in the recognition site of a restriction endonuclease. In this example the normal ("wild-type") allele is linked to the shorter fragment, and the mutant allele is linked to the longer fragment. **B,** VNTRs are especially useful because multiple alleles (repeat lengths) occur in the population. In this example, the mutant allele of the heterozygote will be transmitted to the children together with the shorter fragment. ↓, Cleavage by the restriction endonuclease; ⊓⊓⊓, probe used to detect the polymorphism.

because they allow an almost 100% accurate determination of paternity—unless the alternative putative fathers are identical twins.

DNA Microarrays Can Be Used for Genetic Screening

Dot blotting is the established method for genetic screening, but it tests for only one or a few mutations or polymorphisms at a time. The ideal method would test for thousands of DNA variants at a time or scan a whole gene for all possible point mutations.

DNA microarrays, also known as **"DNA chips,"** make this possible. In dot blotting, the patient's DNA is immobilized on nitrocellulose paper, and a fluorescent-labeled probe is added. *In DNA microarrays, the reverse strategy is used, with unlabeled probes rather than patient DNA immobilized on the chip.*

An **oligonucleotide microarray** is prepared from a glass slide that is subdivided into thousands of little squares. Through photochemical methods, *an oligonucleotide with a length of at least 20 nucleotides is synthesized on each square.* Each square gets a different oligonucleotide, and each oligonucleotide is complementary to a short stretch of genomic DNA.

Figure 11.15 shows an experimental procedure. First, oligonucleotides whose 3′ terminus is immediately adjacent to a variable site in the target DNA are synthesized. Photochemical methods are employed to synthesize thousands of such oligonucleotides in one sitting, each for a different DNA variant. All these oligonucleotides are hybridized simultaneously to the denatured target DNA.

Incubation with a DNA polymerase and the four *di*deoxyribonucleotides, each labeled with a different fluorescent tag, produces fluorescent-labeled oligonucleotides. The mix of fluorescent oligonucleotides is then applied to the DNA chip. The nucleotide in the variable site of the target DNA is deduced not from binding or nonbinding of the oligonucleotide but from the color of the fluorescence.

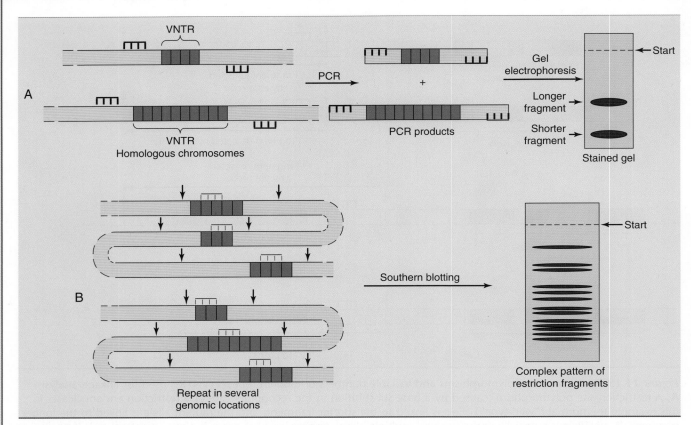

Figure 11.14 Variable numbers of tandem repeats (VNTRs) used for DNA fingerprinting. **A,** Microsatellites consist of dinucleotides, trinucleotides, or tetranucleotide repeats. They are used for single-locus DNA fingerprinting with the polymerase chain reaction (PCR). Even if the repeat is present in many places throughout the genome, the use of the primers ensures that only one of them is amplified. The two homologous chromosomes in each individual will produce two PCR products, and in most cases these will be of different lengths. This method does not require a probe because the PCR products can be identified directly by staining the gel after electrophoresis. **B,** Minisatellites consist of longer repeat units: for example, (AGGGCTGGAGG)$_n$ or (AGAGGTGGGCAGGTGG)$_n$. They can be used for multilocus DNA fingerprinting, through Southern blotting with a frequently cutting restriction endonuclease (for example, *Hae*III; see Table 11.1). The restriction fragments are detected with a probe that is directed at the repeat sequence itself, and therefore any fragment containing the repeat will be detected. If, for example, the repeat is present in 20 locations (loci) in the genome, up to 40 fragments of different lengths will be seen after gel electrophoresis. ⊓⊓, Primer; ⊓⊓, Probe; ↓, restriction site.

DNA Microarrays Are Used for the Study of Gene Expression

The use of microarrays for large-scale genotyping is still experimental. Another use, however, is well established: the study of gene expression.

Assume, for example, that a physician wants to know which genes have increased or reduced expression in a malignant tumor in relation to the normal cells from which the tumor originated. In this case, the scientist-physician can extract the mRNAs from the two sources. Using the procedure shown in Figure 11.17, the mRNAs are used as templates to make cDNAs. The cDNAs from the normal tissue are synthesized with a green fluorescent tag, and the cDNAs from the tumor are synthesized with a red fluorescent tag.

The two extracts are then mixed, and the mix is applied to a **cDNA microarray.** This type of DNA chip is prepared by applying a different known cDNA (with no fluorescent tag) to each square of the chip. Instead of authentic cDNA, synthetic oligonucleotides with a length of 40 to 60 nucleotides can also be used on the chip. In theory, a chip with 30,000 squares can test for the expression of each of a person's 30,000 genes. Each labeled cDNA from the normal cells and the tumor is complementary to an immobilized cDNA on the chip and will hybridize to that spot on the chip. If the expression of a gene is increased in the tumor, the red fluorescence is stronger than the green fluorescence; if its expression is reduced in the tumor, the green fluorescence is stronger. An example is shown in Figure 11.16.

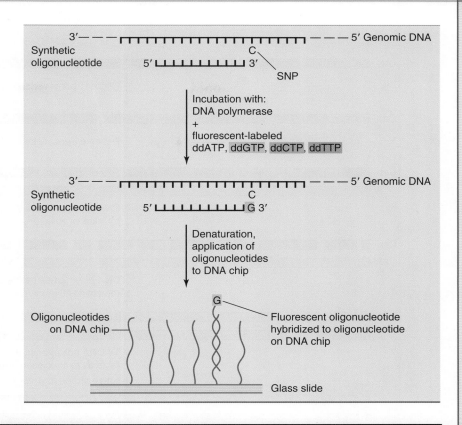

Figure 11.15 An experimental method for microarray-based single-nucleotide polymorphism (SNP) genotyping. Note that the fluorescent-labeled dideoxynucleotides—ddATP, ddCTP, ddGTP, and ddTTP—are incorporated by the DNA polymerase but also cause immediate chain termination, similar to their use in DNA sequencing (see Fig. 11.3). The immobilized oligonucleotides on the DNA chip are complementary to those that were incubated with the genomic DNA.

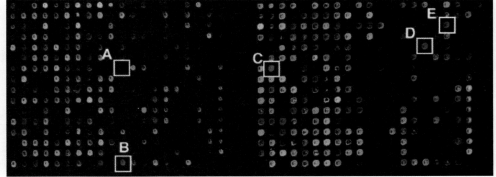

Figure 11.16 Section of a microarray showing a comparison of messenger RNA (mRNA) levels in fibroblasts *(green)* and rhabdomyosarcoma cells *(red).*

Genomic DNA Fragments Can Be Propagated in Bacterial Plasmids

A restriction digest of human genomic DNA contains up to a few million DNA fragments. Single fragments from this broth can be isolated by cloning in bacteria.

This does not require the integration of the DNA into the bacterial chromosome. Genetic engineers insert the foreign DNA in a self-replicating entity called a **cloning vector** instead. The cloning vector can be a plasmid or a bacteriophage. *Cloning requires the covalent joining of the foreign DNA with the vector DNA.*

Figure 11.18 shows the procedure for the cloning of a human DNA with an R-factor plasmid carrying resistance genes for tetracycline and ampicillin. The plasmid and the human DNA are cleaved with

the same highly selective restriction endonuclease. The circular plasmid DNA is cleaved at only one site, and the human DNA is fragmented into pieces of many thousands of base pairs.

Plasmid DNA and human DNA are mixed in the test tube, and their cohesive ends anneal spontaneously. DNA ligase is added, and *plasmid DNA and human DNA are covalently linked into a circle.* The recombinant plasmids are spirited into the bacteria by transformation.

This procedure generates millions of bacteria with recombinant plasmids. *A large collection of transformed bacteria, each containing a random piece of human genomic DNA, is called a* **genomic library.** A genomic library should have each piece of genomic DNA represented in at least one bacterium.

The recovery of the cloned DNA requires the two operations of selection and screening. **Selection**

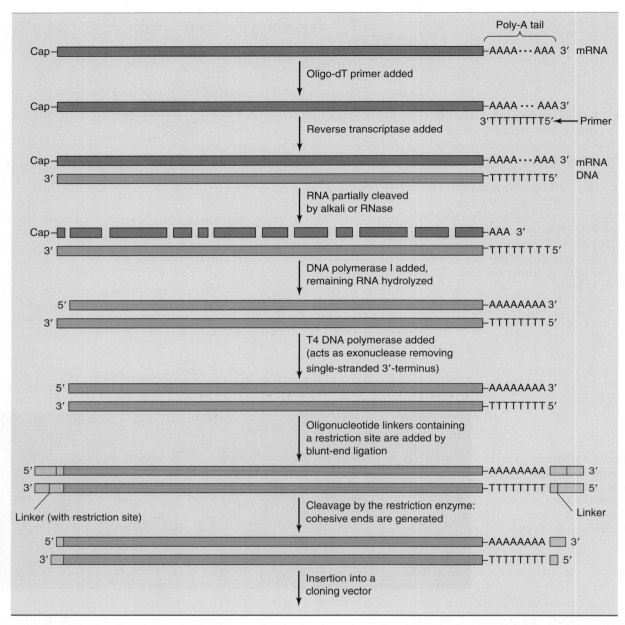

Figure 11.17 Procedure for the synthesis of cDNA for cloning in a plasmid or bacteriophage vector. dT, deoxythymidine.

makes use of the antibiotic resistance gene or genes in the cloning vector. These genes are referred to as **selectable markers.** In the example of Figure 11.18, the tetracycline resistance gene has been disrupted by the insertion of the foreign DNA, whereas the ampicillin resistance gene is still intact. Thus, properly transformed bacteria can grow in the presence of ampicillin but not tetracycline.

The transformed bacteria can be transferred to an agar plate, where each grows into a visible colony. Each colony consists of a **clone** of genetically identical bacteria that carry the same insert of foreign DNA.

The **screening** of a genomic library is performed with a probe for the desired DNA sequence, as shown in Figure 11.19. Once a clone with the desired sequence has been identified, the vector can be recovered and the insert excised with the same restriction endonuclease that had been used for the construction of the recombinant plasmid.

Many cloning vectors have been constructed. Most are derived from plasmids and some from bacteriophages. Some are used to clone small snippets of DNA, whereas others are more suitable for big chunks. **Bacterial artificial chromosomes,** for example, are large recombinant plasmids with a replication origin borrowed from the F factor. They are used to clone DNA pieces of several hundred thousand base pairs.

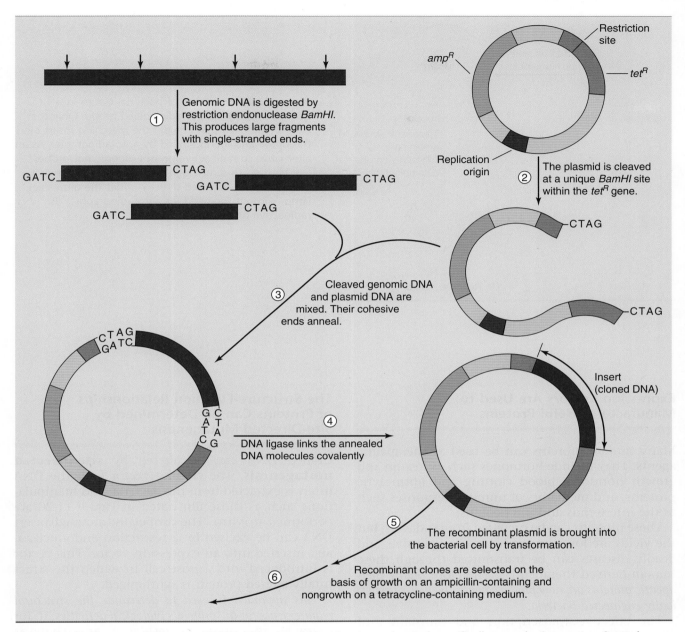

Figure 11.18 The use of plasmid pBR322. This plasmid has been constructed specifically as a cloning vector. Several restriction endonucleases (BamHI in this example) cleave the plasmid at unique sites within either the ampicillin-resistance (amp^R) gene or the tetracycline-resistance (tet^R) gene. In the application shown here, the tet^R gene is destroyed during cloning, whereas the amp^R gene remains intact. Bacteria transformed by a recombinant plasmid can be selected because they can grow in the presence of ampicillin but not of tetracycline.

Complementary DNA Libraries Contain Only Expressed DNA

Only 1.2% of the cloned DNA in genomic libraries codes for proteins. If scientists are interested only in the coding sequences, they have to start with mRNA rather than genomic DNA. The mRNA is extracted from a specific tissue or cell type, such as brain cells, liver cells, embryonic stem cells, or cul-tured fibroblasts, and is converted to a cDNA with the help of reverse transcriptase.

A **cDNA library** is a collection of all the *expressed* DNA of a cell type or tissue. A cDNA library from bone marrow, for example, contains many clones with the cDNAs for hemoglobin α and β chains; a cDNA library from the pancreas contains many cDNAs for pancreatic zymogens.

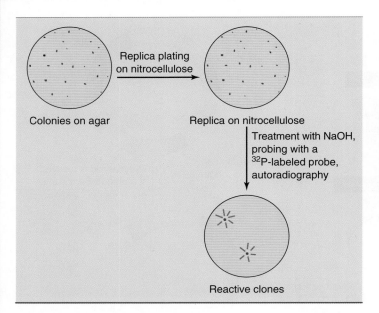

Figure 11.19 Screening of bacterial clones in a genomic library with a radiolabeled probe. Only the clones (colonies) that contain the matching insert bind the probe and are identified by autoradiography. As an alternative to radioactive probes, fluorescent probes can be used to screen genomic libraries. Fluorescent probes can be detected directly under the ultraviolet lamp, without the need for autoradiography. ^{32}P, radioactive phosphorus.

Expression Vectors Are Used to Manufacture Useful Proteins

Many human proteins can be used as therapeutic agents. They include hormones such as insulin and growth hormone, blood clotting and fibrinolytic proteins, and mediators of immune responses such as the interferons and interleukins.

These proteins can be prepared from cadavers, but the yields are low, the products are expensive, and deadly diseases can be transmitted through these human-derived therapeutics. Therefore, *many therapeutic proteins are now produced with the help of genetically engineered bacteria.*

The effective transcription and translation of cloned DNA requires an **expression vector,** and the following conditions have to be met:

1. Only *cDNA but not genomic DNA can be expressed in bacteria.* Bacteria cannot splice introns out of a transcript.
2. *The coding sequence (cDNA) must be joined to a strong bacterial promoter.* This is required for the initiation of transcription.
3. The *5′-untranslated region of the transcript must contain a Shine-Dalgarno sequence.* This is required for the initiation of translation.

Promoter and Shine-Dalgarno sequence are contributed by the expression vector. If a bacterial signal sequence is added as well, the bacteria will secrete the protein into the nutrient medium.

The Structure-Function Relationships of Proteins Can Be Determined by Site-Directed Mutagenesis

Cloned DNA can be altered by **site-directed mutagenesis.** The cloning vector with the DNA insert is extracted from the bacteria, and manipulations such as those illustrated in Figure 11.20 are performed in vitro. The artificially mutated insert DNA can be excised by a restriction endonuclease and inserted into an expression vector. This vector is introduced into a host cell in which the structurally altered protein is synthesized.

This approach is used to determine the structural requirements for the protein's biological activities. If, for example, an amino acid residue in an enzyme is essential for catalysis, then its substitution or deletion will abolish the enzyme's catalytic activity.

Gene Therapy Targets Somatic Cells

Most genetic diseases are caused by the mutational inactivation of an important gene. The most direct treatment for these diseases is the artificial repair of the defective gene or the introduction of a functional gene that can take the place of the defective one.

Somatic gene therapy is being developed for the treatment of genetic diseases and some nongenetic conditions. *This strategy does not manipulate the germline; it manipulates only the patient's somatic*

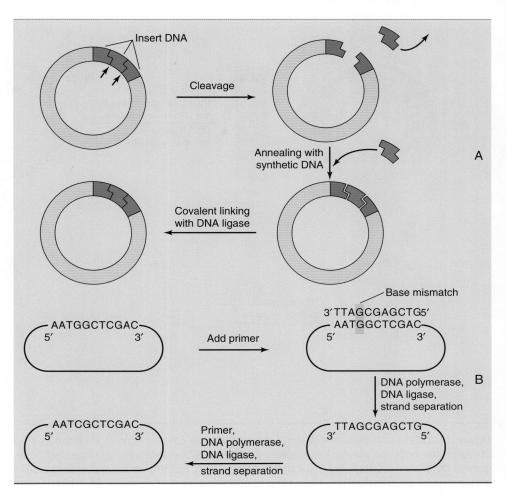

Figure 11.20 Site-directed mutagenesis of cloned DNA in vitro. **A,** A small piece of the cloned DNA is removed by a restriction endonuclease and replaced by a synthetic DNA containing the desired change. ↓, Restriction endonuclease cleavage. **B,** The DNA, inserted into a single-stranded cloning vector, is replicated with a DNA polymerase. The primer is a synthetic oligonucleotide that differs slightly from the original sequence. This primer becomes part of the new DNA strand. In this example, a transversion is achieved.

cells. It does not even attempt to change all somatic cells. For example, in Duchenne muscular dystrophy, an intact dystrophin gene is specifically targeted only to the muscles, and in cystic fibrosis (CF), the intact gene for the CF chloride channel is targeted to the lung epithelium.

Gene therapy is not an easy task. DNA does not cross biological membranes easily, and foreign DNA is rarely incorporated into the genome; it is degraded instead. Before the advent of genetic engineering, most intruding DNAs used to be viruses. Therefore, the cell's border controls are none too friendly to would-be immigrants, with barriers erected along the way and watchful DNases lurking at every corner.

To facilitate cell uptake, the gene can be coated with a lipid bilayer to form a **liposome,** also known as a **lipoplex.** After fusion of the lipid bilayer with the plasma membrane of the target cell, the enclosed gene is released into the cytoplasm (Fig. 11.21A). *Liposome-mediated gene transfer is not cell type specific,* and the DNA of liposomes injected into

the blood is most likely to end up in the endothelial cells lining the blood vessels.

Foreign genes can be taken up by receptor-mediated endocytosis if they are covalently bound to a suitable ligand (see Fig. 11.21B). For example, hepatocytes have a receptor for the uptake of worn-out plasma proteins (asialoglycoproteins). Therefore, a foreign gene that is covalently bound to an asialoglycoprotein is taken up by hepatocytes but not other cells.

Unfortunately, endocytosed macromolecules are usually routed to the lysosomes for degradation. This deplorable outcome can be avoided by including viral proteins in the ligand-DNA complex that disrupt the endosome membrane. Viruses use such proteins to escape from the endosome after endocytosis.

Passage through the nuclear pore complexes is another problem. Unless the DNA is attached to a nuclear localization signal (see Chapter 9), it is unlikely to enter the nucleus. Even if the therapeutic gene reaches the nucleus, however, its stable integration into the genome is unlikely to occur.

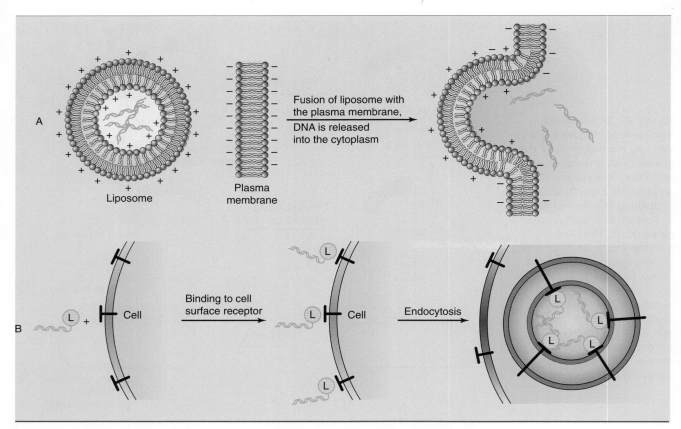

Figure 11.21 Physical methods of gene delivery. **A,** The foreign gene is enclosed in a liposome. To facilitate the fusion of the liposome with the plasma membrane, the liposome is constructed in large part from cationic lipids. **B,** The foreign gene is covalently linked to a ligand that is taken up by receptor-mediated endocytosis. Only cells possessing the receptor for the ligand are transformed. Unless the endosome is disrupted, however, most of the foreign DNA is degraded by lysosomal enzymes. L, ligand; T, receptor.

The foreign DNA remains extrachromosomal, does not replicate, and is eventually degraded by nucleases or diluted out of the cell with successive mitotic divisions.

Viruses Are Used as Vectors for Gene Therapy

Viruses are promising vectors for gene therapy because they are already well designed to bring their genes into the host cell and have their proteins synthesized there. In theory, all that is needed is to replace one or more of the viral genes by the therapeutic **transgene** and have it ferried into the cell by the virus. This process of virus-mediated gene transfer is called **transfection.**

DNA viruses can be used for this purpose. Adenoviruses, for example, are minor respiratory pathogens in humans. When an intact gene for the CF chloride channel is incorporated into the virus DNA in exchange for one or two nonessential viral genes, the virus will bring this transgene into the cells of the respiratory epithelium of CF patients. The gene is expressed in these cells, and the patient gets better as long as the virus is present. Regrettably, *DNA viruses do not normally integrate themselves into the host cell DNA.* Therefore, the therapeutic benefits are transient.

Also, viral proteins and virus particles are still produced by the vector. This damages the cells and alerts the adaptive immune system to produce antibodies against the virus and destroy the virus-infected cells. On the other hand, these vectors can be produced in quantity, and they are able to infect nondividing cells.

Retroviruses Can Splice a Transgene into the Cell's Genome

Unlike DNA viruses, retroviruses integrate themselves into the host cell genome as part of their normal life cycle. Indeed, *retroviral vectors are the*

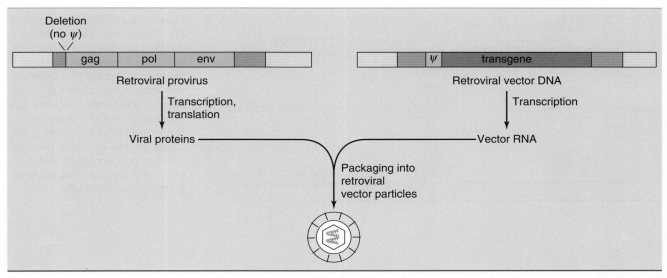

Figure 11.22 Construction of a retroviral vector for gene therapy. Both the retroviral provirus and the retroviral vector DNA are integrated in the producer cell genome. The vector RNA is packaged with the proteins produced by the retroviral provirus. The provirus RNA cannot be packaged because it lacks the packaging signal. ■, Viral genes; ■, long terminal repeat; ■, foreign gene to be transferred; ψ, packaging signal; gag, pol, and env, normal retroviral genes.

most popular vectors for gene therapy because they target the transgene directly to the chromosomes of the cell.

The retroviral vectors that are used for gene therapy contain the long terminal repeats of a "real" retrovirus, but except for a portion of the gag gene that doubles as a packaging signal, *the viral genes are replaced by the transgene.* Retroviral vectors can carry inserts of up to 9000 base pairs, enough to code for a large protein. The transgenes are intronless constructs that are produced from a cDNA or chemically synthesized.

After integration into the cellular genome, the transgene is transcribed from the retroviral promoter in the upstream long terminal repeat (LTR). In other cases, and especially when the regulated expression of the gene is required, an appropriate promoter is spliced into the vector to drive gene expression.

Retroviral vectors produce neither viral proteins nor infectious virus particles. Therefore, they are "clean" vectors that do not damage the cells.

Retroviral vectors are produced in cultured cells that contain the genome of a defective retrovirus. The defective retrovirus expresses the viral genes but is lacking the packaging signal. The gene therapy vector, on the other hand, cannot synthesize viral proteins but has the packaging signal. When the vector is introduced into the cells, it is therefore the vector RNA that is packaged into the virus particles along with retroviral reverse transcriptase and integrase (Fig. 11.22).

Retroviral gene transfer is not very efficient. Even in cell cultures, fewer than 10% of the cells are transfected in most experiments. Also, *most retroviruses cannot infect nondividing cells because they lack a nuclear localization signal to guide them through the nuclear pore complexes. This is true for retroviral vectors as well.* They are therefore poorly suited for gene therapy of nondividing end-stage cells such as neurons and muscle fibers.

The AIDS virus (human immunodeficiency virus [HIV]) does have a nuclear localization signal and can infect nondividing cells. Efforts are therefore under way to construct vectors based on HIV-related viruses.

Gene therapy is still experimental. It is most promising in cases in which transfection of a small number of cells is sufficient to cure the disease and tightly regulated gene expression is not required. For example, clotting factor deficiencies such as hemophilia can potentially be treated by bringing an intact copy of the gene into a small percentage of liver cells.

However, gene therapy for diabetes with a transgene for insulin would be difficult because the expression of the gene would have to be responsive to the blood glucose level, and in hemoglobinopathies, the transgene would have to be brought into a substantial fraction of bone marrow cells in which it would have to be expressed at appropriate levels and during the right stages of erythrocyte maturation.

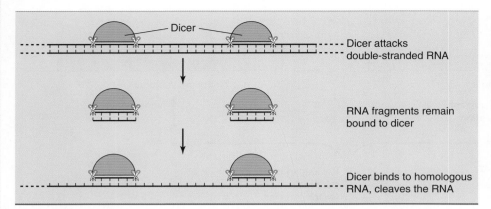

Figure 11.23 RNA interference. The RNase dicer cleaves long double-stranded RNA molecules, including those of RNA viruses. It generates 22–base pair fragments that remain bound to the enzyme and direct it against both single-stranded and double-stranded RNA of the same sequence. For antisense therapy, 22–base pair double-stranded RNA (or a suitable RNA analog) is introduced artificially.

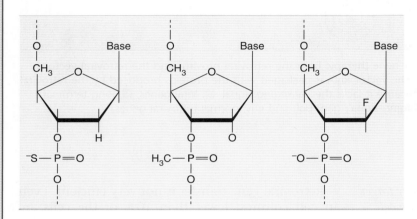

Figure 11.24 Structural modifications in experimentally used antisense oligonucleotides. These modifications are intended to make the oligonucleotides resistant to nucleases, facilitate their uptake into cells, or increase their affinity for their messenger RNA targets.

Antisense Oligonucleotides Can Block the Expression of Rogue Genes

Some diseases are caused not by the lack of a normal gene but by the expression or overexpression of an undesirable gene. In cancers, for example, growth-stimulating genes are either overexpressed or mutated to produce superactive proteins. These genes are called **oncogenes** (see Chapter 18). In theory, *cancer growth can be blocked by inhibiting the expression of oncogenes in the malignant cells.* Similarly, *viral diseases can be treated by inhibiting the expression of essential viral genes.*

Antisense technology makes use of oligonucleotides that are complementary to an undesirable mRNA. *By hybridizing with the mRNA, the antisense oligonucleotide blocks translation.* Antisense oligonucleotides against the 5'-untranslated region or the start codon are especially effective because they block translational initiation.

In addition, *many antisense oligonucleotides induce the cleavage of the mRNA by* **RNase H.** Ordinarily, this cellular enzyme cleaves the RNA strand in a DNA-RNA hybrid. It participates in primer removal during DNA replication, and it is part of the cell's defenses against viral infections.

Antisense agents must have a length of at least 18 to 20 nucleotides to achieve sufficient selectivity for their target sequence, and *nuclease-resistant oligonucleotide analogs are commonly employed.* Figure 11.24 shows some examples. However, even these nuclease-resistant analogs show poor cell uptake and therefore have to be used at high concentrations. This is regrettable because the chemical synthesis of bulk quantities of antisense agents is quite expensive.

Another approach makes use of **RNA interference,** a natural mechanism that evolved as a defense against RNA viruses. Any long double-stranded RNA in the cell is liable to be cleaved into 22–base pair fragments by a cellular RNase complex called **dicer.** The fragments of double-stranded RNA remain bound to the enzyme, and they direct it to single-stranded RNAs with the same sequence. These RNAs are also cleaved (Fig. 11.23).

When a small double-stranded RNA is introduced into the cell, it binds to the dicer complex and directs it against mRNAs with the same sequence. In theory, a single double-stranded RNA molecule can direct the enzyme to destroy thousands of mRNA molecules carrying the same sequence. Effectively, *the antisense oligonucleotide tricks the cell into treating its own mRNA as an invading RNA virus.*

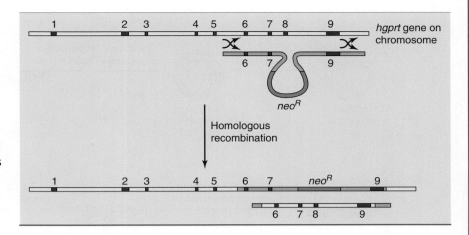

Figure 11.25 The disruption of the gene for hypoxanthine-guanine phosphoribosyltransferase *(hgprt)* in embryonic stem cells. The disrupting DNA is incorporated into the *hgprt* gene through homologous recombination with the chromosomal DNA. A neomycin resistance gene *(neo^R)* is included in the disruption probe as a selectable marker. Only cells that have incorporated this gene are able to grow on a neomycin-containing medium.

Selective Germline Mutations Can Be Produced

Germline cells as well as somatic cells can be manipulated genetically. Genes can be disrupted artificially to produce **knockout mice.** These animals are used in basic research to study the biological importance of genes and to create animal models of human diseases.

Gene disruptions can be achieved with DNA constructs that have sequence homology with the targeted gene, as shown in Figure 11.25. These constructs have to be brought into the cell by injection or electroporation, and their integration into the genome depends on the cellular enzyme systems for homologous recombination.

The introduction of foreign genes results in **transgenic animals.** Transgenic animals are used not only in research but also for "pharming." For example, cattle and sheep that secrete human hormones, clotting factors, or other therapeutic proteins in their milk have been produced.

There are three general methods for the production of genetically modified animals (Fig. 11.26):

1. *The foreign gene is injected into the oocyte.* It can insert randomly anywhere in the genome or by homologous recombination in sites that share sequence homology with the gene construct. Foreign genes can also be introduced in retroviral vectors. After fertilization in the test tube, the zygote is implanted into a foster animal and grown into a genetically modified animal.
2. *The foreign gene is engineered into cultured embryonic stem cells, followed by injection of the engineered stem cells into an embryo at the blastocyst stage.* Because embryonic stem cells are totipotent, they can contribute to all tissues of the developing embryo. The embryos are implanted in foster animals and develop into chimeric animals. *If some of the stem cells enter the germline, the genetic modification can be transmitted to the animal's descendants.* Although the genetic change is initially present in the heterozygous state, it can be made homozygous by classical breeding. This is currently the major method for the production of genetically modified animals.
3. *The gene is engineered into embryonic stem cells whose nuclei are then transferred into enucleated oocytes.* The cloned animals that are produced with this method have the genetic modification in all their cells.

Tissue-Specific Gene Expression Can Be Engineered into Animals

Artificially introduced genes must be linked to an appropriate promoter. For example, a genetic engineer who wants to make humans capable of cellulose digestion could combine a cellulase gene from a snail or a fungus with a signal sequence and the promoter of the gene for trypsinogen or some other pancreatic zymogen. After introduction into the germline, the protein product of this gene is secreted only by the pancreas.

Gene knockouts can be made tissue-specific with the help of **loxP** sites. The loxP site is a 34–base pair palindromic sequence that is recognized by the **Cre recombinase.** This enzyme acts somewhat like a spliceosome but with DNA rather than RNA as a substrate. *Cre recombinase cuts out the DNA between two loxP sites and splices the flanking DNA together.*

Figure 11.27 shows a procedure that has been employed to create knockout mice lacking the gene for the insulin receptor specifically in adipose tissue. The transgenic mice have exon 4 of the insulin receptor gene flanked with loxP sites. They

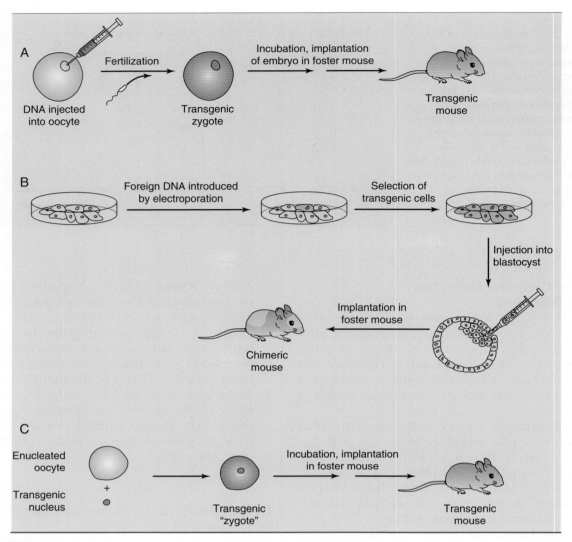

Figure 11.26 Three methods for the production of genetically modified animals. **A,** Foreign DNA is injected into the oocyte. **B,** Cultured embryonic stem cells are genetically modified. These cells are injected in the inner cell mass of a developing embryo at the blastocyst stage to produce a chimeric animal. **C,** Reproductive cloning with the nucleus of a genetically modified embryonic stem cell.

also have the *cre* gene under the control of a tissue-specific promoter that permits gene expression only in adipose tissue.

When the *cre* gene is expressed in adipose tissue, *the Cre recombinase does no harm to normal DNA because the genome does not contain any loxP sites.* Only exon 4 of the insulin receptor gene is cut out of the genome.

The resulting mice cannot make insulin receptors in adipose tissue. Therefore, their adipose tissue cannot respond to insulin. However, they are not diabetic because the insulin receptor is intact in all other tissues. These mice are very lean, and they live longer than normal obese laboratory mice.

Antisense genes offer an alternative to the use of loxP sites. An antisense gene encodes an mRNA that is complementary to the mRNA of the targeted gene. When both genes are expressed in the same cell, the two mRNAs form a double helix that is degraded by dicer or other RNases. For example, an antisense gene for the insulin receptor with an adipose tissue specific promoter would prevent the synthesis of the insulin receptor in adipose tissue without destroying the insulin receptor gene.

The Production of Transgenic Humans Is Technically Possible

In theory, transgenic humans can be produced with the methods described in Figure 11.26. Unfortunately, all these methods are so haphazard that the

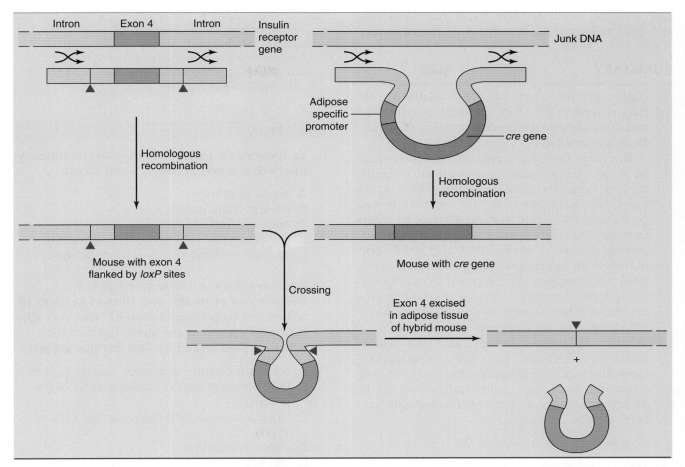

Figure 11.27 A strategy for eliminating the insulin receptor gene selectively in adipose tissue. A strain of mice is created with *loxP* sites (▲) flanking one of the exons (exon 4) of the insulin receptor gene. Another strain is created with the *cre* gene under the control of an adipose tissue selective promoter. When these two strains are crossed to create mice with both kinds of genetic modification, the Cre recombinase excises exon 4 only in adipose tissue.

risk of genetic and developmental abnormalities is unacceptably high.

Human artificial chromosomes are a safer way of making better people. *These chromosomes contain centromeres, telomeres, and replication origins, along with splice sites for the insertion of gene cassettes.* The desired genes are inserted, and the chromosome is injected into the nucleus of the oocyte or zygote during in vitro fertilization. Genes that people might wish to give to their children include the following:

1. *Life-prolonging genes.* Some genetic manipulations in animals, including the adipose-selective insulin receptor knockout shown in Figure 11.27, are known to prolong life.
2. *Tumor suppressor genes.* These are normal genes for DNA repair or negative controls on mitosis whose homozygous inactivation contributes to cancer. In one example, transgenic mice with an extra copy of the tumor suppressor gene *p53* (see

Chapter 18) had a substantially reduced cancer risk. There are many tumor suppressor genes, and having one or two extra copies of each could protect people from cancer.

3. *Genes that antagonize age-related changes.* For example, **Alzheimer disease** is the most common cause of senile dementia. It is caused by the gradual accumulation of a peptide called **β-amyloid** that is derived from a membrane protein called amyloid precursor protein (APP). A brain-expressed antisense gene for APP could reduce the formation of APP and prevent the accumulation of β-amyloid.

Human artificial chromosomes can be equipped with loxP sites left and right of the centromere and a *cre* gene controlled by a germline-specific promoter. In that case, *the centromere will be cut out and the chromosome will be destroyed in the germline, preventing its transmission to the next generation.* When deciding about their children's genes, parents will certainly want to give them not their own outdated chromosome but the most recent model!

SUMMARY

Highly efficient methods are available for the fragmentation of DNA, cloning of the fragments in bacteria, enzymatic amplification, and DNA sequencing.

The most important applications of molecular genetic techniques in medicine are currently for genotyping and the diagnosis of genetic diseases. People can be tested for recessive disease genes and for genes that predispose to multifactorial diseases. Prenatal and preimplantation genetic diagnoses are possible, and whole populations can be screened for problematic genes. DNA microarrays offer the prospect of genotyping people for thousands of mutations and genetic polymorphisms in a single procedure.

Therapeutic applications in the form of somatic cell gene therapy and the use of antisense methods are still experimental. Germline gene modifications have not yet been attempted in humans, although whole armies of knockout mice and transgenic animals have been created.

📖 Further Reading

Blüher M, Kahn BB, Kahn CR: Extended longevity in mice lacking the insulin receptor in adipose tissue. Science 299:572-573, 2003.

Bunney WE, Bunney BG, Vawter MP, et al: Microarray technology: a review of new strategies to discover candidate vulnerability genes in psychiatric disorders. Am J Psychiat 160:657-666, 2003.

Davis ME: Non-viral gene delivery systems. Curr Opin Biotechnol 13:128-131, 2002.

Garcia-Cao I, Garcia-Cao M, Martin-Caballero J, et al: "Super p53" mice exhibit enhanced DNA damage response, are tumor resistant and age normally. EMBO J 21:6225-6235, 2002.

Kuroiwa Y, Tomizuka K, Shinohara T, et al: Manipulation of human minichromosomes to carry greater than megabase-sized chromosome inserts. Nature Biotechnol 18:1086-1090, 2000.

Kurreck J: Antisense technologies. Improvement through novel chemical modifications. Eur J Biochem 270:1628-1644, 2003.

Kwok P-Y: Methods for genotyping single nucleotide polymorphisms. Annu Rev Genomics Hum Genet 2:235-258, 2001.

Pfeifer A, Verma IM: Gene therapy: promises and problems. Annu Rev Genomics Hum Genet 2:177-211, 2001.

Southern E: Blotting at 25. Trends Biochem Sci 25:585-588, 2000.

Stock G: Redesigning Humans. Choosing Our Children's Genes. London: Profile Books, 2002.

Vasquez KM, Marburger K, Intody Z, Wilson JH: Manipulating the mammalian genome by homologous recombination. Proc Natl Acad Sci U S A 98:8403-8410, 2001.

QUESTIONS

1. To sequence a piece of DNA with the dideoxy method, you will probably want to use

   A. A pair of primers.
   B. Reverse transcriptase.
   C. Southern blotting.
   D. Fluorescent-labeled deoxyribonucleotides.
   E. Fluorescent-labeled dideoxyribonucleotides.

2. You have been instructed by the U.S. Department of Health and Human Services to screen the whole population of New York City for the presence of the sickle cell mutation. What method would be best for this project?

   A. Southern blotting with allele-specific probes.
   B. PCR, with electrophoretic separation of the products.
   C. Linkage analysis with closely linked RSPs or VNTRs.
   D. cDNA microarrays.
   E. Dot blotting.

3. Retroviral vectors are more popular for somatic gene therapy than other viral vectors because

   A. They replicate faster than most other viruses.
   B. They contain several copies of their DNA genome in the virus particle.
   C. They can integrate themselves into the host cell DNA.
   D. Their replication is more accurate than that of most other viruses.
   E. Their DNA has extensive sequence homology with normal cellular DNA.

4. The steps of classical Southern blotting include (1) denaturation of DNA with alkali; (2) electrophoresis in a crosslinked agarose or polyacrylamide gel; (3) application of a probe; (4) treatment of DNA with a restriction endonuclease and (5) blotting of DNA to nitrocellulose paper. The correct sequence of these steps is

   A. 1 → 4 → 2 → 5 → 3.
   B. 4 → 3 → 1 → 2 → 5.
   C. 1 → 5 → 2 → 3 → 4.
   D. 4 → 2 → 1 → 5 → 3.
   E. 2 → 1 → 5 → 4 → 3.

5. If you want to use genetically engineered bacteria for the production of human growth hormone, you need all of the following ingredients except

A. A cDNA obtained by the reverse transcription of growth hormone mRNA.
B. A bacterial promoter sequence.
C. A DNA sequence that codes for a bacterial ribosome-binding sequence.
D. Genomic DNA of the growth hormone gene.
E. Restriction endonucleases.

6. PCR-based procedures are often preferred over Southern blotting for the prenatal diagnosis of genetic diseases after amniocentesis or chorionic villus sampling. Why?

A. PCR requires less DNA, and therefore lengthy cell culturing may not be necessary.
B. PCR requires less technical skill than Southern blotting and is therefore less costly.
C. PCR is less sensitive to contamination by extraneous DNA and therefore less prone to false positive results.
D. Unlike Southern blotting, PCR does not require DNA from many family members.
E. Unlike Southern blotting, PCR does not require any knowledge of the DNA sequence in and around the affected gene.

7. The classical PCR procedure (without allele-specific primers and without probes) can be used to

A. Amplify the whole dystrophin gene with its 79 exons and 78 introns in one piece.
B. Diagnose the sickle cell mutation after amniocentesis.
C. Diagnose HIV infection in people with risky lifestyles.
D. Detect point mutations in a gene whose sequence is unknown.
E. Perform all of the above.

8. In order to genotype a skin color gene in DNA from a 30,000-year-old Neanderthal skeleton, you will definitely have to use

A. Southern blotting with allele-specific probes.
B. In situ hybridization.
C. PCR.
D. Oligonucleotide microarrays.
E. Linkage with closely linked VNTR polymorphisms.

9. Linkage studies with closely linked VNTRs are the preferred diagnostic method for the detection of heterozygous carriers of recessive disease genes when

A. There is allelic heterogeneity: Scientists do not know which mutation is present in a known disease gene.
B. There is locus heterogeneity: Scientists do not know which gene is mutated.
C. No case of the disease has so far occurred in the family.
D. Population-wide screening is intended.
E. The exact molecular nature of the mutation is known.

10. In order to compare the expression of a large number of genes in rhabdomyosarcoma cells with gene expression in normal skeletal muscle, you have isolated mRNA from the two sources by affinity chromatography on an oligo-dT column. The most direct method to compare the two mRNA patterns would be

A. PCR with nested primers.
B. Dot blotting.
C. Cloning in bacteria.
D. Southern blotting.
E. Northern blotting.

11. Alternatively, the mRNAs from the tumor and normal cells can be compared using

A. Allele-specific amplification.
B. Expression cloning.
C. In situ hybridization.
D. cDNA miroarrays.
E. RNA interference.

PART THREE

CELL AND TISSUE STRUCTURE

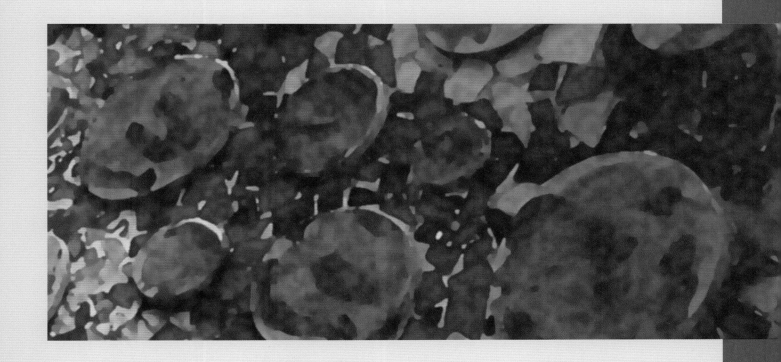

CHAPTER 12

Biological Membranes

All cells are surrounded by a **plasma membrane,** and eukaryotes (but not prokaryotes) have membrane-bounded **organelles** as well.

The terms *plasma membrane* and *cell wall,* so often confused by students, refer to very different structures. The plasma membrane is as thin and fragile as a soap bubble, and yet it forms an effective diffusion barrier. It consists of lipids and proteins.

The cell wall, on the other hand, is strong and stiff and maintains the shape of the cell. Plants and bacteria have a cell wall that is made of tough polysaccharides such as cellulose or peptidoglycan, but humans do not. Human cells are kept in shape by the **cytoskeleton** instead, and human tissues derive mechanical strength from the **extracellular matrix.** This chapter introduces the structure and properties of cellular membranes.

Membranes Consist of Lipid and Protein

Under the electron microscope, a biological membrane in cross-section looks like a railroad track, with a lightly stained layer sandwiched between two deeply stained layers. This structure, with a total diameter of 8 nm, is formed from two layers of lipids.

The membrane lipids are **amphiphilic** or **amphipathic.** This means that *hydrophilic and hydrophobic parts are combined in the same molecule.* **Phospholipids** contain a phosphate group in their hydrophilic part, and **glycolipids** contain covalently attached carbohydrate. On the basis of their chemical building blocks, three classes of membrane lipids can be distinguished: the **phosphoglycerides,** the **sphingolipids,** and **cholesterol.**

Membranes contain proteins as well as lipids. *Lipids form the structural backbone of the membrane, and proteins are in charge of specific functions.* These functions include enzymatic activities, regulated transport, ion permeability and excitability, contact with structural proteins, and the transmission of physiological signals. Therefore, the protein/lipid ratio is highest in membranes with high metabolic activity, such as the inner mitochondrial membrane (Fig. 12.1).

The Phosphoglycerides Are the Most Abundant Membrane Lipids

Phosphoglycerides account for more than one half of all lipids in most membranes (see Fig. 12.1). Their parent compound is **phosphatidic acid,** or **phosphatidate.** It looks similar to a triglyceride but with the third fatty acid of the triglyceride replaced by phosphate:

$$H_2C-O-\overset{\overset{\displaystyle O}{\|}}{C}-R_1$$

$$R_2-\overset{\overset{\displaystyle O}{\|}}{C}-O-CH$$

$$H_2C-O-\overset{\overset{\displaystyle O}{\|}}{C}-R_3$$

Triglyceride

$$H_2C-O-\overset{\overset{\displaystyle O}{\|}}{C}-R_1$$

$$R_2-\overset{\overset{\displaystyle O}{\|}}{C}-O-CH$$

$$H_2C-O-\overset{\overset{\displaystyle O^-}{|}}{\underset{\underset{\displaystyle O}{\|}}{P}}-O^-$$

Phosphatidate

The major membrane phosphoglycerides have a second alcohol bound to the phosphate group in phosphatidic acid, and they are named as derivatives of phosphatidic acid (phosphatidyl-) (Fig. 12.2).

The phosphate group is negatively charged and therefore strongly hydrophilic. Also, the variable alcohol that is bound to the phosphate is either charged or has a high hydrogen bonding potential. *Together with the phosphate, it forms the hydrophilic head group of the molecule, whereas the two fatty acids form two hydrophobic tails.* The fatty acid in position 1 is usually saturated, and that in position 2 is unsaturated.

Two less common phosphoglycerides are shown in Figure 12.3. **Cardiolipin** (diphosphatidyl-glycerol) is common only in the inner mitochondrial membrane. The widespread **plasmalogens,** usually with ethanolamine in their head group, are defined by the presence of an α-β unsaturated fatty alcohol, rather than a fatty acid residue, in position 1.

Dipalmitoyl-Phosphatidylcholine Is the Most Important Component of Lung Surfactant

Most phosphoglycerides are employed only as structural components of biological membranes. **Dipalmitoyl phosphatidylcholine (dipalmitoyl lecithin**), however, plays a special role as the major constituent of **lung surfactant.** This lipoprotein is secreted by type II alveolar cells. *It reduces the surface tension of the thin fluid film that lines the alveolar walls.* Without it, the alveoli collapse and breathing becomes difficult.

This happens in preterm infants who are born with insufficient lung surfactant. They develop **respiratory distress syndrome,** a condition

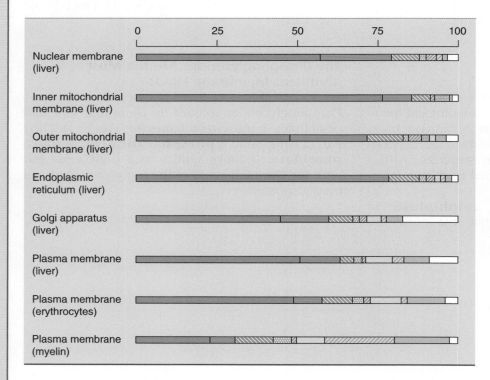

Figure 12.1 The composition of biological membranes. ■, Protein; ▨, phosphatidyl choline; ◹, phosphatidyl ethanolamine; ▨, phosphatidyl serine; ▨, phosphatidyl inositol; ▨, cardiolipin; □, sphingomyelin; ▨, glycolipids; ▨, cholesterol; □, others.

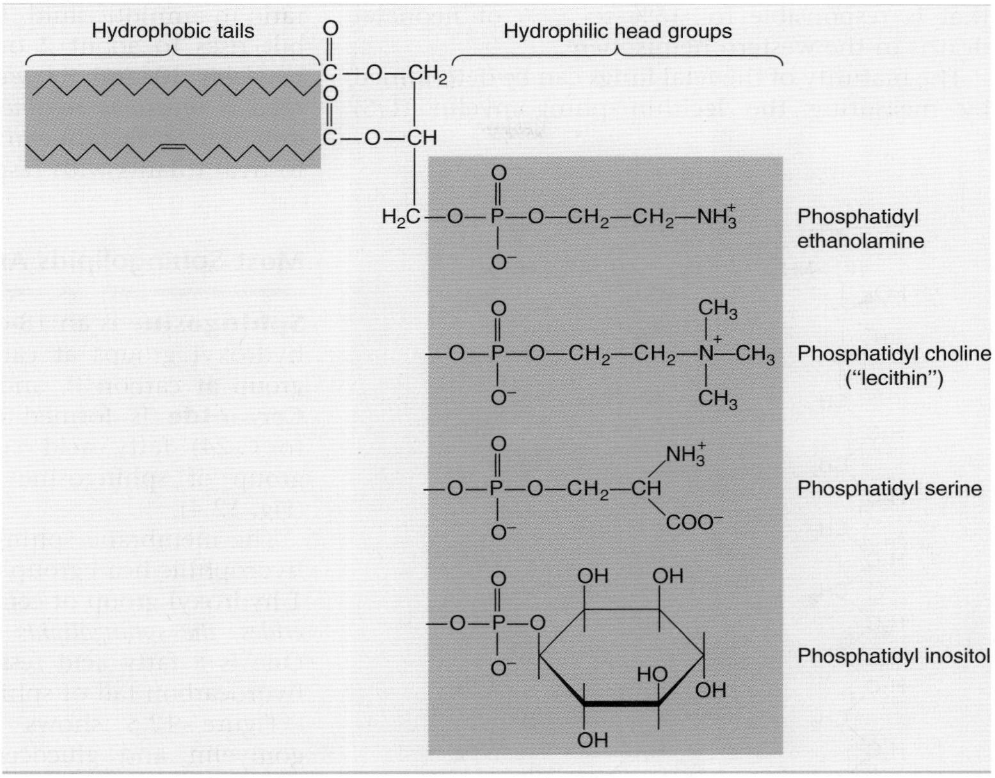

Figure 12.2 Structures of the most common phosphoglycerides.

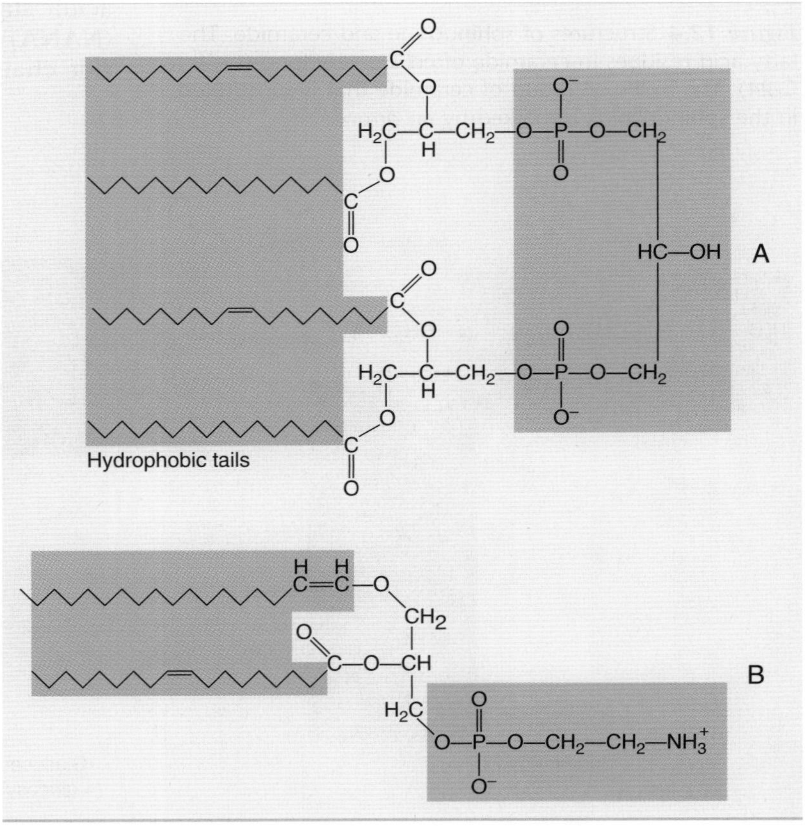

Figure 12.3 Structures of cardiolipin and plasmalogen. **A,** Cardiolipin, a major lipid of the inner mitochondrial membrane. **B,** Ethanolamine plasmalogen. Plasmalogens account for up to 10% of the phospholipid in muscle and nervous tissue and are present in most other tissues as well.

that is responsible for 15% to 20% of neonatal deaths in the western hemisphere.

The maturity of the fetal lungs can be determined by measuring the lecithin/sphingomyelin (L/S) ratio in amniotic fluid. The L/S ratio is initially low but rises to about 2 or a little higher sometime between 30 and 34 weeks of gestation. *The L/S ratio is measured routinely for the timing of elective deliveries.* Surfactant can be administered by inhaler to treat infants with respiratory distress syndrome.

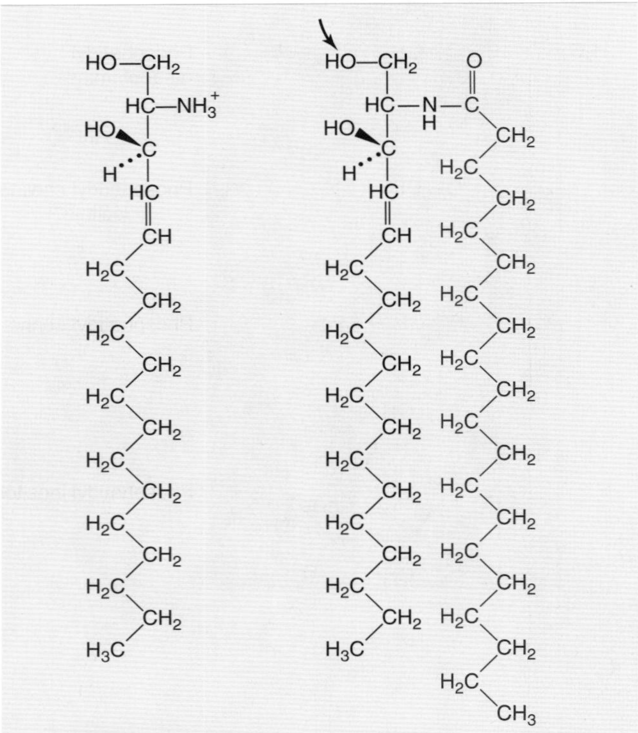

Most Sphingolipids Are Glycolipids

Sphingosine is an 18-carbon amino alcohol with hydroxyl groups at carbons 1 and 3, an amino group at carbon 2, and a long hydrocarbon tail. **Ceramide** is formed when a long-chain (C-18 to C-24) fatty acid combines with the amino group of sphingosine through an amide bond (Fig. 12.4).

The membrane sphingolipids contain a variable hydrophilic head group covalently bound to the C-1 hydroxyl group of ceramide. *Like the phosphoglycerides, the sphingolipids have two hydrophobic tails.* One is a fatty acid residue, and the other is the hydrocarbon tail of sphingosine.

Figure 12.5 shows the structures of sphingomyelin and glucocerebroside. Sphingomyelin, which has the same head group as phosphatidylcholine (see Fig. 12.2), qualifies as a phospholipid. All other sphingolipids are glycolipids. The most complex glycosphingolipids are the **gangliosides.** They contain between one and four residues of the acidic sugar derivative **N-acetylneuraminic acid** (**NANA**) in terminal positions of their oligosaccharide chain:

Figure 12.4 Structures of sphingosine and ceramide. The fatty acid residues in ceramide often are very long (C-20 to C-24). The hydroxyl group of ceramide that is substituted in the sphingolipids is marked by an *arrow*.

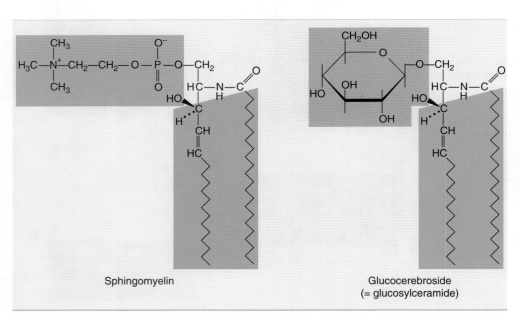

Figure 12.5 Two types of sphingolipid. Sphingomyelin is a phosphosphingolipid, and glucocerebroside is a glycosphingolipid.

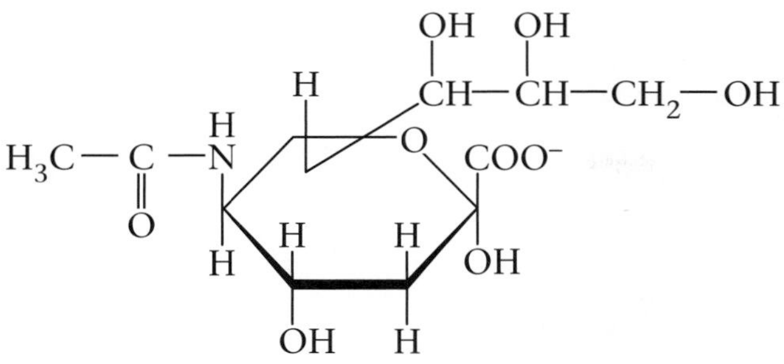

N-Acetylneuraminic acid
(NANA)

Glycosphingolipids are most abundant in the outer leaflet of the plasma membrane, where their carbohydrate heads face the extracellular environment. Sphingomyelin and galactocerebroside (the latter partly in a sulfated form) are important constituents of myelin, and gangliosides and galactocerebroside are abundant in the gray matter of the brain.

Cholesterol Is the Most Hydrophobic Membrane Lipid

Cholesterol is structurally more rigid than the other membrane lipids, with a stiff **steroid ring system** instead of wriggly hydrocarbon tails. Also, instead of a stately hydrophilic head group, there is only a puny hydroxyl group at one end of the molecule:

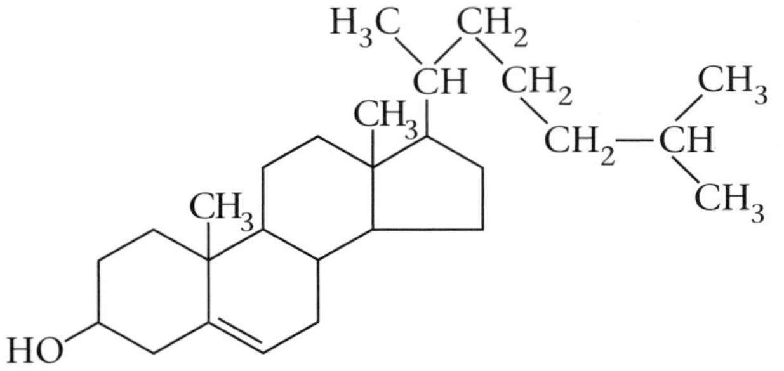

With this structure, *cholesterol is by far the least water-soluble membrane lipid.* Also, unlike the other membrane lipids, *cholesterol alone cannot form membrane-like structures, but it occurs only as a minor component in membranes whose basic structure is formed by other lipids.*

Cholesterol accounts for 10% or more of the total lipid in the plasma membrane and the Golgi membrane, but it is less abundant in other membranes. It is prominent only in animals. Plants have **phytosterols** instead, and most bacteria have no sterols at all. Therefore, *a vegan diet is cholesterol free.*

Membrane Lipids Form a Bilayer

The hydrophilic head groups of the membrane lipids interact with water, whereas the hydrophobic tails avoid water. Rather than dissolving in water as individual molecules, the membrane lipids form aggregates as shown in Figure 12.6.

Globular **micelles** are formed by most polar lipids, including ordinary detergents. **Monolayers** form only at aqueous/nonaqueous interfaces—for example, between water and air—whereas **bilayers** are surrounded by water on both sides. *All biological membranes contain a lipid bilayer as their structural backbone.* The bilayer is a noncovalent structure that is held together by hydrophobic interactions between the hydrocarbon tails of the membrane lipids.

The geometry of the lipid molecules determines whether a bilayer or a globular micelle forms. *A bilayer is formed only if the cross-sectional area of the head groups matches that of the hydrophobic tails.* If, for example, one of the fatty acids is removed from phosphatidylcholine (lecithin) by the enzyme **phospholipase A₂,** the hydrophobic portion becomes too thin. The resulting **lysolecithin** no longer fits into a bilayer but forms micelles instead. Phospholipase A₂ occurs in some snake venoms. It can cause hemolysis by hydrolyzing phosphoglycerides in the red blood cell membrane.

The Lipid Bilayer Is a Two-Dimensional Fluid

A lipid bilayer cannot exist as a flat sheet because its hydrophobic core would be exposed to the surrounding water at the edges. Therefore, *pieces of lipid bilayer tend to close in on themselves to form vesicles.* For the same reason, any tear or hole in the bilayer is energetically unfavorable and is liable to close spontaneously. As a result, *membranes are self-sealing.*

Lipid bilayers are easily deformed even by slight forces. Also, the hydrophobic tails of the lipids can merrily wriggle around, and *each molecule is free to diffuse laterally in the plane of the bilayer.* Lateral diffusion proceeds at a speed of about 2 μm/second in artificial bilayers.

Transverse diffusion, however, is difficult. To flip-flop from one leaflet of the bilayer to the other, the polar head group has to abandon its interactions with water molecules and neighboring head groups to dive across the hydrophobic core. Breakage of these interactions requires so much energy that *transverse diffusion of the more polar membrane lipids is extremely rare in artificial lipid bilayers.* It is occasionally observed in "real" membranes in which proteins assist the flip-flopping lipids.

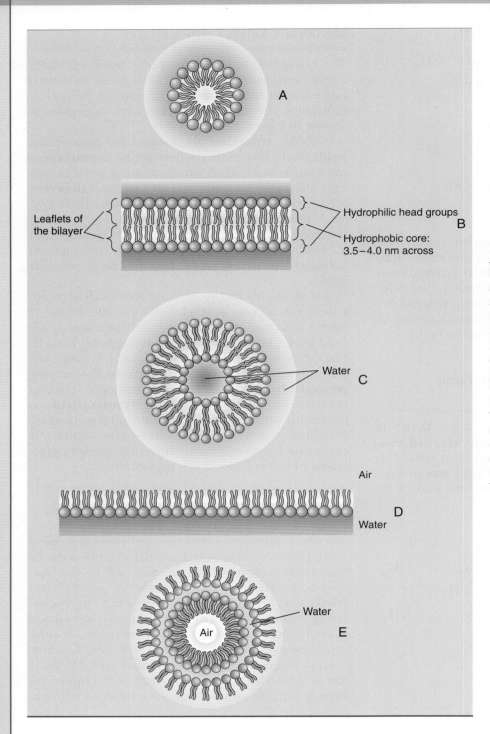

Leaflets of the bilayer

Hydrophilic head groups

Hydrophobic core: 3.5–4.0 nm across

Water — C

Air

Water — D

Water

Air — E

Figure 12.6 Behavior of polar lipids in water. **A,** A *micelle* is a small, spherical structure with a hydrophilic surface and a hydrophobic core. **B,** A *bilayer* is the prototype of a biological membrane. As in the micelle, the hydrophilic head groups are on the surface and the hydrophobic tails are buried in the center. **C,** A *liposome* is the prototype of a membrane-bounded vesicle. It forms spontaneously from a lipid bilayer. **D,** A *monolayer* forms at the interface between water and air. **E,** A *soap bubble* consists of two monolayers enclosing a thin water film.

When a synthetic lipid bilayer that contains only one lipid is cooled, it "freezes" at a well-defined temperature. Above the phase transition, the lipids move around like people on a busy town square, and below the transition, they are immobile, like a platoon of soldiers standing at attention.

Real membranes contain a mixture of many different lipids along with proteins, and the phase transition is gradual. *At ordinary body temperature, membranes behave like a viscous liquid.*

Long, saturated fatty acid chains in the membrane lipids make the membrane more rigid because they align themselves in parallel, forming multiple van der Waals interactions. Unsaturated fatty acids disturb this orderly array because their *cis* double bonds introduce kinks in the hydrocarbon chain. This destabilizes the alignment of the hydrophobic tails (Fig. 12.7). Therefore, *a high content of unsaturated fatty acid residues makes the membrane more fluid.*

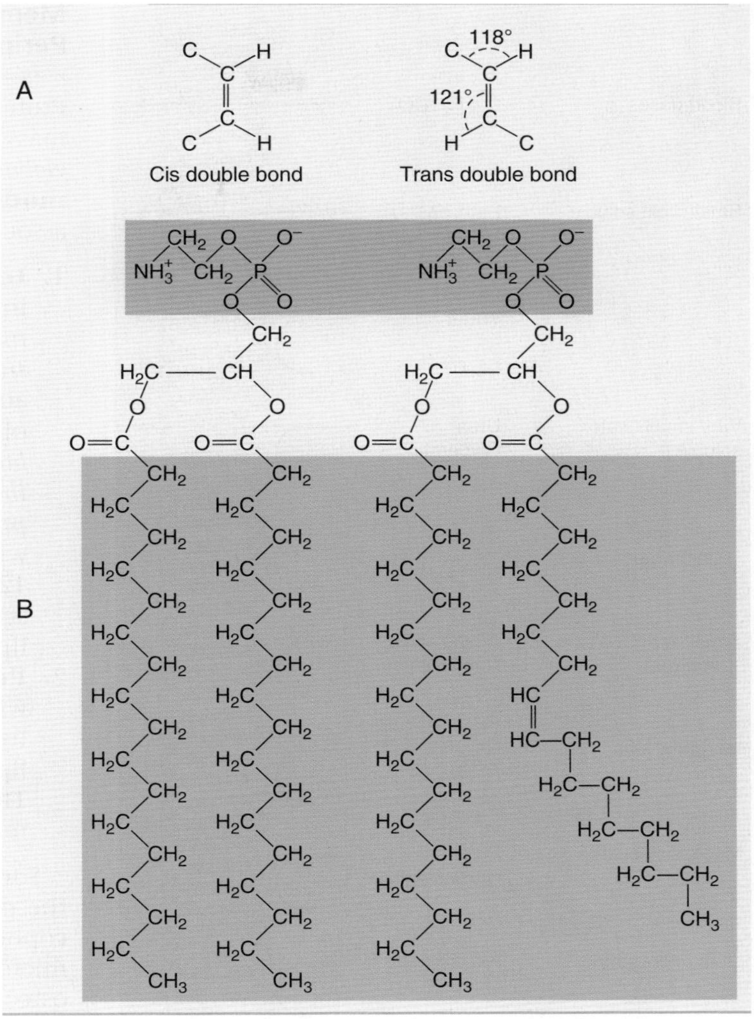

Figure 12.7 Effect of a *cis* double bond on the array of fatty acid chains in the hydrophobic core of the lipid bilayer. **A,** The geometry of *cis* and *trans* double bonds. There is no free rotation around the bond, and all four substituents of the double-bonded carbons are in the same plane. The double bonds in natural fatty acids are always in *cis* configuration. **B,** An unsaturated fatty acid in the lipid bilayer.

Animals can adjust their membrane fluidity by varying the fatty acid composition of their membrane lipids. For example, cold-water fish have more unsaturated fatty acids in their membranes than do tropical fish. This maintains optimal membrane fluidity at frigid temperatures, and it makes cold-water fish a valuable dietary source of polyunsaturated fatty acids.

Because of its stiff ring system, *cholesterol tends to make membranes more rigid*. However, it also inserts itself between the fatty acid chains and prevents their crystallization. In this respect, it acts like an impurity that decreases the melting point of a chemical.

The Lipid Bilayer Is a Diffusion Barrier

To penetrate a lipid bilayer, a substance has to pass from the aqueous solution through the region of the hydrophilic head groups, then across the hydrophobic core and out between the head groups on the opposite side.

Water-soluble substances such as inorganic ions, sugars, amino acids, and proteins cannot penetrate the bilayer because they do not dissolve in lipid. Breakage of their interactions with water would require too much energy. Triglycerides and other water-insoluble lipids also cannot pass, because they form fat droplets that are repelled by the hydrophilic head groups. Only small molecules that are soluble both in lipid and in water can pass freely.

Gases such as oxygen and carbon dioxide diffuse freely across membranes, but *most nutrients, metabolic intermediates, and coenzymes are water soluble and cannot cross the lipid bilayer* (Fig. 12.8). Also, because inorganic ions cannot cross, *the electrical conductivity of lipid bilayers is very low*. In real membranes, resting membrane potential and excitability

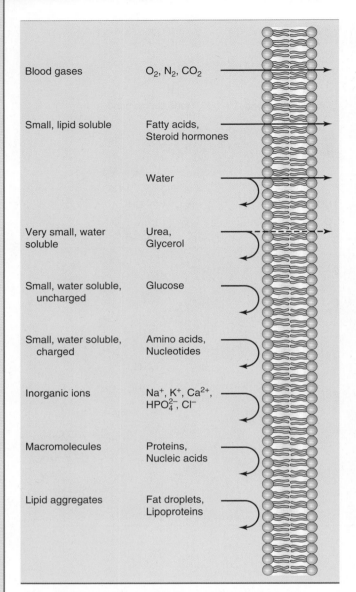

Blood gases	O_2, N_2, CO_2	
Small, lipid soluble	Fatty acids, Steroid hormones	
	Water	
Very small, water soluble	Urea, Glycerol	
Small, water soluble, uncharged	Glucose	
Small, water soluble, charged	Amino acids, Nucleotides	
Inorganic ions	Na^+, K^+, Ca^{2+}, HPO_4^{2-}, Cl^-	
Macromolecules	Proteins, Nucleic acids	
Lipid aggregates	Fat droplets, Lipoproteins	

Figure 12.8 Permeability properties of a typical lipid bilayer.

are regulated by ion channels that are formed by membrane proteins.

Many nutrients and metabolic products are transported by specially designed membrane carriers, but *most drugs have to rely on passive diffusion across the lipid bilayer.* Many water-soluble drugs cannot enter cells or penetrate the blood-brain barrier. *When a drug contains ionizable groups, only the uncharged form crosses membranes.* Some very small lipophilic molecules, however, dissolve in the lipid bilayer and increase its fluidity. Inhalation anesthetics such as ether, chloroform, halothane, and even ethanol have this property.

Membranes Contain Integral and Peripheral Membrane Proteins

Proteins account for about one half of the total mass in most membranes. *Membrane proteins are globular proteins.* According to the **fluid-mosaic model** of membrane structure (Fig. 12.9), they associate with the lipid bilayer in different ways:

1. **Integral membrane proteins** are embedded in the lipid bilayer. In most cases, *the polypeptide traverses the lipid bilayer by means of a **transmembrane helix.*** This is a stretch of α helix, about 25 amino acids long, that consists mainly of hydrophobic amino acid residues. *The nonpolar side chains of these amino acids interact with the membrane lipids.* Some integral membrane proteins traverse the lipid bilayer only once, whereas others crisscross several times (Fig. 12.10). Integral membrane proteins can be solubilized only with treatments that destroy the lipid bilayer.
2. **Peripheral membrane proteins** interact with integral membrane proteins or the hydrophilic head groups of the membrane lipids, but they do not traverse the lipid bilayer. They can be detached from the membrane by manipulating pH or salt concentration.

Some proteins are tethered to the outer surface of the plasma membrane by a covalently bound glycophospholipid anchor. Trehalase on intestinal microvilli (see Chapter 19), alkaline phosphatase on osteoblasts (see Chapter 14) and carcinoembryonic antigen (a tumor marker) are prominent examples. Some proteins on the cytoplasmic surface of the plasma membrane and the organelle membranes achieve the same result with covalently bound fatty acids or isoprenoids (Fig. 12.11).

Membranes Are Asymmetrical

Membrane proteins can diffuse laterally in the plane of the membrane, although their mobility is often restricted by binding to structural proteins. Transverse diffusion ("flip-flop") of membrane proteins has never been observed. In erythrocytes, for example, the asymmetrical orientation of the membrane proteins is maintained throughout the 120-day life span of the cell.

Even membrane lipids flip-flop so rarely that their distribution in the membrane is asymmetrical. Plasma membranes, for example, contain most of their phosphatidylethanolamine, phosphatidylserine, and phosphatidylinositol in the cytoplasmic leaflet and most of their glycolipids, phosphatidylcholine, and sphingomyelin in the exoplasmic leaflet (Fig. 12.12).

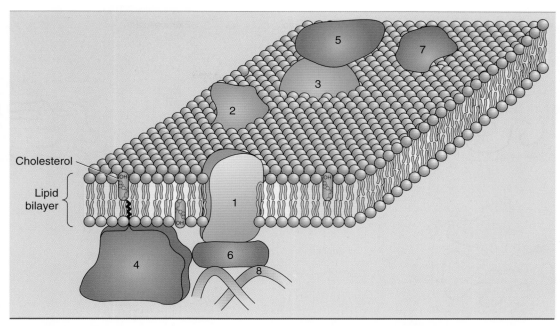

Figure 12.9 The fluid-mosaic model of membrane structure. *1, 2, 3,* Integral membrane proteins traversing the lipid bilayer; *4,* protein anchored by a covalently bound lipid (myristyl, farnesyl, or geranylgeranyl); *5, 6,* peripheral membrane proteins bound to integral membrane proteins; *7,* peripheral membrane protein adsorbed to the head groups of membrane lipids; *8,* cytoskeletal protein attached to a peripheral membrane protein.

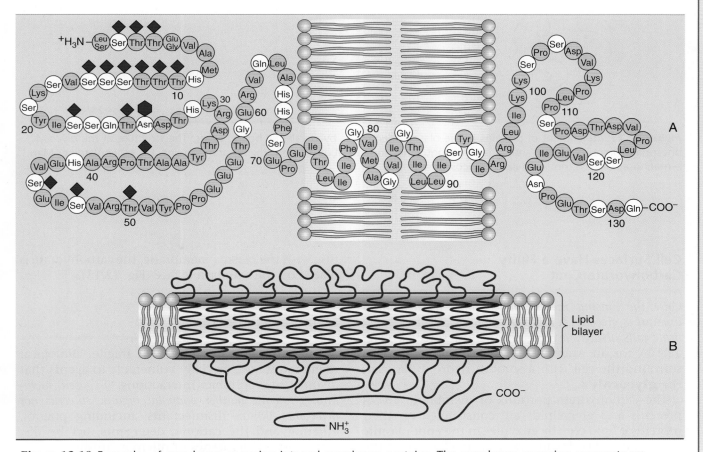

Figure 12.10 Examples of membrane-spanning integral membrane proteins. The membrane-spanning segments are formed by nonpolar α helices. **A,** Glycophorin A, a major protein of the erythrocyte membrane and carbohydrate. ○, nonpolar residues; ◯, charged residues. ◆, O-linked carbohydrate; ⬣, N-linked carbohydrate. **B,** Band 3 protein, another major protein of the red blood cell membrane. The polypeptide consists of 929 amino acid residues and traverses the membrane approximately a dozen times. It is present in a dimeric form, functioning as an anion channel and as an attachment point for cytoskeletal proteins.

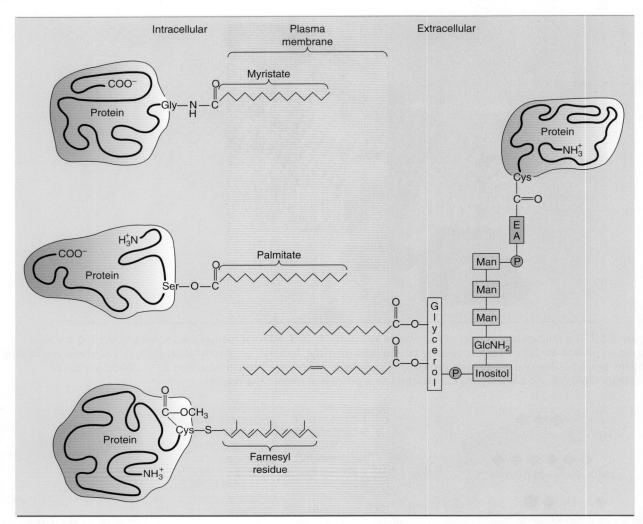

Figure 12.11 Attachment of proteins to the plasma membrane by covalently bound lipids. The structure of the glycosyl phosphatidylinositol anchor shown on the right varies somewhat in different membrane proteins. EA, ethanolamine; Man, D-mannose; GlcNH₂, non-acetylated glucosamine.

Cell Surfaces Have a Fluffy Carbohydrate Coat

Only the plasma membrane contains a substantial amount of glycolipids and glycoproteins. Their carbohydrate tails always face the extracellular space (see Fig. 12.10A for an example). These carbohydrate tails surround the cell with a smooth hydrophilic coat, the **glycocalyx.**

The carbohydrate portions of membrane glycoproteins and glycolipids are constructed on their protein or lipid core by enzymes in the endoplasmic reticulum and Golgi apparatus. Being located in the lumen of these organelles, *the enzymes form the carbohydrates only on the noncytoplasmic surface of the membrane.* When Golgi apparatus–derived vesicles

fuse with the plasma membrane, the carbohydrate is placed on the exoplasmic face (Fig. 12.13).

Membranes Are Fragile

All noncovalent structures are fragile. Biological membranes are especially vulnerable to agents that disrupt hydrophobic interactions. *Exposed membranes tolerate neither nonpolar organic solvents nor detergents.* Many disinfectants, including phenol, ethanol, and the cationic detergents, act by disrupting the membranes of microorganisms.

Mechanical insults by crystalline materials are injurious as well. Crystals of hemoglobin S damage the erythrocyte membrane in sickle cell disease (see

Chapter 10), and crystals of sodium urate damage the membranes of phagocytic cells in patients with gouty arthritis (see Chapter 28). Also, *slow freezing is not tolerated by animal and human cells,* in part because of osmotic stress and in part because the relentlessly growing ice crystals pierce the membranes.

Quick-freezing of dispersed cells or small tissue samples in the presence of antifreeze avoids the formation of large ice crystals. For sperm banking, the samples are frozen quickly in 10% glycerol. Cryopreservation is fairly easy for embryos but difficult for oocytes. The meiotic spindle is even more fragile than the membranes.

Human bodies cannot be cryopreserved in a viable state because the large heat capacity of the body makes quick-freezing impossible. A patient with an incurable disease would be ill-advised to jump into liquid nitrogen in the hope that somebody will thaw him someday when a cure for his disease is found.

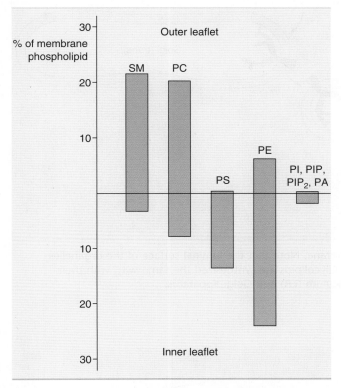

Figure 12.12 Distribution of phospholipids in the outer and inner leaflets of the erythrocyte membrane.
PA, phosphatidic acid; PC, phosphatidylcholine;
PE, phosphatidylethanolamine; PI, phosphatidylinositol;
PIP, phosphatidylinositol 4-phosphate;
PIP_2, phosphatidylinositol 4,5-bisphosphate;
PS, phosphatidylserine; SM, sphingomyelin.

Membrane Carriers Form Channels across the Lipid Bilayer

A few biological membranes, most notably the outer mitochondrial membrane, are riddled with large pores that allow the passage of all small, water-soluble molecules. In most membranes, however, **passive diffusion** is limited to lipid-soluble molecules.

*Water-soluble molecules require **carrier-mediated transport*** (Table 12.1). Membrane carriers are integral membrane proteins that form a **gated channel** across the lipid bilayer. Unlike a simple pore, *the gated channel has a specific binding site for the transported molecule.* The channel undergoes conformational changes that allow the substrate to bind on one side and dissociate on the opposite side of the membrane.

Facilitated diffusion is a type of carrier-mediated transport in which an external energy source is not used. Therefore, the net transport of the substrate is always down its electrochemical gradient. For example, the glucose carrier in the erythrocyte membrane is a gated channel with a binding site for glucose (Fig. 12.14). Most cells in the human body take up glucose by this cost-efficient mechanism. The transport of a single

Table 12.1 Transport of Small Molecules and Inorganic Ions across Biological Membranes.

Type of transport	Carrier Required	Transport Against Gradient	Metabolic Energy Required	ATP Hydrolysis	Example
Passive diffusion	−	−	−	−	Steroid hormones, many drugs
Facilitated diffusion	+	−	−	−	Glucose in RBCs and blood-brain barrier
Active transport	+	+	+	+	Na^+, K^+-ATPase, Ca^{2+}-ATPase
Secondary active transport	+	+	+	−	Sodium cotransport of glucose in kidney and intestine

RBC, red blood cell.

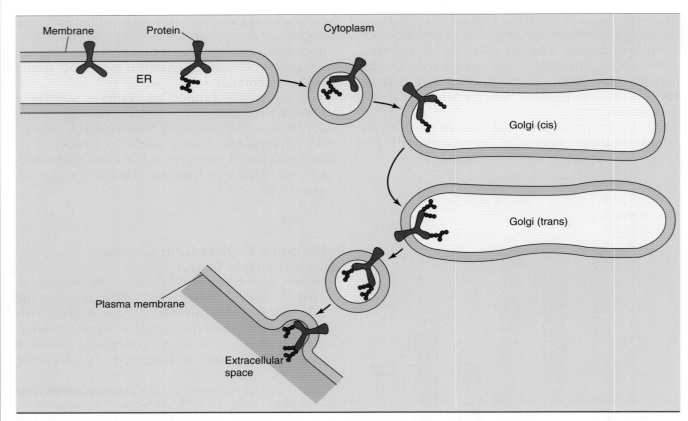

Figure 12.13 Placement of a glycoprotein in the plasma membrane. Note that the luminal surface of the organelles corresponds to the exoplasmic face of the plasma membrane. Glycolipids are synthesized the same way, with their carbohydrate initially facing the lumen of the endoplasmic reticulum (ER) and Golgi apparatus.

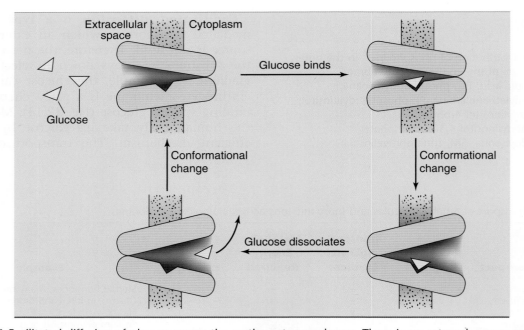

Figure 12.14 Facilitated diffusion of glucose across the erythrocyte membrane. There is no external energy source, and so the net transport is down the concentration gradient. Actually, all steps in this cycle are reversible. A net transport of glucose into the cell takes place only because glucose is consumed in the cell, thereby maintaining a concentration gradient.

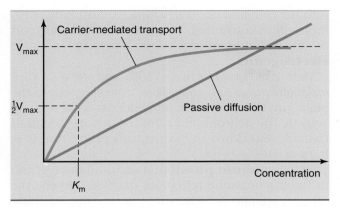

Figure 12.15 Saturability of carrier-mediated transport. We assume that the substrate moves from a compartment with variable concentration (concentration on the x axis) to a compartment where its concentration is zero. This corresponds to the assumption of negligible product concentration in Michaelis-Menten kinetics. Compare this graph with Figure 4.6. V_{max} depends on the number of carriers in the membrane and the number of molecules transported per second. K_m, Michaelis constant; V_{max}, maximal reaction rate.

substrate by a membrane carrier, as in the facilitated diffusion of glucose, is called **uniport**.

Carrier-Mediated Transport Is Substrate-Specific and Saturable and Can Be Selectively Inhibited

Carrier-mediated transport is distinguished from simple diffusion by three important features:

1. **Substrate specificity:** To be transported, the substrate has to bind noncovalently to the carrier. Therefore, *transport depends on the proper fit between substrate and carrier*. The glucose transporter in red blood cells, for example, transports D-glucose but not L-glucose, and it has markedly reduced affinities for other hexoses such as D-mannose and D-galactose.

2. **Saturability:** The rate of passive diffusion is directly proportional to the concentration gradient, but *carrier-mediated transport shows the same saturation kinetics as enzymatic reactions* (Fig. 12.15).

3. **Specific inhibition and physiological regulation:** Carriers, like enzymes, can be inhibited. Glucose transport into erythrocytes, for example, is competitively inhibited by various glucose analogs. Membrane transport can also be a rate-limiting and regulated step in metabolic pathways. For example, the carrier that brings glucose into muscle and adipose tissue (but not erythrocytes) is activated by insulin.

Transport against an Electrochemical Gradient Requires Metabolic Energy

The uphill transport of a substrate against a gradient requires energy-dependent **active transport**. Like chemical reactions, *membrane transport is driven by the free energy change* ΔG (see equation 5 in Chapter 4). However, the situation is less complex because *there is no enthalpy change ($\Delta H = 0$), and the process is purely entropy driven*. For an uncharged molecule, the driving force ΔG for the transfer of a molecule from a compartment with the concentration c_1 to a compartment with the concentration c_2 is given by the equation

1 $$\Delta G = R \times T \times \ln \frac{c_2}{c_1} = 2.303 \times R \times T \times \log \frac{c_2}{c_1}$$

where R is the gas constant (1.987×10^{-3} kcal $\times$ mol$^{-1} \times$ K^{-1}) and T is the absolute temperature. It is now possible to calculate the energy required to pump 1 mol of an uncharged molecule against a 10-fold concentration gradient ($c_2/c_1 = 10$) at 25°C ($298K$):

$$\Delta G = 2.303 \times 1.987 \times 10^{-3} \frac{kcal}{mol \times K} \times 298\ K \times \log 10$$

$$= +1.36\ kcal/mol$$

For an ion, the energy requirement depends not only on the concentration gradient but also on the membrane potential:

2 $$\Delta G = \left[2.303 \times R \times T \times \log \frac{c_2}{c_1} \right] + \left[Z \times F \times \Delta V \right]$$

where Z is the charge of the ion, F is the Faraday constant (23.062 kcal $\times$ V$^{-1} \times$ mol^{-1}), and ΔV is the membrane potential in volts.

By substituting the values of Figure 12.16 into equation 2, it is possible, for example, to calculate the energy required to pump a sodium ion out of the cell:

$$\Delta G = 2.303 \times 1.987 \times 10^{-3} \frac{kcal}{mol \times K} \times 298\ K$$

$$\times \log \frac{137}{10} + 1 \times 23.062 \frac{kcal}{V \times mol} \times 0.06\ V$$

$$= 1.545 \frac{kcal}{mol} + 1.384 \frac{kcal}{mol} = +2.929\ kcal/mol$$

Equation 2 defines the **electrochemical gradient** for ions. The electrochemical gradient is large for such ions as Na$^+$ and Ca^{2+}, for which the two components of equation 2 have the same sign, and small for such ions as K$^+$ and Cl$^-$, for which they have opposite signs.

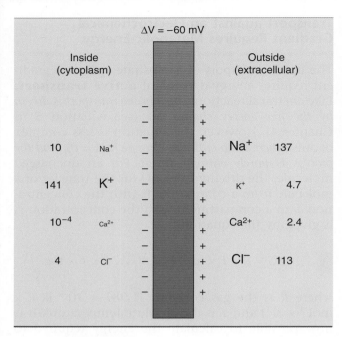

Figure 12.16 Typical ion distributions across the plasma membrane. All concentrations are in (mmol/liter). ΔV, Membrane potential.

Active Transport Consumes ATP Triphosphate

The **sodium-potassium (Na⁺,K⁺) pump** maintains the normal gradients of sodium and potassium across the plasma membrane. It is a glycoprotein with two α subunits and two β subunits. Each α subunit has about 10 transmembrane α helices, and three of them participate in the formation of the gated channel. These three helices are amphipathic, with hydrophobic amino acid residues facing the lipid bilayer and hydrophilic ones lining the channel.

The transport cycle is described in Figure 12.17. In its "inside-open" conformation, the gated channel exposes three Na⁺-binding sites to the cytoplasm. Na⁺ binding triggers the phosphorylation of an aspartate side chain, which flips the channel into the "outside-open" conformation. This conformation has a low affinity for Na⁺ and a high affinity for K⁺. Therefore, the three Na⁺ ions diffuse into the extracellular space, and two K⁺ ions bind. This triggers the dephosphorylation of the aspartate side chain. The channel flips back into the inside-open conformation, which has a low affinity for K⁺ and a high affinity for Na⁺. K⁺ is released into the cytoplasm, Na⁺ again binds, and the process is repeated.

During each transport cycle, three Na⁺ ions are transported out of the cell, 2 K⁺ ions are transported

into the cell, and one adenosine triphosphate (ATP) molecule is consumed. Because of the net transport of an electrical charge, this transport is called **electrogenic.**

Most cells spend between 10% and 40% of their metabolic energy for sodium-potassium pumping. In the brain, in which sodium movements into the cell activate the neurons and form the action potentials that are sent down the axons, this proportion is as high as 70%.

In the **calcium pump** that accumulates calcium in the sarcoplasmic reticulum of muscle fibers, the same transport mechanism as in the sodium-potassium pump is used. It constitutes almost 90% of the total membrane protein in the sarcoplasmic reticulum of skeletal muscle and consumes close to 10% of the total metabolic energy in resting muscle.

Many Molecules Are Transported into the Cell by Sodium Cotransport

The coupled transport of two substrates by the same carrier is called **cotransport.** If, as in the case of the sodium-potassium pump, the two substrates are transported in opposite directions, the mechanism is called **antiport.** If they are transported in the same direction, it is called **symport.**

In **sodium cotransport,** the carrier transports a molecule or inorganic ion into the cell together with a sodium ion. Sodium moves down its steep electrochemical gradient, and this drives the uphill transport of the cotransported substrate. *This type of transport does not hydrolyze ATP, but it depends on the maintenance of the sodium gradient by the sodium-potassium pump.* Therefore, it is characterized as **secondary active transport.**

Sodium cotransport is used for the absorption of glucose and amino acids in the intestinal mucosa and their reabsorption in the kidney tubules (Fig. 12.18). Indeed, the kidneys and intestines often use the same sodium cotransporter, and many inherited transport defects are therefore expressed in both organs.

The Sodium-Potassium Pump Is Inhibited by Cardiotonic Steroids

The contraction of the myocardium, like that of skeletal muscle, is triggered by calcium. *The higher the intracellular calcium concentration, the greater is the force of contraction.* Myocardial cells regulate their intracellular calcium stores by pumping calcium out

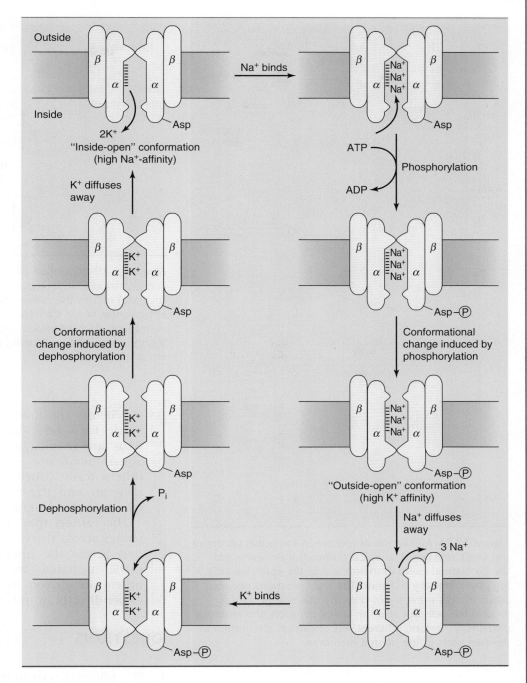

Figure 12.17 The transport cycle of Na+,K+-ATPase. Asp, aspartate.

of the cell in exchange for sodium. Thus, *the extrusion of excess calcium from the cell requires a sodium gradient* (Fig. 12.19).

The sodium gradient depends on the sodium-potassium pump. *Steroidal glycosides from the plant Digitalis purpurea L. inhibit the sodium-potassium pump, weaken the sodium gradient, and thereby impair the removal of calcium from the cell.* The excess calcium is pumped into the sarcoplasmic reticulum,

which stores it for release into the cytoplasm during contraction. This results in an increased force of myocardial contraction.

Digitalis glycosides are still used for the treatment of congestive heart failure, but they are very toxic at high doses. All excitable cells depend on an adequate sodium gradient, and excessive inhibition of the sodium-potassium pump leads to cardiac arrhythmias.

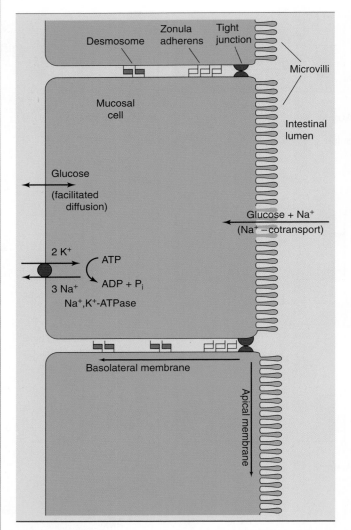

Figure 12.18 Absorption of glucose in the brush border of the small intestine. The apical (luminal) membrane and the basolateral (serosal) membrane of the epithelial cells are physiologically different. The tight junctions between adjacent cells prevent not only the diffusion of solutes around the cells but also the lateral diffusion of membrane proteins. Therefore, different sets of carriers are present in the two parts of the plasma membrane.

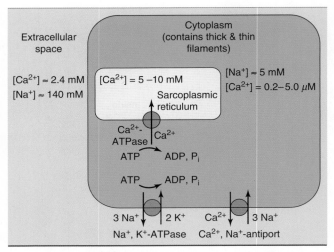

Figure 12.19 Regulation of the intracellular calcium concentration in myocardial cells. Cardiotonic steroids (digitalis) reduce the sodium gradient and therefore the effectiveness of the Ca^{2+}/Na^+ antiporter in the plasma membrane. ADP, adenosine diphosphate; ATP, adenosine triphosphate; mM, millimoles; μM, micromoles; P_i, inorganic phosphate.

Whereas the lipid bilayer forms a diffusion barrier for water-soluble solutes, membrane proteins are in charge of specialized functions. Some membrane proteins are enzymes, and others form structural links with the cytoskeleton and the extracellular matrix or are components of signaling pathways.

The carriers that transport hydrophilic substrates across the membrane form gated channels across the lipid bilayer. Some types of carrier-mediated transport are passive and others are driven by the hydrolysis of ATP, either directly or indirectly.

QUESTIONS

1. The selective transport of molecules and inorganic ions across the membrane requires a "gated channel" across the lipid bilayer. The most typical structural feature of these gated channels is

   A. Several segments of antiparallel β-pleated sheet structure.
   B. Glycolipids forming the inner lining of the channel.
   C. Lipids that form a covalent bond with the transported solute.
   D. Several amphipathic α helices forming the channel.
   E. Nonpolar α helices forming the channel.

SUMMARY

Biological membranes are diffusion barriers and sites of regulated transport. Their structural core is a bilayer that consists of amphipathic lipids: phosphoglycerides, sphingolipids, and cholesterol. Integral membrane proteins are embedded in the lipid bilayer, whereas peripheral membrane proteins are attached to its surface. Most integral membrane proteins traverse the lipid bilayer in the form of a transmembrane α helix.

2. **Which of the following characteristics applies to the lipids in biological membranes?**

    A. Triglycerides and phosphoglycerides are the most abundant lipids in most membranes.
    B. Most glycerol-containing lipids are glycolipids.
    C. Cholesterol is common in the nuclear and inner mitochondrial membranes but not in the plasma membrane of most cells.
    D. The glycolipids of the plasma membrane are found in the outer leaflet of the bilayer.
    E. Membranes in the brain have a high phosphoglyceride content but only very small amounts of sphingolipids.

3. **The transport of glucose across the capillary endothelium of cerebral blood vessels ("blood-brain barrier") is achieved by facilitated diffusion. This means that**

    A. Specific inhibition of cerebral glucose uptake is not possible.
    B. The cerebral glucose uptake is always directly proportional to the concentration gradient for glucose across the endothelium.
    C. The inhibition of ATP synthesis in the endothelial cells will prevent glucose uptake into the brain.
    D. As long as glucose is only consumed but not produced in the brain, the cerebrospinal fluid glucose concentration is always less than the blood glucose concentration.
    E. There is no upper limit to the amount of glucose that can be taken up by the brain.

4. **Many properties of biological membranes depend on the structure of the lipid bilayer. Typical features of lipid bilayers include**

    A. Impermeability for small inorganic ions such as sodium and protons.
    B. Rapid exchange of phospholipids between the two leaflets of the bilayer.
    C. High electrical conductivity.
    D. Lack of lateral mobility of membrane lipids at normal body temperature.
    E. Permeability for proteins.

CHAPTER 13

The Cytoskeleton

Membranes alone are not sufficient to maintain the cell's shape, give it resilience to mechanical forces, or make it contract and move. Structural strength and motility require a network of intracellular fibers that is known as the **cytoskeleton.** It has several components:

1. **Microfilaments** are thin (7-nm) fibers that are formed by the globular protein actin. The reversible polymerization and depolymerization of actin determines the physical consistency of the cytoplasm, and actin microfilaments participate in cell motility and muscle contraction.
2. **Intermediate filaments** are somewhat thicker than the microfilaments (8 to 12 nm). They provide mechanical support for the cell.
3. **Microtubules** are polymers of the globular protein tubulin. With a diameter of 24 nm, they are the thickest and strongest elements of the cytoskeleton. They are important for the maintenance of cell shape, for intracellular transport, and as the structural backbone of cilia and flagella.

The Erythrocyte Membrane Is Reinforced by a Spectrin Network

Erythrocytes travel about 300 miles during their 120-day life, part of this through tortuous capillaries in which they suffer mechanical deformation. *The cells can survive this ordeal only because they possess a meshwork of supporting fibers right under their plasma membrane.*

These fibers consist of **α-spectrin** and **β-spectrin,** two long polypeptides that are folded into **spectrin repeats.** The spectrin repeat is a sequence of 106 amino acids that forms a coiled coil of three intertwined α helices. It is repeated (with variations) 20 times in the α chain and 17 times in the β chain (Fig. 13.1).

Spectrin forms an antiparallel dimer, with an α chain and a β chain lying side by side. These α-β dimers condense head to head to form a tetramer: a long, wriggly, wormlike molecule with a contour length of 200 nm and a diameter of 5 nm. The ends of the spectrin tetramer are bound noncovalently to short (35-nm) actin filaments. This interaction is facilitated by two other proteins: **band 4.1 protein** (so named after its migration in gel electrophoresis) and **adducin.** By binding several spectrin tetramers, *the actin filaments form the nodes of a two-dimensional network* that can be likened to a fishing net or a piece of very thin, flexible chicken wire (Fig. 13.2B).

The spectrin network is anchored to the membrane by the peripheral membrane protein **ankyrin,** which is itself bound to the integral membrane protein **band 3 protein.** This binding is stabilized by **band 4.2 protein** (pallidin). Also, the actin microfilaments interact with the membrane, mainly through **band 4.1 protein** and the integral membrane protein **glycophorin.**

Defects of the Erythrocyte Membrane Skeleton Cause Hemolytic Anemia

Hereditary spherocytosis (HS) is the most common type of inherited hemolytic anemia in northwestern Europe, with a prevalence of about 1 per 5000. Affected patients have small erythrocytes with a round rather than biconcave shape. *These spherocytes are fragile, and they are easily trapped and destroyed in the spleen.*

HS is a heterogeneous group of disorders with varying clinical severity, inherited as an autosomal dominant trait in about 75% of cases. The primary defect can be in the genes for spectrin, ankyrin, or band 3 protein. A reduced amount of spectrin is

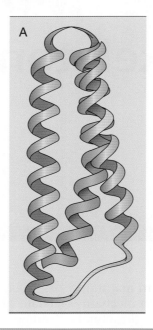

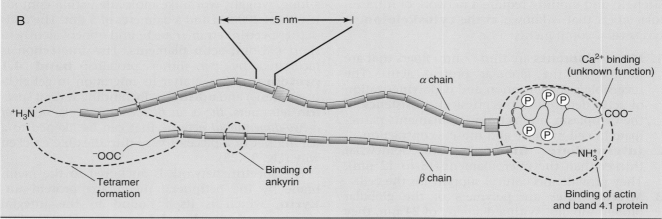

Figure 13.1 **A,** The spectrin repeat consists of three α-helical coiled coils with a total of 106 amino acid residues. **B,** Structure of a spectrin dimer.

common to all forms, probably because any spectrin that is not tied into the membrane skeleton falls prey to proteolytic enzymes during red blood cell maturation. The severity of the disease is proportional to the spectrin deficiency. Splenectomy cures the anemia in most patients.

In **hereditary elliptocytosis (HE)**, the erythrocytes are ellipsoidal rather than spherical. Most affected patients have mutations in the genes for band 4.1 protein or α-spectrin.

Muscular Dystrophies Are Caused by Defects in Structural Proteins of Skeletal Muscle

Dystrophin is a distant relative of spectrin that is found under the plasma membrane of skeletal,

cardiac, and smooth muscle and, to a lesser extent, in the brain. It has 3685 amino acids, with an actin-binding domain, 24 spectrin repeats, a calcium-binding domain, and a carboxyl terminal domain for membrane attachment (Fig. 13.3). Like spectrin, dystrophin appears to form antiparallel dimers.

Dystrophin constitutes only 0.002% of the total muscle protein, but its absence causes **Duchenne muscular dystrophy (DMD).** This is the deadliest and most common form of inherited muscle disease. Inherited as an X-linked recessive trait, it affects about 1 per 4000 males. The patients develop muscle weakness and muscle wasting in early childhood, are wheelchair-bound by age 10 to 12, and die of respiratory or cardiac failure at about age 20.

Most patients with DMD have deletions that eliminate one or more exons of the dystrophin

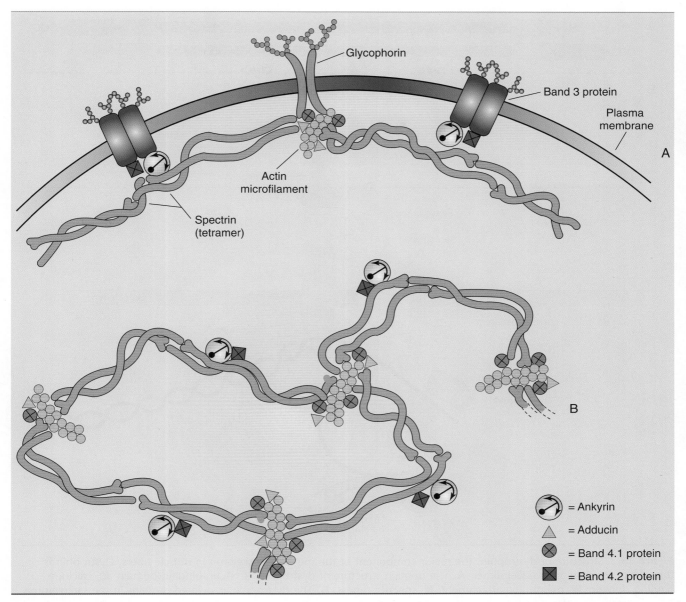

Figure 13.2 Hypothetical model of the membrane skeleton in red blood cells. **A,** In transverse section. **B,** In tangential section.

gene. The gene has 79 exons, and the mutation rate is therefore quite high. Because affected male patients do not reproduce and the gene can be transmitted only through unaffected female carriers, a high proportion of patients have a new mutation. Milder mutations in the dystrophin gene that permit survival into adulthood are diagnosed as **Becker muscular dystrophy.**

Dystrophin binds to a set of membrane proteins that are known as the **dystroglycan complex.** These membrane proteins interact with **laminin** and other proteins of the basal lamina. *They form*

the link between the cytoskeleton and the extracellular matrix. Inherited defects of some of these membrane proteins cause muscle diseases that are clinically distinguishable from DMD (see Fig. 13.3B).

Patients with DMD are prime candidates for gene therapy. Skeletal muscle fibers have multiple nuclei, and getting the gene into only one or a few of them might well be sufficient. However, the large size of the gene makes the construction of vectors difficult. Also, the commonly used retroviral vectors require dividing cells and are therefore not good at transfecting skeletal muscle.

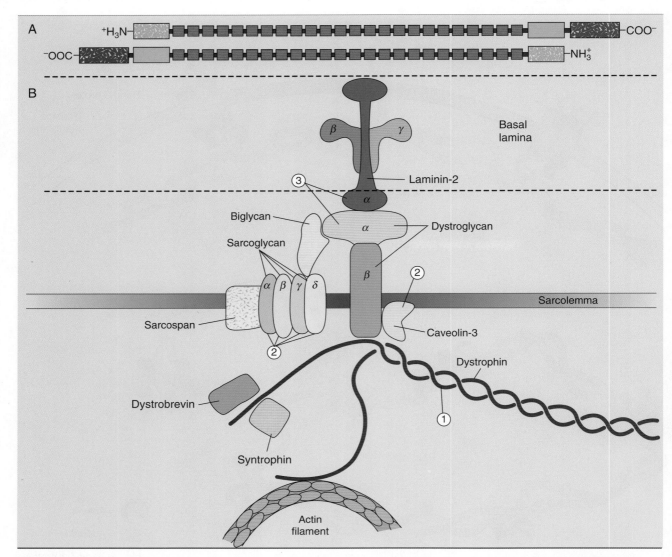

Figure 13.3 Structure of dystrophin, the major component of the membrane skeleton in muscle fibers. Dystrophin is thought to form an antiparallel dimer. **A,** The domain structure of dystrophin. ▨, Actin-binding domain; ▪, calcium-binding domain; ▨, membrane attachment; ■, spectrin repeat. **B,** The dystrophin-associated proteins in the sarcolemma. These proteins link the cytoskeleton to the extracellular matrix. Disease associations: ① Duchenne and Becker muscular dystrophies; ② limb girdle muscular dystrophy; ③ congenital muscular dystrophy.

The Keratins Are the Most Important Structural Proteins of Epithelial Tissues

Intermediate filaments are present in cytoplasm and nucleus of most cells, but the most conspicuous class is the **keratin** filaments of epithelial tissues. Hair, fingernails, and the horny layer of the skin are formed from the keratin cytoskeletons of dead cells.

Keratin contains long stretches of α helix interrupted by short nonhelical segments (Fig. 13.4). There are two different types of keratin: the acidic (type I) and the basic (type II) keratins. Each comes in about 15 different variants. *They form het-erodimers, with a type I polypeptide forming a **coiled coil** with a type II polypeptide* (see Fig. 13.4). The contacts between the two α helices are formed by hydrophobic amino acid side chains on one edge of each helix. Typical keratin fibrils contain between 12 and 24 of these heterodimers in a staggered array.

Different keratins are expressed in different cell types. In the basal layer of the epidermis, for example, K14 is the major type I keratin and K5 is the major type II keratin. In the more mature cells of the spinous and granular layers, keratins K10 and K1 are the major type I and type II keratins, respectively (Fig. 13.5). Single-layered epithelia express

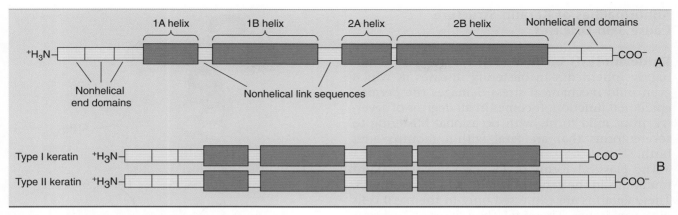

Figure 13.4 Structure of keratin, the major intermediate filament protein of epithelial tissues. **A,** The domain structure of a single polypeptide (type I keratin). The central, mostly α-helical part consists of approximately 310 amino acids. **B,** A parallel heterodimer formed from a type I and a type II keratin polypeptide.

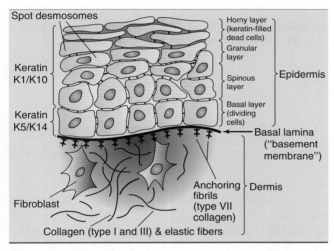

Figure 13.5 The layers of human skin. The epidermal cells are held together by numerous spot desmosomes. These spot desmosomes are attachment points for the intracellular keratin filaments.

keratins 18, 19, and/or 20 (type I) and keratins 7 and 8 (type II), and various other keratin pairs are expressed in the cells that form hair and nails.

Several intermediate filament proteins other than the keratins are expressed in various cell types (Table 13.1). *All of them are dynamic structures that are assembled and disassembled continuously.*

Assembly and disassembly are regulated by proteins that bind either to the ends or to the sides of the filaments. The phosphorylation of the filament proteins can also trigger the disassembly of the filaments. For example, the **lamins** form a supporting fiber network under the nuclear envelope. During mitosis, the lamins become phosphorylated by the cell cycle–induced protein kinase Cdc2. This leads to the disassembly of the fibers and the collapse of the nuclear envelope.

Table 13.1 The Major Types of Intermediate Filament Proteins*

Protein	Tissue or Cell Type
Keratin	Epithelial cells, hair, nails
Vimentin	Embryonic tissues, mesenchymal cells, most cultured cells
Desmin	Myocardium, at Z disk in skeletal muscle
Glial fibrillary acidic protein	Astrocytes, Schwann cells
Peripherin	Neurons of the peripheral nervous system (PNS)
α-Internexin	Neurons of the central nervous system (CNS)
Neurofilament proteins (NF-L, NF-M, NF-H)	Neurons of CNS and PNS
Lamin	Nucleus in all nucleated cells, under the nuclear membrane; this is the only noncytoplasmic intermediate filament protein

* All of these proteins have the general structure depicted in Figure 13.4A for keratin.

Abnormalities of Keratin Structure Cause Skin Diseases

Epidermolysis bullosa (EB) is a group of dominantly inherited skin blistering diseases in which even mild mechanical stress damages the dermal-epidermal junction. It comes in all degrees of severity, from mild forms with occasional blistering to severe forms that are fatal within months after birth.

The classical forms of EB are caused by point mutations in the genes of keratin K14 or keratin K5. These keratins are expressed only in the basal cells of the epidermis. Therefore, *shear forces easily destroy the basal cell layer but leave the overlying cells intact.* The base of the epidermis fills with extracellular fluid, and a blister forms.

Point mutations in the genes for K1 and K10, the major keratins of the spinous and granular cell layers, have been identified as causes of **epidermolytic hyperkeratosis,** a dominantly inherited type of skin disease with scaling, hyperkeratosis, and blistering.

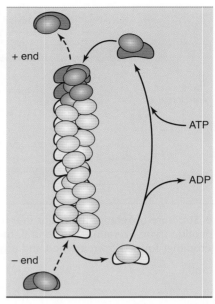

Figure 13.6 Assembly and disassembly of an actin microfilament. The filament grows at the + end and is disassembled at the − end. ◯, Actin monomer with bound ADP; ◖, actin monomer with bound ATP.

Actin Filaments Are Formed from Globular Subunits

Actin microfilaments were previously described as anchoring points for proteins of the membrane skeleton (see Figs. 13.2 and 13.3). Actin is indeed one of the most abundant proteins in the human body, and six different isoforms have been identified in human tissues. In most cells, the microfilaments are concentrated in the cytoplasm underlying the plasma membrane where they form the gel-like cortex of the cytoplasm. *When actin monomers polymerize into microfilaments, the cytoplasm turns into a gel; when they disassemble, the cytoplasm turns into a viscous liquid.*

The globular building blocks of microfilaments are called **G-actin** (molecular weight [MW], 42,000). Each G-actin monomer has a nucleotide binding site that is occupied by ATP or ADP. These subunits can polymerize into a filament in which two strands are coiled gently around one another (Fig. 13.6). *Microfilaments are dynamic structures that can be assembled and disassembled continuously.*

The actin filaments are polar structures. At one end, called the **positive (+) end,** both addition and dissociation of actin monomers are fast. At the opposite end, the **negative (−) end,** both processes are slow. The bound nucleotide is also important. *ATP-actin binds strongly to other actin monomers and tends to add to the microfilament, whereas ADP-actin binds weakly and tends to break away from the microfilament.*

The large majority of free actin monomers in the cytoplasm contain a bound ATP. This form adds to the + end of the microfilament. In the microfilament, however, the ATP is hydrolyzed. When the concentration of G-actin is high, the addition of new actin monomers to the + end is faster than the hydrolysis of the bound ATP. As a result, the last subunits at the + end are in the ATP form, whereas the rest of the microfilament is in the ADP form. *This filament tends to grow at the + end and frizzle away at the − end.*

Cells have a vast bureaucracy of proteins to regulate the formation, growth, and dissolution of microfilaments. Some initiate the formation of a new microfilament, some anchor the filaments to membranes or cytoskeletal structures, and others bundle them into networks or parallel arrays (Table 13.2).

Many specialized cellular functions depend on microfilaments, including

1. Muscle contraction.
2. Ameboid motility.
3. Phagocytosis.
4. Contraction of intestinal microvilli.
5. The formation of the cleavage furrow during mitosis.
6. The shape change of activated platelets.

Table 13.2 Proteins That Regulate Actin Microfilaments

Protein	Function
Thymosin	Binds free actin monomers, making them unavailable for polymerization
Profilin	Delivers actin monomers to growing microfilaments
ARP complex	Nucleates microfilaments at the − end
Tropomyosin	Strengthens microfilaments, regulates their length
Caldesmon Troponin	Prevents myosin from binding to actin/tropomyosin
Spectrin Fodrin Filamin	Link microfilaments into a gel
α-Actinin Fimbrin Villin	Link microfilaments into parallel bundles
Talin Myosin-1 Catenin Vinculin α-Actinin	Link microfilaments to the plasma membrane
Cap Z	Caps and stabilizes the + end of microfilaments
Tropomodulin	Caps and stabilizes the − end of microfilaments
Gelsolin	Cuts microfilaments

7. The outgrowth of dendrites and axons in developing neuroblasts.

Actin-dependent processes are inhibited by **cytochalasin B,** a fungal metabolite that prevents actin polymerization by capping the + end of the growing microfilament. **Phalloidin,** another fungal toxin, prevents the depolymerization of actin filaments. These agents change the shapes of many cells, inhibit cell motility, and prevent the outgrowth of axons from ganglia.

Striated Muscle Contains Thick and Thin Filaments

Ameboid motion, phagocytosis, and muscle contraction all require actin microfilaments in combination with the ATPase myosin. Various forms of myosin are present in most cells, but only the myosin of muscle (myosin-II) forms conspicuous fibers. The myosin filaments of muscle are known as the **thick filaments,** in contrast to the **thin filaments** that are formed from actin.

A skeletal muscle fiber has a diameter of 20 to 50 μm and a length of 1 to 40 mm. It is functionally divided into **myofibrils** that run lengthwise through the muscle fiber (Fig. 13.7A). Each myofibril is cylindrical in shape, about 0.6 μm in diameter, and surrounded by cisternae of the sarcoplasmic reticulum.

The myofibrils are organized into **sarcomeres** by transverse partitions known as **Z disks.** Invaginations of the plasma membrane form the **transverse (T) tubules,** which reach each sarcomere at the level of the Z disk. The T tubules are in close apposition to the cisternae of the sarcoplasmic reticulum that envelope the sides of the sarcomere.

The + ends of the thin filaments (7 nm) are attached to the Z disk, and their capped − ends protrude toward the center of the sarcomere. The thick filaments (16 nm diameter) are suspended in the center of the sarcomere, overlapping with the thin filaments. *The length of the filaments does not change during contraction, but the thick and thin filaments slide along each other* (see Fig. 13.7B and C). This shortens the sarcomere by about 30%.

The thin filaments of skeletal muscle contain tropomyosin and troponin in addition to actin. **Tropomyosin** is a long coiled coil of two α-helical polypeptides that winds along the microfilament near the groove between the two actin strands. **Troponin** consists of the three globular subunits **Tn-T** (tropomyosin binding), **Tn-I** (inhibitory, actin binding) and **Tn-C** (calcium binding). This complex is spaced at regular intervals of 38.5 nm along the thin filament, corresponding to the length of the tropomyosin dimer (Fig. 13.8). *Troponin makes the thin filament sensitive to calcium.*

Myosin Is a Two-Headed Molecule with ATPase Activity

The myosin of skeletal muscle contains one pair of heavy chains (MW, 230,000 each) and two pairs of light chains (MWs, 16,000 and 20,000). The carboxyl terminal 60% of the two heavy chains form an α-helical coiled coil with a length of 130 nm and a diameter of 2 nm. *This coiled coil bundles the myosin into the thick filaments.*

Together with the light chains, the amino terminal ends of the two heavy chains form two globular heads (Fig. 13.9A). *The myosin heads possess ATPase activity, but this activity requires physical contact with actin.* In the presence of actin, ATP is hydrolyzed quickly, but ADP and inorganic phosphate remain tightly bound to the catalytic site and prevent the access of further ATP molecules.

The thick filament contains 300 to 400 myosin molecules whose heads protrude in all directions. In the middle of the filament the molecules are bundled tail to tail, and therefore this central portion has no heads. A hinge region in the myosin tail functions as a joint, allowing the myosin heads to wag back and forth on the surface of the thick filament (see Fig. 13.9).

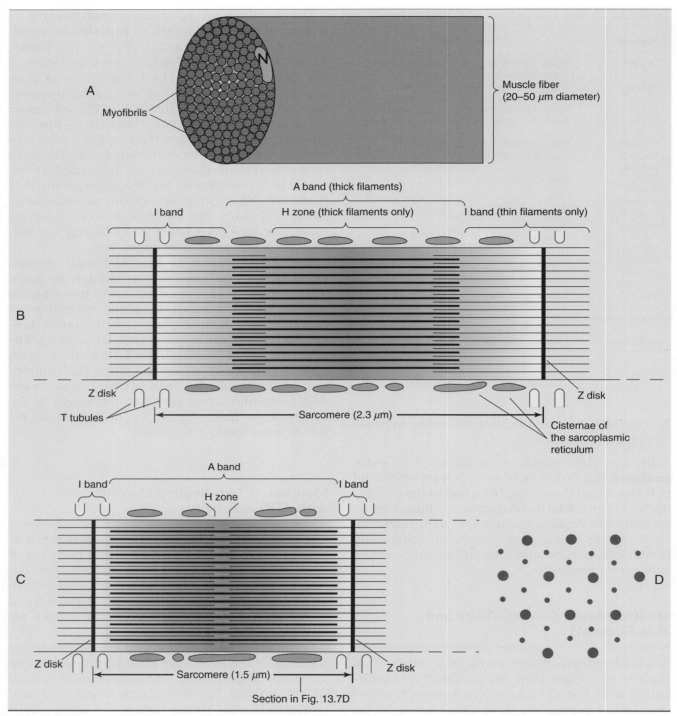

Figure 13.7 Structure of the skeletal muscle fiber. **A,** Section through a muscle fiber. The fiber has a diameter of 20 to 50 μm and is surrounded by the plasma membrane (sarcolemma). Its nuclei (N, up to 100 per fiber) are located peripherally, and the mitochondria are interspersed between the myofibrils. More than 100 myofibrils (0.6 to 1.0 μm diameter) run the length of the muscle fiber. **B,** The sarcomere structure of the myofibril in the relaxed state. **C,** The sarcomere in the contracted state. **D,** A cross section through the overlap zone of thick and thin filaments: The filaments are neatly packed, with each thick filament surrounded by six thin filaments and each thin filament surrounded by three thick filaments.

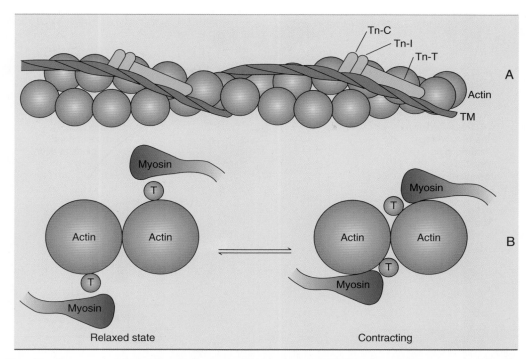

Figure 13.8 The thin filaments of skeletal muscle. **A,** A simplified model of thin filament structure. The troponin complex (Tn-C, Tn-I, and Tn-T) binds to a specific site on the dimeric tropomyosin (TM) molecule. **B,** The position of tropomyosin (T) in the relaxed state (low [Ca^{2+}]) and during contraction (high [Ca^{2+}]). When tropomyosin moves into the groove between the actin monomers, the myosin-binding sites on actin become exposed.

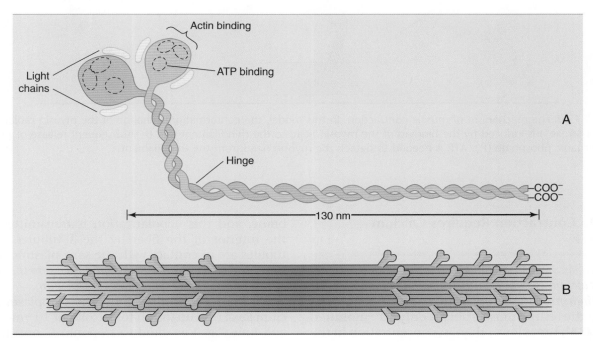

Figure 13.9 Structure of myosin and the thick filaments. **A,** Structure of a single myosin molecule. **B,** Structure of the thick filaments in skeletal muscle. The globular heads of myosin are on the surface of the filament. Its center consists only of the fibrous tails and is therefore without globular heads. The packed tails have a diameter of 10.7 nm.

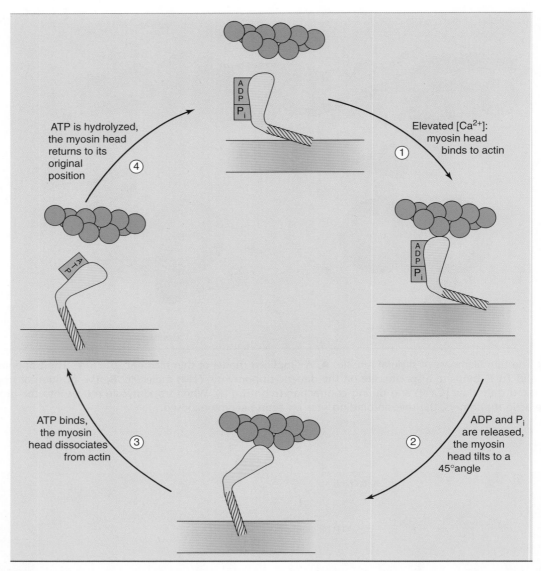

Figure 13.10 The mechanism of muscle contraction. In this model, the conformational change of the myosin molecule ("power stroke") is induced by the binding of the myosin head to the thin filament and the subsequent release of ADP and inorganic phosphate (P_i). ATP is needed to detach the myosin head from the thin filament.

Muscle Contraction Requires Calcium and ATP

The myosin heads can bind to the thin filaments only when calcium is bound to the troponin complex on the thin filament. The cytoplasmic calcium concentration in the resting muscle fiber is only 10^{-7} mol/liter, 1/10,000th times lower than its concentration in the extracellular space. This is not sufficient to engage the troponin complex. Therefore, *muscle contraction requires a rise in the cytoplasmic calcium level.*

This rise in the calcium level is triggered by the neurotransmitter **acetylcholine.** Activation of the acetylcholine receptor depolarizes the plasma mem-

brane, and this depolarization is transmitted into the interior of the fiber by the T tubules. The T tubules are in contact with the sarcoplasmic reticulum, and *membrane depolarization triggers the release of calcium from the sarcoplasmic reticulum.*

Within a few milliseconds, the cytoplasmic calcium level rises up to 100-fold, to about 10^{-5} mol/liter, and four Ca^{2+} ions bind to troponin C on the thin filaments. *This triggers a conformational change in the troponin complex that pulls tropomyosin from the myosin-binding sites of actin* (see Fig. 13.8B).

The myosin heads, each with a tightly bound ADP, can now bind to the exposed actin of the thin filaments (Fig. 13.10). *Actin binding causes the release*

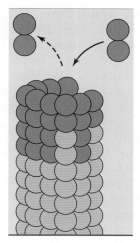

Figure 13.11 The end of a microtubule. GTP-ligated tubulin (⬤) adds to the end of the microtubule. GTP-ligated tubulin has a greater propensity for polymerization than does the GDP-ligated tubulin (⬤) that is formed by the hydrolysis of the bound GTP in the microtubule.

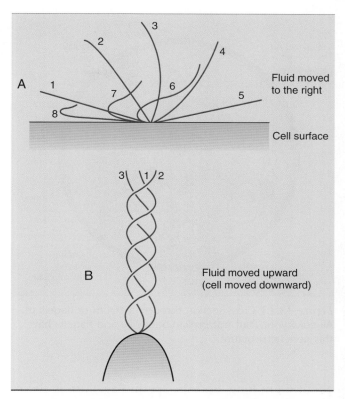

Figure 13.12 The motile patterns of cilia and flagella. **A,** Cilium. **B,** Flagellum. Sperm flagella beat 30 to 40 times per second.

of the bound ADP and phosphate. This triggers a conformational change in the myosin that pulls the thick filament about 7 nm along the thin filament. ATP is required to detach the myosin head from actin but is then rapidly hydrolyzed to ADP and phosphate.

In death, the cytoplasmic Ca^{2+} concentration rises, while ATP is depleted. Therefore, the myosin heads can bind to the thin filaments, but they cannot dissociate in the absence of ATP. The resulting stiffness of the muscles is called **rigor mortis.**

Microtubules Consist of Tubulin

Microtubules are thick hollow tubes with an outer diameter of 24 nm and an inner diameter of 14 nm. They are built from globular subunits of **α-tubulin** and **β-tubulin,** with molecular weights of 53,000 each.

These building blocks polymerize into a helical array with 13 protein subunits per turn (Fig. 13.11). Like the actin microfilaments, microtubules have a + end where new subunits are added and a − end where subunits break off. Like actin, tubulin binds a nucleotide that facilitates polymerization. This nucleotide is not ATP but GTP, and it hydrolyzes to GDP after polymerization. As a result, *microtubules can rapidly be assembled and disassembled as needed.*

Microtubules can reach lengths of several micrometers, and they are present in all nucleated cells. They are important for the *maintenance of cell shape* and for many *intracellular transport processes.* During

mitosis, for example, microtubules are used as ropes to pull the chromosomes to opposite poles of the cell; in neurons, they are used as railroad tracks to ship vesicular organelles from the perikaryon to the nerve terminals.

Microtubule-dependent transport requires accessory proteins that translate the hydrolysis of ATP into sliding movement along the side of the microtubule. During fast axoplasmic transport, for example, the ATPases MAP 1c and kinesin pull vesicles along the microtubules at a speed of 25 cm/day (3 μm/second).

Colchicine, the poison of autumn crocus, blocks the polymerization of tubulin. It inhibits microtubule-dependent processes, including mitosis.

Eukaryotic Cilia and Flagella Contain a 9 + 2 Array of Microtubules

Cilia and flagella are hairlike cell appendages that are capable of beating or swirling motion (Fig. 13.12). Ciliated cells are found in many epithelia, including those of the bronchial tree, upper respiratory tract, and fallopian tubes. The only flagellated cell in humans is the sperm cell. Cilia are

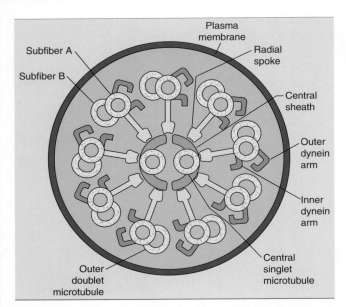

Figure 13.13 Cross section through a cilium or flagellum. All eukaryotic (but not prokaryotic) cilia and flagella have this general structure.

about 6 μm long, and the sperm flagellum is about 40 μm long.

The skin of cilia and flagella is formed by an extension of the plasma membrane, and their skeleton consists of microtubules: two single microtubules in the center and nine double microtubules in the periphery. The double microtubules consist of a circular A fiber and a crescent-shaped B fiber (Fig. 13.13). Unlike the cytoplasmic microtubules that are assembled and dismantled as needed, *the microtubules of cilia and flagella are permanent structures,* held in place by various accessory proteins.

The A subfiber of the doublet microtubules extends two arms that are formed by the protein **dynein.** The outer dynein arm has three globular heads, and the inner arm has either two or three. *The dynein heads use the energy of ATP hydrolysis to walk along the B subfiber of a neighboring doublet microtubule.* Thus dynein plays the same role in flagellar movement that myosin plays in muscle contraction. Even the role of ATP is similar in the two systems. ATP is needed to dissociate the dynein heads from the neighboring B subfiber, as it is needed to dissociate the myosin heads from the thin filament.

Structural Defects of Cilia and Flagella Cause Bronchitis, Sinusitis, and Infertility

Recessively inherited defects in the microtubule-associated proteins of cilia and flagella result in the **immotile cilia syndrome.** This rare disorder (population incidence, 1 per 20,000 to 1 per 60,000) is genetically and biochemically heterogeneous. Some affected patients have missing or abnormal dynein arms, and others have defects in other structural proteins. Cilia and flagella are completely immotile or feebly motile, or they show erratic movements.

Patients with this syndrome suffer from frequent infections of the bronchial tree and the nasal sinuses. In these locations, epithelial cells have to move mucus by coordinated beatings of their cilia. The epithelium of the lower respiratory tract is covered by a mucus blanket with a thickness of about 5 μm. Most inhaled particles and microorganisms get caught on this glue trap and are moved up the bronchi and the trachea by coordinated ciliary beating. This "mucus elevator" removes 30 to 40 g of mucus from the bronchial system every day.

Male patients with this syndrome are infertile because their sperm cells are paralyzed. Even traditional in vitro fertilization is not possible, and intracytoplasmic sperm injection is required. In affected female patients, fertility is reduced, presumably for lack of ciliary movement in the fallopian tubes. The most surprising observation, however, is that 50% of all patients with immotile cilia syndrome have complete situs inversus (left-right inversion of the internal organs). Possibly, the beating of cilia on embryonic epithelia is required for the development of a normal left-right asymmetry.

Cells Form Specialized Junctions with Other Cells and with the Extracellular Matrix

To form a coherent tissue and to respond to signals from their immediate environment, cells must interact with neighboring cells and with structural proteins of the extracellular matrix. This requires specialized sites of contact.

Tight junctions are found in many single-layered epithelia. The intestinal epithelium, for example, has two essential functions: (1) formation of a barrier that prevents the haphazard crossing of molecules into and out of the intestinal lumen and (2) the absorption of nutrients.

The absorptive function requires two sets of membrane carriers: one on the **apical surface** to absorb nutrients from the lumen, and one on the **basolateral surface** to transfer the nutrients from the cell to the extracellular fluid. It is therefore mandatory to prevent the carriers of the apical plasma membrane from diffusing into the basolateral plasma membrane and vice versa.

The tight junctions of the intestinal mucosa form a continuous belt around each epithelial cell. This belt is a network of long strands, formed by the integral membrane proteins **claudin** and **occludin** (Fig. 13.14). *They form a seal that prevents the diffusion of many water-soluble molecules through the narrow clefts between the epithelial cells.* Because the protein strands cut through the lipid bilayer, *they also form the boundary between the apical and basolateral membrane by preventing the lateral diffusion of membrane proteins and membrane lipids.*

The tightness of tight junctions differs in different tissues. For example, those in the intestine are 10,000 times more permeable for small cations such as sodium than are those in the urinary bladder. **Anchoring junctions** link the cytoskeleton either with the cytoskeleton of a neighboring cell or with the extracellular matrix. **Adherens junctions** and **desmosomes** connect the cell with neighboring cells. They contain proteins of the **cadherin** family. Different cadherins are present on different cell types. They bind to cadherins of their own kind, and this ensures that cells of the same kind connect to one another in the tissue. **Focal adhesions** and **hemidesmosomes** connect the cell with the extracellular matrix. They contain proteins of the **integrin** family that link directly to proteins of the extracellular matrix (Table 13.3).

On the cytoplasmic side, *focal adhesions and adherens junctions are linked to microfilaments while desmosomes and hemidesmosomes are linked to intermediate filaments.* These interactions are mediated by specialized anchoring proteins (Fig. 13.15).

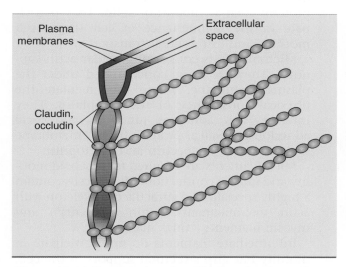

Figure 13.14 The tight junction. The junctional proteins (claudin, occludin) form a tight seal that restricts the diffusion of water-soluble molecules and ions through the narrow clefts of extracellular space between the cells. The proteins prevent the lateral diffusion of membrane proteins and membrane lipids as well. Therefore, the cell can maintain different protein and lipid compositions on the two sides of the tight junction.

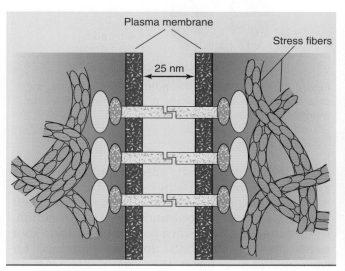

Figure 13.15 The belt desmosome ("adherens junction"). The major adhesive membrane protein is E-cadherin (▢). E-cadherin is bound to β-catenin or plakoglobin (◉) on the cytoplasmic side of the membrane, and these are bound to α-catenin (◉), which interacts with actin microfilaments ("stress fibers"). Spot desmosomes have a similar molecular architecture, but they are linked to intermediate filaments, not to microfilaments.

Table 13.3 The Four Types of Anchoring Junction

	Adherens Junction	**Desmosome**
Contact with	Neighboring cell	Neighboring cell
Transmembrane protein	Cadherin	Cadherin
Cytoskeletal attachment	Microfilaments	Intermediate filaments
Intracellular adapter proteins	Catenin, vinculin, plakoglobin	Desmoplakin, plakoglobin

	Focal Adhesion	**Hemidesmosome**
Contact with	Extracellular matrix	Extracellular matrix
Transmembrane protein	Integrin	Integrin
Cytoskeletal attachment	Microfilaments	Intermediate filaments
Intracellular adapter proteins	Talin, vinculin, filamin	Plectin

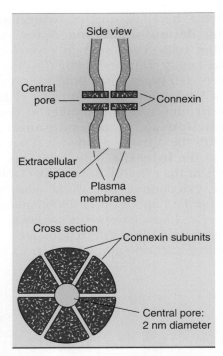

Figure 13.16 The gap junction. In the "open" state, the central pore allows the passage of solutes with molecular weights up to about 1200 D.

The most characteristic adherens junction is the **zonula adherens** of single-layered epithelia. In intestinal mucosal cells, for example, it forms a belt that runs around the cell under the tight junction. Desmosomes do not form a belt, but they form spot welds between the cells. In the epidermis, for example, they connect the keratin filaments of neighboring cells.

Hemidesmosomes and focal adhesions link the cell to collagen, laminin, fibronectin, and other proteins of the extracellular matrix. For example, epidermal cells of the skin are glued to the basal lamina by hemidesmosomes; in the myotendinous junction, the actin filaments of the muscle fiber are linked to the collagen of the tendon through focal adhesions.

Anchoring junctions are affected in some autoimmune diseases. In the skin disease **pemphigus,** for example, antibodies to the desmosomal proteins of the skin cause severe damage.

Gap junctions are clusters of small channels that interconnect the cytoplasm of neighboring cells. Each half-channel is formed by six subunits of the transmembrane protein **connexin** (Fig. 13.16). With a diameter of 2 nm, *gap junctions allow the passage of molecules up to a molecular weight of approximately 1200.* Because they are permeable to inorganic ions, *gap junctions can also transmit membrane depolarization from cell to cell.* Myocardial contrac-

tion, for example, depends on the electrical coupling of the cells by gap junctions.

Gap junctions close when the cytoplasmic calcium level rises. This happens when a cell dies. In this situation, the surrounding cells have to sever their trade relations with the dying neighbor to maintain their own ion gradients and to prevent a unidirectional drain of their metabolites.

Many different connexins occur in human tissues that are encoded by separate genes. For example, mutations in the gene for connexin-26, which is expressed mainly in the inner ear, are the most common cause of recessively inherited deafness.

SUMMARY

Cytoskeletal fibers are formed either by the bundling of fibrous proteins such as keratin or myosin or by the polymerization of globular proteins such as tubulin or actin. They participate in the maintenance of cell shape, cell motility, and intracellular transport.

Microfilaments consist of globular actin subunits. They are most concentrated under the plasma membrane, where they regulate the physical consistency of the cytoplasm. They interact with adherens junctions and focal adhesions, as well as proteins of the "membrane skeleton" such as spectrin and dystrophin.

Microfilaments are required for ameboid motility and muscle contraction. Muscle cells contain a highly specialized contractile cytoskeleton with actin microfilaments ("thin filaments") and myosin filaments ("thick filaments").

Intermediate filaments do not participate in motility but give structural support to the cell. Microtubules are large hollow tubes that are formed by the polymerization of globular tubulin subunits. They participate in intracellular transport processes, and they form the skeleton of cilia and flagella.

📖 Further Reading

Calderwood DA, Shattil SJ, Ginsberg MH: Integrins and actin filaments: reciprocal regulation of cell adhesion and signaling. J Biol Chem 275:22607-22610, 2000.

Goldman YE: Wag the tail: structural dynamics of actomyosin. Cell 93:1-4, 1998.

Korge BP, Krieg T: The molecular basis for inherited bullous diseases. J Mol Med 74:59-70, 1996.

Perez-Moreno M, Jamora C, Fuchs E: Sticky business: orchestrating cellular signals at adherens junctions. Cell 112:535-548, 2003.

Pollard TD, Borisy GG: Cellular motility driven by assembly and disassembly of actin filaments. Cell 112:453-465, 2003.

QUESTIONS

1. **Some cytoskeletal fibers are formed from globular protein subunits. This type of fiber includes the**

   A. Intermediate filaments and actin microfilaments.
   B. Thick and thin filaments of skeletal muscle.
   C. Microtubules and the thick filaments of skeletal muscle.
   D. Keratin filaments in the skin and the thick filaments of skeletal muscle.
   E. Actin microfilaments and microtubules.

2. **Colchicine is a plant alkaloid that prevents the formation of microtubules. This drug is most likely to inhibit**

   A. The mechanical integrity of the horny layer of the skin.
   B. Mitosis.
   C. Muscle contraction.
   D. The electrical coupling between myocardial cells.
   E. The contraction of intestinal microvilli.

3. **The structural integrity of the epidermis depends critically on the presence of**

   A. Keratin filaments and zonula adherens.
   B. Actin microfilaments and tight junctions.
   C. Keratin filaments and desmosomes.
   D. Myosin filaments and gap junctions.
   E. Keratin filaments and tight junctions.

4. **Recurrent respiratory infections in children can have many causes. One possibility that you should consider in a child who presented with repeated bouts of bronchitis and sinusitis is an inherited defect in the protein**

   A. Dynein.
   B. Tropomyosin.
   C. Connexin.
   D. Keratin.
   E. Dystrophin.

CHAPTER 14

The Extracellular Matrix

In soft tissues such as liver, brain, and epithelia, the cells are separated only by narrow clefts about 20 nm wide. *The mechanical properties of these tissues are determined by the cytoskeleton and by specialized cell-cell adhesions.*

Connective tissues, in contrast, consist mainly of extracellular matrix. *The mechanical properties of these tissues are determined by the composition of the extracellular matrix.* Several building materials contribute to the extracellular matrix (Fig. 14.1):

1. **Collagen fibers** are ropelike structures that give the tissue tensile strength.
2. **Elastic fibers** have the properties of rubber bands and give elasticity to the tissue.
3. **Proteoglycans** and **hyaluronic acid** have a gel-like or slimy consistency. They are major constituents of the amorphous ground substance.
4. **Glycoproteins** are the glue that holds fibers and cells together.

Collagen Is the Most Abundant Protein in the Human Body

Collagen accounts for approximately 25% of the body protein in adults and 15% to 20% in children. As shown in Table 14.1, *it is most abundant in strong, tough connective tissues.*

There are at least 14 different collagens that differ in their fiber-forming habits. *Only collagen types I, II, III, V, VI, and XI form fibrils.* Type IV collagen, a major constituent of basement membranes, is the most important nonfibrillar collagen (Table 14.2).

Type I collagen is by far the most abundant collagen in the body. It has a most unusual amino acid composition, with 33% glycine and 10% proline. It also contains nearly 0.5% 3-hydroxyproline, 10% 4-hydroxyproline, and 1% 5-hydroxylysine:

4-hydroxyproline   3-hydroxyproline

5-hydroxylysine

These hydroxylated amino acids are not represented in the genetic code. Therefore, *they have to be synthesized post-translationally from prolyl and lysyl residues in the polypeptide.*

Collagen contains relatively low amounts of some of the nutritionally essential amino acids such as isoleucine, phenylalanine/tyrosine, and the sulfur amino acids. Thus, Jell-O (**gelatin** is denatured collagen) is not a good source of dietary protein.

Collagen contains a small amount of carbohydrate, most of it linked to the hydroxyl group of hydroxylysine in the form of a Glu-Gal disaccharide. The carbohydrate content of the fibrillar collagens is low (0.5% to 1% in types I and III), but it

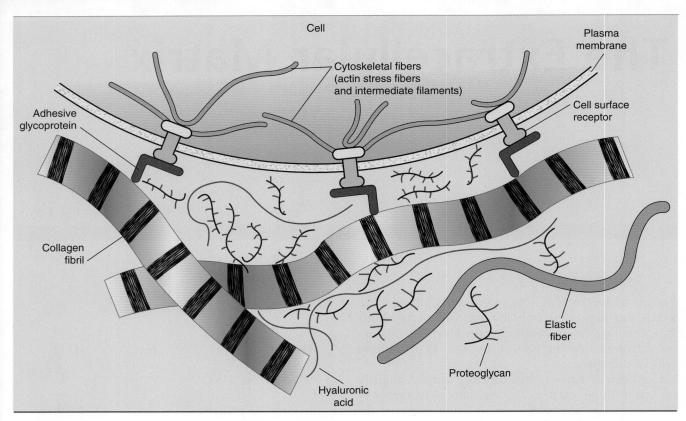

Figure 14.1 Major constituents of the extracellular matrix. Collagen fibers and elastic fibers are required for tensile strength and elasticity, respectively. The amorphous ground substance is formed from proteoglycans, adhesive glycoproteins, and the polysaccharide hyaluronic acid. The extracellular matrix is linked to the cytoskeleton through proteins in the plasma membrane.

Table 14.1 Approximate Collagen Contents of Different Tissues, Expressed as Percentage of the Dry Weight.

Tissue	Collagen Content (%)
Demineralized bone*	90
Tendons	80-90
Skin†	50-70
Cartilage	50-70
Arteries	10-25
Lung	10
Liver	4

* Bone from which the inorganic components (mostly calcium phosphates) have been removed by acid treatment.
† Mostly in the dermis. The major structural proteins of the epidermis are the keratins (see Chapter 13).

is higher in some of the nonfibrillar types (14% in type IV).

The Tropocollagen Molecule Forms a Long Triple Helix

The basic structural unit of collagen fibrils, the **tropocollagen** molecule, consists of three intertwined polypeptides (Fig. 14.2). In the case of type I collagen, this three-stranded rope contains two different polypeptides, each with about 1050 amino acids: two copies of the $\alpha_1(I)$ chain and one copy of the $\alpha_2(I)$ chain. The structural formula is $[\alpha_1(I)]_2\alpha_2(I)$. *These polypeptides have very unusual amino acid sequences, with glycine in every third position.*

Each of the three polypeptides in tropocollagen forms a **polyproline type II helix.** It resembles a helix type that is formed by the synthetic polypeptide polyproline, and it is very different from the familiar α-helix (see Chapter 2). The α-helix is a compact right-handed helix with 3.6 amino acids per turn and a rise per amino acid of 0.15 nm; the polyproline helix, however, is an extended left-handed helix with 3 amino acids per turn and a rise per amino acid of 0.30 nm.

This means that *the polyproline helix is twice as extended as the α-helix.* The glycine residues are found in every third position of the amino acid sequence, and therefore, *all glycine residues are on the same side of the helix.* Unlike the α-helix, the polyproline helix is not stabilized by hydrogen bonds between peptide bonds but by steric repulsion of the bulky proline and hydroxyproline side chains.

Table 14.2 The Collagens

Type	Most Common Composition	Structural Features	Tissue Distribution
I	$[\alpha_1(I)]_2, \alpha_2(I)$	67-nm–banded fibrils	Most abundant type, in most connective tissues
II	$[\alpha_1(II)]_3$	67-nm–banded fibrils	Cartilage, vitreous humor
III	$[\alpha_1(III)]_3$	67-nm–banded fibrils	Fetal tissues, skin, blood vessels, lungs, uterus, intestine, tendons, fresh scars
IV	$[\alpha_1(IV)]_2, \alpha_2(IV)*$	Globular C-terminal end domain; forms a branched network	All basement membranes
V	$[\alpha_1(V)]_2, \alpha_2(V)†$	67-nm–banded fibrils	Most tissues, minor component associated with type I collagen
VI	$\alpha_1(VI), \alpha_2(VI), \alpha_3(VI)$	C- and N-terminal globular domains; forms atypical fibrils	Most tissues, including cartilage
VII	$[\alpha_1(VII)]_3$	Dimer	Anchoring fibrils under basement membranes
VIII	$[\alpha_1(VIII)]_2, \alpha_2(VIII)$	Short helix, globular end domains, no fibril formation	Formed by endothelial cells, in Descemet's membrane
IX	$\alpha_1(IX), \alpha_2(IX), \alpha_3(IX)$	With bound dermatan sulfate	On surface of type II collagen fibrils in cartilage
X	$[\alpha_1(X)]_3$	Similar to type VIII	Calcifying cartilage
XI	$\alpha_1(XI), \alpha_2(XI), \alpha_3(XI)$	67-nm–banded fibrils	Cartilage
XII	$[\alpha_1(XII)]_3$	Many globular domains	On surface of type I collagen fibrils
XIII	$[\alpha_1(XIII)]_3$ (?)	With transmembrane domain	Minor collagen in skin, intestine
XIV	$[\alpha_1(XIV)]_3$ (?)	Nonfibrillar	Like type XII
XV	$[\alpha_1(XV)]_3$ (?)	Nonfibrillar	Many tissues
XVI	$[\alpha_1(XVI)]_3$ (?)	Nonfibrillar	On surface of collagen fibrils
XVII	$[\alpha_1(XVII)]_3$ (?)	With transmembrane domain	Hemidesmosomes of skin
XVIII	$[\alpha_1(XVIII)]_3$ (?)	Nonfibrillar	Liver, kidney, skeletal muscle
XIX	$[\alpha_1(XIX)]_3$ (?)	Nonfibrillar	On surface of collagen fibrils, in rhabdomyosarcomas

* Tissue-specific $\alpha_3(IV)$, $\alpha_4(IV)$, $\alpha_5(IV)$, and $\alpha_6(IV)$ chains also occur.
† A less abundant $\alpha_3(V)$ chain is also often present.

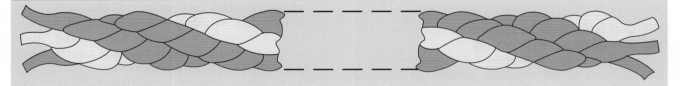

Figure 14.2 The triple-helical structure of collagen. The tropocollagen molecule has a length of approximately 300 nm and a diameter close to 1.5 nm. In the typical fibrillar collagens, only short terminal portions of the polypeptides (the telopeptides) are not triple helical.

The three helical polypeptides of the tropocollagen molecule are wound around each other in a right-handed triple helix. Like the β-pleated sheet (see Chapter 2), this superhelical structure is held together by hydrogen bonds between the peptide bonds of the interacting polypeptides. The contacts are formed by that edge of the polyproline helix that has the glycine residues. Only glycine is small enough to permit close contact between the main chains of the polypeptides. The whole molecule has a length of 300 nm and a diameter of 1.5 nm.

Collagen Fibrils Are Staggered Arrays of Tropocollagen Molecules

The long, ropelike tropocollagen molecules form fibrils by aligning themselves in parallel. They form a characteristic staggered array in which the end of one molecule extends 67 nm beyond that of its neighbor and with gaps of approximately 35 nm between the ends of successive molecules (Fig. 14.3). This staggered array gives collagen a characteristic cross-striated appearance under the electron microscope.

Fibril formation depends on interactions between amino acid side chains in neighboring molecules. Collagen types I, II, III, V, and XI form typical cross-striated fibrils with diameters between 10 and 300 nm that contain hundreds or even thousands of tropocollagen molecules in cross section. More often than not, a single fibril contains more than one type of collagen.

Collagen fibrils have great tensile strength, and a fibril 1 mm in diameter would be able to carry a weight of about 10 kg. This tensile strength is fully exploited in tendons in which the fibrils are

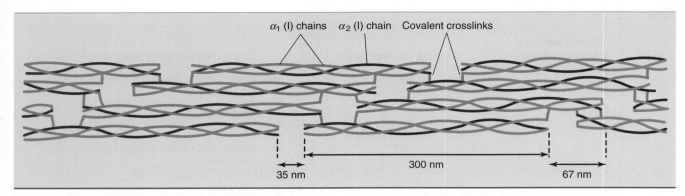

Figure 14.3 The typical staggered array of tropocollagen molecules in the collagen fibril. The telopeptides participate in covalent crosslinking.

arranged in parallel. Collagen is also durable, with life spans ranging from several weeks (blood vessels, fresh scars) to many years (bone).

Collagen degradation is initiated by an extracellular collagenase that cleaves a single peptide bond about three fourths down the length of the triple helix. The resulting fragments unravel spontaneously and are further degraded by other proteases. Intact, triple-helical collagen is very resistant to common proteases such as pepsin and trypsin.

Collagen Is Subject to Extensive Post-translational Processing

Like all extracellular proteins, *collagen is processed through the secretory pathway* (see Chapter 9). The polypeptides that are synthesized by ribosomes on the rough endoplasmic reticulum (ER) are called **pre-procollagen.** In addition to the 1050 amino acids of tropocollagen, they contain amino- (N-) and carboxyl- (C-) terminal extensions that are known as **propeptides.** In the α_1(I) chain of type I collagen, the propeptides measure approximately 170 amino acids at the amino end and 220 at the carboxyl end.

The propeptides have neither the unusual amino acid sequence nor the triple-helical structure of mature collagen. The steps in the processing of type I collagen (Fig. 14.4) are as follows:

1. *A signal sequence of approximately 25 amino acids is removed from the amino ends of the pre-procollagen chains by* **signal peptidase.** *This co-translational reaction converts pre-procollagen to* **procollagen.**
2. *Intrachain disulfide bonds are formed in the N-terminal propeptides of the α_1(I) chain, and inter-chain disulfide bonds are formed between the C-terminal propeptides.*

3. *Some of the prolyl and lysyl side chains become hydroxylated.* This requires three different enzymes: one each for 4-hydroxyproline, 3-hydroxyproline, and 5-hydroxylysine.
4. *Some of the 5-hydroxylysyl residues become glycosylated.* UDP-galactose and UDP-glucose are the precursors.
5. *The triple helix forms in the C→N terminal direction.* The interchain disulfide bonds in the C-terminal propeptides are needed to initiate this process. Because the hydroxylating and glycosylating enzymes act only on the non–triple-helical polypeptides, any delay in triple helix formation or any imperfection of the triple-helical structure is likely to cause overhydroxylation and overglycosylation.
6. *Procollagen is secreted.* Only triple-helical procollagen can be secreted. Improperly coiled molecules are degraded.
7. *The propeptides are removed by extracellular proteases.* This leaves triple-helical tropocollagen molecules with short nonhelical **telopeptides** at both ends. The α_1(I) chains, for example, have a helical sequence of 1014 amino acids (338 Gly-X-Y repeats), an N-terminal telopeptide of 16 amino acids, and a C-terminal telopeptide of 26 amino acids.
8. *The tropocollagen molecules assemble into fibrils.* The propeptides have two different functions:
   • They initiate the formation of the triple helix in the ER.
   • They prevent premature fibril formation.
9. *The molecules in the fibril become crosslinked.* Covalent crosslinking is initiated by **lysyl oxidase.** This oxygen-dependent, copper-containing enzyme acts in the gaps between the ends of the tropocollagen molecules during fibril formation, oxidizing some of the lysyl residues in the telopeptides to allysine and some of the hydroxylysyl residues to hydroxyallysine. The

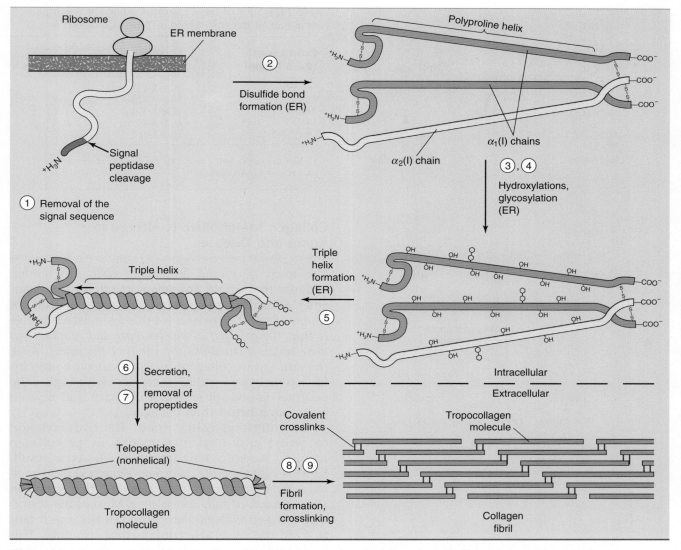

Figure 14.4 Post-translational processing of type I collagen, the most abundant fibrillar collagen. ER, endoplasmic reticulum.

newly created aldehyde groups then react nonenzymatically with other allysyl residues, unmodified lysyl and hydroxylysyl residues, and sometimes histidyl residues. This forms a variety of covalent crosslinks (Fig. 14.5). These crosslinks are essential for the formation of a strong fibril.

Collagen Genes Have Unusual Structures

Unlike the hemoglobin genes (see Chapter 3), collagen genes are not clustered but scattered all over the genome. The exons coding for the triple-helical portions of the collagens are quite remarkable. *They generally start with a codon for glycine and encode a fixed number of Gly-X-Y units.*

As shown in Table 14.3 for the α_1(I) chain of type I collagen, *most exons consist of 54 base pairs (bp) encoding 6 Gly-X-Y units.* The 108- and 162-bp exons were probably created by the fusion of two and three 54-bp exons, respectively. The 45-bp exons probably arose by a 9-bp deletion from the original 54-bp exon, and the 99-bp exons were produced by the fusion of a 45-bp exon with a 54-bp exon.

It is quite likely that the history of the fibrillar collagens started with a microsatellite-like repeat sequence in a gene that became the primordial 54-bp exon. This was followed by exon duplications, exon fusions, and deletions within exons.

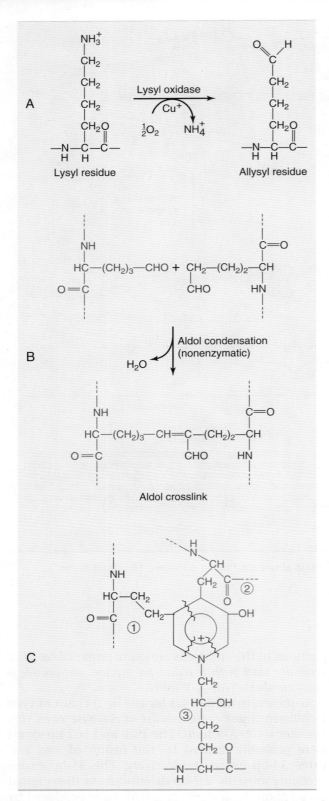

Figure 14.5 Covalent crosslinking of collagen. **A,** The lysyl oxidase reaction. **B,** An aldol crosslink in collagen. **C,** An "advanced" type of covalent crosslink in collagen formed from allysine ①, hydroxyallysine ②, and hydroxylysine ③.

Table 14.3 Sizes of the 41 Exons Coding for the Triple-Helical Part of the $\alpha_1(I)$ Chain in Type I Collagen*.

Exon Length (Base Pairs)	Encoded Sequence	No. of Exons
54	$(Gly\text{-}X\text{-}Y)_6$	21
108	$(Gly\text{-}X\text{-}Y)_{12}$	9
162	$(Gly\text{-}X\text{-}Y)_{18}$	1
45	$(Gly\text{-}X\text{-}Y)_5$	5
99	$(Gly\text{-}X\text{-}Y)_{11}$	5

* Each exon begins with a codon for glycine and encodes a fixed number of Gly-X-Y repeats.

Collagen Metabolism Is Altered in Aging and Disease

The meat of young animals is soft and tender, whereas that of old animals is tough and unpalatable. According to experts, the same is true for human flesh. The reason for this age-related change is that *the collagen of old animals and humans has more covalent crosslinks than that of the young.* Also, the amount of collagen, in relation to the proteins of parenchymal cells, increases with age. The gourmet knows, of course, that actin and myosin taste much better than collagen!

Also, nutrition is important. The hydroxylation of prolyl and lysyl side chains in procollagen requires ascorbic acid (vitamin C). As a result, *patients with vitamin C deficiency **(scurvy)** form a collagen with insufficient hydroxyproline that denatures spontaneously at body temperature.* Most of the abnormal collagen is degraded in the cell because it fails to form the secretable triple-helical structure. This leads to a generalized hemorrhagic tendency, loosening of teeth, poor wound healing, rupture of scar tissue, and other signs of connective tissue weakness.

Collagen synthesis is stimulated by injury, with fibroblasts creeping to the edge of the wound and into the blood clot to form abundant collagen. *Scars consist mainly of types I and III collagen.* The same can happen after the death of parenchymal cells in tissues such as liver, spleen, kidneys and ovaries. In **liver cirrhosis,** for example, dead hepatocytes are replaced by fibrous connective tissue.

Collagen synthesis is also stimulated at sites of bacterial infection. This prevents the spread of the infection, and the bacteria become walled off in a localized **abscess.** This defense mechanism is not always successful. *Some pathogenic bacteria secrete collagenases that degrade tropocollagen.* Some anaerobic bacteria of the genus *Clostridium* use this trick to spread far and wide through the tissues. They cause **gas gangrene,** an especially severe form of wound infection.

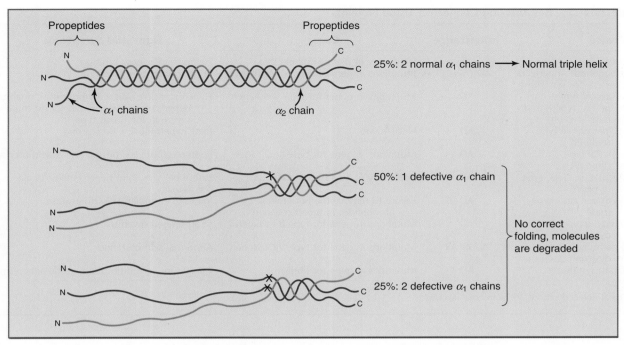

Figure 14.6 Single amino acid substitutions in the α_1 chain of type I collagen are "included" mutations. The abnormal polypeptide initially is included in the molecule, but molecules with at least one abnormal chain are degraded or nonfunctional. Heterozygotes form 50% normal and 50% abnormal α_1 chains, but 75% of the triple-stranded molecules contain at least one abnormal chain and are therefore useless. A similar heterozygous mutation in the gene for the α_2 chain would disrupt only 50% of the molecules and cause a milder disease.

Many Genetic Defects of Collagen Structure and Biosynthesis Are Known

Inherited abnormalities in the structure or post-translational processing of collagen chains are classified according to their phenotypic expression.

Osteogenesis imperfecta (**OI**) is characterized by *brittle bones ("glass bones") and frequent fractures.* It occurs in all degrees of severity. In the mildest forms, there are only occasional pathological fractures, and in the most severe forms, the patient dies shortly after birth with severe fractures and skeletal deformities. Extraskeletal manifestations can include a blue discoloration of the sclera, hearing loss, and poor tooth development. The incidence of OI is about 1 per 10,000, and the inheritance is autosomal dominant in most cases.

OI is caused by mutations in the genes for the α_1 and α_2 chains of type I collagen. More than 200 different OI mutations are known, many of them point mutations that replace a glycine residue by another amino acid. These mutations impair the formation of the triple helix in the ER, and they are most damaging when they occur near the carboxyl end of the triple helix. This is because the triple helix forms in the C→N terminal direction (see Fig. 14.4). The amino acid substitution arrests the coiling process, and this results in overhydroxylation and overgly-cosylation of amino acid residues located in the N-terminal direction from the site of the mutation. This prevents the completion of the triple helix, and the loose polypeptides fall prey to intracellular proteases.

Mutations that affect the α_1 chain are worse than those affecting the α_2 chain. The α_1 chain is present in two copies in the triple helix. Therefore, 75% rather than 50% of the tropocollagen molecules in the heterozygous patient have at least one defective chain and are degraded (Fig. 14.6).

Mutations in the type I collagen genes cause bone diseases because virtually all the collagen in bone is type I collagen. In most other tissues, type I collagen occurs along with type II (cartilage) or type III collagen (skin, blood vessels, hollow viscera).

Ehlers-Danlos syndrome is a group of inherited diseases characterized by *stretchy skin and loose joints.* The "India rubber man" who could bend and twist himself in incredible shapes and package himself into tiny boxes had Ehlers-Danlos syndrome. The price for this virtuosity is a fragile skin that bruises easily. Even small wounds heal poorly, with the formation of characteristic "cigarette paper" scars.

Ehlers-Danlos syndrome is heterogeneous both clinically and biochemically. Mutations in the genes for type V collagen have been demonstrated in some patients, but defects in the removal of the

Table 14.4 Diseases Affecting Connective Tissue Proteins.

Disease	Inheritance	Cause	Signs and Symptoms
Scurvy	—	Deficiency of dietary vitamin C	Hemorrhages, easy bruising
Osteogenesis imperfecta	AD (most)	Mutations in genes for type I collagen	Brittle bones, blue sclera; deafness
Ehlers-Danlos syndrome			
Classical types: gravis (type I) and mitis (type II)	AD	Mutations in genes for type V collagen	Hyperextensible skin, easy bruising, "cigarette paper" scars, hypermobile joints; more severe in the gravis type
Hypermobile type (type III)	AD	Not known	Joint hypermobility, no scarring
Arterial type (type IV)	AD	Mutations in gene for type III collagen	Repture of arteries, bowel, and gravid uterus
Ocular, scoliotic type (type VI)	AR	Deficiency of lysyl hydroxylase	Extensible skin, joint hypermotility, ocular fragility
Arthrochalasis type (type VII)	AD	Failure to remove the N-terminal propeptides in type I collagen	Joint hypermobility, hip dislocation
Spondyloepiphyseal dysplasia	AD	Mutations in gene for type II collagen	Short-limbed dwarfism
Epidermolysis bullosa dystrophica	AD or AR	Mutations in gene for type VII collagen	Abnormal skin blistering
Marfan syndrome	AD	Mutations in gene for fibrillin	Tall stature, lens dislocation, aortic aneurysm

AD, autosomal dominant; AR, autosomal recessive.

N-terminal propeptides from type I procollagen have been described as well (Table 14.4).

Structural defects of type III collagen result in the arterial form of Ehlers-Danlos syndrome. This disease can lead to the rupture of large blood vessels, the colon, or the gravid uterus. These tissues are rich in type III collagen.

Abnormalities of type II, IX, X, and XI collagen result in **chondrodysplasias.** These diseases affect endochondral bone formation and lead to skeletal deformities and dwarfism. As with other dysplasias, there is a wide range of clinical severity. The most important type, diagnosed as **spondyloepiphyseal dysplasia,** leads to dwarfism, joint degeneration, and ocular abnormalities of variable severity.

Type VII collagen forms anchoring fibrils at the dermal-epidermal junction that anchor the basement membrane to the underlying dermis. The absence of this collagen causes the dystrophic variety of **epidermolysis bullosa.** Its clinical manifestations are similar to those of the keratin defects described in Chapter 13.

Elastic Fibers Contain Elastin and Fibrillin

Human tissues must be able to revert to their original shape after mechanical deformation. This requires elastic fibers with properties similar to those of little rubber bands. The elastic fibers of the extracellular matrix have two components: an inner core of amorphous **elastin** and a layer of 10-nm **microfibrils** surrounding the elastin.

Elastin has an aberrant amino acid composition, with high proportions of glycine (31%), alanine (22%), and proline (11%). Some 4-hydroxyproline (1%) is also present, but there is no hydroxylysine. *Like collagen, elastin contains covalent crosslinks that are derived from allysine.* Therefore, lysyl oxidase is required for the synthesis of elastin as well as of collagen. The covalent crosslinks of elastin are similar to those of collagen except for **desmosine,** which is present in elastin but not collagen:

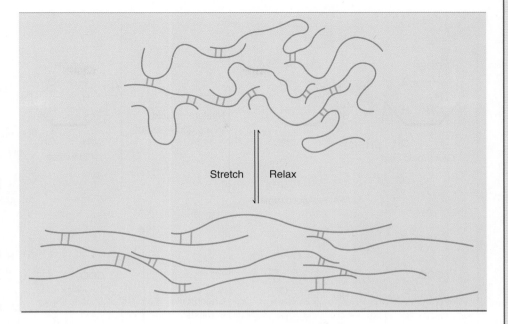

Figure 14.7 A model for the structure of elastin. Elastic recoil during relaxation is thought to depend on hydrophobic interactions between amino acid side chains in the polypeptide.

Little is known about the molecular basis for elastin's elasticity. According to one model, the protein is held in a somewhat disordered but compact shape by weak hydrophobic interactions between amino acid side chains. Stretch loosens these interactions while the elastin network is still held together by the covalent crosslinks (Fig. 14.7).

The amorphous elastin is surrounded by microfibrils. The most important microfibril protein, **fibrillin-1,** is defective in **Marfan syndrome.** Patients with this dominantly inherited condition are unusually tall, with long, spidery fingers (arachnodactyly); the lens is displaced (ectopia lentis); and the media of the large arteries is abnormally weak. Many patients die suddenly in midlife after rupture of their dilated aorta.

Hyaluronic Acid Is a Component of the Amorphous Ground Substance

Glycosaminoglycans (**GAGs**) are unbranched acidic polysaccharides that consist of repeating disaccharide units. One of their building blocks is always an amino sugar. The other is, in most cases, a uronic acid. Uronic acids are hexoses in which the C-6 is oxidized to a carboxyl group (Fig. 14.8).

Hyaluronic acid is an unusually large GAG that consists of more than 10,000 disaccharide units, with a molecular weight up to 10^7 D and a length of up to 10 μm. It contains glucuronic acid and N-acetylglucosamine, held together by β-glycosidic bonds that favor an extended conformation (Fig. 14.9). Its negative charges bind plenty of water and cations, and as a result, *hyaluronic acid forms*

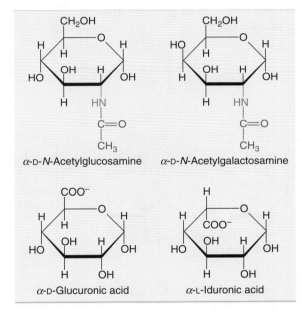

Figure 14.8 Amino sugars and uronic acids are the most common building blocks of the glycosaminoglycans. In the amino sugars, the hydroxyl group at C-2 of the hexose is replaced by an amino group. This amino group is most often acetylated and sometimes sulfated. In the uronic acids, C-6 of the hexose is oxidized to a carboxyl group. N-Acetylglucosamine and N-acetylgalactosamine are the most common amino sugars, and glucuronic acid and iduronic acid (a C-5 epimer of glucuronic acid) are the most common uronic acids. The amino sugars, but not the uronic acids, are also common in glycoproteins and glycolipids. The D and L series of monosaccharides are designated according to the absolute configuration at the asymmetrical carbon farthest away from the carbonyl carbon; hence, the C-5 epimer of D-glucuronic acid belongs to the L series.

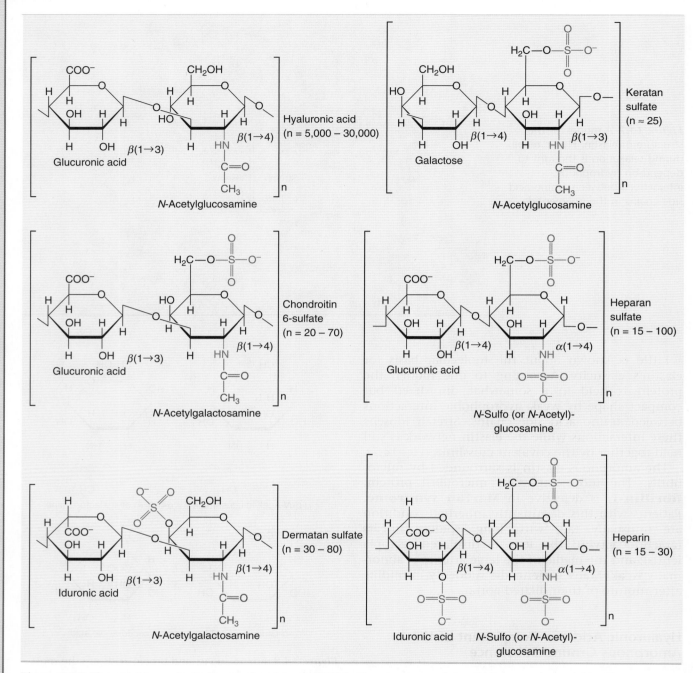

Figure 14.9 The most important glycosaminoglycans (GAGs). The structures of the GAGs are quite variable. Thus, chondroitin 4-sulfate has sulfur on C-4 rather than C-6 of the amino sugar; dermatan sulfate contains some glucuronic acid besides iduronic acid, and the sulfate of the amino sugar may be either on C-4 or on C-6; heparan sulfate contains some iduronic acid besides glucuronic acid; and heparin contains both glucuronic acid and iduronic acid.

viscous solutions at low concentrations and a hydrated gel at high concentrations.

Hyaluronic acid is present in the extracellular matrix of all tissues. **Wharton jelly** in the umbilical cord is a hyaluronate-based gel; the **vitreous body** of the eye is a gel of sodium hyaluronate with an interspersed network of type II collagen fibrils; and **synovial fluid** is a lubricant that contains 0.3% hyaluronic acid along with a glycoprotein.

Sulfated Glycosaminoglycans Are Covalently Bound to Core Proteins

GAGs other than hyaluronic acid carry sulfate groups in the form of sulfate esters and, sometimes, in amide bond with the nitrogen of the amino sugar. These sulfate groups contribute additional negative charges. *The sulfated GAGs are much shorter*

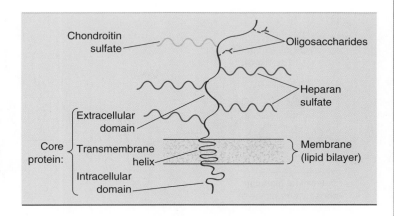

Figure 14.10 Structure of a surface proteoglycan that is present in the plasma membrane of many epithelial cells. Note that more than one glycosaminoglycan (GAG) may be present and that N- or O-linked oligosaccharides may be present as well.

than hyaluronic acid, and they are covalently bound to amino acid side chains in a core protein.

The core protein with its covalently attached GAGs is called a **proteoglycan.** Proteoglycans are found in many places:

1. *They are major components of the amorphous ground substance of connective tissues.*
2. *Some proteoglycans reside in the plasma membrane* (Fig. 14.10). They contain heparan sulfate and, less commonly, chondroitin sulfate.
3. *Mucus contains proteoglycans.* Together with the **mucins** (glycoproteins with abundant O-linked oligosaccharides), proteoglycans are responsible for the slimy consistency of mucus secretions.
4. ***Heparin*** *is formed by mast cells and basophils.* It is a water-soluble product with anticoagulant and lipid-clearing properties. When it is released together with histamine during inflammatory and allergic reactions, the histamine increases vascular permeability and the heparin prevents excessive fibrin formation in the interstitial space.

Cartilage Contains Large Proteoglycan Aggregates

Approximately two thirds of the dry weight of cartilage is collagen (mainly types I and II). Most of the rest is contributed by a large proteoglycan called **aggrecan.** Aggrecan has a core protein of 2316 amino acids. Two globular domains at the amino end are followed by a keratan sulfate domain, a large chondroitin sulfate domain, and finally another globular domain at the carboxyl end (Fig. 14.11).

The aggrecan molecule looks like a test tube brush, with approximately 100 chondroitin sulfate chains and 50 to 80 keratan sulfate chains extending from the core protein in all directions. These GAGs are sprawling, hydrated polysaccharide chains that fill a large volume. In all, aggrecan has

a molecular weight of approximately 2×10^6 D and a length of 400 nm (0.4 μm).

Aggrecan molecules, as their name implies, are gregarious. Large **proteoglycan aggregates** are formed when the N-terminal domains of the core protein bind noncovalently to hyaluronic acid. This binding is reinforced by a small, noncovalently bound link protein (Fig. 14.12). Spaced about 40 nm apart, a single hyaluronic acid molecule binds up to a few hundred aggrecan molecules. These aggregates have a molecular weight of 1 to 5×10^8 D and a length of a few micrometers. The volume occupied by a single proteoglycan aggregate is larger than a bacterial cell!

Proteoglycan aggregates are responsible for the elasticity, resilience, and gel-like properties of cartilage; the collagen fibers that are embedded in the proteoglycan matrix make it resistant to stretch and shear forces.

Bone Consists of Calcium Phosphates in a Collagenous Matrix

Bone consists of approximately 10% water, 20% organic materials, and 70% inorganic salts. *The organic matrix is mainly type I collagen, and the inorganic salts are derived from calcium phosphate [$Ca_3(PO_4)_2$].* **Hydroxyapatite,** $3[Ca_3(PO_4)_2] \cdot Ca(OH)_2$, is the major inorganic component. There are also considerable amounts of Mg^{2+}, Na^+, CO_3^{2-}, F^-, and citrate.

Other metal ions can also be incorporated into this "bone salt." Sr^{2+}, for example, can take the place of Ca^{2+} in the crystal lattice. Radioactive ^{90}Sr, formed during nuclear blasts, can stay in bone for many years, causing damage to the rapidly dividing cells of the neighboring bone marrow.

During bone formation, the organic matrix is deposited first. Mineralization is initiated by the formation of insoluble $CaHPO_4 \cdot 2H_2O$ in the gaps between the ends of tropocollagen molecules in the

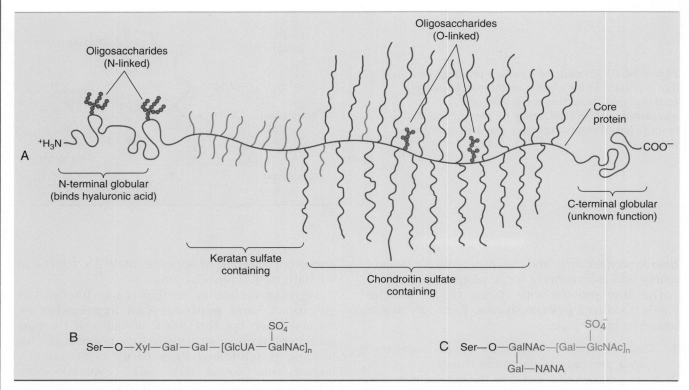

Figure 14.11 Structure of aggrecan, the major proteoglycan of cartilage. **A,** Overall structure (schematic). **B,** Covalent attachment of chondroitin sulfate to serine side chains in aggrecan. The xylose-galactose-galactose linker sequence has been found in several other proteoglycans as well. **C,** Covalent attachment of keratan sulfate to serine (sometimes threonine) side chains in aggrecan. In some other proteoglycans, keratan sulfate is bound N-glycosidically to asparagine rather than O-glycosidically to serine. NANA, *N*-acetylneuraminic acid.

collagen fibrils. This salt is slowly converted into the even less soluble hydroxyapatite.

Plasma and extracellular fluid are supersaturated with the components of bone salt. However, they also contain inorganic pyrophosphate, which prevents crystallization. In bone, pyrophosphate is destroyed by the enzyme **alkaline phosphatase** on the surface of osteoblasts. Patients with a recessively inherited deficiency of alkaline phosphatase suffer from **hypophosphatasia.** They have poor bone mineralization similar to rickets.

In pathological situations, *bones become demineralized whenever either the calcium or the phosphate concentration in the plasma and the extracellular medium is reduced.* This mechanism contributes to the impaired mineralization in **rickets** and **osteomalacia** (vitamin D deficiency; see Chapter 29). **Hypophosphatemia,** also known as **vitamin D–resistant rickets,** is an inherited defect of renal phosphate reabsorption that leads to decreased serum phosphate levels and impaired bone mineralization.

The solubility of the bone salt increases profoundly at low pH. Thus, chronic acidosis leads to bone demineralization. In patients with renal failure, bone demineralization results from a combination of impaired vitamin D metabolism and an incompletely compensated metabolic acidosis. *Poorly mineralized bones have a soft consistency, much like cartilage, and they bend rather than break under stress.*

Impaired formation of the organic matrix leads to brittle bones that break easily. This happens not only in osteogenesis imperfecta but also in **osteoporosis.** This common age-related disorder is associated with impaired synthesis of type I collagen. Low collagen leads to poor mineralization and abnormal fractures. Osteoporosis can be treated with estrogens or androgens and with supplements of calcium and vitamin D.

Metastatic calcification is the inappropriate deposition of insoluble calcium salts in soft tissues. It is caused by prolonged periods of hypercalcemia or hyperphosphatemia.

Basement Membranes Contain Type IV Collagen, Laminin, and Heparan Sulfate Proteoglycans

The "basement membrane" is not a biological membrane but a thin, translucent sheet of extracellular

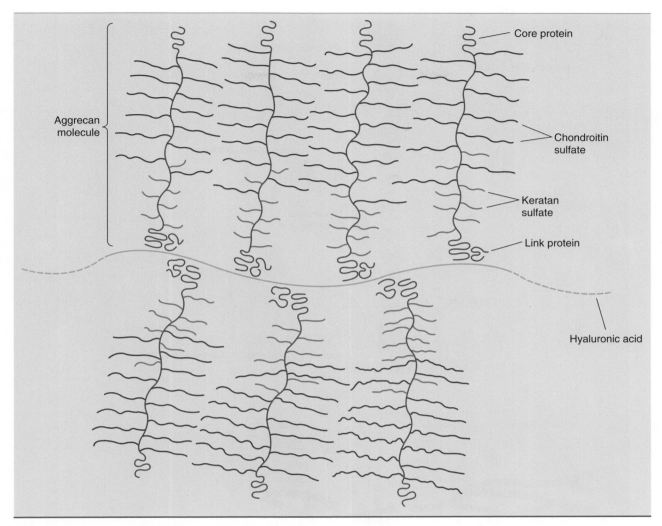

Figure 14.12 Structure of the proteoglycan aggregate in cartilage.

matrix with a thickness of 60 to 100 nm. It consists of a **basal lamina** facing the cells and a **reticular lamina** facing the extracellular matrix. Epithelial cells rest on a basement membrane, and large cells such as muscle fibers and adipocytes are surrounded by it (Fig. 14.13).

Basement membranes contain **type IV collagen.** This collagen contains the familiar triple helix, but it cannot form fibrils because the triple helix is interrupted at about 20 sites. There is also a globular, nonhelical domain at the C-terminus of the polypeptide. *Instead of fibrils, type IV collagen forms an irregular two-dimensional network in the basement membrane.*

Basement membranes also contain **laminin,** a large cross-shaped glycoprotein consisting of three intertwined polypeptides (Fig. 14.14). Laminin has binding sites for integrin receptors on the cell surface, for type IV collagen, heparan sulfate proteoglycans and the basement membrane glycopro-

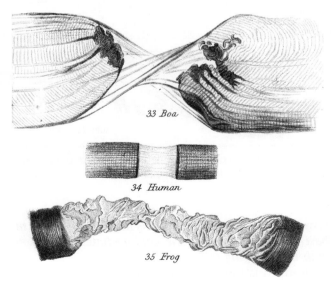

Figure 14.13 Early drawings of severed muscle fibers in the boa constrictor, human, and frog, showing the translucent basement membrane.

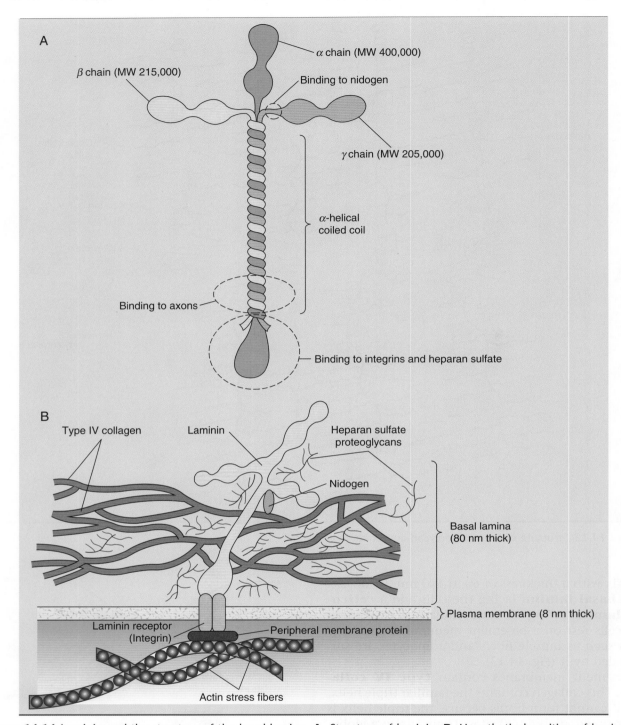

Figure 14.14 Laminin and the structure of the basal lamina. **A,** Structure of laminin. **B,** Hypothetical position of laminin on the cell surface. MW, molecular weight.

tein entactin (nidogen). *It holds the components of the basement membrane together and mediates interactions with the overlying cells.*

Laminin is more than glue, however. *Through the integrin receptors to which it binds, laminin triggers physiological responses in the cells.* Some cell types proliferate or change their shape in response to laminin

binding, and epithelial cells spread on laminin-coated surfaces. In this respect, *laminin acts like a hormone or growth factor that triggers physiological responses by binding to cell surface receptors* (see Chapter 17).

Besides laminin and type IV collagen, basement membranes contain heparan sulfate proteoglycans.

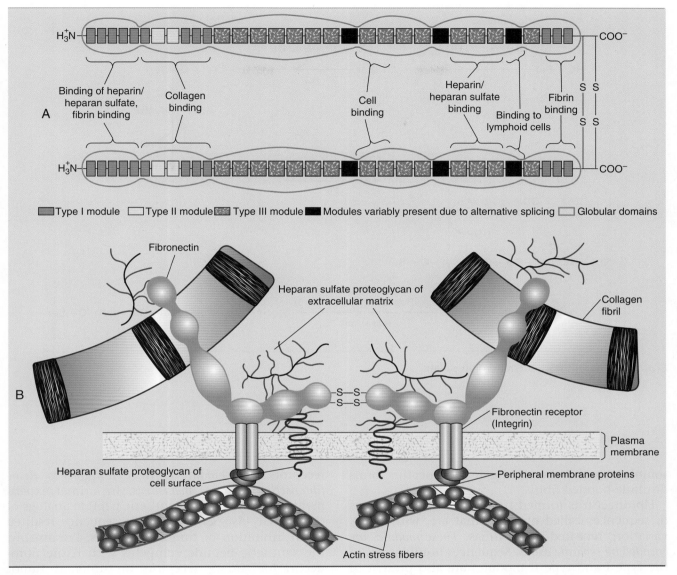

Figure 14.15 Fibronectin and cell-to-fiber adhesion. **A,** Domain structure of fibronectin. The cell-binding site is surprisingly small, with the sequence Arg-Gly-Asp-Ser as the minimal required structure. As a result of alternative splicing, the binding site for lymphoid cells is present in some but not all fibronectins. **B,** Hypothetical position of fibronectin on the cell surface.

These proteoglycans influence the permeability of the basement membrane for soluble proteins. This is most important in the double-thickness basement membrane of the renal glomerulus. *This "membrane" retains the negatively charged plasma proteins, whereas cationic proteins of equal size can pass.* It behaves as if it had pores that are lined by negative charges. Almost all plasma proteins have isoelectric points well below the normal blood pH of 7.4 and are therefore negatively charged.

The glomerular basement membrane of diabetic patients is leaky, and plasma proteins are excreted in the urine. This defect is associated with a reduced heparan sulfate content of the glomerular basement membrane.

Fibronectin Glues Cells and Collagen Fibers Together

Fibronectin is the most abundant multiadhesive protein in connective tissues, and it even circulates in the plasma in a concentration of about 30 mg/100 mL. Like laminin, it is a very large protein. It is formed from two similar polypeptides, each with a length of about 2500 amino acids, which are linked by disulfide bonds near their carboxyl end (Fig. 14.15).

Humans have only one fibronectin gene, but tissue-specific isoforms are formed by differential splicing of the transcript. Plasma fibronectin is a

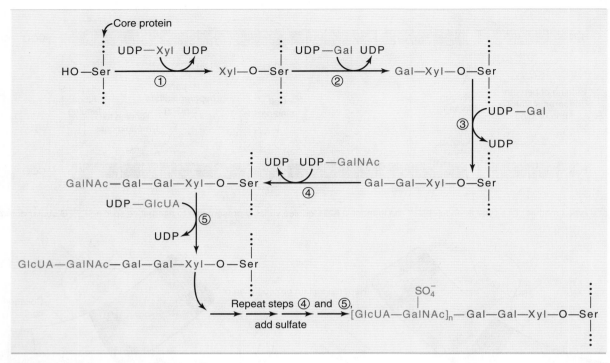

Figure 14.16 Synthesis of chondroitin sulfate.

soluble dimer, whereas tissue fibronectin forms disulfide-bonded fibrils.

Fibronectin is formed from three different types of sequences called modules that are, with much variation, repeated many times. *These modules are encoded by separate exons.* Sequences homologous to the type I and type II modules are also present in some other, unrelated proteins. Apparently, *the fibronectin gene was assembled by exon shuffling and exon duplication.*

Different parts of fibronectin bind to cell surface receptors, heparan sulfate proteoglycans, fibrillar collagens, and fibrin. The binding to cell surface receptors of the integrin type is mediated by the surprisingly short sequence Arg-Gly-Asp-Ser in the 9th and 10th type III modules. *Fibronectin glues the cells to the fibrous meshwork of the extracellular matrix.*

During embryonic development, fibronectin is necessary for the migration of cells along fibrous tracks. During wound healing, it is incorporated into the fibrin clot and even becomes covalently crosslinked to fibrin. This enmeshed fibronectin attracts fibroblasts and endothelial cells during wound healing.

Many malignant cells are devoid of surface-bound fibronectin, although they possess fibronectin receptors. *The binding of these receptors to tissue fibronectin facilitates metastasis.* In animal experiments, treatment with synthetic peptide analogs of the Arg-Gly-Asp-Ser recognition sequence resulted in an inhibition of tumor metastasis. Presumably, the synthetic peptide competes with tissue fibronectin for surface receptors on itinerant tumor cells.

Proteoglycans Are Synthesized in the Endoplasmic Reticulum and Degraded in Lysosomes

Like "ordinary" glycoproteins, proteoglycans are processed through the secretory pathway. *The core protein is made by ribosomes on the rough ER, and the polysaccharides are constructed in the ER and Golgi apparatus.* The precursors of the GAG chains are nucleotide-activated sugars (Fig. 14.16).

Some modifications are introduced in the polysaccharide after the formation of the glycosidic bonds. Iduronic acid is formed by the epimerization of glucuronic acid, and sulfate groups are introduced by the transfer of sulfate from **phospho-adenosine phosphosulfate (PAPS):**

PAPS is biosynthetically derived from ATP. *It provides an activated sulfate for sulfation reactions much as ATP provides an activated phosphate for phosphorylation reactions.*

At the end of their life cycle, *the extracellular proteoglycans undergo endocytosis and are sent to the lysosomes.* Many different enzymes have to cooperate in their degradation. The complete degradation of heparan sulfate, for example, requires three different exoglycosidases, four sulfatases, and an acetyl transferase.

Most of the sulfated GAGs are degraded by the stepwise removal of monosaccharides from the nonreducing end, whereas sulfatases remove the sulfate groups. Only hyaluronic acid and chondroitin sulfate can be degraded by a lysosomal endoglycosidase ("hyaluronidase").

Mucopolysaccharidoses Are Caused by the Deficiency of Glycosaminoglycan-Degrading Enzymes

The deficiency of only one of the required lysosomal enzymes can interrupt the ordered sequence of GAG degradation. As a result, *the undegraded GAGs accumulate in the lysosomes.* Some of the accumulating polysaccharide is processed to smaller fragments by endoglycosidases. These fragments often appear in blood and urine, in which they can be demonstrated in diagnostic tests.

This type of disease is called **mucopolysaccharidosis.** "Mucopolysaccharide" is an obsolete name for GAG, but "glycosaminoglycanosis" does not seem to sound right. The mucopolysaccharidoses are examples of **lysosomal storage diseases.**

Some features of the mucopolysaccharidoses (Table 14.5) should be emphasized:

1. *The enzyme deficiency is generalized, affecting all organ systems.* This is a feature of all lysosomal storage diseases.
2. *The diseases are inherited as autosomal recessive or (type II) X-linked recessive traits.* This means that heterozygotes, who typically have half of the normal enzyme activity, are healthy. Heterozygotes can be identified by measuring the enzyme activity in cultured leukocytes, fibroblasts, or amniotic cells.
3. *Many mucopolysaccharidoses are known both in severe and mild forms.* Patients with severe disease have no detectable enzyme activity, whereas those with less severe disease have an enzyme with abnormally low activity. The difference between types IH and IS shown in Table 14.5 is an example.
4. *Most mucopolysaccharidoses are not apparent at birth.* Signs and symptoms develop gradually as more and more mucopolysaccharide accumulates.
5. *Defects in the degradation of keratan sulfate and dermatan sulfate cause skeletal deformities and other connective tissue abnormalities.* Common manifestations include coarse facial features ("gargoylism"), short stature, corneal clouding, hearing loss, joint stiffness, valvular heart disease, obstructive lung disease, and hepatosplenomegaly. All these problems are caused by the buildup of GAGs in the tissues.
6. Of all the mucopolysaccharide defects, *only those in heparan sulfate degradation cause mental retardation and neurological degeneration.* Heparan sulfate is the only important GAG in the central nervous system.
7. *Chondroitin sulfate and hyaluronic acid do not accumulate* because they can also be degraded by lysosomal hyaluronidase, an endoglycosidase.

The mucopolysaccharidoses are rare diseases, with a combined incidence of approximately 1 per 10,000 to 1 per 20,000. Specific treatment in the form of enzyme replacement has been attempted, but the success was limited because of poor tissue uptake of the injected enzymes and because of immunological responses.

SUMMARY

The extracellular matrix of connective tissue consists of an amorphous ground substance and fibers. The most abundant fiber type is formed from collagen, a long ropelike molecule consisting of three intertwined polypeptides. There

Table 14.5 The Mucopolysaccharidoses

Systematic Name	Common Name	Inheritance	Enzyme Deficiency	GAG(s) Affected	Clinical Features
IH	Hurler	AR	α-L-Iduronidase (complete deficiency)	Dermatan sulfate, heparan sulfate	Skeletal deformities, dwarfism, corneal clouding, hepatosplenomegaly, valvular heart disease, mental retardation, death at ≤10 years
IS	Scheie	AR	α-L-Iduronidase (partial deficiency)	Dermatan sulfate, heparan sulfate	Corneal clouding, stiff joints, normal intelligence and life span
II	Hunter	XR	Iduronate sulfatase	Dermatan sulfate, heparan sulfate	Similar to Hurler but no corneal clouding; death at 10-15 years
IIIA	Sanfilippo A	AR	Heparan-N-sulfatase	Heparan sulfate	Severe to profound mental retardation, mild physical abnormalities
IIIB	Sanfilippo B	AR	α-N-Acetyl-glucosaminidase		
IIIC	Sanfilippo C	AR	Acetyl-CoA: α-glucosaminide acetyltransferase		
IIID	Sanfilippo D	AR	N-Acetylglucosamine 6-sulfatase		
IVA	Morquio A	AR	Galactose 6-sulfatase	Keratan sulfate	Severe skeletal deformities, corneal clouding, normal intelligence
IVB	Morquio B	AR	β-Galactosidase		
VI	Maroteaux-Lamy	AR	N-Acetylgalactosamine 4-sulfatase	Dermatan sulfate	Severe skeletal deformities, corneal clouding, normal intelligence
VII	Sly	AR	β-Glucuronidase	Dermatan sulfate, heparan sulfate	Skeletal deformities, hepatosplenomegaly

AR, Autosomal recessive; CoA, coenzyme A; GAG, glycosaminoglycan; XR, X-linked recessive.

are many types of collagen that differ in their structure, properties, and tissue distribution.

Collagen is synthesized from a larger precursor called procollagen, which is processed in the secretory pathway and extracellularly. Several inherited connective tissue diseases, including OI and Ehlers-Danlos syndrome, are caused by abnormalities of collagen.

The amorphous ground substance consists of proteoglycans, hyaluronic acid, and multiadhesive glycoproteins. Hyaluronic acid and proteoglycans are highly hydrated, with a mucilaginous or gel-like consistency.

Multiadhesive glycoproteins, including laminin and fibronectin, glue cell surfaces and fibrous matrix proteins together. Through cell surface receptors of the integrin type, they link the extracellular matrix with the cytoskeleton and regulate the growth and behavior of the cells.

Mucopolysaccharidoses are caused by deficiencies of lysosomal enzymes for GAG degradation. These diseases cause connective tissue abnormalities and/or mental impairment.

Further Reading

Hynes RO: Integrins: bi-directional, allosteric signaling machines. Cell 110:673-687, 2002.

Malinda KM, Kleinman HK: The laminins. Int J Biochem Cell Biol 28:957-959, 1996.

Parish CR, Freeman C, Hulett MD: Heparanase: a key enzyme involved in cell invasion. Biochim Biophys Acta 1471:M99-M108, 2001.

Sanes JR: The basement membrane/basal lamina of skeletal muscle. J Biol Chem 278:12601-12604, 2003.

Tammi MI, Day AJ, Turley EA: Hyaluronan and homeostasis: a balancing act. J Biol Chem 277:4581-4584, 2002.

Tatham AS, Shewry PR: Elastomeric proteins: biological roles, structures and mechanisms. Trends Biochem Sci 25:567-571, 2000.

Watanabe H, Yamada Y, Kimata K: Roles of aggrecan, a large chondroitin sulfate proteoglycan, in cartilage structure and function. J Biochem 124:687-693, 1998.

QUESTIONS

1. In a home for handicapped children, you see an 11-year-old girl who is only 90 cm tall, is wheelchair bound, and has multiple limb deformities. The nurse tells you that the girl has "glass bones" and had suffered severe fractures on many occasions. Most likely, this girl has a mutation in a gene for

   A. Type I collagen.
   B. Type III collagen.
   C. Elastin.
   D. Fibronectin.
   E. Fibrillin.

2. Besides the ubiquitous type I collagen, cartilage contains large quantities of

   A. Type III collagen and fibronectin.
   B. Type VII collagen and elastin.
   C. Elastin and hyaluronic acid.
   D. Type III collagen and laminin.
   E. Type II collagen and proteoglycans.

3. A first-semester medical student presents with follicular hyperkeratosis (gooseflesh), numerous small subcutaneous hemorrhages, and loose teeth. He reports that for the past 4 months, he has been living only on canned foods, spaghetti, and soft drinks. The process that is most likely impaired in this student is

   A. The removal of propeptides from procollagen.
   B. The hydroxylation of prolyl and lysyl residues in procollagen.

   C. The formation of allysine residues in collagen.
   D. The formation of covalent crosslinks between allysine and lysine residues in collagen.
   E. The formation of desmosine in elastin.

4. Some mucopolysaccharidoses cause only connective tissue problems. In others, however, the patients have mental deficiency. Mental deficiency is most likely to occur in diseases with impaired breakdown of

   A. Hyaluronic acid.
   B. Chondroitin sulfate.
   C. Dermatan sulfate.
   D. Heparan sulfate.
   E. Keratan sulfate.

5. Poor bone mineralization can be expected in all of the following situations *except*

   A. Increased intestinal absorption of dietary calcium.
   B. Increased renal excretion of inorganic phosphate.
   C. A deficiency of alkaline phosphatase in bone.
   D. Chronic acidosis.

PART FOUR

INTEGRATION

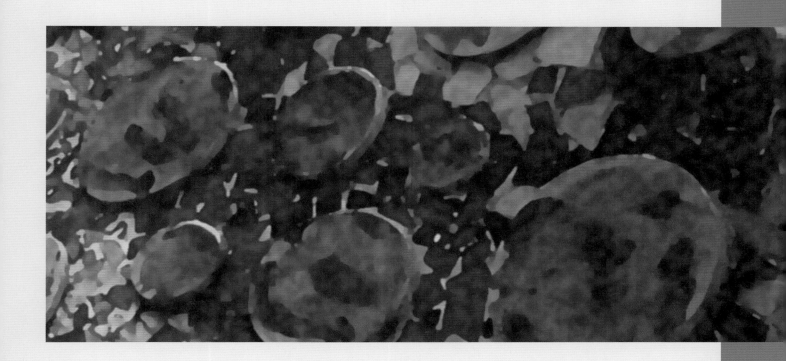

CHAPTER 15

Plasma Proteins

Centrifugation of a blood sample in the presence of an anticoagulant produces a pellet of blood cells that occupies between 40% and 50% of the total volume. The remaining 50% to 60% appears as a clear yellowish fluid called **plasma.** When blood clotting is induced before centrifugation—for example, by stirring the blood with a toothpick in the absence of an anticoagulant—the resulting fluid is called not plasma but **serum.** It has the same composition as plasma except for the absence of fibrinogen and some other clotting factors that are used up during clotting.

Plasma contains approximately 0.9% inorganic ions, 0.8% small organic molecules (more than half of this is lipid), and 7% protein (Table 15.1). A pink coloration of the plasma suggests hemolysis, either in the patient or, more often, in the test tube as a result of careless handling. A milky appearance, or the formation of a fatty layer during centrifugation, shows the presence of chylomicrons: small fat droplets that appear in the plasma after a fatty meal. A turbid appearance in the fasting state suggests a hypertriglyceridemia with elevated very-low-density lipoprotein (VLDL).

Plasma proteins are a mix of about a dozen major and innumerable minor components. They participate in regulation of the blood volume, the transport of nutrients and hormones, blood clotting, and the defense against infections. This chapter describes the most important plasma proteins, their functions, and their abnormalities in disease states.

The Blood pH Is Tightly Regulated

Most biomolecules contain weakly ionizable groups that are subject to protonation and deprotonation. Consequently, *all biological processes depend on the pH value of the environment.* The maintenance of an optimal pH is therefore essential for survival and optimal function.

The pH of plasma is approximately 7.40 in arterial blood and 7.35 in venous blood. This difference is caused by the higher concentration of carbonic acid in venous blood. Carbonic acid is formed spontaneously from carbon dioxide and water, but the reaction is accelerated dramatically by the enzyme **carbonic anhydrase** in erythrocytes:

$$CO_2 + H_2O$$

$$\Updownarrow \text{Carbonic anhydrase}$$

$$H_2CO_3$$

$$\Updownarrow \text{Spontaneous}$$

$$HCO_3^- + H^+$$

At 37° C and a pH of 7.4, there are approximately 800 molecules of dissolved CO_2 and 16,000 molecules of HCO_3^- for every molecule of H_2CO_3. The apparent pK for the overall reaction $CO_2 + H_2O \rightarrow HCO_3^- + H^+$ is 6.1. Thus, the bicarbonate system acts as an effective buffer in the neutral to slightly acidic pH range.

Carbonic acid/bicarbonate is the most important physiological buffer system in the body. It is important because CO_2 and HCO_3^- are present in high concentrations in the body, not only in the plasma but also in the interstitial and intracellular compartments (Fig. 15.1). Also, *the CO_2 level can be regulated by the lungs and the HCO_3^- level by the kidneys.*

Phosphate groups provide an additional buffer system:

$$H_3PO_4 \xrightleftharpoons{\qquad} H_2PO_4^- \xrightleftharpoons[pK = 6.8]{\qquad} HPO_4^{2-} \xrightleftharpoons{\qquad} PO_4^{3-}$$

with H^+ released at each step.

Table 15.1 Reference Values for Some Plasma Constituents

Plasma Constituent	Reference Value
Gases and electrolytes	
pO₂ arterial	95-100 mm Hg
CO₂ arterial	21-28 mmol/L
CO₂ venous	24-30 mmol/L
HCO₃⁻	21-28 mmol/L
Cl⁻	95-103 mmol/L
Na⁺	136-142 mmol/L
K⁺	3.8-5.0 mmol/L
Ca²⁺ (total)	2.3-2.74 mmol/L
Mg²⁺	0.65-1.23 mmol/L
pH	7.35-7.44
Metabolites	
Glucose (fasting)	3.9-6.1 mmol/L (70-110 mg/dL)
Ammonia	7-70 μmol/L (12-120 mg/dL)
Urea nitrogen	2.9-8.2 mmol/L (8-23 mg/dL)
Uric acid	0.16-0.51 mmol/L (2.7-8.5 mg/dL)
Creatinine	53-106 μmol/L (0.6-1.2 mg/dL)
Bilirubin (total)	2-20 μmol/L (0.1-1.2 mg/dL)
Bile acids	0.3-3 mg/dL
Lipids (total)	400-800 mg/dL
Acetoacetic acid	20-100 μmol/L (0.2-1 mg/dL)
Acetone	50-340 μmol/L (0.3-2 mg/dL)
Proteins	
Total protein	6-8 g/dL
Albumin	3.2-5.6 g/dL (52-65% of total)
α₁-Globulins	0.1-0.4 g/dL (2.5-5% of total)
α₂-Globulins	0.4-1.2 g/dL (7-13% of total)
β-Globulins	0.5-1.1 g/dL (8-14% of total)
γ-Globulins	0.5-1.6 g/dL (12-22% of total)

Only $H_2PO_4^-$ and HPO_4^{2-} are present in appreciable quantities at physiological pH values. The phosphate buffer is important only in the intracellular compartments, in which phosphate is the major inorganic anion. Cells also contain much organically bound phosphate with pK values similar to those of inorganic phosphate.

Proteins also participate in pH buffering, mainly through their histidine side chains:

with pK ~ 7.

Serum albumin, for example, has 16 histidine residues with pK values not too far from the blood pH of 7.4. Like phosphate, proteins are more important buffer systems in the cells than in the plasma.

Acidosis and Alkalosis Are Common in Clinical Practice

Even small deviations from the normal blood pH lead to severe clinical disturbances. An arterial pH lower than 7.35 is called **acidemia,** and an arter-

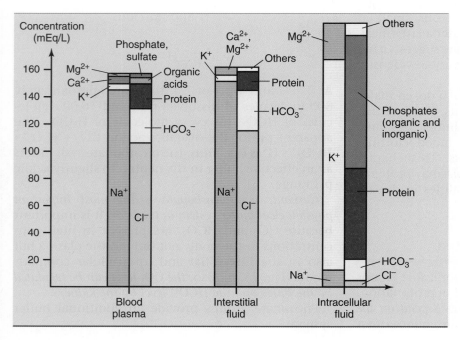

Figure 15.1 The ionic compositions of blood plasma, interstitial fluid, and intracellular fluid.

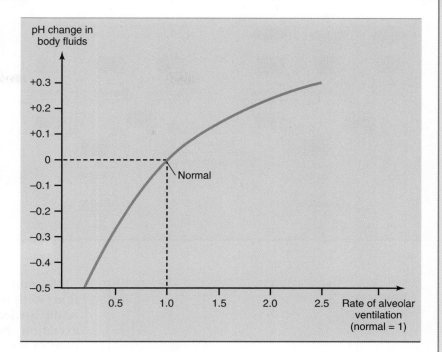

Figure 15.2 The pH change in plasma and extracellular fluids in response to changes in alveolar ventilation.

ial pH exceeding 7.45 is called **alkalemia.** The pathological states leading to these outcomes are called **acidosis** and **alkalosis,** respectively.

Respiratory acidosis is caused by any impairment in the disposal of CO_2. Conversely, **respiratory alkalosis** results from hyperventilation. For example, a doubling in the rate of alveolar ventilation raises the blood pH from 7.40 to 7.62, and a 50% reduction in alveolar ventilation lowers the blood pH from 7.40 to 7.12 (Fig. 15.2).

Metabolic acidosis is caused either by an overproduction of organic acids or by an inability of the kidneys to excrete excess acid. The normal urinary pH varies over a range of 4.0 to 7.0, depending on the need to excrete excess protons. Conversely, **metabolic alkalosis** is caused by the abnormal loss of acids from the body: for example, as a result of excessive vomiting.

In every case, the body employs regulatory systems that are designed to restore the normal blood pH. There are three lines of defense against acidosis and alkalosis:

1. *The buffer systems act immediately to prevent excessive fluctuations of the blood pH.*
2. *Alveolar ventilation increases in acidosis and decreases in alkalosis.* The respiratory center in the medulla oblongata of the brain responds directly to pH and CO_2. This mechanism works on a time scale of minutes.
3. *The kidneys excrete excess H+ in acidosis and excess HCO_3^- in alkalosis.* This is a long-term mechanism that acts on a time scale of hours to days.

The most important laboratory test for the distinction between metabolic and respiratory acidosis is the determination of the plasma total carbon dioxide $(CO_2 + H_2CO_3 + HCO_3^-)$. In respiratory acidosis, the total carbon dioxide is elevated because CO_2 retention is, by definition, the cause of the acidosis; in metabolic acidosis, it is reduced because the patient hyperventilates in an attempt to eliminate excess carbonic acid. The converse applies to alkalosis.

Most Plasma Proteins Are Derived from the Liver

Most plasma proteins are derived from the liver. In all, the liver synthesizes about 25 g of plasma proteins every day, which accounts for nearly 50% of the total protein synthesis in the liver. Only the immunoglobulins are not produced by the liver. They are synthesized by plasma cells.

Most plasma proteins (exception: albumin) are glycoproteins. They circulate for several days and are eventually removed from the circulation when their oligosaccharide chains are worn down. Most of their N-linked oligosaccharides end with sialic acid (*N*-acetylneuraminic acid) bound to galactose. During the lifetime of the plasma protein, the terminal sialic acid residues are gradually chewed off by endothelial neuraminidases (Fig. 15.3). After the loss of the sialic acid, the exposed galactose at the end of the oligosaccharide binds to an **asialogly-**

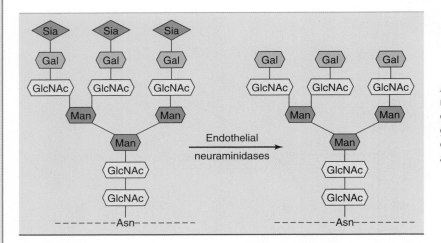

Figure 15.3 Removal of terminal sialic acid residues (Sia) from a typical *N*-linked oligosaccharide in a plasma protein exposes galactose residues that mediate the binding of the protein to the hepatic asialoglycoprotein receptor.

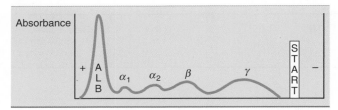

Figure 15.4 Electrophoretic separation of plasma proteins on cellulose acetate foil at pH 8.6, densitometric scan. The electrophoretic pattern depends somewhat on the separation conditions, including support medium, pH, and ionic strength. ALB, albumin.

coprotein receptor on the surface of hepatocytes, followed by receptor-mediated endocytosis and lysosomal degradation.

Albumin Prevents Edema

Electrophoresis is the most important method for the separation of plasma proteins in the clinical laboratory (Fig. 15.4). It is usually performed at a mildly alkaline pH and on a solid or semisolid support such as cellulose acetate foil or an agarose gel. *This separates the proteins by their charge/mass ratio rather than their molecular weight.* The separated protein fractions are identified by staining and densitometric scanning. Most procedures separate the proteins into five fractions: albumin and the α_1, α_2, β, and γ globulins.

Of these five fractions, *only the albumin peak consists of a single major protein.* Albumin is a single tightly packed polypeptide with 585 amino acids, without any covalently bound carbohydrate. Its compact shape minimizes its effect on plasma viscosity. In general, compact proteins do not increase the plasma viscosity to the same extent as more elongated proteins of the same molecular weight.

Albumin has a half-life of 17 days in the circulation. With its molecular weight of 66,000 D and an acidic isoelectric point (pI), it is able to avoid renal excretion, but it does cross the vascular endothelium of most tissues to a limited extent. Therefore, it is present in interstitial fluid and lymph but at lower concentrations than in the plasma.

Because the interstitial fluid volume is far larger than the plasma volume (12% versus 4.5% of the body volume, respectively), the total amount of albumin in the interstitial spaces slightly exceeds that in the vascular compartment. This albumin is returned to the blood by the lymph.

Although albumin accounts for only 60% of the total plasma protein, it provides 80% of the colloid osmotic pressure of the plasma. This is because the colloid osmotic pressure depends on the amount of water and electrolytes that a protein attracts to its surface, and albumin is one of the most hydrophilic plasma proteins.

The colloid osmotic pressure is necessary to prevent edema. In the capillaries, the hydrostatic pressure of the blood forces fluid from the blood into the interstitial spaces. The colloid osmotic pressure of albumin and other plasma proteins is necessary to draw this fluid back into the capillary. Fluid balance across the endothelium is maintained as long as these two forces cancel each other (Fig. 15.5).

Usually, edema develops when the albumin concentration drops below 2.0 g/dL. Edema can also be caused by an increase in capillary permeability, venous obstruction, impaired lymph flow, and congestive heart failure with an increased venous pressure.

Albumin Binds Many Small Molecules

As a binding protein, albumin is extremely versatile, with binding sites for fatty acids, thyroxine,

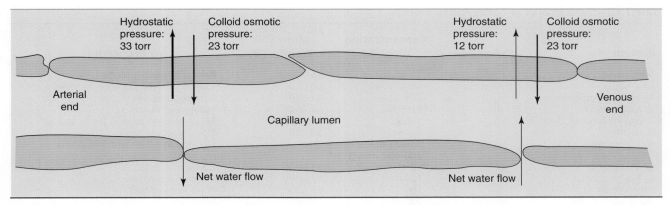

Figure 15.5 Importance of the colloid osmotic pressure for fluid exchange across the capillary wall. A net flow of water into the interstitium is observed at the arterial end of the capillary. This is balanced by a net flow into the capillary at its venous end.

cortisol, heme, bilirubin, and many other metabolites. Even approximately half the serum calcium is albumin bound.

Foreign substances, including many drugs, also bind to serum albumin with varying affinities. *Only the free, unbound fraction of a drug is pharmacologically active.* Being noncovalent, albumin binding is reversible:

$$Albumin \cdot Drug \rightleftharpoons Albumin + Drug$$

The dissociation constant K_D for the release of the drug from albumin is defined as

1
$$K_d = \frac{[Alb] \times [Drug]}{[Alb \cdot Drug]}$$

This can be rearranged as

2
$$\frac{[Drug]}{[Alb \cdot Drug]} = \frac{K_d}{[Alb]}$$

As long as the molar concentration of albumin is far higher than that of the drug, the concentration of free, unbound albumin [Alb] approximates the total serum albumin concentration. Equation 2 indicates that in a patient whose albumin concentration is only half of normal, the ratio of free drug/bound drug is doubled.

This becomes important when the plasma level of a chronically administered drug such as warfarin or a cardiotonic steroid is measured. *If the patient has severe hypoalbuminemia, an otherwise desirable plasma level may actually be in the toxic range* because an increased fraction of the drug is in the biologically active, unbound form. The commonly employed laboratory tests for plasma drug levels do not distinguish between the free and bound fractions.

Some Plasma Proteins Are Specialized Carriers of Small Molecules

Many of the proteins listed in Table 15.2 are binding proteins that ferry endogenous substances through the blood.

Transthyretin, also called **prealbumin** because it moves slightly ahead of albumin during electrophoresis, participates in the transport of retinol from the liver to other tissues. The liver releases retinol bound to **retinol-binding protein (RBP);** retinol in turn binds to transthyretin in the blood. The formation of this ternary complex is important because RBP alone (molecular weight [MW], 21,000 D) is too small to escape renal excretion.

Transthyretin also binds thyroid hormones. However, the major transport protein for these hormones is **thyroxine-binding globulin (TBG),** which binds thyroxine with 100 times higher affinity than does transthyretin. An increased level of transthyretin leads to an increased level of total circulating thyroid hormone, whereas its congenital absence leads to abnormally low levels. In both cases, however, the patient is healthy because the level of the free, unbound hormone is kept in the physiological range by homeostatic mechanisms.

Circulating steroid hormones are also protein bound. Glucocorticoids are bound to **transcortin,** whereas androgens and estrogens have their own **sex hormone–binding globulin.** Because only the unbound fraction of the hormone is biologically active, *variable levels of the binding proteins can complicate the interpretation of hormone levels measured in the clinical laboratory.* What the laboratory measures routinely is the concentration of the total (free + protein-bound) hormone.

Table 15.2 Characteristics of Some Plasma Proteins

Protein	Fraction	Concentration (mg/dL)	Molecular Weight (D)	Properties
Transthyretin	Prealbumin	15-35	55,000	Retinol transport, binds T_4
Albumin	Albumin	4000-5000	66,000	Colloid osmotic pressure, binding protein
Retinol-binding protein	α_1	3-6	21,000	Retinol transport
α_1-Antiprotease	α_1	85-185	54,000	Protease inhibitor
Thyroxine-binding globulin	α_1	1-3.5	58,000	Major binding protein for T_3 and T_4
Transcortin	α_1	3-3.5	52,000	Binds glucocorticoids
α-Fetoprotein	α_1	0.002 (adults) 200-400 (fetus)		Elevated in adults with hepatoma
Ceruloplasmin	α_2	20-40	132,000	Contains copper
α_2-Macroglobulin	α_2	150-400	725,000	Protease inhibitor
Haptoglobin	α_2	100-300	85,000*	Binds hemoglobin
Transferrin	β	200-400	89,000	Binds iron
Hemopexin	β	50-120	60,000	Binds heme
Fibrinogen	β	200-400	340,000	Clot formation
C-reactive protein	γ	1.0	110,000	Acute phase reactant
Immunoglobulins	γ	700-1500	150,000-950,000	Very heterogeneous

* One genetic variant forms higher molecular weight polymers (>200,000 D).
T_3, triiodothyronine; T_4, thyroxine.

The hormone-binding proteins buffer the plasma concentration of the free unbound hormone, in the same way that a pH buffer buffers the concentration of free protons.

Haptoglobin and **hemopexin** are binding proteins with a very different function. After intravascular hemolysis, the hemoglobin that is released from the ruptured erythrocytes dissociates into $\alpha\beta$ dimers that are too small (MW, 33,000 D) to escape renal excretion. *To prevent the loss of hemoglobin with its valuable iron, the hemoglobin binds to haptoglobin, and any free heme binds to hemopexin.* These complexes are cleared by reticuloendothelial cells and hepatocytes, respectively (Fig. 15.6).

Because haptoglobin is degraded along with hemoglobin in this process, *the serum haptoglobin level is depressed in all hemolytic conditions,* sometimes to nearly zero. Haptoglobin does not bind the myoglobin that is released from damaged muscles. Therefore, *the haptoglobin level is normal in muscle diseases.* Because the common laboratory tests for "blood" in the urine do not distinguish between hemoglobin and myoglobin, *serum haptoglobin can be determined to distinguish between hemoglobinuria and myoglobinuria.*

The Deficiency of α_1-Antiprotease Causes Lung Emphysema

In the blood, proteolytic events occur during blood clotting and during immune responses. These processes are modulated by circulating protease inhibitors. Some of these inhibitors are very selective, whereas others inhibit a large number of proteases.

The protease inhibitor α_2-**macroglobulin,** so-called because of its size (MW, 725,000 D), is a major component of the α_2-globulin fraction. It binds and inhibits a wide variety of proteases. The protease-inhibitor complexes are ingested by reticuloendothelial cells, in which they are digested by lysosomal enzymes.

α_2-Macroglobulin is considered a backup protease inhibitor that comes into play when more selective inhibitors fail.

α_1-**Antiprotease** is also known as α_1-**protease inhibitor** or α_1-**antitrypsin.** It inhibits many serine proteases, including elastase from white blood cells. In the laboratory, its activity is measured as the **trypsin inhibitory capacity (TIC).**

More than 50 genetic variants of α_1-antiprotease are known. One of them, the Z allele, codes for a protein that cannot be secreted from the hepatocytes in which it is synthesized, which results in a very low TIC. Whereas heterozygotes are healthy, *homozygosity for the Z allele causes early-onset lung emphysema.*

In lung emphysema, the septa of the lung alveoli degenerate, and the surface area available for gas exchange is reduced. Ordinarily, emphysema is caused by the smoldering inflammation of chronic bronchitis and is seen mainly in long-term smokers.

The observation of early-onset lung emphysema in individuals with α_1-antiprotease deficiency suggests that *excessive proteolytic activity is an important mediator of tissue damage in chronic bronchitis and emphysema.*

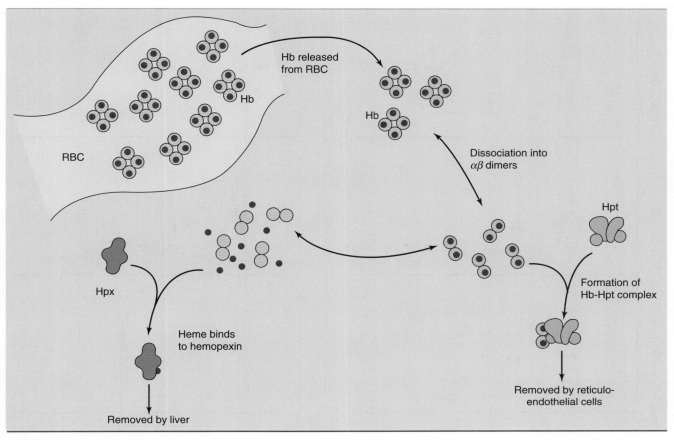

Figure 15.6 The fate of hemoglobin (Hb) after intravascular hemolysis. Hpt, haptoglobin; Hpx, hemopexin; RBC, red blood cell.

Macrophages and neutrophils release lysosomal proteases during phagocytosis. By attacking proteins of the extracellular matrix, these proteases help the phagocytic cell move through the tissue. However, to prevent excessive tissue damage, these proteases must be kept in check by α_1-antiprotease.

α_1-Antiprotease is present not only in the blood but also in bronchial secretions and the interstitial fluid.

The lungs are especially vulnerable to out-of-control proteases because they are exposed to inhaled bacteria and other foreign particles that have to be scavenged continuously by neutrophils and alveolar macrophages.

α_1-Antiprotease can be inactivated by smoking. An essential methionine residue in the protein becomes oxidized to methionine sulfoxide by components of cigarette smoke. This may well contribute to the development of chronic bronchitis and emphysema in smokers, even those without a genetic defect in the protease inhibitor system.

The prevalence of α_1-antiprotease deficiency in the white population of the United States is about 1 per 7000. Of these people, 80% will eventually develop emphysema, many of them at an early age. *The strict avoidance of smoking is essential in the management of these patients.*

Some patients with α_1-antiprotease deficiency develop neonatal hepatitis or infantile cirrhosis. This is, in all likelihood, caused not by a lack of protease inhibition but by the accumulation of nonsecretable α_1-antiprotease in vesicles within the hepatocytes.

The Levels of Plasma Proteins Are Affected by Many Diseases

Plasma protein electrophoresis is a valuable aid in the diagnosis of many diseases. Figure 15.7 summarizes some typical patterns.

Acute-phase reactants are plasma proteins whose levels change within 1 or 2 days after acute inflammation, trauma, or surgery (Table 15.3). Their synthesis appears to be affected by stress hormones and cytokines that are released in these conditions. The albumin peak is reduced, whereas the α_2 peak is often increased because one of its major compo-

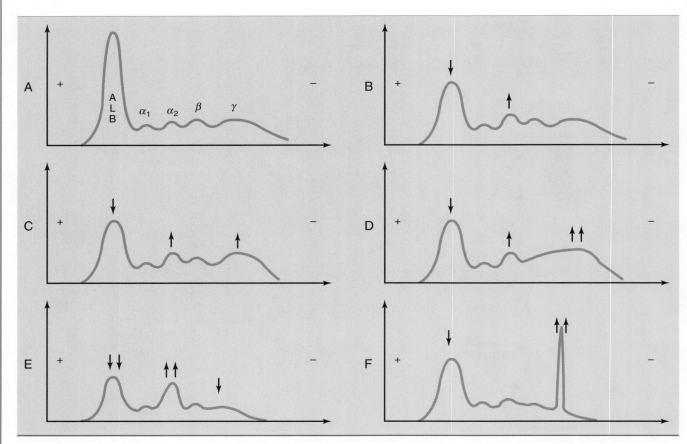

Figure 15.7 Plasma protein electrophoresis in various disease states. **A,** Normal. ALB, albumin. **B,** Immediate response pattern. **C,** Delayed response pattern. **D,** Liver cirrhosis. **E,** Protein-losing conditions (nephrotic syndrome, protein-losing enteropathy). **F,** Monoclonal gammopathy ("paraprotein").

Table 15.3 Acute-Phase Reactants*

Protein	Fraction	Response
Albumin	Albumin	↓
α_1-Acid glycoprotein	α_1	↑↑
α_1-Antiprotease	α_1	↑
Ceruloplasmin	α_2	(↑)
Haptoglobin	α_2	↑↑
α_2-Macroglobulin	α_2	↓
C-reactive protein	β/γ	↑↑↑

*The levels of these plasma proteins are either elevated or reduced in many acute illnesses.

nents, haptoglobin, is a positive acute-phase reactant.

The most sensitive acute-phase reactant, however, is **C-reactive protein.** Its plasma level rises up to 100-fold in bacterial infections and to a lesser degree in some other diseases, after trauma, or after surgery. This protein binds avidly to some bacterial polysaccharides, and it seems to play a role in the immune response against these bacteria.

γ-Globulins are increased in many chronic diseases including infections, malignancies, and liver cirrhosis, apparently by a general stimulation of immunoglobulin synthesis. This condition is called **polyclonal gammopathy.** In **monoclonal gammopathy,** in contrast, a single immunoglobulin is overproduced by an abnormal plasma cell clone.

In **nephrotic syndrome,** the glomerular basement membrane is damaged and plasma proteins are lost in the urine. The protein loss is most severe for small proteins. This depresses the albumin peak and most of the globulin peaks, whereas the α_2 peak is increased. The α_2-macroglobulin in this fraction is so large (MW, 725,000 D) that it is retained, whereas the smaller plasma proteins are lost.

Similar patterns of decreased albumin and increased α_2-globulin are seen in protein-losing enteropathy, when plasma proteins are lost through a large inflamed area in the intestine, and in extensive burns, when plasma proteins seep through the denuded body surface.

Abnormalities in the concentrations of minor plasma proteins cannot be divined from the elec-

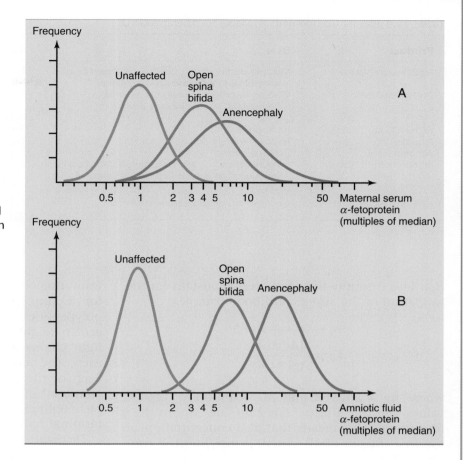

Figure 15.8 The use of α-fetoprotein in amniotic fluid for the diagnosis of neural tube defects in the fetus. Maternal serum can be screened for α-fetoprotein **(A)**, and suspect results are followed up by amniocentesis **(B).**

trophoretic pattern and have to be determined by radioimmunoassay (RIA) (see Chapter 16) or other sensitive methods. **α-Fetoprotein,** for example, is synthesized in the fetal liver but occurs in only trace amounts in normal adult blood. *Its levels are increased in most patients with hepatocellular carcinoma.*

α-*Fetoprotein is also used for the prenatal diagnosis of open neural tube defects.* In these severe malformations, it leaks from the fetal blood into amniotic fluid and even into the maternal blood (Fig. 15.8).

Blood Components Are Used for Transfusions

Blood transfusions necessitate blood group matching, and there is a risk of transmitting acquired immunodeficiency syndrome (AIDS), hepatitis, and other diseases. Also, not every patient requires the same blood component. An anemic patient needs red blood cells, a patient with nephrotic syndrome benefits from albumin, and a patient with a clotting disorder needs clotting factors.

Table 15.4 lists some of the most important plasma products and their uses. Not only plasma products but also red blood cells, platelets, and granulocytes are, of course, available in modern medicine.

Immunoglobulins Bind Antigens Very Selectively

The immunoglobulins make up approximately 20% of the total plasma protein. Most move in the γ-globulin region during electrophoresis, but there are immunoglobulins under the β and α₂ peaks as well.

The immunoglobulins function as **antibodies** that bind tightly to **antigens.** An antigen is, by definition, any molecule that induces the formation of a matching antibody. An antigen must fulfill two requirements:

- *It has to be large,* ideally with a molecular weight of more than 10,000 D.
- *It has to be a foreign molecule.* Except in autoimmune diseases, humans do not form antibodies to components of their own bodies.

The antigen-antibody complex is formed only by non-covalent interactions. This means that antigen-antibody binding is reversible. The tightness of binding is described by the **affinity constant**

Table 15.4 Plasma Components Available for Therapeutic Use

Product	Uses	Comments
Fresh-frozen plasma	Multiple clotting factor deficiencies, liver cirrhosis, disseminated intravascular coagulation	Danger of disease transmission
Cryoprecipitate	Clotting disorders: hypofibrinogenemia, hemophilia, von Willebrand disease	Produced by freezing and thawing of plasma; enriched in fibrinogen, factor VIII, and fibronectin
Factor VIII concentrate	Hemophilia A	Some danger of hepatitis transmission
Albumin 5%	Hypovolemic shock	No danger of hepatitis or AIDS transmission; no blood group antibodies present
Albumin 25%	Cerebral edema	
Immune serum globulin	Immunodeficiency states affecting B cells; passive immunization against hepatitis, tetanus, etc.	For IV or IM injection

AIDS, acquired immunodeficiency syndrome; IM, intramuscular; IV, intravenous.

K_{aff}. This is simply the equilibrium constant for the formation of the antigen-antibody complex:

$$Ag + Ab \rightleftharpoons Ag \cdot Ab$$

$$K_d = \frac{[Ag \cdot Ab]}{[Ag] \times [Ab]}$$

where Ag = antigen and Ab = antibody. Typical values for the affinity constant are 10^7 to 10^{11} liters/mole. This means that at a concentration of the free antigen of 10^{-7} to 10^{-11} mol/liter the concentration of the antigen-antibody complex equals that of the free antibody.

The formation of the antigen-antibody complex is the first step in the elimination of the antigen. Antigen-antibody complexes can undergo endocytosis by reticuloendothelial cells, and antibodies on the surface of a bacterium or a virus are a powerful stimulus for phagocytic cells. The stimulation of phagocytosis is called **opsonization.**

Antibody-labeled cells can also be destroyed by the **complement system,** which consists of soluble plasma proteins. The first component of the complement system binds to the antigen-antibody complex on the cell surface. This triggers a proteolytic cascade and, eventually, formation of a cytolytic complex that creates a gap junction ("drills a hole") in the membrane.

The most astounding property of antibodies is their diversity. *Every person has at least 1 million structurally different antibodies, each with its own unique antigen-binding specificity.* This diversity enables the body to recognize and eliminate almost any imaginable antigen.

Antibodies Consist of Two Light Chains and Two Heavy Chains

Despite their diverse antigen-binding specificities, all antibodies have the same general structure.

Immunoglobulins of the G1 class (IgG1) (Fig. 15.9), for example, consist of four disulfide-bonded polypeptides: two identical heavy chains with molecular weights of 53,000 D each and two identical light chains with molecular weights of 23,000 D each. The molecule has the shape of the letter Y. Each of the two arms of the Y is formed by the amino-terminal half of a heavy chain and a complete light chain. The stem consists of the carboxyl-terminal halves of the two heavy chains.

The light chain has two globular domains, and the heavy chain has four. All domains have a similar higher order structure, with approximately 110 amino acid residues folded into two blanket-like antiparallel β-pleated sheets (Fig. 15.10). The two "blankets" are held together by a disulfide bond.

The heavy chain also contains a less compact **hinge region** between the second and third domains, in which disulfide bonds are formed between the two heavy chains.

The second, third, and fourth domains of the heavy chains are the same in all IgG1 molecules. These are the **constant domains,** and they define the γ_1 **chain.** The second domain of the light chain is also constant, but there are two types: the κ (**kappa**) and λ (**lambda**) light chains. *Each immunoglobulin molecule has either two κ chains or two λ chains but never one of each.*

Only the amino-terminal domains of both the heavy and the light chains are variable. If a very skilled biochemist could isolate hundreds of IgG1 molecules and determine their amino acid sequences individually, she would rarely ever find two molecules with exactly the same amino acid sequence in the variable domains. Most of the variability is concentrated in **hypervariable regions.** There are three hypervariable regions in the variable domain of the light chain and either three or four in the variable domain of the heavy chain. They are the major sites of contact with the antigen.

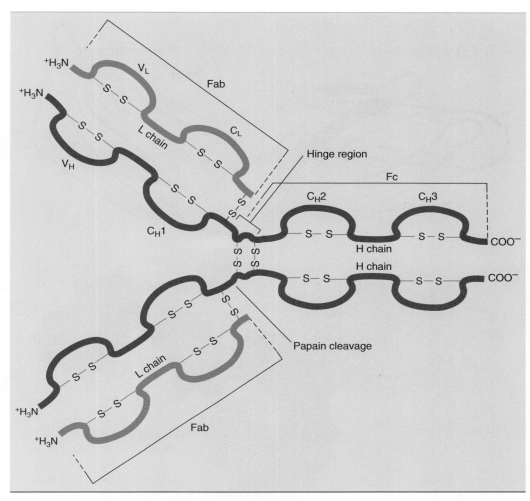

Figure 15.9 Structure of human immunoglobulin G1 (IgG1). Each domain (V_L and C_L in the light [L] chains; V_H, C_H1, C_H2, and C_H3 in the heavy [H] chains) is a globular portion of the molecule, stabilized by an intrachain disulfide bond. Fab, antigen-binding fragment; Fc, crystallizable fragment.

The important properties of the immunoglobulins include *antigen binding* and *effector functions.* Effector functions are the events that are triggered by antigen binding: for example, complement activation, opsonization, and the induction of histamine release from mast cells.

The allocation of these functions to different regions of the molecule has been possible by partial proteolysis. Papain, a protease from the latex of the papaya plant, cleaves a single peptide bond in the hinge region of IgG1. This generates two types of fragments: two identical **antigen binding (F_{ab}) fragments,** containing a complete light chain and the amino-terminal half of a heavy chain, and one **crystallizable (F_c) fragment,** consisting of the carboxyl-terminal halves of the two heavy chains. *The F_{ab} fragment binds the antigen, and the F_c fragment is in charge of the effector functions.*

There are two antigen-binding regions in the immunoglobulin molecule, each consisting of the variable domain of a light chain and the variable domain of a heavy chain. This facilitates the formation of large insoluble aggregates of interconnected antigen and antibody molecules. Therefore, *the reaction between a soluble antigen and an antibody results in **precipitation.*** Precipitation works best with equimolar concentrations of antigen and antibody (Fig. 15.11).

When the antigen is on a cell surface, the two antigen-binding sites can combine with antigen on different cells, effectively gluing the cells together. This is called **agglutination.** It can be observed when blood cells are mixed with an antiserum to a blood group antigen.

Different Immunoglobulin Classes Have Different Properties

There are five major classes of heavy chains which define the class of the immunoglobulin: immunoglobulin G (IgG) has γ chains; immunoglobulin M

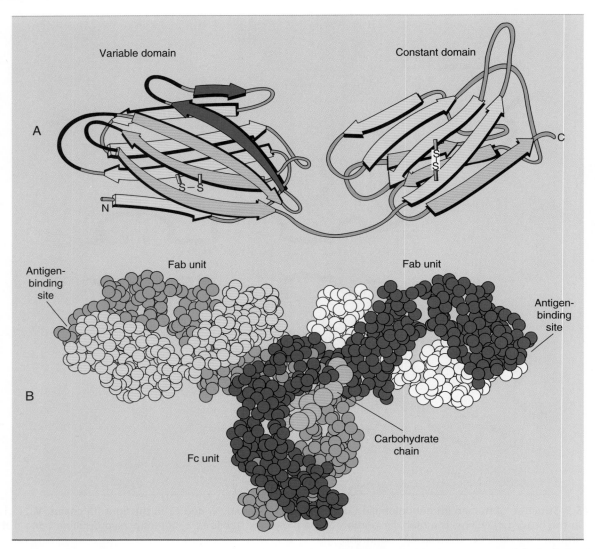

Figure 15.10 The three-dimensional structure of immunoglobulins. **A,** Ribbon model of an immunoglobulin light chain. Each domain contains two "blankets" formed from antiparallel β-pleated sheets (⇨ and ⇾). The interfaces of the two blankets are formed by hydrophobic amino acid side chains, and the structure is reinforced by a single disulfide bond. The variable domain contains two additional β-pleated sheet sequences not present in the constant domain (⇨). The antigen binds to three loops (━) that are formed by the hypervariable regions. **B,** The three-dimensional structure of an immunoglobulin G molecule. In this immunoglobulin class, *N*-linked oligosaccharides participate in the interactions between the heavy chains.

(IgM), μ chains; immunoglobulin A (IgA), α chains; immunoglobulin D (IgD), δ chains; and immunoglobulin E (IgE), ε chains. IgG has four subclasses containing four slightly different γ chains with about 95% sequence homology in the constant domains, and IgA has two subclasses. Figure 15.12 and Table 15.5 summarize the features of the immunoglobulin classes and subclasses.

Some immunoglobulins occur in oligomeric forms. These oligomers contain a small polypeptide known as the **J chain,** and they are stabilized by disulfide bonds. Figure 15.13 shows the structure of **IgM,** which occurs in a pentameric form in the serum.

IgA is the most abundant immunoglobulin in external secretions, including tears, saliva, bronchial mucus, intestinal and genitourinary secretions, and milk. Secretory IgA is synthesized in submucosal lymphatic tissues, including the tonsils in the throat and Peyer's patches in the intestine. It is secreted as a dimer, with a J chain and a noncovalently bound **secretory component.** The secre-

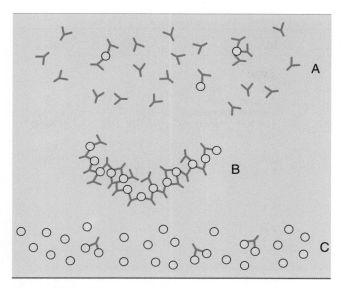

Figure 15.11 Formation of antigen-antibody complexes.
A, Antibody excess: small complexes, no precipitation.
B, Equivalence zone: large complexes, precipitation.
C, Antigen excess: small complexes, no precipitation.

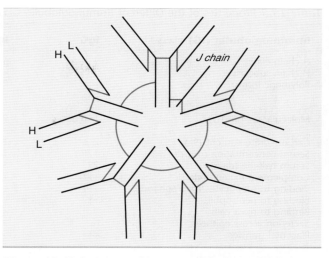

Figure 15.13 Structure of immunoglobulin M (IgM), which is present as a pentamer of molecular weight 900,000 D in the serum. IgM on the surface of B cells, however, is present in a monomeric form. H, heavy chain; L, light chain. —, Disulfide bonds.

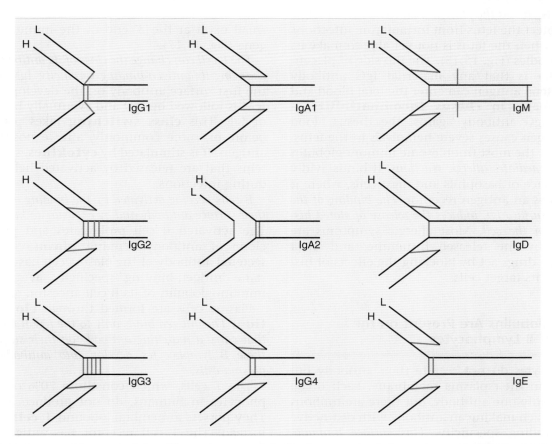

Figure 15.12 Structural features of the different immunoglobulin classes and subclasses. Immunoglobulins M (IgM) and E (IgE) have four rather than three constant domains. Note the variability in the locations of the interchain disulfide bonds. H, heavy chain; IgA, IgD, and IgG, immunoglobulins A, D, and G; L, light chain. —, Disulfide bonds.

Table 15.5 Properties of the Different Immunoglobulin Classes

Immunoglobulin (IG) class	IgG	IgM	IgA	IgD	IgE
H chain class	γ	μ	α	δ	ε
H chain subclasses	γ₁, γ₂, γ₃, γ₄	—	α₁, α₂	—	—
Polymeric forms	—	Pentamer	Monomer, dimer, or trimer (serum), dimer (secreted)	—	—
Molecular weight (D)	150,000	950,000	180,000 (monomer) 400,000 (secreted)	180,000	190,000
Carbohydrate content (%)	2-3	12	7-11	9-14	12
Serum concentration (mg/dL)	1200	120	200	3	0.005
Serum half-life (days)	21	5	6	3	2
Complement fixation (classic)	++*	+++	−	−	−
Binding to monocytes/macrophages	++†	+	−	−	+
Binding to neutrophils	+‡	—	++	−	−
Binding to mast cells	−	−	−	−	+++
Secretion across epithelia	−	−	+++	−	−
Placental transfer	+++	−	−	−	−

Binding to monocytes/macrophages and neutrophils is important for the stimulation of phagocytosis, and binding to mast cells is important for the stimulation of histamine release during allergic responses.
* Except IgG4.
† Except IgG2.
‡ IgG1 and IgG3 only.

tory component is derived from the membrane receptor that triggers transcytosis of the IgA across the mucosa (Fig. 15.14).

*Only **IgG** crosses the placental barrier.* Maternal IgG has to protect the fetus from intrauterine infections at a time when the fetus is not yet able to make its own antibodies (Fig. 15.15). The flip side of placental transfer is that any maternal IgG antibody against a fetal antigen can enter the fetal blood and cause damage. In **rhesus incompatibility,** a maternal IgG antibody against the rhesus blood group antigen causes severe hemolysis in the fetus.

However, the most troublesome immunoglobulin is IgE. *IgE mediates allergic reactions.* It binds avidly to the surface of basophils and mast cells, where it functions as an antigen receptor. *The binding of the antigen to surface IgE induces the release of stored histamine from the cell.* Most allergic symptoms are mediated by the released histamine, and most antiallergic drugs act by blocking the effects of histamine on its target cells.

Immunoglobulins Are Present on the Surface of B Lymphocytes

B lymphocytes do not secrete their antibody but deposit it in their plasma membrane. Each B cell produces only one antibody, but there are millions of B cells, each making an antibody with distinctive antigen-binding specificity. *This surface immunoglobulin makes the B cell responsive to antigen, much as a hormone receptor makes a cell responsive to a hormone* (Fig. 15.16).

The membrane-bound antibody contains a transmembrane helix near the C-terminus of the heavy chain that is missing in the secreted antibody. This structural feature results from the optional use of a small exon at the 3′ end of the immunoglobulin gene (Fig. 15.17).

The B cell can change the class of its antibody without changing its antigen-binding specificity. IgM is always the first surface antibody on the developing B cell. IgM is followed by IgD and eventually by IgG, IgA, or IgE. This **class switching** takes place either before or, more commonly, after exposure to the antigen. It is stimulated by **cytokines,** soluble proteins that are released by activated helper T cells during infections.

B cells become activated by the binding of antigen to their surface antibody and by exposure to helper T cells. The activated B cell proliferates and produces a clone of antibody-secreting **plasma cells.** The secreted antibody of the plasma cell has exactly the same antigen-binding specificity as the surface immunoglobulin of its B cell ancestor.

Plasma cells are formed through **clonal selection:** *The antigen binds only to the few B lymphocytes that carry a matching antibody on their surface. Only these B lymphocytes develop into antibody-secreting plasma cells.*

The T cells, which constitute 70% of the lymphocytes in humans, do not produce antibodies. They possess a membrane-bound **T cell receptor** instead. The T cell receptor has antigen-binding domains and is functionally equivalent to the surface antibodies of B cells. *Only B lymphocytes and T lymphocytes possess antigen receptors on their surface*

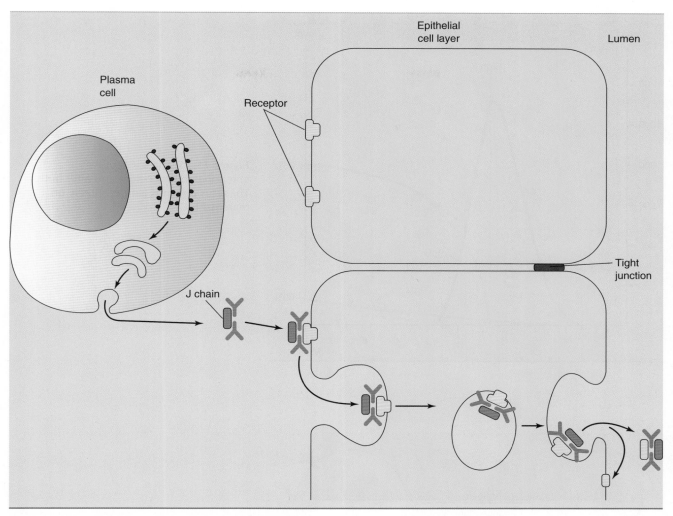

Figure 15.14 Synthesis of secretory immunoglobulin A (IgA). The dimeric form of IgA, which is derived from plasma cells in submucosal lymphatic tissue, is transported across the epithelial cell by transcytosis after binding to a cell surface receptor. On the luminal surface, the extracellular domain of the receptor is cleaved from the membrane-spanning domain and remains bound to the secreted IgA as the "secretory component."

that enable them to respond specifically to a matching antigen.

The Immunoglobulin Genes Are Rearranged during B Cell Development

How can humans make millions of different antibodies although they have only 30,000 genes in their genome? This task is not as formidable as it seems because the antigen-binding site is formed by two polypeptides. In theory, 1000 different heavy chains and 1000 different light chains, encoded by a total of 2000 genes, would be sufficient to make one million different antibodies.

The immunoglobulin chains are encoded by three separate gene clusters: one for κ light chains (on chromosome 2), one for λ light chains (on chro-

mosome 22), and one for heavy chains (on chromosome 14). *Each gene cluster contains separate genes for the variable and constant domains.* During B cell development, *these separate genes have to be combined into a single transcription unit that codes for a complete light chain or heavy chain.*

Figure 15.18 shows the gene cluster for the κ light chain. A single gene codes for the constant domain, which starts with amino acid 109. Amino acids 1 to 95 of the variable domain are encoded by a **variable (V) gene,** and amino acids 96 to 108 are encoded by a tiny **joining (J) gene.** The germline contains a library of 5 J genes and about 50 V genes.

During B cell development, *one of the V genes is selected at random from the library of V genes and spliced to one of the J genes.* This forms a complete variable domain gene that is transcribed along with the constant domain gene. The sequence

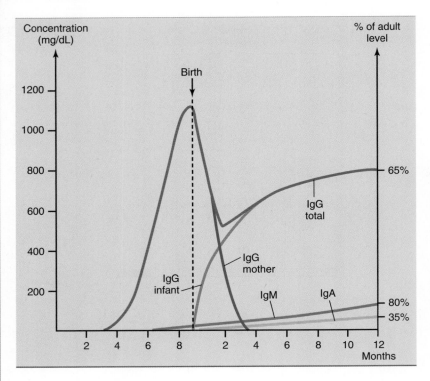

Figure 15.15 The levels of immunoglobulins before and after birth. The fetus depends almost entirely on maternal IgG.

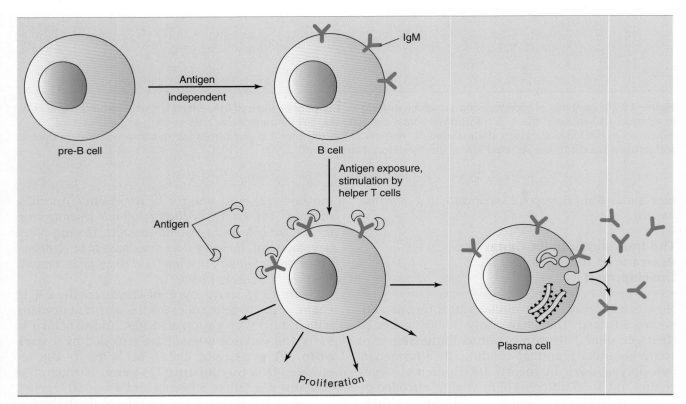

Figure 15.16 Differentiation of a B lymphocyte. Class switching can occur either before or after antigen exposure. IgM, immunoglobulin M.

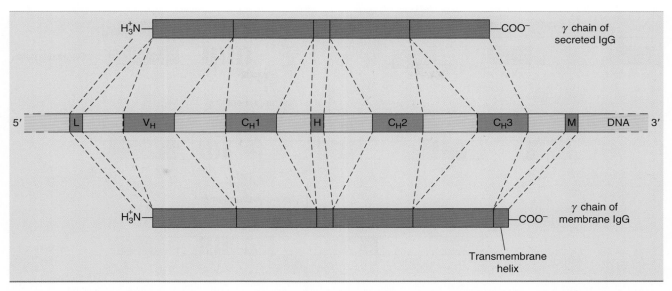

Figure 15.17 The intron-exon structure of a γ chain gene is shown schematically. The signal sequence, the four domains, and the hinge region are encoded by separate exons. The exon for the membrane attachment region (M) is included in membrane-bound immunoglobulin G (IgG) but not in secreted IgG. Exon L (for leader) encodes the signal sequence.

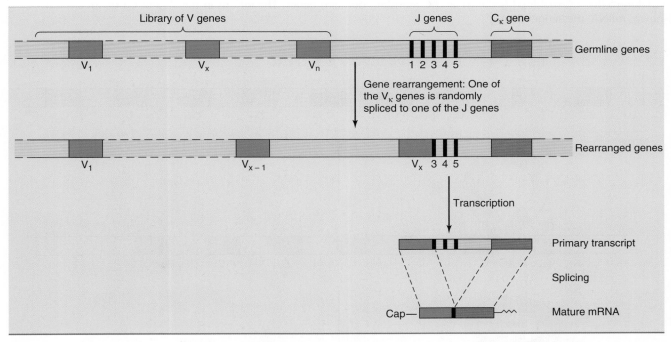

Figure 15.18 Rearrangement and expression of the κ light chain genes. The gene rearrangement takes place early in the development of B lymphocytes, before any antigen exposure. During the gene rearrangement, the intervening DNA (in this case, the DNA between genes V_x and J3) is deleted. mRNA, messenger RNA.

between the J gene and the constant domain gene is treated as an intron and spliced out of the primary transcript.

The heavy chain genes are assembled the same way, but the heavy chain gene cluster contains a set of approximately 30 **diversity (D) genes** in addition to the V, J, and C_H genes (Fig. 15.19). During class switching, the complete variable domain gene (V + D + J) is successively joined to different constant domain genes (Fig. 15.20). This produces antibodies with the same variable domains, but different constant domains.

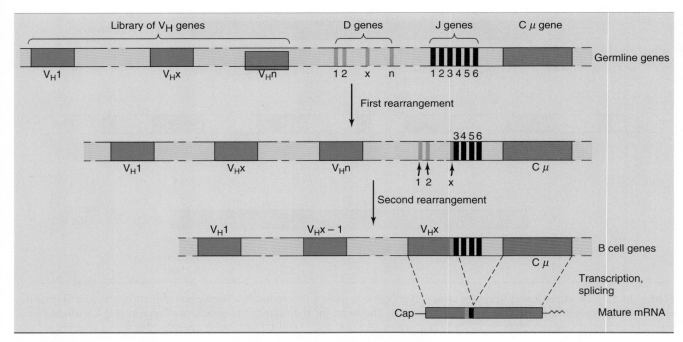

Figure 15.19 Rearrangements of heavy chain genes in developing B lymphocytes. The process is similar to the rearrangement of κ light chains shown in Figure 15.18, but an additional small gene, the D (diversity) gene, contributes in addition to the V (variable), J (joining), and C (constant domain) genes. The introns in the V$_H$ and Cμ genes are not shown. mRNA, messenger RNA.

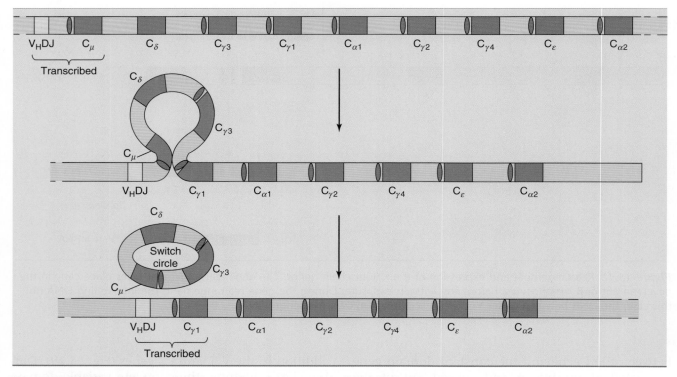

Figure 15.20 Class switching, in this case from immunoglobulin M (μ chain) to immunoglobulin G1 (γ$_1$ chain). Class switching takes place after the rearrangements shown in Figures 15.18 and 15.19. It can be triggered by cytokines that are released from activated T lymphocytes, and it can occur either before or after antigen exposure. The intervening genes (in this case, μ, δ, and γ$_3$) are released as a cyclic product known as a "switch circle." Each gene is preceded by a switch region (•). Recombination takes place between the switch regions of two C$_H$ genes.

Monoclonal Gammopathies Are Neoplastic Diseases of Plasma Cells

Broad elevations of γ-globulins **(polyclonal gammopathy)** are seen in infectious diseases and also in many other chronic diseases, whereas reductions are typical for inherited immune deficiency.

Monoclonal gammopathy can be traced to the abnormal proliferation of a single plasma cell. The descendants of this out-of-control cell all produce the same antibody. This antibody forms a sharp **"paraprotein"** peak in the γ-globulin fraction or, less commonly, in the β- or $α_2$-globulin fraction (see Fig. 15.7F).

Multiple myeloma is a malignant disease with an overproduced IgG, IgA, or IgD antibody. In some patients, the malignant cells overproduce not a complete immunoglobulin but loose κ or λ light chains that are eventually excreted in the urine. These overproduced light chains are known as **Bence Jones protein.** The malignant plasma cells thrive in the bone marrow, where they cause bone pain and abnormal fractures.

Waldenstrom macroglobulinemia is a malignant disease in which *an IgM antibody is overproduced.* Because of its high molecular weight of 900,000 D, this IgM antibody causes a dangerous increase of the blood viscosity.

In **benign monoclonal gammopathy,** a paraprotein is present but there are no signs of malignant disease. *It is very common in the geriatric age group.* The evaluation of monoclonal gammopathies is one of the most common indications for plasma protein electrophoresis in the clinical laboratory.

Blood Clotting Must Be Tightly Controlled

Blood clotting is essential to prevent excessive blood loss after injuries, but it is not without danger. Inappropriate clotting in an intact blood vessel produces a **thrombus** that can cause vascular occlusion and tissue infarction. Therefore, clotting must be tightly controlled to prevent death from thrombosis as well as death from uncontrolled bleeding. These are the major characters in the drama of blood coagulation:

1. **Endothelial cells** inhibit blood clotting. Their surface is not conducive to platelet adhesion; some of the proteins and heparan sulfate proteoglycans in their membrane inhibit the clotting cascade; and they form prostacyclin, an inhibitor of platelet adhesion and aggregation.

2. **Subendothelial tissues** contain membrane proteins and extracellular matrix proteins that are not normally in contact with the blood. Platelets and clotting factors bind to these proteins when the endothelium is damaged. This helps in the activation of platelets and clotting factors.

3. **Platelets** release proteins and vasoactive amines after binding to exposed subendothelial tissue. Clotting factors become activated on the surface of these activated platelets.

4. **Clotting factors** are plasma proteins that form a proteolytic cascade, activating each other by selective proteolytic cleavage. This cascade ends with the formation of insoluble fibrin from soluble fibrinogen. The clotting factors are designated by Roman numerals. The subscript letter "a" denotes the proteolytically activated form of the clotting factor.

Platelets Adhere to Exposed Subendothelial Tissue

Platelets adhere to the exposed extracellular matrix whenever the endothelial lining of a blood vessel is destroyed. Platelet adhesion is mediated by **von Willebrand factor (vWF),** a protein that is present both in the plasma and the extracellular matrix. vWF binds both to a receptor on the platelet membrane and to collagen fibers in the tissue (Fig. 15.21).

Platelet activation invariably occurs in the adherent platelets. It is stimulated by agents that increase the calcium concentration in platelets, including thrombin and thromboxane.

Activated (but not resting) platelets release a wealth of chemicals: ADP; ATP; 5-hydroxytryptamine; calcium; and various proteins, including fibrinogen, vWF, factor V, factor XIII, platelet-derived growth factor (PDGF), and platelet factor 4. The released clotting factors contribute to the formation of the fibrin clot, PDGF helps in wound healing, and platelet factor 4 prevents the formation of an active thrombin inhibitor from heparin and antithrombin III (see later discussion).

During activation, a receptor for fibrinogen becomes exposed on the platelet membrane. *Fibrinogen binds to this receptor and glues the platelets together.* This process is called **platelet aggregation.**

Even the membrane lipids become rearranged during platelet activation. Phosphatidyl serine, in particular, which is normally concentrated in the inner leaflet of the plasma membrane, flip-flops to the outer leaflet, where it helps in the binding of prothrombin and other clotting factors.

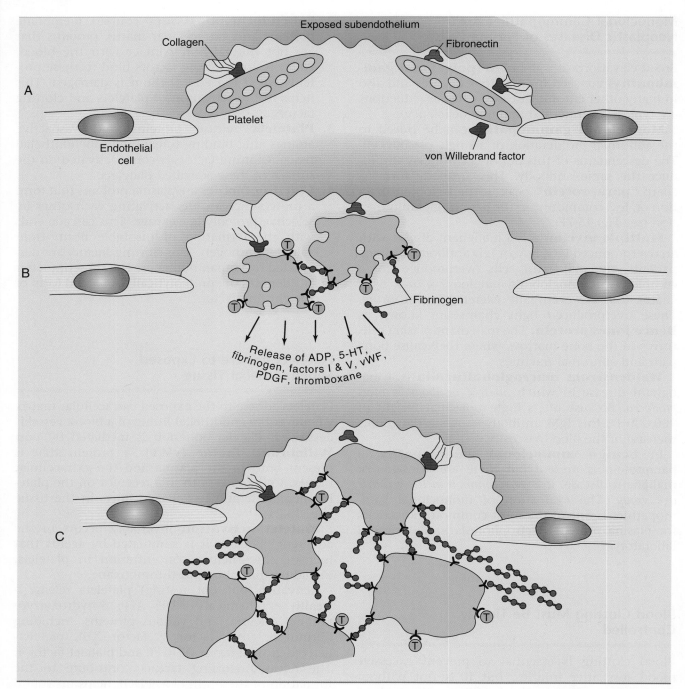

Figure 15.21 Formation of the platelet plug. **A,** Platelets adhere to exposed subendothelium. The binding is mediated by von Willebrand factor (vWF), but direct binding to tissue fibronectin or other tissue components may be important as well. **B,** Platelets become activated after binding to the subendothelial tissue and exposure to thrombin (T), resulting in shape change and degranulation. Functional fibrinogen receptors are assembled on the cell surface. **C,** Continued thrombin exposure, together with some of the released mediators (ADP, thromboxane), activates more and more platelets. The platelets are glued together by fibrinogen, and the platelet plug forms. The action of thrombin on fibrinogen forms insoluble fibrin, and the platelets become enmeshed in the fibrin clot. ADP, adenosine diphosphate; 5-HT, 5-hydroxytryptamine; PDGF, platelet-derived growth factor.

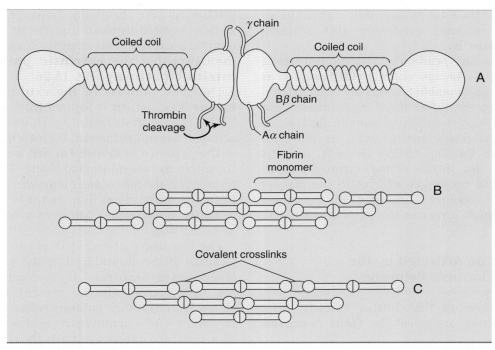

Figure 15.22 Structure of fibrinogen. **A,** Schematic representation of fibrinogen. The coiled coil regions, each 150 to 160 nm in length, are formed by three α-helical portions of the Aα, Bβ, and γ chains. **B,** Aggregation of fibrin monomers. **C,** Transglutaminase (factor XIII$_a$) strengthens the clot by forming covalent crosslinks.

The importance of the platelet plug is shown by the observation that *patients with unusually low platelet counts (<40,000/μL) develop spontaneous hemorrhages.* Normal platelet counts range between 100,000 and 400,000/μL.

Insoluble Fibrin Is Formed from Soluble Fibrinogen

The platelet plug alone is sufficient to seal very small lesions, but larger injuries require the formation of a fibrin clot. **Fibrin** is not a constituent of normal blood, but its precursor **fibrinogen** is present at concentrations averaging 300 mg/dL. With a molecular weight of 340,000 D, it is larger than most plasma proteins, and it is more elongated, with dimensions of 9 × 45 nm. Its three polypeptides, designated Aα, Bβ, and γ, are present in two copies each. The overall structure of fibrinogen is shown in Figure 15.22.

*The protease **thrombin** converts fibrinogen to fibrin.* Thrombin cleaves two peptide bonds near the amino termini of the Aα and Bβ chains, releasing two small peptides: fibrinopeptides A (20 amino acids) and B (18 amino acids). The remaining protein is called a **fibrin monomer.** Once formed, the fibrin monomers aggregate into fibrous structures.

Fibrinogen is more soluble than fibrin because the fibrinopeptides are studded with negative charges on aspartate and glutamate side chains. These negative charges keep fibrinogen molecules apart and prevent the formation of fibrous aggregates.

Although insoluble, the fibrin monomers form only a soft gel rather than a solid clot. For structural strength, *fibrin requires covalent crosslinking.* Crosslinking is catalyzed by the enzyme **transglutaminase** (also known as **clotting factor XIII$_a$**), which links glutamine and lysine side chains in fibrin (Fig. 15.23).

Thrombin Is Derived from Prothrombin

Thrombin converts fibrinogen into fibrin. Because fibrin must never be formed in an intact blood vessel, *thrombin formation must be restricted to the site of the injury.* Indeed, active thrombin is formed from its inactive precursor **prothrombin** by the protease **factor X$_a$** (Fig. 15.24). The reaction produces thrombin (308 amino acids) and a catalytically inactive amino-terminal fragment of 274 amino acids.

This amino-terminal fragment contains 10 residues of **γ-carboxyglutamate**. This nonstandard amino acid is formed during the processing of prothrombin in the endoplasmic reticulum of hepatocytes. The enzyme catalyzing this reaction requires **vitamin K.**

Unlike glutamate, γ-carboxyglutamate is a strong calcium chelator. *Through γ-carboxyglutamate and its bound calcium, prothrombin becomes anchored to phosphatidyl serine on the surface of activated platelets.* Also factor X_a contains γ-carboxyglutamate and binds to activated platelets, along with its activator protein **factor Va** (Fig. 15.25). *Factor X_a activates prothrombin on the surface of the activated platelet.* Active thrombin no longer adheres to the platelet lipids, but it becomes enmeshed in the fibrin network, in which it retains its enzymatic activity.

Factor X Can Be Activated by the Extrinsic and Intrinsic Pathways

The last reactions of the clotting cascade, from factor X_a to fibrin, are called the **final common pathway.** Like thrombin, however, factor X_a has to be generated from an inactive precursor by proteolytic cleavage. This activation can be achieved through either the **extrinsic pathway** or the **intrinsic pathway** (Fig. 15.26).

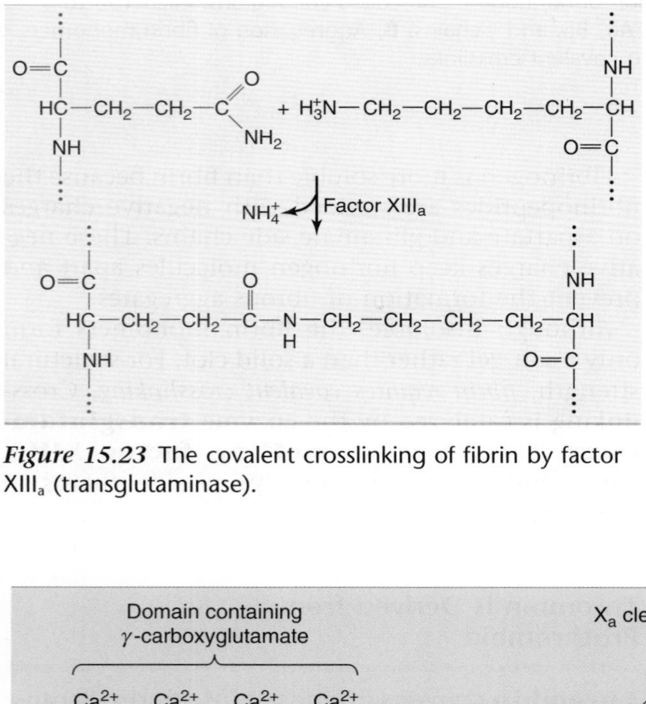

The only protease of the extrinsic pathway is **factor VII_a,** which is formed from inactive factor VII by thrombin or factor X_a. However, proteolytic activation is not sufficient. Factor VII_a is active only in the presence of **tissue factor,** a membrane glycoprotein in subendothelial tissue. *Tissue factor and factor VII come into contact only after vascular injury.* In the presence of calcium, factor VII quickly binds to tissue factor, either before or after its activation to factor VII_a.

The intrinsic pathway derives its name from the fact that it can be induced in the test tube in the absence of an "extrinsic" tissue component, requiring only factors already present in the blood. However, *the intrinsic pathway becomes activated only on contact with a negatively charged surface.* The glass of a test tube offers a negatively charged surface, and so does the exposed extracellular matrix in the body.

The initiating reactions of the intrinsic pathway are known as **contact-phase activation.** They require the two proteases, **kallikrein** and **factor XII_a,** which activate each other on the exposed extracellular matrix. Also, the activator protein **high–molecular weight kininogen (HMWK)** is required.

Factor XII_a activates factor XI, factor XI_a activates factor IX, and factor IX_a activates factor X. This last reaction requires the activator protein **factor VIII_a.**

γ-Carboxyglutamate is present not only in prothrombin and factor X but also in factors VII and IX. Therefore, all these clotting factors are targeted to activated platelets. This design keeps clotting

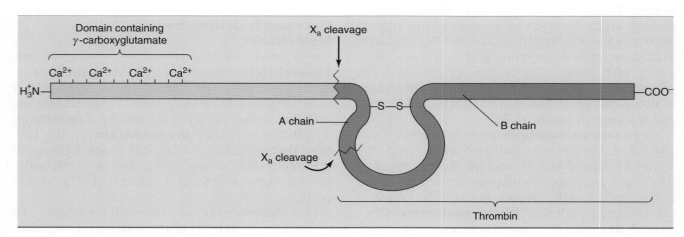

Figure 15.23 The covalent crosslinking of fibrin by factor XIII_a (transglutaminase).

Figure 15.24 Structure of prothrombin.

highly localized. *The initiating reactions are triggered by components of the exposed subendothelial tissue, and the final steps require activated platelets.*

Negative Controls Are Necessary to Prevent Thrombosis

Figure 15.26 shows that the clotting cascade has several elements of *positive feedback:* kallikrein and factor XII_a activate each other, factor XI_a acts on its own precursor to produce more XI_a, and thrombin activates several clotting factors (V, VII, VIII, XI) in the earlier steps of the cascade. These positive feedback loops permit a quick response to injury, but without inhibitory controls, the process would progress until all blood vessels were filled with solid fibrin.

Protease inhibitors provide negative controls by inactivating clotting factors that have escaped from the site of injury. Most clotting factors can be inactivated by the nonselective protease inhibitors α_1-antiprotease and α_2-macroglobulin. More important is **antithrombin III** (Fig. 15.27), which is present at a concentration of approximately 15 mg/dL in the plasma.

Antithrombin III is stimulated by the glycosaminoglycan **heparin.** A specific positioning of sulfate groups on the polysaccharide chains of heparin is necessary for antithrombin III activation. This required structure is present in about 30% of all heparin molecules and also in a small proportion of the heparan sulfate chains on the surface of endothelial cells. *It is therefore likely that the action of antithrombin III is facilitated by contact with intact endothelial cells in vivo.* Most proteases of the intrinsic and final common pathway are inhibited by heparin/antithrombin III (Table 15.6).

A different anticoagulant mechanism is employed by **thrombomodulin** (Fig. 15.28), a protein on the surface of endothelial cells that binds circulating thrombin. Once bound to thrombomodulin, thrombin is no longer able to act on fibrinogen, factor VIII, factor V, or factor XIII. It activates **protein C** instead. The activated form of this protease acts as a powerful anticoagulant by degrading factors V_a and VIII_a. Because thrombomodulin is present only on intact endothelium, *this*

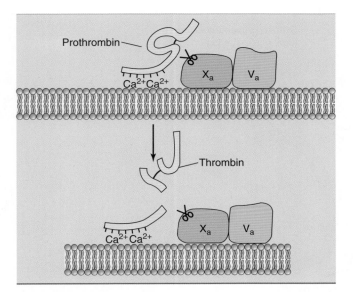

Figure 15.25 Activation of prothrombin by factor X_a on the surface of the platelet membrane. The membrane phospholipids facilitate the reaction by bringing prothrombin and factor X_a together on the surface of the lipid bilayer, and factor V_a enhances the catalytic activity of factor X_a.

Table 15.6 Properties of the Blood Clotting Factors

Factor	Functions in	Protease Precursor	Molecular Weight (D)	Plasma Concentration (mg/dL)	Vitamin K– Dependent	Heparin Inhibited	Activated by
Fibrinogen (I)	Common pathway	No	330,000	150-400	No	No	Thrombin
Prothrombin (II)	Common pathway	Yes	72,000	8-9	Yes	Yes	X_a
V	Common pathway	No	330,000		No	No	Thrombin
X	Common pathway	Yes	59,000	0.6	Yes	Yes	IX_a, VII_a
XIII	Common pathway	No*	320,000		No	No	Thrombin
VII	Extrinsic pathway	Yes	50,000	0.05	Yes	No	Thrombin, X_a
VIII	Intrinsic pathway	No	330,000	0.02	No	No	Thrombin,
IX	Intrinsic pathway	Yes	57,000	0.4	Yes	Yes	XI_a, VII_a
XI	Intrinsic pathway	Yes	160,000	0.5	No	Yes	Thrombin, XI_a, XII_a
XII	Intrinsic pathway	Yes	76,000	3	No	Yes	Kallikrein
Prekallikrein	Intrinsic pathway	Yes	82,000	4	No	No	XII_a
High-molecular-weight kininogen	Intrinsic pathway	No	108,000	7-10	No	No	—

* Yields a fibrin-crosslinking enzyme.

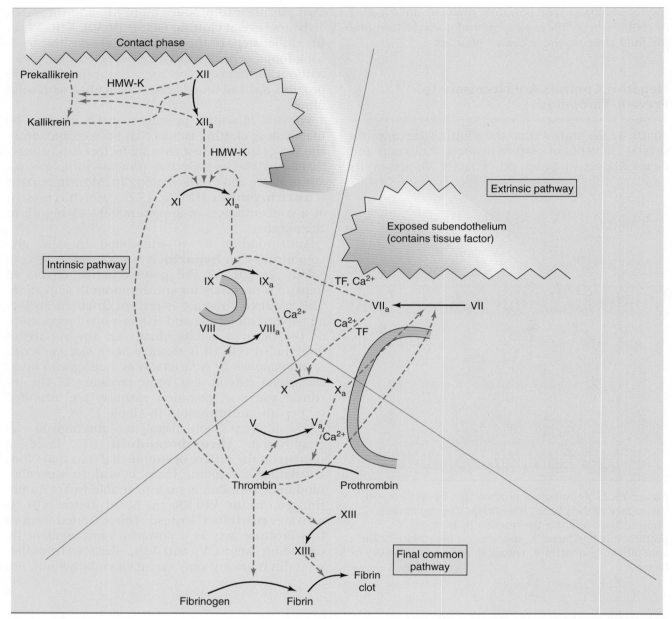

Figure 15.26 The blood clotting system. *Dashed arrows* indicate proteolytic activation. B, surface of activated platelets; HMWK, high–molecular weight kininogen; TF, tissue factor.

mechanism prevents the encroachment of clot formation on areas with an intact endothelial lining.

Some patients with thrombotic disorders have inherited deficiencies of anticoagulant proteins. Deficiencies of antithrombin III and protein C have been observed repeatedly. They cause thrombotic disease even in heterozygotes, who still possess 50% of the normal amount of the affected protein.

Plasmin Degrades the Fibrin Clot

A blood clot is an ephemeral structure that has to be removed during wound healing. The major enzyme of fibrin degradation is the protease **plasmin.** Its inactive precursor **plasminogen,** which circulates in the plasma in a concentration of 10 to 20 mg/dL, binds with high affinity to the fibrin clot. This fibrin-bound plasminogen can be activated by **tissue-type plasminogen activator (tPA),** a serine protease that also binds avidly to fibrin. tPA does not require proteolytic activation, but its activity is minimal in the absence of fibrin. Therefore, *active plasmin is formed only in the fibrin clot where it is needed* (Fig. 15.29).

Plasminogen can also be activated by **urokinase,** a kidney-derived protein that is present in normal urine. **Streptokinase** is a bacterial

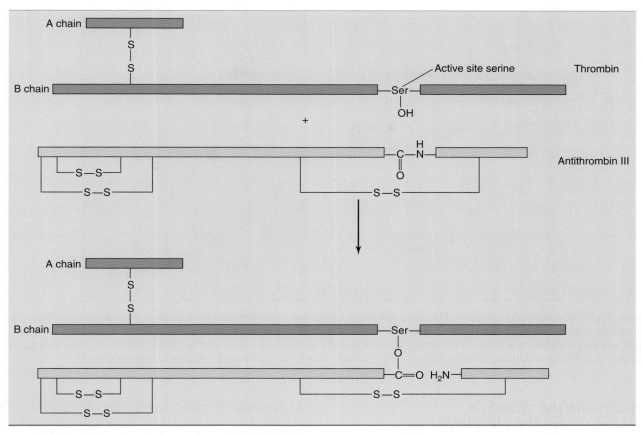

Figure 15.27 Proposed mechanism for the inhibition of thrombin by antithrombin III.

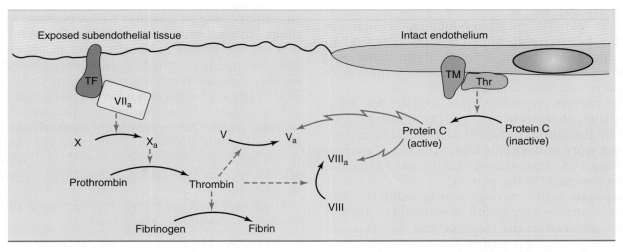

Figure 15.28 The roles of intact endothelium and exposed subendothelial tissue are evident when the effects of tissue factor and thrombomodulin are compared. Tissue factor triggers the clotting system through the extrinsic pathway (compare Fig. 15.26); thrombomodulin blocks the process. Thrombin, which is otherwise a "procoagulant," becomes effectively an "anticoagulant" after binding to thrombomodulin. *Dashed arrows* indicate proteolytic activation; *jagged arrows*, proteolytic inactivation. TF, tissue factor; Thr, thrombin; TM, thrombomodulin.

protein (from streptococci) that activates plasminogen allosterically, without making a proteolytic cleavage.

Streptokinase, urokinase, and tPA are used as thrombolytic agents. For example, most cases of acute myocardial infarction are caused by a thrombus formed on an atherosclerotic plaque in a coronary artery. In affected patients, thrombolytic therapy can limit the size of the infarction if it is administered within an hour after vascular occlusion, before the damage has become irreversible.

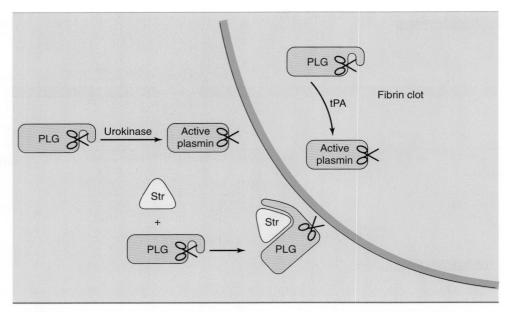

Figure 15.29 The fibrinolytic system. Plasminogen (PLG) is a circulating zymogen that binds to the fibrin clot. Tissue-type plasminogen activator (tPA) also binds to the clot, where it activates plasminogen by proteolytic cleavage, exposing its active site (✂). Urokinase activates circulating plasminogen by proteolysis, whereas the bacterial protein streptokinase (Str) activates plasminogen without proteolytic cleavage, by inducing a conformational change in the zymogen.

Heparin and the Vitamin K Antagonists Are the Most Important Anticoagulants

Blood clotting can be inhibited by the removal of calcium ions. All γ-carboxyglutamate containing clotting factors (prothrombin, VII, IX, X) depend on calcium. The catalytic activity of thrombin also requires calcium, although thrombin no longer contains γ-carboxyglutamate.

The calcium chelators citrate, oxalate, and ethylenediaminetetraacetic acid (EDTA) all can be used to inhibit clotting in the test tube, but this strategy cannot work in the living body. The blood calcium level must be constant, and a high dose of a calcium chelator would kill the patient.

Heparin, acting through antithrombin III, is an effective anticoagulant both in vivo and in vitro. It is not absorbed in the intestine and therefore not orally active, but *it is used as a short-acting injectable anticoagulant.*

Coumarin, warfarin, and **dicumarol** act by an entirely different mechanism. As competitive inhibitors of vitamin K, *they prevent the formation of γ-carboxyglutamate* during the post-translational processing of prothrombin and of factors VII, IX, and X in the endoplasmic reticulum of hepatocytes.

These drugs do not prevent clotting in the test tube. And because the vitamin K–dependent clotting factors have plasma half-lives of 1 to 5 days, several days of treatment are required before the old, normal clotting factors are replaced by the abnormal, uncarboxylated factors that are produced in the presence of the drug.

Coumarin-type anticoagulants are used not only for the long-term management of patients with thrombotic disease but also as rat poisons. These drugs have no immediate toxicity. Therefore, rats will eat the poison repeatedly until death ensues from internal hemorrhage. Poisons with immediate toxicity invariably cause a conditioned taste aversion in rats after a first exposure to a nonlethal dose.

The accidental ingestion of coumarin-based rat poisons should be treated with **menadione,** an injectable form of vitamin K. If abnormal clotting develops (as determined by the prothrombin time, see below), the transfusion of fresh-frozen plasma may be required.

The function of the blood clotting system can be assessed with various clotting tests:

1. **Bleeding time:** Bleeding time is measured after a standardized small skin prick lesion in fingertip or earlobe. *It is prolonged in platelet disorders.*
2. **Activated partial thromboplastin time:** Citrated plasma is treated with a combination of kaolin, a phospholipid preparation, and excess calcium. The kaolin activates the contact factors of the intrinsic pathway, and the phospholipid substitutes for platelet membranes. *This procedure tests the functioning of the intrinsic and final common pathways.* It can be used to monitor the heparin effect.

3. **Prothrombin time:** A tissue factor–containing extract from the brain or lungs is added to citrated plasma along with excess calcium. *The prothrombin time is prolonged in deficiencies of the extrinsic and final common pathways.* It is used routinely to monitor patients on treatment with coumarin-type anticoagulants.

Table 15.7 Plasma Half-Lives of Some Enzymes

Enzyme	t½ (Days)
Plasma cholinesterase*	12-14
Lactate dehydrogenase	6.8
Alanine transaminase	6.3
Aspartate transaminase	2.0
Creatine kinase	1.4

* This enzyme normally is secreted into the blood by the liver.

Clotting Factor Deficiencies Cause Abnormal Bleeding

Hemophilia A is an X-linked disease that affects nearly one in 12,000 boys and men. It is a serious bleeding disorder, caused by a *complete or near-complete deficiency of factor VIII,* one of the components of the intrinsic pathway (see Fig. 15.26).

Unlike patients with platelet disorders, hemophiliac patients are rarely plagued by spontaneous hemorrhages. Their problem is prolonged bleeding from small wounds. Repeated bleeding into joints is also common, and this can lead to arthritis in later life. Bleeding episodes can be treated with cryoprecipitate, factor VIII concentrate, or recombinant factor VIII. These treatments are quite expensive.

Factor IX deficiency **(hemophilia B)** causes the same clinical manifestations as hemophilia A. This is not surprising because both factors VIII and IX are required for the same reaction. Factor XI deficiency causes a milder bleeding disorder, and deficiencies of factor XII, prekallikrein, or HMWK do not cause abnormal bleeding, although the activated partial thromboplastin time is prolonged.

Deficiencies in the final common pathway tend to be more serious than those in the intrinsic pathway. The absence of fibrinogen **(afibrinogenemia)** causes a severe clotting disorder that is often fatal in childhood. The same is true for deficiencies of prothrombin, factor V, and factor X. These clotting factor deficiencies are inherited as recessive disorders.

Von Willebrand disease is an autosomal dominant disorder with impaired platelet adhesion and reduced factor VIII level. Normally, vWF circulates in a noncovalent complex with factor VIII, and its deficiency leads to the premature degradation of factor VIII. Platelet disorders can also be caused by defects of the receptors for vWF or fibrinogen on the platelet membrane.

Tissue Damage Causes the Release of Cellular Enzymes into the Blood

Most metabolic enzymes are intracellular. They leak out of the cell during cell death, and trace amounts of them are therefore always present in the plasma. In the clinical laboratory, these enzymes can be measured in the blood along with other cellular proteins.

Cell death is the most common cause of elevated plasma levels of cellular enzymes. In other cases, metabolic stress raises the permeability of cellular membranes. Enzymes leak out, although the cells do not die. Cancerous tumors can also raise enzyme levels. The tumor cells provide an expanded tissue source of the enzyme. Tumor-invaded tissues are also destroyed, and areas of tumor necrosis can develop when the tumor outgrows its blood supply.

Once released into the blood, the tissue enzymes have half-lives between 1 day and 1 week (Table 15.7).

Those enzymes that are present only in one organ or tissue are the most useful for diagnosis, but few enzymes meet this requirement. The enzymes of the major metabolic pathways, in particular, are present in most cells of the body. Fortunately, *many enzymes occur as tissue-specific* **isoenzymes.**

Isoenzymes are structurally different enzymes that catalyze the same reaction. They can be separated from each other by electrophoresis, differ in kinetic properties and sensitivity to inhibitors, and are in most cases encoded by different genes.

In the clinical laboratory, the enzyme is incubated with saturating concentrations of its substrates at fixed temperature and pH. Its maximal reaction rate (V_{max}) is determined either by the decrease in substrate concentration or by the formation of the product. V_{max} is proportional to the amount of the enzyme in the enzyme solution (see Chapter 4). Enzyme activities can be expressed in **international units** (**IU**). *One IU corresponds to the amount of enzyme that catalyzes the conversion of one micromole (μmol) of substrate to product per minute.*

Serum Enzymes Are Used for the Diagnosis of Many Diseases

The levels of only a limited number of enzymes are determined on a routine basis in most clinical lab-

Table 15.8 Changes in Serum Enzyme Levels in Different Diseases

| | Change in Enzyme Level in | | | | | Neoplastic Disease Metastasis to | | |
Enzyme	Viral Hepatitis	Biliary Obstruction	Muscular Dystrophy	Acute Myocardial Infarction	Acute Pancreatitis	Liver	Bone	Other
Plasma cholinesterase	↓↓	— or ↓	—	—	—	↓↓	—	Organophosphate poisoning
Alanine transaminase	↑↑↑	↑	— or ↑	— or ↑	—	↑	—	
Aspartate transaminase	↑↑↑	↑	↑	↑↑	—	↑↑	—	
Alkaline phosphatase	↑	↑↑↑	—	—	—	↑↑	↑↑↑	Bone diseases, fractures
Acid phosphatase	—	—	—	—	—	—	— or ↑	Prostatic carcinoma
Lactate dehydrogenase	↑	↑	↑↑	↑↑	—	↑↑↑	— or ↑	Megaloblastic anemia, shock
Creatine kinase	—	—	↑↑↑	↑↑	—	—	—	
Lipase	—	—	—	—	↑↑↑	—	—	Perforation of the small intestine
Amylase	—	—	—	—	↑↑↑	—	—	
γ-Glutamyltransferase	↑	↑↑↑	—	—	—	↑↑	—	

—, No change; ↑, increased; ↓, decreased.

oratories (Table 15.8). The most important of these are as follows.

PLASMA CHOLINESTERASE

This is one of the few diagnostically important enzymes whose major place of residence is in the plasma. It differs from the acetylcholinesterase at cholinergic synapses (see Chapter 16) by its broader substrate specificity. Its physiological role is uncertain, but it participates in the metabolism of some drugs, including succinylcholine and cocaine.

Succinylcholine is a short-acting muscle relaxant that is used as an adjunct in general anesthesia. This drug is inactivated by plasma cholinesterase but not by the tissue enzyme. *Some otherwise normal people have a deficiency of plasma cholinesterase. They are at risk for fatal apnea after a standard dose of the drug.* Therefore, a determination of plasma cholinesterase may be prudent before the patient is exposed to succinylcholine.

Plasma cholinesterase is decreased in severe liver diseases, including viral hepatitis and liver cirrhosis. More important is its use in the diagnosis of **organophosphate poisoning.** Organophosphates, which are widely used in pesticides and nerve gases, inhibit not only the action of acetylcholinesterase at cholinergic synapses but also that of the plasma cholinesterase.

ALANINE TRANSAMINASE (ALT) AND ASPARTATE TRANSAMINASE (AST)

These enzymes are most abundant in the liver. They are not secreted into the blood, and therefore any elevation of their plasma levels is due to leakage from damaged cells.

The transaminase levels are used for the diagnosis of liver diseases. In viral hepatitis, the plasma levels of both enzymes can easily be 20 to 100 times above the upper limit of the normal range. The enzyme elevations are proportional to the extent of the ongoing tissue damage, and they can be demonstrated before fever and jaundice develop. The transaminase levels are only mildly elevated in patients with liver cirrhosis. Elevation of the ALT level is quite specific for liver damage, but the AST level is also elevated in muscle diseases and acute myocardial infarction.

ALKALINE PHOSPHATASE (ALP)

This enzyme is abundant in bone, placenta, intestine, and the hepatobiliary system. Each of these organs contains a different isoenzyme. The bone and liver enzymes are the most abundant in normal serum.

The bone enzyme is derived from osteoblasts (see Chapter 14). *Its serum level rises in bone conditions with*

Table 15.9 Occurrence of Lactate Dehydrogenase Isoenzymes in Different Tissues

Isoenzyme no.*	Composition	Presence in				
		Myocardium	Erythrocytes	Skeletal Muscle	Liver	Kidney
1	H_4	++++	+++	–	–	+
2	H_3M	++++	+++	–	–	+
3	H_2M_2	+	+	+	+	++
4	HM_3	–	–	++	++	++
5	M_4	–	–	++++	++++	++

* Enzyme 1 has the highest, and enzyme 5 the lowest, anodic mobility on electrophoresis at slightly alkaline pH values. H, heart; M, muscle.

increased osteoblastic activity: rickets, osteomalacia, hyperparathyroidism, osteitis deformans, neoplastic diseases with bone metastases, and healing fractures. The liver enzyme level is increased in patients with biliary obstruction. The bone and liver enzymes can be distinguished by electrophoresis or by heat inactivation. During heating at 56° C for 15 minutes, the bone enzyme is destroyed to a greater extent than is the liver enzyme.

γ-GLUTAMYL TRANSFERASE (GGT)

This is an enzyme of uncertain function that participates either in amino acid transport or in the metabolism of the "natural antioxidant" glutathione. Although present in most tissues, it is most abundant in liver and kidney.

In the clinical laboratory, GGT is used as a sensitive indicator of biliary obstruction. In this condition, it is elevated along with ALP. GGT synthesis in the liver is also induced by many drugs and other foreign compounds, including alcohol. Therefore, elevations of GGT are seen in many alcoholics and in patients taking certain drugs, such as phenobarbital.

ACID PHOSPHATASE (ACP) AND PROSTATE-SPECIFIC ANTIGEN (PSA)

These are tumor markers, used for the diagnosis and follow-up of patients with prostatic cancer.

ACP was originally described in 1925 as a constituent of normal urine. It soon became evident that its concentration was far higher in male than female urine and that its major source was the prostate gland. Red blood cells, platelets, the liver, and bone also contain various forms of ACP.

ACP is present in seminal fluid, and its determination in vaginal specimens has been used forensically to substantiate allegations of rape. Also, the enzyme is remarkably stable and can be determined in stains even after several weeks.

ACP is not elevated in the early stages of prostatic cancer, and its main use is in the follow-up of patients with established disease. PSA is elevated at earlier stages and is therefore useful for initial diagnosis as well as for later follow-up. PSA is a serine protease that is normally secreted into seminal fluid.

LACTATE DEHYDROGENASE (LDH)

This is an enzyme of anaerobic glycolysis that is present in all tissues. Therefore, its plasma level is elevated in a wide variety of diseases. Fortunately, LDH has tissue-specific isoenzymes. The active enzyme is a tetramer of four equivalent subunits, and there are two different subunits: H (heart) and M (muscle). These subunits can combine to form five different isoenzymes (Table 15.9). Isoenzyme 1 (H_4) is fastest, and isoenzyme 5 (M_4) is slowest during electrophoresis at pH 8.6.

The isoenzyme patterns of the tissues depend on the relative amounts of H and M subunits produced by the cells. Myocardium and bone marrow produce mainly H subunits, and liver and skeletal muscle produce mainly M subunits. Most other tissues produce both.

Differential diagnosis requires either the separate determination of the isoenzymes or the simultaneous determination of other enzymes. For example, elevations of isoenzymes 1 and 2, measured 1 or 2 days after an episode of chest pain, suggest myocardial infarction, whereas elevations of isoenzymes 3, 4, and 5 have to be expected after pulmonary infarction. Also, combined increases of LDH, AST, and creatine kinase (CK) levels suggest myocardial infarction, whereas elevated LDH level with more or less normal AST and CK levels is typical for pulmonary infarction.

CREATINE KINASE

This enzyme occurs in muscle tissue where it catalyzes the reversible reaction

$$\text{Creatine} + \text{ATP} \rightleftharpoons \text{Creatine phosphate} + \text{ADP}$$

Creatine phosphate serves as a store of high-energy phosphate bonds for contracting muscles (see Chapter 30). Other than muscle tissue, only the brain contains appreciable amounts of CK.

CK is a dimer of two equivalent subunits. Two slightly different monomers occur in the tissues: M subunits in skeletal muscle, and B subunits in the brain. The myocardium contains mainly M but also some B subunits. The two subunits can form three isoenzymes: BB (CK-1), MB (CK-2), and MM (CK-3) (Table 15.10).

Table 15.10 Isoenzymes of Creatine Kinase (CK)

Isoenzymes	Subunit Structure	Electrophoretic Mobility	Present in
CK-1	BB	Fast	Brain
CK-2	BM	Medium	Myocardium
CK-3	MM	Slow	Skeletal muscle, myocardium

H, heart; M, muscle.

CK is used for the diagnosis of muscle diseases. Along with LDH, AST, and myoglobin levels, the CK level is elevated in dermatomyositis, polymyositis, and the muscular dystrophies. It even rises after injuries, intramuscular injections, and vigorous physical exercise. CK levels are normal or near normal in patients with neurological motor disorders such as myasthenia gravis, peripheral neuropathy, and Parkinson disease.

Elevations of CK-2 (along with CK-3) are seen after acute myocardial infarction. *CK, LDH, and AST are the most useful enzymes for the diagnosis of acute myocardial infarction.* The typical time courses for these enzymes are shown in Figure 15.30.

In the diagnosis of acute myocardial infarction, enzyme determinations can provide only estimates of the extent of the damage, whereas electrocardiography (ECG) can locate the site of the infarction. However, ECG does not distinguish between old defects and a recent infarction, whereas enzyme elevations are diagnostic for recent and ongoing tissue damage.

LIPASE AND AMYLASE

Levels of these digestive enzymes are elevated in acute pancreatitis, and their main use is *the differential diagnosis in patients who present with severe abdominal pain of sudden onset.* In these abdominal emergencies, acute pancreatitis has to be differentiated from a variety of other disorders, including peptic ulcer disease and cholelithiasis.

Amylase and lipase levels are elevated in some extrapancreatic diseases as well, including intestinal infarction or perforation, and in peritonitis. Amylase levels may even be elevated in patients with mumps or other forms of parotitis.

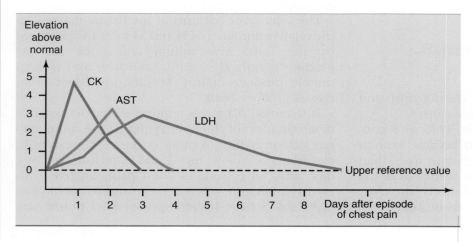

Figure 15.30 Enzyme elevations after acute myocardial infarction. AST, aspartate transaminase; CK, creatine kinase; LDH, lactate dehydrogenase.

SUMMARY

The blood has to make sure that the cells in the body are bathed in a solution with constant levels of electrolytes and a constant pH. Fluid balance between the blood and the interstitial spaces depends on the colloid-osmotic pressure of the plasma proteins, and a constant pH is maintained with the help of the bicarbonate buffer system that is controlled by the lungs and kidneys.

The transport of some nutrients and hormones also depends on plasma proteins. There are specialized proteins for the transport of steroid and thyroid hormones and even for vitamins and trace minerals, including retinol and iron. The hormone-binding proteins buffer the concentration of the free, unbound hormone in the same way that pH buffers buffer the concentration of free protons.

Immunoglobulins (antibodies) are designed for the binding and inactivation of foreign macromolecules (antigens). Millions of different antibodies with diverse antigen-binding specificities are produced by B lymphocytes. However, only the few that encounter a matching antigen are mass-produced after their B lymphocytes metamorphose into antibody-secreting plasma cells.

The blood clotting system is a cascade of proteolytic activations that culminate in the formation of a fibrin clot from soluble fibrinogen. Blood clotting is subject to complex regulation to ensure that clotting remains limited to areas of injury.

The plasma also contains trace amounts of enzymes and other proteins that are usually intracellular. During tissue damage, these proteins are released into the blood, in which they can be assayed for diagnostic purposes.

📖 Further Reading

Bassing CH, Swat W, Alt FW: The mechanism and regulation of chromosomal V(D)J recombination. Cell 109:S45-S55, 2002.

Burtis CA, Ashwood ER (eds): Tietz Textbook of Clinical Chemistry, 3rd ed. Philadelphia: WB Saunders, 1999.

Koj A: Initiation of acute phase response and synthesis of cytokines. Biochim Biophys Acta 1317:84-94, 1996.

Melchers F, Rolink AG, Schaniel C: The role of chemokines in regulating cell migration during humoral immune responses. Cell 99:351-354, 1999.

Potempa J, Korzus E, Travis J: The serpin superfamily of proteinase inhibitors: structure, function, and regulation. J Biol Chem 269:15957-15960, 1994.

QUESTIONS

1. **A complete IgG molecule contains**

   A. Two antigen-binding regions.
   B. A hinge region between the variable domain and the first constant domain of the heavy chain.
   C. One κ light chain and one λ light chain.
   D. A J chain.
   E. Disulfide bonds between the two light chains.

2. **During a routine checkup of an asymptomatic middle-aged woman, the level of haptoglobin is found to be extremely low. Other blood values are normal. This finding could indicate:**

   A. Chronic damage to skeletal muscle.
   B. Either liver damage or biliary obstruction.
   C. An acute-phase response.
   D. Mild chronic hemolysis.
   E. Multiple myeloma.

3. **A 35-year-old man complains about a chronic cough and poor exercise tolerance. Abnormal breath sounds suggest the presence of emphysema. The man used to smoke moderately for several years but gave up smoking 5 years ago. Which blood test should be performed in this situation?**

   A. Transferrin saturation.
   B. Serum creatine kinase.
   C. Serum α-fetoprotein.
   D. TIC.
   E. Bence-Jones protein.

4. **Classical hemophilia is caused by an inherited deficiency of clotting factor VIII. This deficiency blocks**

   A. The intrinsic pathway of blood clotting.
   B. The extrinsic pathway of blood clotting.
   C. The final common pathway of blood clotting.
   D. The fibrinolytic system.
   E. Contact-phase activation.

5. **Patients with nephrotic syndrome have deficiencies of most plasma proteins, but one plasma protein fraction is actually increased. This fraction is**

   A. Albumin.
   B. α_1-Globulin.
   C. α_2-Globulin.
   D. β-Globulin.
   E. γ-Globulin.

CHAPTER 16

Extracellular Messengers

Cells must respond to their environment. Attachments to neighboring cells and the surrounding extracellular matrix provide signals from the immediate environment, but signals from distant sources have to be transmitted by soluble extracellular messenger molecules.

Hormones are synthesized either by specialized endocrine glands or by "ordinary" tissues such as heart, kidney, intestine, and adipose tissue. They are transported by the blood and induce physiological responses in distant targets.

Paracrine messengers are not transported by the blood but act on neighboring cells in their tissue of origin. Many paracrine messengers also act on the synthesizing cell itself. This is called **autocrine** signaling.

Neurotransmitters are released by neurons at specialized cell-cell contacts called synapses. They do not broadcast a message but establish contact between two individual cells.

This chapter is concerned with the metabolism of extracellular messengers. The actions of these agents on their target cells is discussed in Chapter 17.

Steroid Hormones Are Made from Cholesterol

The steroids are classical hormones: synthesized in endocrine glands and transported by the blood. The adrenal steroids regulate energy metabolism (glucocorticoids) and mineral balance (mineralocorticoids), and the gonadal steroids are concerned with sex. Table 16.1 shows representatives of the major classes of steroid hormones.

All steroid hormones are synthesized from cholesterol. Structural changes that are introduced during hormone synthesis include the following:

1. *The side chain at carbon 17 of cholesterol is either shortened to two carbons (progestins, corticosteroids) or lost entirely (androgens, estrogens). This requires* **side chain cleavage reactions** *during steroid hormone biosynthesis.*
2. *The steroid hormones contain hydroxyl groups and/or keto groups. Only the oxygen atom at C-3 is inherited from cholesterol. Those at C-11 (corticosteroids), C-17 (glucocorticoids, androgens, estrogens), and C-21 (corticosteroids) have to be introduced by* **hydroxylation reactions.**
3. ***Mineralocorticoids*** *have an aldehyde group at C-18.*
4. ***Estrogens*** *are distinguished by the aromatic nature of ring A.*

Progestins Are the Biosynthetic Precursors of All Other Steroid Hormones

The *precursor relationships* of the steroid hormones can be summarized as follows:

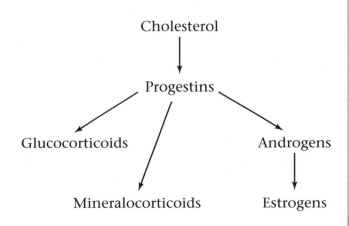

Cholesterol → Progestins → Glucocorticoids, Mineralocorticoids, Androgens → Estrogens

Table 16.1 Structures of Some Representative Steroids

Steroid Class	Source	Synthesis Stimulated by	Example
Cholesterol	Ubiquitous	—	Cholesterol
Progestins	Corpus luteum,* placenta	LH	Progesterone
Glucocorticoids	Adrenal cortex	ACTH	Cortisol
Mineralocorticoids	Adrenal cortex (zona glomerulosa)	Angiotensin II, ACTH	Aldosterone
Androgens	Leydig cells (major) Adrenal cortex (minor)	LH ACTH	Testosterone
Estrogens	Ovarian follicle (granulosa cells)†	FSH	Estradiol

* Progestins also are released in small quantities by the adrenal cortex and other steroid-producing glands, where they are intermediates in the synthesis of the other hormones.

† Also formed in small quantities in the corpus luteum, and by the aromatization of androgens in nonendocrine tissues.

ACTH; adrenocorticotropic hormone; FSH, Follicle-stimulating hormone; LH, luteinizing hormone.

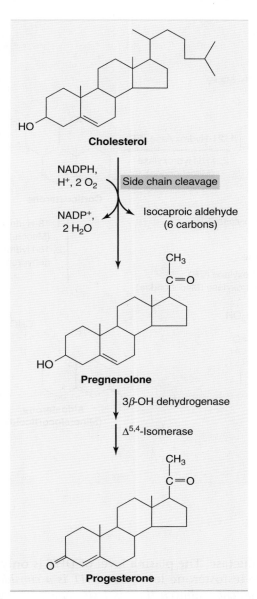

Figure 16.1 Synthesis of progesterone. NADP⁺, NADPH, nicotinamide adenine dinucleotide phosphate.

The synthesis of the progestins (Fig. 16.1) is initiated by the mitochondrial **side chain cleavage enzyme**, also known as **desmolase**. It hydroxylates carbons 20 and 22, followed by cleavage of the carbon-carbon bond. This reaction produces **pregnenolone**, which is converted to **progesterone** by microsomal and cytoplasmic enzymes.

Progesterone is the major end product in the corpus luteum and the placenta, but *the other endocrine glands convert pregnenolone and progesterone to other steroid hormones*. Figure 16.2 shows the synthesis of the major adrenal steroids.

The **corticosteroids** are distinguished from the progestins by the presence of additional hydroxyl groups. These hydroxyl groups are introduced by **monooxygenase reactions** with the overall balance

$$\text{Steroid-H} + O_2 + \text{NADPH} + H^+$$
$$\downarrow \text{P-450}$$
$$\text{Steroid-OH} + \text{NADP}^+ + H_2O$$

*These reactions require **cytochrome P-450** as an intermediate electron carrier.* Various forms of cytochrome P-450 serve as subunits of hydroxylating enzyme systems in the inner mitochondrial membrane and the endoplasmic reticulum (ER) membrane. The micro-somal forms (those in the ER) are reduced by **cytochrome P-450 reductase**, a flavoprotein containing both flavin adenine dinucleotide (FAD) and flavin mononucleotide (FMN). Electrons pass from the reduced form of NADPH to FAD, then to FMN, and finally to an oxygen molecule that is bound to the heme iron of cytochrome P-450. The heme-bound oxygen molecule, activated by the electron transfer, reacts with the substrate:

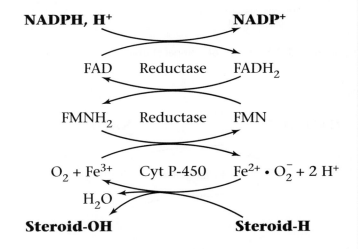

The mitochondrial forms of cytochrome P-450 receive their electrons through an FAD-containing flavoprotein and the iron-sulfur protein **adrenodoxin**:

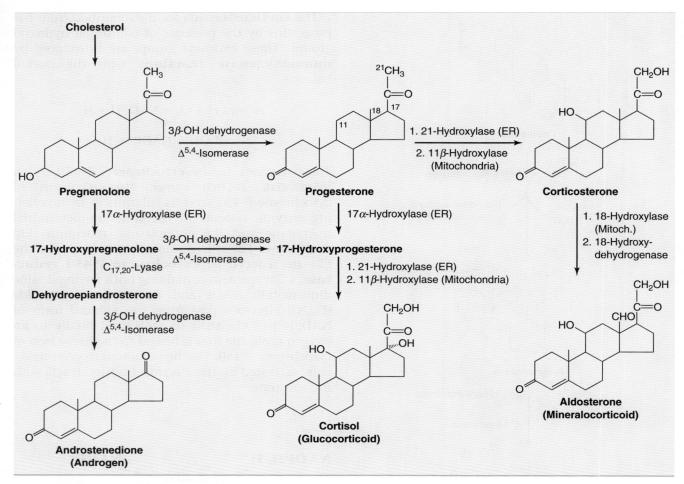

Figure 16.2 Synthesis of adrenal steroids. ER, endoplasmic reticulum.

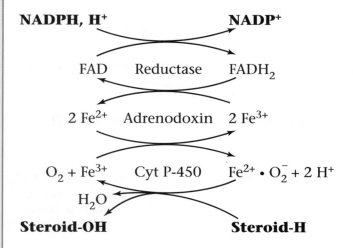

Testosterone is the major testicular androgen. About 5 mg is produced by the Leydig cells in the testis every day. In the target tissues and, to a lesser extent, in the testis itself, testosterone is converted to **dihydrotestosterone (DHT)** by the enzyme 5α-reductase. The plasma level of DHT is only 10% of the testosterone level, but *DHT is a considerably more potent androgen than is testosterone.* Therefore, testosterone acts, in part at least, as a precursor, or *prohormone,* of the active hormone DHT.

Androgens are also synthesized in the adrenal cortex and the theca cells at the periphery of the ovarian follicle (Fig. 16.3; see also Fig. 16.2). **Androstenedione** is produced by the adrenal cortex at a rate of about 3 mg/day. It is far less potent than testosterone, but it is the major source of androgenic activity in girls and women.

Boys and men produce small amounts of estrogen: 65 µg of estrone from androstenedione and 45 µg of estradiol from testosterone. These reactions are catalyzed by the microsomal enzyme system **aromatase.** A small quantity of estradiol is synthesized in the testes, but most estrogens in the male are produced in adipose tissue, the liver, skin, the brain, and other nonendocrine tissues. Therefore, *testosterone is a precursor of two other hormones, DHT and estradiol:*

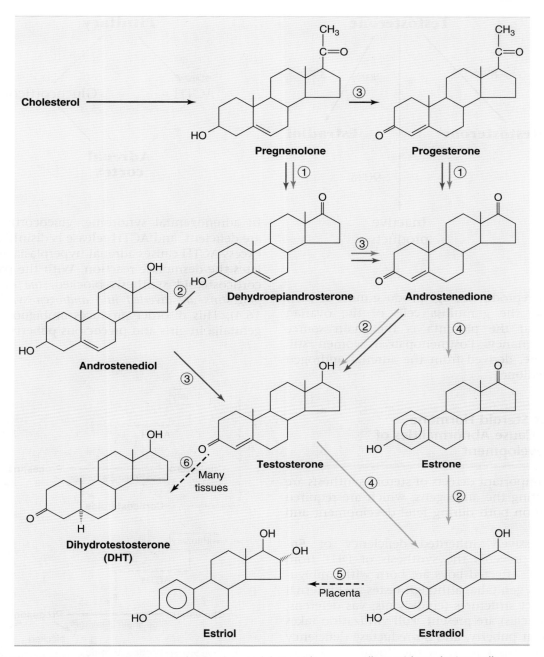

Figure 16.3 The major pathways for the synthesis of gonadal steroids. ⟶, All steroid-producing cells; ⟶, ovary, theca cells; ⟶, ovary, granulosa cells; ⟶, testis. ①, 17α-hydroxylase/C_{17,20}-lyase; ②, 17β-hydroxy-steroid dehydrogenase; ③, 3β-dehydrogenase and $\Delta^{5,4}$-isomerase; ④, aromatase; ⑤, 16α-hydroxylase; ⑥, 5α-reductase.

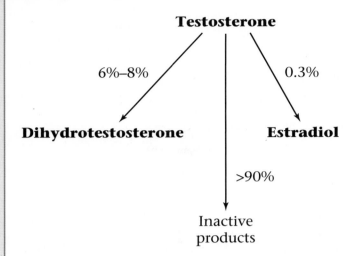

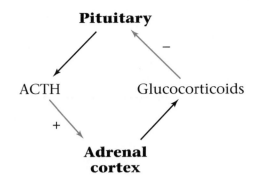

Women of reproductive age produce most of their estrogen in the granulosa cells of the ovarian follicles, and the placenta is the main source during pregnancy. Postmenopausal women still have estrone, derived from the adrenal androgen androstenedione.

Defects of Steroid Hormone Synthesis Cause Abnormalities of Sexual Development

The most important defects of steroid synthesis are those affecting the androgens, which are required for virilization both during fetal development and at puberty.

The recessively inherited deficiency of **5α-reductase** prevents the synthesis of DHT from testosterone. Affected boys are born with ambiguous external genitalia, although testes and internal wolffian duct structures (epididymis, vas deferens, seminal vesicles) are present. Full virilization takes place only at puberty, and 5α-reductase deficiency is therefore also known as the "penis-at-12 syndrome." This rare disorder shows that *DHT is required for the prenatal development of the external male genitalia.*

Congenital adrenal hyperplasia, also known as **adrenogenital syndrome** (incidence, 1 per 10,000), is caused by the deficiency of either 21-hydroxylase or 11β-hydroxylase. These two enzymes are required for the synthesis of corticosteroids but not androgens (see Fig. 16.2).

Ordinarily, the desmolase reaction in the adrenal cortex is stimulated by adrenocorticotropic hormone (ACTH), a pituitary hormone, whereas the glucocorticoids inhibit ACTH release:

In adrenogenital syndrome, glucocorticoid levels are deficient, and ACTH release is disinhibited. The excess ACTH causes adrenal hyperplasia and stimulates the desmolase reaction. With the pathway of corticosteroid synthesis blocked, *the overproduced progestins are diverted into androgen synthesis* (Fig. 16.4). This disorder produces ambiguous external genitalia in girls and precocious puberty in boys.

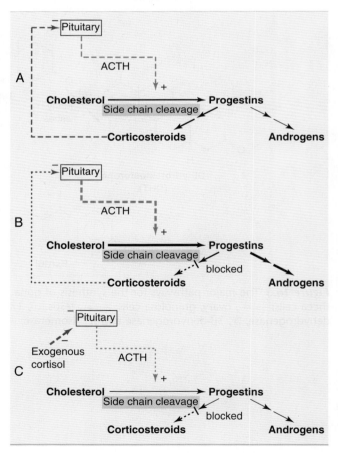

Figure 16.4 Adrenal steroid synthesis in adrenogenital syndrome. **A,** Normal. **B,** Untreated adrenogenital syndrome. **C,** Adrenogenital syndrome treated with cortisol (+ mineralocorticoid). ACTH, adrenocorticotropic hormone.

A partial deficiency of either 11β- or 21-hydroxy-lase causes only virilization, but complete deficiencies cause life-threatening hyponatremia and hyperkalemia as well. Glucocorticoids are optional, but mineralocorticoids are essential for life. Both the virilization and the electrolyte imbalance can be cured by orally administered corticosteroids.

Thyroid Hormones Are Synthesized from Protein-Bound Tyrosine

The thyroid hormones are the only constituents of the human body that contain organically bound iodine:

Triiodothyronine
(T_3)

Thyroxine
(T_4)

Food supplies about 100 μg of iodine per day in the form of the iodide ion (I^-). Its plasma concentration is only 0.2 μg/dL, but the thyroid gland accumulates iodide by means of sodium cotransport. Iodide uptake is a rate-limiting step for the synthesis of the thyroid hormones. From the follicular cell, iodide can enter the lumen of the thyroid follicle by facilitated diffusion (Fig. 16.5).

The second ingredient for thyroid hormone synthesis, besides iodine, is **thyroglobulin.** This large glycoprotein, formed from two subunits with molecular weights of 330,000 D each, is secreted into the lumen of the thyroid follicle by the follicular cells. Up to 40 tyrosine side chains in this protein become iodinated, but only 8 to 10 of these are processed to the active hormones.

The iodination of the tyrosine side chains requires the oxidation of iodide to iodine by **thyroperoxidase,** a heme-containing enzyme on the apical (luminal) surface of the plasma membrane

(see Fig. 16.5). The iodine reacts with tyrosine side chains, and the coupling of two iodinated tyrosines produces the protein-bound hormones (Fig. 16.6).

The thyroid follicle stores the hormones in the form of thyroglobulin. *Their release requires the pinocytotic uptake of thyroglobulin into the follicular cell, followed by the degradation of the whole molecule by lysosomal proteases.* The iodinated but uncoupled tyrosine from thyroglobulin is deiodinated in the cell, and the iodine is recycled.

More than 99% of triiodothyronine (T_3) and more than 99.9% of thyroxine (T_4) are bound to plasma proteins in the blood. This extensive protein binding protects the hormones from enzymatic attack and renal excretion, and therefore their biological half-lives are remarkably long: 6.5 days for T_4 and 1.5 days for T_3. The T_4 level in the plasma is 50 times higher than the T_3 level (80 ng/mL versus 1.5 ng/mL), but the concentrations of free, unbound hormone are more balanced because T_3 is less extensively bound to plasma proteins than is T_4.

Of the hormone released from the thyroid gland, about 90% is T_4 and 10% is T_3. In the target tissues, some T_4 is converted to active T_3, and some is converted to the inactive reverse T_3 (Fig. 16.7).

Indeed, two thirds of the circulating T_3 do not come directly from the thyroid gland but are produced from T_4 in peripheral tissues. Of the two hormones, T_3 is about four times more potent than T_4 in most bioassays. Therefore, *T_4 is a prohormone for the more potent T_3, much as testosterone is a prohormone for the more potent DHT.*

Both Hypothyroidism and Hyperthyroidism Are Common Disorders

The deficiency of thyroid hormone is called **hypothyroidism.** In adults it leads to **myxedema,** with widespread subcutaneous edema, decreased basal metabolic rate, bradycardia, and sluggish thinking. Hypothyroidism in infants leads to **cretinism,** with severe and irreversible mental deficiency, stunted growth, and multiple physical deformities.

Congenital hypothyroidism afflicts about 1 per 4000 newborns. Because the dire consequences of this condition can readily be prevented by the oral administration of T_4, *neonatal screening for congenital hypothyroidism is routinely performed in many parts of the world.*

Iodine deficiency causes hypothyroidism in mountainous areas of the world where the soil and the plants grown on it are deficient in this mineral. In the Alps, the condition was common until the

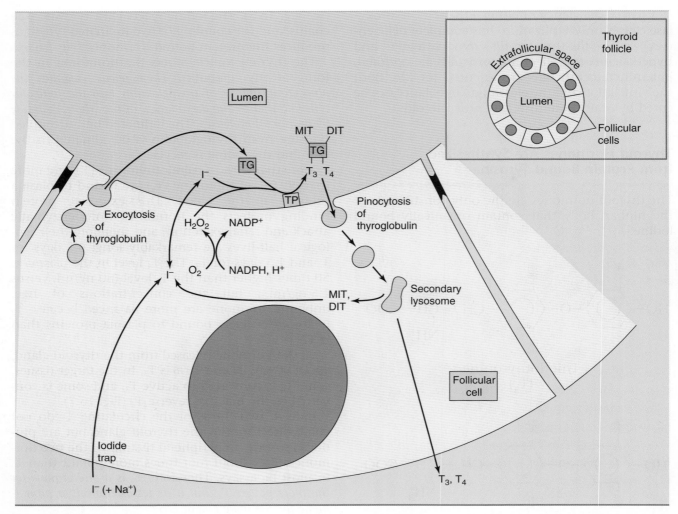

Figure 16.5 Cellular compartmentation of thyroid hormone synthesis. DIT, diiodotyrosine; MIT, monoiodotyrosine; NADP$^+$, NADPH, nicotinamide adenine dinucleotide phosphate; TG, Thyroglobulin; TP, thyroperoxidase.

early years of the 20th century. Iodine deficiency is now rare in most countries because of the routine use of iodized salt, although there is still an extensive "goiter belt" in the Himalaya mountains.

The thyroid gland is stimulated by thyroid stimulating hormone (TSH), a pituitary hormone. TSH release from the pituitary gland, in turn, is suppressed by thyroid hormones:

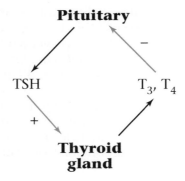

This feedback loop maintains a constant level of thyroid hormone under ordinary conditions. In iodine deficiency, however, the thyroid gland cannot make its hormones. Therefore, the thyrotrophs of the pituitary gland are disinhibited, and the TSH level soars. TSH not only stimulates the biochemical steps in thyroid hormone synthesis but also causes hyperplasia of the follicular cells and the excessive accumulation of uniodinated thyroglobulin. This condition is called **goiter.**

Graves disease, which afflicts about 0.4% of the population (mainly women), is the most common cause of **hyperthyroidism.** It is an autoimmune disease in which an abnormal IgG antibody binds to the TSH receptor. The antibody stimulates the receptor, causing excessive hormone secretion **(thyrotoxicosis)** and enlargement of the gland.

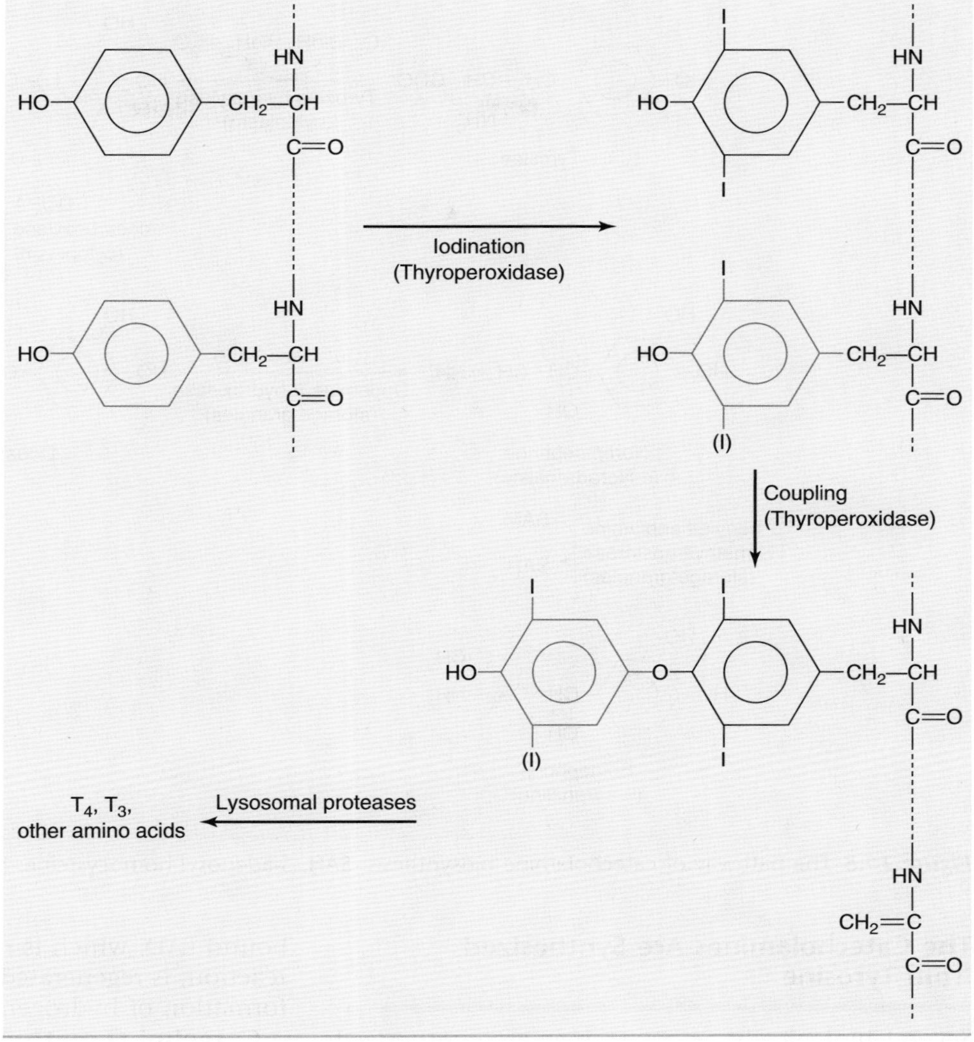
HN
HO
CH2
CH
C=O
I
Iodination
(Thyroperoxidase)
(I)
Coupling
(Thyroperoxidase)
O
T4, T3,
other amino acids
Lysosomal proteases
CH2=C

Figure 16.6 Synthesis of thyroid hormones from iodinated tyrosine residues in thyroglobulin. These reactions take place on the luminal surface of the follicular cells in the thyroid gland. T_3, triiodothyronine; T_4, thyroxine.

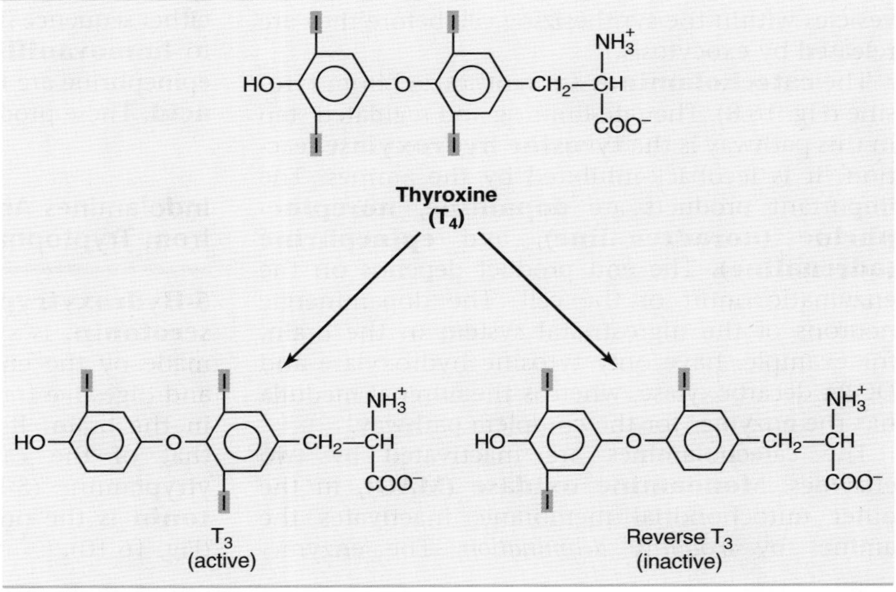
I
HO
O
CH2
CH
NH3+
COO−
Thyroxine
(T4)
T3
(active)
Reverse T3
(inactive)

Figure 16.7 In its target tissues, thyroxine (T_4) is converted to either the more active triiodothyronine (T_3) or to inactive reverse T_3.

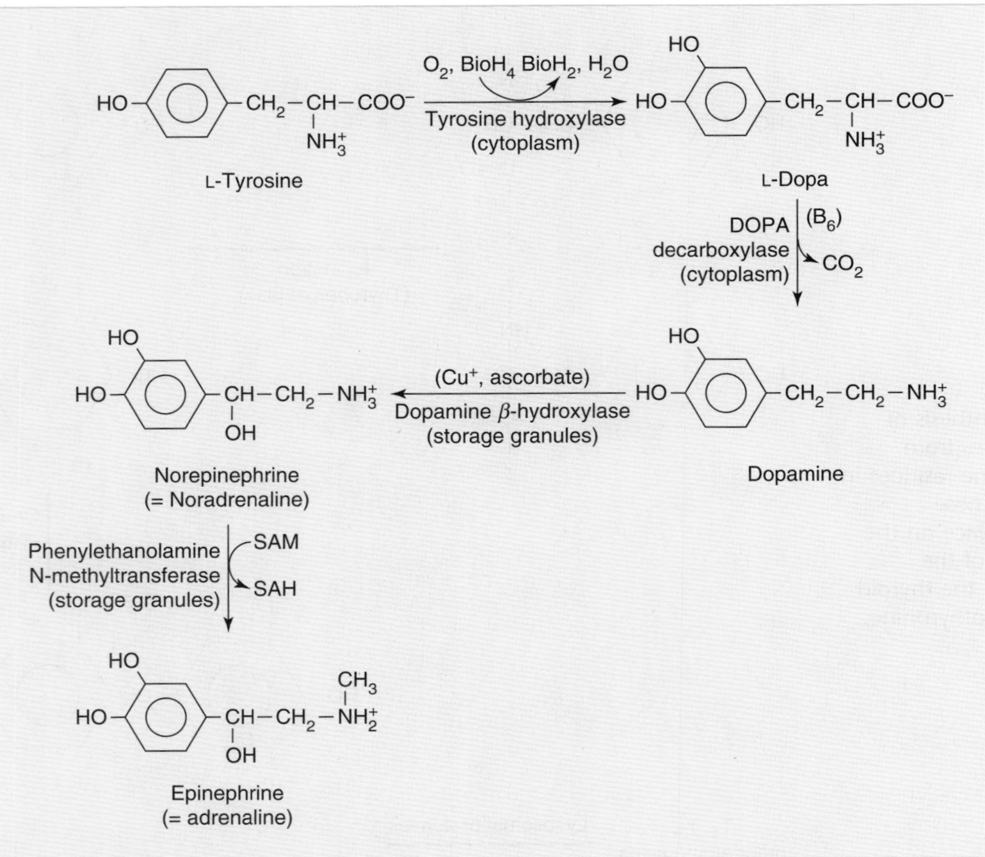

Figure 16.8 The pathway of catecholamine biosynthesis. SAH, *S*-adenosyl homocysteine; SAM, *S*-adenosyl methionine.

The Catecholamines Are Synthesized from Tyrosine

Several biologically active amines are synthesized by the decarboxylation of aromatic amino acids. *These amino acid decarboxylations always depend on pyridoxal phosphate (vitamin B₆).* Being water soluble, biogenic amines are stored in membrane-bounded vesicles within the synthesizing cell before they are released by exocytosis.

The **catecholamines** are synthesized from tyrosine (Fig. 16.8). The rate-limiting and regulated step in this pathway is the **tyrosine hydroxylase** reaction. It is feedback-inhibited by the amines. The important products are **dopamine, norepinephrine (noradrenaline),** and **epinephrine (adrenaline).** The end product depends on the enzymatic outfit of the cell. The dopaminergic neurons of the nigrostriatal system in the brain, for example, have only tyrosine hydroxylase and DOPA decarboxylase, whereas the adrenal medulla has the enzymes for the complete pathway.

The catecholamines are inactivated by two enzymes. **Monoamine oxidase (MAO),** in the outer mitochondrial membrane, inactivates the amines by *oxidative deamination.* The enzyme-bound FAD, which is reduced to $FADH_2$ during the reaction, is regenerated by molecular oxygen under formation of hydrogen peroxide (H_2O_2).

Catechol-*O*-methyltransferase (COMT) inactivates catecholamines by *S-adenosyl methionine (SAM)–dependent methylation* of one of the ring OH groups. Both MAO and COMT have broad substrate specificities, and the two reactions can occur in either sequence (Fig. 16.9). Dopamine is metabolized to **homovanillic acid,** and norepinephrine and epinephrine are metabolized to **vanillylmandelic acid.** These products are excreted in the urine.

Indolamines Are Synthesized from Tryptophan

5-Hydroxytryptamine (5-HT), also known as **serotonin,** is synthesized from tryptophan. It is made by the enterochromaffin cells of the lungs and digestive tract, in platelets, and some neurons in the brain. Its biosynthetic pathway resembles that of the catecholamines. Besides 5-hydroxytryptamine (5-HT), the pineal hormone **melatonin** is the only other indoleamine in humans (Fig. 16.10).

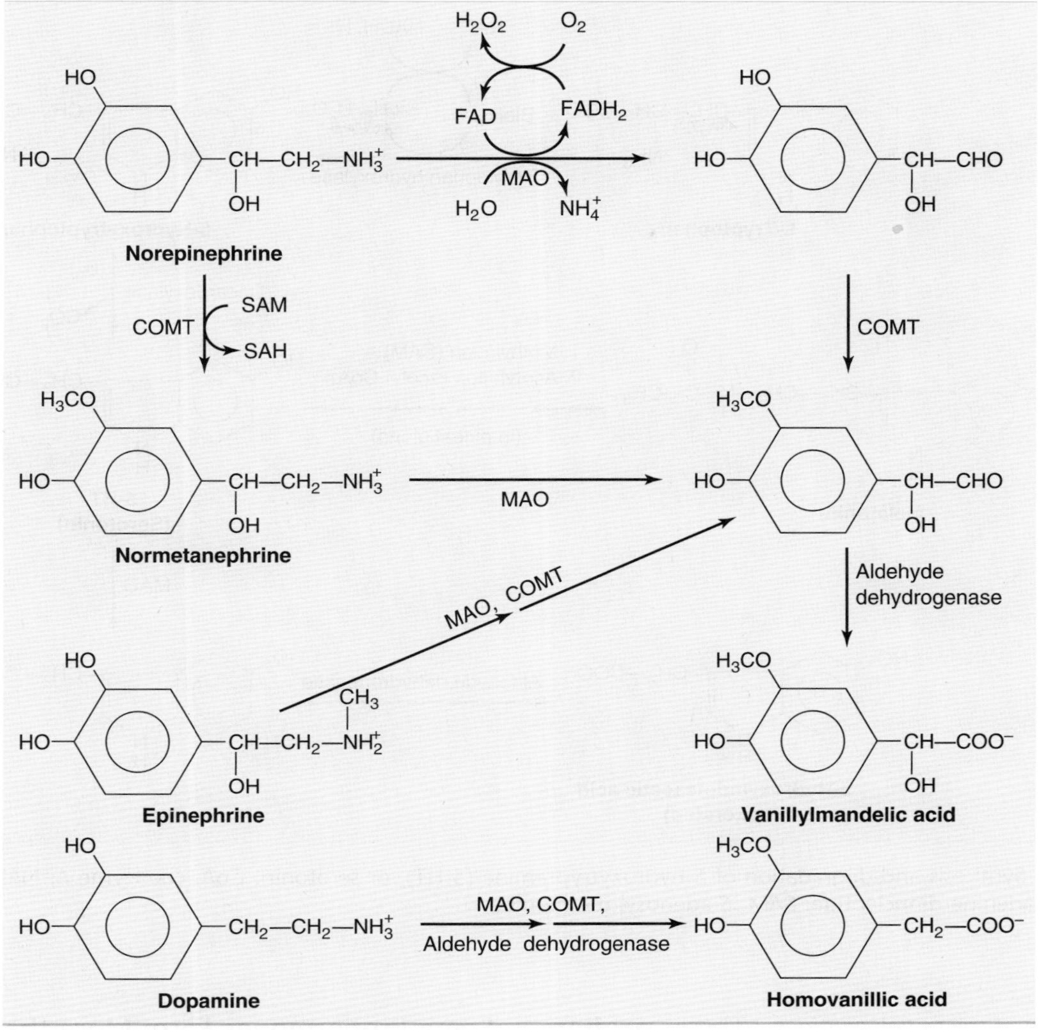

Figure 16.9 Enzymatic inactivation of catecholamines. Besides enzymatic inactivation, which is mostly intracellular, the rapid uptake of catecholamines into the cell is critically important for the termination of their biological actions. COMT, catechol-*O*-methyltransferase; FAD, FADH$_2$, flavin adenine dinucleotide; MAO, monoamine oxidase; SAH, *S*-adenosyl homocysteine; SAM, *S*-adenosyl methionine.

Serotonin is inactivated by MAO but not by COMT. Humans have two isoenzymes of MAO. **MAO-A** acts on serotonin, and **MAO-B** acts on dopamine. Norepinephrine is inactivated by both.

Histamine Is Produced by Mast Cells and Basophils

As a major mediator of allergic responses, *histamine is released by circulating basophils and their sedentary cousins, the mast cells.* Histamine dilates small blood vessels, increases capillary permeability, contracts bronchial and intestinal smooth muscle, stimulates gastric acid secretion and nasal fluid discharge, and regulates the cells of the immune system. Its syn-

thesis and degradation are summarized in Figure 16.11.

Insulin Is Released Together with the C-Peptide

Most extracellular messengers are either proteins or small oligopeptides. They include many hormones and neurotransmitters, growth factors, and the cytokines that are released by white blood cells during inflammation.

All extracellular signaling proteins are made on the assembly line of the secretory pathway: from ER-bound ribosomes through the ER, Golgi apparatus, and secretory vesicles. *Small peptide hormones are*

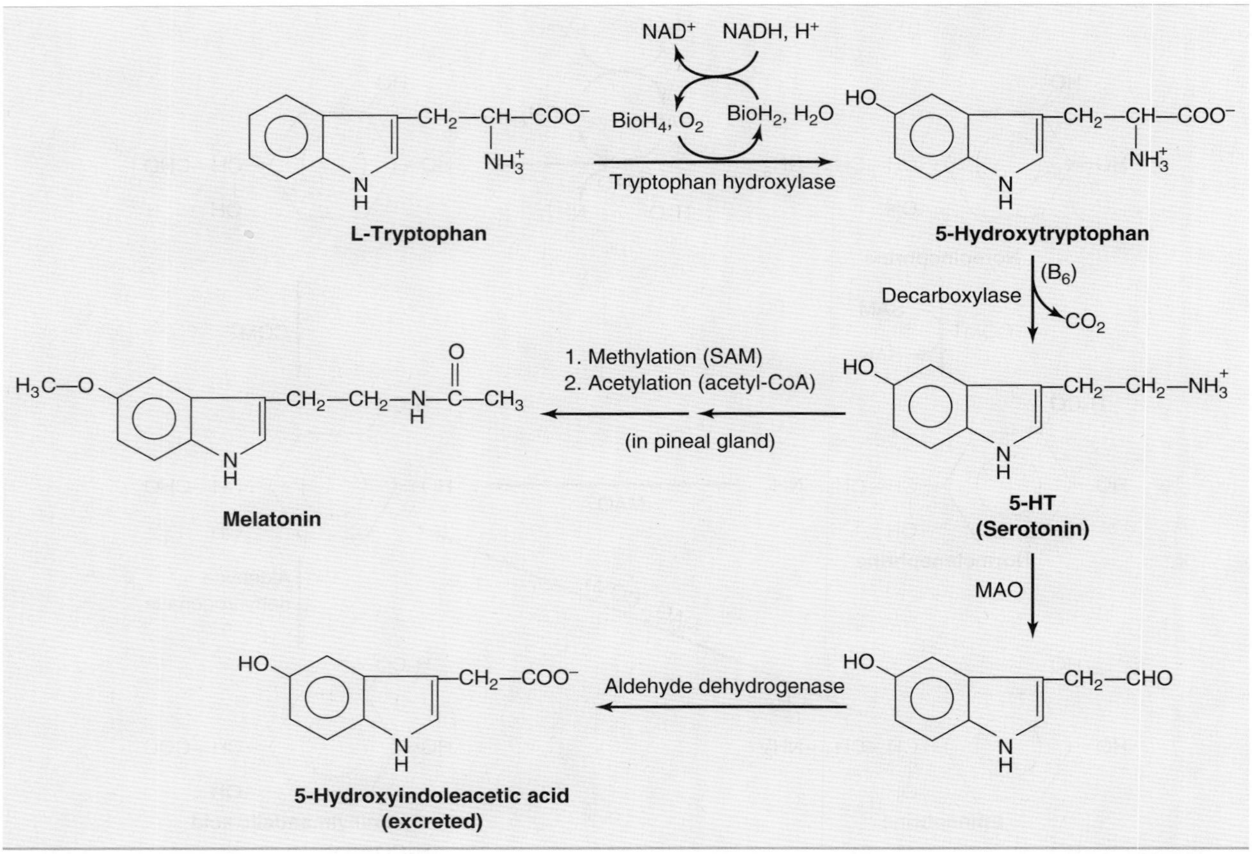

Figure 16.10 Synthesis and degradation of 5-hydroxytryptamine (5-HT), or serotonin. CoA, coenzyme A; NAD⁺, NADH, nicotinamide adenine dinucleotide; SAM, S-adenosyl methionine.

derived from larger polypeptides. These **prohormones** are processed by endopeptidases in the ER, Golgi apparatus, or secretory vesicles.

The synthesis of insulin in the pancreatic β cells is a typical example. Mature insulin consists of two disulfide-bonded polypeptides: the A chain with 21 amino acids, and the B chain with 30 amino acids (Fig. 16.12).

Insulin is derived from **preproinsulin,** a single polypeptide with 103 amino acids. The first 24 amino acids at the amino terminus are the signal sequence. They are removed by signal peptidase in the ER. The remaining structure, known as **proinsulin,** is cleaved at paired basic amino acid residues by enzymes in the secretory granules. These cleavages release a hormonally inactive fragment, the **C-peptide** (C = connecting).

Being formed in the same secretory vesicle, insulin and C-peptide are released together into the blood. The serum C-peptide level can be determined in the clinical laboratory. Unlike insulin, C-peptide can be used to assess β cell function in diabetic patients who receive insulin injections.

Some Prohormones Form More than One Active Product

All small peptide hormones and peptide neurotransmitters are produced by the processing of larger precursor proteins. One example is the **enkephalins:**

Tyr-Gly-Gly-Phe-Met (Met-enkephalin)
Tyr-Gly-Gly-Phe-Leu (Leu-enkephalin)

The enkephalins belong to a family of peptides that are known as **opioid peptides** or **endorphins,** because they act on the same receptors as the opiates and induce opiate-like effects. They are neurotransmitters in the brain, spinal cord, and peripheral nerve plexuses.

*The precursor **proenkephalin A** contains 6 copies of the met-enkephalin sequence and one copy of the leu-enkephalin sequence,* each flanked on both sides by pairs of basic amino acid residues (Fig. 16.13). As in proinsulin, these pairs of basic amino acid residues are preformed cleavage sites for prohormone processing.

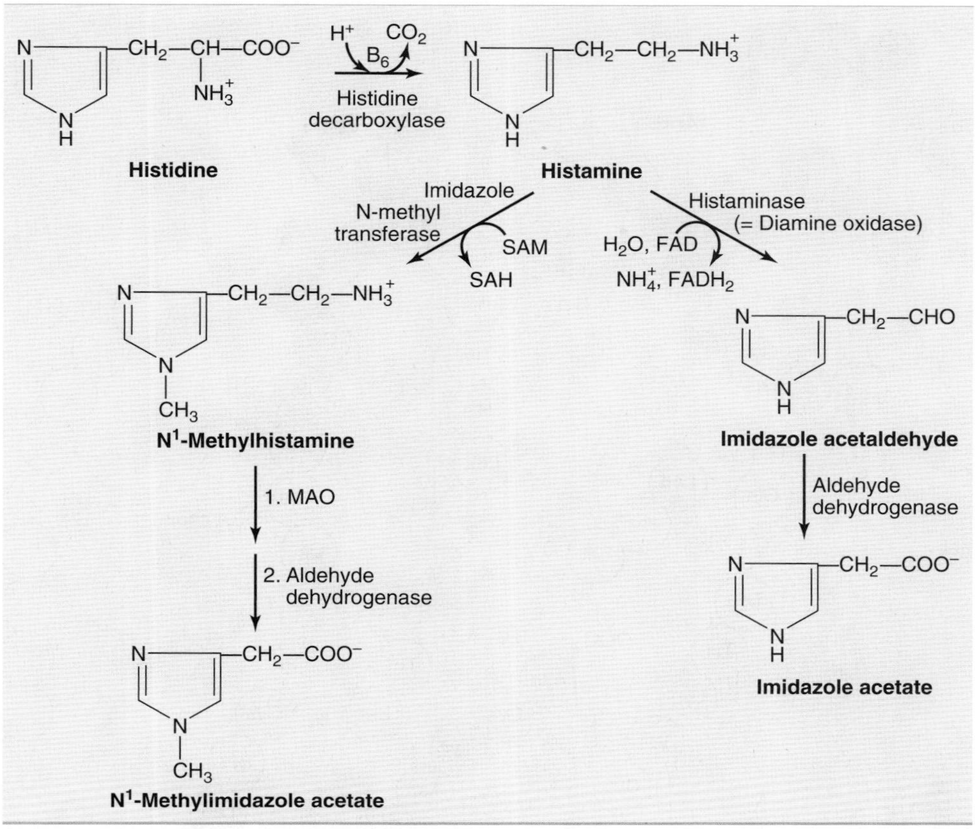

Figure 16.11 Synthesis and degradation of histamine. FAD, flavin adenine dinucleotide; $FADH_2$, reduced form of FAD; MAO, monoamine oxidase; SAH, *S*-adenosyl homocysteine; SAM, *S*-adenosyl methionine.

Proopiomelanocortin is a prohormone in the anterior pituitary gland. It is a precursor of ACTH, β-endorphin, various forms of melanocyte-stimulating hormone (MSH), and some lipotropic hormones that stimulate fat breakdown in adipose tissue.

The processing of proopiomelanocortin is tissue-specific (Fig. 16.14). ACTH and β-endorphin are the main products in the anterior pituitary gland. They are stored in the same vesicles and released together in response to the same stimuli. In the pars intermedia of the pituitary gland, ACTH is further processed to α-MSH.

In humans, most MSH activity is contained in the larger fragments β-lipotropin, γ-lipotropin, and ACTH. In patients with **Cushing disease** (an adenoma of the pituitary corticotrophs) or **Addison disease** (destruction of the adrenal glands), hyperpigmentation is caused by the excessive release of these peptides.

Angiotensin Is Formed from Circulating Angiotensinogen

Some hormones are produced by proteases in the blood. The vasoconstrictor peptide **angiotensin,** for example, is derived from the plasma protein **angiotensinogen.** When the blood pressure in the kidneys is too low, the juxtaglomerular cells release the protease **renin.** Renin cleaves angiotensinogen to form the 10–amino acid peptide **angiotensin I.**

Angiotensin I is biologically inactive. It has to be processed to active **angiotensin II** by **angiotensin-converting enzyme,** a protease on the surface of endothelial cells in the lungs. Cleavage by renin is the rate-limiting step in this sequence (Fig. 16.15).

Angiotensin II raises the blood pressure by a direct action on vascular smooth muscle, and indirectly by enhancing the release of norepinephrine

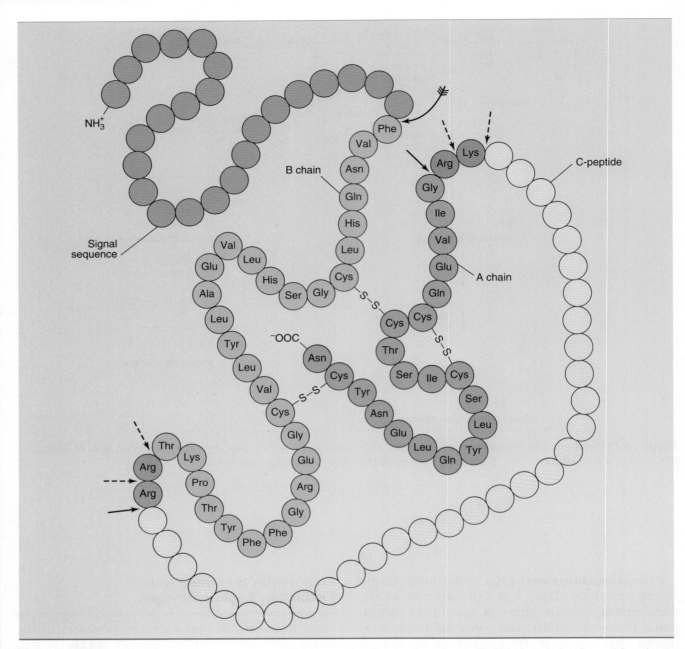

Figure 16.12 Synthesis of insulin from pre-proinsulin. Mature insulin consists of two disulfide-bonded polypeptides, the A chain and the B chain. During prohormone processing, the signal sequence (⚫⚫) and the C-peptide (⚪⚪) are removed proteolytically. The proteolytic cleavages are performed by the signal peptidase in the rough endoplasmic reticulum (ER) (⫸⟶) and by prohormone convertases (⟶) in secretory granules that cleave proinsulin at two sites on the C-terminal side of dibasic residues (Arg-Arg and Lys-Arg). The basic residues are then removed sequentially by carboxypeptidase E/H (--➤).

from sympathetic nerve endings. It also stimulates aldosterone secretion from the adrenal cortex. Aldosterone causes a delayed rise in blood pressure by preventing the renal excretion of sodium. Good renin inhibitors are not currently available, but **captopril** and other converting enzyme inhibitors are among the most important antihypertensive drugs.

Angiotensin II is degraded by endothelial peptidases in less than 1 minute. *Most biologically active peptides are rapidly degraded.* Very small peptides, in particular, are easy prey for peptidases on the surface of capillary endothelial cells. The life spans of oxytocin and vasopressin (nine amino acids), for example, are in the 1- to 10-minute range, and injected enkephalins (five amino acids) are

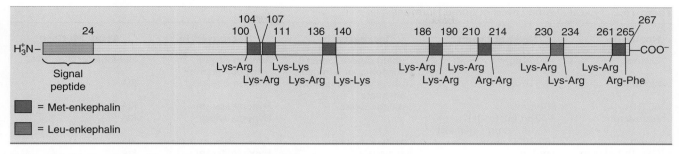

Figure 16.13 Structure of human (pre-) proenkephalin A.

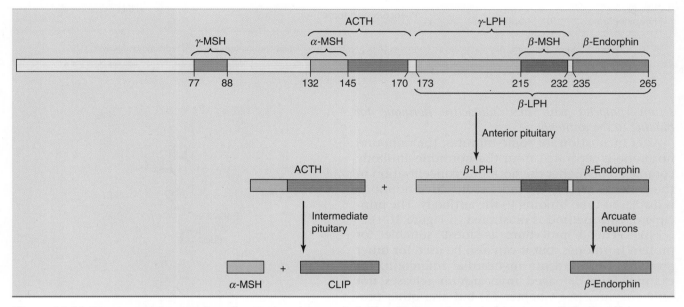

Figure 16.14 Structure and processing of proopiomelanocortin in the pituitary gland. As in proenkephalin (see Fig. 16.13), the active fragments are in most cases framed by pairs of basic amino acid residues (not shown here). ACTH, adrenocorticotropic hormone; CLIP, a hormonally inactive fragment; LPH, lipotropic hormone; MSH, melanocyte-stimulating hormone.

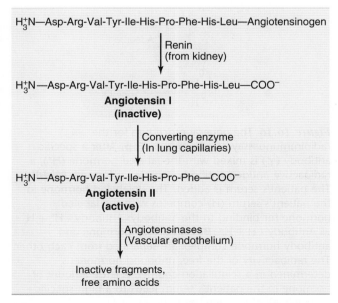

Figure 16.15 Synthesis of angiotensin II from circulating angiotensinogen.

degraded within seconds. Even circulating insulin survives for only 1 to 5 minutes.

Radioimmunoassay Is the Most Versatile Method for the Determination of Hormone Levels

The plasma concentrations of most hormones are extremely low (Table 16.2), and very sensitive methods are therefore required for the measurement of hormone levels in the clinical laboratory.

The most widely used procedure for hormone determinations is **radioimmunoassay (RIA).** It requires a specific antibody to the hormone and a radiolabeled version of the hormone containing tritium, radioactive iodine, or some other suitable isotope. When the patient's serum is added to a complex of the antibody with the radiolabeled hormone, *the (unlabeled) hormone in the patient's*

Table 16.2 Typical Plasma Levels of Some Hormones

Hormone	Normal Levels	Increased in	Decreased in	Assay Method
Cortisol	50-250 ng/mL	Cushing disease, adrenal adenoma, or iatrogenic	Addison disease, hypopituitarism	Fluorometric, RIA, HPLC
Aldosterone	40-310 pg/mL	Cushing disease, adrenal adenoma	Addison disease	RIA
ACTH	50 pg/mL	Cushing disease	Hypopituitarism	RIA
Testosterone	3-12 ng/mL (male) 0.3-0.9 ng/mL (female)		Hypogonadism	RIA
Insulin	180-1000 pg/mL	Obesity, insulinoma	Type I diabetes mellitus	RIA
Growth hormone	1 ng/mL	Acromegaly	Hypopituitarism	RIA
Vasopressin	1-5 pg/mL	Inappropriate ADH secretion	Diabetes insipidus	RIA
Epinephrine	≤140 pg/mL	Pheochromocytoma		HPLC
Norepinephrine	70-1500 pg/mL			

ACTH, adrenocorticotropic hormone; ADH, antidiuretic hormone; HPLC, high-pressure liquid chromatography; RIA, radioimmunoassay.

serum competes with the radioactive hormone for binding to the antibody.

After incubation for some minutes, the unbound hormone is separated from the hormone-antibody complex. The higher the hormone concentration in the patient's serum, the more radioactive hormone is displaced from binding to the antibody. The principle of this method is illustrated in Figure 16.16.

This general procedure is most suitable for protein hormones, but it can also be used for other proteins. During acute myocardial infarction, for example, the damaged myocardium releases not only enzymes (see Chapter 15) but also other proteins, including myoglobin and troponin. The determination of these proteins by RIA is a valuable aid in the diagnosis of myocardial infarction.

Arachidonic Acid Is Converted to Biologically Active Products

The **eicosanoids** (Greek εἴκοσα = "20") are biologically active lipids that are derived from polyunsaturated 20-carbon fatty acids. Any of the three fatty acids in Figure 16.17 can be used as a precursor, but *arachidonic acid is most important simply because it is far more abundant than the others*. In the cell, these fatty acids are encountered in position 2 of membrane phosphoglycerides, from which they are released by the action of **phospholipase A₂** (Fig. 16.18).

Free arachidonic acid can be salvaged by an acyl–coenzyme A (CoA) synthetase for reesterification. Alternatively, it can be processed to biologically active products by either of two pathways. The **cyclooxygenase pathway** produces prostaglandins, prostacyclin, and thromboxane, and the **lipoxygenase pathway** produces leukotrienes (Fig. 16.19).

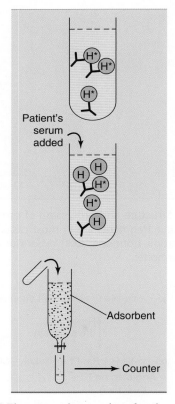

Figure 16.16 The general procedure for the radioimmunoassay of a hormone. **Top,** After a specific antibody (Y) is mixed with the labeled hormone (H*), a radioactive antigen-antibody complex is formed. **Middle,** The patient's serum is added. The unlabeled hormone in the patient's serum (H) competes with the labeled hormone for binding to the antibody: Antibody · H* + H ⇌ Antibody · H + H*. **Bottom,** Free hormone and antibody-hormone complex are separated from each other. The radioactivity of the free, unbound hormone is determined in a scintillation counter. A large amount of hormone in the patient's serum leads to a high specific radioactivity of the free hormone.

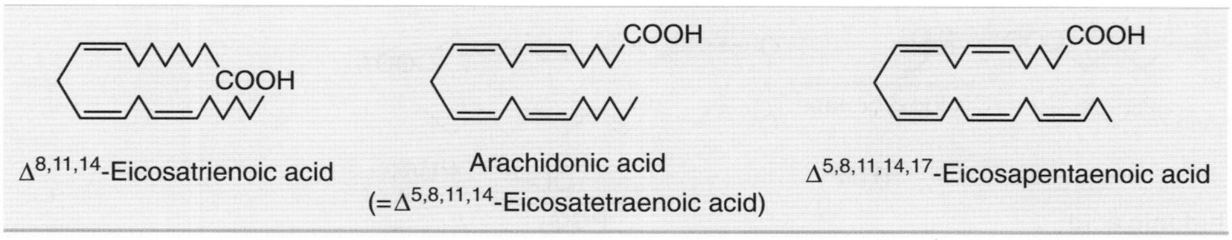

$\Delta^{8,11,14}$-Eicosatrienoic acid

Arachidonic acid
$(=\Delta^{5,8,11,14}$-Eicosatetraenoic acid)

$\Delta^{5,8,11,14,17}$-Eicosapentaenoic acid

Figure 16.17 The three 20-carbon fatty acids pictured are the precursors of prostaglandins, leukotrienes, and other biologically active products.

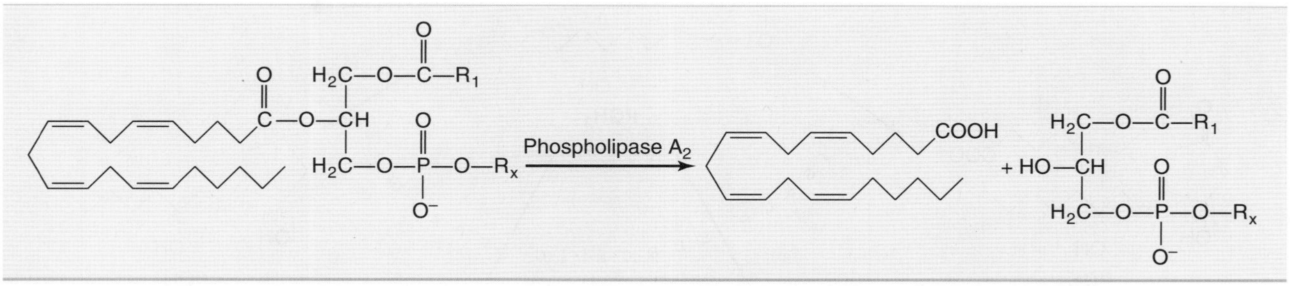

Phospholipase A$_2$

Figure 16.18 The release of free arachidonic acid from membrane phosphoglycerides.

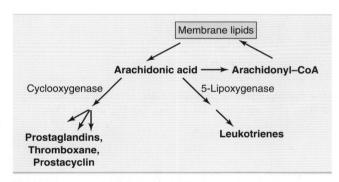

Figure 16.19 The major fates of arachidonic acid. Cyclooxygenase and 5-lipoxygenase are the key enzymes for the synthesis of the biologically active eicosanoids. CoA, coenzyme A.

Prostaglandins Are Synthesized in Almost All Tissues

Prostaglandins and related products are formed by the microsomal **cyclooxygenase complex,** which consists of cyclooxygenase and peroxidase components. Its name indicates that it uses molecular oxygen as an oxidant and that it creates a ring structure in its substrate.

Two isoenzymes of cyclooxygenase are present in the body. **Cyclooxygenase 1 (COX-1)** is a constitutive enzyme that is present in most cells except erythrocytes, and **cyclooxygenase 2 (COX-2)** is an inducible enzyme in white blood cells but also in epithelial cells and smooth muscle cells. *COX-2 is induced by proinflammatory stimuli.*

The prostaglandin H that is formed by the cyclooxygenase complex is converted to other products by tissue-specific enzymes (Fig. 16.20). *Each cell type makes only one or a few major products.* For example, the platelets make thromboxane, and vascular endothelial cells make prostaglandins E and I.

Prostaglandins are named with a capital letter according to the nature of the substituent on the cyclopentane ring, and a subscript indicates the number of double bonds outside the ring (Fig. 16.21).

The types of prostaglandin, as designated by the capital letter, have different and sometimes antagonistic biological effects. The number of double bonds, on the other hand, affects the potency of the product but not the kind of effect on a particular target tissue.

The Prostanoids Participate in Many Physiological Processes

Almost every cell in the human body responds to one or more products of the cyclooxygenase pathway. Only a few of the more interesting actions can be mentioned here:

1. *Aggregating platelets release thromboxane A$_2$ (TXA$_2$).* This prostaglandin derivative causes vasoconstriction and platelet activation. Its actions are short lasting, because it is hydrolyzed to an inactive product within 30 to 60 seconds. The actions of TXA$_2$ on platelets and blood vessels are antagonized by prostaglandin I$_2$

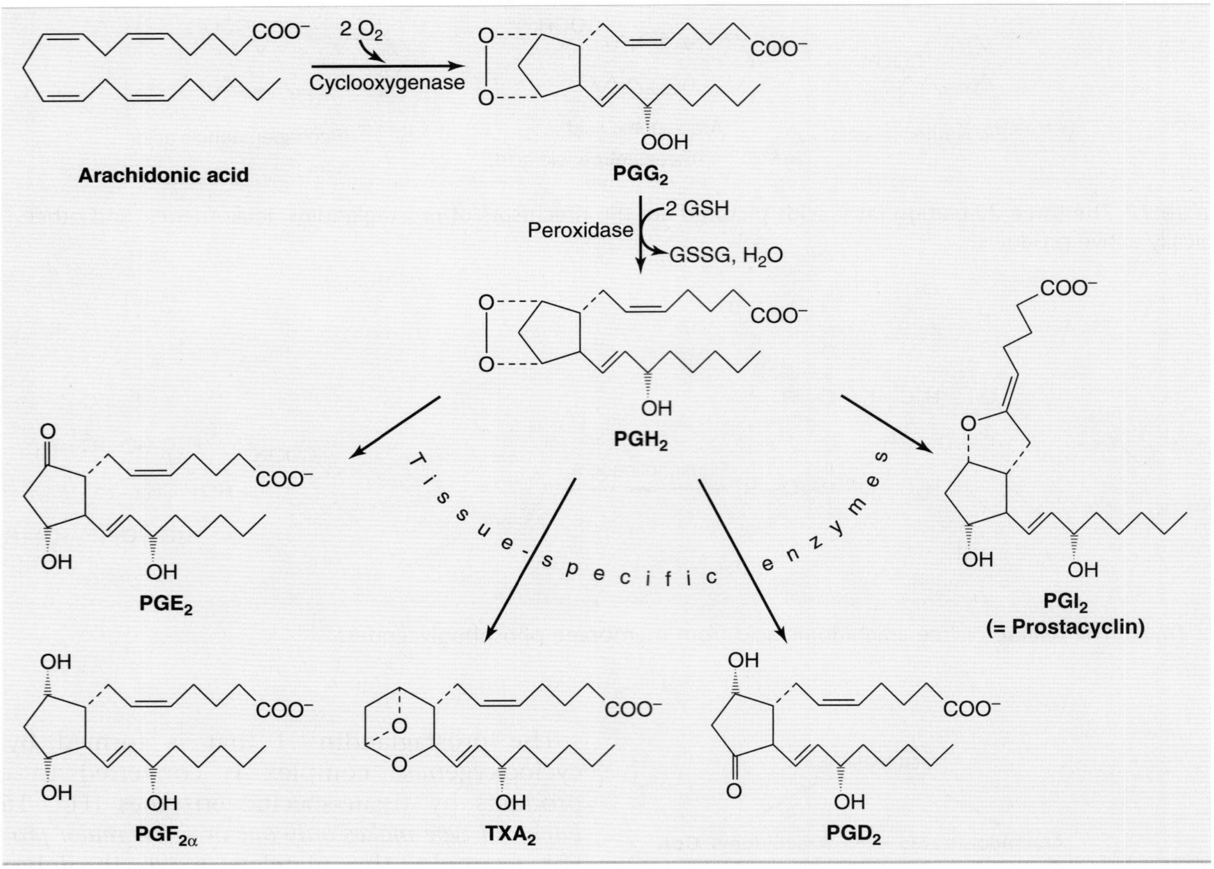

Figure 16.20 Synthesis of prostaglandins and thromboxanes by the cyclooxygenase pathway. GSH, reduced glutathione; GSSG, oxidized glutathione; PGD_2, PGE_2, $PGF_{2\alpha}$, PGG_2, PGH_2, and PGI_2, prostaglandins D_2, E_2, $F_{2\alpha}$, G_2, H_2, and I_2; TXA_2, thromboxane A_2.

(PGI_2, or prostacyclin) from endothelial cells. PGI_2 has a half-life of 3 minutes.

2. *Prostaglandin E_2 (PGE_2) and PGI_2 are vasodilators that are formed by endothelial cells.* They cannot be used as antihypertensives because of their rapid inactivation and numerous extravascular effects, but *PGE_1 can be used in infants with pulmonary stenosis to maintain the patency of the ductus arteriosus* until surgical correction can be performed.

3. *Prostaglandin E formed by the gastric mucosa suppresses gastric acid secretion.* Consequently, it reduces the risk of gastric and duodenal ulcer.

4. *PGE_2 and prostaglandin $F_{2\alpha}$ ($PGF_{2\alpha}$), synthesized in the endometrium, induce uterine contraction.* Their levels in amniotic fluid are low during pregnancy but increase massively at parturition. Together with oxytocin, *they participate in the induction of labor.* Unlike oxytocin, the prostaglandins contract the uterus not only at term of pregnancy but at all times. Therefore, *they can be used for the induction of abortion* by intravenous, intravaginal, or intra-amniotic

administration. Outside of pregnancy, the excessive formation of prostaglandins contributes to menstrual cramps.

5. *PGE_2 and TXA_2 are formed by white blood cells as mediators of inflammation.* Together with histamine, bradykinin, leukotrienes, and cytokines, they mediate the cardinal signs of inflammation.

6. *Fever is mediated by the cytokine **interleukin-1 (IL-1)**,* a product from activated monocytes and macrophages. IL-1 binds to vascular receptors in the preoptic area of the hypothalamus, where it induces the formation of PGE_2. Diffusing across the blood-brain barrier, PGE_2 causes fever by a direct action on the thermoregulatory center.

The Leukotrienes Are Produced by the Lipoxygenase Pathway

Humans have at least five different molecular forms of lipoxygenase that oxidize arachidonic acid at carbons 5, 12, or 15. The **hydroperoxyeicosatetraenoic acids (HPETEs)** formed in these reac-

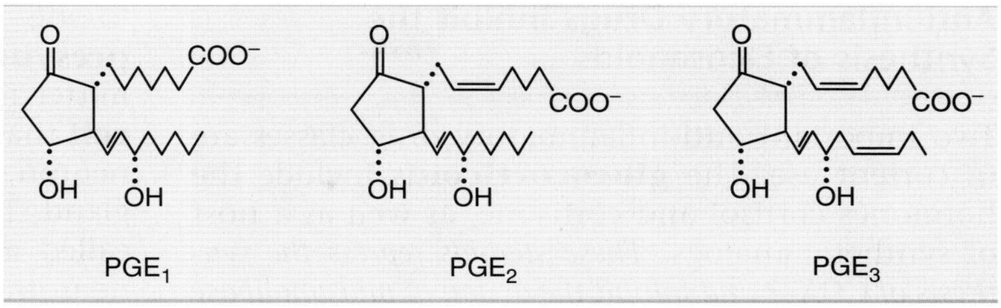

Figure 16.21 Three molecular forms of prostaglandin E (PGE). PGE$_1$ is synthesized from eicosatrienoic acid, PGE$_2$ from arachidonic acid, and PGE$_3$ from eicosapentaenoic acid.

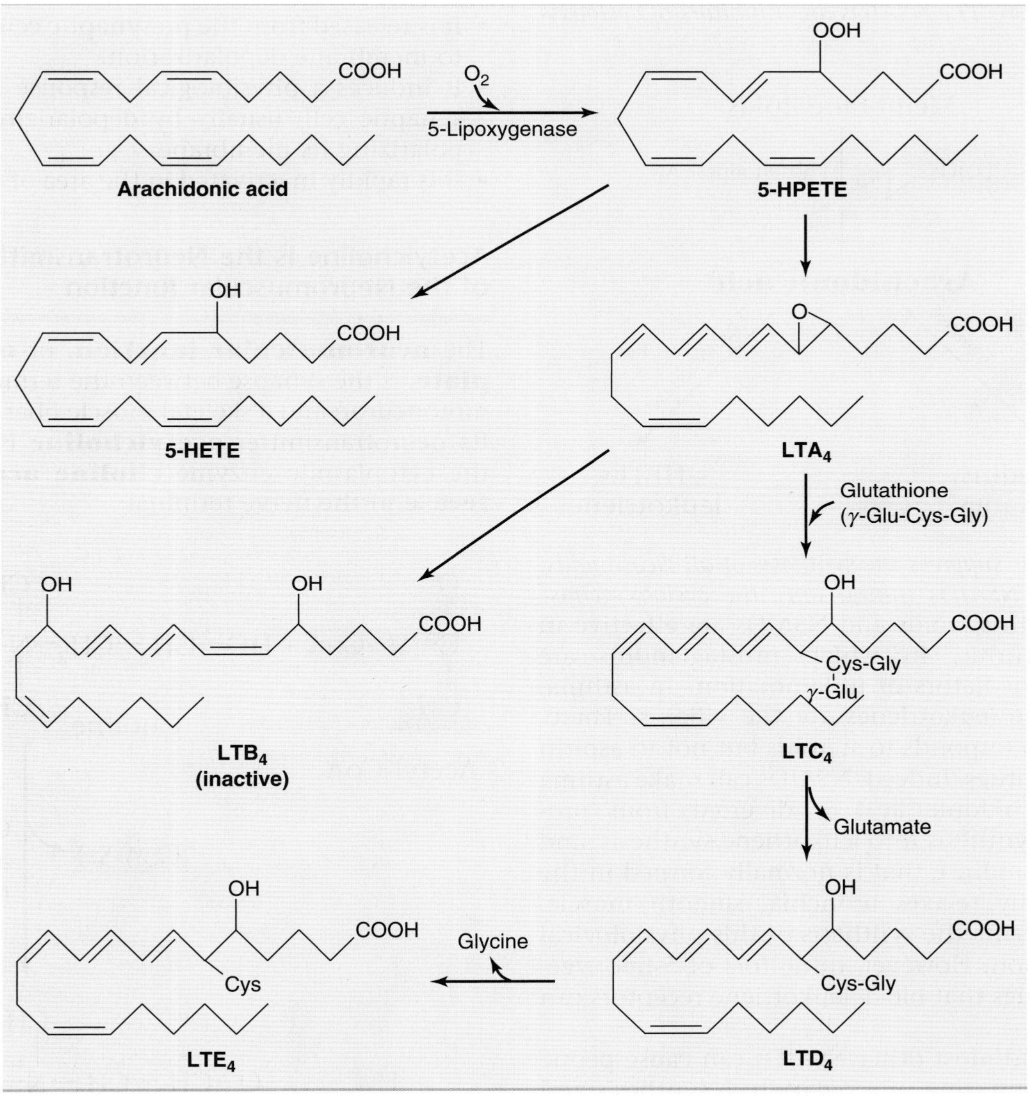

Figure 16.22 The products of 5-lipoxygenase: hydroperoxyeicosatetraenoic acid (HPETE), hydroxyeicosatetraenoic acid (HETE), and the leukotrienes (LTA$_4$, LTB$_4$, LTC$_4$, LTD$_4$, and LTE$_4$).

tions are rapidly reduced to the more stable **hydroxyeicosatetraenoic acids (HETEs),** which function as chemoattractants for white blood cells.

5-HPETE is converted to the **leukotrienes** in white blood cells and some other cells (Fig. 16.22). Leukotrienes are powerful constrictors of bronchial and intestinal smooth muscle, and they increase capillary permeability. Unlike the other eicosanoids, *the leukotrienes survive for some hours in the tissue.* Leukotrienes C$_4$, D$_4$, and E$_4$ (LTC$_4$, LTD$_4$, and LTE$_4$), which were originally characterized as the **slow-reacting substance of anaphylaxis,** are responsible for the protracted bronchoconstriction in asthma.

Anti-inflammatory Drugs Inhibit the Synthesis of Eicosanoids

Two important anti-inflammatory drug classes are in current use. The **glucocorticoids** include the hormones cortisol and cortisone, as well as a host of synthetic analogs. *These steroids repress the synthesis of COX-2 and inhibit the action of phospholipase A₂.* The **nonsteroidal anti-inflammatory drugs** (**NSAIDs**) include aspirin, indomethacin, and ibuprofen. *The NSAIDs are inhibitors of cyclooxygenase:*

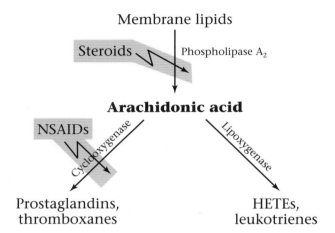

The steroids suppress the synthesis of all eicosanoids, whereas the NSAIDs inhibit only the cyclooxygenase pathway. Both steroids and NSAIDs are effective in treating arthritis, in which prostaglandins are important mediators of inflammation. In asthma, however, the leukotrienes are the villains. Therefore, asthma responds to steroids but not to aspirin and related drugs. Indeed, NSAIDs can make asthma worse. Arachidonic acid is diverted from prostaglandin synthesis into leukotriene synthesis, and the prostaglaudin E that is normally formed in the lungs actually relaxes bronchial smooth muscle. Aspirin prevents the synthesis of this physiological bronchdilation. However, inhibitors of 5-lipoxygenase and drugs that block leukotriene receptors can be effective.

Aspirin and most other NSAIDs can cause peptic ulcer by suppressing prostaglandin E synthesis and thereby increasing acid secretion in the stomach. *Selective inhibitors of COX-2 avoid this problem because they prevent prostaglandin synthesis in white blood cells but not in the stomach.*

Neurotransmitters Are Released at Synapses

While hormones and paracrine messengers broadcast their message, neurotransmitters establish one-to-one communication between two cells. The **presynaptic cell** that synthesizes the neurotransmitter is always a neuron, but the **postsynaptic cell** that responds to the neurotransmitter can be a neuron, a muscle cell, or an epithelial cell in a gland. The site of contact between the two cells is called a **synapse.** The attributes of a "classical" neurotransmitter are as follows:

- It is synthesized in the presynaptic cell.
- It is stored in membrane-bounded vesicles.
- It is released from the presynaptic cell in response to membrane depolarization.
- It induces a physiological response in the postsynaptic cell, usually by depolarizing or hyperpolarizing its membrane.
- It is rapidly inactivated in the area of the synapse.

Acetylcholine Is the Neurotransmitter of the Neuromuscular Junction

The **neuromuscular junction,** or **motor endplate,** is the synapse between the terminal of an α-motoneuron and a skeletal muscle fiber (Fig. 16.23). Its neurotransmitter **acetylcholine** is formed by the cytoplasmic enzyme **choline acetyl transferase** in the nerve terminal:

where CoA-SH = uncombined coenzyme A. Acetylcholine is packaged in synaptic vesicles (diameter, 40 nm) in the nerve terminal. When an action potential (a reversal of the membrane potential, caused by the opening of voltage-gated sodium channels) arrives in the nerve terminal, a voltage-gated calcium channel opens to allow the influx of

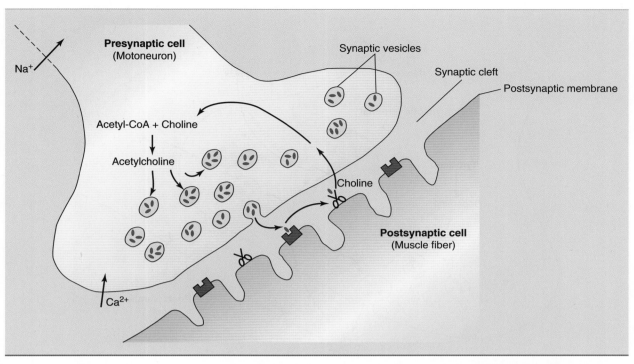

Figure 16.23 The neuromuscular junction: an example of a cholinergic synapse. ●, Acetylcholine; ■, acetylcholine receptor; ✂, acetylcholinesterase. CoA, coenzyme A.

calcium. Calcium triggers the exocytosis of acetylcholine by inducing the fusion of synaptic vesicles with the plasma membrane. *The release of neurotransmitters is always triggered by calcium.*

Within 1 millisecond, acetylcholine diffuses across the synaptic cleft, a distance of 50 nm. It binds to a receptor in the postsynaptic membrane, but *within a few milliseconds, acetylcholine is degraded by **acetylcholinesterase,** an enzyme in the basal lamina.* The catalytic mechanism of this enzyme resembles that of the serine proteases (see Chapter 4):

$$
\text{Enzyme—Ser—OH} + \underset{\text{Acetylcholine}}{\text{H}_3\text{C}-\overset{\overset{\text{CH}_3}{|}}{\underset{\underset{\text{CH}_3}{|}}{\text{N}^+}}-\text{CH}_2-\text{CH}_2-\text{O}-\overset{\overset{\text{O}}{\|}}{\text{C}}-\text{CH}_3}
$$

$$\downarrow$$

$$
\text{Enzyme—Ser—O}-\overset{\overset{\text{O}}{\|}}{\text{C}}-\text{CH}_3 \quad + \quad \underset{\text{Choline}}{\text{H}_3\text{C}-\overset{\overset{\text{CH}_3}{|}}{\underset{\underset{\text{CH}_3}{|}}{\text{N}^+}}-\text{CH}_2-\text{CH}_2-\text{OH}}
$$

$$\downarrow \text{H}_2\text{O} \quad \searrow \text{H}^+$$

$$
\text{Enzyme—Ser—OH} + {}^-\text{O}-\overset{\overset{\text{O}}{\|}}{\text{C}}-\text{CH}_3
$$

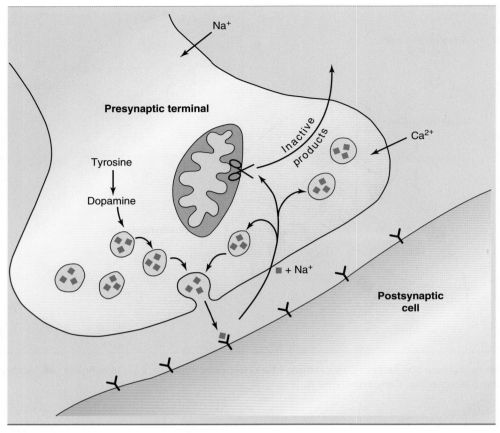

Figure 16.24 A noradrenergic synapse. The transmitter is taken up into the presynaptic nerve terminal by sodium-dependent, high-affinity uptake. Once in the nerve terminal, it is either recycled into the synaptic vesicles or degraded by monoamine oxidase (MAO). Υ, Postsynaptic receptor; ■, norepinephrine; ✕, MAO.

This reaction takes place in the synaptic cleft. The breakdown products, choline and acetate, are rapidly taken up into the nerve terminal, where they are used for the resynthesis of acetylcholine.

There Are Many Neurotransmitters

Catecholamines, 5-HT, and histamine are also used as neurotransmitters. Like acetylcholine, they are stored in synaptic vesicles and released by a depolarization-induced, calcium-dependent mechanism.

Their synaptic inactivation, however, is different. Unlike acetylcholine, *the biogenic amines are not degraded in the synaptic cleft but removed from their receptors by sodium-dependent, high-affinity uptake back into the nerve terminal.* Once back in its home cell, the amine can be repackaged into synaptic vesicles. Alternatively, it is degraded by MAO, the major inactivating enzyme in nervous tissue (Fig. 16.24).

Only 1% to 2% of the neurons in the brain use a catecholamine or 5-HT as their neurotransmitter, and perhaps another 2% use acetylcholine. Amino acids are far more popular. **Glutamate** and **aspartate** are the major excitatory neurotransmitters in the central nervous system, and **glycine** is an important inhibitory neurotransmitter in the spinal cord and brain stem. These amino acids are recruited as neurotransmitters simply by being packaged into synaptic vesicles. *Their actions are terminated by sodium-dependent, high-affinity uptake* without the need for synthesizing and inactivating enzymes.

γ-Aminobutyric acid (GABA) is the most important inhibitory neurotransmitter in the brain. It is produced by the decarboxylation of glutamate. Its use in the nerve terminal is described in Figure 16.25.

Small peptides, such as the enkephalins, are also used as neurotransmitters. Their high-molecular-weight precursors are synthesized at the rough ER

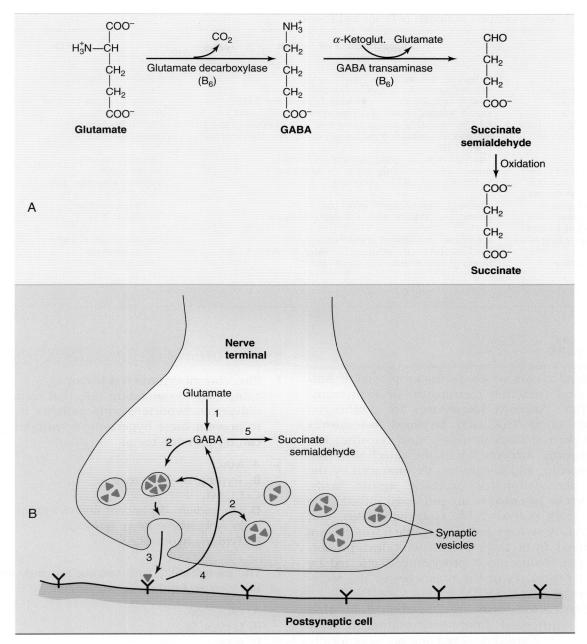

Figure 16.25 Metabolism of γ-aminobutyric acid (GABA). **A,** Reactions. **B,** Compartmentation. ①, Glutamate decarboxylase; ②, vesicular storage; ③, release by exocytosis; ④, sodium-dependent, high-affinity uptake; ⑤, GABA transaminase. ▼, GABA; Υ, postsynaptic receptors.

in the perikaryon, packaged into vesicles, and transported to the nerve endings by fast axoplasmic transport. En route, the active transmitter is released from its precursor protein by proteolytic cleavages. Peptide neurotransmitters are inactivated by enzymes on the surface of neurons and glial cells.

Neurotransmitter systems mediate the actions of many drugs and toxins. Some examples are listed in Table 16.3.

Table 16.3 Neurotrasmitters as Targets of Drugs and Toxins

Agent	Mechanism of Action	Effects
Drugs		
L-Dopa	Catecholamine precursor	Antiparkinsonian
MAO inhibitors	Inhibit degradation of catecholamines and 5-HT	Antidepressant
Reserpine	Inhibits vesicular storage of catecholamines and 5-HT	Antihypertensive, sedative, depressant
Tricyclics	Inhibit synaptic uptake of norepinephrine and/or 5-HT	Antidepressant
Cocaine	Inhibits synaptic uptake of dopamine, norepinephrine, and 5-HT	Psychostimulant
Amphetamine	Releases nonvesicular (cytoplasmic) dopamine, norepinephrine, and 5-HT	Psychostimulant
Opiates	Agonist action on opiate (endorphin) receptors	Narcotic analgesic
Neuroleptics	Antagonist action on D_2 dopamine receptors	Antipsychotic
Benzodiazepines	Sensitization of GABA-A receptors	Sedative, anxiolytic, anticonvulsant
Bacterial toxins		
Tetanus toxin	Inhibits glycine release in spinal cord	Lockjaw, convulsions
Botulinum toxin	Inhibits acetylcholine release at motor endplate	Flaccid paralysis
Chemical toxins		
Organophosphates	Irreversible inhibition of acetylcholinesterase	Autonomic nervous effects, CNS effects
Curare	Blocks acetylcholine receptors in neuromuscular junction	Flaccid paralysis
Strychnine	Blocks glycine receptors in spinal cord	Convulsions

CNS, central nervous system; GABA, γ-aminobutyric acid; 5-HT, 5-hydroxytryptamine; MAD, monoamine oxidase.

SUMMARY

Several classes of agents are employed as hormones, paracrine messengers, or neurotransmitters. **Steroid hormones** are synthesized from cholesterol, and **thyroid hormones** are derived from protein-bound tyrosine. The **biogenic amines,** including catecholamines, serotonin, and histamine, are produced by the decarboxylation of aromatic amino acids. **Protein hormones** are processed through the secretory pathway: ER, Golgi apparatus, and secretory vesicles. Smaller peptide hormones are derived from large precursors called prohormones. Prohormone processing is effected by endopeptidases in the organelles of the secretory pathway.

The **eicosanoids** are 20-carbon lipids that are synthesized from polyunsaturated fatty acids. Most are short-lived and act only locally in their tissue of origin. They are important mediators of inflammation, and agents that inhibit their synthesis are important anti-inflammatory drugs.

Neurotransmitters transmit signals at synapses. Acetylcholine, the biogenic amines, some amino acids, and a variety of peptides are used as neurotransmitters.

📖 Further Reading

Funk CD: Prostaglandins and leukotrienes: advances in eicosanoid biology. Science 294:1871-1875, 2001.

QUESTIONS

1. **Pheochromocytoma is a tumor of catecholamine-secreting cells that causes dangerous hypertension in patients. In order to prevent these hypertensive episodes, you can try an inhibitor of**

   A. MAO.
   B. Tryptophan hydroxylase.
   C. COMT.
   D. The sodium-dependent norepinephrine carrier in sympathetic nerve terminals.
   E. Tyrosine hydroxylase.

2. **The pancreatic β cells secrete not only insulin but also an equimolar amount of**

   A. Glucagon.
   B. C-peptide.
   C. Renin.
   D. Proopiomelanocortin.
   E. Enkephalin.

3. **The adrenal cortex contains a sizable collection of enzymes for steroid hormone synthesis. Two of these enzymes are required for the synthesis of glucocorticoids but not androgens, and therefore their deficiency leads to an overproduction of adrenal androgens. These two enzymes are**

   A. Cyclooxygenase and 17-hydroxylase.
   B. Desmolase and cytochrome P-450.
   C. 11β-Hydroxylase and 21-hydroxylase.
   D. 17-Hydroxylase and adrenodoxin.
   E. 18-Hydroxylase and aromatase.

4. Inhibitors of lipoxygenase can be used for the treatment of asthma because they prevent the formation of

   A. Prostaglandins.
   B. GABA.
   C. Thromboxanes.
   D. Prostacyclin.
   E. Leukotrienes.

CHAPTER 17

Intracellular Messengers

A key is useless without a matching lock, and a hormone or other extracellular signaling molecule is useless without a matching receptor. The receptor is an allosteric protein that changes its conformation when it binds the signaling molecule. Messengers that do not enter the cell activate receptors in the plasma membrane, and those that can enter activate receptors in the cytoplasm or nucleus (Fig. 17.1).

Receptor binding triggers an intracellular signaling cascade with protein-protein interactions and enzymatic reactions. *The phosphorylation of cellular proteins by protein kinases is a recurrent feature of hormonally induced signaling cascades.* Eventually, the cascade has to impinge on genes, ion channels, and/or metabolic enzymes to induce a physiological response. This chapter describes the most important receptor mechanisms and signaling cascades.

Receptor-Hormone Interactions Are Noncovalent, Reversible, and Saturable

Like the binding of a substrate to its enzyme (see Chapter 4) or an antigen to its antibody (see Chapter 15), *hormone-receptor binding is always noncovalent.* Being noncovalent, it is reversible. The receptor-hormone complex ($R \cdot H$) can easily dissociate back into free receptor (R) and free hormone (H):

$$R \cdot H \underset{k_1}{\overset{k_1}{\rightleftharpoons}} R + H$$

The **dissociation constant K_D** of the receptor-hormone complex is defined as

$$K_D = \frac{[R] \times [H]}{[R \cdot H]} = \frac{k_1}{k_{-1}}$$

$$\frac{K_D}{[H]} = \frac{[R]}{[R \cdot H]}$$

The K_D corresponds to the hormone concentration [H] at which half the receptor molecules are converted to receptor-hormone complex. Thus, it describes the affinity between hormone and receptor, just as the Michaelis constant describes the affinity between enzyme and substrate. Dissociation constants between 10^{-9} and 10^{-11} mol/liter are typical for hormone-receptor interactions.

Hormone binding shows *saturation kinetics* (Fig. 17.2). At a hormone concentration far above the K_D, almost all receptors are occupied. The physiological response is near maximal and cannot be augmented by adding even more hormone. This is equivalent to zero-order kinetics for enzymes. The **maximal binding (B_{max})** corresponds to the number of receptor molecules in the cell.

Many Neurotransmitter Receptors Are Ion Channels

The job of a neurotransmitter is to change the membrane potential of the postsynaptic cell and to do it fast. Rather than triggering lengthy signaling cascades, the transmitter should act as directly as possible on the ion channels that determine the membrane potential. *The fastest and most direct mechanism is the binding of the neurotransmitter to a ligand-gated ion channel in the plasma membrane.*

The **nicotinic acetylcholine receptor** in the neuromuscular junction, for example, is a channel for the monovalent cations sodium and potassium (Fig. 17.3). It consists of five membrane-spanning

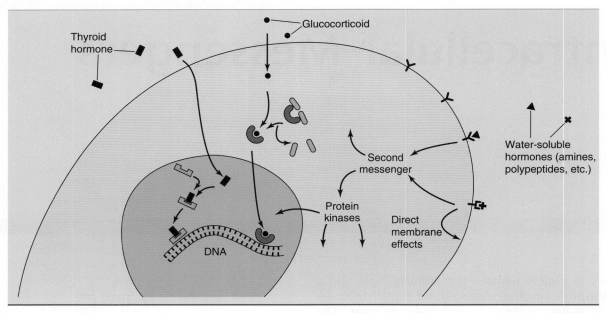

Figure 17.1 Cellular locations of receptors for hormones and other extracellular messengers. ▭, Thyroid hormone receptor; ◡, glucocorticoid receptor; Ψ and Y, cell surface receptors.

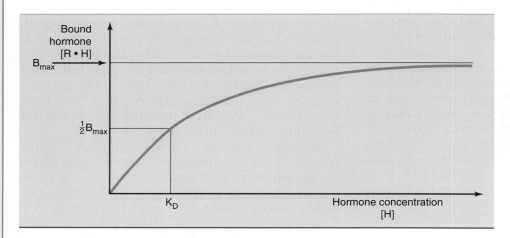

Figure 17.2 Receptor (R) binding at various hormone (H) concentrations. The maximal binding B_{max} corresponds to the total number of receptors.

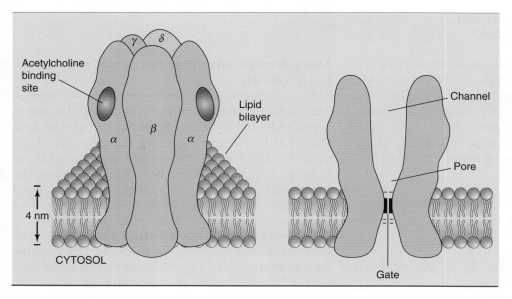

Figure 17.3 Structure of the nicotinic acetylcholine receptor in the neuromuscular junction. This receptor is a ligand-gated channel for small cations (Na^+, K^+). Acetylcholine binds with positive cooperativity to the two α subunits. Each of the five polypeptides traverses the membrane four times, and one of the transmembrane helices in each subunit contributes to the "gate" in the channel.

subunits with the subunit structure α_2, β, γ, and δ. Each of the subunits has four transmembrane helices, and one helix of each subunit lines the central pore of the channel. The α subunits contain binding sites for acetylcholine facing the extracellular space. *The channel is closed in the resting state, opening only when acetylcholine binds.* Opening of the channel allows the influx of sodium into the cell, which depolarizes the membrane.

There is a whole family of ligand-gated ion channels. They all consist of five subunits but differ in their ligand-binding specificities and ionic selectivities. In most cases, *excitatory neurotransmitters open sodium or calcium channels, and inhibitory neurotransmitters open chloride or potassium channels.*

The ligand-gated ion channels come in many different variants. The subunits of the nicotinic acetylcholine receptors in the brain, for example, are slightly different from those of the receptor in the neuromuscular junction. Indeed, different populations of neurons possess different combinations of subunits that are either encoded by separate genes or obtained by alternative splicing.

This diversity is important for drug development. **Nicotine,** for example, stimulates nicotinic receptors in the brain but not in the neuromuscular junction, and the arrow poison **curare** blocks nicotinic receptors in the neuromuscular junction but not in the brain. A drug that activates a receptor is called an **agonist,** and a drug that blocks a receptor is called an **antagonist.** *Like enzymes, receptors are subject to competitive, noncompetitive, and irreversible inhibition by drugs and toxins.*

The Receptors for Steroid and Thyroid Hormones Are Transcription Factors

Unlike neurotransmitters, the steroid and thyroid hormones can diffuse across membranes and activate receptors in the cytoplasm or the nucleus. For example, the glucocorticoid receptor resides in the cytoplasm, complexed to cytoplasmic proteins that mask its DNA-binding domain. These proteins are released when the hormone binds.

Along with the bound hormone, *the activated receptor translocates to the nucleus, where it binds to **hormone response elements (HREs)** in the promoters and enhancers of genes.* Approximately 1% of all genes have glucocorticoid response elements in their regulatory sites. This implies two levels of targeting: *Only cells that possess the receptor can respond to the hormone, and within the cell, only genes that possess the appropriate response element are regulated by the hormone.*

The receptors for steroid hormones, thyroid hormones, retinoic acid, and calcitriol all belong to the same superfamily of hormone-regulated transcription factors. All are zinc finger proteins that bind their response elements in a dimeric form, although the details of their subcellular location and receptor activation are different in different cases. For example, unstimulated thyroid hormone receptors are intranuclear rather than cytoplasmic.

An inherited deficiency of a receptor makes the cells unable to respond to the matching hormone. A defective androgen receptor, for example, causes **testicular feminization.** Genetically male individuals with this condition are externally female, and their psychosexual development is also feminine. However, they possess testes rather than ovaries, and the müllerian duct structures (uterus and fallopian tubes) are absent. Although they have androgens both during fetal development and in later life, they develop as phenotypically female because the target tissues cannot respond to the male hormones.

The Seven-Transmembrane Receptors Are Coupled to G Proteins

Being unable to enter their target cells, water-soluble hormones have to deliver their message at the cell surface. Their receptors are integral membrane proteins with three functional domains. The *extracellular domain* binds the hormone; one or several *transmembrane α-helices* penetrate the lipid bilayer; and the *intracellular domain* is coupled with an effector mechanism.

Most hormone receptors belong to a family of membrane proteins with seven membrane-spanning α-helices (Fig. 17.4). These criss-crossing proteins do not form a channel or possess enzymatic activities. They trigger signaling cascades by activating a guanine nucleotide–binding protein, or **G protein.**

The G protein is loosely bound to the cytoplasmic surface of the plasma membrane, and it consists of three subunits designated α (molecular weight [MW], 45,000), β (MW, 35,000) and γ (MW, 7000). The α subunit has a nucleotide binding site that can accommodate either GDP or GTP. β and γ subunits function as a single unit, but the α subunit is only loosely associated with $\beta\gamma$.

The function of the G protein is described in Figure 17.5. The inactive G protein is associated with the unstimulated receptor, with GDP bound to the α subunit. Hormone binding induces a conformational change both in the receptor and the attached G protein. This conformational change greatly reduces the affinity of the α subunit for GDP. GDP dissociates away and is quickly replaced by GTP.

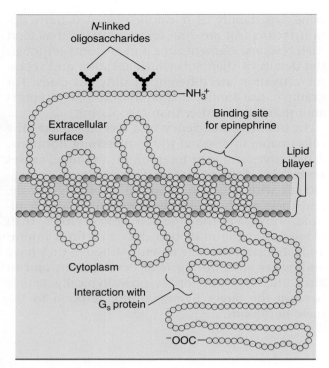

Figure 17.4 The β-adrenergic receptor is an integral membrane protein with seven membrane-spanning α helices. Note that the binding site for β-adrenergic agonists is on the extracellular side, whereas the binding site for the G_s protein is on the cytoplasmic side of the plasma membrane. All G protein–coupled receptors resemble the β-adrenergic receptor in their amino acid sequence and membrane topography.

Once GTP is bound, the G protein leaves the receptor and breaks up into the α-GTP subunit and the βγ complex. Both the α-GTP subunit and βγ complex diffuse along the inner surface of the plasma membrane, where they bind to target proteins that are known as **effectors.** *The components of the activated G protein are membrane-bound messengers that transmit a signal from the receptor to the effector.*

The α subunit possesses a GTPase activity that is stimulated by its interaction with the effector. As a result, *the α subunit quickly hydrolyzes its bound GTP to GDP and inorganic phosphate.* GDP remains bound to the α subunit, but the α-GDP complex no longer acts on the effector. Rather than transmitting a signal, it returns home to the βγ complex and the hormone receptor. *All G proteins exist in two forms: an active GTP-bound form that acts on the effector and an inactive GDP-bound form that does not.*

The α, β, and γ subunits come in many different molecular forms that are encoded by separate genes and are expressed in various combinations in different cells. G protein are classified according to the structure and function of their α subunit. For example, in the G_s proteins, the α subunit–GTP complex stimulates adenylate cyclase, and in the G_i proteins, it inhibits adenylate cyclase.

However, the βγ subunits can also transmit signals. The myocardium, for example, has a muscarinic acetylcholine receptor that is linked to a G_i protein. The βγ-complex of this G_i protein binds to a potassium channel in the plasma membrane, opening it and thereby hyperpolarizing the membrane. Through this mechanism, the acetylcholine released from the vagus nerve slows down the heart.

Adenylate Cyclase Is Regulated by G Proteins

Hormone-activated G proteins carry messages along the plasma membrane, but they do not travel across the cytoplasm. *To send a signal into the interior of the cell, the G protein has to induce the synthesis of a small, diffusible molecule known as a* **second messenger.**

One of the more important second messengers is **cyclic adenosine monophosphate (cAMP)**. It is synthesized from adenosine triphosphate (ATP) by **adenylate cyclase,** a hormone-controlled enzyme in the plasma membrane:

$$\text{ATP} \xrightarrow[\text{(plasma membrane)}]{\text{Adenylate cyclase}} \text{cAMP} + \text{PP}_i$$

The rapid hydrolysis of pyrophosphate (PP_i) by cellular pyrophosphatases makes this reaction irreversible. Humans have nine isoenzymes of adenylate cyclase with somewhat different regulatory properties, each encoded by a different gene. All are integral membrane proteins with 12 transmembrane helices. *The adenylate cyclases are stimulated by the $α_s$ subunit of the G_s proteins.*

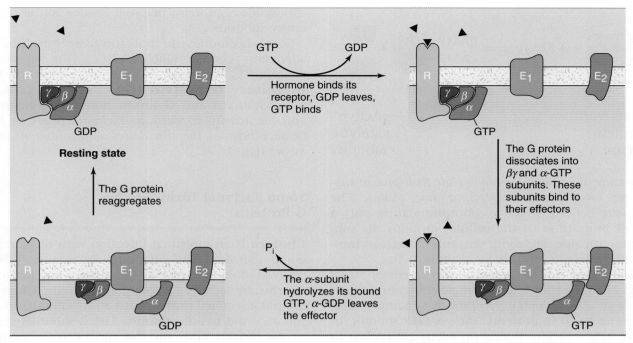

Figure 17.5 Coupling of a hormone receptor (R) to effector proteins (E_1, E_2) in the plasma membrane through a G protein. By an allosteric mechanism, the activation of the receptor causes GDP–GTP exchange and the dissociation of the heterotrimeric G protein into βγ and α-GTP subunits. These subunits act allosterically on the effectors. The action on the effector is terminated when the α subunit hydrolyzes its bound GTP. The most important effectors of hormone-regulated G proteins are second messenger–synthesizing enzymes such as adenylate cyclase and phospholipase C, but some calcium and potassium channels also are regulated by this mechanism.

cAMP is degraded by a group of enzymes that are collectively known as **phosphodiesterases:**

cAMP

H₂O → Phosphodiesterase

AMP

The human genome contains at least 20 different phosphodiesterase genes, and because of differential splicing, humans have no fewer than 50 different phosphodiesterases in all. Most of them are inhibited by **methylxanthines,** including caffeine, theophylline, and aminophylline. These drugs potentiate the effects of cAMP. After a person drinks a cup of coffee, for example, the level of plasma free fatty acids rises because fat breakdown in adipose tissue is stimulated by cAMP.

*The most important target of cAMP is **protein kinase A.*** In the absence of cAMP, two catalytic subunits of this enzyme are tightly bound to two regulatory subunits. This form of the enzyme is inactive. The two regulatory subunits have no enzymatic activity, but they can bind up to four cAMP molecules. This induces a conformational change that leads to the release of active catalytic subunits as shown on the following page:

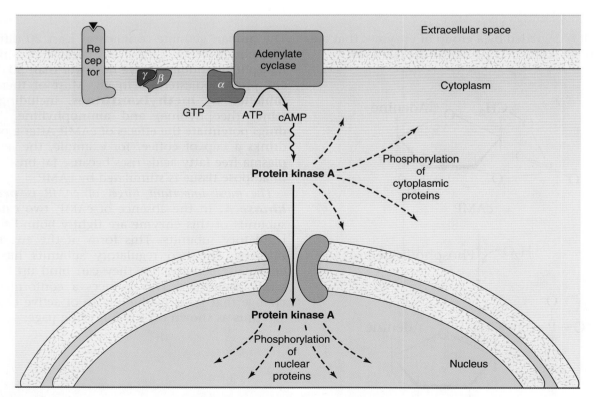

$$\text{R C} \;/\; \text{R C} \;+\; 4\ \text{cAMP} \;\rightleftharpoons\; \begin{matrix}\text{cAMP}-\text{R}\\\text{cAMP}-\text{R}\end{matrix} \;+\; \begin{matrix}\text{C}\\\text{C}\end{matrix}$$

Inactive
protein
kinase A

Active
catalytic
subunits

The catalytic subunits phosphorylate their protein substrates on serine and threonine side chains. The enzyme is quite selective, phosphorylating only a small proportion of the cellular proteins. Its substrates include metabolic enzymes, nuclear transcription factors, and many other proteins.

The cAMP cascade amplifies the hormonal signal (Fig. 17.6). The binding of a single epinephrine molecule to a β-adrenergic receptor, for example, activates up to 20 G_s proteins. Each α_s-GTP subunit, in turn, acts sufficiently long on adenylate cyclase to cause the synthesis of hundreds of cAMP molecules. Although four cAMP molecules are sufficient to activate two catalytic subunits of protein kinase A, each active subunit phosphorylates hundreds or thousands of proteins before it returns to the regulatory subunits.

Some hormones do not stimulate but inhibit adenylate cyclase (Table 17.1). This negative coupling is mediated by the α_i subunit of an **inhibitory G protein (G_i).** Most cells possess both G_s-linked and G_i-linked hormone receptors, and *the activity of adenylate cyclase depends on the balance between the stimulatory and inhibitory hormones* (Fig. 17.7).

Some Bacterial Toxins Modify G Proteins

Cholera is an intestinal infection with life-threatening diarrhea. The offending bacterium, *Vibrio cholerae,* does not invade the tissues but induces diarrhea by secreting a potent enterotoxin. Cholera toxin is a secreted protein with an A_1 subunit, an A_2 subunit, and five B subunits. The B subunits bind to ganglioside GM_1 on the surface of intestinal mucosal cells. The A_1 subunit then enters the cell, where it acts as an enzyme, catalyzing the covalent modification of an arginine side chain in the α subunit of the G_s protein:

Figure 17.6 The cyclic adenosine monophosphate (cAMP) cascade. Receptor and adenylate cyclase are coupled by the stimulatory G protein (G_s), which consists of the α_s, β, and γ subunits. All known cAMP effects in humans are mediated by protein kinase A. This protein kinase phosphorylates a variety of proteins in the cytoplasm and the nucleus.

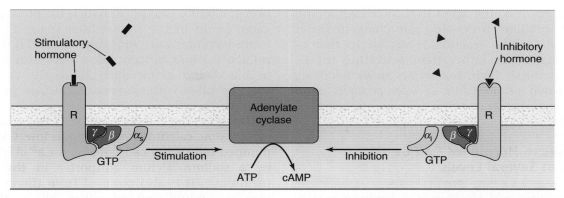

Figure 17.7 Regulation of adenylate cyclase by the α subunits of the stimulatory and inhibitory G proteins. Some isoforms of adenylate cyclase are affected by βγ-complexes of the G proteins as well. R, Receptor.

Table 17.1 Roles of Cyclic Adenosine Monophosphate (cAMP) in Different Tissues

Tissue/Cell Type	Agents Increasing cAMP	Agents Decreasing cAMP	Effects of Elevated cAMP
Liver	Glucagon, epinephrine	Insulin*	Glycogen degradation, gluconeogenesis
Skeletal muscle	Epinephrine	—	Glycogen degradation, glycolysis
Adipose tissue	Epinephrine	Insulin*	Lipolysis
Renal tubular epithelium	Antidiuretic hormone	—	Water reabsorption
Intestinal mucosa	Vasoactive intestinal polypeptide, adenosine, epinephrine	Endorphins	Water and electrolyte secretion
Vascular smooth muscle	Epinephrine (β receptor)	Epinephrine (α_2 receptor)	Relaxation, growth inhibition
Bronchial smooth muscle	Epinephrine (β receptor)	—	Relaxation
Platelets	Prostacyclin, prostaglandin E	ADP	Maintenance of inactive state
Adrenal cortex	ACTH	—	Hormone secretion
Melanocytes	MSH	Melatonin	Melanin synthesis
Thyroid gland	TSH	—	Hormone secretion

* Insulin does not act through a G protein; it decreases cAMP levels by alternative routes.
ACTH, adrenocorticotropic hormone; MSH, melanocyte-stimulating hormone; TSH, thyroid-stimulating hormone.

$$\alpha_s - \text{Arg} + \begin{array}{cc} \text{Nicotinamide} & \text{Adenine} \\ | & | \\ \text{Ribose} - \text{P} - \text{P} - \text{Ribose} \end{array}$$

$$\downarrow$$

$$\begin{array}{c} \alpha_s \\ | \\ \text{Arg} \\ | \\ \text{Ribose} \\ | \\ \text{P} \\ | \\ \text{P} \\ | \\ \text{Nicotinamide} + \text{Ribose} - \text{Adenine} \end{array}$$

The modified α subunit can still bind GTP and stimulate adenylate cyclase, but its GTPase activity is lost. As a result, *the G_s protein is locked in the active, GTP-bound form.* With continued stimulation of adenylate cyclase, *the cell is soon flooded with cAMP.*

Fortunately, cholera toxin is not carried to distant organs but its effects remain confined to the intestine. In the intestinal mucosa, however, the overabundance of cAMP causes the profuse secretion of water and electrolytes.

One of the toxins of enterotoxigenic *Escherichia coli* also acts by covalent modification of the G_s protein. This bacterium causes the dreaded traveler's diarrhea, known locally under names like Tehranitis, Kabulitis, and Montezuma's revenge. The best treatment for traveler's diarrhea is opium taken by mouth. Opiate receptors are coupled to the G_i protein (see Table 17.1). Through the G_i protein, opium antagonizes the out-of-control G_s protein.

The inhibitory G protein is the target of another bacterial toxin. **Pertussis toxin** is produced by

Bordetella pertussis, the agent that causes whooping cough. It modifies a cysteine side chain in the α subunit of G_i. The reaction is similar to that of cholera toxin, but rather than activating the G_i protein, pertussis toxin inactivates it. *By inhibiting the inhibition of adenylate cyclase, pertussis toxin causes overproduction of cAMP.*

Responses to Hormones Can Be Blocked at Several Levels

The pharmacological blockage of a hormone receptor prevents the hormone from acting on the cell. β-Adrenergic receptor blockers, for example, make adipose cells unable to form cAMP and to break down their stored fat in response to epinephrine. However, if the cell possesses receptors for other G_s-coupled hormones such as adrenocorticotropic hormone (ACTH), glucagon, or β-lipotropin, then these hormones can still induce cAMP synthesis and fat breakdown.

A defective or inhibited G_s or G_i protein, on the other hand, makes the cell unable to respond to *any* hormone that is coupled to the faulty G protein. This occurs in **pseudohypoparathyroidism.** Patients with this inherited disorder have hypocalcemia, like patients with true hypoparathyroidism, but their parathyroid hormone (PTH) level is either normal or elevated.

Some of these patients have an abnormal G_s protein that couples poorly between the PTH receptor and adenylate cyclase. Many patients with this disorder have associated abnormalities, including short stature and poor intellectual development, because the actions of many other hormones are impaired as well.

The abnormal activation of a G protein can also lead to problems. In the thyroid gland, thyroid-stimulating hormone (TSH) stimulates hormone synthesis and cell proliferation through cAMP. On occasion, a thyroid follicular cell undergoes a somatic mutation that makes the α subunit of the G_s protein unable to hydrolyze its bound GTP. This abnormal G_s protein is always in the active form and keeps stimulating adenylate cyclase. The result is a **toxic nodule:** a small benign tumor that secretes an inordinate amount of thyroid hormone.

Cytoplasmic Calcium Is an Important Intracellular Signal

The extracellular calcium concentration is of the order of 2 mmol/liter, but its cytoplasmic concentration is only 0.2 μmol/liter. The most elementary reason for maintaining this 10,000-fold concentra-

tion gradient is that phosphate is the principal inorganic anion in the intracellular space. Phosphate forms insoluble salts with calcium, and if the intracellular calcium concentration were similar to that in blood and extracellular fluid, the cell would soon be filled with obnoxious calcium phosphate crystals.

Therefore, the cell goes out of its way to keep the cytoplasmic calcium concentration low. Calcium is pumped out of the cell both by a Ca^{2+}-ATPase and by a sodium-calcium antiporter in the plasma membrane. It is also pumped from the cytoplasm into the endoplasmic reticulum (ER) by the Ca^{2+}-ATPase. Indeed, the calcium concentration in the ER approximates that in the extracellular fluid.

External signals can trigger a transient rise of the cytoplasmic calcium concentration. They can achieve this by several mechanisms:

1. *The extracellular messenger opens a ligand-gated calcium channel in the plasma membrane.* The *N*-methyl-D-aspartate (NMDA) type of glutamate receptor in the brain is a ligand-gated calcium channel.
2. *A receptor-coupled G protein opens a calcium channel in the plasma membrane.* Myocardial cells, for example, possess a voltage-gated calcium channel that is positively regulated by the α subunit of the G_s protein in response to norepinephrine.
3. *A stimulus depolarizes the plasma membrane, thereby opening voltage-gated calcium channels.* In nerve terminals, for example, depolarization induces transmitter release by opening voltage-gated calcium channels in the plasma membrane of the nerve terminal (see Chapter 16). Also, the plasma membrane of smooth muscle cells is riddled with voltage-gated calcium channels. They are the targets of the **calcium channel blockers.** These drugs are used for the treatment of hypertension, vasospastic disorders, angina pectoris, and cardiac arrhythmias.
4. *A hormone induces the release of calcium from the ER.* This mechanism is discussed as follows.

Phospholipase C Generates Two Second Messengers

Most calcium-elevating hormones trigger the release of calcium from the ER. The signaling cascade starts with a hormone receptor of the 7-transmembrane type that is coupled to a G protein of the G_q family. This type of G protein does not act on adenylate cyclase; instead it activates a **phospholipase C** that is specific for inositol-containing phosphoglycerides.

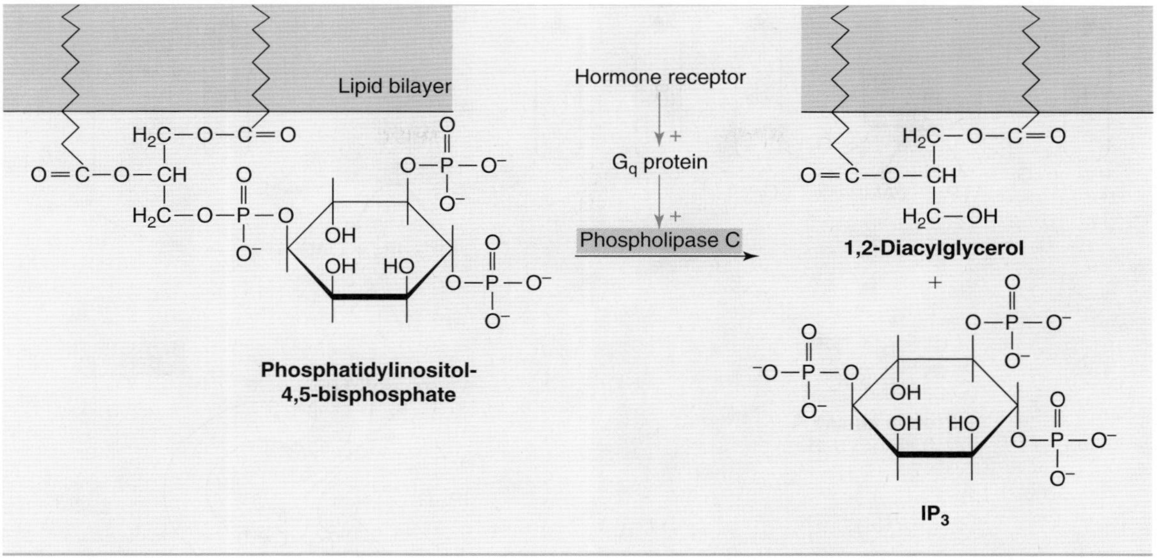

Figure 17.8 Formation of the second messengers 1,2-diacylglycerol and inositol-1,4,5-trisphosphate (IP$_3$) from phosphatidylinositol-4,5-bisphosphate. The *green arrows* represent allosteric stimulation.

The hormone-stimulated phospholipase C acts on phosphatidylinositol and related lipids in the inner leaflet of the plasma membrane. Phosphatidylinositol-4,5-bisphosphate is the most important substrate because its cleavage forms the second messengers **1,2-diacylglycerol** and **inositol-1,4,5-trisphosphate** (**IP$_3$**) (Fig. 17.8).

1,2-Diacylglycerol remains membrane bound but diffuses laterally in the inner leaflet of the lipid bilayer. In the presence of calcium and phosphatidylserine, it activates the membrane-associated enzyme **protein kinase C** (Fig. 17.9). Like protein kinase A, protein kinase C phosphorylates serine and threonine side chains in proteins. Although some proteins can be phosphorylated by both, the substrate specificities of the two kinases are quite different.

Protein kinase C promotes the proliferation of many cells. **Phorbol esters,** which are naturally present in croton oil, act as tumor promoters by activating protein kinase C.

IP$_3$ is a soluble messenger that can diffuse across the cytoplasm. *It raises cytoplasmic calcium by opening a calcium channel in the ER membrane.* IP$_3$ is inactivated by successive dephosphorylations, either directly or after an initial phosphorylation to inositol-1,3,4,5-tetrakisphosphate.

Calcium induces its effects by binding to specific regulatory proteins. **Troponin C** has already been described as a calcium sensor on the thin filaments of striated muscle (see Chapter 13). The structurally related **calmodulin** (MW, 17,000) is present in all nucleated cells. In a Ca^{2+} concentration range of 10^{-7} mol to 10^{-6} mol, *calmodulin forms a calcium complex that functions as an activator of many enzymes.* The Ca^{2+}-calmodulin–regulated enzymes include a family of protein kinases that phosphorylate serine and threonine side chains but with substrate specificities different from those of protein kinases A and C.

Both cAMP and Calcium Regulate Gene Transcription

The catalytic subunits of protein kinase A are able to translocate to the nucleus, where they phosphorylate several transcription factors, including the **cAMP response element–binding (CREB) protein.** These transcription factors form homodimers and heterodimers that bind to the **cAMP response element,** a palindromic sequence (TGACGTCA) in the promoters and enhancers of the cAMP-regulated genes. CREB is always bound to the response element, but *it stimulates transcription only after the phosphorylation of a single serine residue (Ser^{133}) by protein kinase A* (Fig. 17.10).

The calcium-dependent **calmodulin kinase II (CaMK II)** phosphorylates a different serine residue (Ser^{142}) in CREB, but this phosphorylation prevents transcriptional activation. Both CaMK II and another Ca^{2+}-calmodulin–dependent protein kinase, CaMK IV, can also phosphorylate Ser^{133} and thereby activate transcription. As a result, *calcium can act either synergistically or antagonistically with cAMP in the regulation of gene expression,* depending on the Ca^{2+}-calmodulin–regulated protein kinases that are present in the cell.

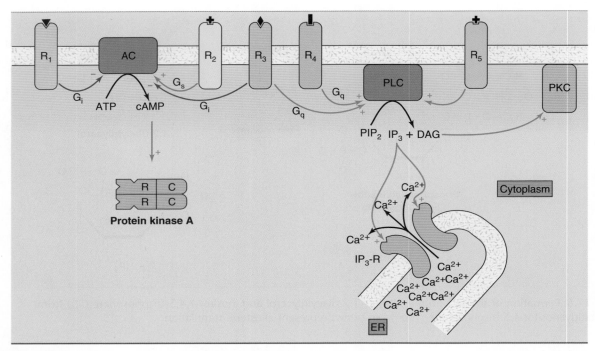

Figure 17.9 G protein–coupled receptors (R$_1$, R$_2$, and so forth) and their second messenger systems. Note that more than one hormone receptor can couple to an effector in the plasma membrane (●). The effector produces the second messenger, and the second messenger stimulates intracellular targets (▭). Note also that some receptors can couple to more than one G protein (G$_i$ and G$_q$ in the case of R$_3$) and thereby act on different effectors. AC, adenylate cyclase; ATP, adenosine triphosphate; cAMP, cyclic adenosine monophosphate; DAG, 1,2-diacylglycerol; IP$_3$, inositol-1,4,5-trisphosphate; IP$_3$-R, IP$_3$ receptor (an IP$_3$-regulated calcium channel in the endoplasmic reticulum [ER]); PIP$_2$, phosphatidylinositol-4,5-bisphosphate; PLC, phosphatidylinositol-specific phospholipase C; PKC, protein kinase C.

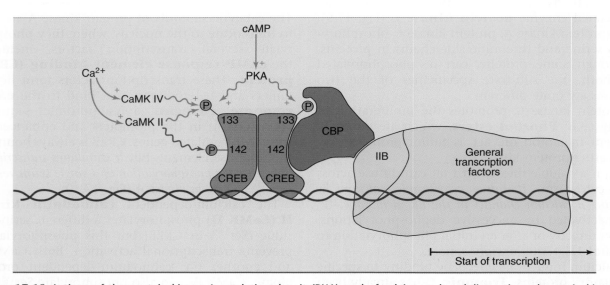

Figure 17.10 Actions of the protein kinase A catalytic subunit (PKA) and of calcium-calmodulin–activated protein kinases (CaMK II, CaMK IV) on the cyclic adenosine monophosphate (cAMP) response element–binding (CREB) protein, which mediates cAMP effects on transcription. The phosphorylation of Ser[133] is thought to induce transcription through a CREB-binding protein (CBP) that binds both to phosphorylated CREB and to transcription factor IIB in the transcriptional initiation complex. The phosphorylation of Ser[142] is thought to prevent this interaction. *Straight arrow* indicates allosteric stimulation; *green wavy arrow,* activating phosphorylation; *red wavy arrow,* inhibitory phosphorylation.

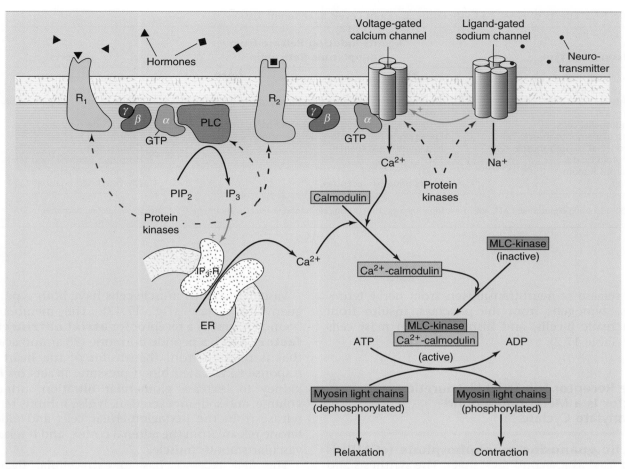

Figure 17.11 Regulation of smooth muscle contraction by calcium. Calcium enters the cytoplasm either from the extracellular space through voltage-gated calcium channels or through the inositol-1,4,5-trisphosphate (IP_3)–operated channel in the ER (IP_3-R). Voltage-gated calcium channels are regulated indirectly by neurotransmitters that act on ligand-gated ion channels. However, they also are regulated by hormone-operated G proteins, and they can be phosphorylated by protein kinases that are themselves under the control of second messengers. MLC-kinase, myosin light-chain kinase; PIP_2, phosphatidylinositol-4,5-bisphosphate; PLC, phospholipase C; R_1 and R_2, G protein–linked hormone receptors.

Muscle Contraction and Exocytosis Are Triggered by Calcium

Muscle contraction is always calcium dependent. Striated muscle contraction requires the binding of calcium to troponin C on the thin filaments, but smooth muscle cells do not have troponin. *The calcium-sensing protein in smooth muscle is calmodulin, not troponin C* (Fig. 17.11). The Ca^{2+}-calmodulin complex activates the enzyme **myosin light chain kinase,** which causes contraction by phosphorylating a pair of light chains on the globular head of myosin.

cAMP decreases the calcium concentration in many types of smooth muscle, probably by inducing the phosphorylation of proteins involved in calcium homeostasis. Also, a direct action of the α_s-GTP subunit on voltage-gated calcium channels has

been described in some types of smooth muscle. Therefore, *most types of smooth muscle are contracted by agents that raise cytoplasmic calcium levels and relaxed by agents that raise cytoplasmic cAMP levels* (Tables 17.1 and 17.2).

Bronchial smooth muscle, for example, is contracted by the calcium-elevating agents histamine (through H_1 receptors) and acetylcholine (through muscarinic receptors), and it is relaxed by epinephrine, which raises cAMP levels through β-adrenergic receptors. Therefore, epinephrine and other β agonists can be used for the treatment of asthma and other obstructive pulmonary diseases. Asthma can also be treated with the phosphodiesterase inhibitors theophylline and aminophylline.

Also, the release of water-soluble products by exocytosis is always triggered by calcium. Examples include

Table 17.2 Effects of Elevated Cytoplasmic Calcium Levels in Different Tissues

Tissue/Cell Type	Agents Inducing Release from Endoplasmic Reticulum	Effects
Pancreatic acinar cells	Cholecystokinin, acetylcholine	Zymogen secretion
Intestinal mucosa	Acetylcholine	Water and electrolyte secretion
Platelets	Thromboxane, collagen, thrombin, platelet-activating factor, ADP	Shape change, degranulation
Endothelial cells	Histamine, bradykinin, ATP, acetylcholine, thrombin	Nitric oxide synthesis
Vascular smooth muscle cells	Epinephrine (α_1 receptor), angiotensin II, vasopressin	Contraction
Bronchial smooth muscle cells	Histamine, leukotrienes	Contraction
Thyroid gland	TSH	Hormone synthesis and release
Corpus luteum	LHRH	Hormone synthesis
Liver	Epinephrine (α_1 receptor)	Glycogen degradation

ADP, adenosine diphosphate; ATP, adenosine tripnosphate; LHRH, luteinizing hormone–releasing hormone; TSH, thyroid-stimulating hormone.

the release of neurotransmitters from nerve terminals, zymogens from the pancreas, insulin from pancreatic β-cells, and histamine from mast cells (see Table 17.2).

The Receptor for Atrial Natriuretic Factor Is a Membrane-Bound Guanylate Cyclase

Cyclic guanosine monophosphate (cGMP) is also used as a second messenger. The synthesis and degradation of cGMP are analogous to the corresponding steps in cAMP metabolism:

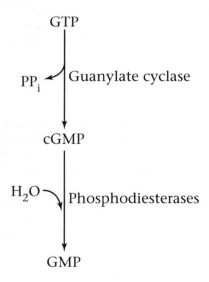

Unlike the adenylate cyclases, guanylate cyclases are not activated by hormone-coupled G proteins. There are two families of guanylate cyclases: membrane-bound enzymes that are activated directly by extracellular ligands, and soluble enzymes in the cytoplasm that respond to small diffusible molecules.

Vascular smooth muscle cells have both types of guanylate cyclase (Fig. 17.12). The membrane-bound enzyme is a receptor for **atrial natriuretic factor (ANF)**, a peptide hormone (28 amino acids) that is released from the atrium of the heart in response to elevated blood pressure. It acts on the kidney to increase glomerular filtration, urinary volume, and sodium excretion. It also inhibits renin release from the juxtaglomerular cells and aldosterone release from the adrenal cortex, and it relaxes vascular smooth muscle.

The ANF receptor has an extracellular ligand-binding domain, a single transmembrane helix, and an intracellular guanylate cyclase domain, all on the same polypeptide. *The guanylate cyclase domain is active only when ANF is bound to the extracellular domain.*

Like cAMP, *cGMP induces most or all of its effects by activating a protein kinase.* This kinase is conveniently named **protein kinase G.** The cyclic nucleotides are not entirely specific for their respective protein kinases. Thus, cAMP in vascular smooth muscle cells can dilate the vessel by activating protein kinase G. In the intestinal mucosa, high levels of cGMP can cause fluid secretion and diarrhea by an action on protein kinase A.

Nitric Oxide Stimulates a Soluble Guanylate Cyclase

Although some vascular beds are relaxed by ANF, the major guanylate cyclase of vascular smooth muscle is a soluble, cytoplasmic enzyme that is activated by **nitric oxide (NO)**. NO is synthesized by a Ca^{2+}-calmodulin–activated **nitric oxide synthase** in endothelial cells. Being small and lipid soluble, it diffuses rapidly to the underlying smooth muscle cells, in which it activates the soluble guanylate cyclase. NO is chemically unstable and decom-

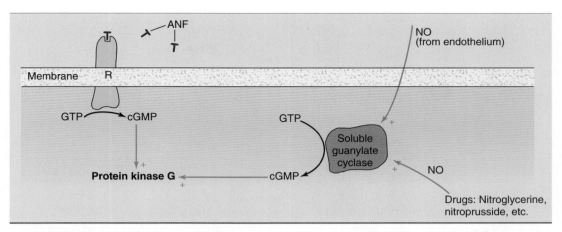

Figure 17.12 Formation of cyclic GMP (cGMP) in vascular smooth muscle cells. The atrial natriuretic factor (ANF) receptor is present not only in vascular smooth muscle but in the kidneys and some other tissues as well. Nitric oxide (NO) acts as "endothelium-derived relaxing factor." The *straight green arrows* indicate allosteric stimulation. GTP, guanosine triphosphate; R, ANF receptor.

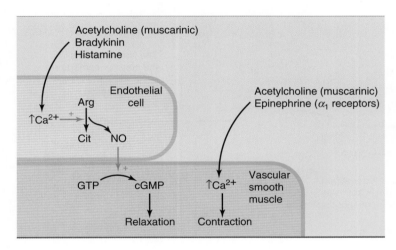

Figure 17.13 The roles of endothelium and vascular smooth muscle in the regulation of vascular tone. Agents that raise the calcium level in endothelial cells relax vascular smooth muscle because they stimulate the synthesis of nitric oxide (NO).

poses within a few seconds, without the need for degrading enzymes. Before its chemical nature was known, NO had been described as the "endothelium-derived relaxing factor."

Because the endothelial NO synthase is stimulated by calcium-calmodulin, *vascular smooth muscle is contracted by agents that raise calcium levels in the smooth muscle cells but is relaxed by agents that raise calcium levels in the endothelial cells* (Fig. 17.13).

Nitroglycerin is a fast-acting vasodilator that is used to treat acute attacks of angina pectoris:

It is effective because it is rapidly metabolized to produce NO.

In the corpora cavernosa of the penis, there is a vascular bed that is expected to respond to parasympathetic nerve stimulation with profound vasodilation. Several neurotransmitters share in this important task, but NO is the most important mediator. In this tissue, NO is formed mainly in the nerve terminals and only to a lesser extent in the vascular endothelium. As in other vascular beds, however, it acts by stimulating the soluble guanylate cyclase in the smooth muscle cells.

Sildenafil (Viagra) and related drugs induce their effect by inhibiting phosphodiesterase-5. This cGMP-specific phosphodiesterase is responsible for the degradation of cGMP in the vascular smooth muscle cells of the penis.

Nitroglycerine

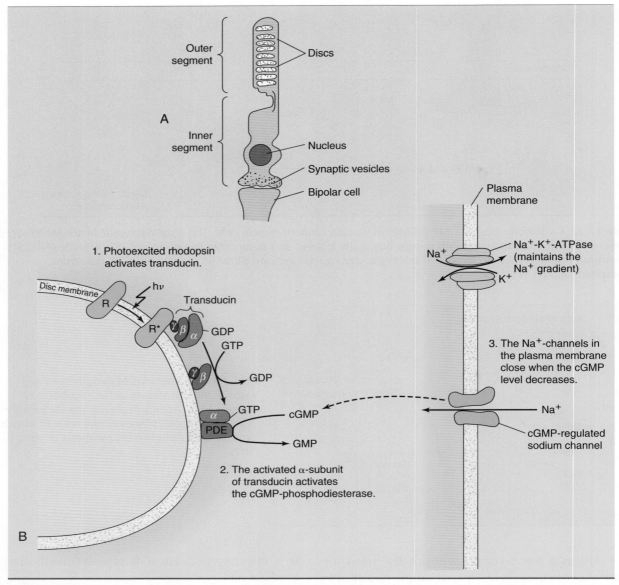

Figure 17.14 Signal transduction in the retinal rod cell. **A,** Structure of the retinal rod cell. **B,** The visual cascade. cGMP, cyclic guanosine monophosphate; hv, visible light; PDE, cGMP phosphodiesterase; R, Rhodopsin; R*, photoexcited rhodopsin.

cGMP Is a Second Messenger in Retinal Rod Cells

The task of the retinal rod cell is to register light and transmit the information to the next cell in the neural signaling chain. As shown in Figure 17.14, the receptive part of the cell is its outer segment—actually a vastly modified cilium—that is filled with flattened membrane stacks.

Embedded in these membranes is the light-absorbing protein **rhodopsin.** Ordinary proteins do not absorb visible light, but rhodopsin employs a light-absorbing prosthetic group in the form of **retinal.** When retinal absorbs light, the 11-*cis* double bond in retinal is isomerized into the *trans* configuration, leading to a substantial steric change not only in retinal but in the whole rhodopsin molecule:

11-*cis* retinal in
unexcited rhodopsin

All-*trans* retinal in
photoexcited rhodopsin

All-*trans* retinal + Opsin

This photoisomerization switches rhodopsin to an activated, "photoexcited" conformation known as **metarhodopsin II (R*)**. The bond between all-*trans* retinal and the apoprotein in R* hydrolyzes, and all-*trans* retinal dissociates from the apoprotein.

Rhodopsin is an integral membrane protein with seven transmembrane α helices. Not only does it look like a G protein–linked hormone receptor, but it also functions like one. It is coupled to the G protein **transducin,** switching it to the active GTP form after light exposure.

In the dark, the membrane of the rod cell is always half depolarized because a sodium channel in the plasma membrane is kept in a half-open state by a tightly bound molecule of cGMP. *The light-activated transducin stimulates a phosphodiesterase.* cGMP is hydrolyzed, and the sodium channel loses its bound cGMP. Closure of the sodium channel hyperpolarizes the membrane, and the cell stops releasing its neurotransmitter.

This cascade amplifies the stimulus enormously. A single photoexcited rhodopsin molecule activates about 500 transducin molecules, each transducin-activated phosphodiesterase molecule hydrolyzes about 1000 cGMP molecules per second, and the removal of cGMP from a single sodium channel prevents the influx of thousands of sodium ions. Therefore, a single photon can hyperpolarize the cell by about 1 mV.

Receptors for Insulin and Growth Factors Contain a Protein Tyrosine Kinase Domain

Growth factors in the widest sense are soluble proteins that regulate mitosis, cell differentiation, cell migration, and programmed cell death. They help in determining cell fate during embryonic and fetal development, and they regulate cell turnover and regeneration throughout life. Although growth factors induce most of their effects at the level of gene transcription, their receptors are in the plasma membrane.

The intracellular domain of most growth factor receptors is a ligand-activated, tyrosine-specific protein kinase (Fig. 17.15). The predilection of these receptor kinases for tyrosine side chains is unusual. In resting cells, most protein-bound phosphate is on serine and threonine side chains, and less than 0.1% is on tyrosine side chains. The substrate specificity of these receptors is also unusual. After ligand binding, *the receptors aggregate in the membrane and phosphorylate each other.* This is called **autophosphorylation.**

Tyrosine protein kinase receptors can autophosphorylate on multiple tyrosine side chains, sometimes more than a dozen. Autophosphorylation has two effects: *It stimulates the receptor kinase activity towards external substrates,* and *it creates docking sites for cytoplasmic and membrane-associated proteins.* Most of these proteins bind to tyrosine-phosphorylated sites through a specialized domain, the **SH2 domain** (SH = src homology). Because each protein tyrosine kinase receptor has a unique combination of autophosphorylation sites, *each receptor can interact with a unique set of SH2-containing proteins.* Binding to the autophosphorylated receptor can have several consequences:

1. *Soluble cytoplasmic proteins are recruited to the plasma membrane.* Some are enzymes that are brought in contact with their membrane-bound substrates, and others are recruited as allosteric links in signaling pathways.
2. *Receptor binding induces allosteric changes in the bound molecules.* Some enzymes, for example, are allosterically activated by binding to the autophosphorylated receptor.
3. *Some of the bound proteins become tyrosine-phosphorylated by the receptor.* This changes their biological properties.

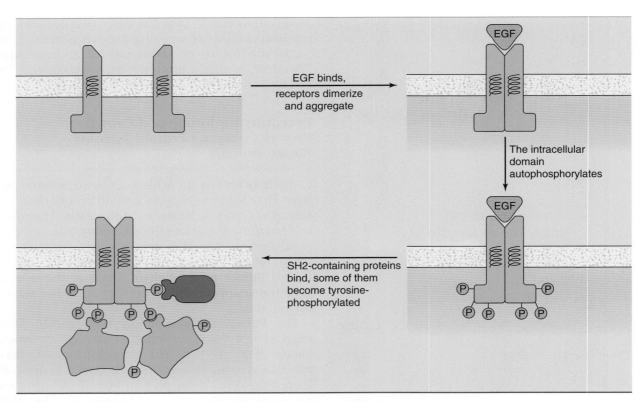

Figure 17.15 Receptor for epidermal growth factor (EGF). Ligand binding induces dimerization or oligomerization of the receptor, followed by autophosphorylation on tyrosine side chains. Most growth factors act by this general mechanism. Their actions are terminated by tyrosine-specific protein phosphatases that dephosphorylate the receptor and its substrates.

The insulin receptor is also a tyrosine-specific protein kinase (Fig. 17.16). In this case, the receptor phosphorylates a small set of receptor-associated proteins. The most important of these, **insulin receptor substrate 1 (IRS-1)**, becomes phosphorylated on about 20 tyrosine residues. *These phosphotyrosine residues are docking sites for SH2-containing proteins.*

Growth Factors and Insulin Trigger Multiple Signaling Cascades

Although growth factor signaling and insulin signaling have a common evolutionary origin, *in vertebrates, growth factors stimulate growth and mitosis, whereas insulin stimulates the utilization of nutrients.* Nevertheless, there is extensive overlap in the signaling cascades of the two types of hormone.

Figure 17.17 shows how growth factors can stimulate the IP_3 second messenger system. The key enzyme in this cascade, phospholipase C, comes in several isoforms. One group of isoforms, called **phospholipase Cβ,** is activated by the α subunits of G_q proteins, as shown in Figures 17.9 and 17.11.

Another type, **phospholipase Cγ,** associates with growth factor receptors and becomes activated by tyrosine phosphorylation.

Figure 17.18 shows another cascade. The activated tyrosine kinase receptor initiates a bucket brigade of allosteric protein-protein interactions to convert the G protein **Ras** into the active GTP-bound form. Like the heterotrimeric G proteins that are coupled to 7-transmembrane receptors, the Ras protein cycles between an inactive GDP-bound form and an active GTP-bound form. However, Ras consists of a single subunit.

In yet another pathway (Fig. 17.19), the autophosphorylated receptor recruits the enzyme **phosphatidylinositol 3–kinase (PI3K)** to the membrane. PI3K is allosterically activated by binding to the autophosphorylated growth factor receptor or to tyrosine-phosphorylated IRS-1. Alternatively, it is activated by Ras-GTP. PI3K phosphorylates inositol lipids in the plasma membrane in position 3. For example, it converts phosphatidylinositol-4,5-bisphosphate into phosphatidylinositol-3,4,5-trisphosphate. The 3-phosphorylated inositol lipids recruit a set of proteins to the membrane that contain a **pleckstrin homology (PH) domain.**

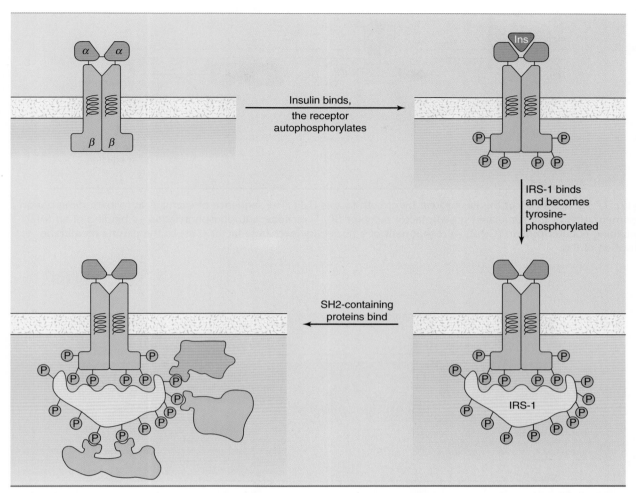

Figure 17.16 The insulin receptor. Unlike the growth factor receptors, which are monomers in the unstimulated state, the insulin receptor is a disulfide-bonded tetramer. Also, the insulin receptor does not bind SH2-containing signaling proteins itself but rather recruits insulin receptor substrate 1 (IRS-1) for this purpose.

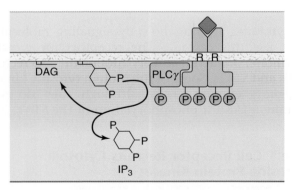

Figure 17.17 The activation of phospholipase Cγ (PLCγ) by growth factor receptors (R). PLCγ is activated by binding to the autophosphorylated receptor and by tyrosine phosphorylation. DAG, 1,2-diacylglycerol; IP_3, inositol-1,4,5-trisphosphate.

One of these proteins is **protein kinase B,** also known as **Akt.** Once anchored to the membrane, protein kinase B becomes activated by phosphorylations on serine and threonine side chains. One of the two protein kinases that are required for these phosphorylations is activated by 3-phosphorylated inositol lipids, and the other one is activated by integrins in focal adhesions.

Humans have three isoforms of protein kinase B: one mediating the growth-promoting and anti-apoptotic effects of growth factors, one mediating insulin effects, and one of unknown function. These kinases phosphorylate their substrates on serine and threonine side chains.

Some Receptors Recruit Tyrosine-Specific Protein Kinases to the Membrane

Another signaling cascade is used by the receptors for cytokines, including the interferons and inter-

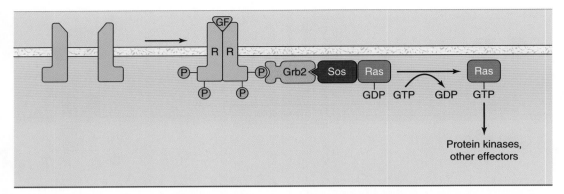

Figure 17.18 Activation of the Ras protein by growth factors (GF). The sequence of events is as follows: dimerization or oligomerization of the stimulated growth factor receptor (R) → receptor autophosphorylation → binding of an SH2-containing adapter protein (Grb2) → recruitment of a nucleotide exchange factor (Sos) to the plasma membrane → activation of Ras.

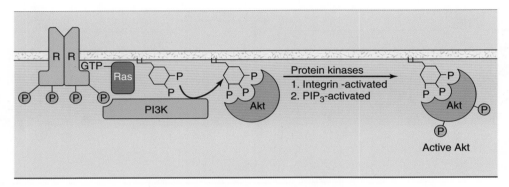

Figure 17.19 The activation of protein kinase B (Akt) by tyrosine protein kinase receptors. The autophosphorylated receptor (R) recruits the SH2 protein phosphatidylinositol 3–kinase (PI3K). This enzyme can also be recruited by Ras-GTP. The 3-phosphorylated inositol lipids formed by PI3K recruit Akt. After activating phosphorylations on serine and threonine, Akt phosphorylates serine and threonine side chains in its substrates. GTP, guanosine triphosphate; PIP_3, phosphatidylinositol-3,4,5-trisphosphate.

leukins. These proteins are secreted by white blood cells during inflammatory responses to coordinate the immune response.

Cytokine receptors have no intrinsic enzymatic activity. However, the ligand-activated form of the receptor binds and thereby activates a **Janus kinase** (also called **JAK,** for "just another kinase"). There are several JAKs that associate with different receptors. *The receptor-bound kinases phosphorylate both each other and the receptor on tyrosine side chains* (Fig. 17.20).

Next, *the tyrosine-phosphorylated receptor attracts a protein of the* **signal transducer and activator of transcription (STAT)** *family*. There are several STATs that associate selectively with different receptors by means of an SH2 domain. The STAT becomes phosphorylated by the receptor-bound JAK and then moves to the nucleus, in which it binds to response elements in promoters and enhancers to regulate transcription.

Cytokines are not the only signaling molecules that use this cascade. The receptors for growth hormone, prolactin, and erythropoietin also recruit JAKs and STATs. Some of the protein tyrosine kinase receptors employ STATs, although they do not require a JAK for phosphorylation of the STAT.

The T Cell Receptor Recruits Cytosolic Tyrosine Protein Kinases

In the presence of cytokines from helper T cells, lymphocytes respond to an unusual class of growth factors: antigens. B cells proliferate and differentiate into plasma cells when an antigen binds to their surface immunoglobulin. At least some of these effects are mediated by JAKs and STATs.

T cells proliferate when an antigen binds to their functional equivalent of surface immunoglobulin, the **T cell receptor.** The T cell receptor has two

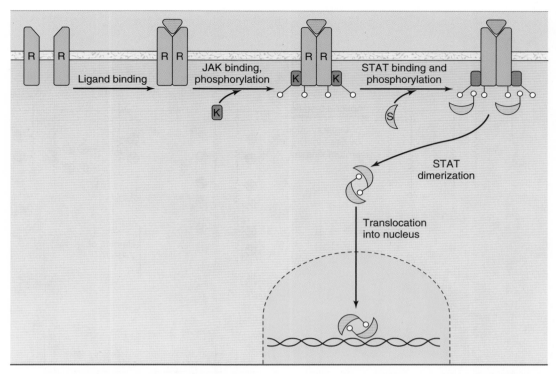

Figure 17.20 Signaling through cytokine receptors. The ligand-activated receptor (R) attracts a Janus (JAK) kinase (K). This kinase tyrosine-phosphorylates both itself and the receptor. A signal transducer and activator of transcription (STAT) protein (S) binds to the tyrosine-phosphorylated receptor-kinase complex. After being phosphorylated by the Janus kinase, the STATs form active dimers that translocate into the nucleus to regulate transcription. ∂, Phosphotyrosine groups.

antigen-binding polypeptides called α and β that end in highly variable antigen-binding domains. Each T cell expresses only one combination of these variable domains. In addition to the α and β chains, the receptor contains a dimer of two ζ chains, as well as the **CD3** complex, consisting of a γ chain, a δ chain, and two ε chains (Fig. 17.21).

Antigen binding induces a conformational change that exposes the cytoplasmic tails of the γ, δ, ε, and ζ chains to the action of a tyrosine-specific protein kinase of the **Src** family (named after avian sarcoma, a virus-induced cancer in chickens). These protein kinases are attached to the inner surface of the plasma membrane by a covalently bound myristoyl group. Besides Src itself, there are eight different Src-related protein kinases in different cells. Two of them, known as Lck and Fyn, are the major kinases phosphorylating the T cell receptor.

Once the tyrosines are phosphorylated by the Src family kinases, the T cell receptor binds a second type of tyrosine protein kinase, known as **zeta-associated protein 70 (ZAP-70)**. ZAP-70 anchors itself to the tyrosine-phosphorylated receptor and phosphorylates target proteins. One of these target proteins, phospholipase Cγ, mediates mitogenesis through 1,2-diacylglycerol, IP$_3$, and calcium.

An inherited deficiency of ZAP-70 has been identified as a cause of severe combined immunodeficiency in some patients. Although signaling through the surface immunoglobulin of B cells does not require ZAP-70, B cells are crippled as well because their activation requires activated helper T cells in addition to antigen.

Many Receptors Become Desensitized after Overstimulation

Many cells lose their responsiveness when they are exposed to high concentrations of a messenger molecule. This **desensitization** can occur rapidly, within seconds to minutes, or gradually, in the course of hours or days.

The receptors of many G protein–linked receptors become desensitized because *the intracellular domain of the receptor becomes phosphorylated after agonist exposure.* The G$_s$ protein–linked β-adrenergic receptor, for example, can be desensitized in two ways. It can be phosphorylated by protein kinase A, and this phosphorylation prevents the interaction of the receptor with the G$_s$ protein. *This type of desensitiza-*

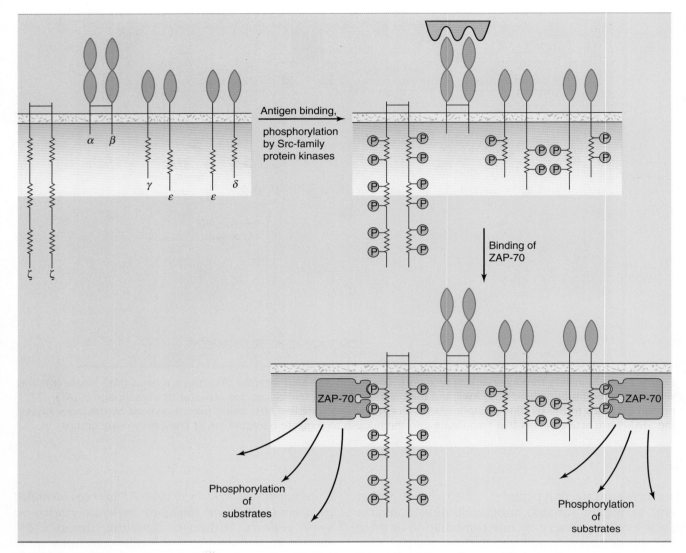

Figure 17.21 Signaling through the T cell receptor. The intracellular tails of the γ, δ, ε, and ζ chains possess antigen-recognition activation motifs (ARAMs; ‑ᴡᴡᴡ‑) that become tyrosine-phosphorylated by tyrosine protein kinases of the Src family. The extracellular portions of the α, β, γ, and δ chains contain immunoglobulin-like domains, but only the α and β chains have variable domains for antigen recognition. T cells can respond specifically to an antigen on the surface of a presenting cell. Like many other signal transducing proteins, zeta-associated protein 70 (ZAP-70) has SH2 domains (⧈) that bind to tyrosine-phosphorylated sites.

tion can be reversed by the action of protein phosphatases that remove the phosphate from the receptor.

The receptor can also be phosphorylated by a specific **β-adrenergic receptor kinase (BARK)**. BARK phosphorylates only the stimulated but not the unstimulated receptor. The protein **arrestin** binds to the phosphorylated receptor, and this prevents the receptor from activating the G$_s$ protein. It can even trigger the endocytosis of the receptor (Fig. 17.22). The receptors are either stored in the membranes of intracellular vesicles or directed to the lysosomes for degradation. *In cases in which receptors are degraded, desensitization can be reversed only by the synthesis of new receptors.*

Some tyrosine kinase receptors also undergo endocytosis in response to overstimulation. For example, overeating leads to excessive insulin release. The overstimulated insulin receptors are prone to endocytosis, and some of the endocytosed receptors are destroyed by lysosomal enzymes. Some overeaters can balance this loss by making more insulin receptors, but others cannot. In type II diabetes, which occurs most frequently in obese people, insulin receptor number is decreased. However, most of the "insulin resistance" seen in this disease is caused not by a decrease in the number of receptors but by defects in downstream signaling components that are still being identified.

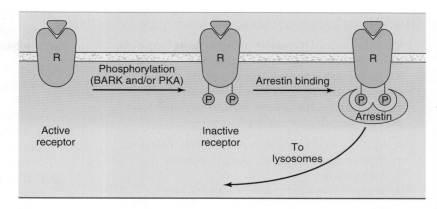

Figure 17.22 The desensitization of the β-adrenergic receptor (R). Phosphorylation by protein kinase A prevents the interaction of the receptor with the G$_s$ protein. Alternatively, the ligand-activated receptor is phosphorylated by a specialized β-adrenergic receptor kinase (BARK). The cytoplasmic protein arrestin binds to the phosphorylated receptor, preventing the activation of the G$_s$ protein and triggering receptor endocytosis. PKA, protein kinase A.

Nevertheless, weight loss in obese patients with type II diabetes can reduce the insulin level, minimize receptor endocytosis, and restore a normal insulin response.

SUMMARY

Receptor binding is always the first step in the action of an extracellular messenger molecule on its target cells. Receptors are allosteric proteins that bind their ligand with high affinity and selectivity. The receptors for steroid hormones, thyroid hormones, calcitriol, and retinoic acid are ligand-regulated transcription factors, but water-soluble agents to bind to receptors on the cell surface.

Many neurotransmitters manipulate the membrane potential of their target cell directly, by opening a ligand-gated ion channel in the plasma membrane. Water-soluble hormones, however, trigger lengthy signaling cascades. Most hormone receptors activate a G protein, and the activated G protein triggers the synthesis of a second messenger. cAMP, cGMP, IP$_3$ (acting through Ca^{2+}), and 1,2-diacylglycerol are most important. The second messengers activate protein kinases, including kinases A (cAMP-activated), C (Ca^{2+}-diacylglycerol–activated), and G (cGMP-activated), and the calmodulin-dependent protein kinases (Ca^{2+}-activated).

The receptors for insulin and many growth factors are protein tyrosine kinases. They autophosphorylate in response to ligand binding and can also phosphorylate other proteins. The receptors for cytokines, some hormones, and some growth factors are not enzymatically active but recruit protein kinases along with the substrates for these kinases.

Further Reading

Brazil DP, Hemmings BA: Ten years of protein kinase B signalling: a hard Akt to follow. Trends Biochem Sci 26:657-664, 2001.

Fujisawa H: Regulation of the activities of multifunctional Ca^{2+}/calmodulin–dependent protein kinases. J Biochem 129:193-199, 2001.

Fukami K: Structure, regulation, and function of phospholipase C isozymes. J Biochem 131:293-299, 2002.

Kraus WL, Wong J: Nuclear receptor-dependent transcription with chromatin. Is it all about enzymes? Eur J Biochem 269:2275-2283, 2002.

McKenna NJ, O'Malley BW: Combinatorial control of gene expression by nuclear receptors and coregulators. Cell 108:465-474, 2002.

Mehats C, Andersen CB, Filopanti M, et al: Cyclic nucleotide phosphodiesterases and their role in endocrine cell signaling. Trends Endocrinol Metab 13:29-35, 2002.

Rhee SG: Regulation of phosphoinositide-specific phospholipase C. Annu Rev Biochem 70:281-312, 2001.

Rizzuto R, Pozzan T: When calcium goes wrong: genetic alterations of a ubiquitous signaling route. Nat Genet 34:135-141, 2003.

Roymans D, Slegers H: Phosphatidylinositol 3–kinases in tumor progression. Eur J Biochem 268:487-498, 2001.

Shirai Y, Saito N: Activation mechanisms of protein kinase C: maturation, catalytic activation, and targeting. J Biochem 132:663-668, 2002.

QUESTIONS

1. Vascular smooth muscle contracts in response to increased cytoplasmic calcium. Nevertheless, many natural agents that stimulate the IP_3/calcium system (including acetylcholine, histamine and bradykinin) are potent vasodilators. Why?

   A. In the vascular smooth muscle cell, calcium rapidly equilibrates across the plasma membrane.
   B. The calcium-calmodulin complex blocks voltage-gated calcium channels in vascular smooth muscle.
   C. Calcium is transferred from endothelial cells to vascular smooth muscle through gap junctions.
   D. The calcium-calmodulin complex stimulates NO synthase in endothelial cells.
   E. The calcium-calmodulin complex inhibits adenylate cyclase in vascular smooth muscle cells.

2. The activation of the IP_3/calcium system leads to growth stimulation in many cells, including cancer cells. In order to inhibit this second messenger system, you could try to develop a drug that

   A. Inhibits the dephosphorylation of IP_3.
   B. Stimulates protein kinase C.
   C. Reacts chemically with the α subunits of the G_q proteins, thereby making them unable to activate phospholipase C.
   D. Inhibits the GTPase-activity of the G_q proteins.
   E. Inhibits the active transport of calcium in the plasma membrane.

3. cAMP regulates the transcription of many genes. What is the major mechanism for this action?

   A. It induces the phosphorylation of transcription factors.
   B. It binds directly to cAMP response elements in promoters and enhancers.
   C. It mediates this effect by increasing the calcium concentration in the cytoplasm and the nucleus.
   D. It binds directly to nuclear transcription factors.
   E. It induces the phosphorylation of STAT proteins, thus enabling them to translocate into the nucleus.

4. Most growth factor receptors are able to phosphorylate tyrosine side chains of proteins. Although the substrates of the activated receptors differ, one protein always becomes tyrosine-phosphorylated. This protein is

   A. Adenylate cyclase.
   B. Inositol trisphosphate.
   C. Protein kinase C.
   D. Protein kinase A.
   E. The receptor itself.

5. A drug that inhibits the hydrolysis of 3-phosphorylated inositol lipids (e.g., phosphatidylinositol-3,4,5-trisphosphate) is likely to increase the cell's responsiveness to some of the effects of

   A. Glucocorticoids.
   B. Hormones acting through G_s protein–coupled receptors.
   C. Hormones acting through G_i protein–coupled receptors.
   D. Insulin.
   E. NO.

CHAPTER 18

Cellular Growth Control and Cancer

The human body is produced from the fertilized ovum in a succession of mitotic cell divisions. Each mitotic cycle consists of an orderly sequence of events, including growth, DNA replication, and cell division.

As they go through repeated rounds of cell division, the cells of the embryo metamorphose into the differentiated cells of the mature body: blood cells, neurons, muscle cells, and so forth. Cell growth, mitotic rate, and cell differentiation are controlled by external stimuli. These stimuli include nutrients, hormones, growth factors, and contacts with neighboring cells and the extracellular matrix.

Derangements in the controls on the cell's proliferation, differentiation, and survival cause cancer. This chapter describes the elements of cell cycle control, the proliferative responses of the cell to external stimuli, and the aberrations in these processes in cancer.

The Cell Cycle Is Controlled at Two Checkpoints

Under the microscope only two phases of the cell cycle can be distinguished: **interphase** and **mitosis** (Fig. 18.1). Mitosis is the stage of cell division and takes approximately 1 hour. All of the rest is interphase. Chromosomes are visible as distinct entities only during mitosis, when the DNA has to be packaged for relocation into the daughter cells. During interphase, there is only dispersed chromatin all over the nucleus.

Interphase is subdivided into G_1, **S,** and G_2 phases. During G_1 (G = gap), the genome is in the **diploid** state, with two copies of each chromosome. This is followed by S (synthesis) phase, during which the DNA is replicated, and finally by G_2. *S phase can be identified by feeding the cells with radiolabeled thymidine.* Cells in S phase incorporate a large amount of the thymidine into DNA (but not RNA). Outside S phase, only a small amount of **unscheduled DNA synthesis** takes place during DNA repair.

The cell makes two important all-or-none decisions during the cell cycle. At the **G_1 checkpoint** in late G_1, it decides about the *entry into S phase.* DNA replication should be initiated only when the cell is ready to progress through the complete cell cycle and only after any DNA damage that may have been sustained has been thoroughly repaired.

At the **G_2 checkpoint** in late G_2, the cell decides about the *entry into mitosis.* Mitosis should be initiated only after the completion of DNA replication and only if the replicated chromosomes are structurally intact.

Nondividing cells are said to be in **G_0.** Some nondividing cells, including neurons and skeletal muscle fibers, are in G_0 forever. Others, including fibroblasts, hepatocytes, and lymphocytes, are usually in G_0 but can be coaxed into the cell cycle by external agents: fibroblasts by platelet-derived growth factor (PDGF) during wound healing, and lymphocytes by antigen along with cytokines from helper T cells.

Cells Can Be Grown in Culture

The cell cycle is most easily studied in cultured cells. Leukocytes, fibroblasts, and many other cells (but not neurons) can be induced to grow and divide in culture. Typical features of these cultured cells include the following:

1. *Cell growth is mitogen dependent.* Human cells are programmed to proliferate only when told to do

so by soluble mitogens that are normally present in the body.

2. *Cell growth is anchorage dependent.* Cells in the body are attached to the extracellular matrix, and they proliferate only as long as these attachments are maintained. Cultured cells other than white blood cells need a solid or semisolid surface to substitute for the extracellular matrix.

3. *Cell growth is contact inhibited.* In the body, cells must stop proliferating once the available space is filled; and in the test tube, they stop dividing as soon as a continuous cell layer has been formed.

4. *Cells are mortal.* Cultured fibroblasts, for example, divide between 30 and 80 times until they succumb to senility. Fibroblasts from a baby have a higher life expectancy in culture than do those from an elderly person.

These limitations on cell growth apply only to normal cells and not to cancer cells. Cancer cells are mitogen independent and anchorage independent, are not subject to contact inhibition, and are immortal.

The Cyclins Play Key Roles in Cell Cycle Control

The cell cycle requires both *regulation of protein synthesis* and *regulation of preexisting proteins by phosphorylation.* These processes are coordinated by the **cyclin-dependent kinases (Cdks)** in the nucleus and by their regulatory subunits, the **cyclins.** Most of the cyclins and some of the Cdks have half-lives of 1 hour or less. Therefore, their concentrations in the cell can change rapidly with the cell cycle (Fig. 18.2).

Only cyclin D is not controlled by the cell cycle; it is controlled by mitogens. It is the first cyclin to rise when the cell approaches the G_1 checkpoint. Through its catalytic subunits, **Cdk4** and **Cdk6,** cyclin D induces the synthesis of **cyclin E,** followed shortly by **cyclin A.** Cyclins E and A activate the kinase **Cdk2.**

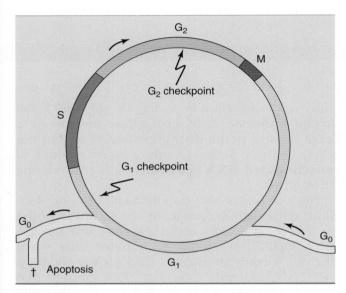

Figure 18.1 The cell cycle. G_1, S, and G_2 constitute interphase. The DNA is replicated during the S (synthesis) phase; the chromosomes segregate during mitosis (M). Nondividing cells are in the G_0 phase.

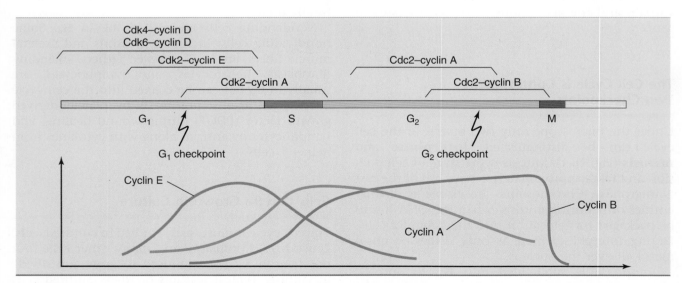

Figure 18.2 Cyclins and cyclin-dependent kinases (Cdks, Cdc, cell division cycle gene products) during the cell cycle. Most cyclins are short lived, and their levels fluctuate with the stages of the cell cycle. The cyclin-dependent kinases and cyclin D, on the other hand, are present throughout the cell cycle. G_1, S, G_2, and M are the stages of the cell cycle (see Fig. 18.1).

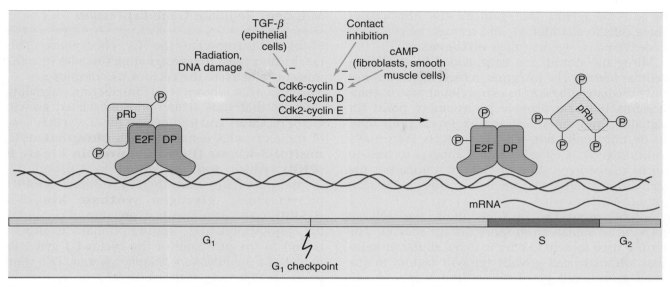

Figure 18.3 Function of the retinoblastoma protein (pRb) in the control of the G_1 checkpoint. The phosphorylation of pRb by cyclin-dependent protein kinases (Cdks) releases the transcription factor E2F/DP from inhibitory control, thus enabling the transcription of genes for cell cycle progression. Growth-inhibiting stimuli prevent pRb phosphorylation indirectly by increasing the activity of cyclin/Cdk inhibitors. cAMP, cyclic adenosine monophosphate; mRNA, messenger RNA; P, phosphate groups; TGF-β, transforming growth factor-β.

Finally, **cyclin B** accumulates during G_2 but is abruptly degraded during mitotic metaphase. Working with the catalytic subunit **Cdc2** (Cdc = cell division cycle [gene product]), it prepares the cell for entry into mitosis and executes the early steps of mitosis. It condenses the chromosomes by phosphorylating chromosomal scaffold proteins and histone H_1, and it triggers the breakdown of the nuclear envelope by phosphorylating and thereby destabilizing the lamin network under the inner nuclear membrane.

The cyclin-dependent protein kinases are controlled not only by cyclins. They are also subject to multiple phosphorylations, some with stimulatory and others with inhibitory effects. Antimitotic agents can also induce the synthesis of **Cdk inhibitors** that form catalytically inactive complexes with the Cdks.

The Retinoblastoma Protein Guards the G_1 Checkpoint

The kinases that are controlled by cyclins D and E can push the cell through the G_1 checkpoint by phosphorylating the **retinoblastoma protein (pRb)** (Fig. 18.3).

pRb does not bind to DNA, but it has a binding pocket for the transcription factor **E2F.** Along with its dimerization partner, **DP,** *E2F activates the transcription of genes for cell cycle progression and DNA synthesis,* including the genes for cyclins D1 (there

are several closely related D-cyclins), E and A, Cdc2, thymidine kinase, dihydrofolate reductase, DNA polymerase α, the proto-oncogenes *c-myc* and *N-myc,* and even the E2F gene itself.

Throughout G_0 and early G_1, pRb is tightly bound to E2F. It prevents gene expression by masking the transcriptional activation domain of E2F and by recruiting a histone deacetylase. At the checkpoint, however, both pRb and E2F become phosphorylated by the kinase complexes of cyclins D and E. The phosphorylated pRb falls off the transcription factor, and the genes can be transcribed.

These events are all-or-none because they incorporate an element of *positive feedback.* Once the activity of the cyclin D/Cdk complexes has passed a threshold, the cyclin genes become derepressed. Even more cyclin/Cdk is formed, pushing the cell through the G_1 checkpoint.

Cell Proliferation Is Regulated by External Stimuli

During embryonic development, cell proliferation is tightly linked to cell differentiation. In general, immature stem cells divide more or less continuously, but *once the cell develops into a specialized cell type, it withdraws from the cell cycle.* For some cells, including neurons and skeletal muscle fibers, the withdrawal into G_0 is final. Others, however, including hepatocytes and fibroblasts, behave like Sleeping Beauty: They can be restored to reproductive life by external agents. The "prince's kiss" that causes these cells to abandon G_0 and reenter the cell cycle is delivered by agents called **mitogens.**

Mitogenic stimuli can be provided by the extracellular matrix. The integrins in focal adhesions not only mediate adhesion to extracellular matrix components but also provide an assembly point for signaling molecules. Cell-matrix interactions tend to be mitogenic, but cell-cell contacts are usually antimitogenic. Cell-cell contact appears to lead to an increased expression of Cdk inhibitors, but the signaling cascades that mediate contact inhibition are not well known.

Soluble **growth factors** allow the cell to respond to signals from more distant sources. The term is used loosely to refer to extracellular proteins that stimulate cell growth (growth factors in the strict sense), cell proliferation (mitogens), or cell survival (survival factors). Examples of growth factors include the following:

1. **PDGF** is present in the α granules of platelets from which it is released during platelet activation. Acting on fibroblasts, smooth muscle cells, and other cells, *PDGF participates in wound healing.* The discovery of PDGF followed the observation that added serum but not plasma stimulates the proliferation of cultured cells. The serum effect could be traced to PDGF, which is released from activated platelets during blood clotting.
2. **Epidermal growth factor (EGF)** stimulates the proliferation of epithelial cells. It acts primarily in its tissues of origin.
3. **Fibroblast growth factor (FGF)** occurs in at least 21 molecular variants in humans. It stimulates not only fibroblasts but also many other cells. Genetic defects in FGF receptors have been identified as causes of several syndromes with dwarfism or skeletal deformities.
4. **Insulin-like growth factor–1 (IGF-1)** is released from the liver in response to growth hormone. Pygmies are said to have as much growth hormone as taller people, but they release less IGF-1 in response to growth hormone.
5. **Erythropoietin** is released from the kidney in response to hypoxia. Acting on a JAK-STAT coupled receptor (see Chapter 17), it stimulates specifically the development of red blood cell precursors in the bone marrow.
6. **Nerve growth factor (NGF)** stimulates the growth and differentiation (but not mitosis) of postganglionic sympathetic neurons. Being released by sympathetically innervated tissues during embryonic development, it also acts as a chemoattractant that guides the growing axons to their proper destinations.

Mitogens Regulate Gene Expression

Mitogens manipulate the G_1 checkpoint. This means they must trigger signaling cascades into the nucleus to activate the cyclin-Cdk complexes.

Figure 18.4 shows two interacting signaling cascades that start at autophosphorylated growth factor receptors and impinge on the G_1 cyclins. One of these cascades signals through **phosphatidylinositol 3–kinase (PI3K)** and **protein kinase B (PKB),** which was introduced in Chapter 17. It phosphorylates and thereby inhibits another protein kinase, **glycogen synthase kinase–3 (GSK3).** GSK3 inhibits the expression of cyclin D1 by phosphorylating transcriptional regulators bound to the promoter of the cyclin D1 gene. *By inhibiting these inhibitory phosphorylations, PKB stimulates the expression of the cyclin D1 gene.*

The other mitogenic cascade shown in Figure 18.4 is the **mitogen-activated protein (MAP) kinase cascade.** It starts with the activated Ras protein at the cytoplasmic surface of the plasma membrane. In Chapter 17, the Ras protein was described as a small monomeric G protein that is activated by growth factor receptors.

The Ras protein assists in the activation of cytoplasmic serine/threonine kinases, including **Raf-1.** Once at the plasma membrane in association with Ras, Raf-1 becomes activated by phosphorylation. Some isoenzymes of protein kinase C can activate Ras-bound Raf.

Raf phosphorylates and thereby activates the protein kinase **MAPK/ERK kinase (MEK).** MEK phosphorylates a third set of kinases known as **extracellular signal–regulated kinases (ERKs)** on threonine and tyrosine residues in the sequence Thr-Glu-Tyr. The ERKs belong to a family of serine-threonine kinases known as the **MAP kinases.**

The activated MAP kinases phosphorylate proteins in the cytoplasm, but they also translocate into the nucleus. They regulate transcription factors by phosphorylation, and they also work indirectly by phosphorylating nuclear protein kinases. The products of some of the activated genes are themselves transcriptional regulators. These mitogen-induced transcription factors include the products of the *jun, fos,* and *myc* proto-oncogenes.

There are many negative controls on mitogenic signaling. One obvious mechanism is the *dephosphorylation of proteins by protein phosphatases* at all levels, from the autophosphorylated growth factor receptors to the phosphorylated transcription factors. Another negative control is the *hydrolysis of its bound guanosine triphosphate (GTP) by the Ras protein.* The GTPase activity of Ras is stimulated by various regulatory proteins, including **Ras-GAP**

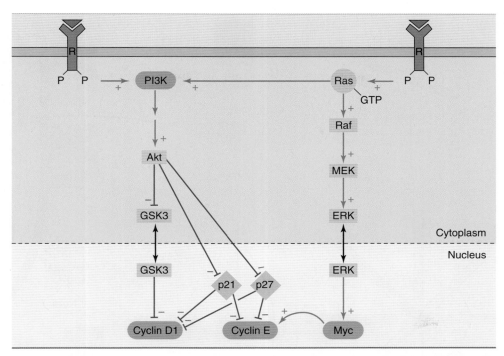

Figure 18.4 Two mitogenic signaling cascades. On the left side, the activated growth factor receptor (R) activates phosphatidylinositol 3–kinase (PI3K). Through the 3-phosphorylated inositol lipids that it produces, PI3K assists in the activation of the protein kinase B (Akt). Akt inhibits glycogen synthase kinase–3 (GSK3) by phosphorylation. GSK3 inhibits the synthesis of cyclin D1 by phosphorylating transcriptional regulator proteins. The right side shows the mitogen-activated protein (MAP) kinase pathway. The small monomeric G protein Ras triggers a phosphorylation cascade through Raf and MEK (MAP/ERK kinase) to the ERKs (extracellular signal–regulated kinases). Myc is a promitogenic transcription factor, and p21 and p27 are cyclin-Cdk inhibitors.

(GAP = GTPase activating protein) and **neurofibromin,** the product of the *NF-1* tumor suppressor gene.

The MAP kinase pathway is quite complex. There are, for example, three different isoforms of Ras and three different isoforms of Raf. MEK can be activated not only by Raf but also by a whole set of **MEK kinases (MEKKs).** There are no fewer than four different MEKKs in some cells. Also, there are two isoforms of MAP kinases with different regulatory properties and substrate specificities.

Cells Can Commit Suicide

Cells can also commit suicide by programmed cell death, or **apoptosis.** Apoptosis is common during normal embryonic development, but in adults it occurs mainly in response to severe cellular damage, viral infections, and somatic mutations. *Apoptosis eliminates many virus-infected and genetically altered cells.* These cells must be prevented from evolving into cancer cells.

Apoptotic stimuli destroy the cell through a death squad of proteases that are collectively known as **caspases.** Caspases are synthesized as inactive precursors that have to be activated by a proteolytic cascade. The initiating caspases activate themselves in response to pro-apoptotic stimuli. They then proceed to activate the downstream caspases, which in turn kill the cell by destroying vital proteins.

There are two routes to apoptosis. In the mitochondrial pathway, pro-apoptotic and antiapoptotic proteins act on the outer mitochondrial membrane to regulate the release of **cytochrome c** and other pro-apoptotic proteins from the intermembranous space. **Bax** and related proteins favor apoptosis, whereas **Bcl2** and related proteins inhibit apoptosis. A whole swarm of other proteins participate in this process, often by binding and inactivating Bcl2 and its relatives.

Whereas cytochrome *c* appears to associate with the scaffold protein **Apaf-1** and the precursor of the initiator caspase **Casp-9,** other mitochondrion-derived proteins are inhibitors of cytoplasmic caspase inhibitors. The procaspase-9 molecules that are incorporated in the "apoptosome" activate each other to form active Casp-9. The activated Casp-9 then proceeds to activate the effector caspase **Casp-3** (Fig. 18.5).

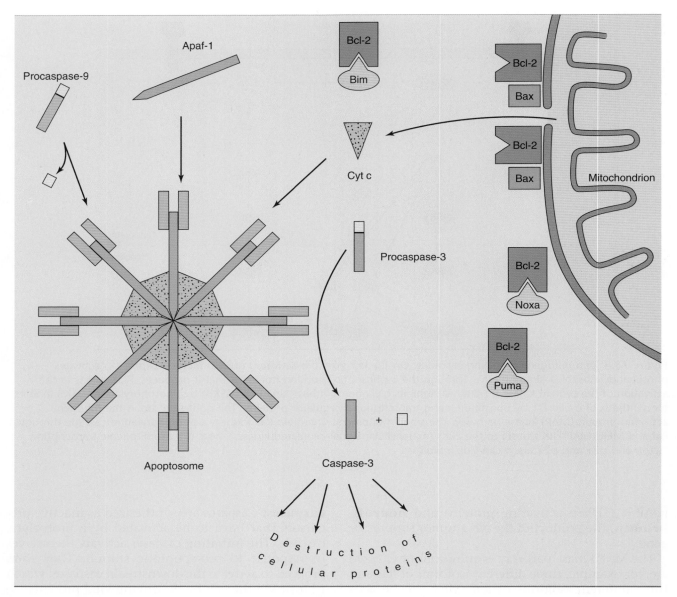

Figure 18.5 The induction of apoptosis by the mitochondrial pathway. The intermembranous space contains pro-apoptotic proteins, including cytochrome *c.* The release of these proteins into the cytoplasm is regulated by several related families of pro-apoptotic and antiapoptotic proteins (*red/pink* and *green,* respectively). In this model, antiapoptotic Bcl-2 competes with pro-apoptotic Bax, whereas proteins with such names as Puma, Noxa, and Bim help Bax by binding Bcl-2. In the cytoplasm, an "apoptosome" is constructed by the scaffold protein Apaf-1 with the help of proteins released from the mitochondrion. Procaspase-9 activates itself in the apoptosome, and the activated caspase-9 activates procaspase-3.

An alternative pathway is triggered by extracellular mediators, such as the cytokine **tumor necrosis factor (TNF).** The intracellular portion of the TNF receptor contains a **death domain** that is common to all apoptosis-mediating cell surface receptors. It is a docking site for various adapter proteins and for the precursor of the initiator caspase **Casp-8.** This receptor-assembled complex allows procaspase-8 to convert itself into active Casp-8 (Fig. 18.6). Once activated, Casp-8 proceeds to activate Casp-3 and other downstream caspases.

DNA Damage Causes Either Growth Arrest or Apoptosis

Cells with damaged DNA are not merely sick. They can also become dangerous because somatic mutations can lead to cancerous growth. In this situation, the cell practices triage: cells with good DNA proceed through the cell cycle; those with remediable damage are prevented from DNA replication until the damage is repaired; and irreversibly

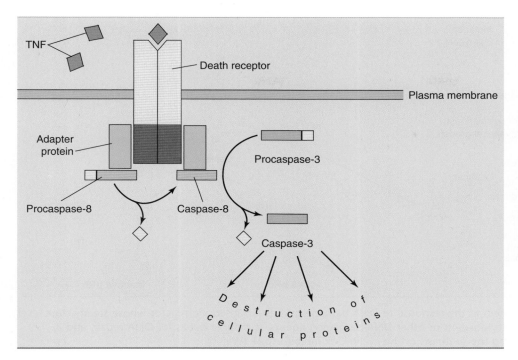

TNF

Death receptor

Plasma membrane

Adapter protein

Procaspase-3

Procaspase-8

Caspase-8

Caspase-3

Destruction of cellular proteins

Figure 18.6 The induction of apoptosis through death receptors, including those for tumor necrosis factor (TNF) and the Fas ligand. The system consists of a receptor *(pink)* with a death domain *(red)*, adapter proteins that bind to the death domain while recruiting procaspase-8, and the caspases.

damaged cells are liquidated altogether, either by the immune system or by apoptosis.

DNA damage activates protein kinases, either directly or in short signaling cascades. For example, DNA double-strand breaks activate the **"ataxia-telangiectasia mutated" (ATM)** protein kinase, so-called because this protein kinase is mutated in the recessively inherited disease **ataxia-telangiectasia.** Without a functioning ATM kinase, affected patients are unable to activate the appropriate DNA repair enzymes and to delay S phase until the damage is repaired. This leads to neurological degeneration, abnormalities of peripheral blood vessels, immunodeficiency, sterility, and increased cancer susceptibility. There are several damage-sensing proteins other than ATM, each responsive to a different type of DNA damage.

Responses to DNA damage are coordinated by the nuclear phosphoprotein **p53,** named after its molecular weight (MW) of 53,000 D. *p53 is a transcription factor that drives the expression of genes for growth arrest, DNA repair, and apoptosis.* It is present in low concentrations at all times, with a half-life of less than 1 hour in unstressed cells. DNA damage activates several protein kinases, including ATM, and these kinases phosphorylate p53 at up to 12 sites. These phosphorylations cause p53 to accumulate in the nucleus, and they stabilize it against degradation by the ubiquitin-proteasome system (see Chapter 9). Oxidative stress, hypoxia, the inhibition of transcription, and telomere erosion can also activate p53, either through protein kinases or through allosteric protein-protein interactions.

p53 induces the synthesis of several pro-apoptotic proteins, thereby tilting the delicate balance between pro-apoptotic and antiapoptotic proteins in favor of apoptosis. It also induces cell cycle arrest by inducing the synthesis of the Cdk-inhibitor **p21,** a nuclear phosphoprotein (MW, 21,000 D) that inhibits various cyclin-Cdk complexes, including those that phosphorylate pRb (Fig. 18.7).

By preventing DNA replication until all DNA damage has been repaired, and by driving irreversibly damaged cells into apoptosis, *p53 has antimutagenic properties.* In recognition of these achievements, p53 has been named the "guardian of the genome." p53 is not required for normal development, however. Knockout mice that lack both copies of the *p53* gene develop normally, although they die of cancer during midlife (see Table 18.4). Conversely, transgenic mice with elevated expression of p53 are resistant to cancer but are afflicted by early senility.

Cancers Are Monoclonal in Origin

Because they are genetically identical, the cells of the human body behave unselfishly toward one another. This means that each cell grows and divides only to the extent that it furthers the greater good of the body. Some cells even die dutifully—by apoptosis—once their task has been fulfilled.

Cancer cells, however, have the cellular equivalent of antisocial personality disorder. A cancer cell arises when a somatic mutation creates a "selfish

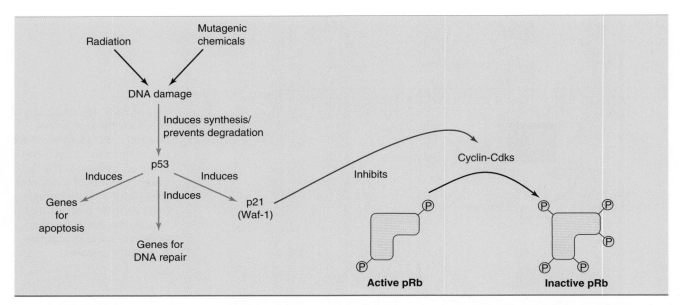

Figure 18.7 Role of the p53 protein in the response to DNA damage. p53 is a transcription factor whose steady-state level increases sharply after exposure to radiation or other DNA-damaging agents. It induces genes for DNA repair, and it causes cell cycle arrest by inducing the synthesis of the cyclin-Cdk inhibitor p21 (Waf-1).

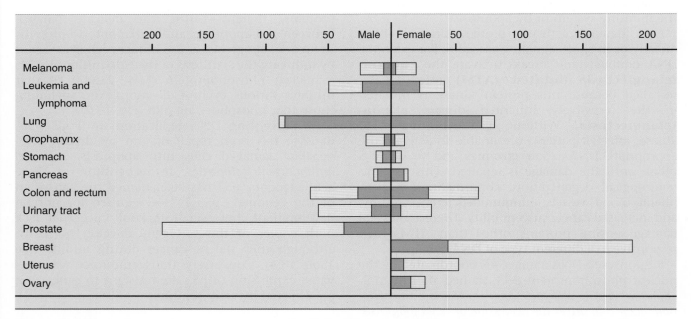

Figure 18.8 The incidence of new cancer cases in the United States in 1998 *(complete bars)* and the annual death rate *(dark-colored portions)*, in thousands per year. Basal cell carcinomas and squamous cell carcinomas of the skin are not included. These skin cancers have a very high incidence, but most are readily cured by resection of the tumor.

gene" that causes the cell to proliferate without regard for the greater good of the organism. This single abnormal cell grows into a cell mass called a **neoplasm** or **tumor.** *Most tumors are monoclonal in origin.* This means that all tumor cells are derived from a single abnormal ancestor. **Benign tumors** limit their growth without doing much harm, but **malignant tumors,** commonly called **cancer,** kill the organism. Cancer causes more than 20% of all deaths in industrialized countries. Figure 18.8 shows the incidence of various kinds of cancer in the United States.

Malignant cells retain morphological and biochemical features typical for their cells of origin. Some tumors of epithelial origin, for example, known as **carcinomas,** still produce keratins; some connective tissue tumors, known as **sarcomas,** still produce constituents of the extracellular matrix; and some endocrine tumors still secrete hormones. However, these specialized features tend to be lost when cancers become more malignant. There are some other characteristic differences between malignant neoplastic cells and the normal cells from which they are derived:

1. *Cancer cells have an abnormally high mitotic rate.* The abundance of mitotic cells in histological specimens is studied diagnostically to estimate the malignant potential of tumors.
2. *Cancer cells show signs of de-differentiation and assume features of immature stem cells.* The cells in epithelial cancers (carcinomas), for example, lose the normal squamous, cuboidal, or columnar shape of their normal progenitors and come to resemble immature embryonic cells.
3. *Cancer cells show disordered growth.* They have no respect for anatomical boundaries but grow as a chaotic mass, spreading and sprawling in all directions. The de-differentiation and disordered growth of cancerous cells are called **anaplasia.** The degree of anaplasia is predictive of the malignant behavior of the cells and, consequently, the patient's chances of survival.
4. *Cancer cells can colonize distant tissues.* They can break loose from the primary tumor to be disseminated by lymph or blood, and they take root in distant tissues to form secondary growths called **metastases.** Metastasis requires poor adherence to neighboring cells in the tumor, attachment to components of distant tissues, the crossing of basement membranes, and the ability to grow in an environment different from the cell's tissue of origin.
5. *Cancer cells are genetically unstable.* They tend to have aberrations in chromosome number, major deletions and translocations, gene amplifications, and even extrachromosomal genetic elements. They keep mutating because their ability to prevent and repair DNA damage is defective.
6. *Cancer cells can grow in the absence of mitogens.* Their mitogenic signaling cascades are switched on permanently, even in the absence of mitogens.
7. *Cancer cells are immortal.* Although many cancer cells do succumb to haphazard mutations, they escape the normal process of senescence. Most neoplastic cells have also lost the ability for apoptosis in response to growth factor deprivation, DNA damage, and other environmental insults.

Cancer Is Caused by the Activation of Growth-Promoting Genes and the Inactivation of Growth-Inhibiting Genes

Some gene products promote cell proliferation, whereas others are inhibitory. Growth factors and their receptors, components of the MAP kinase and PI3K pathways, and the G_1 cyclins are examples of mitogenic gene products, and cyclin-Cdk inhibitors, pRb, and the p53 protein are inhibitory. Therefore, malignant growth can be caused by two types of mutation (Fig. 18.9):

1. *A gene that codes for a promitotic protein becomes abnormally activated.* The normal promitotic gene is called a **proto-oncogene,** and its mutationally activated form is called an **oncogene** (Greek όγκος = "mass"). Mutation in a regulatory site can cause the overproduction of a structurally normal gene product. Even the amplification of proto-oncogenes is not uncommon in malignant tumors. In other cases, a point mutation creates a structurally abnormal "superactive" gene product. Also, many signaling proteins are normally restrained by a regulatory domain. The loss of this domain through a nonsense mutation, frameshift mutation, or partial gene deletion can produce a truncated protein that no longer responds to negative controls. There are even cases in which a proto-oncogene becomes translocated to a site where it is overexpressed under the influence of the enhancers or promoters of other genes or in which an abnormal protein is created by the fusion of two genes (Fig. 18.10).
2. *A gene that codes for a growth-inhibiting product becomes inactivated.* This can involve any mechanism, from point mutation to gene deletion. The normal gene that prevents cancerous growth is called a **tumor suppressor gene.** Oncogene activation changes the cell's growth habits even when only one copy of a proto-oncogene becomes activated. However, the inactivation of a tumor suppressor gene is effective only when both copies of the gene are inactivated and no tumor-suppressing protein at all is produced from the gene. This means that from the cell's point of view, *oncogene activations are expressed as dominant traits, whereas inactivations of tumor suppressor genes are expressed as recessive traits.*

A single mutation is rarely sufficient to convert a cell into malignancy, and common cancers contain a whole assortment of activated oncogenes and inactivated tumor suppressor genes.

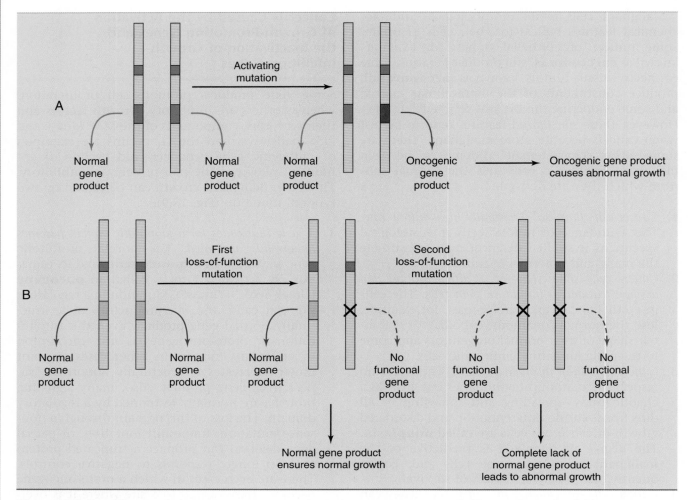

Figure 18.9 The difference between an oncogene and a tumor suppressor gene. **A,** The products of cellular proto-oncogenes (■) are growth-stimulating proteins. A single activating mutation ("gain-of-function" mutation) is sufficient to produce abnormal cell growth. **B,** The products of tumor suppressor genes (□) are growth-inhibiting proteins. Two inactivating mutations ("loss-of-function" mutations) are necessary to produce abnormal cell growth.

Some Retroviruses Contain an Oncogene

Some viruses cause cancer by introducing a **viral oncogene.** As early as 1910, Peyton Rous established the transmissible nature of a rare connective tissue tumor in chickens. Much later the transmissible agent, now known as the **Rous sarcoma virus,** was identified as a retrovirus.

Like all retroviruses, Rous sarcoma virus has a small RNA genome with three major genes that are essential for viral reproduction: *gag, pol,* and *env.* A fourth gene, v-*src* (v = viral, *src* = sarcoma), is not required for viral replication. v-*src* is a *viral oncogene* that causes the abnormal proliferation of the virus-infected cells (Fig. 18.11). It gets inserted into the host cell DNA along with the rest of the viral genome and is expressed at a high rate under the direction of the viral promoter and enhancer in the long terminal repeats.

The v-*src* oncogene is closely related to a normal cellular gene. Both the normal cellular *src* proto-oncogene and the v-*src* oncogene code for a non–receptor tyrosine protein kinase that is loosely bound to cellular membranes through a covalently bound myristic acid residue. The normal cellular Src kinase is controlled by growth factor receptors and by proteins in focal adhesions. It stimulates mitosis by phosphorylating many of the same substrates that are phosphorylated by activated growth factor receptors.

Apparently, the virus acquired its oncogene accidentally during a previous infectious cycle. *This hijacked gene, slightly mutated and grossly overexpressed, turns the virus-infected cell into a cancer cell.* Some other retroviral oncogenes besides v-*src* have

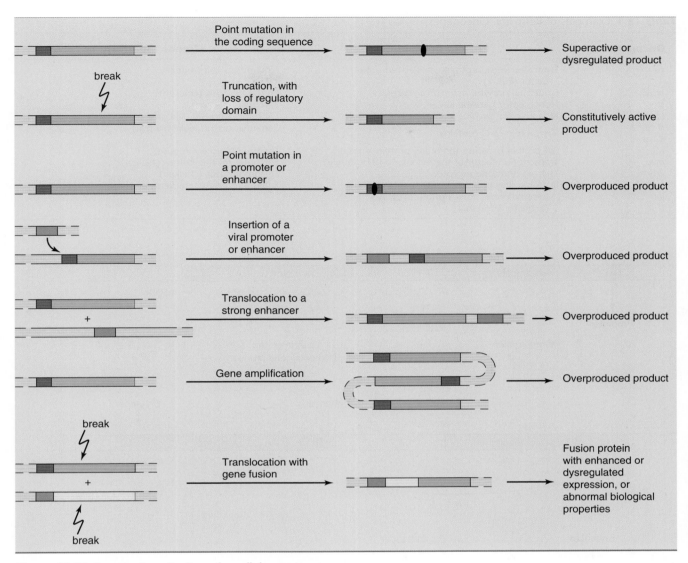

Figure 18.10 Oncogenic activation of a cellular proto-oncogene.

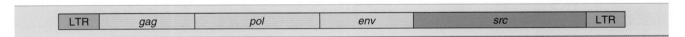

Figure 18.11 The genome of Rous sarcoma virus. Whereas *gag, pol,* and *env* are required for virus replication, *src* causes malignant transformation. The total length of the provirus is approximately 11,000 base pairs. LTR, long terminal repeat.

been identified (Table 18.1). All of them are closely related to normal cellular proto-oncogenes.

Retroviral oncogenes transform cells only after insertion into the cellular genome. Rous sarcoma virus is fully infective, but the other oncogenic retroviruses have lost some of the essential retroviral genes during acquisition of their oncogene. Therefore, they can reproduce only if their host cell is also infected by a second, intact retrovirus that supplies the missing gene products.

Retroviruses Can Also Cause Cancer by Inserting Themselves Next to a Cellular Proto-oncogene

Even retroviruses that do not carry an oncogene can cause cancer. Retroviruses integrate a complementary DNA copy of their genome at more or less random sites in the host cell DNA. On occasion, the virus inserts itself next to a cellular proto-oncogene.

Table 18.1 Examples of Retroviral Oncogenes

Oncogene	Protein Product	Tumor (Species)
sis	Truncated version of platelet-derived growth factor (PDGF)	Simian sarcoma (monkey)
erb-B	Epidermal growth factor (EGF) receptor	Erythroblastosis (chicken)
src	Nonreceptor tyrosine kinase	Sarcoma (chicken)
abl	Nonreceptor tyrosine kinase	Leukemia (mouse), sarcoma (cat)
H-ras *K-ras*	Ras protein (a G protein)	Sarcoma, erythroleukemia (rat)
raf	Raf protein (a serine/threonine protein kinase)	Sarcoma (chicken, mouse)
myc	Transcription factor of the helix-loop-helix family	Sarcoma, myelocytoma (chicken)
erb-A	Thyroid hormone receptor	Erythroblastosis (chicken)
fos *jun*	DNA-binding proteins, components of the heterodimeric transcription factor AP-1 (activator protein 1)	Sarcoma (mouse, chicken), erythroblastosis (chicken)

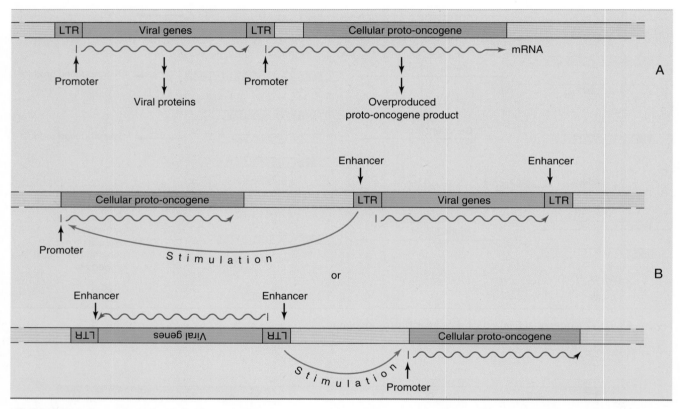

Figure 18.12 Activation of a cellular proto-oncogene by an integrated retrovirus. The two long terminal repeats (LTRs) of the provirus are identical. Note that the proto-oncogene is not damaged during retroviral integration, but its rate of transcription is increased. **A,** Promoter insertion. The promoter in the downstream LTR is used for the transcription of the proto-oncogene. mRNA, messenger RNA. **B,** Enhancer insertion. The viral enhancer stimulates transcription from the normal promoter even if inserted downstream of the proto-oncogene or if inserted with opposite polarity.

This can boost the transcription of the proto-oncogene in two ways (Fig. 18.12):

1. In **promoter insertion,** the retroviral complementary DNA is lodged immediately upstream of the proto-oncogene. This can lead to transcription of the proto-oncogene from the promoter in the downstream long terminal repeat of the virus—at an abnormally high rate and without the usual negative controls.

2. In **enhancer insertion,** the enhancer in the long terminal repeats of the inserted retrovirus stimulates the transcription of a neighboring proto-oncogene. Because enhancers can act over distances of more than 10,000 base pairs, this mechanism works even if the virus is inserted some distance away from the transcriptional start site.

Many Oncogene Products Are Links in Mitogenic Signaling Chains

Ordinarily, cells divide only in response to mitogens. Therefore, abnormal cell proliferation can be expected whenever components of mitogenic signaling cascades become overactive as a result of

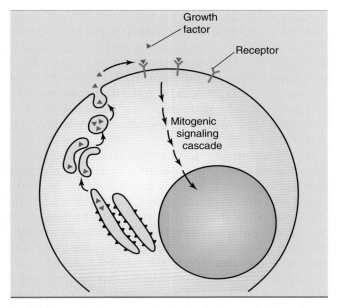

Figure 18.13 Autocrine stimulation of a neoplastic cell. Some tumor cells express both a growth factor and the corresponding receptor, thereby stimulating their own growth.

somatic mutation. Indeed, many oncogenes code for components of mitogenic cascades, described as follows.

GROWTH FACTORS

Growth factors are relatively uncommon as oncogene products. Only one viral oncogene, the **simian sarcoma (*sis*)** oncogene, is known to code for a growth factor. However, *some spontaneous cancers secrete growth factors that stimulate the tumor cells through an autocrine loop* (Fig. 18.13). For example, normal melanocytes respond to FGF although they do not produce it, but many malignant melanomas stimulate their own growth by producing FGF.

RECEPTOR TYROSINE KINASES

Receptor tyrosine kinases are overexpressed or structurally altered in many malignant tumors. The ***erb-B*** oncogene of the avian erythroblastosis virus codes for a truncated version of the EGF receptor that has lost the extracellular ligand-binding domain (Fig. 18.14). The tyrosine protein kinase domain is intact but is no longer controlled by the ligand. It phosphorylates substrates at all times, even in the absence of EGF.

The ***neu*** oncogene, which is found in some spontaneous neuroblastomas, also codes for an aberrant growth factor receptor. It differs from its normal

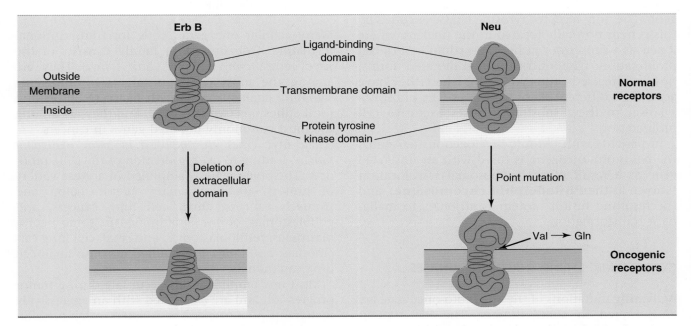

Figure 18.14 Abnormal growth factor receptors as oncogene products. The intracellular protein tyrosine kinase domains of the abnormal receptors are constitutively active, even in the absence of the ligand.

counterpart by only a single amino acid substitution at one end of the transmembrane helix. This point mutation keeps the protein kinase active at all times, even in the absence of the ligand. Constitutively active receptors are one possible reason for mitogen independence in cancer cells.

Besides structurally abnormal receptors, overexpressed receptors are common in various cancers. Many squamous cell carcinomas and glioblastomas, for example, have an overexpressed or amplified gene for the EGF receptor.

NON–RECEPTOR TYROSINE PROTEIN KINASES

Non–receptor tyrosine protein kinases include the **c-src** oncogene. The normal Src protein kinase is inhibited by tyrosine phosphorylation, and under ordinary conditions, more than 90% of Src is in the inactive, tyrosine-phosphorylated form. The inhibitory phosphate is removed by protein phosphatases only after binding of Src to growth factor receptors or focal adhesions.

Some structurally altered oncogenic forms of Src are mutated at the tyrosine phosphorylation site and are therefore permanently activated. Also, the simple overexpression of a structurally normal cellular *src* gene is not uncommon in spontaneous cancers. Because Src relays mitogenic stimuli both from growth factor receptors and focal adhesions, *src* mutations contribute both to the mitogen independence and to the anchorage independence of malignant growth.

A different situation is encountered with the **abl** gene. The non–receptor tyrosine kinase encoded by this gene is normally located in the nucleus, where it acts as a suppressor rather than stimulator of cell proliferation. The oncogenically mutated forms, however, reside in the cytoplasm, where they have access to a different set of substrates. The phosphorylation of these substrates causes excessive cell proliferation.

In patients with chronic myelogenous leukemia, the *abl* proto-oncogene is fused with an unrelated gene as a result of a chromosomal translocation (known as the **Philadelphia chromosome**), and the resulting fusion protein contributes to malignant transformation.

CYTOPLASMIC SERINE/THREONINE KINASES

Activating mutations of the **raf** proto-oncogene are encountered in some tumors. The Raf protein kinase encoded by this gene (see Fig. 18.7) is regulated by phosphorylations at multiple sites, some activating and some inhibitory. Oncogenic forms of Raf frequently have point mutations that destroy negative phosphorylation sites, or they have lost part or all of their regulatory domain. *These mutations leave the kinase in a permanently activated state.*

G PROTEINS

Oncogenic forms of the *ras* gene are found in about 30% of all spontaneous cancers, including 30% to 50% of lung and colon cancers and 90% of pancreatic cancers. Most oncogenic forms of *ras* have point mutations that disrupt the GTPase activity of the encoded Ras protein or make it unresponsive to GTPase-activating proteins. *These oncogenic Ras proteins have lost their "off" switch and remain in the active state at all times.*

Also, heterotrimeric G proteins are involved in some neoplastic conditions. Cyclic adenosine monophosphate (cAMP) is antimitogenic in fibroblasts and smooth muscle cells, but it stimulates the proliferation of many endocrine cells. Mutations in the α subunit of either the G_s or the G_i protein are not uncommon in benign adenomas of the pituitary somatotrophs, the thyroid gland, and the adrenal cortex. These mutations eliminate the GTPase activity of the α_s subunit or prevent the action of the α_i subunit on adenylate cyclase, respectively. As a result, *the affected cells are flooded with cAMP, and they proliferate and secrete excessive amounts of hormone.*

NUCLEAR TRANSCRIPTION FACTORS

Many cellular oncogenes code for transcriptional regulators. One important family consists of the **myc** genes: c-*myc*, N-*myc*, and L-*myc*. They are among the most common targets of mitogenic signaling chains from growth factor receptors and focal adhesions (see Fig. 18.7), and they are among the most commonly mutated genes in cancers.

The myc *genes are amplified in many malignant tumors,* leading to overproduction of the gene products. The c-*myc* gene is amplified in a great variety of tumors, including many breast, colon and stomach cancers, small cell lung cancers, and glioblastomas; N-*myc* is amplified in some neuroblastomas, retinoblastomas, and small cell lung carcinomas; and L-*myc* is amplified in some small cell lung carcinomas.

Most *myc* amplifications occur late during tumor progression and are associated with an aggressively malignant phenotype. The isolated overexpression of a *myc* gene in an otherwise normal cell can lead to abnormal proliferation, but it is also likely to cause apoptosis. Therefore, *myc* overexpression is

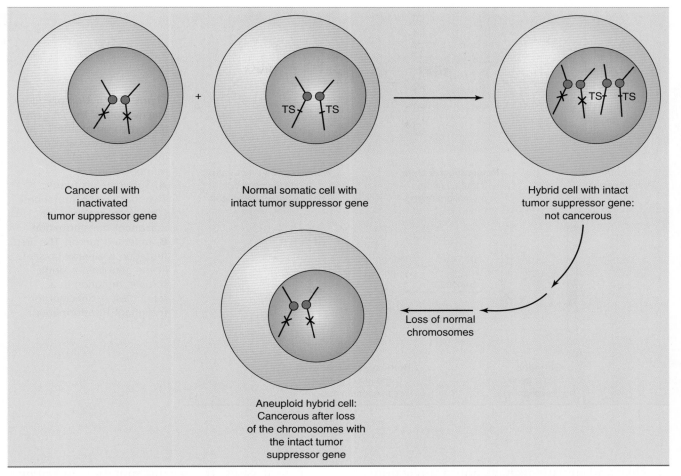

Figure 18.15 The importance of tumor suppressor genes, as demonstrated by somatic cell hybridization. Only the chromosome with the tumor suppressor gene (TS) is shown. The tumorigenicity of the cells can be assessed by injecting them into immunodeficient mice. The original cancer cell is able to cause tumors, but the hybrid cell is not. The hybrid cell becomes tumorigenic only if the chromosomes with the intact tumor suppressor gene are lost during prolonged culturing. The product of the tumor suppressor gene has growth-inhibiting properties; thus, progeny cells that have lost the normal chromosomes with the intact tumor suppressor gene by mitotic nondisjunction gradually outgrow the normal hybrid cells in culture.

most dangerous in aberrant cells that have lost the capacity for apoptosis.

In **Burkitt's lymphoma,** the c-*myc* gene on chromosome 8 is translocated into the locus for immunoglobulin κ chains (on chromosome 2), for λ chains (chromosome 22), or for heavy chains (chromosome 14). *The translocation places the* myc *gene into a transcriptionally active spot of the genome, where it is overexpressed under the influence of local enhancers.*

Retinoblastoma Is Caused by the Inactivation of a Tumor Suppressor Gene

The inactivation of tumor suppressor genes is even more important than the activation of cellular proto-oncogenes in most spontaneous cancers.

Figure 18.15 shows a classical experiment with cultured cells. After fusion of a cancer cell with a normal cell, the resulting hybrid cells grow like normal cells because they possess the product of the intact tumor suppressor gene from the normal cell. If malignant transformation were caused by dominantly acting oncogenes, the hybrid cells would grow like cancer cells. Some cells lose the chromosomes with the intact tumor suppressor genes during prolonged culturing, and these cells become, again, like cancer cells.

Not all cancer-promoting mutations occur in somatic cells. **Retinoblastoma** is a rare malignant tumor of immature retinal cells (retinoblasts) that occurs in 1 per 20,000 children during the first 5 years of life.

About 60% of affected patients have a sporadic form of the disease. No other family members are

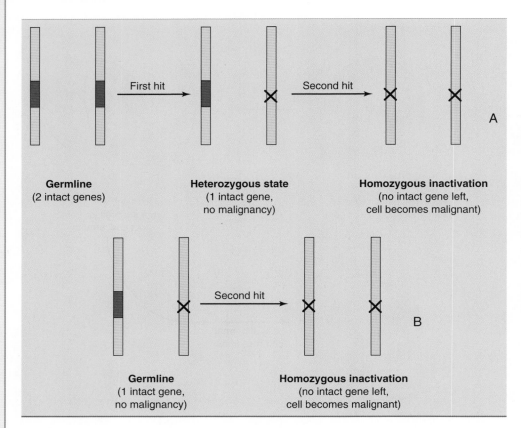

Figure 18.16 Homozygous inactivation of the *Rb* gene (■) on chromosome 13 in the spontaneous and the inherited forms of retinoblastoma. **A,** Spontaneous tumor: Two inactivating mutations ("hits") are required for malignant transformation. **B,** Inherited tumor: The first mutation is already present in the germline. A single somatic mutation in a retinoblast is sufficient for malignant transformation.

Germline
(2 intact genes)

Heterozygous state
(1 intact gene,
no malignancy)

Homozygous inactivation
(no intact gene left,
cell becomes malignant)

First hit

Second hit

A

Second hit

Germline
(1 intact gene,
no malignancy)

Homozygous inactivation
(no intact gene left,
cell becomes malignant)

B

affected, and all patients have only a single primary tumor. The other 40% have a form of the disease that is heritable as an autosomal dominant trait. Most of these familial cases have more than one primary tumor. *These patients are heterozygous for the predisposing mutation.* They have a 90% chance of getting at least one malignant eye tumor.

In both forms of the disease, *the tumor cells are totally deficient in pRb.* Without this "guardian of the G$_1$ checkpoint" (see Fig. 18.3), the cells keep dividing at a breathtaking pace. Only the homozygous inactivation of the *Rb* gene in an immature retinal cell causes malignant transformation. Cells with a single intact copy of the gene are normal. Therefore, *two mutations in the Rb gene are required for malignant transformation* (Fig. 18.16).

In the sporadic form of the disease, both mutations take place in the retinoblast. These mutations are rare events, and sporadic retinoblastoma is indeed a rare disease. However, patients with the inherited form of the disease have only one intact copy of the *Rb* gene in all their cells. Therefore, a single *Rb* mutation in one of the million or so retinoblasts is sufficient to create a malignant cell. There is a strong chance that this occurs in more than one retinoblast, and the tumors in the inherited disease are therefore often multifocal.

In most cases, the second mutation in patients with inherited retinoblastoma is not an independent small mutation but a large deletion, loss of the normal chromosome, or the replacement of the normal gene by the defective one through homologous recombination during mitosis (Fig. 18.17). These events lead to **loss of heterozygosity** both for the *Rb* gene and for genetic markers (restriction fragment length polymorphisms, variable number of tandem repeats, and single-nucleotide polymorphisms) close to it. Loss of heterozygosity in cancer cells is used for the mapping of tumor suppressor genes.

Retinoblastoma is inherited as an autosomal dominant trait at the level of the individual, because people with the cancer susceptibility are heterozygotes. However, the mutation is recessive at the cellular level because the cell becomes malignant only if it loses both copies of the *Rb* gene.

The *Rb* gene is expressed in all nucleated cells. Therefore, it is not surprising that patients who survive familial retinoblastoma in childhood have an increased risk of osteosarcoma (bone cancer) and perhaps other cancers in later life. Somatic mutations of the *Rb* gene are also seen in many spontaneous cancers other than retinoblastoma, including most small cell lung carcinomas and in about one

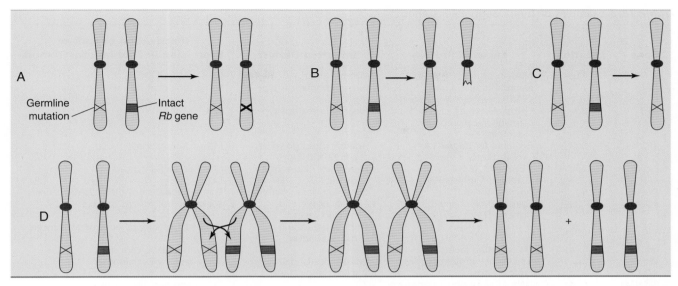

Figure 18.17 Loss of the intact *Rb* gene in patients with inherited retinoblastoma. The mechanisms shown in **B, C,** and **D** (but not **A**) lead to a loss of heterozygosity both for the gene itself and for nearby genetic markers. Mechanism **D** (somatic recombination in mitosis) is the most common for all those tumor suppressor genes that are far away from the centromere.

third of all breast and bladder cancers. This suggests that *in cells other than retinoblasts, the loss of* Rb *gene function can contribute to malignant transformation but is not by itself sufficient to cause cancer.*

Many Tumor Suppressor Genes Are Known

Table 18.2 gives an overview of some of the more important tumor suppressor genes. The products of these genes include the following:

1. *Negative regulators of the G_1 checkpoint.* The most important examples are pRb and the Cdk inhibitor INK4a.
2. *Proteins responsible for the DNA damage response.* p53 and p53-activating proteins (e.g., ATM and Arf) are among the most commonly mutated tumor suppressor genes in spontaneous cancers.
3. *Negative regulators of mitogenic or antiapoptotic signaling cascades.* The lipid phosphatase PTEN, which hydrolyzes the second messenger phosphatidylinositol-3,4,5-trisphosphate, is the most prominent example. Neurofibromin (NF1, an inhibitor of Ras) and APC (an inhibitor of β-catenin signaling) are also negative regulators of signaling cascades.
4. *Cell adhesion molecules.* The loss of E-cadherin, for example, is associated with loss of contact inhibition during the transition from benign tumors to invasive cancer. In many cancers, E-cadherin is not lost by somatic mutation, but its

synthesis is blocked by methylation of the DNA in and around the promoter of its gene.

For many tumor suppressor genes, germline mutations that lead to a dominantly inherited cancer susceptibility syndrome are known. An affected patient's somatic cells are heterozygous for the mutated and the normal ("wild-type") allele. As in the classical example of retinoblastoma, *the cell becomes neoplastic when it loses the wild-type allele.* Inherited cancer susceptibility syndromes are rare, accounting for 4% to 8% of all breast and colon cancers and even fewer for other common cancers.

Components of the Cell Cycle Machinery Are Abnormal in Most Cancers

The mechanisms of cell cycle control are exceedingly complex, and they vary according to the cell type. There are, for example, three different isoforms of cyclin D (D1, D2, and D3); besides pRb, there are two other "pocket proteins," p107 and p130, that bind to transcription factors of the E2F type; and there are six genes for E2F and two for its dimerization partner, DP. With alternative splicing and the use of alternative promoters in some of the genes, the actual number of gene products is even greater.

The cyclin-dependent kinases are controlled by Cdk inhibitors. **p21** is induced by p53 (see Fig.

Table 18.2 Examples of Tumor Suppressor Genes

Gene	Location*	Encoded Protein	Inherited Disease†	Inactivation or Lack of Expression in Spontaneous Tumors
WT-1	11p	Nuclear protein	Wilms' tumor	Rare
NF1	17q	Neurofibromin, a Ras-GTPase–activating protein	Neurofibromatosis type 1	Some tumors of neural crest origin
NF2	5q	Cytoskeleton-associated peripheral membrane protein	Neurofibromatosis type 2	Rare
APC	5q	Required for degradation of β-catenin	Adenomatous polyposis coli (APC)	Most colon cancers
E-cad	16q	E-cadherin, a cell adhesion molecule	Hereditary diffuse gastric cancer	Many epithelial cancers
INK4a	9p	An inhibitor of Cdk4	Some familial melanomas	Some esophageal and pancreatic cancers
BRCA1	17q	Transcription-coupled repair (?)	Familial breast and ovarian cancer	Some sporadic breast cancers
BRCA2	13q	?	Familial breast and ovarian cancer	20%-40% of spontaneous breast cancers
nm23	17q	Transcription factor (?)	?	Many metastatic cancers
VHL	3p	Cell surface protein (?)	von Hippel–Lindau disease	Some renal cell carcinomas
ATM	11q	Protein kinase	Ataxia-telangiectasia	
SMAD4	18q	DNA-binding signal transducer	?	Colon and pancreatic cancers
PTEN	10q	Lipid phosphatase	Cowden disease	30%-50% of spontaneous cancers

*p, Short arm of chromosome; q, long arm.
†These diseases are inherited as autosomal dominant traits.

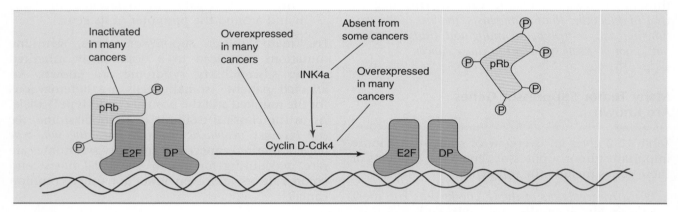

Figure 18.18 Abnormalities of the G_1 checkpoint in human cancers. For explanations, see text. pRb, retinoblastoma protein.

18.7), and the related inhibitor **p27** is induced by many growth-inhibiting stimuli from outside the cell. The complexes of cyclin D with Cdk4 and Cdk6 are inhibited by a whole family of Cdk inhibitors that includes INK4a, INK4b, INK4c, and INK4d (INK4 = inhibitor of kinase 4).

Alterations in the components of the G_1 checkpoint are common in spontaneous cancers (Fig. 18.18; Table 18.3). Of the pocket proteins, only pRb is abnormal in many cancers; p107 and p130 are generally normal.

In the normal cell cycle, pRb is inactivated by cyclin-dependent phosphorylations. Indeed, *cyclin D1 is overexpressed in many cancers.* Amplifications of the cyclin D1 gene have been found in 43% of squamous cell carcinomas of the head and neck, 34% of esophageal cancers, and 10% of small cell lung cancers and liver cancers. More than 50% of breast cancers overexpress cyclin D1, although the gene is in most cases not amplified. Cdk4, the most important catalytic partner of the D-cyclins, is also overexpressed or structurally abnormal in some cancers.

Of the Cdk inhibitors, the p53-induced p21 protein is rarely affected in cancers, but *mutations that inactivate INK4a are very common.* Data indicate that 55% of gliomas and mesotheliomas, 50% of biliary tract cancers, 40% of nasopharyngeal carci-

Table 18.3 Cell Cycle Regulators in Cancer

Protein	Normal Function	Abnormalities in Cancer Cells
Cyclin D1	Major G_1 cyclin; responds to mitogens	Overexpressed in many cancers
Cyclin D2 Cyclin D3	G_1 cyclins	None known
Cyclin E	Entry into S phase	None known
Cyclin A	Entry into S phase and progression toward mitosis	Rarely overexpressed in cancers
Cdk4	Major catalytic partner of the D cyclins	Amplification in sarcomas and gliomas; activating mutations in some melanomas
INK4a	Inhibitor of Cdk4, induced by growth-inhibiting stimuli	Deleted or mutated in many cancers
INK4b INK4c INK4d	Similar to INK4a	None known
pRb	"Pocket protein"; controls E2F	Mutated or deleted in many cancers
p107, p130	Similar to pRb	None known
E2F	Transcription factors; regulated by pocket proteins	None known

nomas and 30% of esophageal cancers and acute lymphocytic leukemias, as well as many sarcomas, bladder and ovarian cancers, have lost functional INK4a. Some patients with familial melanoma were found to have inactivating germline mutations in the INK4a gene.

Interestingly, tumors that overexpress cyclin D1 or are deficient in INK4a usually retain pRb, whereas those with pRb loss express cyclin D1 and INK4a normally. Therefore, it seems that the control of the G_1 checkpoint is defective in most and possibly all cancers, but the molecular defect is variable.

The cyclin-Cdk complexes, Cdk inhibitors, and pocket proteins work mainly through the E2F transcription factors. Therefore, overexpression of E2F in tumor cells might be expected. Actually, however, E2F mutations are not common in human cancers. Cultured cells that are transfected with overexpressed E2F genes do indeed increase their mitotic rate, but this is followed by apoptosis. It is quite possible that activating E2F mutations are not seen in cancers because such mutations lead to apoptosis.

Mutations in the *p53* Tumor Suppressor Gene Are the Most Common Genetic Changes in Spontaneous Cancers

In response to DNA damage and other forms of stress, the nuclear phosphoprotein p53 induces the transcription of genes for growth arrest, DNA repair, and apoptosis (see Fig. 18.7). This pathway is compromised in most if not all cancers, and *mutations in p53 have been identified in 50% to 60% of all spontaneous human cancers,* including 70% of all colorectal cancers, 50% of lung cancers, and 40% of breast cancers. This is the most common genetic change in spontaneous cancers.

Of the *p53* mutations, 70% to 80% are missense mutations. The mutant forms of the p53 protein are conformationally changed, fail to activate gene transcription, and are, in most cases, longer lived than authentic p53, which has a half-life of less than 1 hour in unstressed cells.

Are *p53* mutations carcinogenic because they prevent cell cycle arrest or because they prevent apoptosis? p53-Mediated cell cycle arrest is known to depend on the Cdk inhibitor p21. If p21 prevents tumors, its mutational inactivation is expected to be tumorigenic. Actually, however, such mutations have been found in only a few prostatic cancers and are otherwise rare in malignant tumors. Therefore, the antiapoptotic effect of p53 seems to be more important for cancer prevention than is the inhibition of S phase entry. Without functional p53, aberrant cells can survive and evolve into fully malignant cells. This is important for cancer treatment, because *tumor cells without p53 fail to go into apoptosis after treatment with radiation or DNA-damaging chemicals.*

Many common cancers have lost functional p53 through somatic mutation, but patients with **Li-Fraumeni syndrome** are born with a mutation in one copy of the *p53* gene. This rare (about 1 per 30,000), dominantly inherited condition entails a high risk of sarcomas, breast cancer, leukemias, brain tumors, and adrenocortical carcinomas. Of affected patients, 50% develop invasive cancers by age 30 and 90% by age 70. These cancers develop when the second copy of *p53* is knocked out by a somatic mutation. This is the same two-mutation model described for retinoblastoma (see Fig. 18.16).

Most of the *p53* mutations, both in spontaneous tumors and in the germline of patients with Li-Fraumeni syndrome, lead to single amino acid substitutions in the DNA-binding domain. *These mutant p53 proteins are not necessarily inactive.* Some of them can form transcriptionally inactive com-

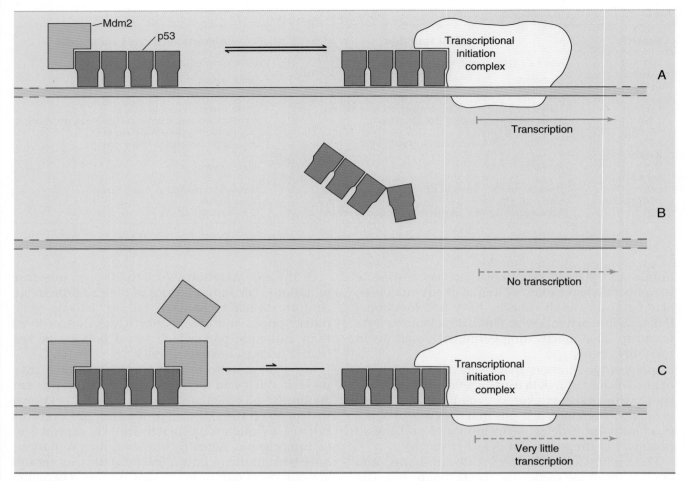

Figure 18.19 Interaction between p53 (■) and Mdm2 (□), the product of the *mdm2* (proto-) oncogene. The transcriptional activation by p53 can be disrupted by *p53* mutations that prevent sequence-specific DNA binding, the formation of transcriptionally active p53 oligomers, or the interaction with the transcriptional machinery. It also can be disrupted by the overexpression of the Mdm2 protein, which binds to p53 and thereby prevents its interaction with the transcriptional initiation complex. **A,** Normal *p53* stimulates gene transcription, and this action is antagonized by Mdm2. **B,** Mutant *p53* fails to bind to its response elements in the promoters of regulated genes and to stimulate transcription. **C,** When the *mdm2* gene is amplified and its product is overexpressed, most of the p53 is tied up in complexes with Mdm2 and is not available for transcriptional activation.

plexes with normal p53, thereby inactivating the normal p53 protein in a heterozygous cell. Normal p53 binds DNA as a tetramer, and the incorporation of mutant p53 in these tetramers disrupts their biological activity. Some mutant p53 proteins even stimulate cell proliferation by unknown mechanisms.

Defects in p53-Regulating Proteins Can Contribute to Cancer

p53 is tightly regulated in the cell. **Mdm2,** the protein product of the *mdm2* gene, binds to a site on p53 that overlaps with the transcriptional acti-

vation domain, thereby inhibiting p53's effect on gene transcription (Fig. 18.19). Besides blocking p53-induced transcription, Mdm2 transports p53 out of the nucleus and it acts as a ubiquitin ligase, attaching ubiquitin to p53 and marking it for destruction by the proteasome. Transcription of the *mdm2* gene is stimulated by p53. This feedback loop prevents the overproduction of p53 in situations in which growth arrest or apoptosis would be inappropriate.

Mdm2 is an essential regulator of p53. Homozygous *p53* knockout mice are viable and have few abnormalities other than cancer susceptibility, but *mdm2* knockouts die as embryos (Table 18.4). Conversely, transgenic mice with a poorly regulated extra copy of *p53* develop early senility, and those

Table 18.4 Abnormalities in Knockout Mice that Are Homozygously Deficient in Cell Cycle Regulators

Protein	Viability of Mice	Tumors
Regulators of the G_1 checkpoint		
Cyclin D1	Viable, but small size and behavioral abnormalities	None
pRb	Death at gestational day 14	—
p27*	Viable, but increased body size and female sterility	Pituitary tumors
INK4a*	Viable	Tumors by 6 months of age
E2F-1[†]	Viable, but T cell hyperplasia	None
Components of the DNA damage response		
p53	Viable, few abnormalities	Tumors by 3 months of age
p21*	Normal	None
Mdm2	Embryos dying at implantation[‡]	—
Mitogenic signal transducers		
N-Ras	Viable, no gross abnormalities	None
c-Src	Viable, but osteoclast malfunction (osteopetrosis)	None
c-Myc	Early death	—

* CDK inhibitors.
† An isoform of E2F that is regulated by pRb but not by p107 and p130.
‡ Mice lacking both Mdm2 and p53 are viable.

with a normally regulated extra copy of *p53* are unusually cancer resistant and age normally.

The *mdm2* gene is a proto-oncogene that is amplified in approximately 30% of all soft tissue sarcomas, as well as in some glial tumors. Although these tumor cells possess normal p53, they show the same phenotypic features as do cells with inactivated p53.

Mdm2 is itself inhibited by the protein Arf, which binds to Mdm2 and prevents it from inactivating p53. Many signaling cascades, including those involving the Ras protein, PKB (protein kinase B, or Akt), and the E2F and Myc transcription factors, impinge on p53 through either Mdm2 or Arf (Fig. 18.20).

The PI3K/Protein Kinase B Pathway Is Activated in Many Cancers

As shown in Figure 18.20, many oncogene products, including Myc, Ras, and E2F, can activate p53. Therefore, *in the presence of intact p53, the mutationally activated oncogenes are likely to induce cell cycle arrest, senescence, or apoptosis.* Only PKB suppresses p53 by phosphorylating and thereby activating Mdm2.

Indeed, *the PKB cascade transmits a survival signal that prevents apoptosis by multiple mechanisms.* As shown in Figure 18.21, it regulates the synthesis of pro-apoptotic and antiapoptotic proteins by phosphorylating several transcription factors, including NFκB and transcription factors of the forkhead family. It also phosphorylates and thereby inactivates the pro-apoptotic protein Bad and the initiator caspase Casp-9.

The genes for both PI3K and PKB are amplified in some cancers. The most common alteration,

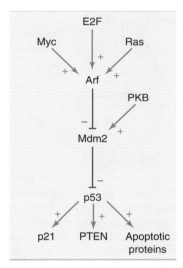

Figure 18.20 The regulation of p53. The p53 inhibitor Mdm2 is itself inhibited by Arf. Note that many oncogenes *(myc, ras, E2F)* can activate p53 through Arf and Mdm2. This tends to suppress cancer because it leads to apoptosis of oncogenically mutated cells. However, protein kinase B (PKB) inhibits p53 by phosphorylating Mdm2, thereby promoting the entry of Mdm2 into the nucleus.

however, is the mutational inactivation of **PTEN.** This lipid phosphatase dampens the signaling cascade by hydrolyzing the phosphatidylinositol-3,4,5-trisphosphate that is generated by PI3K (Fig. 18.22). Without PTEN, levels of this lipid remain permanently elevated and PKB remains active at all times. Apoptosis is suppressed, whereas cell cycle progression is stimulated. Between 30% and 50% of spontaneous cancers have lost PTEN through somatic mutations.

The PTEN gene is itself an important target of p53. Its transcription is stimulated by p53, and the resulting inhibition of the PI3K/PKB pathway contributes to p53-induced apoptosis.

The Products of Some Viral Oncogenes Neutralize the Products of Cellular Tumor Suppressor Genes

Retrovirus-induced cancers are extremely rare in humans. Some of the common cancers, however,

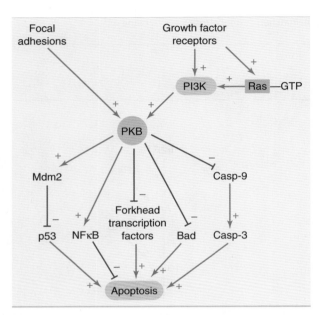

Figure 18.21 The role of phosphatidylinositol 3–kinase (PI3K) and protein kinase B (PKB) in the prevention of apoptosis. This signaling pathway prevents apoptosis by multiple mechanisms that involve nuclear transcription factors (p53, NFκB, forkhead proteins), the protease caspase-9, and the pro-apoptotic protein Bad, which acts as a Bcl2 antagonist in the mitochondrial pathway of apoptosis.

are associated with DNA viruses. Some DNA viruses promote cancer simply by causing chronic tissue damage and a stimulation of cell division in the surviving cells. This increases the pool of mitotic cells that can potentially acquire oncogenic mutations.

Unlike the retroviruses, *DNA viruses do not habitually integrate their DNA into the host cell genome.* The integration of their DNA into a host cell chromosome is a rare accident during viral infection, but when it occurs, it can activate a cellular proto-oncogene by promoter insertion or enhancer insertion. **Hepatitis B virus,** for example, carries no oncogene; nevertheless, chronic hepatitis B infection is a risk factor for liver cancer, probably because the virus can insert at random sites in the genome.

The **human papillomavirus** (wart virus), however, which infects the cells of squamous epithelia in the skin and mucous membranes, has its own oncogenes. This virus is a genetic pauper, with a small circular double-stranded DNA genome of 8000 base pairs that codes for about half a dozen proteins. For its reproduction, the virus depends on DNA polymerases, helicases, and other proteins of the host cell. These host cell proteins are produced only in dividing cells.

Therefore, the virus can reproduce only by driving its host into mitosis, while preventing apoptosis. It achieves these two aims through the products of its two oncogenes, **E6** and **E7.** *The viral oncogene products inactivate the products of the major cellular tumor suppressor genes.* E6 binds tightly to p53, and E7 binds to pRB (Fig. 18.23). These complexes are destroyed by the proteasome system. Untroubled by suicidal thoughts, the virus-infected cell can now sail through the cell cycle, replicating the viral DNA along with its own. Unlike the retroviral oncogenes, the oncogenes of the papillomavirus and other DNA viruses are not related to normal cellular proto-oncogenes.

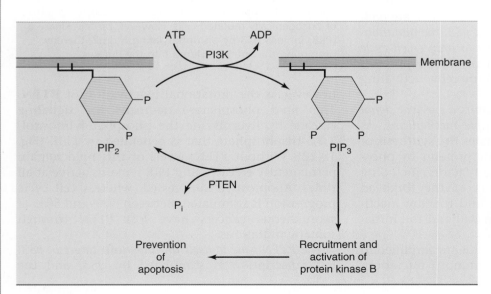

Figure 18.22 The phosphatase PTEN removes a phosphate from phosphatidylinositol-3,4,5-trisphosphate (PIP_3) in the plasma membrane, thereby inactivating this second messenger. PTEN is inactivated in many cancers, and the resulting overactivity of protein kinase B prevents apoptosis. PIP_2, phosphatidylinositol-4,5-bisphosphate.

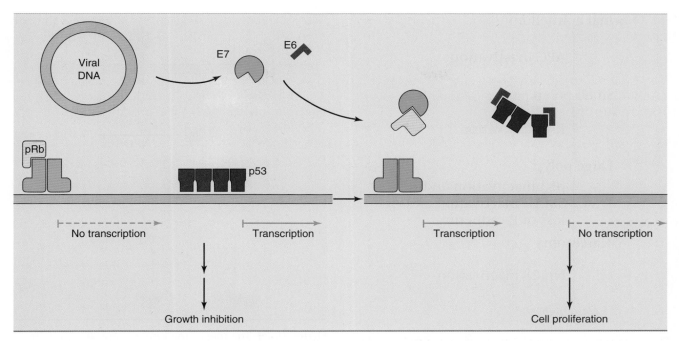

Figure 18.23 The molecular mechanism by which human papillomavirus stimulates the growth of infected cells. The viral *E6* and *E7* proteins bind to the p53 protein and the retinoblastoma protein (pRb), respectively, tying them up in inactive complexes. The resulting changes in gene transcription lead to increased cell proliferation and an increased rate of somatic mutations. In ordinary warts, the viral DNA exists as a plasmid-like episome, but in most cervical cancers, the viral *E6* and/or *E7* genes are integrated in the host cell DNA. Although the product of the *E6* gene acts like the product of the cellular *mdm2* gene (see Fig. 18.19), the two proteins are not structurally related.

Ordinarily the papillomavirus produces a common wart, with abnormally proliferating epithelial cells that contain viral DNA as plasmid-like entities. The abnormal growth is benign, and eventually the infected cells either die or lose their virus. In rare cases, however, snippets of viral DNA containing *E6* and/or *E7* become integrated into a host cell chromosome. *These cells cannot lose the viral DNA, and they are at risk of malignant transformation by additional somatic mutations.*

The papillomavirus plays a sinister role in cancer of the uterine cervix. Of cervical cancers worldwide, 93% contain the viral *E6* and/or *E7* genes, integrated into their genome. The papillomavirus can be transmitted by sexual intercourse, and therefore cervical cancer can be considered a "sexually transmitted cancer." Also, more than 50% of other anogenital cancers, as well as many nonmelanoma skin cancers and some cancers of the oral cavity, contain the viral oncogenes.

Carcinogenesis Is a Multistep Process

Even cancers that are derived from the same cell type vary greatly in their growth habits and clinical behavior, depending on the combination of mutations and epigenetic changes present in the cells. Cancer cells also change their character over time. A benign mole, for example, can turn into a malignant melanoma; a slowly progressive chronic leukemia that had been present for years can suddenly transform into an acute disease ("blast crisis") that kills the patient within weeks; and a long-standing, indolent astrocytoma or oligodendroglioma can mutate into a highly aggressive, rapidly fatal glioblastoma.

These are examples of **tumor progression.** It is seen when a cell in an already abnormal cell population acquires a new mutation that makes it faster growing, more invasive, or more resistant to apoptosis. Tumor progression is evolution in the fast track, with new variants formed continuously and more malignant clones taking over the ecosystem from less malignant clones. Like all other life forms, neoplastic cells are subject to Darwinian selection: *fast-reproducing variants replace slower reproducing variants.* This process is favored by the genetic instability and high mutation rate that are typical for most cancers.

Most colorectal cancers, for example, develop from benign polyps. A typical sequence of mutational events for this cancer is as follows:

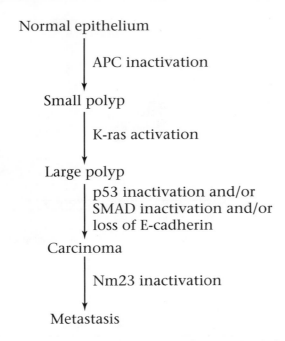

Normal epithelium

↓ APC inactivation

Small polyp

↓ K-ras activation

Large polyp

↓ p53 inactivation and/or
SMAD inactivation and/or
loss of E-cadherin

Carcinoma

↓ Nm23 inactivation

Metastasis

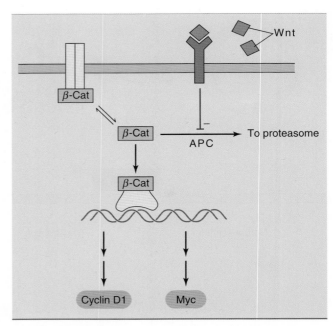

Figure 18.24 The role of the tumor suppressor protein APC in the Wnt signaling cascade. APC is required for the breakdown of β-catenin by the proteasome system. The Wnt pathway prevents the breakdown of β-catenin (β-Cat). This allows β-catenin to reach the nucleus, where it stimulates the expression of promitotic genes. In the absence of functional APC, β-catenin cannot be degraded even in the absence of Wnt signaling. Therefore, the Wnt pathway is switched on at all times.

The homozygous inactivation of the **APC** (adenomatous polyposis coli) gene is sufficient for the formation of a benign polyp. Normal people have occasional intestinal polyps, but in dominantly inherited **adenomatous polyposis coli (APC)**, the colonic mucosa becomes studded with thousands of polyps. Affected patients have a heterozygous loss of *APC* in all their cells, and the inactivation of the single remaining *APC* gene by a somatic mutation is sufficient to create a polyp. Most of these polyps remain benign, but there is an 80% chance that at least one of them will eventually turn malignant. APC accounts for approximately 2% of all colon cancers.

The product of the APC *tumor suppressor gene is a negative regulator in the* **Wnt** *signaling pathway,* as shown in Figure 18.24. This mitogenic signaling cascade uses the multifunctional protein **β-catenin,** which is otherwise a constituent of adherens junctions (see Chapter 13). Normally, any β-catenin that strays away from its adherens junction is scavenged by a protein complex that contains the APC protein along with a protein kinase. Phosphorylation of β-catenin in this complex marks it for ubiquitination and destruction by the proteasome.

The destruction of β-catenin can be prevented by a signaling protein from the mitogenic Wnt signaling pathway. This allows the β-catenin to escape into the nucleus, where it participates in the regulation of gene expression, stimulating transcription from the genes for cyclin D1, the Myc protein, and other mitogenic proteins. *Mutational inactivation of the* APC *gene prevents the destruction of β-catenin,* and the accumulating β-catenin stimulates gene expression permanently.

Like β-catenin, APC is a multifunctional protein. In addition to promoting the degradation of β-catenin, it also interacts with the microtubules of the mitotic spindle. Mutant forms of APC fail to do so, and this leads to frequent errors in chromosome segregation during mitosis. The resulting chromosomal instability favors tumor progression.

Some small polyps have normal APC, but β-catenin is mutated to make it resistant to degradation. These polyps look like those with missing APC, but they rarely progress to a malignant state.

Activating mutations of the **K-ras** proto-oncogene are not seen in small polyps but occur in 40% of large polyps and carcinomas. The loss of a tumor suppressor gene, either **p53, E-cadherin,** or **SMAD,** appears to mark the transition from a benign polyp to a true carcinoma. E-cadherin is a cell adhesion protein that is involved in the contact inhibition of cell growth. SMAD proteins are signal transducers and transcriptional regulators in yet another signaling pathway that is triggered by the antimitotic protein **transforming growth factor β (TGF-β).** The receptor for TGF-β is also mutationally inactivated in about 30% of spontaneous colon cancers.

Little is known about the genetic changes that predispose cancer cells to metastasis. The *nm23* gene seems to be important, inasmuch as it has frequently been found mutated in metastases but not the primary tumor.

Some molecular markers are useful for the prognosis of cancer. The deletion of the long arm of chromosome 18 in the tumor cells, for example, signals a loss of a *SMAD* gene and is associated with decreased survival in patients with colorectal cancer, and a reduction or absence of expression of the *nm23* gene is always associated with a high metastatic potential, not only in colorectal cancers but also in many other malignancies.

Molecular markers can be used for disease prediction, but *they also help with the selection of treatment strategies.* When the genes indicate a poor prognosis, aggressive treatment is indicated; when the markers point to a high metastatic potential, systemic treatments, including chemotherapy, are indicated at an early stage in addition to the local treatments of surgery and radiation.

SUMMARY

Cell cycle progression requires a finely tuned sequence of biochemical events, including transcriptional regulation and protein phosphorylation. Many of these events are coordinated by the Cdks and their regulatory subunits, the cyclins. The cyclins and Cdks bring the cell through the G_1 checkpoint by phosphorylating and thereby inactivating pRb.

Cells can also commit suicide, or apoptosis, under adverse conditions. Apoptosis can be triggered by two pathways, one dependent on mitochondria and the other dependent on the activation of death receptors by extracellular ligands. Both pathways are controlled by a delicate balance between pro-apoptotic and antiapoptotic proteins.

The growth, differentiation, proliferation, and survival of cells are regulated by extracellular signals. Focal adhesions favor survival and mitosis and are responsible for the anchorage dependence of cell growth. Contacts with neighboring cells lead to contact inhibition of cell proliferation, and soluble extracellular signaling proteins can both stimulate and inhibit growth, mitosis, and apoptosis.

Typical mitogenic signaling pathways include the PI3K/PKB cascade and the MAP kinase cascade. Both lead to the phosphorylation of nuclear transcription factors, thereby regulating the expression of genes for cell cycle progression, terminal differentiation, and apoptosis.

Oncogenes are mitogenic or antiapoptotic genes that are abnormally activated in cancer cells, and tumor suppressor genes are antiproliferative genes that are mutationally inactivated in cancers. Inherited defects of tumor suppressor genes can contribute to the development of cancer. Some viruses can also cause cancer. However, most of the genetic alterations in spontaneous cancers are somatic mutations. Cancers tend to become more malignant over time because the cancer cells are subject to frequent mutations and to Darwinian selection acting on the mutant cells.

📖 Further Reading

Appella E, Anderson CW: Post-translational modifications and activation of p53 by genotoxic stresses. Eur J Biochem 268:2764-2772, 2001.

Frame MC: Src in cancer: deregulation and consequences for cell behaviour. Biochim Biophys Acta 1602:114-130, 2002.

Grady WM, Markowitz SD: Genetic and epigenetic alterations in colon cancer. Annu Rev Genomics Hum Genet 3:101-128, 2002.

Hingorani SR, Tuveson DA: Ras redux: rethinking how and where Ras acts. Curr Opin Genetics Dev 13:6-13, 2003.

Lowe SW, Sherr CJ: Tumor suppression by *INK4a-Arf*: progress and puzzles. Curr Opin Genet Dev 13:77-83, 2003.

Lutz W, Leon J, Eilers M: Contributions of Myc to tumorigenesis. Biochim Biophys Acta 1602:61-71, 2002.

Mayo LD, Donner DB: The PTEN, Mdm2, p53 tumor suppressor-oncoprotein network. Trends Biochem Sci 27:462-467, 2002.

Newmeyer DD, Ferguson-Miller S: Mitochondria: releasing power for life and unleashing the machineries of death. Cell 112:481-490, 2003.

Stevens C, La Thangue NB: E2F and cell cycle control: a double-edged sword. Arch Biochem Biophys 412:157-169, 2003.

Venkitaraman AR: Cancer susceptibility and the functions of BRCA1 and BRCA2. Cell 108:171-182, 2002.

QUESTIONS

1. **An activating mutation in the *ras* gene will most likely**

   A. Prevent the autophosphorylation of growth factor receptors.
   B. Inhibit the release of calcium from the endoplasmic reticulum.
   C. Increase the activity of the MAP kinases.
   D. Activate the Src protein kinase.
   E. Reduce the nuclear concentration of cyclin D.

2. **What type of structural/functional change would be most likely in an oncogenically activated variant of the Ras protein?**

   A. Inability to interact with the Raf-1 protein kinase.
   B. Reduced GTPase activity.
   C. A point mutation in a transmembrane helix.
   D. Resistance to the phosphatase PTEN.
   E. An increased ability to tyrosine-phosphorylate proteins.

3. **Most of the cyclins are induced and repressed periodically during the cell cycle. One cyclin, however, is controlled primarily by mitogens rather than the cell cycle machinery. This mitogen-sensing cyclin is**

   A. Cyclin A.
   B. Cyclin B.
   C. Cyclin C.
   D. Cyclin D.
   E. Cyclin E.

4. **pRb is a major control element of the cell cycle. It normally becomes**

   A. Transcriptionally induced at the G_1 checkpoint.
   B. Dephosphorylated at the G_1 checkpoint.
   C. Phosphorylated at the G_1 checkpoint.
   D. Phosphorylated at the G_2 checkpoint.
   E. Transcriptionally induced at the G_2 checkpoint.

5. **The homozygous loss of a cell cycle regulator or signaling molecule can contribute to malignant transformation. This is most likely for the homozygous loss of**

   A. The Cdk4 protein kinase.
   B. Cyclin E.
   C. E-cadherin.
   D. A MAP kinase.
   E. The transcription factor E2F.

6. **The oncogenes of the human papillomavirus**

   A. Bind to the host cell DNA, stimulating the transcription of antiapoptotic genes.
   B. Inactivate the retinoblastoma and p53 proteins.
   C. Activate growth factor receptors in the absence of the normal ligand.
   D. Activate cyclin-dependent kinases by direct binding to the catalytic subunit.
   E. Are protein kinases that phosphorylate many of the same proteins as the MAP kinases.

7. **The entry into mitosis is accompanied by the phosphorylation of histone H1, chromosomal scaffold proteins, and nuclear lamins. The protein kinase that is responsible for these phosphorylations is activated by**

   A. The p53 protein.
   B. Cyclin D.
   C. The Ras protein.
   D. The ERK protein kinases through phosphorylation.
   E. Cyclin B.

8. **Mutations in the p53 gene are the most common aberrations in spontaneous human cancers. The normal p53 protein affects the cell cycle by**

   A. Inducing cell cycle arrest and apoptosis in response to DNA damage.
   B. Inducing the phosphorylation of pRb in response to mitogens.
   C. Directly inhibiting Cdk inhibitors in response to cell-cell contact and other growth-inhibiting stimuli.
   D. Increasing the activity of cyclin-dependent protein kinases by inducing their phosphorylation.
   E. Binding and thereby inactivating the products of many pro-apoptotic genes.

9. **The loss of the lipid phosphatase PTEN is likely to**

   A. Increase the activity of the Ras protein.
   B. Make the cell more vulnerable to apoptosis-inducing stimuli.
   C. Raise the cellular levels of p53.
   D. Activate PKB (Akt).
   E. Lead to the dephosphorylation of pRb.

PART FIVE

METABOLISM

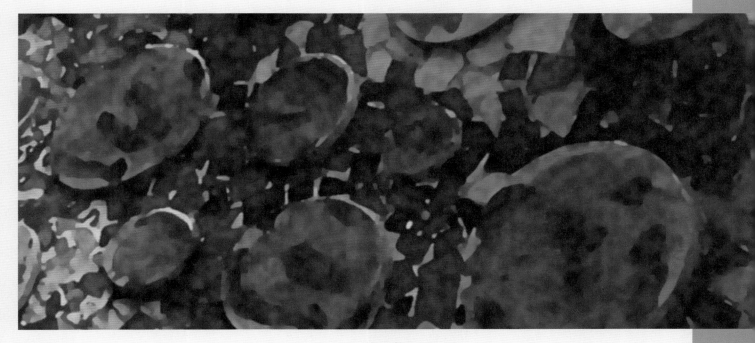

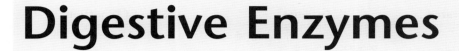

CHAPTER 19

Digestive Enzymes

Most dietary nutrients come in the form of large polymeric structures that cannot be absorbed in the intact state. They have to be hydrolyzed by enzymes in the gastrointestinal (GI) tract, and the breakdown products, including monosaccharides, amino acids, and fatty acids, are absorbed. *The whole process of digestion consists of hydrolytic cleavage reactions.*

Approximately 30 g of digestive enzymes are secreted per day. Because each enzyme has a fairly narrow substrate specificity and hydrolyzes only certain bonds, several enzymes have to cooperate in the digestion of complex nutrients (Table 19.1).

Saliva Contains α-Amylase and Lysozyme

The main function of saliva is not the digestion of nutrients but the conversion of food into a homogeneous mass during mastication. The only noteworthy enzymes in saliva are **α-amylase** and **lysozyme.** Both are **endoglycosidases** that cleave internal glycosidic bonds in a polysaccharide substrate. **Exoglycosidases,** in contrast, cleave glycosidic bonds at the ends.

α-Amylase cleaves α-1,4 glycosidic bonds in starch. Starch occurs in two forms: **amylose** is a linear polymer of glucose, linked by α-1,4 glycosidic bonds; and **amylopectin,** which usually forms the larger part of the starch in plants, is a branched molecule with a variable number of α-1,6 glycosidic bonds in addition to the α-1,4 bonds.

α-Amylase acts only on starch, but not on disaccharides and trisaccharides, and it cleaves only α-1,4 bonds, not α-1,6 bonds. Therefore, it produces **maltose, maltotriose,** and **α-limit dextrins** rather than free glucose (Fig. 19-1). Maltose is a disaccharide and maltotriose is a trisaccharide of glucose residues in α-1,4 glycosidic linkage. α-Limit dextrins are oligosaccharides containing an α-1,6 glycosidic bond.

The salivary α-amylase is active at the normal salivary pH of 6.5 to 7.0 but is rapidly denatured in the acidic environment of the stomach. Therefore, it makes only a minor contribution to starch digestion. Its main function is to keep the teeth clean by dissolving starchy bits of food that remain lodged between the teeth after a meal. In cancer the salivary glands have been destroyed by radiation therapy and are prone to develop rapid tooth decay.

The other salivary endoglycosidase, **lysozyme,** hydrolyzes β-1,4 glycosidic bonds in the bacterial cell wall polysaccharide **peptidoglycan** (Fig. 19.2). *Lysozyme kills some types of bacteria;* others, however, are resistant because their peptidoglycan is protected from the enzyme by other cell wall components or, in the case of gram-negative bacteria, by an overlying outer membrane. Obviously, the members of the normal bacterial flora in the mouth (including those that cause bad breath) are resistant to lysozyme. However, many bacteria from other ecosystems are killed by lysozyme, and animals make use of this effect by licking their wounds. They use their saliva as an antiseptic.

Protein Digestion Starts in the Stomach

With a pH close to 2.0, the stomach is a forbidding place. The proton gradient between gastric juice and the blood—an almost million-fold concentration difference—is the steepest ion gradient anywhere in the body. The gastric acid has three major functions:

Table 19.1 Dietary Nutrients and Their Fates in the Gastrointestinal Tract

Nutrient	Products Generated	Enzymes	Sites of Digestion
Starch, glycogen	Glucose	α-Amylase, disaccharidases, and oligosaccharidases	Saliva, intestinal lumen, brush border
Maltose	Glucose	Glucoamylase, sucrase	
Sucrose	Glucose + fructose	Sucrase	Brush border
Lactose	Glucose + galactose	Lactase	
Proteins	Amino acids, dipeptides, and tripeptides	Pepsin, pancreatic enzymes, brush border enzymes	Stomach, intestinal lumen, brush border
Triglycerides	Fatty acids, 2-monoacylglycerol	Pancreatic lipase	Intestinal lumen
Nucleic acids	Nucleosides, bases	DNAses, RNAses	Intestinal lumen
"Fiber": cellulose, hemicelluloses, lignin, etc.	Acetate, propionate, lactate, H_2, CH_4, CO_2	Only very limited fermentation by colon bacteria	

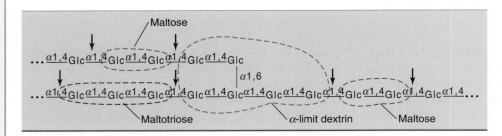

Figure 19.1 The pattern of starch digestion by α-amylase. This enzyme acts strictly as an endoglycosidase. It is unable to cleave the bonds in maltose, maltotriose, and the α-limit dextrins. *Arrows* indicate cleavage sites.

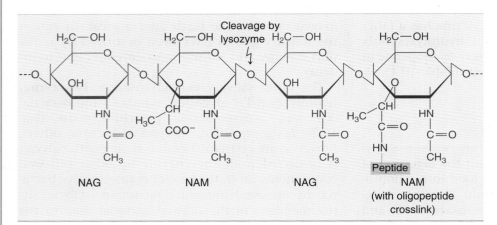

Figure 19.2 Structure of peptidoglycan, the substrate of lysozyme. NAG, *N*-acetylglucosamine; NAM, *N*-acetylmuramic acid.

1. *It kills most microorganisms.* People with achlorhydria (lack of gastric acid) and those who have had a gastrectomy (surgical removal of the stomach) have an increased risk for intestinal infections. Also, pathogens are more likely to establish an intestinal infection when ingested in water or other fluids than in solid food, because solid foods remain in the stomach far longer than fluids.
2. *It denatures dietary proteins.* This helps with protein digestion because it makes the peptide bonds more accessible for proteases.
3. *It is required for the action of **pepsin.*** Pepsin is a protease with an unusually low pH optimum of

2.0. It is considered an **endopeptidase,** but it also cleaves peptide bonds at the ends of the polypeptide. Pepsin cleaves only some peptide bonds, with a preference for bonds formed by the amino groups of large hydrophobic amino acids. Therefore, it produces a mix of oligopeptides along with some free amino acids. This mix is known as **peptone.** Protein digestion has to be completed by other enzymes in the small intestine (Table 19.2).

Neither gastric acid nor pepsin is essential for life, and protein digestion is still possible after total gastrectomy.

Table 19.2 Enzymes of Protein Digestion

Enzyme	Source	Type	Catalytic Mechanism	Cleavage Specificity
Pepsin	Stomach	Endopeptidase	Carboxyl protease	NH side of hydrophobic amino acids
Trypsin	Pancreas	Endopeptidase	Serine protease	CO side of basic amino acids
Chymotrypsin	Pancreas	Endopeptidase	Serine protease	CO side of hydrophobic amino acids
Elastase	Pancreas	Endopeptidase	Serine protease	CO side of small amino acids
Carboxypeptidase A	Pancreas	Carboxypeptidase	Metalloprotease (Zn^{2+})	Hydrophobic amino acids at C-terminus
Carboxypeptidase B	Pancreas	Carboxypeptidase	Metalloprotease (Zn^{2+})	Basic amino acids at C-terminus

The Pancreas Is a Factory for Digestive Enzymes

In the duodenum, the acidic stomach contents are rapidly neutralized by bicarbonate in the pancreatic secretions. The pancreas also supplies a mixture of enzymes, including copious amounts of **α-amylase.** This enzyme is different from the salivary α-amylase, with slightly different structure and encoded by a separate gene. Closely related enzymes that catalyze the same reaction but differ in molecular structure, physical properties, and reaction kinetics are called **isoenzymes.**

The pancreas also supplies the endopeptidases (and exopeptidases) **trypsin, chymotrypsin,** and **elastase.** All three are serine proteases (see Chapter 4), but with different cleavage specificities (see Table 19.2). Their action is complemented by exopeptidases: **Carboxypeptidase A** cleaves nonpolar amino acids from the carboxyl end of peptides, and **carboxypeptidase B** cleaves basic amino acids. Several other enzymes are contributed by the pancreas, including **pancreatic lipase,** various **phospholipases,** and **nucleases.**

Fat Digestion Requires Bile Salts

Triglycerides are almost totally insoluble in water. They form large fat droplets in water that provide only a small surface area for enzymatic attack, and therefore the first task in fat digestion is to disperse the fat into smaller entities with a larger surface/volume ratio.

To some extent, the fat is emulsified with the help of dietary phospholipids and proteins and dispersed in the process of mastication. In the small intestine, **pancreatic lipase** binds to these emulsion droplets with the help of a **colipase,** a small protein that is also derived from the pancreas. Pancreatic lipase hydrolyzes dietary triglycerides to free fatty acids and 2-monoacylglycerol:

Triglyceride

Pancreatic lipase (+ colipase)

2-Monoacylglycerol   Fatty acids

Unlike the triglycerides, *the products of fat digestion are slightly soluble in water.* The efficient absorption of the fatty acids and 2-monoacylglycerol requires **bile salts** as emulsifiers (Fig. 19.3). Between 20 and 50 g of bile salts reach the intestine every day.

Bile acids help with the formation of **mixed micelles** in the intestine; these are lipid aggregates that look like little shreds of lipid bilayer. The products of fat digestion form the two layers of the micelle, and the bile salt covers the hydrophobic edges. *Mixed micelles ferry the lipids rapidly through the unstirred layer overlying the intestinal mucosa.* Being slightly water soluble, fatty acids and 2-monoacylglycerol diffuse from the micelles to the microvilli, where they enter the mucosal cells, probably by passive diffusion across the microvillar membrane (Fig. 19.4).

Bile salts are also needed for the absorption of other dietary lipids, including cholesterol and the fat-soluble vitamins. In general, *lipids with the lowest*

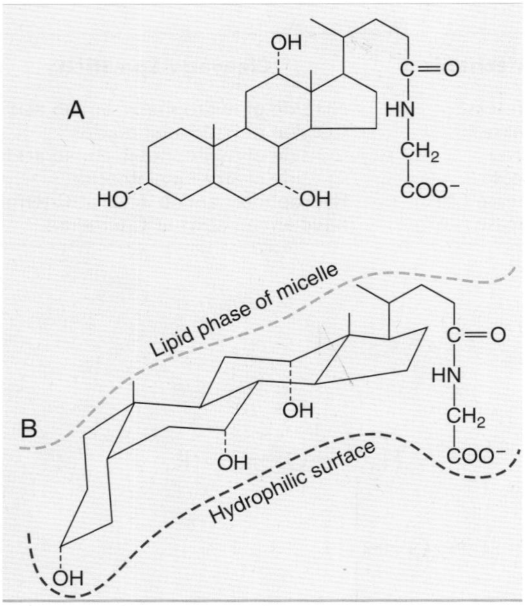

Figure 19.3 Structure of glycocholate, the most abundant bile salt in humans. The protonated forms of the bile salts are called "bile acids." **A**, Structure. **B**, Stereochemistry. Note that the molecule has a hydrophilic surface and a hydrophobic surface.

water solubility are most dependent on bile salts for their absorption.

Fat malabsorption can result from pancreatic failure, lack of bile salts, or extensive intestinal diseases. Pancreatic failure leads to bulky, fatty, floating stools that contain undigested triglycerides. This condition is called **steatorrhea.** Deficiencies of fat-soluble vitamins can occur because the vitamins are excreted in the stools along with the fat rather than being absorbed. A lack of bile salts in patients with biliary obstruction has similar consequences, but in this case most of the "fat" in the stools consists of unabsorbed fatty acids, monoglycerides, and diglycerides.

Fat malabsorption can be treated effectively. Both pancreatic enzymes and bile salts are available in tablet form and are used routinely in patients with pancreatic insufficiency or biliary disease.

Some Digestive Enzymes Are Anchored to the Surface of the Microvilli

The crypts of Lieberkühn in the small intestine secrete between 1 and 2 liters of a watery fluid every day, but this secretion is almost devoid of digestive enzymes. There are, however, enzymes attached to the luminal surface of the intestinal mucosal cells. This surface, known as the **brush border,** mea-

Table 19.3 Disaccharidases and Oligosaccharidases of the Intestinal Brush Border

Enzyme	Cleavage Specificity
Glucoamylase	Maltose, maltotriose; acts as exoglycosidase on α-1,4 bonds at the nonreducing end of starch and starch-derived oligosaccharides
Sucrase	Sucrose, maltose, maltotriose
Isomaltase	α-1,6 Bonds in isomaltose and α-limit dextrins
Lactase*	Lactose; also cellobiose†
Cerebrosidase*	Glucocerebroside and galactocerebroside
Trehalase	Trehalose‡

*The lactase and cerebrosidase activities reside in two different globular domains of the same polypeptide (see Fig. 19.5).
†Cellobiose is a disaccharide of two glucose residues in β-1,4–glycosidic linkage.
‡Trehalose is a disaccharide of two glucose residues in α,α′-1, 1–glycosidic linkage; common only in mushrooms and insects.

sures more than 200 m^2 because of the extensive folding of the villi and the innumerable microvilli. The brush border enzymes are firmly attached to the surface of the microvilli, with their catalytic domains protruding into the intestinal lumen (Fig. 19.5).

There are a large number of different peptidases on brush border membranes, including several types of **aminopeptidases, endopeptidases, carboxypeptidases,** and **dipeptidases** that act on the small oligopeptides formed by pepsin and the pancreatic enzymes. Nevertheless, a sizable portion of the dietary protein is absorbed not in the form of free amino acids but as dipeptides and tripeptides. These are further hydrolyzed to free amino acids by cytoplasmic enzymes in the mucosal cells.

Disaccharidases and **oligosaccharidases** (Table 19.3) hydrolyze sucrose and lactose, as well as the maltose, maltotriose and α-limit dextrins that are formed by the action of α-amylase on starch.

Not Everything Can Be Digested

In comparison with other animals, humans have a substandard digestive system. The digestion of most nutrients is incomplete. About 95% of the dietary fat and variable proportions of other dietary lipids are utilized. Starch is digested with an efficiency of 70% to 90%, depending on the dietary source. Protein digestion is variable. Keratins and some plant proteins, for example, are incompletely digested. Overall, however, not more than 5 to 20 g of protein is excreted in the stools every day. This includes not only dietary protein but also

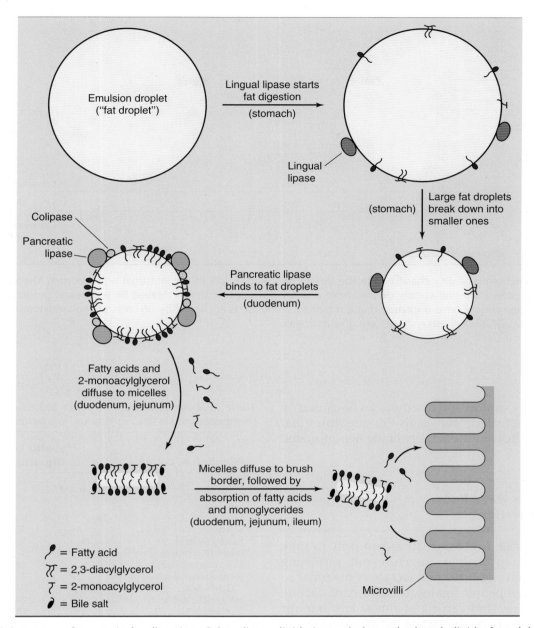

Figure 19.4 Sequence of events in fat digestion. Other dietary lipids (e.g., cholesterol, phospholipids, fat-soluble vitamins) are absorbed by the same mechanism, requiring mixed bile salt micelles for their diffusion to the brush border. Lingual lipase is secreted by glands at the base of the tongue. It produces small amounts of fatty acids, diglycerides, and monoglycerides that act as emulsifiers.

protein from digestive enzymes and desquamated mucosal cells.

Many plant polymers, including cellulose, hemicelluloses, inulin, pectin, lignin, and suberin, are resistant to human digestive enzymes. A small percentage of this undigestible "dietary fiber" is hydrolyzed and anaerobically fermented by the lush bacterial flora of the colon. This bacterial fermentation produces a flammable mixture of the gases **hydrogen, methane,** and **carbon dioxide,** as well as the organic acids **acetate, pro-pionate, butyrate,** and **lactate.** Most of this is absorbed through the colonic mucosa.

Some vegetables contain indigestible carbohydrates that are nevertheless avidly consumed by colon bacteria. Beans and peas, for example, contain raffinose (galactose-glucose-fructose), stachyose (galactose-galactose-glucose-fructose), and other oligosaccharides with galactose residues in α–1,6–glycosidic linkage. These oligosaccharides are rapidly fermented to acids and gas by colon bacteria, with harmless but socially embarrassing flatulence. Also,

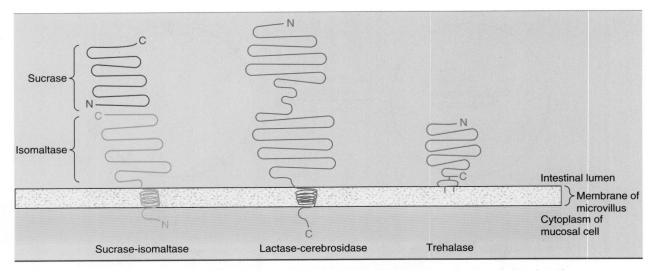

Figure 19.5 Anchoring of disaccharidases to the surface of the microvilli in the intestinal brush border. The sucrase-isomaltase complex is biosynthetically derived from a single polypeptide that is cleaved by pancreatic proteases. Isomaltase and lactase/cerebrosidase have transmembrane α helices; trehalase is anchored by glycosyl phosphatidylinositol (see Fig. 12.11, Chapter 12). All of these enzymes are glycoproteins.

abdominal discomfort and diarrhea can be caused by the irritant effect of the acids on the intestinal mucosa and the osmotic activity of the deprotonated acids.

Many Adults Have Poor Lactose Digestion

The disaccharide **lactose** is abundant only in milk and milk products. It is therefore not surprising that the activity of intestinal lactase is maximal in infants. Some people maintain abundant lactase throughout life. They can digest almost any amount of lactose. In others, the lactase activity declines to only 5% to 10% of the original level. This results in **lactose intolerance:** flatulence and other intestinal symptoms after the consumption of more than 200 to 500 mL of milk.

The symptoms are caused by the osmotic activity of the undigested lactose and the excessive formation of gas and acids by intestinal bacteria. As every student knows only too well, the intestinal bacterium *Escherichia coli* quickly develops a taste for lactose by inducing its lactose operon (see Chapter 6).

Lactose intolerance is not an important clinical problem because most people have enough common sense to adjust their milk consumption to their digestive capacity. It should, however, be routinely considered in patients with ill-defined

Table 19.4 Approximate Prevalence of Lactase Restriction (Nonpersistent Lactase) in Various Populations

Population/Country	% with Low Lactose-Digesting Capacity
Sweden	1
Britain	6
Germany	15
Greece	53
Morocco	78
Tuareg (Niger)	13
Fulani (Nigeria, Senegal)	0–22
Ibo, Yoruba (Nigeria)	89
Saudi Arabia: Bedouins	23
Other Arabs	56
India (different areas)	27–67
Thailand	98
China	93–100
North American Indians	63–95

abdominal complaints ("irritable bowel syndrome"). Various lactase preparations are commercially available. They are either taken in tablet form or mixed with the milk. These products contain lactases of microbial origin.

Lactose intolerance is a recessively inherited mendelian trait. In most parts of the world, a majority of the population is lactose intolerant. Persistent lactase prevails only in Europeans and some desert nomads of Arabia and Africa (Table 19.4). It appears that the persistent variety of lactase became common only in the past 6000 years or so and only in populations in which adults used to drink the milk of their cattle, goats, horses, camels, or reindeer. Thus, a Roman anthropologist reported about the Germans: "They do not eat much cereal food, but live chiefly on milk and meat . . . ." (Caesar, *Gallic War*, 4.1). It appears that in such populations, those who could digest the milk of their animals were slightly more likely to survive and reproduce than were those who could not.

Biochemically, lactose intolerance can be demonstrated in two ways. In the **lactose tolerance test,** the blood glucose level is determined before and after the ingestion of 50 g lactose. A rise in blood glucose of less than 20 mg/100 mL signals a delay in the absorption of lactose-derived glucose and galactose. Alternatively, the hydrogen content of breath can be determined before and after an oral lactose load. Increased hydrogen signals the fermentation of undigested lactose by colon bacteria.

Many Digestive Enzymes Are Released as Inactive Precursors

Among the digestive enzymes, *the proteases and phospholipases are dangerous.* They must be kept chained and muzzled until they reach the lumen of the GI tract, lest they attack proteins and membrane lipids in the cells of their birth.

To prevent self-digestion, the dangerous enzymes (but not lipases and glycosidases) are synthesized and secreted as inactive precursors called **zymogens.** The zymogens are synthesized at the rough endoplasmic reticulum, stored in secretory vesicles, released by exocytosis, and activated by selective proteolytic cleavage in the lumen of the GI tract.

Pepsinogen is secreted from the chief cells of the stomach and subsequently converted to active pepsin by the proteolytic removal of a 44–amino acid peptide from its amino-terminus. This reaction takes place at pH values below 5. At pH values above 2, the cleaved peptide remains bound to pepsin, masking its active site and thereby acting as a pepsin inhibitor. With or without the bound peptide, *pepsin is essentially inactive at pH values close to 7.0.*

The pancreatic zymogens include **trypsinogen, chymotrypsinogen** (Fig. 19.6), **proelastase, procarboxypeptidases,** and **prophospholipases.** *All these zymogens are activated by trypsin in the intestinal lumen.* Trypsinogen itself is activated either by trypsin or by the duodenal enzyme **enteropeptidase.**

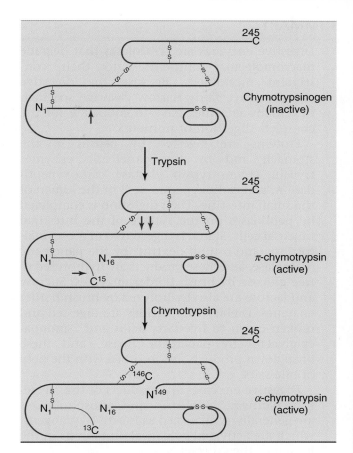

Figure 19.6 Activation of chymotrypsinogen to chymotrypsin. These reactions take place in the duodenum. Although π-chymotrypsin is fully active, α-chymotrypsin is the predominant form in the small intestine.

The pancreas protects itself not only by synthesizing the more dangerous enzymes as inactive zymogens but also by a **trypsin inhibitor.** The pancreatic trypsin inhibitor is a small (6-kD) polypeptide that binds very tightly (but noncovalently) to trypsin. It is present in the cytoplasm of the acinar cells and in the ductal system, in which it inactivates any trypsin that is erroneously activated within the organ.

These protective mechanisms are overwhelmed in **acute pancreatitis,** an often life-threatening condition in which the pancreas digests itself. The enzymes not only wreak havoc within the pancreas but also spill over into the abdominal cavity, in which the pancreatic lipase finds ample substrate in the intra-abdominal adipose tissue. Acute pancreatitis is diagnosed from the determination of lipase or amylase in the blood (see Chapter 15).

SUMMARY

Digestive enzymes are hydrolases that degrade macromolecular nutrients into their constituent monomers. Because the digestive enzymes have fairly narrow cleavage specificities, many enzymes have to cooperate for the complete digestion of nutrients.

Proteins are digested by pepsin in the stomach and by the pancreatic enzymes trypsin, chymotrypsin, elastase, carboxypeptidase A, and carboxypeptidase B in the lumen of the small intestine. Their digestion is completed by peptidases on the surface of the intestinal mucosal cells. Starch is digested to maltose, maltotriose, and α-limit dextrins by the pancreatic α-amylase, and these products are hydrolyzed to free glucose by brush border enzymes. Sucrose and lactose are also hydrolyzed by brush border enzymes. Dietary triglycerides are digested and broken down to free fatty acids and 2-monoacylglycerol by pancreatic lipase, and these breakdown products are absorbed with the help of bile salts.

Digestive enzymes are products of the "secretory pathway." Proteases and phospholipases are generally synthesized as inactive zymogens, which are activated by partial proteolysis in the lumen of the GI tract.

QUESTIONS

1. A Chinese student at a U.S. medical school complains to the school physician that he suffers from bouts of flatulence and diarrhea shortly after each breakfast. His usual breakfast consists of two candy bars, a small bag of peanuts, and three glasses of fresh milk. He never had digestive problems in his home country, where his diet consisted only of vegetables, meat, and rice. He has most likely a low level of:

    A. Pepsin.
    B. Pancreatic lipase.
    C. Lactase.
    D. Trypsin.
    E. α-Amylase.

2. Patients who had a pancreatectomy (surgical removal of the pancreas) should take supplements of digestive enzymes with each meal. These enzyme supplements need *not* contain

    A. α-Amylase.
    B. Proteases.
    C. Lipase.
    D. Disaccharidases.

CHAPTER 20

Introduction to Metabolic Pathways

The metabolic activities of cells are dictated by two major concerns:

1. *The cell has to synthesize its macromolecules.* Proteins have to be synthesized from amino acids; complex carbohydrates from monosaccharides; membrane lipids from fatty acids and other building blocks; and nucleic acids from nucleotides. These biosynthetic processes are called **anabolic.** They require metabolic energy, usually in the form of adenosine triphosphate (ATP).
2. *The cell has to generate metabolic energy.* Nutrients must be oxidized to supply the energy for biosynthesis, active membrane transport, cell motility, and muscle contraction. Degradative processes are called **catabolic** and, when possible, they are coupled to ATP synthesis. Most ATP is produced during the end-oxidation of metabolic intermediates to CO_2 and H_2O in the mitochondria (pathway (5) in Fig. 20.1).

Therefore, an unsuspecting nutrient molecule entering a cell has two alternative fates: Either it is used as a building block for the synthesis of a cellular macromolecule or it is oxidized to carbon dioxide and water for the generation of ATP (see Fig. 20.1).

The biosynthesis of cellular macromolecules has to be balanced by their degradation (pathway (2) in Fig. 20.1). A **steady state** must be maintained in which the rates of synthesis and degradation are balanced and the amount of the biosynthetic product remains constant. Different nutrients can also be interconverted through metabolic intermediates (pathways (3) and (4) in Fig. 20.1). For example, most amino acids can be converted to glucose, and glucose can be converted to amino acids and fatty acids.

Metabolic Processes Are Compartmentalized

The eukaryotic cell is partitioned into organelles, each with its own enzymatic outfit and metabolic activities (Fig. 20.2).

1. The **cytoplasm** contains both biosynthetic pathways and some nonoxidative catabolic pathways, and it is also the place where glycogen and fat are stored as energy reserves.
2. The **endoplasmic reticulum (ER)** and **Golgi apparatus** are concerned with the synthesis and processing of proteins and membrane lipids.
3. **Lysosomes** are filled with hydrolytic enzymes for the degradation of macromolecules. They hydrolyze endocytosed materials and some cellular macromolecules.
4. **Peroxisomes** are specialized organelles for some oxidative reactions.
5. **Mitochondria** are the powerhouses of the cell, generating more than 90% of the cell's ATP by oxidative phosphorylation.

The Free Energy Changes in Metabolic Pathways Are Additive

Complex metabolic transactions, such as the synthesis of glucose from lactate and the oxidation of acetyl–coenzyme A (acetyl-CoA) to carbon dioxide and water, cannot occur in a single step. They require a whole sequence of reactions in the form of a **metabolic pathway.** *The direction in which the pathway proceeds depends on the sum of the free energy changes of the individual reactions.* Consider the simple pathway

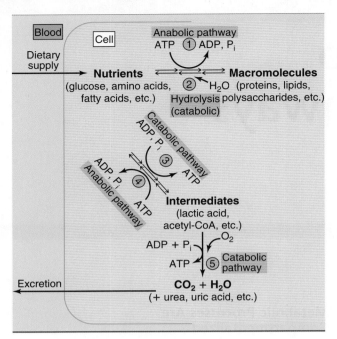

Figure 20.1 The major types of metabolic activity in the cell. ADP, adenosine diphosphate; ATP, adenosine triphosphate; CoA, coenzyme A; P_i, inorganic phosphate.

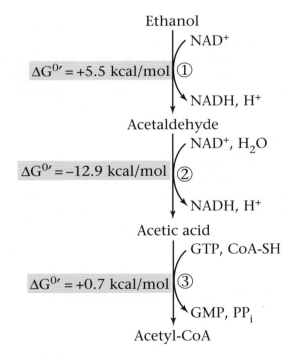

where $\Delta G^{0\prime}$ = standard free energy change, GMP = guanosine monophosphate, GTP = guanosine triphosphate, NAD$^+$ = nicotinamide adenine dinucleotide, NADH = nicotinamide adenine dinucleotide phosphate, and PP_i = inorganic pyrophosphate. Two of the three reactions have an unfavorable equilibrium with a positive $\Delta G^{0\prime}$.

Nevertheless, the sum of the free energy changes is negative: –6.7 kcal/mol. Therefore, under standard conditions, the pathway will turn ethanol into acetyl-CoA, rather than turn acetyl-CoA into ethanol.

However, the actual free energy change is quite different from the standard free energy change. Reaction (1), for example, has a very unfavorable equilibrium. With equal concentrations of NAD$^+$ and NADH, there would be only one molecule of acetaldehyde at equilibrium for every 10,000 molecules of ethanol! (see Chapter 4). However, under aerobic conditions, [NAD$^+$] is always far higher than [NADH]. When NAD$^+$ is 100 times more abundant than NADH, one molecule of acetaldehyde can be expected to be in equilibrium with 100 molecules of ethanol, and with an [NAD$^+$]/[NADH] ratio of 1000, the [ethanol]/[acetaldehyde] ratio is 10. Therefore, this seemingly "irreversible" reaction is actually reversible under cellular conditions. Indeed, it proceeds in the right direction because its product, acetaldehyde, is rapidly mopped up by the next enzyme in the pathway.

Reaction (3) appears freely reversible with its $\Delta G^{0\prime}$ of +0.7 kcal/mol. In the cell, however, the GTP concentration is about 100 times higher than the GMP concentration, and the level of PP_i is extremely low because this product is rapidly cleaved to inorganic phosphate (P_i) by various pyrophosphatases. Therefore, the reaction actually proceeds only in the direction of acetyl-CoA formation.

The terms **freely reversible** and **(physiologically) irreversible** are used to indicate whether a reaction can and cannot, respectively, proceed in both directions under ordinary cellular conditions.

Most Metabolic Pathways Are Regulated

The cells of the human body respond to signals from nutrients and hormones to adjust their metabolism to the physiological needs. They have three options for the regulation of their metabolic pathways:

1. *The amount of the enzyme is adjusted by a change in its rate of synthesis or degradation.* The lactose operon of the bacterium *Escherichia coli* (see Chapter 6) is the classical example for regulated enzyme synthesis, but humans employ similar mechanisms. Metabolic enzymes have life spans ranging from 1 hour to several days, and therefore this is a long-term type of regulation.

2. *Some enzymes are modified covalently, usually by the phosphorylation of amino acid side chains.* Either the phosphorylated or the dephosphory-

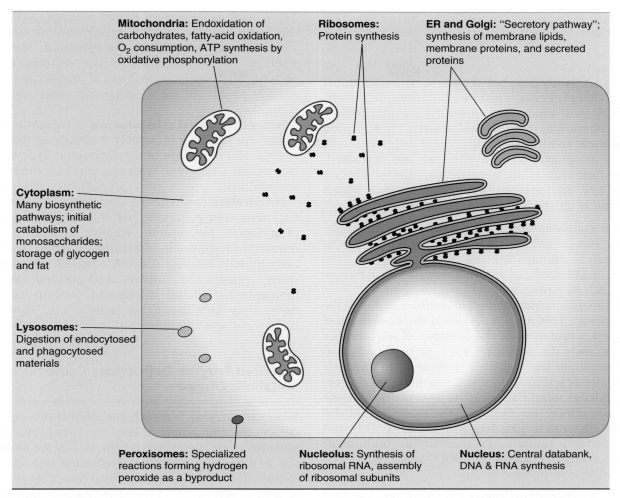

Figure 20.2 The metabolic functions of the major organelles. ATP, adenosine triphosphate; ER, endoplasmic reticulum.

lated enzyme is the catalytically active form. This regulatory mechanism requires a **protein kinase** (phosphorylating enzyme) and a **protein phosphatase** (dephosphorylating enzyme):

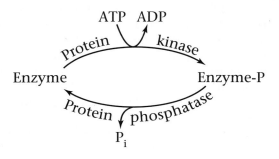

The protein kinases and protein phosphatases are regulated by metabolites or hormones.

3. *Some metabolic enzymes are regulated by allosteric effectors.* In most cases, the allosteric effector is a substrate, intermediate, or product of the pathway. In some regulated enzymes, the equilibrium between active and inactive conformations is affected both by phosphorylation and by allosteric effectors.

Metabolic enzymes are also subject to competitive inhibition in the form of **product inhibition.** This means that the product of the reaction competes with the substrate for the active site of the enzyme.

Feedback Inhibition and Feedforward Stimulation Are the Most Important Regulatory Principles

Consider a biosynthetic pathway in which an important product such as heme, cholesterol, or a purine is synthesized from a simple precursor:

$$\text{Substrate A} \xrightarrow{(1)} \text{B} \xrightarrow{(2)} \text{C} \xrightarrow{(3)} \text{D} \xrightarrow{(4)} \text{Product E}$$

This pathway should be active when the end product E is needed, but it should be switched off when there is enough product E in the cell already. In fact, *most biosynthetic pathways are inhibited by high concentrations of their end product.* This is called **feedback inhibition** (Fig. 20.3A).

Not all enzymes in a pathway are regulated. Short-term regulation, in particular, affects only one or a few enzymes in the pathway. But which enzyme is most suitable for regulation?

1. *A regulated enzyme must be present in lower activity than the other enzymes in the pathway.* It has to catalyze the rate-limiting step.
2. *It should serve an essential function in only one metabolic pathway.*
3. *It should catalyze the first irreversible reaction in the pathway.* This reaction is called the **committed step.** Regulation of the committed step ensures that only the substrate of the pathway accumulates when the regulated enzyme is inhibited. If a later reaction were regulated, metabolic intermediates would accumulate and possibly cause toxic effects. For example, the inhibition of the last enzyme in pathway A in Figure 20.3 would inevitably result in an undesirable buildup of intermediate D and, possibly, intermediates C and B as well.

In energy-producing catabolic pathways (see Fig. 20.3B), the important product is ATP. Therefore,

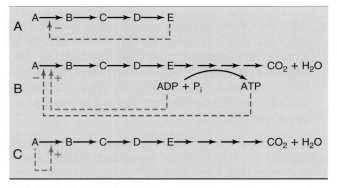

Figure 20.3 Regulation of metabolic pathways. The indicated regulatory influences (⊸, stimulation; --⊸, inhibition) may work through changes in the enzyme concentration (regulation of enzyme synthesis or degradation), by direct allosteric effects, or by effects on protein kinases and protein phosphatases that regulate the phosphorylation state of the enzyme. **A,** Anabolic pathway: feedback inhibition. **B,** Catabolic pathway: regulation by adenosine triphosphate (ATP) and adenosine diphosphate (ADP). P_i, inorganic phosphate. **C,** Catabolic pathway: regulation by feedforward stimulation.

ATP is used as a feedback inhibitor. When ATP is in short supply, the catabolic pathways are stimulated; when it is abundant, they are inhibited. The ATP level is inversely related to the concentrations of ADP and AMP. Indeed, *ADP and/or AMP act opposite to ATP in the regulation of many catabolic pathways.*

In **feedforward stimulation,** a substrate stimulates the pathway by which it is utilized (see Fig. 20.3C). The induction of the *lac* operon of *E. coli* by lactose (see Chapter 6) is an example of feedforward stimulation.

Hormones can regulate both the synthesis and degradation of metabolic enzymes, and their phosphorylation by protein kinases. Hormones are released in response to physiological stimuli such as carbohydrate feeding (insulin), fasting (glucagon), stress (epinephrine, cortisol), and physical exercise (epinephrine). Being distributed throughout the body, they coordinate the activities of different tissues in these situations.

Inherited Enzyme Deficiencies Cause Metabolic Diseases

When an enzyme is missing as a result of a genetic defect, the immediate effects are always the *accumulation of the substrate* and the *lack of the product.*

If a biosynthetic pathway is affected (Fig. 20.4A), *clinical signs and symptoms can be caused by the lack of the end product.* A classical example is **oculocutaneous albinism.** In this benign condition, the dark pigment melanin is not formed because one of the steps in melanin synthesis is genetically deficient: either the enzyme tyrosinase or the membrane carrier that transports the precursor tyrosine into the melanosome. In some other metabolic disorders, however, it is not the lack of the end product but the accumulation of a toxic metabolic intermediate that causes signs of disease.

The deficiency of an enzyme in a major catabolic, ATP-producing pathway is likely to cause serious problems for the cells that depend on that pathway for the generation of their metabolic energy. More commonly, an enzyme deficiency affects only the catabolism of a specialized substrate such as fructose or galactose (see Chapter 22) or the amino acid phenylalanine (see Chapter 26). In these cases, ATP can still be synthesized from other substrates, but *the accumulation of the nutrient or its immediate metabolites can cause problems* (see Fig. 20.4B). Some of these diseases can be treated simply by avoiding the offending nutrient.

In **storage diseases,** the intracellular degradation of a macromolecule by hydrolytic enzymes (pathway (2) in Fig. 20.1) is blocked, and problems

Figure 20.4 Consequences of an enzyme deficiency. **A,** Anabolic pathway: metabolite C accumulates, product E is deficient. C is either excreted or diverted into alternative pathways. Clinical signs and symptoms may be caused either by the deficiency of the product or by the accumulation of C. **B,** Catabolic pathway: a nutrient or one of its metabolites accumulates. Unless the pathway is essential for ATP synthesis (e.g., glycolysis, tricarboxylic acid cycle), the clinical signs are caused not by ATP deficiency but by the accumulation of the nutrient and/or its metabolites. **C,** Degradation of a macromolecule: the undegraded molecule C accumulates, mostly within the cells. The result is a "storage disease."

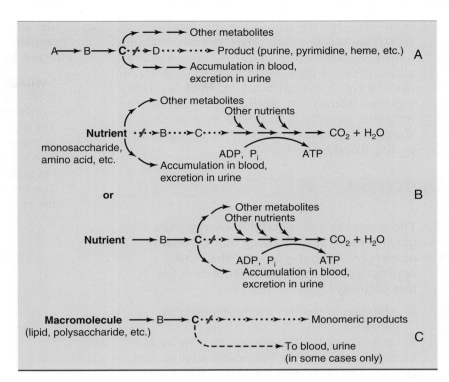

arise through the *abnormal accumulation ("storage") of the nondegradable macromolecule* (see Fig. 20.4C). The mucopolysaccharidoses (see Chapter 14), glycogen storage diseases (see Chapter 22), and lipid storage diseases (see Chapter 14) are the most prominent examples. Many but not all storage diseases are caused by the deficiency of a lysosomal enzyme.

Many metabolic enzymes come in the form of tissue-specific **isoenzymes** that are encoded by different genes. Therefore, *many inherited enzyme deficiencies are expressed only in some tissues but not others.*

Hundreds of enzyme deficiencies have been recognized in inherited metabolic diseases. Most of them are rare, with frequencies of less than 1 per 10,000 in the population. However, they provide valuable information about the normal roles of the affected pathways. Most of these **inborn errors of metabolism** are recessively inherited. This means that the heterozygotes, who still have half of the normal enzyme activity, are healthy. Only the complete loss of the enzyme in homozygotes causes a disease.

Vitamin Deficiencies, Toxins, and Endocrine Disorders Can Also Disrupt Metabolic Pathways

Many **toxins** act by inhibiting metabolic enzymes. For example, lead causes the accumulation of toxic intermediates by inhibiting enzymes of heme biosynthesis, and cyanide blocks cell respiration by inhibiting the mitochondrial cytochrome oxidase.

Vitamin deficiencies can affect multiple metabolic pathways. Many metabolic enzymes require a coenzyme, and many coenzymes are derived from a dietary vitamin (see Chapter 29). Therefore, a vitamin deficiency can prevent a metabolic reaction by depriving it of an essential coenzyme. Most vitamin-derived coenzymes, including NAD, flavin adenine dinucleotide, and CoA, participate in multiple metabolic pathways. All of these pathways are impaired when the vitamin is deficient.

Endocrine disorders are the most complex metabolic diseases because each hormone controls a whole set of metabolic pathways. In diabetes mellitus, for example, insufficient insulin action disrupts a host of pathways in carbohydrate and fat metabolism.

SUMMARY

Anabolic, or biosynthetic, pathways produce complex biosynthetic products from simple precursors. The necessary energy for biosynthesis is generated during catabolic processes, above all by the oxidation of nutrients in the mitochondria.

The direction in which a metabolic pathway proceeds is determined by the sum of the standard free energy changes of the individual reactions and by the cellular concentrations of substrates and products. Enzymes in metabolic pathways can be regulated in three ways: by adjustments of their own synthesis or degradation, by covalent modifications, or by reversibly binding ligands. In feedback inhibition, the regulated enzyme is inhibited by a product of the pathway, and in feedforward stimulation, it is stimulated by a substrate.

QUESTIONS

1. **The generation of metabolic energy from glucose requires a pathway that is known as glycolysis. What would be the most appropriate mechanism of regulation for this pathway?**

   A. Inhibition of the first irreversible step by glucose.
   B. Inhibition of the first irreversible step by ADP.
   C. Inhibition of the last irreversible step by ADP.
   D. Inhibition of the first irreversible step by ATP.
   E. Inhibition of the first irreversible step by carbon dioxide and water.

2. **Under physiological conditions, the "reversibility" of a metabolic reaction is affected by all of the following *except***

   A. Concentrations of the substrates and products.
   B. Concentration of the enzyme.
   C. The energy charge if ATP and ADP participate in the reaction.
   D. The standard free energy change of the reaction.
   E. The pH if protons are formed or consumed in the reaction.

CHAPTER 21

Glycolysis, Tricarboxylic Acid Cycle, and Oxidative Phosphorylation

The human body is a machine fueled by food. During their oxidation to carbon dioxide and water, carbohydrates yield about 4 kcal/g; triglycerides, 9.3 kcal/g; proteins, between 4.0 and 4.5 kcal/g; and alcohol, 7.0 kcal/g. Molecular oxygen is consumed during oxidative metabolism, and carbon dioxide is produced:

$$C_6H_{12}O_6 + 6\ O_2 \rightarrow 6\ CO_2 + 6\ H_2O$$
Glucose

$$C_{51}H_{98}O_6 + 72\tfrac{1}{2}\ O_2 \rightarrow 51\ CO_2 + 49\ H_2O$$
Tripalmitate, a triglyceride

The stoichiometry of O_2 consumption and CO_2 production is described by the **respiratory quotient (RQ):**

$$RQ = \frac{CO_2\ (\text{produced})}{O_2\ (\text{consumed})}$$

The RQ for the oxidation of carbohydrates is 1.0; for fat, about 0.7; and for protein, about 0.8.

Most cells have a choice among alternative substrates, including glucose, fatty acids, and amino acids. Others are more specialized. A few cell types, such as neurons and red blood cells, depend mainly or exclusively on glucose for their energy needs. This chapter traces the fate of glucose through its major catabolic pathways.

Glucose Is the Principal Transported Carbohydrate in Humans

Glucose is the most abundant monosaccharide in dietary carbohydrates. The other dietary monosaccharides, fructose from sucrose and galactose from lactose, can be converted to glucose in the liver (Fig. 21.1). Being small, soluble, and osmotically active, glucose can be transported by the blood, but it cannot be stored in the cells. For storage, it has to be converted to the polysaccharide **glycogen.** Glycogen granules are present in most cells, being most plentiful in liver and muscle tissue.

Because some tissues, including the brain, depend on a supply of glucose at all times, blood glucose must be maintained at an adequate level. The normal fasting blood glucose level is 4.0 to 5.5 mmol/liter (70 to 100 mg/dL), and even after a carbohydrate-rich meal, it rarely rises above 8.5 mmol/liter (150 mg/dL). *In the fasting state, the blood glucose level is maintained by the liver,* first by the breakdown of its stored glycogen and later by the synthesis of glucose from amino acids, lactic acid, and glycerol.

Glucose Uptake into the Cells Is Regulated

Glucose is too water soluble to penetrate membranes by passive diffusion. To enter the cell, it requires specialized carriers in the plasma membrane. Although the intestine absorbs glucose by sodium cotransport, glucose uptake from blood or interstitial fluid is by facilitated diffusion. No fewer than eight facilitated-diffusion carriers for glucose have been identified, encoded by separate genes and expressed in a tissue-specific manner.

In some tissues, including liver and brain, glucose uptake is not a limiting factor for its metabolism. Muscle and adipose tissue, however, have the **GLUT-4 (glucose transporter 4)** type of glucose carrier. *GLUT-4 is controlled by insulin.* In the absence of insulin, most GLUT-4 transporters are in the membranes of intracellular vesicles. By mechanisms that are not yet fully understood, activation of the insulin receptor triggers the fusion of these vesicles with the plasma membrane (Fig. 21.2). Therefore, muscle and adipose tissue take up glucose after a carbohydrate-rich meal, when the insulin level is high, but not during fasting, when the insulin level is low.

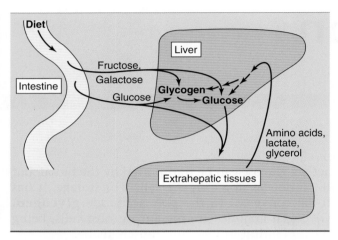

Figure 21.1 The role of glucose as the principal transported carbohydrate in the human body. Note the important role of the liver in glucose metabolism.

Glucose Degradation Begins in the Cytoplasm and Ends in the Mitochondria

The steps in glucose oxidation are summarized in Figure 21.3. The initial reaction sequence, known as **glycolysis,** takes place in the cytoplasm. It turns one molecule of glucose (6 carbons) into two molecules of the three-carbon compound **pyruvate.** All cells of the body are capable of glycolysis.

Under aerobic conditions, pyruvate is transported into the mitochondrion, where it is turned into the two-carbon compound **acetyl–coenzyme A (CoA).** Acetyl-CoA then enters the **tricarboxylic acid (TCA) cycle** by reacting with the four-carbon compound oxaloacetate to form the six-carbon compound citrate. Citrate is converted back to oxaloacetate in the reactions of the TCA cycle.

In these pathways, *the hydrogen of the substrate is transferred to the coenzymes nicotinamide adenine dinucleotide (NAD+) and flavin adenine dinucleotide (FAD)* (see Chapter 5). The reduced coenzymes donate their hydrogen to the **respiratory chain** of the inner mitochondrial membrane, which in turn donates it to molecular oxygen. *The reoxidation of the reduced coenzymes is highly exergonic.* The energy

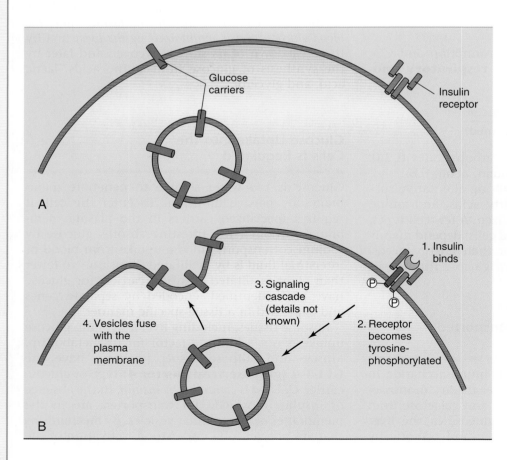

Figure 21.2 Effect of insulin on the glucose carriers in adipocytes. A similar mechanism is thought to operate in skeletal muscle. **A,** In the resting state, most glucose carriers are present in the membrane of intracellular vesicles. **B,** After insulin binding and receptor autophosphorylation, the carrier-containing vesicles fuse with the plasma membrane. This leads to an increased V_{max} of glucose transport across the plasma membrane.

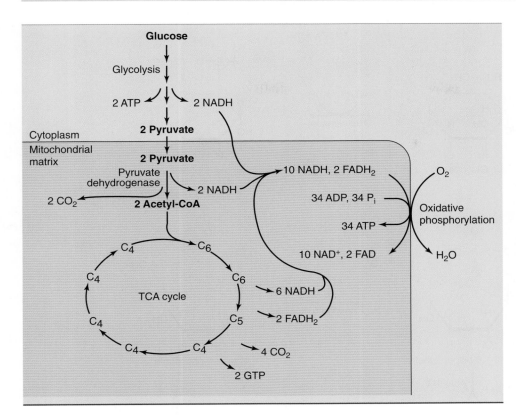

Figure 21.3 The steps in glucose oxidation. The catabolic pathways convert the carbon of the substrate to carbon dioxide. The hydrogen initially is transferred to the coenzymes NAD⁺ and FAD. The reduced coenzymes then are reoxidized by the respiratory chain. Most of the adenosine triphosphate (ATP) is produced in the process of oxidative phosphorylation, which couples the oxidation of the reduced coenzymes to ATP synthesis.

of this process is used for ATP synthesis by **oxidative phosphorylation.** The TCA cycle and oxidative phosphorylation take place in all cells that contain mitochondria.

Glycolysis participates only in carbohydrate metabolism, but acetyl-CoA is also formed in the degradation of fatty acids and amino acids. *The TCA cycle and oxidative phosphorylation are therefore the final common pathway for the oxidation of all major nutrients.*

Glycolysis Begins with ATP-Dependent Phosphorylations

After entering the cell, glucose is phosphorylated to glucose-6-phosphate by **hexokinase** (Fig. 21.4). The reaction is exergonic ($\Delta G^{0\prime}$ = −4.0 kcal/mol) because an energy-rich phosphoanhydride bond in ATP is cleaved, whereas a "low-energy" phosphate ester bond is formed (Table 21.1). In addition, the ATP concentration in a healthy cell is always far higher than the ADP concentration. Therefore, *the hexokinase reaction is irreversible.*

The hexokinase reaction is always the first step in glucose metabolism, whether glucose is being used for glycolysis or for other metabolic pathways. Glucose-6-phosphate cannot leave the cell on a membrane carrier as glucose can. Indeed, *phospho-*

rylated intermediates in general do not cross the plasma membrane.

In glycolysis, glucose-6-phosphate is in equilibrium with fructose-6-phosphate through the reversible **phosphohexose isomerase** reaction. Fructose-6-phosphate is then phosphorylated to fructose-1,6-bisphosphate by **phosphofructokinase** (PFK). This is the first irreversible reaction specific for glycolysis. It is its **committed step.**

The reactions from glucose to fructose-1,6-bisphosphate require two high-energy phosphate bonds in ATP. This initial investment has to be recovered in later reactions of the pathway.

Most Glycolytic Intermediates Have Three Carbons

The six-carbon intermediate fructose-1,6-bisphosphate is cleaved into two triose phosphates by the enzyme **aldolase.** Carbons 1, 2, and 3 of the sugar form dihydroxyacetone phosphate, and carbons 4, 5, and 6 form glyceraldehyde-3-phosphate. The two triose phosphates are interconverted in the reversible **triose phosphate isomerase** reaction.

Aldolase and triose phosphate isomerase establish an equilibrium between fructose-1,6-bisphosphate, dihydroxyacetone phosphate, and glyceraldehyde-

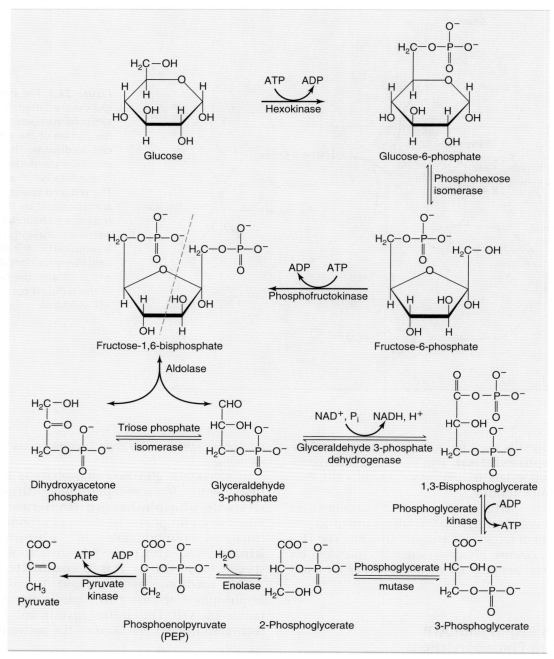

Figure 21.4 The reactions of glycolysis, the major catabolic pathway for glucose. It is active in the cytoplasm of all cells in the human body.

3-phosphate. Although only glyceraldehyde-3-phosphate proceeds through the remaining glycolytic reactions, triose phosphate isomerase ensures that all six glucose-derived carbons can proceed through the pathway.

Glyceraldehyde-3-phosphate is converted to the energy-rich intermediate 1,3-bisphosphoglycerate by **glyceraldehyde-3-phosphate dehydrogen-** **ase.** The enzyme couples the exergonic oxidation of the aldehyde group in the substrate with the endergonic formation of an energy-rich mixed anhydride bond. In this reaction, the phosphate group is derived not from ATP but from inorganic phosphate. The reaction also produces the reduced form of NAD+ (NADH), which is a valuable substrate for oxidative phosphorylation.

Table 21.1 Standard Free Energy Changes of Glycolytic Reactions

Reaction	Enzyme	$\Delta G^{0\prime}$ (kcal/mol)
Glucose $\xrightarrow{\text{ATP ADP}}$ Glucose-6-phosphate	Hexokinase	−4.0
Glucose-6-phosphate $\rightleftharpoons$ Fructose-6-phosphate	Phosphohexose isomerase	+0.4
Fructose-6-phosphate $\xrightarrow{\text{ATP ADP}}$ Fructose-1,6-bisphosphate	Phosphofructokinase	−3.4
Fructose-1,6-bisphosphate $\rightleftharpoons$ Dihydroxyacetone phosphate + Glyceraldehyde-3-phosphate	Aldolase	+5.7
Dihydroxyacetone phosphate $\rightleftharpoons$ Glyceraldehyde-3-phosphate	Triose phosphate isomerase	+1.8
Glyceraldehyde-3-phosphate $\underset{\text{NAD}^+, \text{P}_i \quad\quad \text{NADH, H}^+}{\rightleftharpoons}$ 1,3-bisphosphoglycerate	Glyceraldehyde-3-phosphate dehydrogenase	+1.5
1,3-Bisphosphoglycerate $\underset{\text{ADP ATP}}{\rightleftharpoons}$ 3-Phosphoglycerate	Phosphoglycerate kinase	−4.5
3-Phosphoglycerate $\rightleftharpoons$ 2-Phosphoglycerate	Phosphoglycerate mutase	+1.1
2-Phosphoglycerate $\underset{\text{H}_2\text{O}}{\rightleftharpoons}$ Phosphoenolpyruvate (PEP)	Enolase	+0.4
Phosphoenolpyruvate $\xrightarrow{\text{ADP ATP}}$ Pyruvate	Pyruvate kinase	−7.5

ADP, adenosine diphosphate; ATP, adenosine triphosphate; $\Delta G^{0\prime}$, standard free energy change; NAD$^+$, nicotinamide adenine dinucleotide; NADH, reduced form of NAD; P$_i$, inorganic phosphate.

Simple hydrolysis of the mixed anhydride bond would release 11.8 kcal/mol in the form of heat. To prevent this waste of energy, the cell does not hydrolyze the phosphate but transfers it to ADP, forming ATP. The reaction is catalyzed by **phosphoglycerate kinase.** This strategy of ATP synthesis is called **substrate-level phosphorylation:** the formation of an energy-rich intermediate, which is then used for the synthesis of ATP.

3-Phosphoglycerate is isomerized to 2-phosphoglycerate by **phosphoglycerate mutase.** "Mutase" is an old-fashioned name for isomerases that shift the position of a phosphate group in the molecule. 2-Phosphoglycerate, in turn, is dehydrated to phosphoenolpyruvate (PEP) by **enolase.**

The last enzyme of glycolysis, **pyruvate kinase,** makes substrate-level phosphorylation by transferring the phosphate group of PEP to ADP. Although ATP is synthesized, this reaction is highly exergonic with a standard free energy change ($\Delta G^{0\prime}$) of −7.5 kcal/mol. This implies a free energy content of 14.8 kcal/mol for the phosphate ester bond in PEP. Why is this phosphate ester so unusually energy rich? The initial transfer of phosphate from PEP to ADP is indeed endergonic. However, the enolpyruvate formed in this reaction rearranges almost immediately to pyruvate. This highly exergonic reaction removes enolpyruvate from the equilibrium (Fig. 21.5).

Overall, the reactions of glycolysis produce a net yield of *two ATP molecules and two NADH molecules* for each molecule of glucose (Table 21.2).

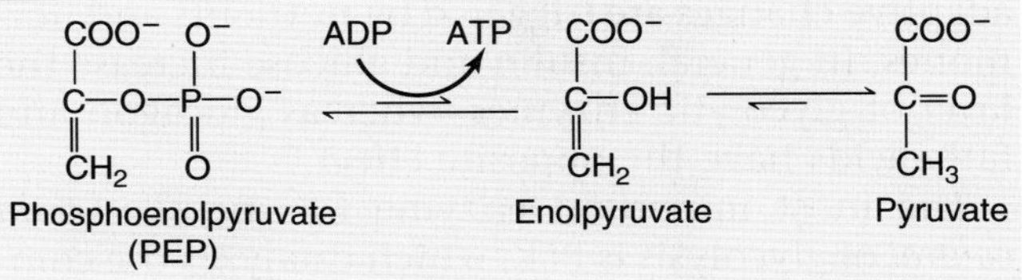

Figure 21.5 The pyruvate kinase reaction. Pyruvate shows keto-enol tautomerism, the keto form being energetically far more stable than the enol form.

Table 21.2 Products Formed during the Conversion of One Molecule of Glucose to Two Molecules of Pyruvate in Aerobic Glycolysis*

Enzyme	Product (Molecules)
Hexokinase	−1 ATP
Phosphofructokinase	−1 ATP
Glyceraldehyde-3-phosphate dehydrogenase	+2 NADH
Phosphoglycerate kinase	+2 ATP
Pyruvate kinase	+2 ATP
	2 ATP + 2 NADH

*Note that all reactions beyond the aldolase reaction occur twice for each glucose molecule.

Only the *hexokinase, PFK,* and *pyruvate kinase* reactions are "irreversible." The aldolase and triose phosphate isomerase reactions have very unfavorable equilibria (see Table 21.1), but they can still proceed because fructose-1,6-bisphosphate is formed in the irreversible PFK reaction and glyceraldehyde-3-phosphate is rapidly consumed in the next reactions of the pathway. The actual equilibrium of the glyceraldehyde-3-phosphate dehydrogenase reaction is far more favorable than suggested by its $\Delta G^{0\prime}$ value of +1.5 kcal/mol, because NAD^+ is far more abundant than NADH in the aerobic cell.

Phosphofructokinase Is the Most Important Regulated Enzyme of Glycolysis

Most tissues glycolyze heavily after a carbohydrate meal but switch to fatty acid oxidation during fasting. The *long-term control* of glycolysis, particularly in the liver, is effected by changes in the amounts of some key glycolytic enzymes. These adaptive changes are triggered by nutrients and hormones. In general, insulin and glucose increase the level of glycolytic enzymes, whereas glucagon and fatty acids have the opposite effect.

The most important enzyme for the *short-term control* of glycolysis is PFK, which catalyzes the committed step of glycolysis. PFK is

- inhibited by ATP and stimulated by AMP and ADP.
- inhibited by low pH.
- inhibited by citrate.
- stimulated by insulin and inhibited by glucagon (in the liver).

The response to adenine nucleotides ensures that *glycolytic activity increases when more ATP is needed:* for example, in contracting muscle. Citrate is a mitochondrial metabolite that signals an abundance of energy and metabolic intermediates; and low pH dampens glycolytic activity when pyruvic and lactic acid, the end products of glycolysis, accumulate to dangerous levels.

Of the important hormones, *insulin rises in response to elevated blood glucose after a meal,* and it stimulates glucose consumption. *Glucagon rises in response to low blood glucose during fasting,* and it reduces glucose consumption in the tissues that are able to switch to alternative fuels.

Some hormone effects are tissue specific. In humans, glucagon is important only in the liver and has little effect on other tissues, and epinephrine is a powerful activator of PFK in muscle but not in most other tissues. In the brain, which depends on glucose metabolism at all times, PFK responds neither to insulin nor to other hormones.

The other irreversible enzymes of glycolysis, hexokinase and pyruvate kinase, also are often regulated. In most tissues (but not the liver), hexokinase is competitively inhibited by its own product, glucose-6-phosphate. This prevents the accumulation of glucose-6-phosphate when the supply of glucose exceeds the capacity of the metabolizing pathways. Glucose-6-phosphate must not be allowed to accumulate because it would tie up the cell's phosphate and thereby impair ATP synthesis. Pyruvate kinase, finally, is inhibited by ATP in many tissues, including the liver.

Lactate Is Produced by Glycolysis under Anaerobic Conditions

Glycolysis produces ATP without consuming oxygen. Does this mean that by turning glucose into pyruvate, humans can synthesize ATP without the need for oxygen? Not quite. The problem is that glycolysis turns NAD^+ into NADH. Without a mechanism to regenerate NAD^+, glycolysis would soon grind to a halt for lack of NAD^+.

The solution to this problem is simple. The hydrogen of NADH is transferred to the keto group of pyruvate, forming lactate:

$$\text{Pyruvate} + \text{NADH} + H^+ \rightarrow \text{Lactate} + NAD^+$$

$$\Delta G^{0\prime} = -6.0\,\text{kcal/mol}$$

This reaction, catalyzed by **lactate dehydrogenase (LDH),** regenerates NAD^+ for the glyceraldehyde-3-phosphate dehydrogenase reaction of glycolysis (Fig. 21.6). The overall balance of anaerobic glycolysis is:

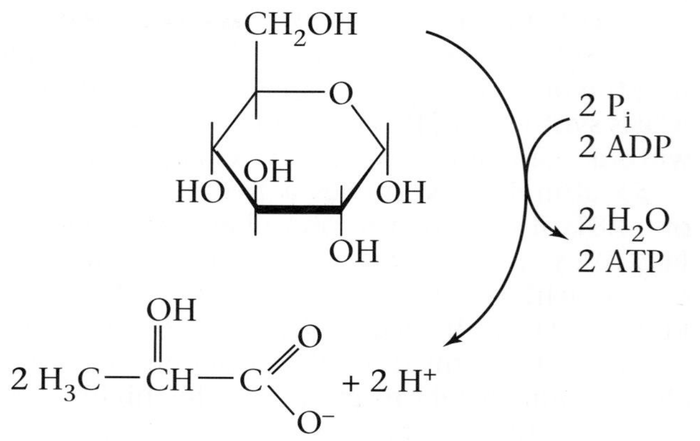

Thus, it is possible to make ATP in the absence of oxygen. *Carbohydrates are the only metabolic substrates that can produce ATP under anaerobic conditions.*

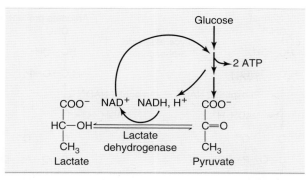

Figure 21.6 Anaerobic glycolysis: lactate dehydrogenase regenerates nicotinamide adenine dinucleotide (NAD⁺) for the glyceraldehyde-3-phosphate dehydrogenase reaction. The conversion of glucose to lactic acid can proceed smoothly with a net synthesis of two adenosine triphosphate (ATP) molecules. NADH, reduced form of NAD.

Table 21.3 Conditions Resulting in Lactic Acidosis

Condition	Mechanism
Physical exercise	Anaerobic glycolysis in muscle
Severe lung disease ⎫ High altitude ⎬ Drowning ⎭	Impaired respiration
Severe anemia ⎫ Carbon monoxide poisoning ⎬ Sickling crisis ⎭	Impaired oxygen delivery
Cyanide poisoning	Inhibition of oxidative phosphorylation
Alcohol intoxication ⎫ von Gierke disease ⎬	Impaired gluconeogenesis Impaired gluconeogenesis
Pyruvate dehydrogenase deficiency	Impaired pyruvate oxidation
Leukemia ⎫ Metastatic carcinoma ⎬	Anaerobic glycolysis by neoplastic cells

However, the protons that are formed along with the lactate anion acidify the environment. This can create a serious pH problem for the cells, and it limits the usefulness of anaerobic glycolysis.

The equilibrium of the LDH reaction favors lactate, but the reaction is physiologically reversible because NAD⁺ is always far more abundant than NADH under aerobic conditions. In fact, *lactate is a metabolic dead end,* and the LDH reaction is the only way to channel lactate back into the metabolic pathways.

The two ATP molecules formed in glycolysis capture only 14.6 kcal of useful energy, whereas the complete oxidation of glucose produces approximately 270 kcal (see Table 21.6). Therefore, anaerobic glycolysis is useful only under certain circumstances; for example:

1. *Mature erythrocytes* have no mitochondria. They do not engage in biosynthetic activity and require ATP only for the maintenance of ion gradients across their membrane. Their energy requirement is so modest that it can be met by the anaerobic glycolysis of 15 to 20 g of glucose per day.

2. *Skeletal muscle* has to increase its ATP production more than 20-fold during bouts of vigorous contraction. During a 100-m sprint, for example, the supply of oxygen by the blood becomes a limiting factor. To keep going, the muscles must turn glucose from the blood and their own stored glycogen into lactic acid. The lactate concentration in the blood rises 5- to 10-fold in this situation.

3. *Ischemic tissues,* which have been cut off from their blood supply, use anaerobic glycolysis for crisis management. The shortage of ATP from oxidative phosphorylation stimulates glycolysis at the level of PFK. A large amount of pyruvate is formed but cannot be oxidized by the mitochondria and is therefore turned into lactate by LDH. Although the ATP from anaerobic glycolysis can tide the cell over for some time, the accumulating lactic acid acidifies the tissue and contributes to cell death.

Lactic Acid Accumulates in Many Metabolic Disorders

The overproduction or underutilization of lactic acid leads to **lactic acidosis.** The most common cause is an *impairment of oxidative metabolism* by respiratory failure, insufficient oxygen transport, or direct inhibition of oxidative phosphorylation. As in tissue ischemia, glycolysis is stimulated by low energy charge, and pyruvate can no longer be oxidized by the mitochondria. Excess pyruvate is turned into lactate.

Without oxygen, the mitochondria cannot oxidize NADH to NAD⁺. As a result, *the accumulating NADH makes the LDH reaction irreversible in the direction of lactate formation.* This happens not only in hypoxia but also in any condition that raises the [NADH]/[NAD⁺] ratio. In alcohol intoxication, for example, the uncontrolled oxidation of alcohol produces a large amount of NADH in the liver. The high [NADH]/[NAD⁺] ratio makes the liver unable to oxidize lactate, and lactate accumulates in the blood. Some causes of lactic acidosis are listed in Table 21.3.

Genetic Defects and Toxins Can Inhibit Glycolysis

A complete deficiency of any glycolytic enzyme would be fatal, at least if it affects cells such as neurons or erythrocytes that depend on glucose as an energy source. However, partial deficiencies of glycolytic enzymes in red blood cells are seen as rare causes of hemolytic anemia.

Recessively inherited **pyruvate kinase deficiency** has a frequency of nearly 1 per 10,000. The erythrocytes of affected individuals have between 5% and 25% of the normal pyruvate kinase activity, and the severity of the hemolytic anemia depends on the residual enzyme activity. An enzyme activity of less than 5% of normal causes fetal death, and an activity of more than 25% of normal is asymptomatic. The affected isoenzyme is present only in erythrocytes. Therefore, glycolysis is unimpaired in other tissues.

Fluoride ions inhibit the enolase reaction of glycolysis. In the clinical laboratory, sodium fluoride is routinely added to blood samples that are used for the determination of the blood glucose level.

Arsenate is a structural analog of phosphate that competes with phosphate in many biochemical reactions. Figure 21.7 shows how arsenate uncouples substrate-level phosphorylation by glyceraldehyde-3-phosphate dehydrogenase and phosphoglycerate kinase. The term "uncoupling" implies that *the pathway can proceed, but without ATP synthesis*. Indeed, the net ATP yield of glycolysis is zero in the presence of arsenate.

Pyruvate Is Decarboxylated to Acetyl-CoA in the Mitochondria

Pyruvate diffuses through the pores in the outer mitochondrial membrane and is transported across the inner mitochondrial membrane. In the mitochondrial matrix, it is oxidatively decarboxylated to acetyl-CoA:

$$\text{Pyruvate} + \text{NAD}^+ + \text{CoA-SH} \rightarrow \text{Acetyl-CoA} + \text{NADH} + \text{CO}_2$$

where CoA-SH = uncombined CoA. This irreversible reaction is catalyzed by **pyruvate dehydrogenase**, a multienzyme complex with three components:

1. The *pyruvate dehydrogenase component* (E_1), which contains **thiamine pyrophosphate** as a prosthetic group.
2. The *dihydrolipoyl transacetylase component* (E_2), which contains **lipoic acid** covalently bound to a lysine side chain.

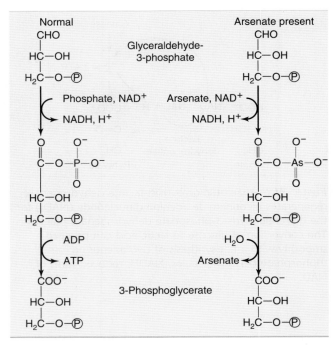

Figure 21.7 Uncoupling of substrate-level phosphorylation in glycolysis by arsenate. An unstable mixed anhydride is formed between arsenate and 3-phosphoglycerate. This anhydride hydrolyzes spontaneously. The pathway can proceed because the product of this hydrolysis, 3-phosphoglycerate, is a normal glycolytic intermediate.

3. The *dihydrolipoyl dehydrogenase component* (E_3), a flavoprotein that contains FAD.

In addition to the tightly bound prosthetic groups, the cosubstrates NAD+ and CoA are required for the reaction.

The structures of thiamine pyrophosphate and lipoic acid are shown in Figure 21.8. Thiamine pyrophosphate acts as a carrier of pyruvate and of the hydroxyethyl group that is formed by its decarboxylation. Lipoic acid participates as a redox system and carrier of the acetyl group. The reaction sequence is shown in Figure 21.9.

Acetyl-CoA Is Formed from Carbohydrates, Fatty Acids, and Amino Acids

All metabolic roads lead to acetyl-CoA. It is formed from carbohydrates through glycolysis and pyruvate dehydrogenase and from fatty acids in the pathway of β-oxidation (see Chapter 23). Even amino acids are degraded to acetyl-CoA, either directly or via pyruvate (Fig. 21.10).

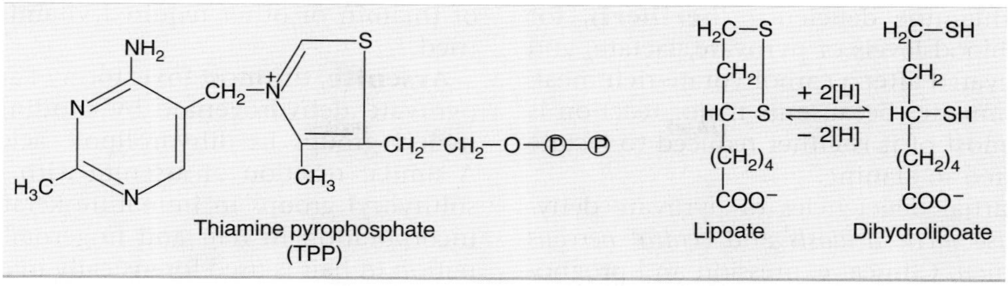

Figure 21.8 Structures of thiamine pyrophosphate and lipoic acid. In the pyruvate dehydrogenase complex, thiamine pyrophosphate is bound noncovalently to the apoprotein, whereas lipoic acid is bound covalently by an amide bond with a lysine side chain.

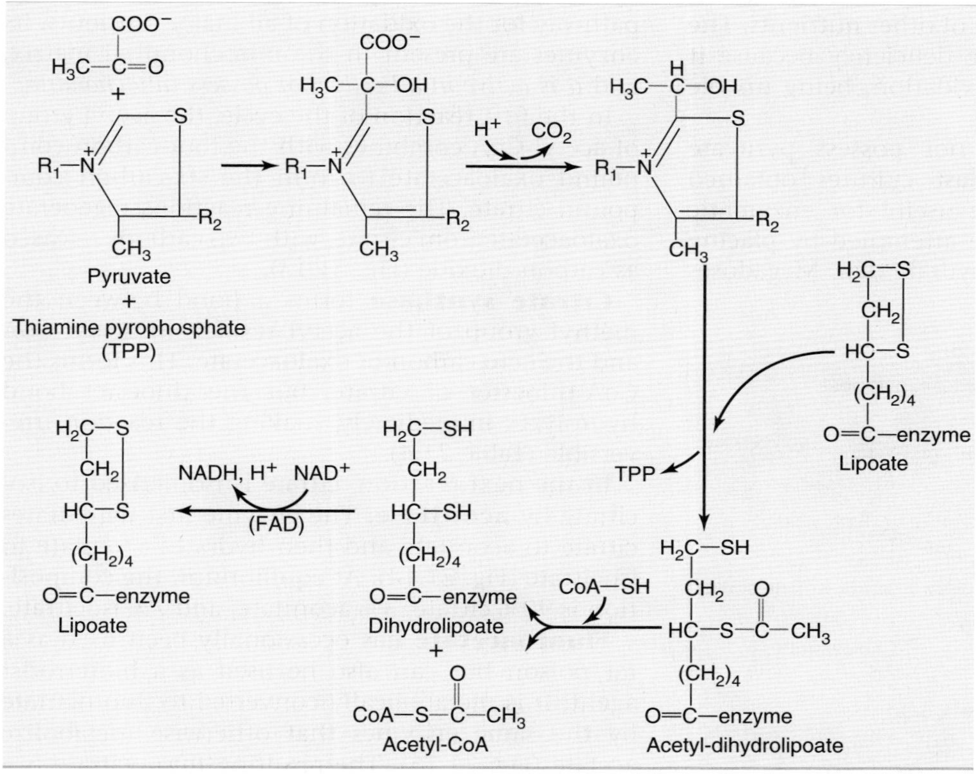

Figure 21.9 The pyruvate dehydrogenase reaction.

Acetyl-CoA can be used for the synthesis of fatty acids, cholesterol, and ketone bodies. After a carbohydrate meal, for example, excess glucose is degraded to acetyl-CoA and the acetyl-CoA is converted to fatty acids and triglycerides. In **acetylation reactions,** acetyl-CoA is used as an activated form of acetate for the synthesis of acetic acid esters and amides (Fig. 21.11). However, the major fate of acetyl-CoA is oxidation in the TCA cycle.

The Pyruvate Dehydrogenase Reaction Is Impaired in Several Diseases

With the exception of lipoic acid, the coenzymes of pyruvate dehydrogenase require vitamins for their synthesis: pantothenic acid (CoA), niacin (NAD), riboflavin (FAD), and thiamine (thiamine pyrophosphate [TPP]). A deficiency of any of these vitamins can impair the pyruvate dehydrogenase reaction. In thiamine deficiency **(beriberi),** for example, the blood levels of pyruvate, lactate, and alanine are elevated after a carbohydrate-rich meal. Pyruvate accumulates because its major reaction is blocked, and most of it is either reduced to lactate or transaminated to alanine.

Inherited partial deficiencies of pyruvate dehydrogenase cause *lactic acidosis* and *central nervous system dysfunction*. Clinical expression and prognosis depend on the residual enzyme activity. With severe deficiencies (<40% of normal), symptoms appear in early infancy and often include mental retardation, microcephaly, optical atrophy, and severe motor dysfunction. In less severe cases, the major manifestation is a slowly progressive spinocerebellar ataxia (motor incoordination).

The brain is prominently involved because pyruvate dehydrogenase is needed for carbohydrate oxidation but not the oxidation of other nutrients. The brain suffers most from the deficiency because it depends on carbohydrate oxidation, being unable to oxidize alternative fuels.

Mature erythrocytes do not possess pyruvate dehydrogenase, but fibroblast cultures obtained from the patient's skin are useful for enzymatic diagnosis. Treatment can be attempted by placing the patient on a low-carbohydrate diet. Megadoses of thiamin or other required vitamins can also be tried.

Arsenite, the most toxic form of arsenic, poisons pyruvate dehydrogenase by binding to the sulfhydryl groups in dihydrolipoic acid (Fig. 21.12). A similar reaction of arsenite with closely spaced sulfhydryl groups in immature keratin leads to its incorporation in hair and fingernails. Its determination in hair is used forensically in cases of alleged arsenic poisoning.

The TCA Cycle Produces Two Molecules of Carbon Dioxide for Each Acetyl Residue

The **TCA cycle,** also known as the **citric acid cycle** or **Krebs cycle,** is the final common pathway for the oxidation of all major nutrients. Its enzymes are present in the mitochondrial matrix, and *it is active in all cells that possess mitochondria.*

In the first reaction of the cycle, the acetyl group of acetyl-CoA combines with the four-carbon compound oxaloacetate to form the six-carbon compound citrate. The remaining reactions regenerate oxaloacetate from citrate, with two carbons released as carbon dioxide (Fig. 21.13).

Citrate synthase forms a bond between the methyl group of the acetyl residue in acetyl-CoA and the keto carbon of oxaloacetate. This forms the CoA-thioester of citrate, but the thioester bond hydrolyzes immediately, making the reaction irreversible (Table 21.4).

In the next reaction, citrate is isomerized to isocitrate by **aconitase.** The enzyme first dehydrates citrate to aconitate and then hydrates aconitate to isocitrate (Fig. 21.14). At equilibrium, the composition is 90% citrate, 3% aconitate, and 7% isocitrate.

Fluoroacetate has occasionally been used as a rat poison but can also be used as a bioterrorist agent. It is metabolically converted to fluorocitrate by the same enzymes that otherwise metabolize acetate (Fig. 21.15). The resulting fluorocitrate is a potent inhibitor of aconitase.

Isocitrate is oxidatively decarboxylated to α-ketoglutarate (2-oxoglutarate) by **isocitrate dehydrogenase** (Fig. 21.16). Oxalosuccinate is an enzyme-bound intermediate in this reaction. The

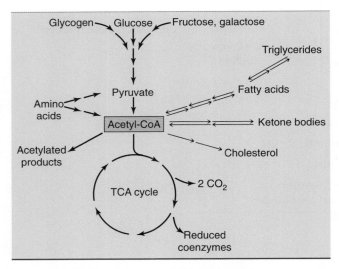

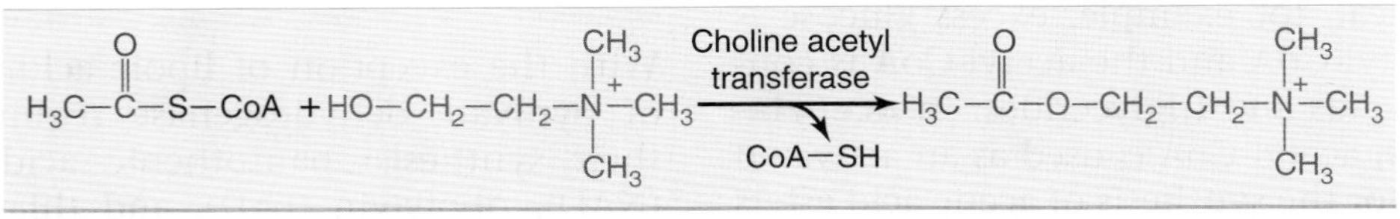

Figure 21.10 The sources and fates of acetyl–coenzyme A (acetyl-CoA).

Figure 21.11 Synthesis of acetylcholine in cholinergic neurons. This is an example of an acetylation reaction. CoA-SH, in combined coenzyme A.

isocitrate dehydrogenase of the TCA cycle is an NAD-linked enzyme.

The next enzyme of the cycle, α-**ketoglutarate dehydrogenase,** resembles pyruvate dehydrogenase in structure and reaction mechanism. However, it works on α-ketoglutarate rather than pyruvate and produces succinyl-CoA rather than acetyl-CoA. The coenzyme requirements of the two multienzyme complexes are identical.

In the reversible **succinyl-CoA synthetase** (also known as **succinyl thiokinase**) reaction, the hydrolysis of the energy-rich thioester bond in succinyl-CoA is coupled to the synthesis of GTP. This is yet another example of substrate-level phosphorylation, in which an energy-rich bond in a metabolic intermediate is used for the synthesis of an energy-rich nucleotide. GTP is equivalent to ATP,

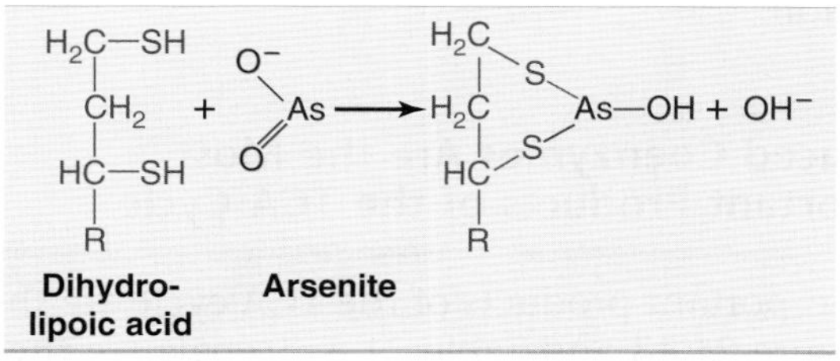

Figure 21.12 Reaction of arsenite with dihydrolipoic acid.

Table 21.4 The Standard Free Energy Changes ($\Delta G^{0'}$) of the Pyruvate Dehydrogenase Reaction and the TCA Cycle Reactions

Enzyme	$\Delta G^{0'}$ (kcal/mol)	Products
Pyruvate dehydrogenase	−8.0	CO_2, NADH
Citrate synthase	−8.5	
Aconitase	+1.6	
Isocitrate dehydrogenase	−2.0	CO_2, NADH
α-Ketoglutarate dehydrogenase	−8.0	CO_2, NADH
Succinyl-CoA synthetase	−0.7	GTP
Succinate dehydrogenase	~0	$FADH_2$
Fumarase	−0.9	
Malate dehydrogenase	+7.1	NADH

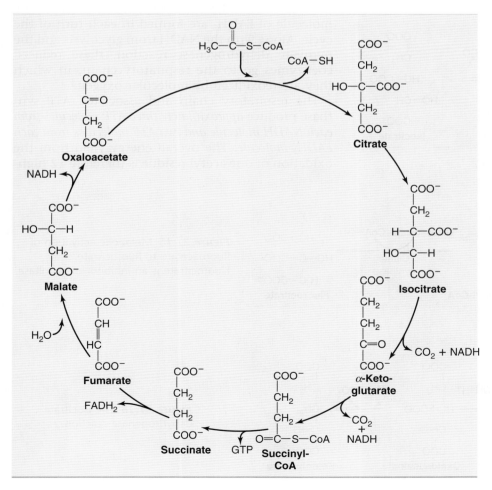

Figure 21.13 Summary of the reactions of the tricarboxylic acid (TCA) cycle, showing carbon intermediates and key products.

with which it is in equilibrium through the nucleoside diphosphate kinase reaction:

$$GTP + ADP \rightleftharpoons GDP + ATP$$

Succinate is a four-carbon dicarboxylic acid. In the remaining reactions, two hydrogen atoms of succinate have to be replaced by oxygen to complete the cycle with the formation of oxaloacetate.

The enzyme **succinate dehydrogenase (SDH)** abstracts two hydrogen atoms from succinate to form fumarate. The hydrogen atoms are first parked on the FAD prosthetic group of SDH and then quickly passed on to the respiratory chain. Unlike the other TCA cycle enzymes, which are soluble in the mitochondrial matrix, SDH is an integral protein of the inner mitochondrial membrane.

Why does SDH use enzyme-bound FAD rather than soluble NAD^+ to abstract hydrogen from its substrate? The reason is that FAD has the higher affinity for hydrogen. If NAD^+ were used, the reaction would be irreversible in the direction of succinate formation, but with FAD it is freely reversible.

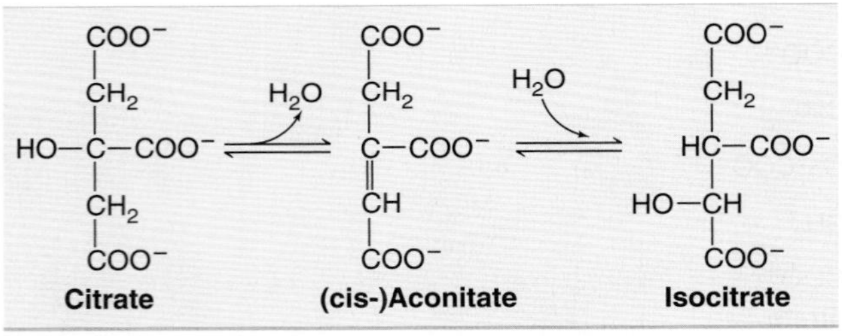

Fumarate is hydrated to L-malate by **fumarase.** Like the enolase reaction of glycolysis, this is a freely reversible lyase reaction.

Malate is finally oxidized to oxaloacetate in the NAD^+-dependent **malate dehydrogenase** reaction. Like lactate dehydrogenase (LDH), malate dehydrogenase equilibrates an α-hydroxy acid with its corresponding α-keto acid. Also as in the LDH reaction, the equilibrium favors the hydroxy acid (see Table 21.4). The reaction can nevertheless proceed toward oxaloacetate because the $[NAD^+]/[NADH]$ ratio in the mitochondrion is very high under aerobic conditions and because oxaloacetate is consumed in the irreversible citrate synthase reaction.

Reduced Coenzymes Are the Most Important Products of the TCA Cycle

The important products of the TCA cycle are shown in Figure 21.13 and Table 21.4. To balance the two carbons that enter the cycle from acetyl-CoA, each turn of the cycle releases two carbons as carbon dioxide. The excess hydrogen in the substrate does not form water, but *it is transferred to the coenzymes NAD^+ and FAD.* Three molecules of NADH and one molecule of $FADH_2$ are formed in each turn of the cycle. Along with the NADH from glycolysis and the pyruvate dehydrogenase reaction, these reduced coenzymes go to the respiratory chain, in which they are reoxidized by molecular oxygen.

The respiratory chain and associated ATP synthase produce *approximately three ATP molecules from each NADH molecule and two ATP molecules from each $FADH_2$ molecule.* The overall energy yield from the oxidation of one acetyl residue is therefore 12 high-

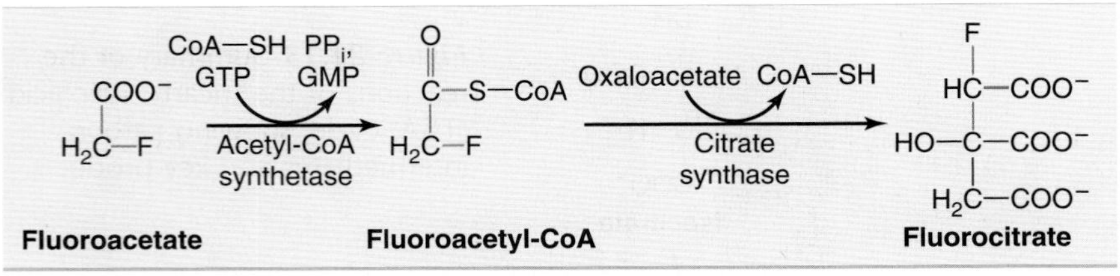

Figure 21.14 The aconitase reaction.

Figure 21.15 Metabolic activation of fluoroacetate to fluorocitrate. Fluorocitrate is an inhibitor of aconitase.

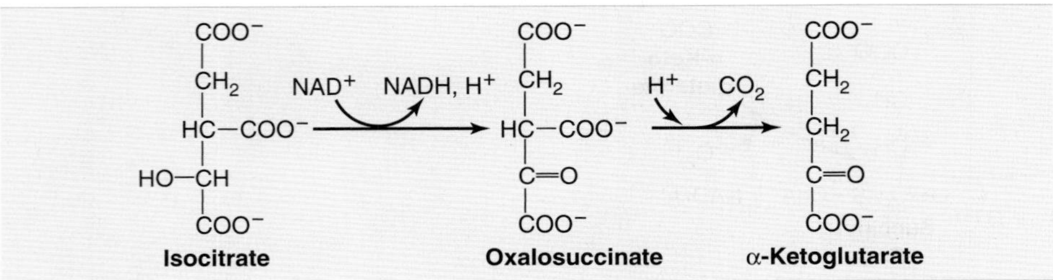

Figure 21.16 The isocitrate dehydrogenase reaction.

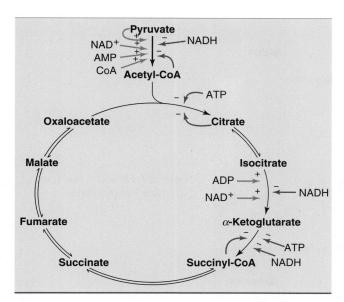

Figure 21.17 Regulatory effects on pyruvate dehydrogenase and the tricarboxylic acid cycle. Note the importance of both energy charge and the [NADH]/[NAD⁺] ratio, and note the product inhibition of the irreversible reactions. →, stimulation; →, inhibition.

energy phosphate bonds: one from substrate-level phosphorylation and 11 by the reoxidation of the reduced coenzymes.

There is no alternative to the respiratory chain for the oxidation of the reduced coenzymes in the mitochondrion. Therefore, unlike glycolysis, *the TCA cycle cannot function under anaerobic conditions.* Without molecular oxygen, the cycle soon grinds to a halt for lack of NAD⁺ and FAD.

The Oxidative Pathways Are Regulated by Energy Charge and [NADH]/[NAD⁺] Ratio

The oxidative pathways produce NADH directly and ATP indirectly through the oxidation of NADH. Therefore, it comes as no surprise that most of the regulated enzymes in these pathways are inhibited by an elevated [ATP]/[ADP] ratio and an elevated [NADH]/[NAD⁺] ratio. This ensures that a constant ATP level is maintained at all times and that NADH production matches the rate of NADH oxidation in the respiratory chain. There is also more direct feedback inhibition of the irreversible reactions to avoid an undesirable accumulation of metabolic intermediates, as summarized in Figure 21.17.

Pyruvate dehydrogenase, which is outside the TCA cycle, is important because *it channels carbohydrate-derived carbons irreversibly into acetyl-CoA.* It is inhibited by its products NADH and acetyl-CoA and stimulated by AMP. It is also inactivated by the phosphorylation of a single serine side chain, and reactivated by dephosphorylation.

The protein kinase that phosphorylates the enzyme complex is allosterically activated by the same factors that also inhibit pyruvate dehydrogenase allosterically: high energy charge, high [NADH]/[NAD⁺] ratio, and high [acetyl-CoA]/[CoA] ratio. It is also inhibited by pyruvate. The action of the protein kinase is opposed by a protein phosphatase that removes the bound phosphate.

In the TCA cycle, **citrate synthase** is inhibited by ATP. More important, however, is the availability of oxaloacetate. The Michaelis constant (K_m) of citrate synthase for this substrate is on the same order of magnitude as its intramitochondrial concentration ($\approx$10 μmol/liter). Citrate inhibits the reaction by competing with oxaloacetate for the active site of the enzyme.

Isocitrate dehydrogenase is inhibited by high energy charge and high [NADH]/[NAD⁺] ratio. Citrate accumulates along with isocitrate when isocitrate dehydrogenase is inhibited. It can leave the mitochondrion to act as an allosteric effector in the cytoplasmic pathways of glycolysis, gluconeogenesis (see Chapter 22), and fatty acid biosynthesis (see Chapter 23). Therefore, elevations of mitochondrial energy charge and [NADH]/[NAD⁺] ratio can affect these cytoplasmic pathways by inhibiting isocitrate dehydrogenase.

α-Ketoglutarate dehydrogenase, like pyruvate dehydrogenase, is inhibited by its own products (succinyl-CoA and NADH) and by high energy charge, but, unlike pyruvate dehydrogenase, it is not regulated by phosphorylation/dephosphorylation.

Except in anoxia, the mitochondrial [NAD⁺]/[NADH] ratio is so high that NAD⁺ is not a limiting factor as a substrate for the dehydrogenase reactions. However, the equilibrium of the NAD⁺-dependent malate dehydrogenase reaction is so unfavorable (see Table 21.4) that an elevated [NADH]/[NAD⁺] ratio seriously impairs the formation of oxaloacetate. As a result, citrate synthase suffers from a shortage of its substrate oxaloacetate.

The TCA Cycle Provides an Important Pool of Metabolic Intermediates

The TCA cycle is not only the final common pathway for the oxidation of metabolic fuels; it is also a source of precursors for biosynthetic reactions, as summarized in Figure 21.18. Most of

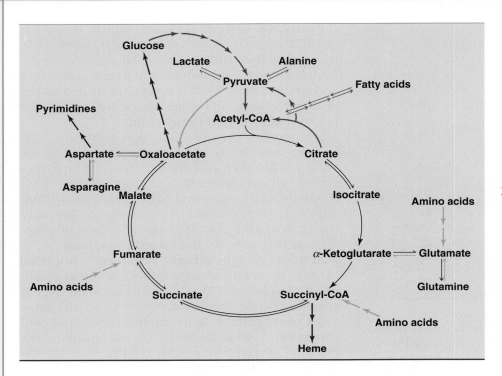

Figure 21.18 Some reactions of TCA cycle intermediates.

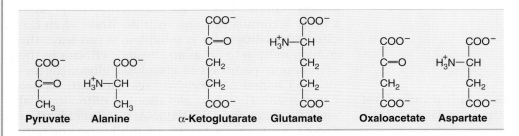

Figure 21.19 α Keto acids and their corresponding α amino acids.

these reactions are tissue specific. For example, the synthesis of glucose from oxaloacetate occurs only in the liver and kidneys, and the synthesis of heme from succinyl-CoA is most active in the bone marrow.

The removal of TCA cycle intermediates for biosynthesis creates a problem: the failure to regenerate oxaloacetate as a substrate for the citrate synthase reaction. Therefore, *biosynthetic reactions that consume TCA cycle intermediates must be balanced by reactions that produce them.* This latter type of reaction is called **anaplerotic** (from the Greek word for "to fill up").

The three α keto acids pyruvate, α-ketoglutarate, and oxaloacetate are structurally related to the amino acids alanine, glutamate, and aspartate (Fig. 21.19). When the amino acids are in demand, they can be synthesized from the α keto acids. Under most conditions, however, excess dietary amino acids are metabolized to their corresponding α keto acids. Also, most other amino acids are degraded to TCA cycle intermediates.

Another important anaplerotic reaction is the synthesis of oxaloacetate from pyruvate by **pyruvate carboxylase.** This *ATP-dependent carboxylation* introduces a carboxyl group from inorganic bicarbonate. The reaction requires enzyme-bound **biotin,** and it proceeds in two steps (Fig. 21.20). First, CO_2 binds to a nitrogen atom in biotin to produce **carboxy-biotin.** This endergonic reaction ($\Delta G^{0\prime} = +4.7$ kcal/mol) is fueled by the hydrolysis of ATP to ADP + phosphate ($\Delta G^{0\prime} = -7.3$ kcal/mol), resulting in an overall free energy change of -2.6 kcal/mol ($4.7 - 7.3$ kcal/mol). In the next step, the "activated carboxyl group" of carboxy-biotin is transferred to pyruvate to form oxaloacetate.

Pyruvate carboxylase is a strictly mitochondrial enzyme. It requires manganese or magnesium for its activity, and acetyl-CoA is a positive allosteric effector. When the citrate synthase reaction is impaired by a lack of oxaloacetate, acetyl-CoA accumulates in the mitochondrion and activates pyruvate carboxylase. Patients with a genetic deficiency of pyruvate carboxylase (a rare recessively inherited

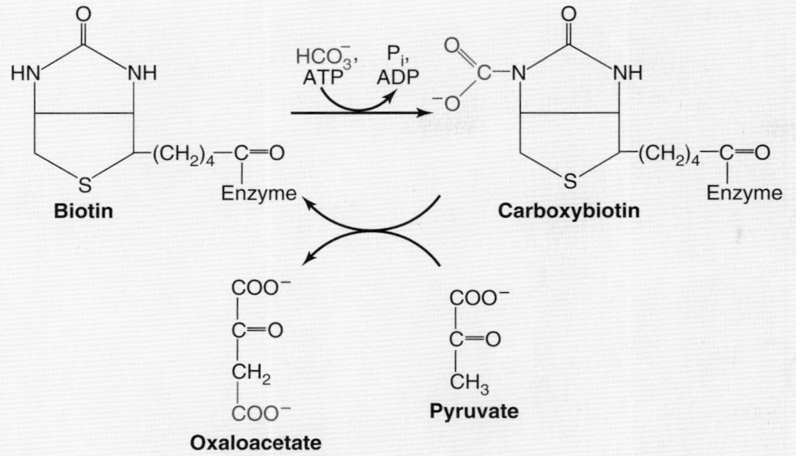

Figure 21.20 The pyruvate carboxylase reaction. This general mechanism applies to all biotin- and ATP–dependent carboxylations.

condition) suffer from lactic acidosis and central nervous system dysfunction.

Most Intermediates of Mitochondrial Metabolism Can Be Transported across the Inner Mitochondrial Membrane

The import and export of metabolites is essential for mitochondrial function. Pyruvate is transported into the mitochondrion, TCA cycle intermediates are transported to the cytoplasm for use in biosynthetic reactions, and ADP and inorganic phosphate enter the mitochondrion while ATP leaves.

The outer mitochondrial membrane is not a barrier against small water-soluble molecules because it is riddled with small pores, but transport across the inner mitochondrial membrane requires specific carriers. Most of the important metabolic intermediates, with the exceptions of acetyl-CoA, oxaloacetate, fumarate, NAD^+, and NADH, have carriers in the inner mitochondrial membrane. ATP and ADP (but not the other nucleotides) are also transported, as are pyruvate and phosphate. The amino acids that are directly derived from pyruvate, α-ketoglutarate, and oxaloacetate are transported as well.

The mitochondrial translocases, summarized in Figure 21.21, are antiporters. They do not hydrolyze ATP, but energy is consumed in cases in which actively maintained ion gradients or the membrane potential are dissipated. The membrane potential (positive outside, negative inside) is needed for oxidative phosphorylation. For example, the transport of hydroxyl ions out of the mitochondrion by the phosphate carrier dissipates an actively maintained proton gradient. The ATP/ADP exchange also weakens the membrane potential because ADP has

about three negative charges at physiological pH, whereas ATP has about four.

NADH can donate its hydrogen to the respiratory chain only from the mitochondrial matrix, not from the cytoplasm. This creates a problem for the use of the cytoplasmic NADH produced in glycolysis, because neither NADH nor NAD^+ is transported across the inner mitochondrial membrane. The problem is solved by the use of two shuttle systems: the **glycerol phosphate shuttle** and the **malate-aspartate shuttle** (Fig. 21.22).

The glycerol phosphate shuttle transfers the hydrogen first to dihydroxyacetone phosphate, forming glycerol phosphate, and then to the FAD prosthetic group of the mitochondrial glycerol phosphate dehydrogenase, an integral protein of the inner mitochondrial membrane. Like succinate dehydrogenase, this enzyme regenerates its FAD by the direct transfer of electrons to the respiratory chain, *producing two ATP molecules.*

The malate-aspartate shuttle transfers hydrogen from cytoplasmic NADH to oxaloacetate, forming malate. Malate is transported into the mitochondrion, where it donates its hydrogen to NAD^+, forming NADH. This NADH is oxidized by the respiratory chain, *producing three ATP molecules.*

The Respiratory Chain Uses Molecular Oxygen to Oxidize NADH and $FADH_2$

All major catabolic pathways form NADH and/or $FADH_2$. These reduced coenzymes must be reoxidized to NAD^+ and FAD, which are needed as substrates of the pathways. This requires the **respiratory chain** in the inner mitochondrial membrane. The overall reactions in the respiratory chain are simple enough:

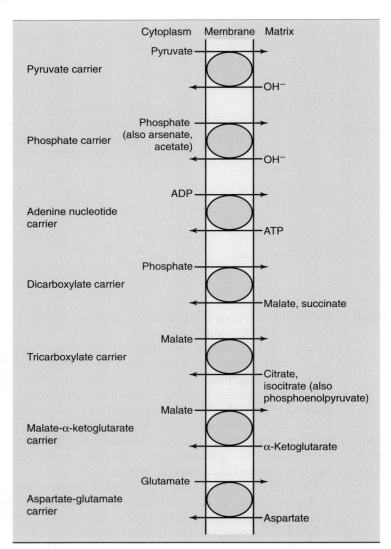

Figure 21.21 Translocases that transport metabolites across the inner mitochondrial membrane. ADP, adenosine diphosphate; ATP, adenosine triphosphate.

$$NADH + H^+ + \tfrac{1}{2} O_2 \rightarrow NAD^+ + H_2O$$

$$FADH_2 + \tfrac{1}{2} O_2 \rightarrow FAD + H_2O$$

The free energy changes, however, are enormous. The oxidation of NADH + H$^+$ releases 52.6 kcal/mol under standard conditions. This corresponds to the free energy content of seven phosphoanhydride bonds in ATP! Oxidation of the FADH$_2$ in mitochondrial flavoproteins yields approximately 40 kcal/mol.

In **oxidative phosphorylation,** some of this energy is harvested as ATP. First, *the oxidations are broken down into sequential reactions with smaller free energy changes.* In these reactions, the components of the respiratory chain accept and donate electrons, either with or without accompanying protons. A simple hydrogen transport chain looks somewhat like this:

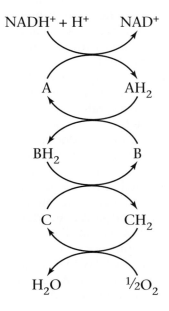

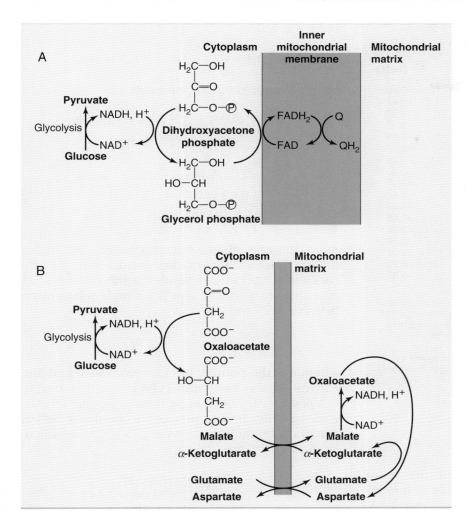

Figure 21.22 The glycerol phosphate shuttle **(A)** and the malate-aspartate shuttle **(B).** Both of these shuttles are active in most cell types. **A,** The mitochondrial glycerol phosphate dehydrogenase is an integral protein of the inner mitochondrial membrane, whose glycerol phosphate-binding site is on the cytoplasmic surface. Therefore, glycerol phosphate need not cross the membrane. The flavin adenine dinucleotide (FAD) prosthetic group of the enzyme is regenerated by transfer of its hydrogen to ubiquinone (Q), a component of the respiratory chain. QH_2, ubi-hydroquinone. **B,** Because oxaloacetate is not transported across the inner mitochondical membrane, its carbons are shuttled out of the mitochondrion in the form of aspartate. The *arrows* indicate the direction in which the shuttle proceeds during the transport of cytoplasmic hydrogen into the mitochondrion. Actually, the shuttle is freely reversible and can transport hydrogen out of the mitochondrion in some situations.

The individual reactions in this chain are as follows:

1. $NADH + H^+ + A \rightarrow NAD^+ + AH_2$
2. $AH_2 + B \rightarrow A + BH_2$
3. $BH_2 + C \rightarrow B + CH_2$
4. $CH_2 + \frac{1}{2} O_2 \rightarrow C + H_2O$

These four reactions add up to the overall reaction:

$$NADH + H^+ + \tfrac{1}{2} O_2 \rightarrow NAD^+ + H_2O$$

Electron carriers can react with "hydrogen" carriers because a hydrogen atom consists of an electron and a proton. Protons are readily exchanged with the solvent during redox reactions; for example:

$$FADH_2 + 2\ Fe^{3+} \rightarrow FAD + 2\ Fe^{2+} + 2\ H^+$$

Fe^{2+}, in turn, can donate an electron to a hydrogen carrier:

$$2\ Fe^{2+} + \tfrac{1}{2} O_2 + 2\ H^+ \rightarrow 2\ Fe^{3+} + H_2O$$

The Standard Reduction Potential Describes the Tendency to Donate Electrons

Redox reactions are electron transfers by definition. This implies the participation of two substrates: a reduced substrate, or **reductant,** which donates electrons (e^-) and becomes oxidized during the reaction, and an oxidized substrate, or **oxidant,** which accepts electrons and becomes reduced.

A substance that can exist in oxidized and reduced forms is called a **redox couple.** FAD/$FADH_2$, Fe^{3+}/Fe^{2+}, and $\frac{1}{2} O_2/H_2O$ are redox couples. During a redox reaction, each redox couple undergoes a "half-reaction"; for example:

$$FAD + 2\ H^+ + 2e^- \rightleftharpoons FADH_2$$

$$Fe^{3+} + e^- \rightleftharpoons Fe^{2+}$$

$$\tfrac{1}{2} O_2 + 2\ H^+ + 2e^- \rightleftharpoons H_2O$$

Table 21.5 Standard Reduction Potentials of Some Biologically Important Redox Couples

Oxidant/Reductant	$E^{0\prime}$ (volt)
Acetate/acetaldehyde	−0.60
2 H⁺/H₂	−0.42*
NAD⁺/NADH + H⁺	−0.32
NADP⁺/NADPH + H⁺	−0.32
Lipoate/dihydrolipoate	−0.29
Acetoacetate/β-hydroxybutyrate	−0.27
Glutathione oxidized/reduced	−0.23
Acetaldehyde/ethanol	−0.20
Pyruvate/lactate	−0.19
Oxaloacetate/malate	−0.17
Fumarate/succinate	+0.03
Cytochrome b Fe³⁺/Fe²⁺	+0.08
Dehydroascorbate/ascorbate	+0.08
Ubiquinone/ubiquinol	+0.10
Cytochrome c Fe³⁺/Fe²⁺	+0.22
Fe³⁺/Fe²⁺	+0.77†
½ O₂/H₂O	+0.82

*The reduction potential of the hydrogen electrode is set at zero for "chemical" standard conditions, with a proton concentration of 1 M. The shift into the negative range is caused by the far lower proton concentration under "biological" standard conditions (at a pH of 7.0).
†Standard reduction potential of inorganic iron. The reduction potentials of the iron in heme proteins and iron-sulfur proteins may be markedly different.

The reduction potential, also called the redox potential, is a measure for the tendency of a redox couple to donate electrons. It can be determined experimentally by allowing the two half-reactions of a redox reaction to proceed in separate compartments and measuring the resulting electron motive force in volts.

The (biological) **standard reduction potential $E^{0\prime}$**, also called the **standard redox potential,** is determined under standard conditions, with a temperature of 25° C and reactant concentrations of 1 mol/liter, but with the proton concentration fixed at 10^{-7} mol/liter (pH = 7.0). These are the same "biological" standard conditions that are used for the definition of standard free energy changes.

A low $E^{0\prime}$ means that the reduced form of the redox couple has a strong tendency to donate electrons, or a great "reducing power." Therefore, *electrons are transferred from the redox couple with the lower reduction potential to the redox couple with the higher reduction potential.* Table 21.5 shows the standard reduction potentials of some redox couples.

Under standard conditions, the equilibrium of a redox reaction is determined by the difference between the standard reduction potentials of the participating redox couples ($\Delta E^{0\prime}$):

$$\Delta E^{0\prime} = E^{0\prime}_{\text{oxidant}} - E^{0\prime}_{\text{reductant}}$$

For the reaction

$$NADH + H^+ + \tfrac{1}{2} O_2 \rightarrow NAD^+ + H_2O$$

the standard reduction potentials are

$$NAD^+/NADH + H^+ : E^{0\prime} = -0.32 \text{ volt}$$

$$\tfrac{1}{2} O_2 + 2H^+/H_2O : E^{0\prime} = +0.82 \text{ volt}$$

$$\Delta E^{0\prime} = E^{0\prime}{}_{\frac{1}{2}O_2+2H^+/H_2O} - E^{0\prime}{}_{NAD^+/NADH+H^+}$$
$$= 0.82 \text{ volt} - (-0.32 \text{ volt})$$
$$= +1.14 \text{ volt}$$

As in the case of free energy changes, the actual driving force of the reaction under nonstandard conditions (ΔE) also depends on the relative reactant concentrations. There is a simple relationship between $\Delta G^{0\prime}$ and $\Delta E^{0\prime}$:

$$\Delta G^{0\prime} = -n \times F \times \Delta E^{0\prime}$$

where n is the number of electrons transferred and F is the Faraday constant (23.06 kcal $\times V^{-1} \times$ mol⁻¹). *A positive $\Delta E^{0\prime}$, like a negative $\Delta G^{0\prime}$, signifies an exergonic reaction.* In the previous example of NADH oxidation by molecular oxygen, $\Delta G^{0\prime}$ can be calculated as

$$\Delta G^{0\prime} = -n \times F \times \Delta E^{0\prime}$$
$$= -2 \times 23.06 \times 1.14$$
$$= -52.6 \text{ kcal/mol}$$

The Respiratory Chain Contains Flavoproteins, Iron-Sulfur Proteins, Cytochromes, Ubiquinone, and Protein-Bound Copper

Because none of the functional groups in "ordinary" proteins can transfer hydrogen or electrons easily, the components of the respiratory chain have to employ metal ions and coenzymes.

The FAD or flavin mononucleotide (FMN) in the **flavoproteins** can transfer two electrons (+ protons) at a time, but single-electron transfers are possible as well: for example, when the flavin coenzyme donates an electron to protein-bound iron (Fig. 21.23). The standard reduction potentials of the flavoproteins are intermediate between NAD⁺/NADH and the cytochromes. Therefore, *they accept hydrogen/electrons from NADH and donate it to the cytochromes.*

The **iron-sulfur proteins,** also known as **nonheme iron proteins,** contain iron complexed to cysteine side chains. *This iron transfers electrons by switching between the ferrous (Fe²⁺) and*

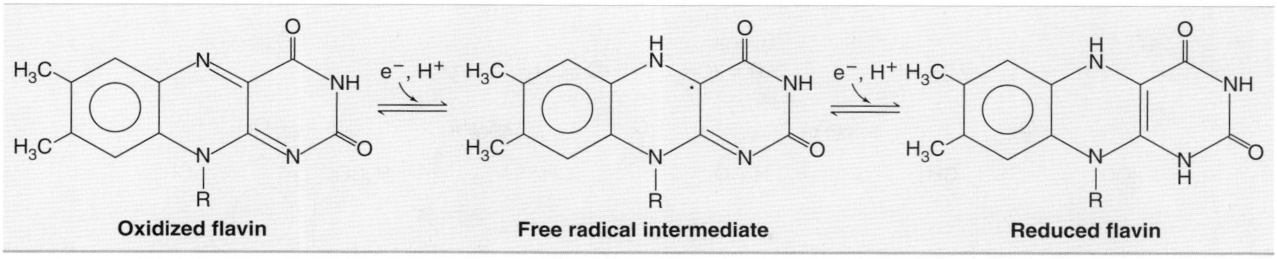

Figure 21.23 Structures of oxidized and reduced flavins. e⁻, electron.

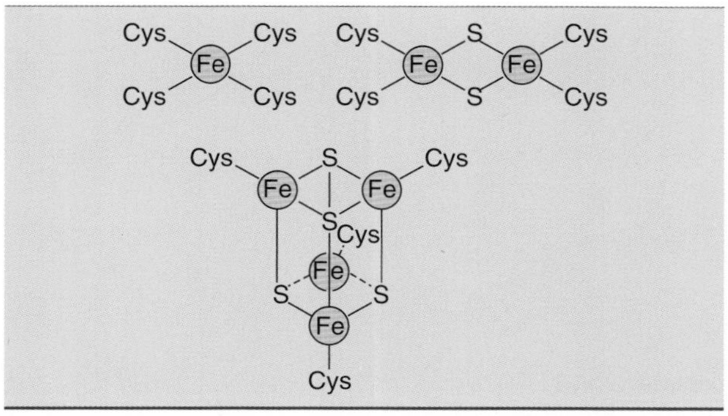

Figure 21.24 Iron-sulfur complexes in proteins. The iron in these complexes can change its oxidation state reversibly between the ferrous (Fe^{2+}) and ferric (Fe^{3+}) forms.

ferric (Fe^{3+}) states. Many iron-sulfur proteins contain inorganic sulfide as well (Fig. 21.24). The standard reduction potentials depend on the polypeptide environment of the nonheme iron. Both the iron-sulfur proteins and the flavoproteins of the respiratory chain are integral membrane proteins.

The **cytochromes** contain iron in the form of an iron-porphyrin, usually the heme group. In contrast to hemoglobin and myoglobin where the iron is always in the ferrous state, *the heme iron of the cytochromes switches back and forth between Fe^{2+} and Fe^{3+}.* Also, in most cytochromes (but not cytochrome a/a_3), the heme iron is bound to two amino acid side chains rather than one. This prevents the binding of molecular oxygen, carbon monoxide, and other potential ligands.

Whereas the heme group of cytochrome b is bound to the apoprotein by noncovalent interactions, it is bound covalently in cytochromes c and c_1. Cytochromes a and a_3 contain **heme a** rather than "ordinary" heme. In this iron-porphyrin, a methyl group of heme is oxidized to a formyl group and a hydrophobic isoprenoid chain is attached to one of the vinyl groups. With the exception of cytochrome c, the cytochromes of the respiratory chain are integral membrane proteins.

Ubiquinone, also known as **coenzyme Q,** is a mobile hydrogen carrier that is not permanently associated with an apoprotein. A long hydrocarbon tail of 10 isoprene (branched 5-carbon) units makes it strongly hydrophobic and confines it to the lipid bilayer of the inner mitochondrial membrane. Like the flavin coenzymes, ubiquinone carries two hydrogen atoms but can act in one-electron transfers by forming a somewhat unstable intermediate (Fig. 21.25).

Protein-bound **copper** participates in the last reaction of the respiratory chain, the transfer of electrons to molecular oxygen. It switches between the Cu^{1+} and Cu^{2+} forms during these electron transfers.

The Respiratory Chain Contains Large Multiprotein Complexes

Four members of the respiratory chain are freely diffusible: NADH, ubiquinone, cytochrome c, and molecular oxygen. NADH is in the mitochondrial matrix, ubiquinone is mobile in the lipid bilayer, and cytochrome c is loosely bound to the outer surface of the inner mitochondrial membrane. Molecular oxygen, freely diffusible across membranes, receives electrons and protons on the matrix side of the inner mitochondrial membrane.

The other components of the respiratory chain are organized in large protein complexes that are arranged asymmetrically in the membrane (Fig. 21.26):

1. The **NADH–Q reductase complex,** also called **NADH dehydrogenase** or "complex I," transfers electrons from NADH to ubiquinone. It contains FMN and several iron-sulfur centers. Electrons are transferred from NADH to FMN, then through a succession of iron-sulfur centers to ubiquinone.

2. The **QH₂–cytochrome c reductase complex,** also called **cytochrome reductase** or "complex III," transfers electrons from ubiquinone to cytochrome c. It contains

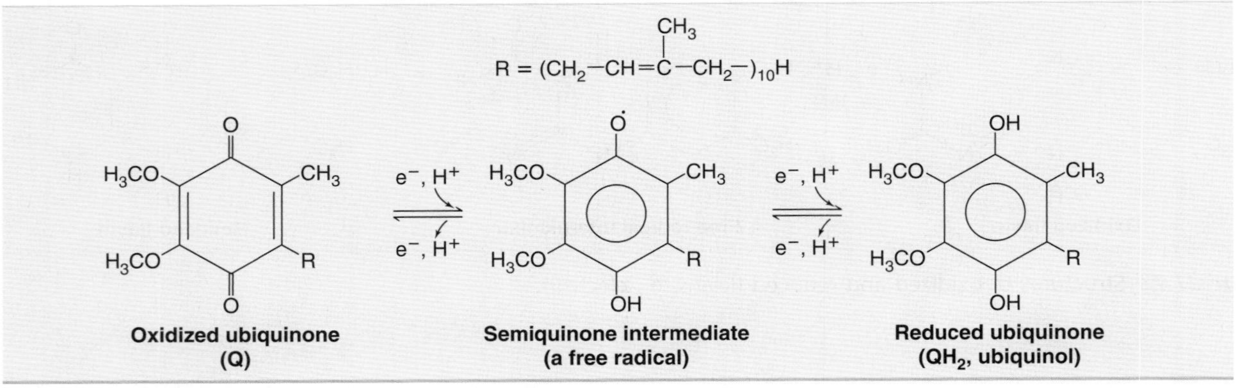

R = $(CH_2-CH=\overset{\overset{\displaystyle CH_3}{|}}{C}-CH_2-)_{10}H$

Oxidized ubiquinone (Q)

Semiquinone intermediate (a free radical)

Reduced ubiquinone (QH₂, ubiquinol)

e^-, H^+

Figure 21.25 Structure of ubiquinone (coenzyme Q). e^-, electron.

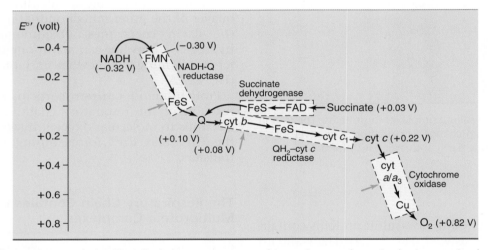

Figure 21.26 The respiratory chain. The *shaded structures* are multiprotein complexes in the inner mitochondrial membrane. The reduced form of icotinamide adenine dinucleotide (NADH) and succinate are in the matrix space, ubiquinone (Q) is in the lipid bilayer of the membrane, and cytochrome c is a peripheral membrane protein, bound to the outer surface of the inner mitochondrial membrane. The standard redox potentials are shown for some components. The *arrows* indicate sites of proton pumping ("phosphorylation sites"). cyt, cytochrome; FAD, flavin adenine dinucleotide; FeS, iron-sulfur protein; FMN, flavin mononucleotide; QH₂, ubihydroquinone.

cytochrome *b*, an iron-sulfur protein, and cytochrome c_1.

3. The **cytochrome oxidase complex** ("complex IV") contains two heme *a* groups (heme *a* and heme a_3), each located near a copper ion. O_2 is tightly bound between heme a_3 and copper, to be released only after its complete reduction to H_2O by the sequential transfer of four electrons. Cytochrome oxidase has a very high affinity for molecular oxygen. This ensures a near-maximal rate of oxidative phosphorylation even at very low oxygen partial pressure.

Mitochondrial flavoproteins, including SDH ("complex II") and the mitochondrial glycerol phosphate dehydrogenase, bypass the NADH–Q reductase complex. They transfer their electrons directly to ubiquinone.

The Respiratory Chain Creates a Proton Gradient

Oxidative phosphorylation proceeds in two steps (Fig. 21.27):

1. *Protons are pumped out of the mitochondrion.* Proton pumping is driven by the redox reactions in the respiratory chain, and it creates a steep electrochemical gradient across the inner mitochondrial membrane.

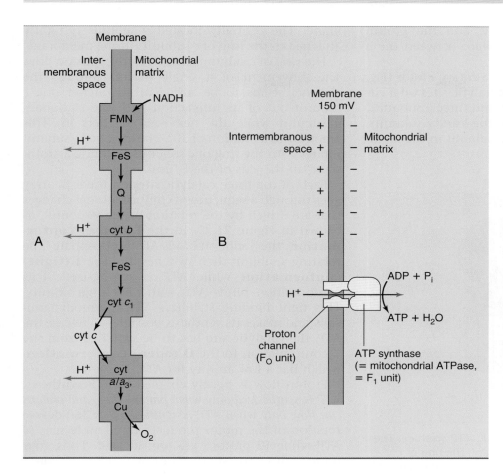

Figure 21.27 The two steps in oxidative phosphorylation. The inner mitochondrial membrane acts like a storage battery that is charged by the proton pumps of the respiratory chain. **A,** Protons are pumped out of the mitochondrial matrix. Proton pumping is fueled by the exergonic redox reactions in the respiratory chain. cyt, cytochrome; FeS, iron-sulfur protein; FMN, flavin mononucleotide. **B,** Protons move back into the matrix space through a specific proton channel. This proton channel is coupled to an ATP–synthesizing enzyme (the F_1F_o-ATP synthase). ATP synthesis is fueled by the flow of protons down their electrochemical gradient.

2. *Protons are admitted back into the mitochondrion through a proton channel.* This entropically favored process drives ATP synthesis.

Protons are pumped in each of the three protein complexes (see Figs. 21.26 and 21.27). Approximately four protons are pumped by the NADH–Q reductase complex and another four by the QH_2–cytochrome c reductase complex. Also, cytochrome oxidase removes four protons from the mitochondrial matrix, translocating two to the intermembranous space and consuming the other two in the reduction of O_2.

The passage of a pair of electrons through each of these "phosphorylation sites" leads to the synthesis of approximately one ATP molecule. Therefore, the **P/O ratio,** defined as the number of high-energy phosphate bonds formed for each oxygen atom (or each pair of electrons) consumed, is conventionally stated as 3 for the oxidation of NADH and 2 for the oxidation of $FADH_2$. However, it seems to be a bit lower than this under "real-world" conditions.

The respiratory chain creates a proton gradient of about one pH unit, inside alkaline. It also helps to maintain a membrane potential of 100 to 200 mV, inside negative. Concentration gradient and electrical potential add up to a steep electrochemical gradient for protons, amounting to 4 to 6 kcal/mol.

To maintain this gradient, the inner mitochondrial membrane must be impermeable to protons and also to other inorganic ions (which would dissipate the membrane potential). It has already been shown (see Fig. 21.21) that most translocases of the inner mitochondrial membrane make electroneutral exchanges, thereby minimizing the effects of substrate transport on the membrane potential.

The Proton Gradient Drives ATP Synthesis

The proton gradient fuels the **mitochondrial ATP synthase,** also known as **F_1F_o-ATP synthase.** The **F_1 unit** (F_1 = "coupling factor 1") of the enzyme is a protein complex of subunit structure $\alpha_3\beta_3\gamma\delta\epsilon$ and a molecular weight of 380 kD. It is visible under the electron microscope as small buttons on the inner surface of the inner mitochondrial membrane. The F_1 unit is attached to the **F_o unit** (F_o = oligomycin-sensitive factor), an integral membrane protein with the subunit structure a,b_2,c_{12}. The c

subunits form a circular array, and the proton channel is formed by the interface between the *a* and *c* subunits.

The ATP synthase works like a rotary motor (Fig. 21.28). The F$_1$ unit has three catalytic sites on a circular array of three α subunits and three β subunits. This array is kept stationary by the *b* and δ subunits, which attach it firmly to the *a* subunit in the mem-

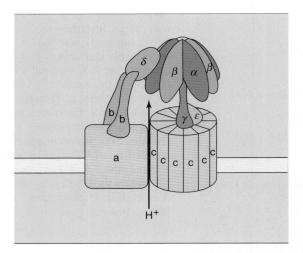

Figure 21.28 The structure of the F$_1$F$_o$–ATP synthase. The a, b, δ, α, and β subunits are stationary. The ring of c subunits with the attached γ and ε subunits rotates when protons move through the channel. The rotation of γ induces sequential changes in the conformation of the catalytic α$_3$β$_3$ "button." These conformational changes drive ATP synthesis.

brane. The centrally located γ subunit is tightly attached to the ring of *c* subunits in the membrane.

The ring of *c* subunits rotates during proton flow. The movement of a single proton through the channel seems to be sufficient to ratchet one *c* subunit out of its interaction with the stationary *a* subunit while the next one ratchets in. This amounts to a rotation of 30°. The attached γ subunit rotates with the ring of *c* subunits, forming a "rotor stalk" in the axis of the F$_1$ unit.

Each of the three catalytic sites on the α$_3$β$_3$ array goes through a sequence of conformational changes that are driven by the rotation of the γ subunit, as shown in Figure 21.29. In the **L (loose) conformation,** the β subunit binds ADP + phosphate. The rotating γ subunit then switches it to the **T (tight) conformation** while ATP is synthesized. This conformation binds ATP with very high affinity. This tight binding stabilizes ATP thermodynamically and makes its synthesis possible. To release the ATP, the catalytic site has to be switched from the T conformation to the **O (open) conformation,** which has a low affinity for ATP.

Proton flow is tightly coupled to ATP synthesis. *ATP is synthesized only when protons flow, and protons can flow only when ATP is synthesized.* A 360-degree rotation of the motor produces three molecules of ATP while 12 protons are translocated. Thus, four protons drive the synthesis of one ATP molecule.

In the absence of a sufficient proton gradient, the ATP synthase does not synthesize but rather hydrolyzes ATP, as shown in the experiment of Figure 21.30. Therefore, the term **mitochondrial**

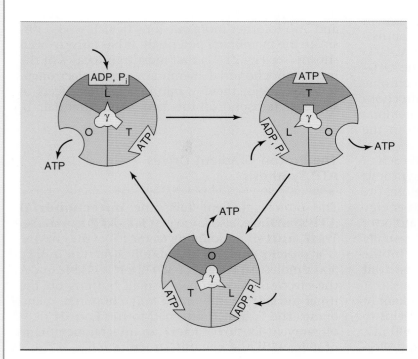

Figure 21.29 The sequence of reactions in the synthesis of ATP by the F$_1$F$_o$-ATP synthase in the inner mitochondrial membrane. The array of α and β subunits forming the three catalytic sites remains stationary, and the conformational transitions between the tight (T), open (O), and loose (L) conformations are driven by the rotating γ subunit.

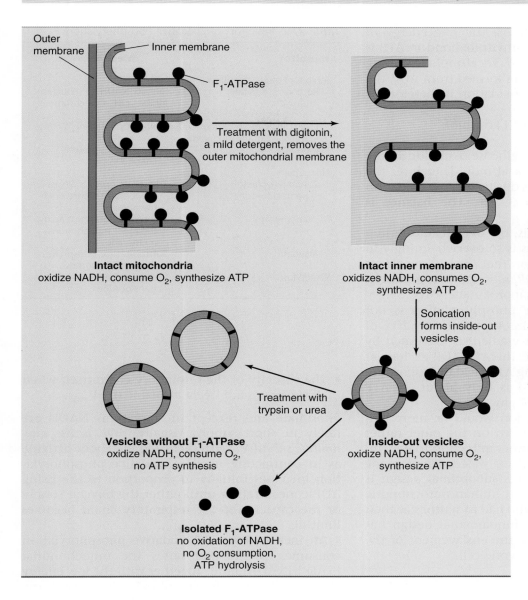

Intact mitochondria
oxidize NADH, consume O₂, synthesize ATP

Treatment with digitonin,
a mild detergent, removes the
outer mitochondrial membrane

Intact inner membrane
oxidizes NADH, consumes O₂,
synthesizes ATP

Sonication
forms inside-out
vesicles

Treatment with
trypsin or urea

Vesicles without F₁-ATPase
oxidize NADH, consume O₂,
no ATP synthesis

Inside-out vesicles
oxidize NADH, consume O₂,
synthesize ATP

Isolated F₁-ATPase
no oxidation of NADH,
no O₂ consumption,
ATP hydrolysis

Figure 21.30 Isolation of the F₁-ATPase. Note that the isolated ATP synthase does not synthesize but rather hydrolyzes ATP. This enzyme therefore is often called the "mitochondrial ATPase" or "F₁-ATPase." An intact membrane with a steep proton gradient is an absolute requirement for ATP synthesis.

ATPase is sometimes applied to the ATP-synthesizing complex.

The Efficiency of Glucose Oxidation Is Close to 40%

It is now possible to examine the efficiency of ATP synthesis from the oxidation of glucose, assuming an ATP yield of three molecules for each NADH and two for each $FADH_2$ oxidized in the respiratory chain. As shown in Table 21.6, 36 to 38 high-energy phosphate bonds are generated. Only four of them are produced by substrate-level phosphorylation in glycolysis and TCA cycle; the rest are from oxidative phosphorylation. Anaerobic glycolysis, on the other hand, yields only two molecules of ATP.

Table 21.6 Energy Yield from Glucose Oxidation

Pathway	Yield (Molecules)
Glycolysis	2 ATP
	2 NADH → 4 or 6 ATP*
Pyruvate dehydrogenase	2 NADH → 6 ATP
TCA cycle	2 GTP → 2 ATP
	6 NADH → 18 ATP
	2 FADH₂ → 4 ATP
	36 or 38 ATP

*The energy yield from cytoplasmic NADH depends on the shuttle system used.

Under standard conditions, the free energy of hydrolysis for a phosphoanhydride bond in ATP is conventionally defined as 7.3 kcal/mol. Assuming that 37 molecules of ATP are formed from ADP, the energy yield from glucose oxidation is therefore

$$37 \times 7.3 = 270.1 \, \text{kcal/mol}$$

The total heat released by glucose oxidation in the bomb calorimeter is 686 kcal/mol. Therefore, the efficiency of ATP synthesis during glucose oxidation is 270.1/686 = 0.394 = 39.4%. The balance is released as heat.

Even with ATP synthesis, the overall equilibrium of the oxidative pathways is so overwhelmingly in favor of substrate oxidation that *the cells are able to maintain a high [ATP]/[ADP] ratio*. In resting muscle, for example, this ratio is approximately 100 : 1.

Nevertheless, oxidative phosphorylation is not quite as efficient as it looks. Approximately 20% of the energy in the proton gradient is dissipated by the phosphate carrier and the ATP/ADP exchanger in the membrane, reducing ATP yield in proportion. Thus, the true ATP yield is only about 30 ATP molecules per molecule of glucose.

Oxidative phosphorylation would be more efficient if ATP were synthesized on the outer rather than inner surface of the inner mitochondrial membrane, obviating the need for wasteful membrane carriers. The reason for this suboptimal design is that the ancestors of current human mitochondria were free-living bacteria who had to synthesize their ATP inside the cell. This fundamental design has never been changed since the enslavement of the mitochondria by the eukaryotic cell.

Oxidative Phosphorylation Is Limited by the Supply of ADP

Respiratory control is based on a tight coupling between electron flow in the respiratory chain and ATP synthesis. *ATP cannot be synthesized without electron flow, and electrons cannot flow without ATP synthesis.* Unless the proton gradient is dissipated through the F_1/F_o-ATP synthase, it will build up to such proportions that the redox reactions in the respiratory chain grind to a halt, being unable to pump against the overwhelming gradient.

There is no "rate-limiting step" in oxidative phosphorylation, but its rate depends on substrate availability. Possible limiting factors include

- NADH
- Oxygen
- ADP
- Phosphate

Table 21.7 Inhibitors of Oxidative Phosphorylation

Inhibitor	Mechanism
Inhibitors of electron flow	
Rotenone, amytal	Inhibits NADH–Q reductase
Antimycin A	Inhibits QH_2–cytochrome c reductase
Cyanide, azide, hydrogen sulfide, carbon monoxide	Inhibits cytochrome oxidase
Oligomycin	Inhibits the F_o proton channel
Uncouplers	
2,4-Dinitrophenol, pentachlorophenol	Transports protons across the inner mitochondrial membrane
Valinomycin	Transports potassium across the inner mitochondrial membrane
Arsenate	Substitutes for phosphate during ATP synthesis
Atractyloside	Inhibits ATP-ADP translocation

- The capacity of the respiratory chain itself when all substrates are freely available (its V_{max}).

Phosphate and (except in starvation) NADH are rarely in short supply. Usually, *ADP is the rate-limiting substrate*. With increased metabolic activity, as in contracting muscle, oxidative phosphorylation increases initially in proportion to the rising ADP concentration until either the oxygen supply or the capacity of the respiratory chain becomes limiting.

An increased rate of oxidative phosphorylation consumes NADH and raises the mitochondrial $[NAD^+]/[NADH]$ ratio. Together with the low energy charge that raised the rate of oxidative phosphorylation in the first place, the high $[NAD^+]/[NADH]$ ratio stimulates pyruvate dehydrogenase and the regulated enzymes of the TCA cycle. NADH production is thereby adjusted to NADH consumption in the respiratory chain.

Oxidative Phosphorylation Is Inhibited by Many Poisons

Electron flow through the respiratory chain can be blocked by *site-specific inhibitors* (Table 21.7). **Rotenone,** obtained from the roots of some tropical plants, inhibits electron flow from the iron-sulfur complexes in the NADH–Q reductase complex to ubiquinone. It is a very effective poison for fish, which take it up through their gills. Humans can eat the poisoned fish with impunity because rotenone is absorbed poorly by the intestine. Rotenone is also in favor as a "natural" insecticide.

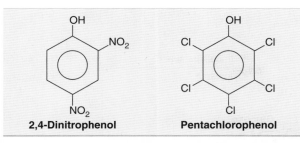

Figure 21.31 Structures of 2,4-dinitrophenol and pentachlorophenol. These chemicals are highly diffusible, acidic substances that can penetrate the inner mitochondrial membrane, even in the negatively charged deprotonated form. They uncouple oxidative phosphorylation by transporting protons across the membrane.

Some **barbiturates** also inhibit electron flow through the NADH–Q reductase complex. This action is unrelated to their sedative-hypnotic properties, which are mediated by an effect on a γ-aminobutyric acid (GABA)–operated chloride channel in the brain, but it can play a role in barbiturate poisoning.

Antimycin A, an antibiotic produced by a streptomycete, blocks electron flow through the QH_2–cytochrome *c* reductase complex.

In the cytochrome oxidase complex, several inhibitors bind to the heme iron in cytochrome a/a_3, whose sixth coordination position is otherwise reserved for oxygen. **Cyanide** and **azide** bind to the ferric form of the iron, and **carbon monoxide** binds to the ferrous form. **Hydrogen sulfide** is another potent inhibitor. Whereas carbon monoxide binds more tightly to hemoglobin than to cytochrome oxidase, the other agents induce their toxic effects by inhibiting electron flow.

Uncouplers of oxidative phosphorylation prevent ATP synthesis despite continuing electron flow. Most uncouplers disrupt the proton gradient across the inner mitochondrial membrane. **2,4-Dinitrophenol** and **pentachlorophenol** (Fig. 21.31) are diffusible, lipid-soluble organic acids. *They dissipate the proton gradient by ferrying protons across the inner mitochondrial membrane.* ATP can no longer be synthesized, but electron flow actually increases because the respiratory chain no longer has to pump protons against a steep gradient.

Some endogenous compounds, including free fatty acids and bilirubin, can also act as uncouplers at high concentrations. Bilirubin can cause brain damage in infants with severe hyperbilirubinemia (see Chapter 27), possibly by uncoupling oxidative phosphorylation.

Valinomycin is a transport antibiotic that makes the inner mitochondrial membrane permeable for potassium. This dissipates the membrane potential, which is an essential component of the proton-motive force.

Arsenate is a structural analog of phosphate. After getting a free ride into the mitochondrion on the phosphate transporter, it competes with phosphate for ATP synthesis. The resulting γ-arsenate analog of ATP is unstable and hydrolyzes spontaneously to ADP and arsenate.

Oligomycin is an antibiotic that prevents ATP synthesis by blocking the proton channel in the F_1F_o-ATP synthase. A steep proton gradient builds up and inhibits electron flow through the respiratory chain.

The plant product **atractyloside** blocks the ATP/ADP antiporter in the inner mitochondrial membrane. The resulting lack of ADP in the mitochondrial matrix stops both ATP synthesis and electron flow.

Oxygen Deficiency Is Rapidly Fatal

The ATP concentration in different tissues is only 1 to 5 g/kg, but at least 70 kg of ATP are synthesized in the human body every day. This means that the average ATP molecule has a life span of only 1 to 5 minutes, and most cells will be depleted of ATP within minutes after the cessation of oxidative phosphorylation.

The most common cause for a failure of oxidative phosphorylation is **hypoxia** (insufficient oxygen) or **anoxia** (complete lack of oxygen). Acute oxygen deficiency is usually caused by **ischemia** (interruption of the blood supply). Ischemic anoxia causes cell death within a few minutes (neurons), half an hour to 2 hours (myocardium, liver, kidney), or several hours (fibroblasts, epidermis, skeletal muscle). Cells in the hair follicles are so resistant to anoxia that a beard keeps growing for 2 or 3 days after death. Some important events in ischemia (Fig. 21.32) are as follows:

- *The failure of ATP-dependent ion pumps causes osmotic imbalances.* The cells swell, and so do membrane-bounded organelles, including lysosomes and mitochondria.
- *Glycolysis is stimulated by low energy charge.* PFK is activated by low energy charge, as is the glycogen-degrading enzyme glycogen phosphorylase. The cells try to survive by turning their stored glycogen into lactic acid, but lactic acid acidifies the tissue and contributes to cell death. The stimulation of glycolysis under anaerobic conditions is known as the **Pasteur effect.**
- *Plasma membrane and organelle membranes become leaky* as a result of osmotic stress and high acidity.

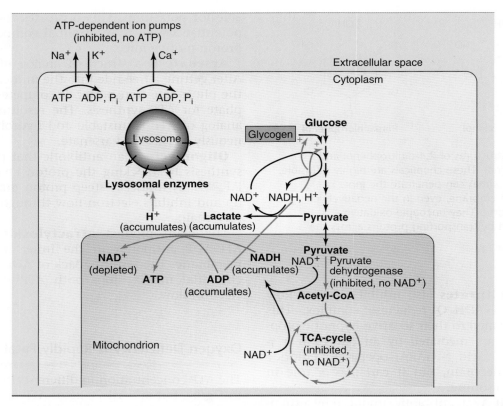

Figure 21.32 The metabolic consequences of hypoxia. A decreased energy charge and decreased [NAD$^+$]/[NADH] ratio are the initial results of oxygen deficiency. The mitochondrial oxidative pathways are arrested for lack of NAD$^+$. The regulated enzymes of glycolysis and glycogen degradation (phosphofructokinase and glycogen phosphorylase) are stimulated by low energy charge. The accumulation of lactic acid acidifies the cell. Both the plasma membrane and the organellar membranes are damaged by the increased acidity and by osmotic imbalances that result from the failure of ATP-dependent ion pumps. Lysosomal enzymes, which are active at low pH, initiate autolysis.

Cellular enzymes leak into the interstitial space and finally appear in the blood. Lysosomal enzymes are spilled into the acidified cytoplasm, in which they attack cellular proteins, glycoproteins, glycolipids, phosphate esters, and other substrates.

Ischemia is worse than hypoxia. In animal experiments, the cells survive "pure" anoxia, without interruption of the blood flow, far longer than ischemic anoxia. This shows that the accumulation of metabolic products, such as lactic acid, contributes to ischemic cell injury.

In ischemia, *loss of function always precedes cell death.* Ischemic myocardial tissue, for example, can survive for 30 to 60 minutes, but it loses its contractility in less than 1 minute. Although neurons survive for some minutes, consciousness is lost almost immediately after a sudden interruption of blood flow to the brain. Presumably, this is the case after decapitation on the guillotine.

Inhibitors of Oxidative Phosphorylation Also Can Be Rapidly Fatal

Cyanide (CN$^-$) blocks the respiratory chain by binding to the ferric iron in cytochrome a/a_3. Although not particularly potent (the lethal dose of hydrogen cyanide in humans is about 1 mg/kg), cyanide is absorbed rapidly from the gastrointestinal tract, and the effect of inhaled hydrogen cyanide gas is almost instantaneous, forestalling any effective measures of treatment. It is used for the extermination of rodents, insects, and, in some states, murderers.

The metabolic derangements of cyanide poisoning resemble those of hypoxia. Hyperventilation develops rapidly, not because of hypoxia but because of massive lactic acidosis. Being unable to synthesize ATP by oxidative phosphorylation, *all tissues switch to anaerobic glycolysis and release lactic acid into the blood.* Acidosis is a powerful stimulus for the respiratory center in the brain. The oxygen saturation of hemoglobin is actually increased in cyanide poisoning.

The treatment of cyanide poisoning is aimed at the removal of the poison from cytochrome oxidase. Sodium nitrite, in moderate doses, is given to induce methemoglobin formation. The ferric iron in methemoglobin binds cyanide avidly, thereby removing it from the ferric iron in cytochrome a/a_3. Sodium thiosulfate is also given, which reacts with cyanide to form the far less toxic thiocyanate. This reaction is catalyzed by the enzyme rhodanase in the liver.

Pentachlorophenol (see Fig. 21.30) is a wood preservative that kills termites, fungi, bacteria, and occasionally humans by uncoupling their oxidative phosphorylation. As in cyanide poisoning, failure of oxidative phosphorylation leads to lactic acidosis. In contrast to cyanide poisoning, however, *NADH oxidation and oxygen consumption are increased.* High [NAD^+]/[$NADH$] ratio and low energy charge stimulate the oxidative pathways, but without ATP synthesis, *the energy of fuel oxidation is released as heat.* Hyperthermia is therefore a prominent sign in pentachlorophenol poisoning.

Mutations in Mitochondrial DNA Can Cause Disease

Any complete malfunction of mitochondrial oxidation is fatal, but milder impairments are seen occasionally. Most inherited mitochondrial diseases are caused by mutations in the mitochondrial DNA.

The mitochondrial genome (see Chapter 8) consists of 16,569 base pairs that encode 13 polypeptides, 22 transfer RNAs, and the two RNAs of the mitochondrial ribosomes (12S and 16S). The mitochondria-encoded polypeptides include 7 (of 42) subunits of NADH–Q reductase, 1 subunit (of 11) of QH_2–cytochrome *c* reductase, 3 (of 13) subunits of cytochrome oxidase, and 2 subunits of ATP synthase. All other mitochondrial proteins are encoded by nuclear genes and synthesized by cytoplasmic ribosomes.

Leber hereditary optic neuropathy (LHON) is characterized by the sudden onset of blindness in young adults, caused by degeneration of the optic nerve. The most common mutation in patients with this disease is a single-base substitution at base pair 11,778 of the mitochondrial DNA, in the gene for one of the subunits of NADH–Q reductase. Other patients have point mutations in genes for subunits of NADH–Q reductase, QH_2–cytochrome *c* reductase, or cytochrome oxidase.

All these mutations impair electron flow through the respiratory chain and reduce ATP synthesis. They lead to blindness because the optic nerve has a high energy demand and depends almost entirely on oxidative phosphorylation for its ATP supply. Because all mitochondria are derived from the ovum and none from the sperm, LHON is transmitted from an affected mother to all her children, but not from an affected father.

Mutations in the genes for ATP synthase subunits and for mitochondrial transfer RNAs have been described as well. These mutations lead to neurological deficits, abnormalities of red muscle fibers, cardiomyopathy, and/or retinal degeneration. These tissues are especially vulnerable because they have a high energy demand and rely heavily on oxidative metabolism. In some cases, the disease-producing mutation is present in all mitochondria; in other cases, some mitochondria are unaffected, whereas others bear the mutation, even in the same cell. The latter case is called **heteroplasmy.** Most cells have hundreds to thousands of mitochondria, and each mitochondrion has several copies of the mitochondrial genome.

Mitochondrial DNA has a higher mutation rate than nuclear DNA. Therefore, mitochondrial mutations accumulate, and the oxidative capacity declines, with advancing age. Deletions in the mitochondrial DNA are especially likely to accumulate because they favor rapid replication of the mitochondrial DNA, provided that the replication origin is spared. The gradual decline of mitochondrial function with age explains why many inherited mitochondrial mutations become symptomatic only at an advanced age, when the combined effects of the inherited mutation and of acquired somatic mutations depress oxidative phosphorylation below a critical threshold.

Reactive Oxygen Derivatives Are Formed during Oxidative Metabolism

The reduction of one molecule of oxygen to two molecules of water requires four electrons and four protons. The partial reduction of oxygen by less than four electrons is possible, but the products are very reactive. The transfer of a single electron to molecular oxygen produces **superoxide:**

$$O_2 + e^- \rightarrow \underset{\text{Superoxide}}{O_2^-}$$

Superoxide is both an anion and a **free radical.** Free radicals are molecular terrorists that are dangerous because they possess a highly reactive unpaired electron. Because it is very reactive, superoxide is short lived. It initiates chain reactions by bumping into another molecule and converting it to a free radical, which in turn reacts with a third molecule, and so forth. It also forms other reactive oxygen species:

$$O_2^{\overline{\cdot}} \rightleftharpoons HO_2^{\cdot}$$

with H^+

| Superoxide radical | Hydroperoxide radical |

$$H_2O_2 \rightleftharpoons 2\,{}^{\cdot}OH$$

via $HO_2^{\cdot}$, O_2

| Hydrogen peroxide | Hydroxyl radical |

The superoxide radical is thought to be formed in small quantity by many oxygenases, but the most important source is probably cytochrome oxidase.

Hydrogen peroxide is also formed by many flavoproteins. Unlike NADH and NADPH, $FADH_2$ and the reduced form of FMN ($FMNH_2$) are tightly bound prosthetic groups. After being reduced in a dehydrogenase reaction, the flavin coenzyme cannot be reoxidized by diffusing away and participating in a different enzymatic reaction. Flavoproteins of the inner mitochondrial membrane, including SDH and the mitochondrial glycerol phosphate dehydrogenase, donate their hydrogen to ubiquinone:

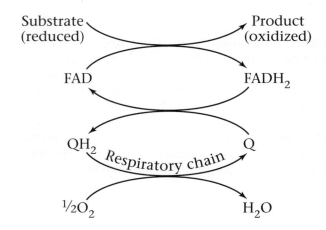

Flavoproteins in other locations transfer their hydrogen directly to molecular oxygen, forming hydrogen peroxide:

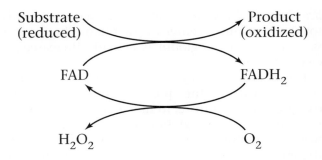

Several enzymes have evolved to destroy reactive oxygen derivatives. **Superoxide dismutase** eliminates the superoxide radical:

$$2\,O_2^{\overline{\cdot}} + 2\,H^+ \xrightarrow[\text{dismutase}]{\text{Superoxide}} H_2O_2 + O_2$$

It is present in the cytoplasm and mitochondria of all cells. The mitochondrial enzyme is activated by manganese, and the cytoplasmic enzyme contains copper and zinc. *Superoxide dismutase is required for aerobic life.* It is present in all aerobic organisms but not in obligate anaerobes.

The heme-containing enzyme **catalase** destroys hydrogen peroxide:

$$2\,H_2O_2 \xrightarrow{\text{Catalase}} 2\,H_2O + O_2$$

It is present in blood and tissues, accounting for 40% of the total protein in peroxisomes. Because of catalase, hydrogen peroxide bubbles when it is applied to wounds.

Peroxidases destroy hydrogen peroxide by reacting it with an organic substrate. The most important of them, **glutathione peroxidase,** uses the sulfhydryl-containing tripeptide glutathione (see Chapter 22):

$$2\,\text{Glutathione-SH} + H_2O_2 \rightarrow \begin{array}{c}\text{Glutathione-S}\\ |\\ \text{Glutathione-S}\end{array} + 2\,H_2O$$

Some vitamins and metabolites can terminate free radical chain reactions by scavenging free radicals. Water-soluble antioxidants, including bilirubin, uric acid, and ascorbate, patrol the aqueous compartments, and the fat-soluble vitamins A and E do police duty in the membranes.

Reactive oxygen derivatives can initiate the nonenzymatic oxidation of polyunsaturated fatty acid residues in membrane lipids and triglycerides (see Chapter 23). They are also likely to cause other types of cellular damage, including somatic mutations. The mitochondria, in particular, are badly polluted with reactive oxygen species. This is a likely reason for the high mutation rate of mitochondrial DNA.

Oxygen derivatives may also play specific roles in some diseases. The formation of toxic H_2O_2 by monoamine oxidase (MAO) (see Chapter 16) is thought to contribute to the destruction of dopamine neurons in Parkinson disease. These neurons have high MAO activity, and treatment with MAO inhibitors has been claimed not only to relieve the symptoms in the short term but also to delay the progression of the disease.

Reactive oxygen derivatives are also the likely culprits in acute oxygen toxicity. The administration of pure oxygen is required in some situations but can also lead to serious toxicity. Experimental animals die in an atmosphere of pure oxygen, and premature infants have developed retrolental fibroplasia with resulting blindness after oxygen treatment.

SUMMARY

Glycolysis produces two molecules of the three-carbon compound pyruvate from the six carbons of glucose. It also produces two molecules of ATP and two molecules of NADH. Under aerobic conditions, pyruvate then enters the mitochondrion, in which it is oxidatively decarboxylated to the two-carbon acetyl group in acetyl-CoA. Acetyl-CoA is formed not only from carbohydrates but also from fatty acids and amino acids.

The tricarboxylic acid (TCA) cycle oxidizes acetyl-CoA, forming carbon dioxide and reduced coenzymes. In the first reaction of the cycle, acetyl-CoA reacts with the four-carbon compound oxaloacetate to form the six-carbon compound citrate. Citrate is then converted back to oxaloacetate in the remaining reactions. Each round of the cycle produces two molecules of carbon dioxide, one of GTP, three of NADH, and one of $FADH_2$ from the acetyl residue.

The reduced coenzymes are reoxidized by molecular oxygen in the respiratory chain. These reactions create a proton gradient across the inner mitochondrial membrane that fuels ATP synthesis by the mitochondrial ATP synthase. The efficiency of ATP synthesis during glucose oxidation is close to 40%. Oxidative phosphorylation is the principal energy source for most tissues, and inhibitors of oxidative phosphorylation can be rapidly fatal.

Oxidative phosphorylation is controlled by the availability of ADP for ATP synthesis, while most of the regulated enzymes in the oxidative pathways are stimulated by low energy charge and a high $[NAD^+]/[NADH]$ ratio. These mechanisms ensure that an adequate cellular ATP pool is maintained at all times.

Under anaerobic conditions, the pyruvate formed in glycolysis is reduced to lactate by LDH. Anaerobic glycolysis produces only two molecules of ATP for each glucose molecule. It can tide the cell over during brief periods of hypoxia, but only cells with very low energy needs can subsist on anaerobic glycolysis permanently.

Further Reading

Schon EA: Mitochondrial genetics and disease. Trends Biochem Sci 25:555-560, 2000.
Senior AE, Nadanaciva S, Weber J: The molecular mechanism of ATP synthesis by F_1F_0-ATP synthase. Biochim Biophys Acta 1553:188-211, 2002.

QUESTIONS

1. **Some enzymes of the TCA cycle are physiologically regulated. The most common regulatory effect on these enzymes is**

   A. Inhibition by ATP.
   B. Inhibition by ADP.
   C. Inhibition by NAD^+.
   D. Stimulation by citrate.
   E. Inhibition by acetyl-CoA.

2. **Some individuals are born with a partial deficiency of pyruvate dehydrogenase in all tissues. What tissue suffers most from this abnormality?**

   A. Liver tissue.
   B. Muscle tissue.
   C. Erythrocytes.
   D. Adipose tissue.
   E. Brain tissue.

3. **What biochemical changes take place in brain cells shortly after decapitation?**

   A. The rate of glycolysis is reduced.
   B. TCA cycle activity is increased.
   C. The [lactate]/[pyruvate] concentration ratio is increased.
   D. All electron carriers in the respiratory chain are converted to the oxidized state.
   E. The potassium concentration in the cells increases, and the sodium concentration decreases.

4. Assume that the concentration of one of the glycolytic enzymes is reduced to 50% of normal as a result of a heterozygous mutation. The reduced activity of which enzyme would decrease overall glycolytic activity to the greatest extent?

   A. Hexokinase.
   B. PFK.
   C. Aldolase.
   D. Enolase.
   E. Pyruvate kinase.

5. Assume that the NADH–Q reductase complex is inhibited by the fish poison rotenone. A likely result of this inhibition will be

   A. The mitochondria can no longer oxidize succinate to fumarate.
   B. Most or all of the mitochondrial NAD will be in the oxidized state.
   C. Most or all of the mitochondrial ubiquinone will be in the oxidized state.
   D. The proton gradient across the inner mitochondrial membrane will be very steep.
   E. PFK will be inhibited.

6. Following the advice of her biochemistry professor, an overweight medical student goes on a sawdust diet (it fills the stomach but cannot be digested). She should make sure that the sawdust is not from wood that has been treated with the uncoupler pentachlorophenol. Pentachlorophenol would cause

   A. Weight gain.
   B. Reduced oxygen consumption (while she is still alive).
   C. Reduced TCA cycle activity.
   D. Hyperthermia.
   E. An increased [NADH]/[NAD$^+$] concentration ratio.

7. Muscle contraction causes an *immediate* increase in the rate of oxidative phosphorylation because it

   A. Decreases the pH.
   B. Increases the NAD$^+$ concentration.
   C. Increases the activity of PFK.
   D. Decreases the activity of pyruvate dehydrogenase.
   E. Increases the ADP concentration.

CHAPTER 22

Carbohydrate Metabolism

The most important functions of carbohydrate metabolism are as follows:

1. *The generation of metabolic energy by the catabolism of glucose.* The glycolytic pathway and its mitochondrial sequels are described in Chapter 21.
2. *The maintenance of a normal blood glucose level.* Glucose is required at all times. In the fasting state, the liver has to provide glucose by the degradation of stored glycogen or by synthesis from noncarbohydrates.
3. *The utilization of dietary monosaccharides other than glucose.* Fructose and galactose, in particular, have to be channeled into the major metabolic pathways of glucose.
4. *The provision of specialized monosaccharides as biosynthetic precursors:* ribose for the synthesis of nucleotides and nucleic acids, and amino sugars and acidic sugar derivatives for the synthesis of glycolipids, glycoproteins, and proteoglycans.

An Adequate Blood Glucose Level Must Be Maintained at All Times

Some cells and tissues, including brain and erythrocytes, depend on glucose because they cannot oxidize alternative fuels. The brain alone consumes nearly 120 g of glucose per day. Therefore, a blood glucose level of 4.0 to 5.5 mmol/liter (70 to 100 mg/dL) must be maintained at all times. Dietary carbohydrates provide glucose for only a few hours after a meal. In the fasting state, the liver has to produce glucose by two pathways:

1. *Glycogen degradation* is fast and requires no metabolic energy, but the glycogen reserves of the liver rarely exceed 100 g and are therefore depleted within 24 hours. Only liver glycogen,

but not the glycogen of muscle and other tissues, can be used to maintain the blood glucose level.
2. *Gluconeogenesis* produces glucose from amino acids, lactic acid, and glycerol. It is the only source of glucose during prolonged fasting. Only the liver and kidneys have a complete gluconeogenic pathway. On a weight basis, the gluconeogenic capacity of the renal cortex equals that of the liver, but because the liver is so much larger than a kidney, it produces 10 times more glucose.

Three Irreversible Reactions of Glycolysis Must Be Bypassed in Gluconeogenesis

The easiest strategy for glucose synthesis would be to reverse glycolysis by making glucose from pyruvate. However, a simple reversal of glycolysis is not possible, because three of the glycolytic reactions are physiologically irreversible: those catalyzed by **hexokinase, phosphofructokinase,** and **pyruvate kinase.** *These three reactions must be bypassed in gluconeogenesis* (Fig. 22.1).

The pyruvate kinase reaction of glycolysis is irreversible despite ATP synthesis. Reversing this reaction by going back from pyruvate to phosphoenolpyruvate (PEP) requires 14.8 kcal/mol: at least two high-energy phosphate bonds.

This feat is accomplished in a sequence of two reactions, as shown in Figure 22.2. First, pyruvate is carboxylated to oxaloacetate by pyruvate carboxylase. This mitochondrial reaction was earlier characterized as an anaplerotic reaction of the TCA cycle. It requires ATP in addition to enzyme-bound biotin. The second reaction, catalyzed by **PEP-carboxykinase,** converts oxaloacetate into PEP. It requires GTP. The two reactions combined have a standard free energy change ($\Delta G^{0'}$) of +0.2 kcal/mol, but in the cell, they proceed only from pyruvate to PEP because of the high cellular concentration ratios of [ATP]/[ADP], [GTP]/[GDP], and [Pyruvate]/[PEP].

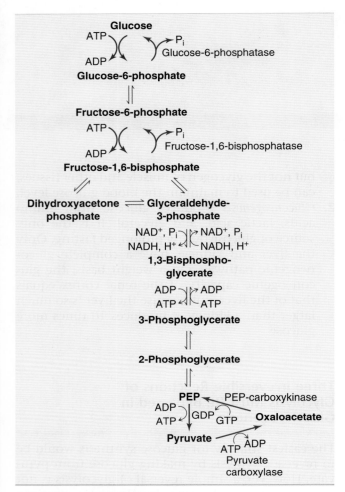

Figure 22.1 The reactions of glycolysis and gluconeogenesis. ADP, adenosine diphosphate; ATP, adenosine triphosphate; GDP, guanosine diphosphate; GTP, guanosine triphosphate; NAD$^+$, nicotinamide adenine dinucleotide; NADH, reduced form of NAD; PEP, phosphoenolpyruvate; P$_i$, inorganic phosphate.

While pyruvate carboxylase is strictly mitochondrial, PEP-carboxykinase is both mitochondrial and cytoplasmic. PEP is transported across the inner mitochondrial membrane, whereas oxaloacetate is shuttled into the cytoplasm after being reduced to malate or transaminated to aspartate.

PEP is processed to fructose-1,6-bisphosphate through the reversible reactions of glycolysis. The irreversible phosphofructokinase reaction is bypassed by **fructose-1,6-bisphosphatase,** which hydrolyzes the phosphate from carbon 1 of its substrate (Fig. 22.3).

The hexokinase reaction is also bypassed by the hydrolytic cleavage of the phosphate ester, catalyzed by **glucose-6-phosphatase.** Unlike the other gluconeogenic enzymes, which are cytoplasmic (except pyruvate carboxylase), this enzyme resides on the inner surface of the endoplasmic reticulum membrane. The fructose-1,6-bisphosphatase and glucose-6-phosphatase reactions are irreversible.

Gluconeogenesis requires *six phosphoanhydride bonds* for the synthesis of one glucose molecule from two molecules of pyruvate or lactate. Pyruvate carboxylase consumes two ATP molecules, PEP-carboxykinase consumes two GTP molecules, and phosphoglycerate kinase consumes two ATP molecules in the reversal of substrate-level phosphorylation.

Fatty Acids Cannot Be Converted into Glucose

Lactate and **alanine** are convenient substrates of gluconeogenesis because they are readily converted to pyruvate by lactate dehydrogenase and by transamination, respectively (Fig. 22.4). **Oxaloacetate** is not only a gluconeogenic intermediate but also a member of the TCA cycle. This is important because most amino acids are degraded to TCA cycle intermediates. Through the TCA cycle, these *"glucogenic" amino acids* feed into gluconeogenesis.

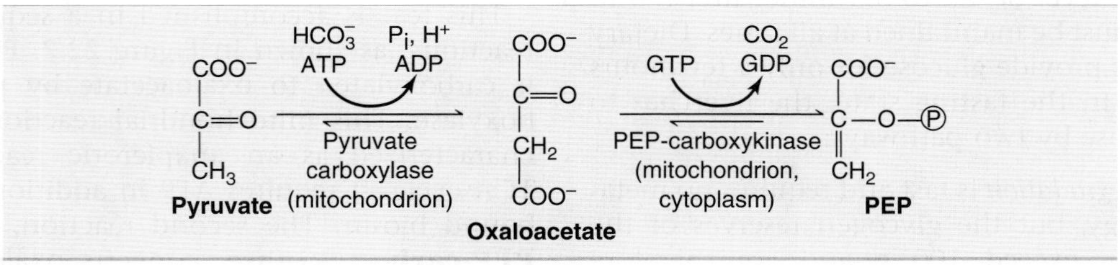

Figure 22.2 The first bypass of gluconeogenesis: from pyruvate to phosphoenolpyruvate (PEP).

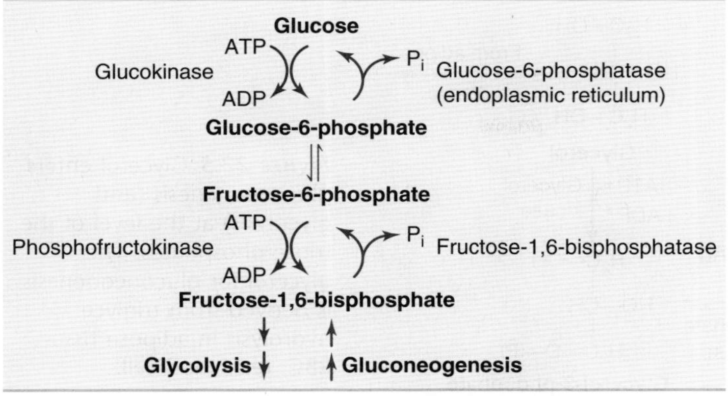

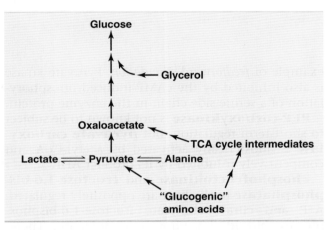

Figure 22.3 The second and third bypasses of gluconeogenesis.

Figure 22.4 The most important substrates of gluconeogenesis. Although acetyl-CoA enters the TCA cycle, it is not a substrate of gluconeogenesis because the citrate synthase reaction does not involve the net synthesis of a TCA cycle intermediate.

Glycerol is another substrate of gluconeogenesis. It enters the pathway at the level of the triose phosphates (Fig. 22.5).

Acetyl–CoA cannot be converted to glucose. The pyruvate dehydrogenase reaction is irreversible, and there are no alternative reactions to channel acetyl-CoA into gluconeogenesis. Fatty acids are degraded to acetyl-CoA. The fatty acids that are released from adipose tissue during fasting can be oxidized by most tissues, but they cannot be turned into glucose. Gluconeogenesis depends on amino acids and, to a lesser extent, on lactic acid and glycerol.

Hormones Are Important for the Regulation of Glycolysis and Gluconeogenesis

A simultaneous activity of glycolysis and gluconeogenesis would be counterproductive because it would achieve nothing but ATP hydrolysis. To avoid such a **futile cycle,** it is mandatory to control the irreversible reactions at all three bypasses: between pyruvate and PEP, between fructose-1,6-bisphosphate and fructose-6-phosphate, and between glucose-6-phosphate and glucose.

In addition to nutrients and metabolites, several hormones participate in the regulation of hepatic glycolysis and gluconeogenesis:

1. **Insulin** is released from pancreatic β cells in response to hyperglycemia (increased blood glucose level). Its plasma concentration is up to 10 times higher after a carbohydrate-rich meal than during prolonged fasting. In addition to regulating gene expression, insulin reduces the cyclic adenosine monophosphate (cAMP) level in the liver, probably by activating a cAMP-degrading phosphodiesterase. By stimulating the glucose-*consuming* pathways and inhibiting the glucose-*producing* pathways in the liver, *insulin lowers the blood glucose level.*

2. **Glucagon** is a polypeptide hormone from the α-cells of the endocrine pancreas. It is released in response to hypoglycemia (decreased blood glucose level), and its plasma level is therefore higher in the fasting state than after a carbohydrate meal. By stimulating the glucose-producing pathways and inhibiting the glucose-consuming pathways in the liver, *glucagon raises the blood glucose level.* The glucagon effects are mediated by cAMP and protein kinase A, and they involve both the phosphorylation of cytoplasmic enzymes and the regulation of gene expression.

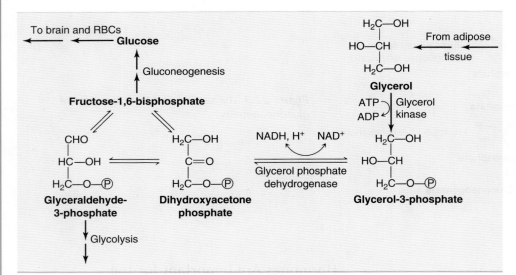

Figure 22.5 Glycerol enters gluconeogenesis (and glycolysis) at the level of the triose phosphates. The glycerol for gluconeogenesis is derived from triglyceride hydrolysis in adipose tissue. RBC, red blood cell.

3. **Epinephrine** and **norepinephrine** are stress hormones that are released during physical exertion and cold exposure and in psychological emergencies, including school biochemistry examinations. Their task is to provide fuel for contracting muscles. In the liver, *they favor gluconeogenesis over glycolysis* by inducing a modest rise of cAMP.

4. **Glucocorticoids** are stress hormones that affect gene transcription directly. By inducing the synthesis of gluconeogenic enzymes, *the glucocorticoids stimulate gluconeogenesis.*

The hormones regulate the synthesis of the distinctive glycolytic and gluconeogenic enzymes at the level of transcription (Fig. 22.6A). Because this involves the synthesis of new enzyme protein and most of the enzymes have life spans of a few days in the cell, this type of regulation works on a time scale of days rather than minutes.

Glycolysis and Gluconeogenesis Are Fine-Tuned by Allosteric Effectors and Hormone-Induced Enzyme Phosphorylations

The short-term control of glycolysis and gluconeogenesis is shown in Figure 22.6B.

The glycolytic enzyme **pyruvate kinase** is the most important regulated enzyme in the PEP-pyruvate cycle. It is allosterically inhibited by ATP and alanine and activated by fructose-1,6-bisphosphate. The concentration of fructose-1,6-bisphosphate is high when phosphofructokinase is activated and when fructose-1,6-bisphosphatase is inhibited. Its effect on pyruvate kinase is an example of *feedforward stimulation.* Pyruvate kinase is also inhibited by the cAMP-induced phosphorylation of a serine side chain in the enzyme protein.

PEP-carboxykinase is not known to be subject to short-term regulation, but **pyruvate carboxylase** is allosterically activated by acetyl-CoA and competitively inhibited by its product ADP.

Phosphofructokinase and **fructose-1,6-bisphosphatase** in the liver are oppositely regulated. ATP and citrate stimulate fructose-1,6-bisphosphatase but inhibit phosphofructokinase. Therefore, *high energy charge and the availability of metabolites favor gluconeogenesis over glycolysis.*

The most potent modulator of these two enzymes, however, is **fructose-2,6-bisphosphate.** This regulatory metabolite, not to be confused with the glycolytic intermediate fructose-1,6-bisphosphate, is an *allosteric activator of phosphofructokinase* and a *competitive inhibitor of fructose-1,6-bisphosphatase.*

Fructose-2,6-bisphosphate is both synthesized from and degraded to fructose-6-phosphate by a unique bifunctional enzyme that combines the activities of a 6-phosphofructo-2-kinase (PFK-2) and a fructose-2,6-bisphosphatase on the same polypeptide.

This bifunctional enzyme is phosphorylated by the cAMP-activated protein kinase A (see Chapter 17). The dephosphorylated enzyme acts as a kinase that makes fructose-2,6-bisphosphate, and the phosphorylated form acts as a phosphatase that breaks it down (Fig. 22.7). Therefore, the level of fructose-2,6-bisphosphate in the liver is high when glucagon and its second messenger cAMP are low, and it is low when glucagon and cAMP are high. Insulin opposes glucagon by lowering the cellular cAMP concentration and by stimulating the protein

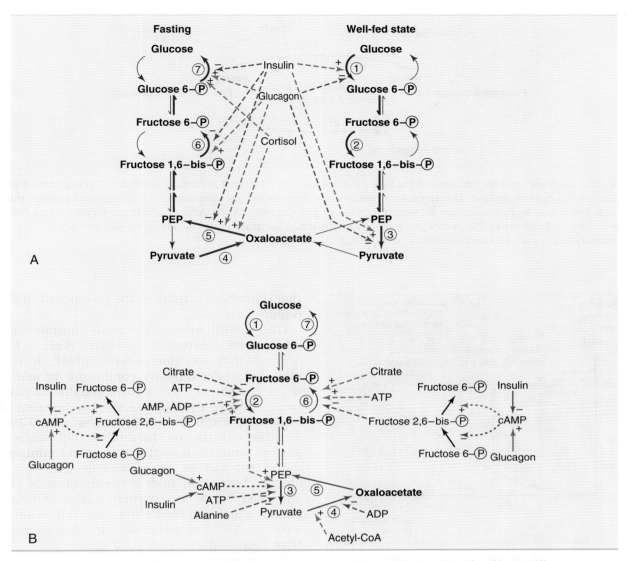

Figure 22.6 The reciprocal regulation of glycolysis and gluconeogenesis in the liver. (1), Glucokinase; (2), phosphofructokinase; (3), pyruvate kinase; (4), pyruvate carboxylase; (5), phosphoenolpyruvate (PEP)–carboxykinase; (6), fructose-1,6-bisphosphatase; (7), glucose-6-phosphatase. $\xrightarrow{+}$, Stimulation; $\xrightarrow{-}$, inhibition. **A,** Substrate flow during fasting and in the well-fed state, and the effects of hormones on the amounts of glycolytic and gluconeogenic enzymes. Regulation of enzyme synthesis and degradation is the most important long-term (hours to days) control mechanism. In most cases, the hormone acts by changing the rate of transcription or by affecting the stability of the messenger RNA. Some of the insulin effects shown here require the presence of glucose. **B,** Short-term regulation of glycolysis and gluconeogenesis by reversibly binding effectors and by phosphorylation/dephosphorylation. $---\!\!\blacktriangleright$, Allosteric and competitive effects; $\cdots\cdots\!\blacktriangleright$, phosphorylation. Only pyruvate kinase and phosphofructo-2-kinase/fructose-2,6-bisphosphatase are regulated by cyclic adenosine monophosphate (cAMP)–dependent phosphorylation.

phosphatase that dephosphorylates the bifunctional enzyme.

Through fructose-2,6-bisphosphate, insulin and glucagon regulate glycolysis and gluconeogenesis on a minute-to-minute time scale. In addition to hormonal control, fructose-6-phosphate stimulates the kinase activity and inhibits the phosphatase activity by an allosteric mechanism.

The enzymes of the glucose/glucose-6-phosphate cycle are regulated mainly by substrate availability.

The glucose-phosphorylating enzyme in the liver is hexokinase 4, an isoenzyme of hexokinase that is better known as **glucokinase.** The most important kinetic difference between glucokinase and the other isoenzymes of hexokinase is the Michaelis constant (K_m) for glucose. Whereas the other forms of hexokinase have K_m values near 0.1 mmol/liter (2 mg/dL), glucokinase has a K_m near 10 mmol/liter (200 mg/dL). Glucokinase also shows a sigmoidal rather than hyperbolic relationship

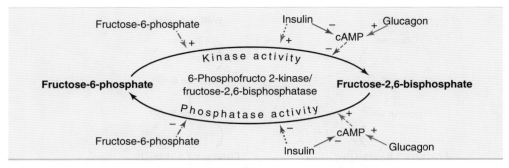

Figure 22.7 Synthesis and degradation of fructose-2,6-bisphosphate, the most important regulator of phosphofructokinase and fructose-1,6-bisphosphatase. This regulatory metabolite is synthesized and degraded by a bifunctional enzyme that combines the kinase and phosphatase activities on the same polypeptide. cAMP–induced phosphorylation inhibits the kinase activity and stimulates the phosphatase activity of the bifunctional enzyme. --►, Phosphorylation; ···►, dephosphorylation; ---►, allosteric effect; ─►, stimulation; ─►, inhibition.

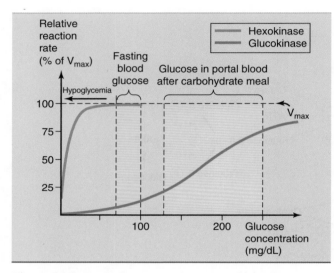

Figure 22.8 Approximate reaction rates of hexokinase (isoenzymes 1, 2, and 3) and glucokinase at different substrate concentrations. The sigmoidal relationship between reaction rate and substrate concentration for glucokinase accentuates the increase of the reaction rate with increased glucose level. V_{max}, maximal reaction rate.

between glucose concentration and reaction rate (Fig. 22.8).

The steep part of the curve is in the range of physiological glucose concentrations, and the reaction rate therefore varies substantially with alterations of the glucose level. The concentration of glucose is far higher in the portal vein than in the systemic blood after a carbohydrate meal, and glucose readily equilibrates across the hepatocyte membrane by a high-capacity bidirectional transporter.

Glucokinase is inhibited by the CoA-thioesters of long-chain fatty acids. These products are most abundant during fasting, when the liver metabolizes large amounts of fatty acids from adipose tissue. Glucokinase is also regulated by a protein that inhibits its activity in the presence of fructose-6-phosphate.

Like glucokinase, glucose-6-phosphatase is affected by substrate availability. With a K_m of 3 mmol/liter for glucose-6-phosphate, it is not saturated under ordinary conditions. In addition, it is inhibited by phosphatidylinositol-3,4,5-trisphosphate, a product of the insulin-stimulated enzyme phosphoinositide-3-kinase (see Chapter 17). Through this mechanism, insulin can reduce glucose production by the liver within minutes.

The stimulation of gluconeogenesis by high energy charge and high concentrations of citrate and acetyl-CoA is counterintuitive. Gluconeogenesis is active in the fasting state. Why would the levels of ATP and metabolites be increased rather than decreased in a starving organism?

The reason is that gluconeogenesis takes place almost exclusively in the liver, and the liver receives large quantities of fatty acids from adipose tissue during fasting. Fatty acid oxidation is less tightly controlled by feedback inhibition than is glucose oxidation. Therefore, the levels of ATP and acetyl-CoA in the liver are actually elevated during fasting. Thus, *the energy for gluconeogenesis is supplied by fatty acid oxidation.*

Carbohydrate Is Stored as Glycogen

Glycogen granules are seen in many cell types, but the most important stores are in liver and skeletal muscle. In the well-fed state, the glycogen content of the liver is up to 8% of the fresh weight: 100 to 120 g in the adult. The glycogen concentration in skeletal muscle is 1% or a bit less, but because most people have more muscle than liver, the total amount of muscle glycogen exceeds that in the liver.

Glycogen is a branched polymer of between 10,000 and 40,000 glucose residues held together by

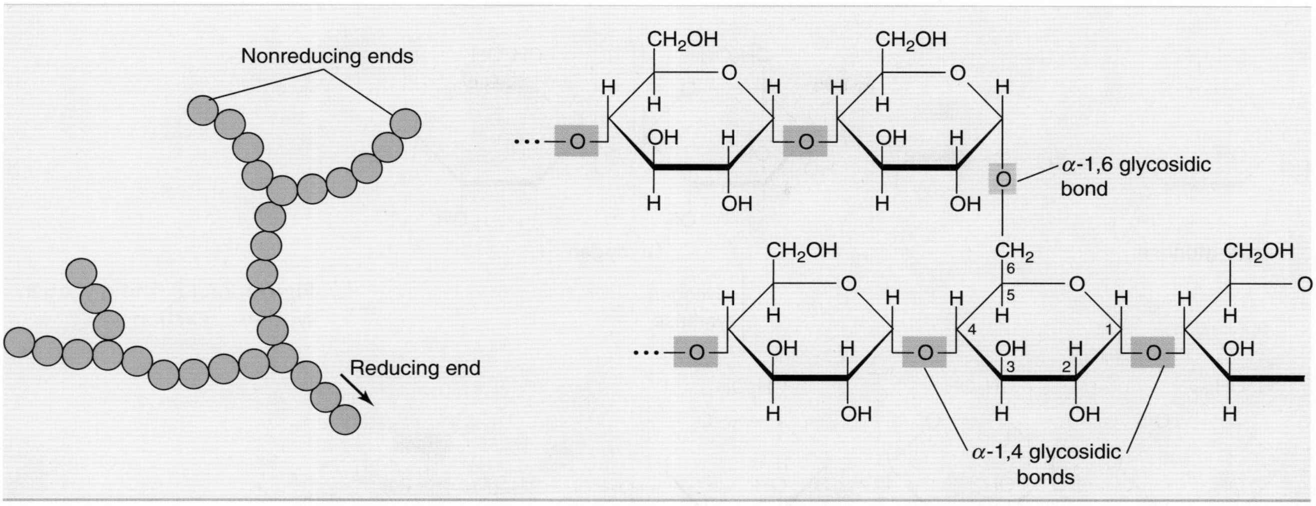

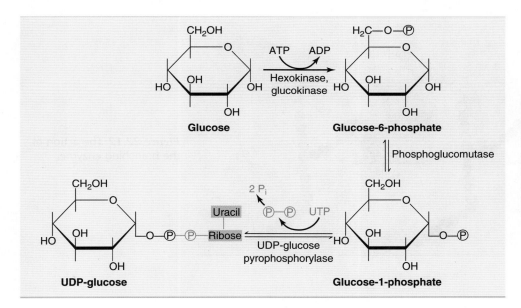

Figure 22.9 Structure of glycogen. *Left,* Overall structure. Note the large number of nonreducing ends, which are required as substrates for the enzymes of glycogen metabolism. *Right,* The structure around a branch point.

Figure 22.10 Synthesis of uridine diphosphate (UDP)–glucose. UDP-glucose is the activated form of glucose for glycogen synthesis, but also for the synthesis of other complex carbohydrates (see Table 9.3, Chapter 9).

α-1,4 glycosidic bonds. Approximately one in 12 glucose residues serves as a branch point by forming an α-1,6 glycosidic bond with another glucose residue (Fig. 22.9). With a molecular weight between 10^6 and 10^7 D, it is as big as a complete human ribosome (4.2×10^6 D).

Theoretically, the molecule has only one reducing end with a free hydroxyl group at carbon 1 but a large number of nonreducing ends with a free hydroxyl group at carbon 4. The enzymes of glycogen synthesis and glycogen degradation are nested between the outer branches of the molecule and act only on the nonreducing ends. Therefore, *the many nonreducing end branches of glycogen facilitate its rapid synthesis and degradation.*

Glycogen Is Readily Synthesized from Glucose

The steps in the synthesis of glycogen from glucose are outlined in Figures 22.10 and 22.11. Glucose-6-phosphate is isomerized to glucose-1-phosphate by **phosphoglucomutase.** At equilibrium, there are about 20 molecules of glucose-6-phosphate for every molecule of glucose-1-phosphate. Glucose-1-phosphate then reacts with uridine triphosphate (UTP) to form **UDP–glucose.** This otherwise reversible reaction is driven to completion by the subsequent hydrolysis of pyrophosphate. *UDP-glucose is the activated form of glucose for biosynthetic reactions.*

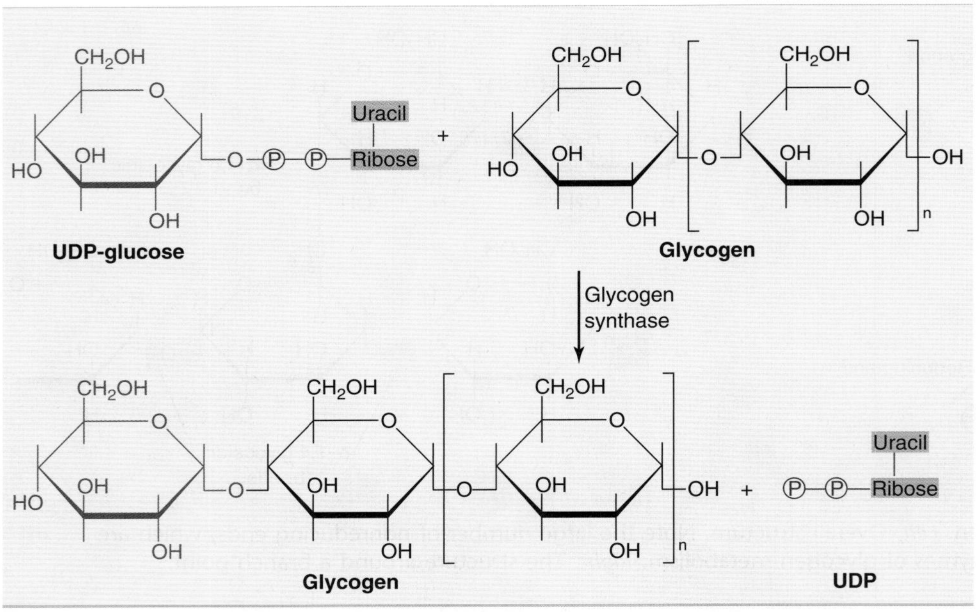

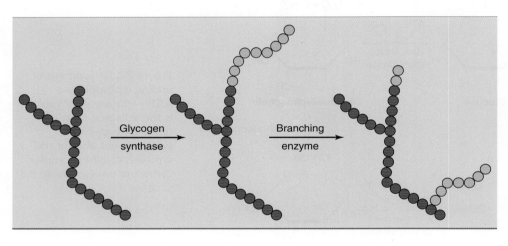

Figure 22.11 The glycogen synthase reaction.

Figure 22.12 The action of the branching enzyme.

UDP is attached to C-1 of glucose, and it is therefore this carbon that forms the glycosidic bond. The bond between glucose and UDP is energy rich. With a free energy content of 7.3 kcal/mol, it rivals the phosphoanhydride bonds in ATP. The free energy content of an α-1,4 glycosidic bond in glycogen is only 4.5 kcal/mol.

Glycogen synthase creates the α-1,4 glycosidic bonds in glycogen by transferring the glucose residue from UDP-glucose to the 4-hydroxyl group at the nonreducing end of the glycogen molecule, elongating the outer branches of glycogen by one glucose residue at a time (see Fig. 22.11).

Glycogen synthase cannot form the α-1,6 glycosidic bonds at the branch points. Branching requires a **branching enzyme,** which transfers a string of about seven glucose residues from the end of an unbranched chain to C-6 of a glucose residue in a more interior location (Fig. 22.12).

Glycogen synthesis from glucose consumes *two phosphoanhydride bonds for each glucose residue:* one in ATP for the hexokinase reaction, and one in UTP for the formation of UDP-glucose.

Glycogen Is Degraded by Phosphorolytic Cleavage

The glycogen-degrading enzyme **glycogen phosphorylase** uses inorganic phosphate to cleave a glucose residue from the nonreducing end of glycogen. This produces glucose-1-phosphate rather than free glucose (Fig. 22.13). The reaction is reversible, with 3.6 molecules of inorganic phosphate for every

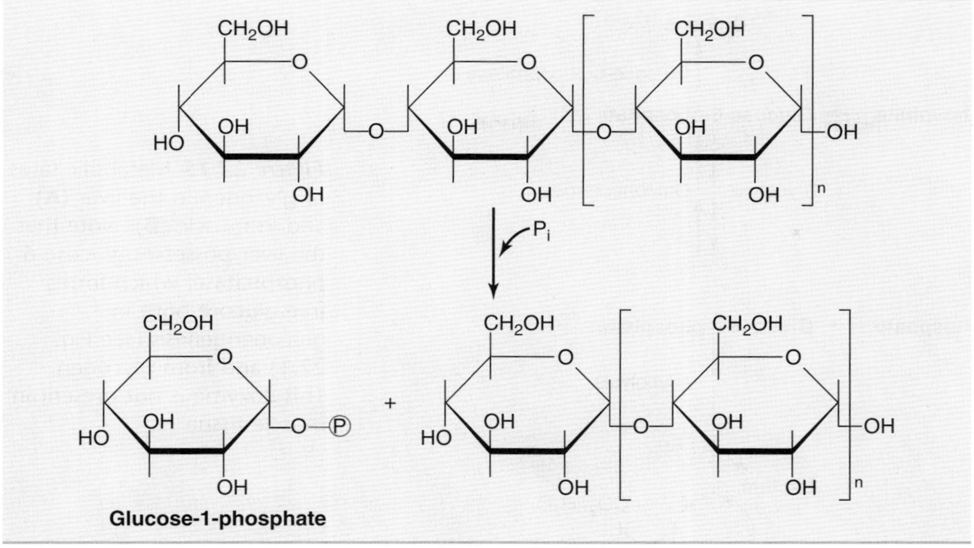

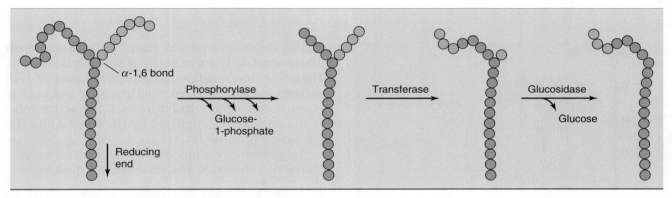

Figure 22.13 The glycogen phosphorylase reaction.

Glucose-1-phosphate

Figure 22.14 The action of the debranching enzyme.

molecule of glucose-1-phosphate at equilibrium. In the living cell, however, it proceeds only in the direction of glycogen breakdown because the cellular [phosphate]/[glucose-1-phosphate] ratio is at least 100.

Glycogen phosphorylase does not cleave the α-1,6 glycosidic bonds at the branch points. It does not even go near the branch points, stopping four residues before. At this point, the **debranching enzyme** has to take over. It first transfers a block of three glucose residues from the end of the chain to the C-4 end of another chain. This leaves only a single glucose at the branch point. This last glucose residue is hydrolyzed off the branch point by the debranching enzyme, producing a molecule of free glucose. Thus, the debranching enzyme has two enzymatic activities: a transferase activity and a hydrolase activity (Fig. 22.14). Overall, *about 92% of the glucose residues in glycogen form glucose-1-phosphate, and 8% form free glucose.* Glucose-1-phosphate is in equilibrium with glucose-6-phosphate through the phosphoglucomutase reaction.

Glycogen breakdown serves different purposes in liver and muscle. *The liver synthesizes glycogen after a carbohydrate meal and degrades it to free glucose during fasting.* The glucose-6-phosphate from glycogen breakdown is cleaved to free glucose by glucose-6-phosphatase. The liver releases this glucose into the blood for use by needy tissues, including brain and blood cells (Fig. 22.15).

Skeletal muscle synthesizes glycogen at rest and degrades it during exercise. Muscles cannot produce free glucose because they have no glucose-6-phosphatase. Unlike glucose, glucose-6-phosphate cannot leave the cell and is therefore metabolized by glycolysis in the muscle fiber. Because glycogen degradation produces glucose-6-phosphate without consuming any ATP, *anaerobic glycolysis from glycogen produces three rather than two molecules of ATP for each glucose residue.*

Liver glycogen is synthesized and degraded in response to feeding and fasting, and its level therefore fluctuates widely in the course of a typical day (Fig. 22.16). Muscle glycogen, in contrast, is fairly

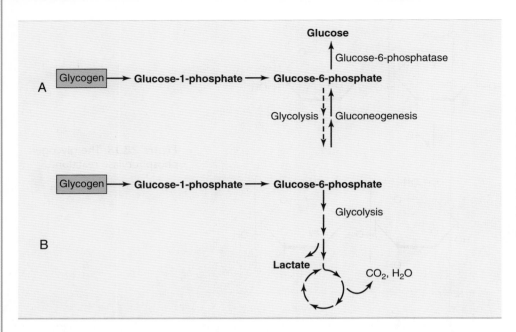

Figure 22.15 Metabolic fates of glycogen in the liver (**A**) and in muscle (**B**). Note that the liver possesses glucose-6-phosphatase, which forms free glucose both in gluconeogenesis (see Fig. 22.1) and from glycogen. This enzyme is not present in muscle tissue.

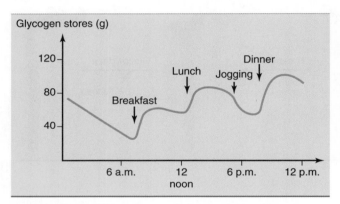

Figure 22.16 Changes in the glycogen stores of the liver in the course of a day. Glycogen metabolism in the liver regulates the blood glucose level in the short term, and gluconeogenesis is important for the long-term regulation after more than 12 to 24 hours of fasting.

constant and becomes depleted only during vigorous and prolonged physical exercise.

Glycogen Metabolism Is Regulated by Hormones and Metabolites

Glycogen synthesis and glycogen degradation should not be active at the same time to avoid an ATP-consuming futile cycle. This is achieved by the phosphorylation of the key enzymes glycogen synthase and glycogen phosphorylase (Fig. 22.17). Both enzymes are phosphorylated in response to the same stimuli, but glycogen synthase is active

in the dephosphorylated state, whereas glycogen phosphorylase is active in the phosphorylated state. Therefore, *the simultaneous phosphorylation of both enzymes switches the cell from glycogen synthesis to glycogen degradation.* In both cases, the active form of the enzyme is designated by the letter *a* and the less active form by *b*.

The phosphorylation state of the enzymes is regulated by hormones and their second messengers.

1. **Insulin** stimulates glycogen synthesis both in the liver and in skeletal muscle. It ensures that excess carbohydrate is stored away as glycogen after a meal.
2. **Glucagon** stimulates glycogen degradation in liver but not muscle during fasting when the blood glucose level is low.
3. **Norepinephrine** and **epinephrine** are powerful activators of glycogen breakdown both in muscle and liver. They mobilize glycogen when glucose is needed to fuel muscle contraction.

Glucagon and the catecholamines induce the phosphorylation of the regulated enzymes, and insulin induces their dephosphorylation. Superimposed on the hormonal actions are the effects of the allosteric effectors glucose, glucose-6-phosphate, and AMP. Figure 22.18 shows the complexity of these regulatory mechanisms.

Glucagon raises the cAMP level through the G_s protein (see Chapter 17) and the cAMP-activated protein kinase A phosphorylates and thereby inactivates glycogen synthase. It also phosphorylates and activates **phosphorylase kinase.** This protein kinase phosphorylates both glycogen phos-

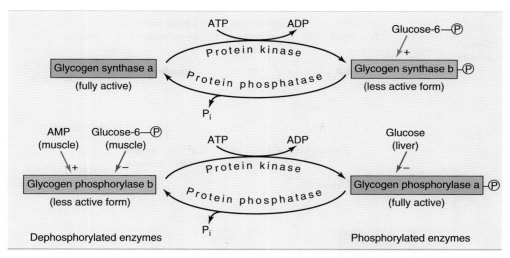

Figure 22.17 Regulation of glycogen synthase and glycogen phosphorylase by covalent modification and allosteric effectors. Note that the simultaneous phosphorylation of the two enzymes leads to glycogen degradation, and their dephosphorylation leads to glycogen synthesis. ⇢, Allosteric activation; ⇢, allosteric inhibition.

phorylase and glycogen synthase. *All regulated enzymes of glycogen metabolism become phosphorylated by the cAMP-induced phosphorylation cascade.*

Norepinephrine and epinephrine can stimulate cAMP synthesis by an action on β-**adrenergic receptors,** and they can raise the cytoplasmic calcium concentration by acting on α₁-**adrenergic receptors.** α₁-adrenergic receptors prevail in the liver, whereas β-adrenergic receptors are more important in muscle tissue. Calcium stimulates phosphorylase kinase synergistically with cAMP, and it also stimulates several other protein kinases. Some of these protein kinases can phosphorylate and thereby inactivate glycogen synthase.

Insulin affects glycogen metabolism by at least three mechanisms:

- *It reduces the level of cAMP,* probably by activating a cAMP-degrading phosphodiesterase.
- *It inhibits glycogen synthase kinase–3* (GSK3), one of several protein kinases that phosphorylate and inactivate glycogen synthase. GSK3 is subject to inhibitory phosphorylation by the insulin-activated protein kinase B.
- *It stimulates protein phosphatase-1.* This enzyme dephosphorylates glycogen synthase, glycogen phosphorylase, and phosphorylase kinase.

Phosphatase-1 is a key enzyme in the regulation of glycogen metabolism. It is activated by an insulin-triggered phosphorylation, but it can also be phosphorylated at a different site by protein kinase A. This latter phosphorylation does not activate the enzyme but removes it from the glycogen granule to which it is otherwise bound through a glycogen-binding subunit. Like glycogen synthase and glycogen phosphorylase, phosphatase-1 is normally nested between the outer branches of the glycogen molecule. Phosphatase-1 is also allosterically inhibited by the cAMP-activated phosphoprotein **inhibitor-1** and stimulated by glucose-6-phosphate (see Fig. 22.18B).

The allosteric effector **glucose-6-phosphate** stimulates both glycogen synthase *b* and phosphatase-1, and in muscle tissue it inhibits glycogen phosphorylase directly. Glycogen phosphorylase in muscle and other extrahepatic tissues is also allosterically activated by **AMP.** This ensures that *glycogen is rapidly degraded in metabolic emergencies,* especially in hypoxia, in which it is required as a substrate of anaerobic glycolysis.

Glycogen phosphorylase in the liver, finally, is inhibited by glucose. In addition to inhibiting the enzyme, the binding of glucose exposes the covalently bound phosphate to the action of the protein phosphatase. The intracellular glucose concentration in the liver approximates the blood glucose level. Therefore, *a high blood glucose level inhibits glycogen breakdown in the liver.*

The effects of the second messengers on glycogen metabolism are similar in muscle and liver, but the stimuli that regulate them are different. Epinephrine, but not glucagon, raises cAMP in skeletal muscle; and whereas calcium levels in the liver are raised by epinephrine through α₁-adrenergic receptors, the cytoplasmic calcium concentration in the muscle fiber depends on calcium release from the sarcoplasmic reticulum during muscle contraction.

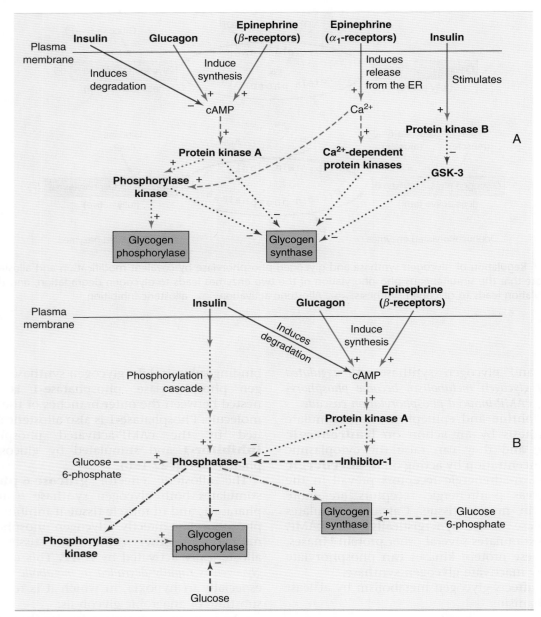

Figure 22.18 Regulation of glycogen metabolism in the liver. Note that the hormones affect glycogen synthase and glycogen phosphorylase through the protein kinases and the protein phosphatase (phosphatase-1) that regulate their phosphorylation state. - - - ►, Allosteric effects; ·······►, phosphorylation; ······►, dephosphorylation; —·±·►, activation; —·−·►, inhibition. **A,** Hormonal effects on the phosphorylation of the glycogen-metabolizing enzymes by protein kinases in the liver. ER, endoplasmic reticulum; GSK3, glycogen synthase kinase–3; **B,** Hormonal effects on the dephosphorylation of the glycogen-metabolizing enzymes by protein phosphatase-1, and the effects of allosteric effectors.

Glycogen Accumulates in Several Enzyme Deficiencies

Deficiencies of glycogen-degrading enzymes lead to **glycogen storage diseases,** with the abnormal accumulation ("storage") of glycogen in liver and/or muscle. Except for X-linked phosphorylase kinase deficiency, these rare diseases (overall incidence, 1 per 40,000) are inherited as autosomal recessive traits. Because different isoenzymes are present in different tissues, a deficiency is usually limited to one or a few organ systems. Clinically, it is possible to distinguish among *hepatic, myopathic,* and *generalized* types of glycogen storage disease (Table 22.1).

The hepatic types are characterized by *hepatomegaly and fasting hypoglycemia*. In **von Gierke disease,** the deficiency of glucose-6-phos-

Table 22.1 Glycogen Storage Diseases

Type	Enzyme Deficiency	Organ(s) Affected	Clinical Course
I (von Gierke disease)	Glucose-6-phosphatase	Liver, kidney	Severe hepatomegaly, severe hypoglycemia, lactic acidosis, ketosis, hyperuricemia
II (Pompe disease)	α-1,4-Glucosidase ("acid maltase")	All organs	Death from cardiac failure in infants
III (Cori disease)	Debranching enzyme	Muscle, liver	Like type I but much milder
IV (Andersen disease)	Branching enzyme	Liver, myocardium	Death from liver cirrhosis usually before age 2
V (McArdle disease)	Phosphorylase	Muscle	Muscle cramps and pain on exertion, easy fatigability, normal life expectancy
VI (Hers disease)	Phosphorylase	Liver	Like type I but milder, with less severe hypoglycemia
VII (Tarui disease)	Phosphofructokinase	Muscle, red blood cells	Like type V
VIII	Phosphorylase kinase*	Liver	Mild hepatomegaly and hypoglycemia

*There is also an X-linked form of phosphorylase kinase deficiency affecting muscle and several autosomal recessive forms affecting liver, muscle + liver, or muscle + heart. The enzyme contains four different subunits, and one of these is encoded by a gene on the X chromosome.

phatase leads to severe hypoglycemia within 2 to 4 hours after the last meal. This has to be expected because glucose-6-phosphatase is required for the formation of glucose by glycogen breakdown as well as gluconeogenesis. Affected patients can be kept alive only by regular carbohydrate feeding day and night. Von Gierke disease shows that *without the synthesis of glucose by the liver, humans would die of hypoglycemia within hours after the last meal.*

McArdle disease is caused by a deficiency of glycogen phosphorylase in skeletal muscle but not the liver. Although otherwise in good health, affected patients complain about muscle weakness and painful cramps on exertion. Some patients experience acute episodes of myoglobinuria, and some develop persistent muscle weakness and muscle wasting as they grow older. This disease shows that *muscle glycogen is not essential for life but is necessary for normal performance during physical exercise.*

Patients with McArdle disease do not show the expected rise in the blood level of lactic acid after muscular activity. This demonstrates that *the most important source of lactic acid during muscular activity is not glucose from the blood but stored muscle glycogen.*

Pompe disease is a generalized glycogen storage disease. Surprisingly, the deficient enzyme is lysosomal. In all tissues, a small amount of glycogen is normally taken up by lysosomes, in which it is degraded by a lysosomal α-glucosidase ("**acid maltase**"). Lysosomes are thought to ingest glycogen granules incidentally during the uptake of other cellular macromolecules. Pompe disease is fatal: Affected infants develop severe cardiomegaly and die of cardiac failure before 3 years of age.

Fructose Is Channeled into Glycolysis/Gluconeogenesis

Free fructose is present in honey and in many fruits, but most of the dietary fructose comes in the form of the disaccharide sucrose (table sugar). This dietary fructose has to be channeled into the major pathways of glucose metabolism.

Fructose is less rapidly absorbed from the intestine than is glucose, but once in the blood, it is more rapidly metabolized. Its plasma half-life after intravenous injection was found to be only half that of glucose (18 minutes versus 43 minutes). Some of the fructose is phosphorylated to the glycolytic intermediate fructose-6-phosphate by hexokinase. But because the K_m of hexokinase for fructose is more than 3 mmol/liter, this pathway is important only when the fructose concentration is very high.

Most of the dietary fructose is phosphorylated by **fructokinase** in the liver, kidneys, and intestines. The liver alone accounts for almost half of the total fructose metabolism. Fructokinase produces fructose-1-phosphate, which is not a glycolytic intermediate (Fig. 22.19). Fructose-1-phosphate is cleaved to dihydroxyacetone phosphate and glyceraldehyde by **aldolase B,** an isoenzyme of aldolase that can cleave both fructose-1,6-bisphosphate and fructose-1-phosphate. The products of aldolase B are further metabolized by glycolysis or gluconeogenesis.

Excess Fructose Is Toxic

The activity of fructokinase exceeds that of aldolase B (Table 22.2), and therefore *fructose-1-phosphate tends to accumulate.* This metabolite is a potent

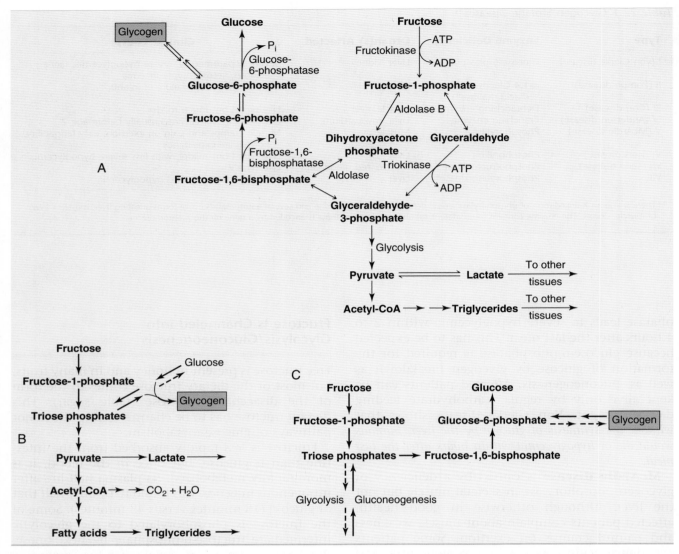

Figure 22.19 Metabolism of fructose in the liver. **A,** Pathways. **B,** Substrate flow after a good meal. **C,** Substrate flow when the blood glucose level is low.

Table 22.2 Kinetic Properties of Fructose-Metabolizing Enzymes in the Liver, and, for Comparison, the Glucose-Metabolizing Enzyme Glucokinase

Enzyme	V_{max} (μmol/min per g of tissue)	K_m for the Carbohydrate Substrate (mmol/liter)
Glucokinase	1*	10
Fructose carrier (in plasma membrane)	30	67-200[†]
Fructokinase	10	0.5
Aldolase B		
Cleavage of fructose-1-phosphate	2-3	1
Cleavae of fructose-1,6-bisphosphate	2-3	0.004-0.012
Triokinase	2	0.01
Fructose-1,6-bisphosphatase	4*	1[‡]
Glucose-6-phosphatase	10*	2.5-3[†]

*Depends on the nutritional state.

[†]After a sweet meal, the fructose concentration in the portal vein reaches approximately 2 to 3 mmol/liter. The usual glucose-6-phosphate concentration in the liver is approximately 0.2 mmol/liter (higher during fasting; lower after a meal).

[‡]Depends on the allosteric effectors.

allosteric effector of several enzymes of carbohydrate metabolism. For example, it activates glucokinase by binding to the previously mentioned glucokinase-regulating protein. Because it does not stimulate phosphofructokinase, fructose-1-phosphate directs dietary glucose into glycogen synthesis.

The liver metabolizes fructose faster than glucose (compare the activities of glucokinase and fructokinase in Table 22.2). Both glucokinase and phosphofructokinase are bypassed by fructose, and pyruvate kinase is stimulated by fructose-1-phosphate as it is by fructose-1,6-bisphosphate (see Fig. 22.6B).

The tissue concentration of fructose-1-phosphate in the liver can reach 10 µmol/g after a sugary meal. This ties up a substantial portion of the inorganic phosphate in the cell, leading to an impairment of oxidative phosphorylation and, possibly, liver damage.

Fructose has been used as a substitute for glucose in parenteral nutrition. Diabetic diets were also formulated in which a large portion of the dietary carbohydrate is supplied as fructose, based on the reasoning that the insulin-dependent phosphofructokinase reaction is bypassed. It was soon found, however, that excess fructose is apt to damage the liver and to raise the plasma levels of lactic acid, triglycerides, and uric acid.

Excess fructose can be metabolized to lactic acid in the liver. Part of the fructose is also used for fatty acid synthesis via acetyl-CoA. The fatty acids are esterified into triglycerides in the liver, and released into the blood in the form of very-low-density lipoprotein (ULDL). Uric acid is increased because fructose raises the level of glucose-6-phosphate in the liver.

Inborn Errors of Fructose Metabolism Cause Hypoglycemia and Liver Damage

Deficiencies of fructose-metabolizing enzymes are seen occasionally. Fructokinase deficiency leads to **essential fructosuria,** with fructose appearing in the urine after a fructose- (or sucrose-) containing meal. This asymptomatic condition is sometimes detected incidentally during urinalysis when "reducing sugar" (fructose) is present, although enzymatic glucose tests are negative. Most of the fructose is eventually metabolized by hexokinase in muscle and adipose tissue.

Aldolase B deficiency causes **hereditary fructose intolerance.** It leads to nausea and vomiting after a meal containing fructose or sucrose, along with signs of hypoglycemia: weakness, trembling, and sweating. Liver damage can develop in untreated cases. Hypoglycemia and liver damage are both attributed to the accumulation of fructose-1-phosphate in the liver. Besides tying up phosphate and thereby impairing ATP synthesis, fructose-1-phosphate inhibits aldolase, phosphohexose isomerase, and glycogen phosphorylase activity, and it stimulates glucokinase activity.

Fructose is transported across the plasma membrane, but fructose-1-phosphate is a strictly intracellular metabolite. Therefore, fructose levels, but not fructose-1-phosphate levels, are elevated in the blood and urine of patients with fructose intolerance. Most monosaccharides, including glucose, fructose, and galactose, are transported across the plasma membrane, but *phosphorylated sugar derivatives are confined to the intracellular compartment.*

A deficiency of the gluconeogenic enzyme fructose-1,6-bisphosphatase results in fructose intolerance similar to aldolase B deficiency, but affected patients also have fasting hypoglycemia. They can form glucose from stored glycogen, but gluconeogenesis is blocked. Therefore, they develop dangerous hypoglycemia after more than 12 to 18 hours of fasting, when the liver glycogen is depleted.

Fructose intolerance is treated by excluding fructose from the diet. Indeed, affected children spontaneously avoid sweets. This is an example of a *conditioned taste aversion,* which develops to the offending food when illness and malaise are experienced after eating. It is an evolved learning predisposition that protects humans from poisonous food. On the bright side: Adults with fructose intolerance have excellent teeth.

Galactose Is Channeled into the Pathways of Glucose Metabolism

Like fructose, dietary galactose is metabolized mainly in the liver. The main pathway is outlined in Figure 22.20. **Galactokinase** phosphorylates galactose to galactose-1-phosphate, which then reacts with UDP-glucose to form UDP-galactose. UDP-galactose is epimerized to UDP-glucose. This pathway amounts to the *ATP-dependent conversion of galactose to glucose-1-phosphate.* Because of its reversibility, the epimerase reaction is also useful as an endogenous source of UDP-galactose for the synthesis of glycolipids, glycoproteins, and proteoglycans.

Classical galactosemia, an autosomal recessive disease with an estimated population incidence of 1 per 40,000, is caused by a deficiency of galactose-1-phosphate-uridyl transferase. It leads to the accumulation of galactose and galactose-1-phosphate after the ingestion of milk and other galactose-containing foods.

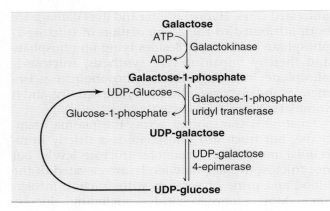

Figure 22.20 Galactose metabolism. ADP, adenosine diphosphate; ATP, adenosine triphosphate; UDP, uridine diphosphate.

Signs of the disease are evident within weeks after birth. The accumulation of galactose-1-phosphate causes liver damage and vomiting after feeding because it ties up inorganic phosphate in the liver. Untreated patients can develop liver cirrhosis, cataracts (clouding of the lens), and mental deficiency. The cataracts are caused by galactose. Aldose reductase, the same enzyme that reduces glucose to sorbitol (see Fig. 22.23), reduces galactose to galactitol in the lens. The galactitol accumulates and damages the lens, presumably through its osmotic activity. Patients with a deficiency of galactokinase get cataracts, although they do not suffer from liver damage.

The diagnosis is suggested by the presence of reducing material (galactose) in the urine and negative results of enzymatic tests for glucose, and it is confirmed by the absence of galactose-1-phosphate-uridyl transferase in red blood cells. The patients have zero enzyme activity, and unaffected heterozygotes have approximately 50% of the normal enzyme activity. Early diagnosis is essential because all clinical manifestations can be avoided by placing the patient on a milk-free diet.

The Pentose Phosphate Pathway Supplies NADPH and Ribose-5-Phosphate

The "minor" pathways of carbohydrate metabolism provide specialized products for biosynthesis. The cytoplasmic **pentose phosphate pathway,** also known as the **hexose monophosphate shunt,** makes two important products: ribose-5-phosphate and NADPH.

Ribose-5-phosphate is a precursor for the synthesis of purine and pyrimidine nucleotides, and

NADPH is a coenzyme for redox reactions. NADPH has the same standard redox potential as NADH, but its functions are different. Unlike NADH, NADPH does not feed its hydrogen into the respiratory chain but uses it for two other purposes instead: the *reductive biosynthesis* of fatty acids, cholesterol, and other products and the *defense against oxidative damage.*

The **oxidative branch** of the pentose phosphate pathway is concerned with the synthesis of NADPH (Fig. 22.21). **Glucose-6-phosphate dehydrogenase** catalyzes the committed and rate-limiting step. The reaction sequence is irreversible, and this enables the cell to maintain a high [NADPH]/[NADP$^+$] ratio. Well-fed liver cells, for example, contain 50 to 100 times more NADPH than NADP$^+$, although they contain more than 100 times more NAD$^+$ than NADH. For this reason, *the cells employ NADPH rather than NADH whenever a strong reducing agent is required.*

The **nonoxidative branch** of the pentose phosphate pathway links ribulose-5-phosphate, the product of the oxidative branch, to the glycolytic and gluconeogenic pathways (Fig. 22.22). The most important enzymes in this reversible reaction sequence are **transketolase** and **transaldolase.** Transketolase transfers a two-carbon unit, and transaldolase transfers a three-carbon unit. Transketolase (but not transaldolase) contains enzyme-bound thiamine pyrophosphate, which functions as a transient carrier of the two-carbon unit.

The overall balance of the pentose phosphate pathway, as described in Figures 22.21 and 22.22, can be written as:

$$3 \text{ Glucose-6-phosphate} + 6 \text{ NADP}^+$$

$$\downarrow$$

$$2 \text{ Fructose-6-phosphate} + \text{Glyceraldehyde-3-phosphate} + 6 \text{ NADPH} + 6 \text{ H}^+ + 3 \text{ CO}_2$$

In addition to the glycolytic intermediates, *two molecules of NADPH are formed for each carbon released as CO$_2$.* Actually, however, the pentose phosphate pathway can run in different modes, according to the relative needs of the cell for NADPH and ribose-5-phosphate:

1. When the cell needs more ribose-5-phosphate than NADPH, ribose-5-phosphate is formed not only through the oxidative branch but also by a reversal of the reactions in the nonoxidative branch.
2. When the cell needs more NADPH than ribose-5-phosphate, the oxidative and nonoxidative branches work in series to form fructose-6-phosphate and glyceraldehyde-3-phosphate. These

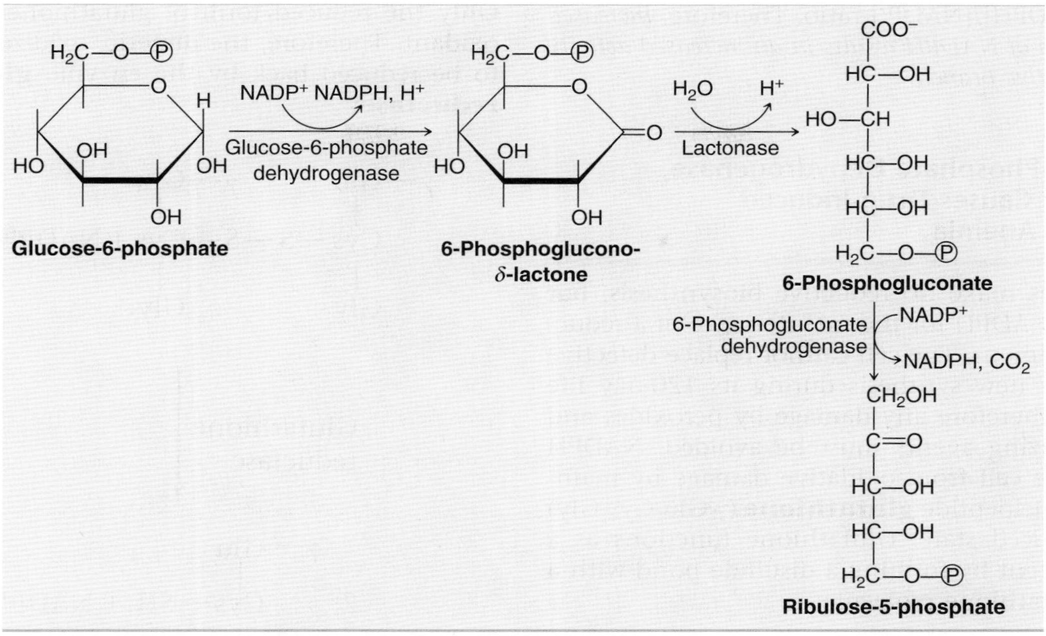

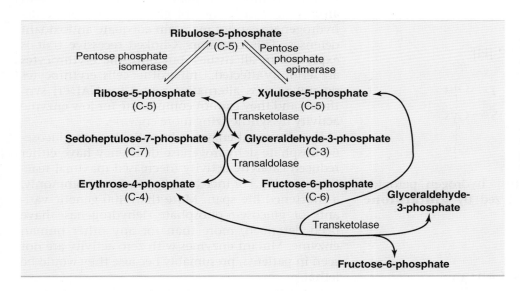

Figure 22.21 The oxidative branch of the pentose phosphate pathway.

Figure 22.22 The nonoxidative branch of the pentose phosphate pathway in adipose tissue.

products are recycled to glucose-6-phosphate in the gluconeogenic reactions. In this mode, the whole glucose molecule can theoretically be oxidized to CO_2 and NADPH.

Pentose phosphate pathway activity is minimal in muscle and the brain, in which almost all the glucose is degraded by glycolysis. But it accounts for a significant portion of the total glucose oxidation in tissues with active fatty acid or cholesterol synthesis, including the liver, adipose tissue, the adrenal cortex, and the lactating (but not the nonlactating) mammary gland. The pentose phosphate pathway is also important in cells that are exposed to a high oxygen partial pressure. In the cornea of the eye, for example, it accounts for 60% of the total glucose consumption.

The amounts of glucose-6-phosphate dehydrogenase and phosphogluconate dehydrogenase are increased in the well-fed state, and this effect is probably mediated by insulin. In the short term, glucose-6-phosphate dehydrogenase is inhibited by a high [NADPH]/[NADP⁺] ratio. Therefore, *increased consumption of NADPH results in an increased activity of the oxidative branch.*

Glucose-6-Phosphate Dehydrogenase Deficiency Causes Drug-Induced Hemolytic Anemia

Erythrocytes make no reductive biosynthesis, but they need NADPH for the maintenance of a reducing environment. The cell cannot replace defective proteins by new synthesis during its 120-day life span, and therefore any damage by peroxides and other oxidizing agents must be avoided. NADPH protects the cell from oxidative damage by maintaining the tripeptide **glutathione** (γ-Glu-Cys-Gly) in the reduced state. Glutathione functions as a reducing agent by forming a disulfide bond with a second glutathione molecule:

$$
\begin{array}{cc}
\gamma—\text{Glu} & \gamma—\text{Glu} \\
| & | \\
\text{Cys—SH} + \text{HS—Cys} \\
| & | \\
\text{Gly} & \text{Gly}
\end{array}
$$

$$2\,[\text{H}] \nearrow \!\!\!\Big\updownarrow\!\!\! \searrow 2\,[\text{H}]$$

$$
\begin{array}{cc}
\gamma—\text{Glu} & \gamma—\text{Glu} \\
| & | \\
\text{Cys—S—S—Cys} \\
| & | \\
\text{Gly} & \text{Gly}
\end{array}
$$

It can, for example, destroy hydrogen peroxide in a reaction that is catalyzed by **glutathione peroxidase:**

$$
2\quad
\begin{array}{c}
\gamma—\text{Glu} \\
| \\
\text{Cys—SH} + \text{H}_2\text{O}_2 \\
| \\
\text{Gly}
\end{array}
$$

Glutathione peroxidase $\downarrow$

$$
\begin{array}{cc}
\gamma—\text{Glu} & \gamma—\text{Glu} \\
| & | \\
\text{Cys—S—S—Cys} + 2\text{H}_2\text{O} \\
| & | \\
\text{Gly} & \text{Gly}
\end{array}
$$

Only the reduced form of glutathione is an antioxidant. Therefore, the dimeric, oxidized form has to be reduced back by the enzyme **glutathione reductase:**

$$
\begin{array}{cc}
\gamma—\text{Glu} & \gamma—\text{Glu} \\
| & | \\
\text{Cys—S—S—Cys} + \text{NADPH} + \text{H}^+ \\
| & | \\
\text{Gly} & \text{Gly}
\end{array}
$$

Glutathione reductase $\downarrow$

$$
2\quad
\begin{array}{c}
\gamma—\text{Glu} \\
| \\
\text{Cys—SH} + \text{NADP}^+ \\
| \\
\text{Gly}
\end{array}
$$

Because glutathione reductase depends on NADPH from the pentose phosphate pathway, patients with an inherited deficiency of glucose-6-phosphate dehydrogenase cannot maintain adequate antioxidant defenses. This common X-linked recessive trait is expressed in all tissues, but only the erythrocytes are seriously affected. Unlike other cells, erythrocytes do not possess alternative routes for NADPH synthesis, and they cannot compensate for low enzyme activity by synthesizing more enzyme.

The abnormal enzymes in patients with glucose-6-phosphate dehydrogenase deficiency have either reduced catalytic activity (decreased maximal reaction rate [V_{max}] or increased K_m) or, more commonly, a shortened life span. More than 400 genetic variants of glucose-6-phosphate dehydrogenase have been described, more than for any other human enzyme. Mutant enzymes with zero activity are not seen in patients, presumably because they would be lethal.

The deficiencies that are seen are harmless under ordinary conditions. Problems arise only during oxidative stress, especially after exposure to drugs that are either oxidants or give rise to oxidizing products during their metabolism. A large amount of glutathione becomes oxidized by the drug, and a large amount of NADPH is required to reduce it. In such situations, the mutant glucose-6-phosphate dehydrogenase cannot keep up with the increased demand. Without sufficient NADPH and reduced glutathione, membrane proteins become covalently crosslinked, aggregates of oxidized hemoglobin (known as **Heinz bodies**) become visible in the

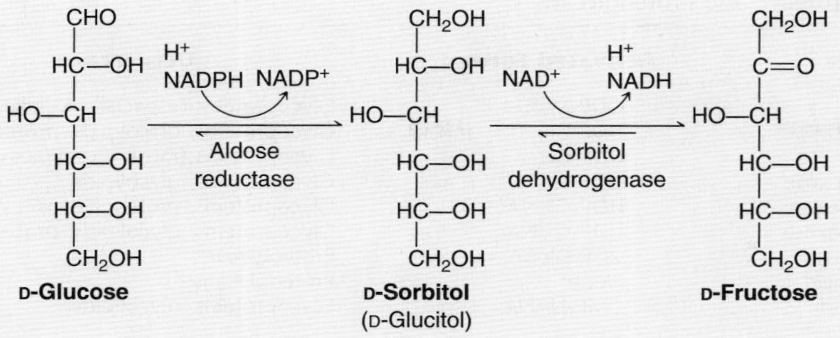

Figure 22.23 The polyol pathway.

cells, and a hemolytic crisis develops within 2 or 3 days after the initial exposure to the drug.

The offending drugs include the antimalarial primaquine, the sulfonamides sulfanilamide and sulfamethoxazole, acetanilid (a minor analgesic), nalidixic acid (an antimicrobial drug), and nitrofurantoin (a urinary antiseptic). Hemolytic attacks can also occur during infections. Even broad beans (*Vicia faba*) are dangerous, causing severe attacks of hemolysis within 1 or 2 days of eating the beans ("favism"). Even in the 6th century B.C., Pythagoras strongly advised against the eating of beans, possibly because of the high prevalence of favism in Greece.*

Glucose-6-phosphate dehydrogenase deficiency affects more than 100 million people (mainly male) worldwide, especially in Africa, the Mediterranean, the Middle East, India, and Southeast Asia, but not central and northern Europe. Of the black male U.S. population, 11% are affected. This high incidence is related to a partial protection of female heterozygotes (but not male hemizygotes) against malarial infection. Thus, the mutations benefit women but hurt men.

Fructose Is the Principal Sugar in Seminal Fluid

Seminal fluid contains up to 11 mmol/liter (200 mg/dL) of free fructose. It is the major energy source for the sperm cells in their all-important race for the ovum. The advantage of fructose over glucose may be that bacteria, which compete with the sperm cells for the available nutrient, often prefer glucose to other energy sources.

However, trying to boost male fertility by eating fructose would be futile. The fructose in seminal fluid comes not from the diet but from synthesis in the seminal vesicles by the **polyol pathway** (Fig. 22.23).

Glucose is reduced by NADPH, and sorbitol is oxidized by NAD+. Therefore, the high ratios of [NADPH]/[NADP+] and [NAD+]/[NADH] in the cell ensure that the pathway proceeds from glucose to fructose rather than from fructose to glucose. This pathway is active not only in seminal vesicles but in many other tissues as well, including the lens, retina, blood vessels, and peripheral nerves.

Amino Sugars and Sugar Acids Are Made from Glucose

The carbohydrate in glycolipids, glycoproteins, and proteoglycans is derived from nucleotide-activated precursors (Table 22.3). These "activated" sugar derivatives are made from glucose. The synthesis of the activated **amino sugars** is described in Figure 22.24.

UDP-glucuronic acid, required for the synthesis of proteoglycans and for conjugation reactions in the liver, is made by the NAD+-dependent oxidation of carbon 6 in UDP-glucose (Fig. 22.25). The free glucuronic acid that is produced during the degradation of proteoglycans (reaction 3 in Fig. 22.25) is metabolized to an intermediate of the pentose phosphate pathway.

Most mammals can convert the intermediate gulonic acid to **ascorbic acid** (**vitamin C**). Only primates, guinea pigs, and fruit bats cannot make their own vitamin C and are therefore prone to scurvy. Ancestors of modern humans could afford this genetic defect because they had a dependable supply of ascorbic acid from the fruits they ate.

Essential pentosuria is caused by an enzymatic block in the conversion of L-xylulose to xylitol (reaction 6 in Fig. 22.25). This harmless inherited condition is sometimes misdiagnosed as diabetes mellitus because the L-xylulose that the patients excrete in the urine yields a positive test

---

*According to some scholars, however, Pythagoras' injunction against beans stems from the belief that beans contain the souls of dead people. Pythagoras was one of the first European philosophers to believe in the transmigration of the soul.

Table 22.3 Sugars in Glycolipids, Glycoproteins, and Proteoglycans

Sugar	Type	Activated Form	Occurrence
Mannose	Hexose	GDP-Man	Glycoproteins (especially *N*-linked)
Galactose	Hexose	UDP-Gal	Glycoproteins, glycolipids, proteoglycans
Glucose	Hexose	UDP-Glc	Glycoproteins (rare), glycolipids
Fucose	Deoxyhexose	GDP-Fuc	Glycoproteins, glycolipids
N-acetylglucosamine	Aminohexose	UDP-GlcNAc	Glycoproteins, proteoglycans
N-acetylgalactosamine	Aminohexose	UDP-GalNAc	Glycoproteins, glycolipids, proteoglycans
Glucuronic acid	Uronic acid	UDP-GlcUA	Proteoglycans
Iduronic acid	Uronic acid	None*	Proteoglycans
N-acetylneuraminic acid	Sialic acid	CMP-NANA	Glycoproteins, glycolipids

*Formed by the epimerization of glucuronic acid in the proteoglycan.

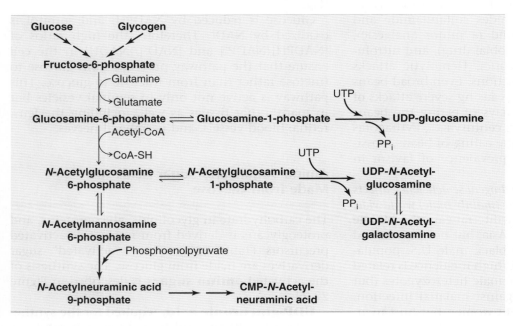

Figure 22.24 Synthesis of amino sugars.

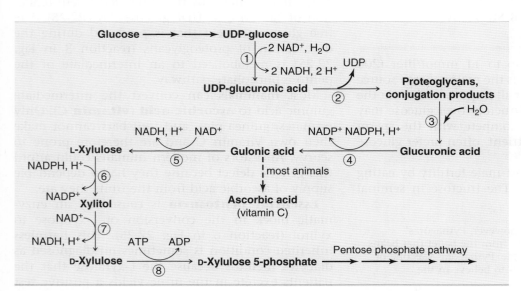

Figure 22.25 The uronic acid pathway.

result for "reducing sugar." Enzymatic tests, such as the glucose oxidase method, are necessary to distinguish between the sugars.

SUMMARY

Glucose is an important metabolic substrate for most tissues, and it is a required fuel for brain and erythrocytes. Therefore, the normal blood glucose level of 70 to 100 mg/dL has to be maintained at all times. In the fasting state, the liver has to produce glucose by gluconeogenesis and glycogen degradation.

Gluconeogenesis produces glucose from amino acids, lactate, and glycerol. This pathway uses the reversible reactions of glycolysis while bypassing the irreversible ones. It is the only source of glucose during long-term fasting.

Glycogen degradation in the liver is the major source of blood glucose during short-term fasting. Extrahepatic tissues use their glycogen not for blood glucose regulation but as an energy reserve during oxygen deficiency, and in skeletal muscle it is a backup fuel that is used during strenuous exercise.

Glucose metabolism is regulated by hormones. Insulin stimulates the glucose-consuming pathways of glycolysis and glycogen synthesis, whereas glucagon and epinephrine stimulate the glucose-producing pathways of gluconeogenesis and glycogen degradation.

The dietary monosaccharides fructose and galactose are channeled into glycolysis. These reactions take place mainly in the liver. The "minor pathways" of carbohydrate metabolism supply specialized products: The *pentose phosphate pathway* provides ribose-5-phosphate and NADPH, and other specialized reaction sequences produce fructose, galactose, amino sugars, and sugar acids.

📖 Further Reading

Ali M, Rellos P, Cox TM: Hereditary fructose intolerance. J Med Genet 35:353-365, 1998.

Bollen M, Keppens S, Stalmans W: Specific features of glycogen metabolism in the liver. Biochem J 336:19-31, 1998.

Foufelle F, Ferré P: New perspectives in the regulation of hepatic glycolytic and lipogenic genes by insulin and glucose: a role for the transcription factor sterol regulatory element binding protein–1c. Biochem J 366:377-391, 2002.

Jitrapakdee S, Wallace JC: Structure, function and regulation of pyruvate carboxylase. Biochem J 340:1-16, 1999.

Nordlie RC, Foster JD, Lange AJ: Regulation of glucose production by the liver. Annu Rev Nutr 19:379-406, 1999.

Watford M: Small amounts of dietary fructose dramatically increase hepatic glucose uptake through a novel mechanism of glucokinase activation. Nutr Rev 60:253-264, 2002.

QUESTIONS

1. **Ischemic tissues have an increased rate of glycolysis. Most of this is not fueled by glucose but by locally stored glycogen that is degraded in response to ischemia. This response depends on the activation of glycogen phosphorylase by**

   A. ATP.
   B. AMP.
   C. Low pH.
   D. Carbon dioxide.
   E. Glucose-6-phosphate.

2. **Several inborn errors of carbohydrate metabolism can cause fasting hypoglycemia. The *most severe* fasting hypoglycemia has to be expected in deficiencies of**

   A. Phosphofructokinase.
   B. Aldolase.
   C. Glycogen phosphorylase.
   D. Fructose-1,6-bisphosphatase.
   E. Glucose-6-phosphatase.

3. **A medical student of Middle Eastern ethnic background develops an episode of hemoglobinuria 24 hours after injecting himself with a street drug of unknown composition. He probably has a low activity of the red blood cell enzyme**

   A. Glucose-6-phosphate dehydrogenase.
   B. Hexokinase.
   C. Phosphofructokinase.
   D. Fructokinase.
   E. Glucose-6-phosphatase.

4. **Liver glycogen is normally synthesized after a meal and degraded during fasting. What pharmacological manipulation would enhance glycogen degradation in the liver?**

   A. An inhibitor of α-adrenergic receptors.
   B. An inhibitor of β-adrenergic receptors.
   C. The injection of insulin.
   D. A drug that activates protein phosphatase 1.
   E. A drug that inhibits the degradation of cAMP.

5. Glycogen degradation is an important energy source for exercising muscle. How many high-energy phosphate bonds are synthesized by converting one glucose residue in glycogen to lactic acid?

A. 1.
B. 2.
C. 3.
D. 4.
E. 5.

CHAPTER 23

The Metabolism of Fatty Acids and Triglycerides

Triglycerides (fat) supply 35% to 40% of the total calories in typical Western diets. Of this energy, 95% is contributed by the fatty acids and only 5% by the glycerol. Triglycerides are also the principal storage form of energy in the body, and most people carry between 5 and 20 kg of fat in their adipose tissue. With a basal metabolic rate of 1800 kcal/day, a 10-kg store of fat (93,000 kcal) can keep a human alive for 52 days without food. Therefore, fat metabolism includes several processes:

1. The digestion, absorption and transport of dietary fat.
2. The generation of metabolic energy from this fat.
3. The storage of excess fat in adipose tissue.
4. The metabolic links between triglycerides and other biomolecules, including carbohydrates and ketone bodies.

Fatty Acids Differ in Their Chain Length and the Number of Carbon-Carbon Double Bonds

A "standard" fatty acid is an unbranched hydrocarbon chain with a carboxyl group at one end. Most naturally occurring fatty acids have an even number of carbons; chain lengths of 16 and 18 are the most common.

In **saturated fatty acids,** the carbons are linked exclusively by single bonds. Of the fatty acids in Table 23.1, **acetic acid** does not occur in natural fats and oils, but vinegar contains about 5% of free (unesterified) acetic acid. **Butyric acid** is also rare in natural fats except milk fat. It is notorious for its smell, which resembles that of malodorous feet. In the production of some types of cheese, butyric acid is released from milk fat by the action of microbial lipases and contributes to the flavor of

the product. **Myristic acid** is abundant in nutmeg, coconut, and palm kernel oil and **palmitic acid** and **stearic acid** are the most common saturated fatty acids in animal and human fat, accounting for 30% to 40% of the fatty acids in human adipose tissue.

The carbons of the fatty acids are numbered, starting with the carboxyl carbon. Alternatively, they are designated by Greek letters. As in the amino acids, the α-carbon is the one next to the carboxyl carbon, the β-carbon is carbon 3, and so forth. The last carbon in the chain is the ω carbon, as in the example of stearic acid:

$$\omega\ \overset{17\ \ 15\ \ 13\ \ 11\ \ 9\ \ 7\ \ 5\ \ 3}{\underset{18\ \ 16\ \ 14\ \ 12\ \ 10\ \ 8\ \ 6\ \ 4\ \ 2}{\wedge\!\wedge\!\wedge\!\wedge\!\wedge\!\wedge\!\wedge}}\ \underset{\delta\ \gamma\ \beta\ \alpha}{}\ COOH$$

Monounsaturated fatty acids have one carbon-carbon double bond, and **polyunsaturated fatty acids** have more than one. The double bonds of the polyunsaturated fatty acids are always three carbons apart, with a single methylene ($—CH_2—$) group in between. The positions of the double bonds are specified by their distance from the carboxyl end. A Δ^9 double bond, for example, is between carbons 9 and 10. Alternatively, the distance from the ω carbon can be specified.

The latter designation is useful because fatty acids can be elongated and shortened only at the carboxyl end. If, for example, oleic acid (Table 23.2) is elongated by two carbons at the carboxyl end, the product is no longer a Δ^9 fatty acid but Δ^{11}, but it is still an ω^9 fatty acid. *Humans cannot introduce new double bonds beyond Δ^9.* Therefore, some of the polyunsaturated fatty acids, notably linoleic acid and possibly α-linolenic acid, are *nutritionally essential.* As shown in Table 23.2, the structures of unsaturated fatty acids can be described by a formula

Table 23.1 Structures of Some Naturally Occurring Saturated Fatty Acids

No. of Carbons	Fatty Acid	Structure	
2	Acetic acid	$H_3C{-}COOH$	
4	Butyric acid	$H_3C{-}(CH_2)_2{-}COOH$	
14	Myristic acid	$H_3C{-}(CH_2)_{12}{-}COOH$	
16	Palmitic acid	$H_3C{-}(CH_2)_{14}{-}COOH$	
18	Stearic acid	$H_3C{-}(CH_2)_{16}{-}COOH$	
20	Arachidic acid	$H_3C{-}(CH_2)_{18}{-}COOH$	
22	Behenic acid	$H_3C{-}(CH_2)_{20}{-}COOH$	
24	Lignoceric acid	$H_3C{-}(CH_2)_{22}{-}COOH$	

Table 23.2 Structures of Some Unsaturated Fatty Acids

Fatty Acid	Biosynthetic Class	Formula	Structure	Nutritionally Essential
Palmitoleic acid	ω7	16:1;9	$H_3C{-}(CH_2)_5{-}CH{=}CH{-}(CH_2)_7{-}COOH$	No
Oleic acid	ω9	18:1;9	$H_3C{-}(CH_2)_7{-}CH{=}CH{-}(CH_2)_7{-}COOH$	No
Linoleic acid	ω6	18:2;9,12	$H_3C{-}(CH_2)_3{-}(CH_2{-}CH{=}CH)_2{-}(CH_2)_7{-}COOH$	Yes
α-Linolenic acid	ω3	18:3;9,12,15	$H_3C{-}(CH_2{-}CH{=}CH)_3{-}(CH_2)_7{-}COOH$	Yes
Arachidonic acid	ω6	20:4;5,8,11,14	$H_3C{-}(CH_2)_3{-}(CH_2{-}CH{=}CH)_4{-}(CH_2)_3{-}COOH$	No*

*Can be synthesized from dietary linoleic acid.

indicating the chain length, the number of double bonds, and their locations.

There is no free rotation around the carbon-carbon double bond, and the substituents are fixed in *cis* or *trans* configuration:

cis   or   *trans*

Whereas the *trans* configuration favors an extended shape of the hydrocarbon chain, a *cis* double bond forms an angle of 120°:

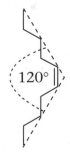

Only fatty acids with cis *double bonds are common in nature.* The properties of the fatty acids can be predicted from their structures:

1. With a pK close to 4.8, *the carboxyl group is 99% deprotonated at the typical cellular pH of 6.8.*
2. *Long-chain fatty acids are slightly water soluble in the deprotonated but not the protonated state.*
3. *Double bonds decrease the melting points of the fatty acids.* Stearic acid, for example, has a melting point of 70° C; oleic acid, of 16° C; linoleic acid, of −5° C; and α-linolenic acid, of −11° C, even though these 18-carbon fatty acids all have about the same molecular weight. The same is true for fats and oils. Those that are solid at room temperature contain mainly saturated (or *trans*-unsaturated) fatty acids, and those that remain liquid even in the refrigerator contain mainly unsaturated fatty acids.

Chylomicrons Transport Triglycerides from the Intestine to Other Tissues

The main products of fat digestion are *2-monoacyl-glycerol* and *free fatty acids* (see Chapter 19). After their absorption, the fatty acids are activated to **acyl–coenzyme A** in the endoplasmic reticulum (ER) of the intestinal mucosal cell:

$$R\text{—}COO^- + HS\text{—}CoA$$

Acyl-CoA synthetase

ATP

AMP, PP$_i$

$$R\text{—}\overset{\displaystyle O}{\overset{\|}{C}}\text{—}S\text{—}CoA$$

This is always the first reaction of a fatty acid after entering a cell, much as phosphorylation by hexokinase is always the first reaction of intracellular glucose metabolism. Like the phosphorylated sugars, *the CoA-activated fatty acids are strictly intracellular metabolites.* They do not cross the plasma membrane and are not transported in the blood.

The synthesis of acyl-CoA is made irreversible by the hydrolysis of the inorganic pyrophosphate that is formed in the reaction. The acyl-CoA then reacts

with 2-monoacylglycerol to form triglyceride (Fig. 23.1).

Why are triglycerides hydrolyzed in the intestinal lumen only to be resynthesized in the mucosal cell? The reason is that triglycerides are too insoluble. Only free fatty acids and monoglycerides are sufficiently water soluble to diffuse to the cell surface for absorption.

In the ER of the intestinal mucosal cell, the triglycerides are assembled into small fat droplets (diameter, 1 µm). These droplets, known as **chylomicrons,** also contain other dietary lipids and a small amount of ER-synthesized proteins. They pass through the secretory pathway and are released into the extracellular space. Because the endothelium of intestinal capillaries has no fenestrations, *chylomicrons are collected by the lymph rather than by the blood.* They are carried to the left brachiocephalic vein by the thoracic duct.

The triglycerides in chylomicrons are utilized by adipose tissue, heart, skeletal muscle, and the lactating mammary gland and, to a lesser extent, by

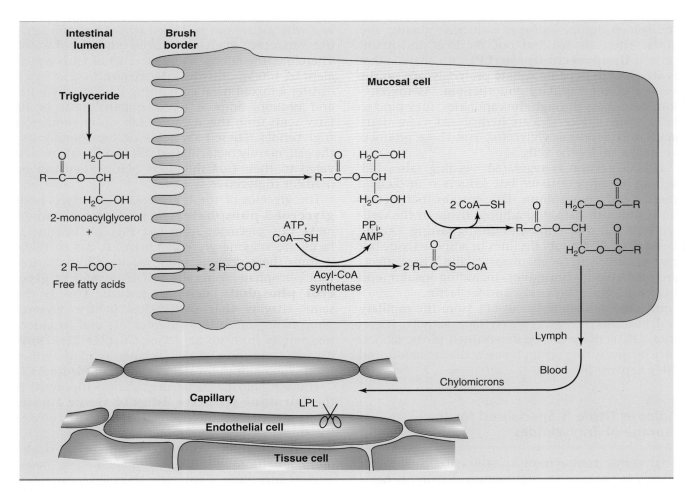

Figure 23.1 Absorption and transport of dietary fat.

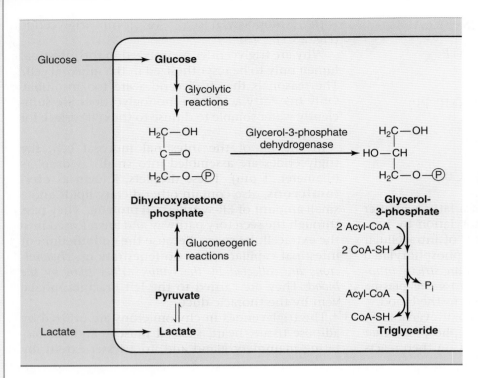

Figure 23.2 The sources of glycerol 3-phosphate for fat synthesis in adipose tissue. After a carbohydrate meal (high insulin), most glycerol phosphate is derived from glucose. Glyceroneogenesis from pyruvate is the major source during fasting, leading to substantial futile cycling.

the spleen, lungs, kidneys, endocrine glands, and aorta. These tissues (but not the liver and brain) possess **lipoprotein lipase** (**LPL**), an enzyme that is attached to heparan sulfate proteoglycans on the surface of the capillary endothelium. As the chylomicrons pass through the capillaries, they bind to LPL. Their triglycerides are hydrolyzed to free fatty acids and 2-monoacylglycerol, and these products are taken up by the cells.

LPL expression is regulated. Feeding raises LPL activity in adipose tissue but reduces it in skeletal muscle and myocardium. This ensures that dietary fat is directed mainly to adipose tissue in the well-fed state but to the muscles during fasting. During lactation, LPL activity declines in adipose tissue but rises massively in the mammary gland. These effects are mediated by hormones, including insulin, epinephrine, glucocorticoids, and prolactin.

Injected heparin detaches LPL from the capillary wall and also increases its enzymatic activity. Therefore, LPL activity can be determined in the laboratory by measuring serum lipase activities before and after heparin injection.

Adipose Tissue Is Specialized for the Storage of Triglycerides

Triglyceride is the most suitable storage form of energy because of its high energy density. It has a caloric value of 9.3, as opposed to 4.0 for glycogen,

and whereas fat can be stored without accompanying water, each gram of glycogen binds 2 g of water. Therefore, the energy value of 15 kg of fat is equivalent to 100 kg of hydrated glycogen.

After a mixed meal containing fat, carbohydrate, and protein, adipose tissue obtains most of its fatty acids from the action of LPL on chylomicron triglycerides. These fatty acids are transported into the cell, mainly by facilitated diffusion, and are activated to their CoA-thioesters before they can be used for triglyceride synthesis.

The glycerol of the triglycerides is derived from **glycerol-3-phosphate.** Adipose tissue cannot make this precursor from free glycerol because it lacks the enzyme glycerol kinase. It has to make it from the glycolytic intermediate dihydroxyacetone phosphate, using the NADH–dependent **glycerol phosphate dehydrogenase.** This is the same enzyme that participates in the glycerol phosphate shuttle (see Chapter 21) and in gluconeogenesis from glycerol (see Chapter 22). Dihydroxyacetone phosphate, in turn, is made either from glucose or pyruvate, as shown in Figure 23.2.

The key enzyme in fat degradation (lipolysis) is the **hormone-sensitive adipose tissue lipase.** Along with other intracellular lipases, it converts the stored fat into glycerol and fatty acids.

Unlike liver and intestine, *adipose tissue releases lipid not in the form of lipoproteins but as "free" (unesterified) fatty acids.* These fatty acids are transported to distant sites in reversible binding to serum

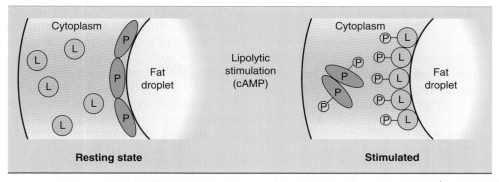

Figure 23.3 The hormonal stimulation of lipolysis (fat breakdown) in adipose tissue. Both the hormone-sensitive lipase (L) and the fat-associated protein perilipin (P) become phosphorylated by the cAMP–dependent protein kinase A. This enables the lipase to bind to the fat droplet and hydrolyze the triglycerides.

albumin. These albumin-bound fatty acids have a plasma half-life of only 3 minutes. While the fatty acids provide energy, the glycerol can be used for gluconeogenesis by the liver.

There is a good deal of futile cycling in fat metabolism. Approximately 40% of the fatty acids that are released by lipolysis during fasting do not leave the tissue but are resynthesized into storage triglyceride. Most of the glycerol phosphate required for fat synthesis during fasting is derived from pyruvate.

Fat Metabolism in Adipose Tissue Is under Hormonal Control

The synthesis and degradation of fat in adipose tissue must be adjusted to the energy demands of the body.

Norepinephrine (noradrenaline) from sympathetic nerve terminals and **epinephrine** (adrenaline) from the adrenal medulla are released during physical exercise and stress. They stimulate lipolysis through β-receptors and the cyclic AMP system. Figure 23.3 shows the mechanism. In the resting state, the hormone-sensitive lipase is cytoplasmic, whereas the surface of the fat droplet is covered by the protein **perilipin.** The cAMP-stimulated protein kinase A phosphorylates both perilipin and the lipase. As a result, perilipin detaches from the fat droplet, whereas the lipase binds, thus bringing the lipase in contact with its substrate.

Synaptically released norepinephrine is more important than circulating epinephrine. In animal experiments, sympathetic denervation causes excessive fat accumulation in the denervated portions of adipose tissue. This is most obvious under conditions of food deprivation or cold exposure, when fat is degraded in the surrounding innervated tissue.

Insulin is released by glucose and amino acids after an opulent meal. A high insulin level signals the abundance of dietary nutrients that are eligible for storage. Conversely, a low insulin level signals a shortage of nutrients during fasting and a need for fat breakdown.

A major effect of insulin on adipose tissue is the *inhibition of the hormone-sensitive lipase.* This effect is mediated by the activation of a cAMP-degrading phosphodiesterase. Another effect is an *increased uptake of glucose into the cell.* Glucose enters the cell by facilitated diffusion, using the GLUT-4 type of glucose transporter. In the absence of insulin, most GLUT-4 carriers are sequestered in intracellular vesicles, where they are useless. Insulin induces the fusion of these vesicles with the plasma membrane. Once in the plasma membrane, the carriers can transport glucose into the cell.

Other insulin effects that facilitate fat synthesis are the stimulation of LPL in the capillaries of adipose tissue and the induction of glycerol phosphate-acyl transferase, the enzyme that adds the first fatty acid to glycerol phosphate in the biosynthetic pathway (see Fig. 23.2).

Glucocorticoids, growth hormone, and the **thyroid hormones** facilitate lipolysis by inducing the synthesis of lipolytic proteins. Glucocorticoids induce the de novo synthesis of the hormone-sensitive lipase and thereby augment the lipolytic response to the catecholamines. They also reduce the reesterification of free fatty acids by *repressing* phosphoenolpyruvate (PEP) carboxykinase in adipose tissue, although they *induce* this enzyme in the liver. This reduces futile cycling in times of stress and fasting, when these hormones are released.

Not all kinds of adipose tissue respond to glucocorticoids. Patients with Cushing syndrome (excess glucocorticoids) lose fat in the extremities but develop truncal obesity and a "buffalo hump."

Fatty Acids Are Transported into the Mitochondrion

Neurons and erythrocytes depend on glucose because they cannot oxidize fatty acids. For most other cells, however, fatty acid oxidation by the mitochondrial pathway of **β-oxidation** is a major energy source.

After being activated to their CoA-thioesters by enzymes on the ER membrane and the outer mitochondrial membrane, the "activated" fatty acids have to be shuttled into the mitochondrion. The hole-riddled outer mitochondrial membrane is no serious barrier, but transport across the inner mitochondrial membrane requires **carnitine:**

$$H_3C-\overset{\overset{\displaystyle CH_3}{|}}{\underset{\underset{\displaystyle CH_2}{|}}{N^+}}-CH_3$$
$$HO-CH$$
$$CH_2$$
$$COO^-$$

Carnitine

On the outer surface of the inner mitochondrial membrane, the fatty acid is transferred from coenzyme A to carnitine, forming acyl-carnitine:

$$H_3C-(CH_2)_{14}-\overset{\overset{\displaystyle O}{\|}}{C}-O-\overset{\overset{\displaystyle CH_3}{|}}{\underset{\underset{\displaystyle CH_2}{|}}{\overset{|}{CH}}}$$

Palmitoyl-carnitine

Acyl-carnitine crosses the membrane in exchange for free carnitine, and in the mitochondrial matrix, the fatty acid is transferred back to coenzyme A. The reversible enzymatic reactions are catalyzed by two carnitine-acyl transferases (Fig. 23.4).

Fatty acids with a chain length of 12 carbons or fewer do not depend on carnitine. They diffuse passively across the membrane and are subsequently activated in the mitochondrion. However, long-chain fatty acids can be directly activated to their CoA-thioesters only in the cytoplasm, but not in the mitochondrion.

β-Oxidation Produces Acetyl-CoA, NADH, and FADH₂

The major pathway of fatty acid oxidation is called β-oxidation because it oxidizes the β-carbon (carbon 3). Eventually, it cuts the whole fatty acid into two-carbon fragments in the form of acetyl-CoA. As shown in Figure 23.5, each cycle of β-oxidation produces NADH and FADH₂, in addition to acetyl-CoA. These reduced coenzymes are fuel for the respiratory chain.

The stoichiometry for the β-oxidation of palmitate is as follows:

$$\text{Palmitoyl-CoA} + 7\ \text{FAD} + 7\ \text{NAD}^+ + 7\ \text{CoA} + 7\ \text{H}_2\text{O}$$

$$\downarrow$$

$$8\ \text{Acetyl-CoA} + 7\ \text{FADH}_2 + 7\ \text{NADH} + 7\ \text{H}^+$$

The energy yield can be calculated as:

$$8\ \text{acetyl-CoA} \rightarrow\ \ 96\ \text{ATP}$$
$$7\ \text{FADH}_2 \rightarrow\ \ \ \ \ \ 14\ \text{ATP}$$

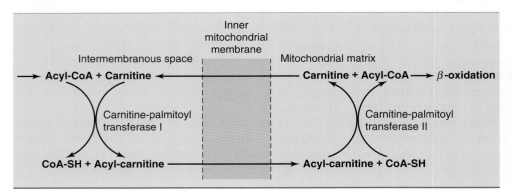

Figure 23.4 Transport of long-chain fatty acids into the mitochondrion. The carnitine-palmitoyl transferase reaction is freely reversible.

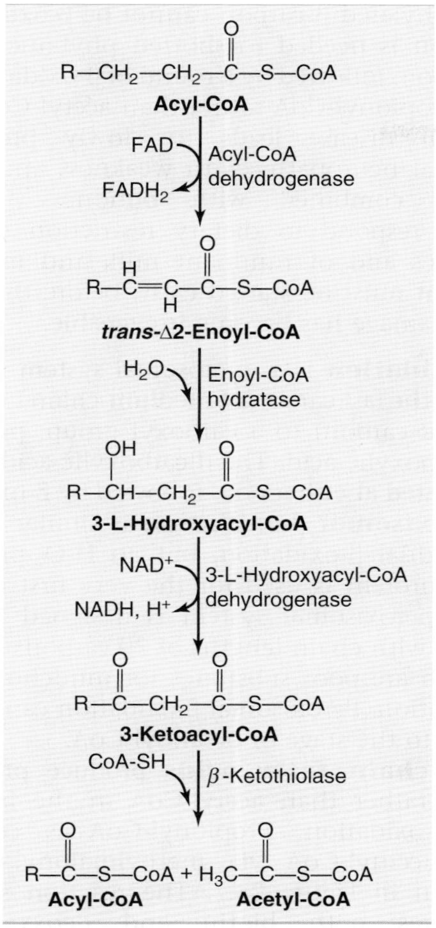

In addition, carnitine-palmitoyl transferase is allosterically inhibited by malonyl-CoA. Malonyl-CoA is formed in the regulated step of fatty acid biosynthesis (see section "Fatty acids are Synthesized from Acetyl-CoA"). Therefore, *fatty acid oxidation is inhibited when fatty acid synthesis is active.* This prevents excessive futile cycling.

Special Fatty Acids Require Special Reactions

Mitochondrial β-oxidation oxidizes unbranched saturated fatty acids with an even number of carbons and a chain length up to 18 or 20 carbons. Fatty acids that do not fit this description require additional enzymatic reactions.

1. **Unsaturated fatty acids** require modifications of their double bonds before β-oxidation, as shown for linoleic acid in Figure 23.6.
2. **α-Oxidation** is a minor pathway in the ER, mitochondria, and peroxisomes. It oxidizes carbon 2 (the α-carbon) and releases carbon 1 as CO_2, thereby shortening the fatty acid by one carbon at a time. α-Oxidation is needed for the degradation of methylated fatty acids.

In **Refsum disease,** a recessively inherited defect of peroxisomal α-oxidation causes the accumulation of **phytanic acid.** This branched-chain fatty acid is derived from the alcohol phytol, a constituent of chlorophyll in green vegetables that accumulates in the fat of ruminants:

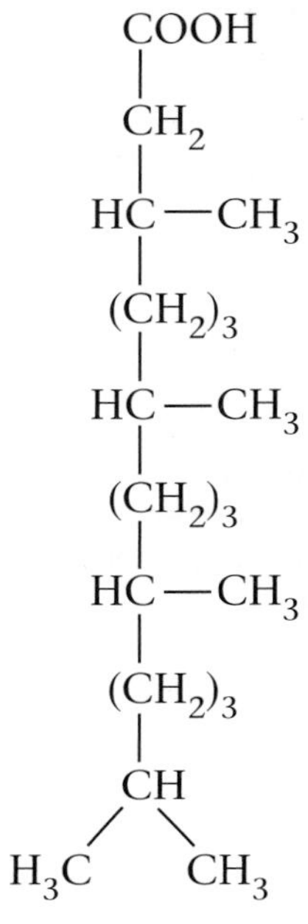

Figure 23.5 Reaction sequence of β-oxidation. These reactions take place in the mitochondrial matrix of most cells.

7 NADH → 　21 ATP
131 ATP
− 2 ATP
129 ATP

Two ATP molecules are subtracted because the initial activation of palmitate to palmitoyl-CoA requires two high-energy phosphate bonds in ATP. *The energy yield is close to 40%,* about the same as for glucose oxidation.

Within rather wide limits, the use of fatty acids by the tissues is proportional to the plasma free fatty acid level. Therefore, *fatty acid oxidation is regulated mainly at the level of the hormone-sensitive adipose tissue lipase.*

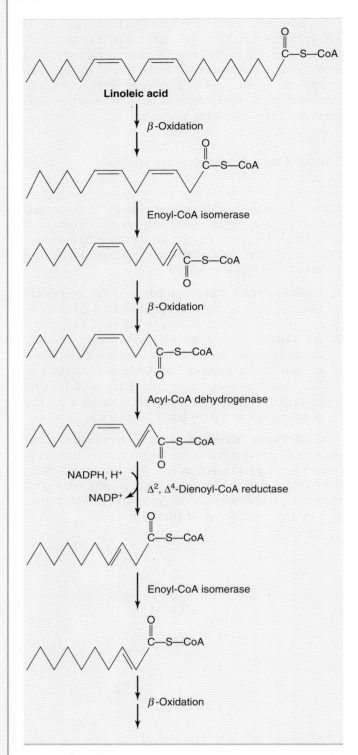

Figure 23.6 The β-oxidation of linoleic acid. Note that the Δ² double bond that is formed in each round of β-oxidation is in *trans* configuration, whereas those in the original fatty acid are in *cis*.

The methylated β carbon cannot be β-oxidized. α-Oxidation is needed to shorten phytanic acid by one carbon, followed by a round of β-oxidation that yields propionyl-CoA rather than acetyl-CoA.

Refsum disease leads to slowly progressive peripheral neuropathy with weakness and muscle wasting, combined with blindness. Affected patients respond to dietary restriction of green vegetables and of ruminant milk and meat, but treatment must be started early, before the neurological damage has become irreversible.

3. **ω-Oxidation** is a microsomal system that oxidizes the last carbon of medium-chain fatty acids (the ω-carbon) to a carboxyl group, producing dicarboxylic acid. The dicarboxylic acids can be activated at either end, followed by β-oxidation.

4. **Peroxisomal β-oxidation** is similar to mitochondrial β-oxidation, but an H_2O_2-producing flavoprotein is used for the very first reaction. The peroxisomal system is designed for fatty acids with chain lengths of 20 carbons or more, which are poor substrates for mitochondrial β-oxidation. Peroxisomal β-oxidation can proceed only to the stage of octanoyl-CoA.

5. **Odd-chain fatty acids** produce propionyl-CoA rather than acetyl-CoA in the last cycle of β-oxidation. Propionyl-CoA is converted to succinyl-CoA via methylmalonyl-CoA, as shown in Figure 23.7. The reaction sequence requires both biotin and deoxyadenosylcobalamin, a coenzyme form of vitamin B_{12}. Unlike acetyl-CoA, propionyl-CoA is a substrate of gluconeogenesis.

The Liver Converts Excess Fatty Acids to Ketone Bodies

The ketone bodies include the three biosynthetically related products **acetoacetate, β-hydroxybutyrate,** and **acetone.** *Ketone bodies are formed only in the liver.* The pathway of ketogenesis in liver mitochondria is shown in Figure 23.8.

A very small amount of acetone is formed by the nonenzymatic decarboxylation of acetoacetate. It serves no recognized biological function and is exhaled through the lungs. In diabetic ketoacidosis, *acetone imparts a characteristic smell to the patient's breath.*

Acetoacetate and β-hydroxybutyrate, however, are useful products. They are sent from the liver to other tissues for oxidation. Even the brain can cover part of its energy requirement from ketone bodies during fasting. The tissues that oxidize the ketone bodies use succinyl-CoA to activate acetoacetate to acetoacetyl-CoA, an intermediate of β-oxidation:

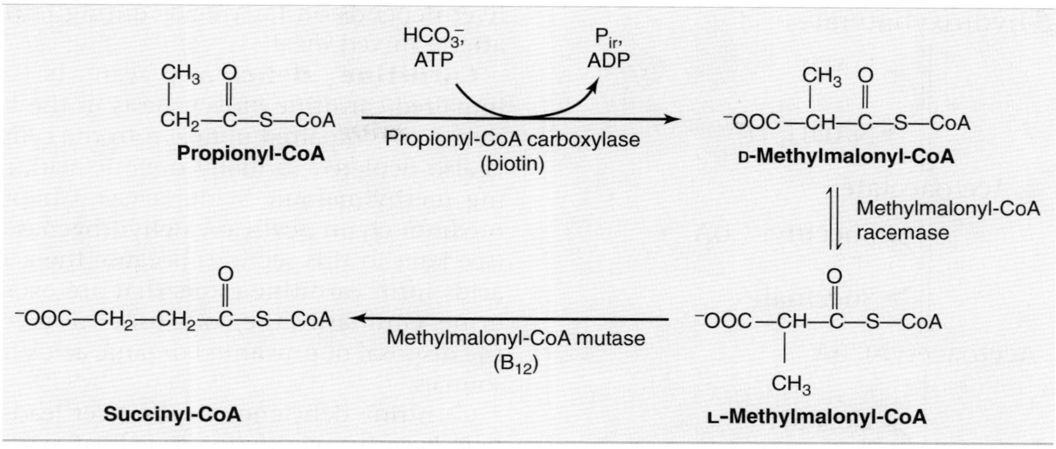

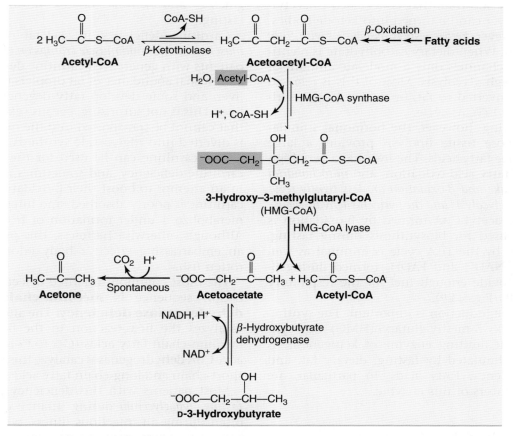

Figure 23.7 The reactions that channel propionyl–CoA into the tricarboxylic acid (TCA) cycle.

Figure 23.8 Formation of ketone bodies in liver mitochondria.

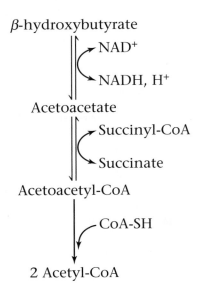

β-hydroxybutyrate

NAD⁺

NADH, H⁺

Acetoacetate

Succinyl-CoA

Succinate

Acetoacetyl-CoA

CoA-SH

2 Acetyl-CoA

In theory, any substrate that is degraded to acetyl-CoA in the liver can be turned into ketone bodies. Actually, however, *ketogenesis is associated with fatty acid oxidation.* When dietary carbohydrate is plentiful, the liver channels only a moderate amount of glucose through glycolysis. Most of this is released as lactate, converted to fat, or oxidized in the tricarboxylic acid (TCA) cycle.

During fasting, however, the hormonal stimulation of adipose tissue lipolysis provides a large amount of free fatty acids. The liver has a very high capacity for fatty acid oxidation, and *mitochondrial fatty acid uptake and β-oxidation are less tightly regulated than are glycolysis and the pyruvate dehydrogenase reaction.* The acetyl-CoA formed by β-oxidation is not readily used for biosynthesis during fasting. Its oxidation by the TCA cycle is minimal as well because the NADH and FADH₂ formed during β-oxidation provide enough fuel for the respiratory chain already (Fig. 23.9).

Also enzyme induction is important. The synthesis of 3-hydroxy-3-methylglutaryl (HMG)–CoA synthase, the rate-limiting enzyme of ketogenesis, is powerfully stimulated by fasting, dietary fat, and insulin deficiency. Fatty acids, in particular, are excellent inducers of this enzyme.

Defects of β-Oxidation Cause Muscle Weakness and Fasting Hypoglycemia

Defects of β-oxidation compromise tissues that depend heavily on fatty acids for their metabolic energy. Skeletal muscle covers a major portion of its energy needs from fatty acids at all times. The liver depends on fatty acids during fasting but not after a mixed meal.

Carnitine deficiency can be caused by impaired carnitine biosynthesis in the kidneys and liver or by impaired uptake into the cells. Carnitine is also depleted in many organic acidurias, including methylmalonic aciduria (see Chapter 26) and medium-chain acyl-CoA dehydrogenase deficiency (see later in this section) because the accumulating acids form carnitine esters that are excreted in the urine. Ordinarily, the body uses this mechanism for the disposal of unwanted organic acids from dietary sources.

Carnitine deficiency in the liver leads to *hypoketotic hypoglycemia during periods of extended fasting.* During fasting, β-oxidation is needed to produce acetyl-CoA for ketogenesis and ATP for gluconeogenesis. Therefore, both pathways are compromised in carnitine deficiency. The combined deficiency of ketone bodies and glucose is especially bad for the brain, because the brain depends on a mix of glucose and ketone bodies during prolonged fasting.

Carnitine deficiency in skeletal muscle causes *muscle weakness and muscle cramps on exertion.* Many patients with generalized carnitine deficiency show an unusual abundance of fat droplets in muscle and liver, and some develop fatty degeneration of the liver. This is not surprising, because excess acyl-CoA that cannot be transported into the mitochondrion is diverted into triglyceride synthesis.

Oral carnitine can be used for the treatment of carnitine deficiency, and sometimes athletes use it in an attempt to boost their β-oxidation. However, carnitine is poorly absorbed, and intestinal bacteria metabolize it under formation of trimethylamine. Although otherwise harmless, this product causes an embarrassing effect: a body odor like that of rotten fish.

The most common inherited defect in the β-oxidation sequence is **medium-chain acyl-CoA dehydrogenase deficiency.** The affected enzyme catalyzes the first reaction in the β-oxidation of medium-chain fatty acids (C-5 to C-12). Two other acyl-CoA dehydrogenases catalyze this reaction with short-chain and long-chain fatty acids, respectively.

Most patients with this deficiency present with *fasting hypoglycemia* during infancy or childhood, often during an infectious illness, when the child eats little. Many cases go undiagnosed, but some infants die of their first hypoglycemic attack under circumstances suggestive of sudden infant death syndrome. The condition is most common in northwestern Europe, where a single mutation accounts for nearly 90% of cases. Therefore, early diagnosis by neonatal screening is an attractive

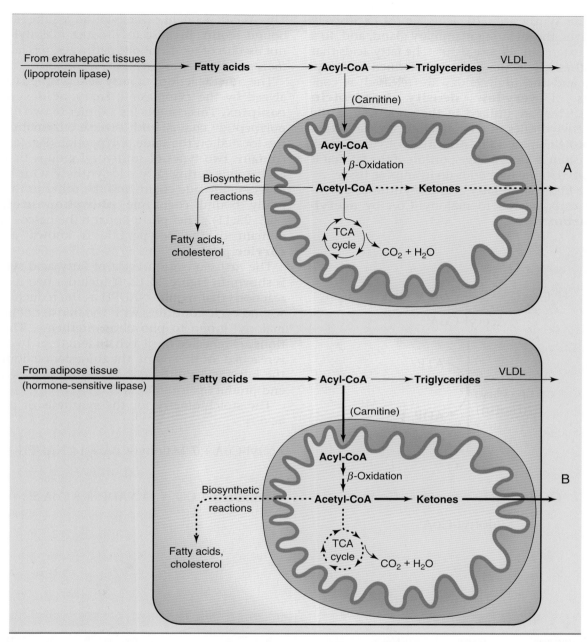

Figure 23.9 The fates of fatty acids and acetyl–coenzyme A (CoA) in the liver when the plasma free fatty acid level is low (after a carbohydrate-rich meal) and during fasting. **A,** After a carbohydrate-rich mixed meal. VLDL, very-low-density lipoprotein. **B,** During fasting.

option. Once the condition is diagnosed, patients can be kept healthy simply by avoiding excessive fasting.

One final way of blocking β-oxidation is by traveling to Jamaica and eating the local ackee fruit. The heat-labile alkaloid hypoglycin in this fruit causes fasting hypoglycemia by blocking the acyl-CoA dehydrogenases of β-oxidation. Market vendors in Jamaica warn the unwary tourist that this fruit must be cooked well because it is poisonous when eaten raw.

Fatty Acids Are Synthesized from Acetyl-CoA

Fatty acids cannot be converted into carbohydrates, but carbohydrates can be converted into fat. Therefore, people can get fat on a carbohydrate-rich diet. This is achieved by turning glucose into acetyl-CoA, and acetyl-CoA into fatty acids. Fatty acid synthesis is important only on a high-carbohydrate diet, in which excess energy from dietary carbohydrate is stowed away as fat.

Humans synthesize fatty acids almost exclusively in the liver, the lactating mammary gland, and, to a limited extent, in adipose tissue. The fatty acids that are synthesized in the liver are esterified to triglycerides, and the triglycerides are released as constituents of **very-low density lipoprotein** (**VLDL**). They are utilized in the same way as the dietary triglycerides in chylomicrons, by the action of lipoprotein lipase (LPL). After a carbohydrate meal, when insulin is high, a large portion of the fat that is synthesized in the liver ends up in adipose tissue.

In the first step of fatty acid biosynthesis, acetyl-CoA is carboxylated to malonyl-CoA by **acetyl-CoA carboxylase:**

$$H_3C-\overset{\overset{\text{O}}{\|}}{C}-S-CoA + HCO_3^-$$

Acetyl-CoA

Acetyl-CoA carboxylase (biotin)

ATP

ADP, P_i

$$^-OOC-CH_2-\overset{\overset{\text{O}}{\|}}{C}-S-CoA$$

Malonyl-CoA

This ATP-dependent carboxylation requires enzyme-bound biotin. Because its product malonyl-CoA is not used in other metabolic pathways, *this reaction is the committed step of fatty acid biosynthesis.*

The other reactions of fatty acid synthesis are catalyzed by the cytoplasmic **fatty acid synthase complex.** This complex is a dimer of two identical polypeptide chains, with diverse enzymatic activities located on the same polypeptide (Fig. 23.10). It contains two types of sulfhydryl groups that carry acyl groups during fatty acid synthesis. One belongs to a cysteine side chain, and the other to the covalently bound coenzyme **phosphopantetheine** (Fig. 23.11). The phosphopantetheine-containing domain of the polypeptide is known as **acyl carrier protein.**

The first elongation cycle of fatty acid synthesis is shown in Figure 23.12. It includes two reductive reactions that require NADPH as the reductant. The second cycle continues with the transfer of another malonyl group to phosphopantetheine. The reactions are repeated until a chain length of 16 carbons is reached. At this point, the thioesterase domain of the fatty acid synthase catalyzes the release of the end product palmitic acid.

The stoichiometry for the synthesis of palmitic acid is

Acetyl-CoA + 7 Malonyl-CoA + 14 NADPH + 14 H⁺

↓

Palmitate + 7 CO_2 + 14 NADP⁺ + 8 CoA-SH + 6 H_2O

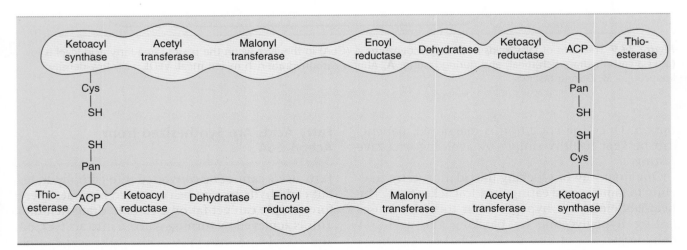

Figure 23.10 Structure of the mammalian fatty acid synthase complex. During fatty acid synthesis, acyl groups are transferred between the cysteine side chain of one subunit and the phosphopantetheine group of the other subunit. ACP, acyl carrier protein.

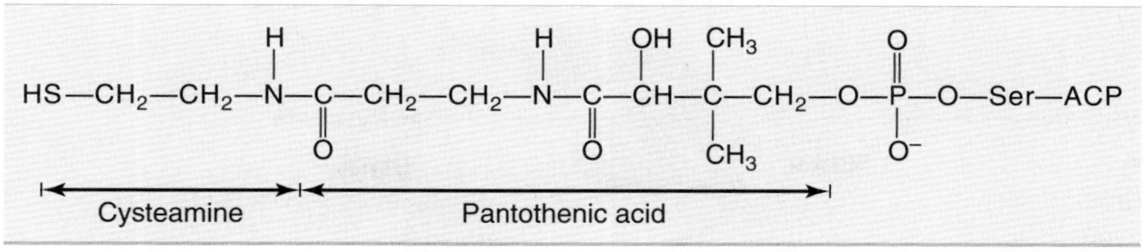

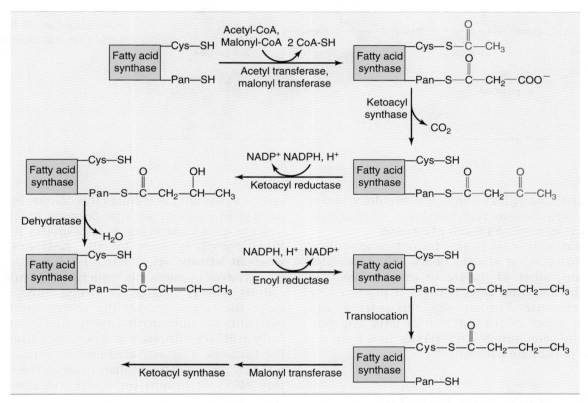

Figure 23.11 The phosphopantetheine group in the fatty acid synthase complex. It resembles coenzyme A in its structure and in its ability to form a thioester bond with organic acids. ACP, acyl carrier protein.

Figure 23.12 Reactions of the first elongation cycle in fatty acid biosynthesis. The cysteine side chain and the phosphopantetheine group actually belong to two separate polypeptides in the fatty acid synthase complex.

Malonyl-CoA is formed from acetyl-CoA in the reaction

$$\text{Acetyl-CoA} + CO_2 + \text{ATP} + H_2O$$

$$\downarrow$$

$$\text{Malonyl-CoA} + \text{ADP} + P_i + H^+$$

Therefore, the overall reaction can be written as

$$8 \text{ Acetyl-CoA} + 7 \text{ ATP} + 14 \text{ NADPH} + 6 H^+ + H_2O$$

$$\downarrow$$

$$\text{Palmitate} + 14 \text{ NADP}^+ + 8 \text{ CoA-SH} + 7 \text{ ADP} + 7 P_i$$

Most naturally occurring fatty acids have an even number of carbons simply because they are patched together from two-carbon units.

Acetyl-CoA Is Shuttled into the Cytoplasm as Citrate

Fatty acids are synthesized from acetyl-CoA in the cytoplasm, but acetyl-CoA is produced in the mitochondrion. Unlike most other mitochondrial metabolites, however, *acetyl-CoA cannot cross the inner mitochondrial membrane*. Citrate, in contrast, can cross. To get it from the mitochondrion into the cytoplasm, acetyl-CoA is therefore converted to

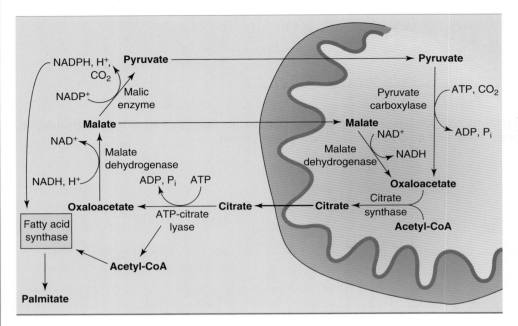

Figure 23.13 Transport of acetyl units from the mitochondrion to the cytoplasm. The inner mitochondrial membrane has carriers for citrate, pyruvate, and malate but not for acetyl-CoA and oxaloacetate.

citrate first. Citrate leaves the mitochondrion and is then cleaved back to acetyl-CoA and oxaloacetate by the cytoplasmic **ATP-citrate lyase.**

Whereas acetyl-CoA is used for fatty acid synthesis, oxaloacetate is shuttled back into the mitochondrion either as malate or as pyruvate (Fig. 23.13). In the latter case, NADPH is produced by **malic enzyme.** Theoretically, this reaction can supply one half of the NADPH for fatty acid synthesis. The remaining NADPH has to come from the pentose phosphate pathway.

Fatty Acid Synthesis Is Regulated by Hormones and Metabolites

On a day-to-day basis, fatty acid synthesis is regulated by adjustments in the synthesis of acetyl-CoA carboxylase, fatty acid synthase, ATP-citrate lyase, and glucose-6-phosphate dehydrogenase. These enzymes are induced by carbohydrate feeding and repressed by a fat-based diet and starvation.

The minute-to-minute control of fatty acid synthesis takes place at the level of acetyl-CoA carboxylase. This enzyme is allosterically activated by citrate and inhibited by the CoA-thioesters of long-chain fatty acids. The well-fed liver has a higher citrate level and a lower acyl-CoA level than does the fasting liver.

In addition, *acetyl-CoA carboxylase is stimulated by insulin and inhibited by glucagon and epinephrine.* The effects of glucagon and epinephrine are mediated by the cAMP-dependent protein kinase A, which phosphorylates and inactivates acetyl-CoA car-

boxylase. Insulin antagonizes this cascade by inducing a phosphodiesterase that degrades cAMP.

Acetyl-CoA carboxylase is also subject to inhibitory phosphorylation by the **AMP-activated protein kinase.** As its name implies, this kinase is activated in metabolic emergencies when the cellular energy charge is dangerously low. It helps the cell to survive the energy shortage by switching off nonessential biosynthetic pathways. Fatty acid biosynthesis is one of these pathways. In the liver, the AMP-activated protein kinase is inhibited by insulin. This mediates part of the stimulatory effect of insulin on acetyl-CoA carboxylase (Fig. 23.14).

Most Fatty Acids Can Be Synthesized from Palmitate

The fatty acid synthase complex produces palmitate, a saturated 16-carbon fatty acid. The fatty acids in human triglycerides and membrane lipids, however, have chain lengths of up to 24 or 26 carbons, C-18 fatty acids being the most common. Also, only about 50% of human fatty acids are saturated; another 40% are monounsaturated, and perhaps 10% are polyunsaturated. Most of these fatty acids can be synthesized from palmitate in the human body.

Chain elongation takes place in both the ER and the mitochondrion. Like the fatty acid synthase complex, *the elongation systems add two carbons at a time.* The mitochondrial system prefers fatty acids with fewer than 16 carbons, but microsomal chain

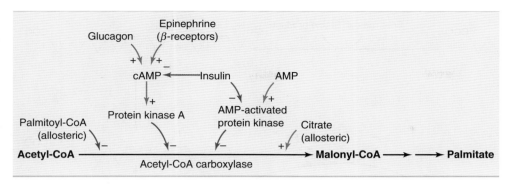

Figure 23.14 Regulation of acetyl-CoA carboxylase by allosteric effectors and hormones. *Green arrow,* stimulation; *red arrow,* inhibition. AMP, adenosine monophosphate; cAMP, cyclic AMP.

elongation works best with palmitate. Both unsaturated and saturated fatty acids can be elongated.

Desaturation requires membrane-bound desaturase enzymes in the ER. The desaturases are monooxygenases that use molecular oxygen as the oxidant and either NADH or NADPH as a cofactor.

The first double bond is introduced in position Δ^9 of palmitic or stearic acid, producing palmitoleic acid or oleic acid, respectively. Oleic acid is the most abundant unsaturated fatty acid in human lipids. Additional double bonds can be introduced between the carboxyl group and the first double bond, but not beyond Δ^9. Most polyunsaturated fatty acids can be synthesized from dietary palmitic or stearic acid by a combination of desaturation and chain elongation. These belong to the ω^7 and ω^9 classes.

Linoleic acid (18:2;9,12) and **α-linolenic acid** (18:3;9,12,15, see Table 23.2) are the parent compounds of the ω^6 and ω^3 classes of polyunsaturated fatty acids, respectively. They cannot be synthesized in the human body and are therefore *nutritionally essential.*

Essential fatty acid deficiency is characterized by dermatitis and poor wound healing. It has been observed in patients who were kept on total parenteral nutrition for long time periods, in patients suffering from severe fat malabsorption, and in infants fed low-fat milk formulas.

Fatty Acids Can Regulate Gene Expression

The synthesis of metabolic enzymes has to be adjusted to the supply of dietary nutrients. Dietary carbohydrates induce most of their gene-regulatory effects indirectly, by stimulating the release of insulin. The insulin signaling pathways, in turn, impinge on nuclear transcription factors to induce the enzymes of carbohydrate metabolism.

Dietary fatty acids use a more direct route, by *binding to nuclear transcription factors.* This mecha-nism resembles the effects of steroid hormones. However, the receptors for dietary lipids are less selective for their ligands than are the hormone receptors. This makes it difficult to be certain which lipids are the physiologically most important ligands. Indeed many lipid-binding nuclear receptors are described as **orphan receptors** because their physiological ligands are not known with any certainty.

The **peroxisome proliferators–activated receptors** (**PPARs**), as their name implies, cause the proliferation of peroxisomes and of the lipid-metabolizing peroxisomal pathways. However, they have many other metabolic effects as well.

PPAR-α is expressed mainly in the liver. It is activated by many monounsaturated and polyunsaturated fatty acids, as well as some oxidized arachidonic acid derivatives from both the cyclooxygenase and lipoxygenase pathways (see Chapter 16). Binding of these ligands to PPAR-α stimulates the peroxisomal pathways profoundly and mitochondrial β-oxidation to a lesser extent.

Knockout mice without PPAR-α have grossly abnormal lipid metabolism with excessive fat accumulation in the liver. Conversely, lipid-lowering drugs of the **fibrate** class (benzafibrate, gemfibrozil) are potent activators of PPAR-α.

PPAR-γ is expressed in many tissues, with important effects especially in adipose tissue. Its activation by polyunsaturated fatty acids induces the synthesis of proteins that are involved in fat synthesis in adipose tissue, including lipoprotein lipase and the membrane protein CD36, which carries fatty acids across the plasma membrane.

The activation of PPAR-γ sensitizes the cells to many effects of insulin. In theory, a diet high in polyunsaturated fatty acids could therefore be used to treat insulin resistance in type II diabetes. Actually, however, highly potent synthetic agents of the **glitazone** class (e.g., rosiglitazone) are used for this purpose. The glitazones are among the most useful drugs for the treatment of type II diabetes.

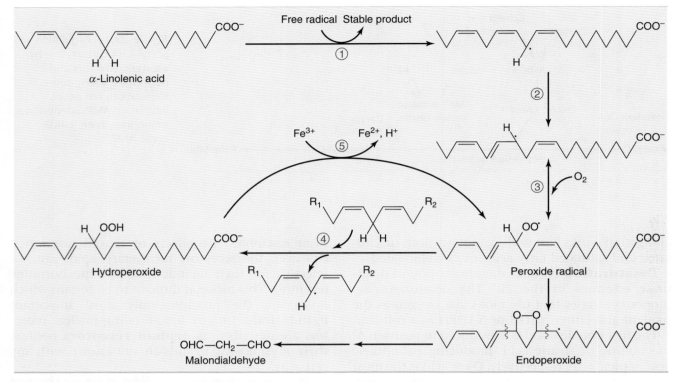

Figure 23.15 Auto-oxidation ("peroxidation") of polyunsaturated fatty acids.

Polyunsaturated Fatty Acids Can Be Oxidized Nonenzymatically

In the presence of oxygen, polyunsaturated fatty acids are subject to nonenzymatic **auto-oxidation** or **peroxidation.** When this occurs outside the body, it causes fat to become rancid. In the body, it can damage the cells.

Polyunsaturated fatty acids auto-oxidize when a hydrogen atom is abstracted from the methylene group between two double bonds (reaction (1) in Fig. 23.15). The initiator is a free radical that is derived either from another polyunsaturated fatty acid (reaction (4) in Fig. 23.15) or from partially reduced oxygen, such as the superoxide radical:

$$O_2^- \xrightarrow[\text{Reaction (1) (Fig. 23.15)}]{\text{[H] from fatty acid}} O_2H^- \xrightarrow{H^+} H_2O_2$$

The initiator can also be a peroxide radical generated from hydrogen peroxide with the aid of a metal ion:

$$H_2O_2 + Fe^{3+} \longrightarrow HOO^{\bullet} + Fe^{2+} + H^+$$

$$HOO^{\bullet} \xrightarrow[\text{Reaction (1) (Fig. 23.15)}]{\text{[H] from fatty acid}} H_2O_2$$

By the same mechanism, hydroperoxide derivatives of polyunsaturated fatty acids can be converted back into reactive peroxide radicals (reaction (5) in Fig. 23.15). This implies the possibility of *a branching chain reaction leading to an avalanche of free radicals.*

The fatty acid itself can finally be fragmented into smaller products. If at least three double bonds (which are always three carbons apart) are present, **malondialdehyde** is a prominent product. Malondialdehyde is chemically reactive. It crosslinks proteins and other molecules, resulting in membrane damage and the accumulation of yellow **lipofuscin,** a poorly degradable polymeric product formed from partially decomposed fatty acids and crosslinked, denatured proteins. It accumulates as "age pigment" in the lysosomes of elderly persons. Most types of lipofuscin are harmless, but other products and intermediates of lipid peroxidation are potentially mutagenic.

The body's defenses against lipid peroxidation include the enzymes **catalase, superoxide dismutase,** and **glutathione peroxidase.** They destroy dangerous products of oxidative metabolism. Some vitamins and metabolites are also protective because they react with free radicals with the formation of harmless products. They include **vitamin E,** the **retinoids, uric acid,** and **vitamin C.**

SUMMARY

The products of intestinal fat digestion are used for the resynthesis of triglycerides in the intestinal mucosa. These triglycerides are transported to other tissues as constituents of chylomicrons. Their utilization by the tissues depends on the endothelial enzyme lipoprotein lipase (LPL).

Adipose tissue is an important destination for dietary triglycerides. Under the influence of insulin, the adipose cells use the products of LPL for the synthesis of storage fat. Conversely, the hydrolysis of the stored fat by the hormone-sensitive adipose tissue lipase is stimulated by norepinephrine and epinephrine but inhibited by insulin. Thus, storage fat is synthesized after a meal, when the insulin level is high, and degraded during fasting, when insulin is low, and during physical exertion, when the catecholamines are high. Fatty acids from adipose tissue are the most important energy source for the body during fasting.

Fatty acids are oxidized by the pathway of β-oxidation, which is active in the mitochondria of most cells. β-Oxidation produces acetyl-CoA for the TCA cycle. The fasting liver, however, converts a major portion of the fatty acids into ketone bodies. The ketone bodies are released into the blood and oxidized in extrahepatic tissues.

On a high-carbohydrate, low-fat diet, carbohydrates are converted into fat by the sequential action of glycolysis, pyruvate dehydrogenase, and fatty acid biosynthesis. This sequence is most active in the liver. The endogenously synthesized fat is transported from the liver to adipose tissue in VLDL.

Further Reading

Carling D: The AMP-activated protein kinase cascade—a unifying system for energy control. Trends Biochem Sci 29:18-24, 2004.

Gregersen N, Bross P, Andresen BS: Genetic defects in fatty acid β-oxidation and acyl-CoA dehydrogenases. Eur J Biochem 271:470-482, 2004.

Hajri T, Abumrad NA: Fatty acid transport across membranes: relevance to nutrition and metabolic pathology. Annu Rev Nutr 22:383-415, 2002.

Jump DB: The biochemistry of n-3 polyunsaturated fatty acids. J Biol Chem 277:8755-8758, 2002.

Mead JR, Irvine SA, Ramji DP: Lipoprotein lipase: structure, function, regulation, and role in disease. J Mol Med 80:753-769, 2002.

Reshef L, Olswang Y, Cassuto H, et al: Glyceroneogenesis and the triglyceride/fatty acid cycle. J Biol Chem 278:30413-30416, 2003.

Yeaman SJ: Hormone-sensitive lipase—new roles for an old enzyme. Biochem J 379:11-22, 2004.

QUESTIONS

1. **Like many other tissues, the myocardium can use the triglycerides in chylomicrons for its own energy needs. The utilization of these triglycerides requires the enzyme**

   A. Acetyl-CoA carboxylase.
   B. Glucose-6-phosphate dehydrogenase.
   C. Phospholipase A$_2$.
   D. LPL.
   E. Hormone-sensitive lipase.

2. **The excessive formation of ketone bodies occurs in many diseases. The *most important* regulated step determining the rate of ketogenesis is catalyzed by**

   A. Acyl-CoA dehydrogenase.
   B. Pyruvate kinase.
   C. Hormone-sensitive adipose tissue lipase.
   D. Acetyl-CoA carboxylase.
   E. Glucose-6-phosphate dehydrogenase.

3. **Medium-chain acyl-CoA dehydrogenase deficiency is the most common inherited defect of β-oxidation. Most patients with this condition present initially with**

   A. Liver cirrhosis.
   B. Fasting hypoglycemia.
   C. Ketoacidosis.
   D. Hypertriglyceridemia.
   E. Slowly developing ataxia (poor motor coordination).

4. **A pharmaceutical company wants to develop an antiobesity drug that acts directly on adipose tissue metabolism. The most promising drug type would be agents that**

A. Stimulate β-adrenergic receptors.
B. Inhibit adenylate cyclase.
C. Stimulate glucose uptake into adipose cells.
D. Inhibit the hormone-sensitive adipose tissue lipase.
E. Stimulate insulin receptors in adipose tissue.

CHAPTER 24

The Metabolism of Membrane Lipids

Biological membranes contain phosphoglycerides, sphingolipids, and cholesterol. All of these membrane lipids can be synthesized in the body, and most are made in the cells in which they are used. However, considerable quantities are also transported in the blood as constituents of plasma lipoproteins. This chapter is concerned with the biosynthesis and degradation of the membrane lipids.

Phosphatidic Acid Is an Intermediate in Phosphoglyceride Synthesis

Phosphoglycerides are synthesized in the cytoplasm and endoplasmic reticulum (ER) of all cells. **Phosphatidic acid,** synthesized from glycerol phosphate, is the key intermediate. Its biosynthesis is shown in Figure 24.1.

There are two pathways for the de novo synthesis of phosphoglycerides. In the **phosphatidic acid pathway,** phosphatidate is activated as cytidine diphosphate (CDP)–diacylglycerol. This strategy is used for the synthesis of phosphatidylinositol (Fig. 24.2) and cardiolipin.

In the **salvage pathway,** the alcohol that becomes bound to phosphatidate is activated as the CDP derivative. Phosphatidylcholine (Fig. 24.3) and phosphatidylethanolamine are synthesized this way. The principle is similar to the activation of glucose for glycogen synthesis, but cytidine triphosphate (CTP) rather than uridine triphosphate (UTP) is used. Also, in the case of the phosphoglycerides, one of the two phosphates in the CDP derivative remains in the product.

Phosphoglycerides Are Remodeled Continuously

Phosphoglycerides are degraded by **phospholipases.** These ubiquitous enzymes are named according to their cleavage specificity:

Phospholipases are used to remodel the phosphoglycerides by changing the fatty acids in positions 1 and 2 (Fig. 24.4).

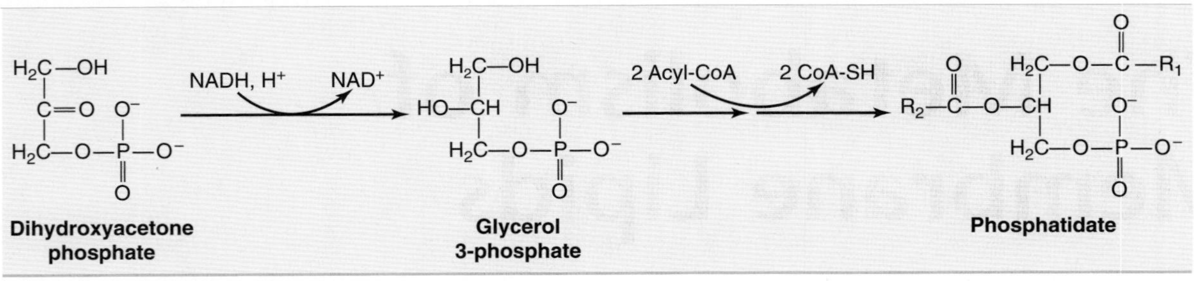

Figure 24.1 The synthesis of phosphatidic acid.

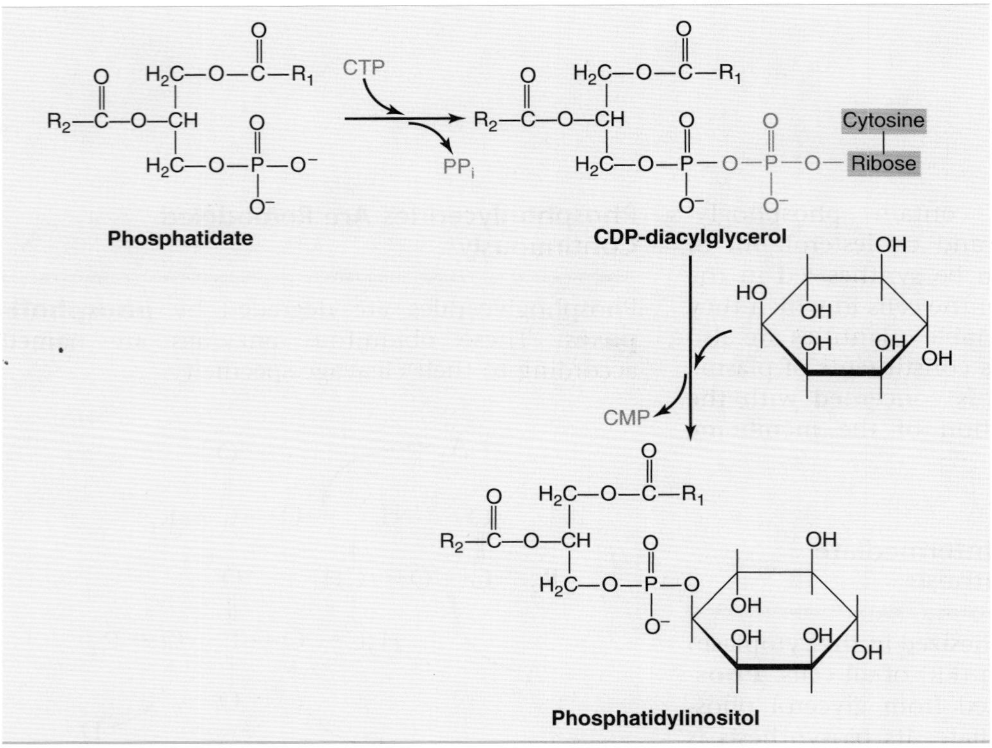

Figure 24.2 Synthesis of phosphatidylinositol by the phosphatidic acid pathway.

The acyltransferases that replace the cutout fatty acid are selective for the lysophosphoglyceride and the fatty acid. They usually place a saturated fatty acid in position 1 and an unsaturated fatty acid in position 2. The unsaturated fatty acid is most often arachidonic acid for phosphatidylinositol and oleic acid or linoleic acid for the other phosphoglycerides.

The alcoholic substituent of phosphatidic acid is also exchangeable. Most phosphatidylserine is synthesized by base exchange with ethanolamine in human tissues:

Phosphatidylethanolamine + Serine

↓

Phosphatidylserine + Ethanolamine

Phosphatidylethanolamine can be made by the decarboxylation of phosphatidylserine; phosphatidylcholine, by the methylation of phosphatidylethanolamine (Fig. 24.5).

Plasmalogens, which constitute up to 10% of the phosphoglycerides in muscle and brain, are synthesized from dihydroxyacetone phos-

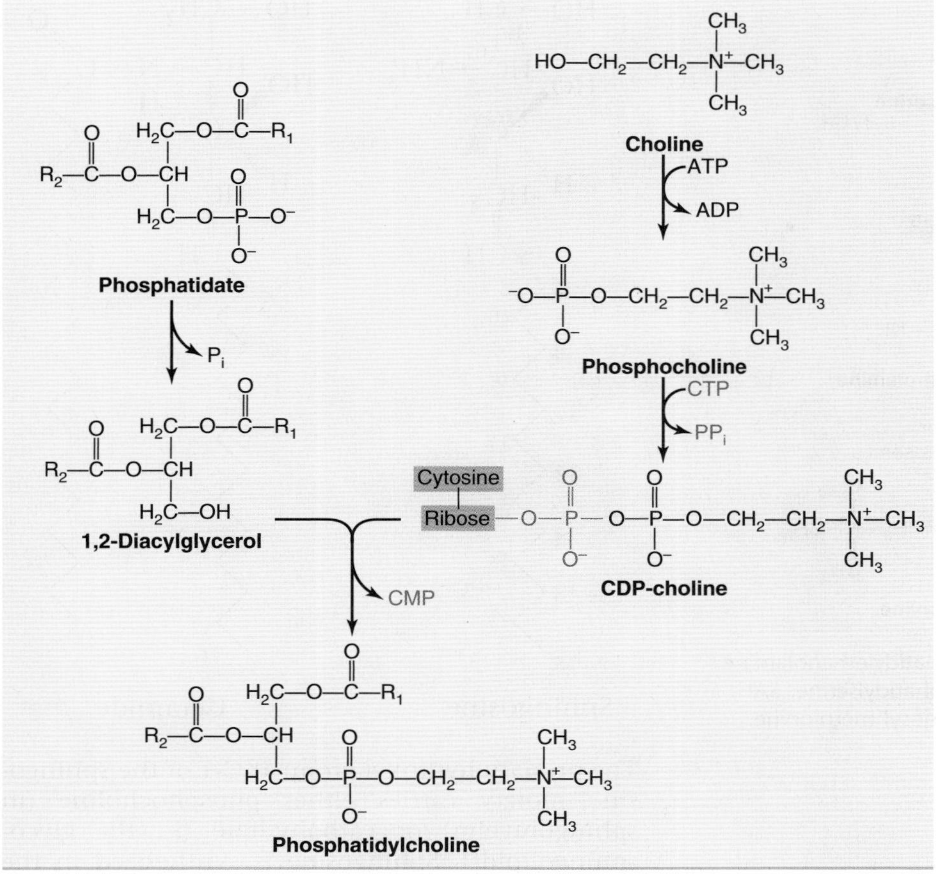

Figure 24.3 Synthesis of phosphatidylcholine by the salvage pathway.

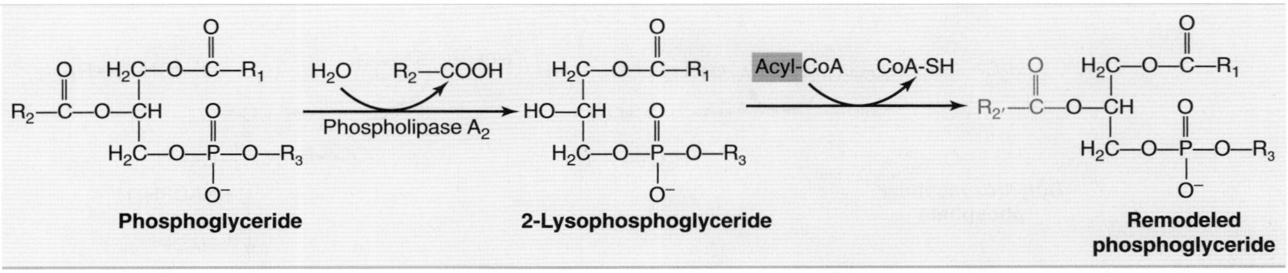

Figure 24.4 The exchange of a fatty acid in a phosphoglyceride by the successive action of phospholipase A$_2$ and an acyl transferase. CoA, coenzyme A; CoA-SH, uncombined CoA.

phate (Fig. 24.6). Most plasmalogens contain ethanolamine.

Platelet-activating factor (**PAF**) (see Fig. 24.6) is formed by white blood cells and acts as a mediator of hypersensitivity reactions and acute inflammation. In concentrations as low as 10^{-11} to 10^{-10} mol/liter, it induces platelet adhesion, vasodilation, and chemotaxis of polymorphonuclear leukocytes. The presence of an acetyl group in position 2, instead of a long-chain acyl group,

makes PAF sufficiently water soluble to diffuse through an aqueous medium.

Sphingolipids Are Synthesized from Ceramide

Ceramide, consisting of sphingosine and a long-chain fatty acid, is the core structure of the sphingolipids:

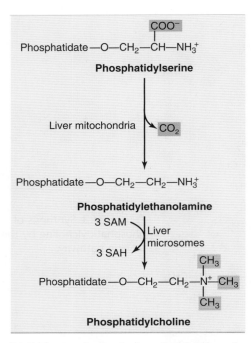

Figure 24.5 The synthesis of phosphatidylethanolamine and phosphatidylcholine from phosphatidylserine. SAH, S-adenosyl homocysteine; SAM, S-adenosyl methionine.

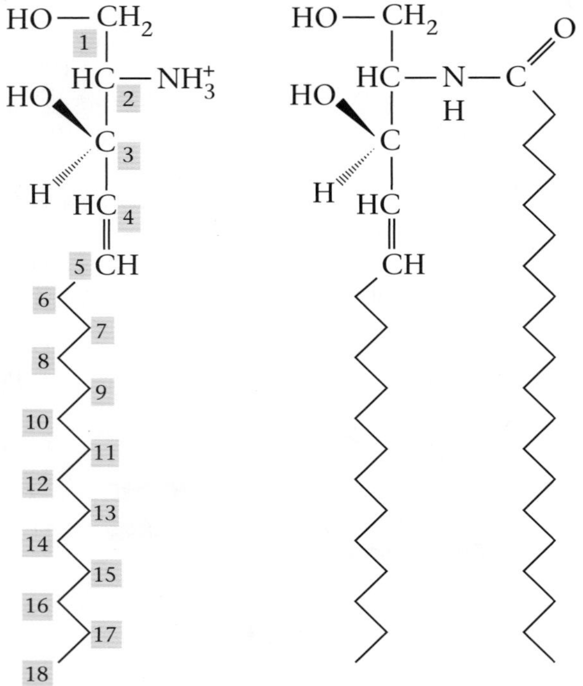

Sphingosine   **Ceramide**

The primary hydroxyl group at C-1 of the sphingosine moiety carries either phosphocholine (in sphingomyelin) or carbohydrate (in the glycosphingolipids). Sphingosine is synthesized in the ER of most cells from palmitoyl–CoA and serine,

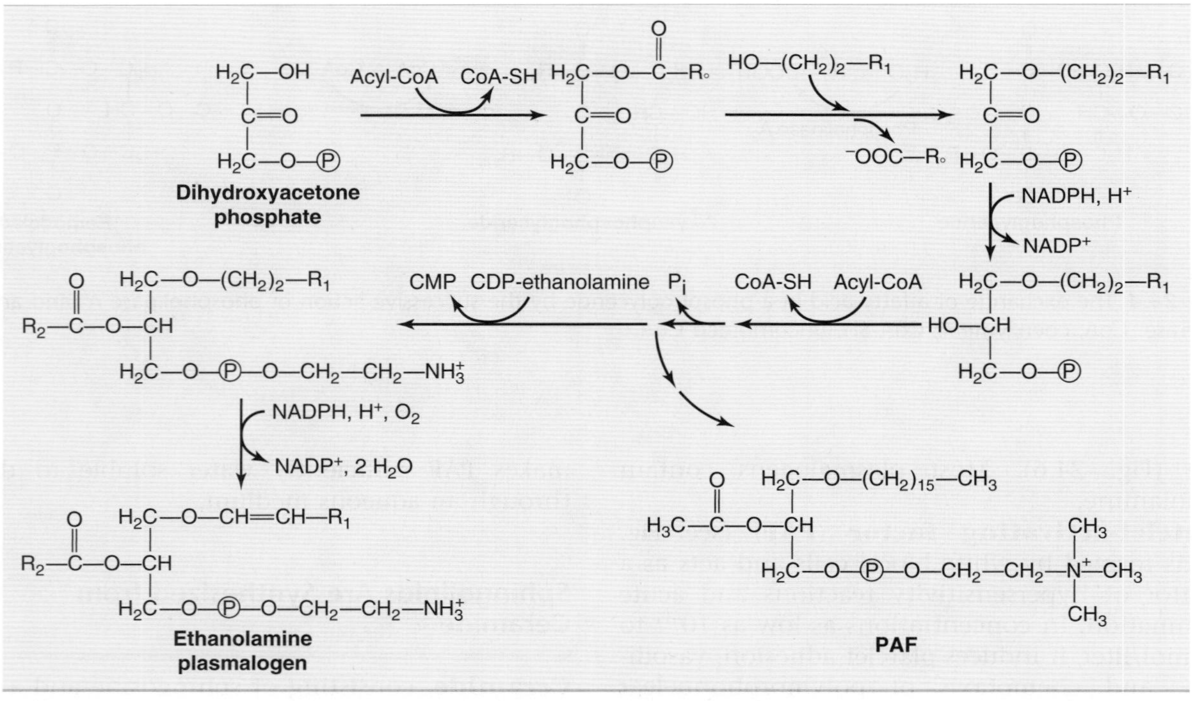

Dihydroxyacetone phosphate

Ethanolamine plasmalogen

PAF

Figure 24.6 Synthesis of plasmalogens and platelet-activating factor (PAF). CDP, cytidine diphosphate; CMP, cytidine monophosphate; CoA, coenzyme A; CoA-SH, uncombined CoA; NADP+, nicotinamide adenine dinucleotide phosphate; NADH, reduced form of NADP; P_i, inorganic phosphate.

and the fatty acid is introduced from its CoA-thioester. The fatty acid is usually saturated and can be very long, with 22 or 24 carbons.

During the synthesis of the sphingolipids in the ER and Golgi apparatus, *the hydroxyl group at C-1 of sphingosine is not activated, but its substituent is introduced from an activated precursor.* Sphingomyelin is synthesized with the help of phosphatidylcholine:

Ceramide + Phosphatidylcholine

↓

Sphingomyelin + 1,2-Diacylglycerol

The oligosaccharide chains of the glycosphingolipids are synthesized by the stepwise addition of monosaccharides from their activated precursors.

The ABO Blood Group Substances Are Oligosaccharides in Glycosphingolipids

Blood group substances are genetically polymorphic antigens on the surface of the erythrocyte membrane. People cannot form antibodies to their own blood group substances, but they can form antibodies against those of other people. This can result in dangerous transfusion reactions.

The antigens of the ABO blood group system are glycosphingolipids. Their antigenic specificities are caused by variations in the terminal sugar of the oligosaccharide (Fig. 24.7).

The glycosyl transferase that adds the last monosaccharide comes in three alleles. The A allele codes for an enzyme that adds *N*-acetylgalactosamine; the B allele codes for an enzyme that adds galactose; and the O allele has a nonsense mutation and produces no enzyme. Only the A and B substances are effective antigens. Genetically, the A and B alleles are codominant, and the O allele is recessive.

In other cases, however, blood group substances arise from variations in the amino acid sequence of a membrane protein. The antigens of the MN blood group system, for example, are variants of the membrane protein glycophorin A that differ in the amino acid residues at positions 1 and 5.

Deficiencies of Sphingolipid-Degrading Enzymes Cause Lipid Storage Diseases

Sphingolipids are degraded in the lysosomes. The breakdown of complex glycosphingolipids requires lysosomal exoglycosidases to remove sugars from the end of the oligosaccharide. Each of these enzymes is specific for the monosaccharide that it removes and the type of glycosidic bond that it cleaves. Figure 24.8 shows the degradation of the most important sphingolipids.

A deficiency of any of these enzymes leads to an accumulation of its substrate in the lysosomes. The resulting disease is called a **lipid storage disease** or **sphingolipidosis.** *The enzyme deficiency is expressed in all tissues.* Complete deficiencies lead to severe disease, with the progressive accumulation of the nondegradable lipid. The nervous system is seriously affected in essentially all cases because of its high sphingolipid content and turnover. Hepatosplenomegaly is also common in these conditions because phagocytic cells in the spleen and liver remove erythrocytes from the circulation and nondegradable lipid from the red blood cell membrane accumulates in these tissues.

For diagnosis, enzyme activities are determined in cultured leukocytes, skin fibroblasts, or, for prenatal diagnosis, amniotic cells. The inheritance is autosomal recessive except for Fabry disease, which is X-linked recessive. In the more severe diseases, affected homozygotes have near-zero enzyme activ-

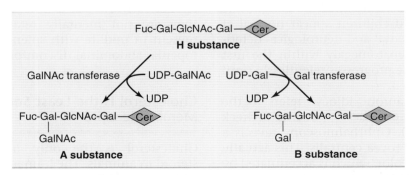

Figure 24.7 The synthesis of the ABO blood group substances. The *N*-acetylgalactosamine (GalNAc) transferase (present in people with blood group A) and the galactose (Gal) transferase (in people with blood group B) are encoded by allelic variants of the same gene. A third variant of this gene does not produce an active enzyme. Homozygosity for this nonfunctional allele produces blood group O (only the H substance is present). Cer, ceramide; Fuc, fucose.

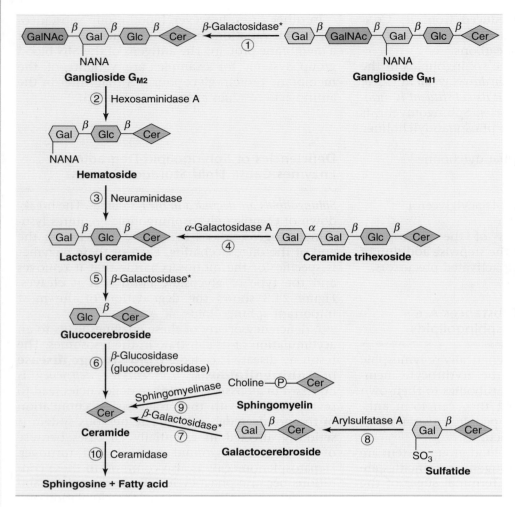

Figure 24.8 Lysosomal degradation of sphingolipids. The numbered reactions refer to the storage diseases in Table 24.1. *There are two different β-galactosidases, one for ganglioside G_{M1} and the other for galactocerebroside. Lactosyl ceramide (Cer) is degraded by both. Gal, galactose; GalNAc, N-acetylgalactosamine; Glc, glucose; NANA, N-acetylneuraminic acid.

ity. These diseases are fatal. In milder variants of lipid storage diseases, affected homozygotes have greatly reduced but not completely absent enzyme activity.

Also, heterozygotes can be identified because their enzyme activity is reduced to about one half of normal.

Tay-Sachs disease is caused by a complete deficiency of hexosaminidase A (reaction (2) in Fig. 24.8), leading to an accumulation of ganglioside G_{M2}. Although affected children appear normal at birth, they develop mental and neurological deterioration along with hepatomegaly within the first year of life. The disease progresses relentlessly until death at or before age 3.

The old name "amaurotic idiocy" refers to the apparent blindness of these patients (Greek αμαυροσ = "obscure"). Ophthalmoscopy reveals a cherry-red spot in the fovea centralis. This actually represents its normal color, which is accentuated by the gray appearance of the surrounding lipid-laden ganglion cells. This finding is not diagnostic for Tay-Sachs disease, however, because it is seen in some other lipid storage diseases as well. Tay-Sachs disease is very rare except among Ashkenazi Jews, in whom it occurs with a frequency of 1 per 3600 births.

Table 24.1 shows some examples of lipid storage diseases. The most common of them is the adult-onset form of Gaucher disease. Like Tay-Sachs disease, it is most prevalent among Ashkenazi Jews. Affected patients still have a residual enzyme activity between 10% and 20% of normal. Therefore, they are not mentally retarded. They typically present in midlife with splenomegaly, thrombocytopenia, abdominal discomfort, and bone erosion.

Cholesterol Is the Least Soluble Membrane Lipid

Cholesterol is the only important membrane steroid in animals. The human body contains about 140 g, most of it in the form of "free" (unesterified) cholesterol in cellular membranes. It is most abundant in tissues that also contain large amounts of

Table 24.1 Examples of Lipid Storage Diseases

Disease	Enzyme Deficiency*	Incidence	Clinical Course
Generalized gangliosidosis	1	Unknown	Mental retardation, hepatomegaly, skeletal abnormalities
Tay-Sachs	2	1 per 3600 (Ashkenazi Jews)	Mental retardation, blindness, hepatosplenomegaly, death in infancy
Gaucher	6	Infantile: rare; adult: 1 per 600 (Ashkenazi Jews)	Infantile form: similar to Tay-Sachs; adult-onset form: without mental retardation
Fabry	4	1 per 40,000	Skin rash, renal failure
Krabbe (globoid leukodystrophy)	7	1 per 50,000 (Sweden); lower elsewhere	Mental retardation, myelin nearly absent
Metachromatic leukodystrophy	8	1 per 100,000	Demyelination, mental deterioration; different degrees of severity
Niemann-Pick	9	Rare	Hepatosplenomegaly, mental retardation, early death
Farber	10	Rare	Hoarse voice, mental retardation, dermatitis, skeletal abnormalities, early death

*The numbers refer to the numbered reactions of Figure 24.8.

other membrane lipids, especially the nervous system. Therefore, brain is considered an unhealthy kind of food.

Cholesterol contains a condensed 4-ring system, known as the **cyclopentanoperhydrophenanthrene,** or **steroid,** ring system. This ring system is decorated with a hydroxyl group, two methyl groups, and a branched hydrocarbon chain.

The molecule contains eight asymmetrical carbons, but only 1 of the 256 possible stereoisomers occurs in nature. Substituents of the steroid nucleus can be in α or β configuration. Those in β configuration, indicated by wedge-shaped lines, face upward from the plane of the steroid ring. Those in α configuration, indicated by broken lines, point behind the plane of the ring:

Cholesterol

Cholesterol has very low water solubility. Only 0.2 mg dissolves in 100 mL of water at 25° C. The concentration of unesterified cholesterol that circulates in the plasma in the form of lipoproteins is 300 times higher than this.

For storage and transport, cholesterol is esterified with long-chain fatty acids. These cholesterol esters are even less soluble than cholesterol itself. In some cells, especially those of steroid-producing endocrine glands, stored cholesterol esters form lipid droplets in the cytoplasm. Also, 70% of the cholesterol in plasma lipoproteins is esterified.

Only animals form significant amounts of cholesterol. Plants contain **phytosterols** instead. Ergosterol (in fungi) and β-sitosterol (in higher plants) are examples of phytosterols. They are poorly absorbed from dietary sources and are therefore present in only small amounts in the human body. Bacteria do not produce steroids. *A vegan diet is essentially cholesterol free.*

Cholesterol Is Derived from Both Endogenous Synthesis and the Diet

Endogenous cholesterol synthesis amounts to 0.5 to 1 g per day, depending on the dietary supply. All nucleated cells can synthesize cholesterol, but the liver accounts for at least 50% of the total. Steroid-producing endocrine glands, including the adrenal cortex and the corpus luteum, have very high rates of cholesterol synthesis.

Humans also get some cholesterol from the diet. Most people in modern societies eat close to 1 g of cholesterol per day. In the presence of bile salts, approximately one half of this is absorbed in the intestine.

In the intestinal mucosa, most of the absorbed cholesterol is converted to cholesterol esters by the microsomal enzyme **acyl-CoA–cholesterol acyl transferase** (**ACAT**). Together with triglycerides,

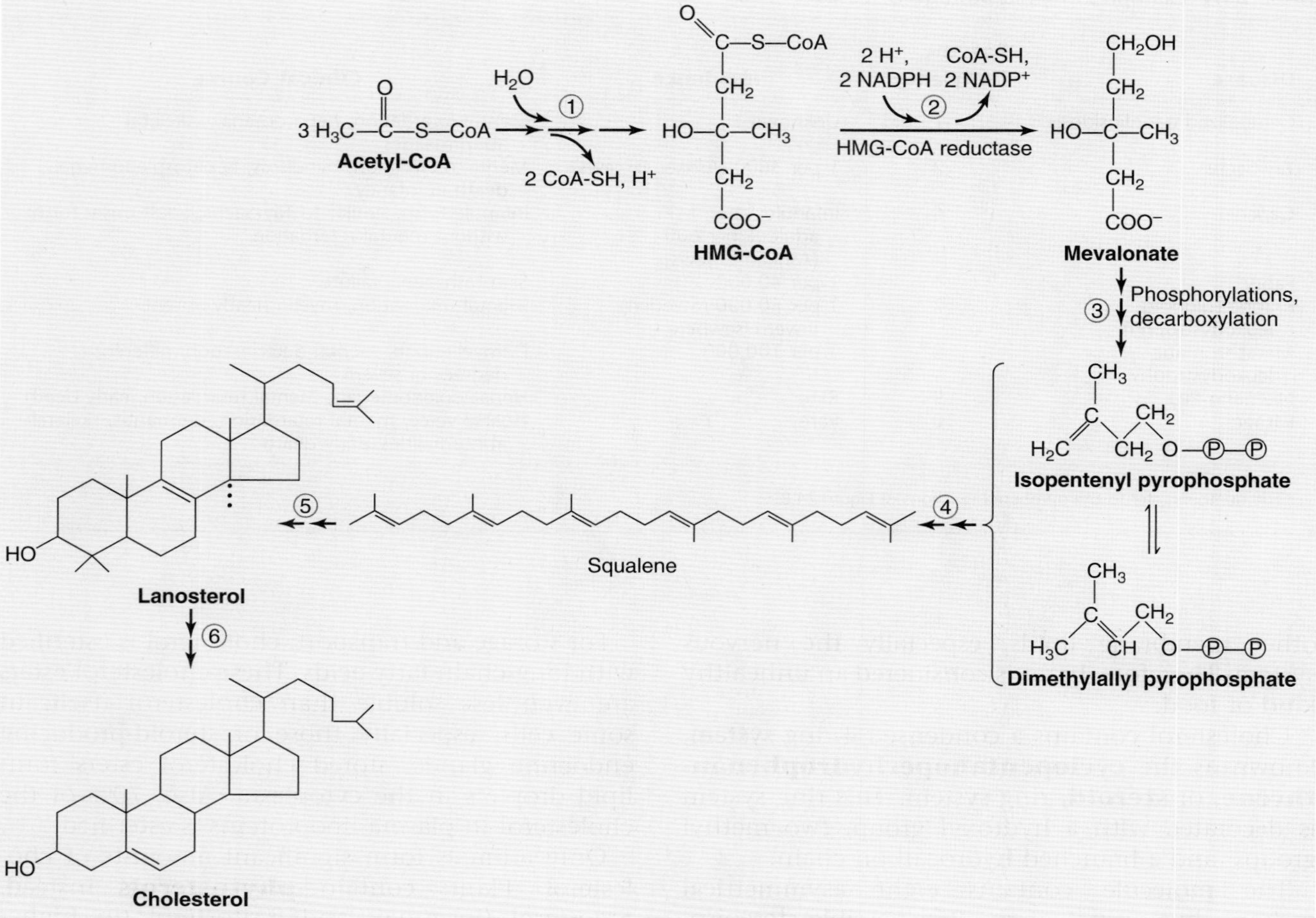

Figure 24.9 The stages of cholesterol synthesis. HMG, 3-hydroxy-3-methylglutaryl.

some free cholesterol, and other dietary lipids, *the cholesterol esters are packaged into chylomicrons.*

Most of the triglyceride is removed by lipoprotein lipase in peripheral tissues, and the cholesterol-rich remnant particles thus formed are taken up by the liver. Thus, *most of the dietary triglyceride goes to extrahepatic tissues, but most of the cholesterol goes to the liver.*

The liver releases cholesterol as a constituent of very-low-density lipoprotein (VLDL), which becomes remodeled into low-density lipoprotein (LDL) in the blood. *LDL is the principal external source of cholesterol for most cells.* The transport of cholesterol from the extrahepatic tissues to the liver requires high-density lipoprotein (HDL) along with other lipoproteins. Details of lipoprotein function and metabolism are described in Chapter 25.

Cholesterol Biosynthesis Is Regulated at the Level of HMG-CoA Reductase

All 27 carbons of cholesterol are derived from the acetyl group in acetyl-CoA. The enzymes of the biosynthetic pathway, which number close to 30, are in the cytosol and the ER. Figure 24.9 shows the pathway in a very abbreviated form. The first reactions, up to 3-hydroxy-3-methylglutaryl (HMG–CoA), are shared with the synthesis of ketone bodies. However, ketogenesis is mitochondrial, whereas the HMG-CoA synthase of cholesterol synthesis is cytoplasmic.

The formation of mevalonate by HMG-CoA reductase (reaction (2) in Fig. 24.9), which is dependent on NADPH, is the committed and regulated step of cholesterol synthesis. *HMG-CoA reductase is feedback-inhibited by free cholesterol.* This effect is mediated both at the transcriptional and the post-transcriptional levels. HMG-CoA reductase has a life span of approximately 4 hours, and a change in its rate of synthesis or degradation can therefore affect cholesterol synthesis rather rapidly.

Insulin stimulates HMG-CoA reductase, and this effect is thought to be mediated by the AMP–activated protein kinase. Like acetyl-CoA carboxy-lase (see Chapter 23), HMG-CoA reductase is phos-phorylated and inactivated by this insulin-inhibited enzyme.

The Isoprenoids Are Derived from the Pathway of Cholesterol Biosynthesis

Products that are synthesized from the branched-chain, five-carbon compounds isopentenyl pyro-phosphate and dimethylallyl pyrophosphate (see Fig. 24.9) are collectively called **isoprenoids.** Besides cholesterol and the other steroids, a few other isoprenoids are synthesized in the human body:

1. The side chain of **ubiquinone** (see Chapter 21).
2. **Dolichol,** which participates in the synthesis of the N-linked oligosaccharides in glycoproteins (see Chapter 9).
3. The side chain of **heme *a*,** the prosthetic group of cytochrome a/a_3.
4. **Farnesyl** and **geranylgeranyl** groups, which are used to anchor some proteins to membranes.

Plants produce a more interesting collection of isoprenoids, including the fat-soluble vitamins. Phytanic acid, which accumulates in patients with Refsum disease (see Chapter 23), also shows the typical isoprenoid structure.

Bile Acids Are Synthesized from Cholesterol

The steroid nucleus of cholesterol cannot be degraded in the human body. *Cholesterol has to be disposed of by the biliary system, either as such or after conversion to bile acids.*

Bladder bile contains approximately 400 mg/dL of nonesterified cholesterol. Because only approxi-mately half of this is absorbed by the intestine, *nearly 500 mg of unmetabolized cholesterol can be elim-inated from the body per day.* Intestinal bacteria metabolize cholesterol to various "neutral sterols."

Approximately one half of the cholesterol is eventually metabolized to the **primary bile acids** in the liver. They include **cholic acid** and **che-nodeoxycholic acid,** cholic acid being the more abundant. The liver secretes the bile acids not in the free form but as conjugation products with glycine or taurine (Fig. 24.10). The ratio of glycine conju-gates to taurine conjugates is about 3 : 1. Bile acids are not useless excretory products; they serve a vital function in lipid absorption (see Chapter 19).

Bile Acid Synthesis Is Feedback-Inhibited

The committed step in bile acid synthesis is cat-alyzed by the microsomal enzyme **7α-hydroxy-lase** (Fig. 24.11). This monooxygenase reaction requires molecular oxygen, NADPH, and cyto-chrome P-450. Ascorbate also seems to be involved. Ascorbate deficiency (scurvy) impairs the formation of bile acids and causes cholesterol accumulation and atherosclerosis, at least in guinea pigs.

Bile acids reduce the level of 7α-hydroxylase by inhibiting the transcription of its gene. Interestingly, bile acids also reduce the activity of HMG-CoA reductase. Cholesterol, in contrast, induces 7α-hydroxylase synthesis in addition to inhibiting HMG-CoA reductase. These regulatory effects ensure the maintenance of an adequate pool of free cholesterol in the liver.

Thyroid hormones induce the synthesis of 7α-hydroxylase. This effect contributes to the in-creased plasma cholesterol level in patients with hypothyroidism.

Bile Acids Are Subject to Extensive Enterohepatic Circulation

As the primary bile acids reach the lower parts of the small intestine, they are modified by bacterial enzymes. First, the glycine or taurine is cleaved off. This is followed by the reductive removal of the 7α-hydroxyl group. The **secondary bile acids** formed in these reactions are **deoxycholic acid** and **lithocholic acid** (Fig. 24.12).

Of the bile acids, 96% are absorbed by a sodium cotransport mechanism in the ileum and returned to the liver. The liver conjugates these bile acids and secretes them again in the bile. Because of this *enterohepatic circulation* (Fig. 24.13), both primary and secondary bile acids are present in the bile.

The enterohepatic circulation of the bile acids ensures that humans have enough of them for fat absorption. Only 0.5 g is synthesized per day, and between 3 and 5 g is present in liver, bile, and intestines at any time. Overall, however, 20 to 30 g

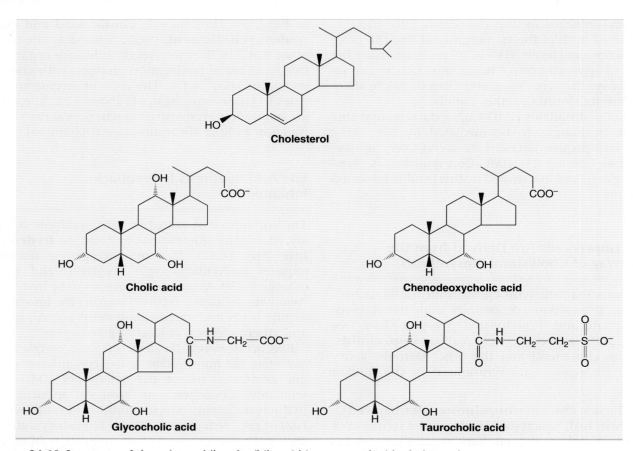

Figure 24.10 Structures of the primary bile salts (bile acids), compared with cholesterol.

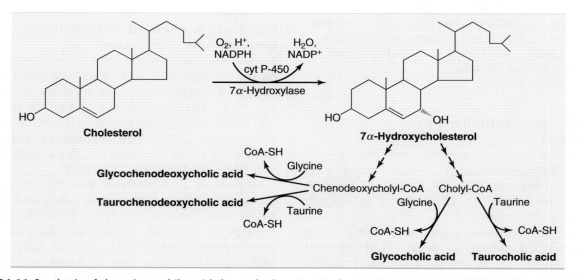

Figure 24.11 Synthesis of the primary bile acids by endoplasmic reticulum–associated enzymes in hepatocytes. cyt, cytochrome.

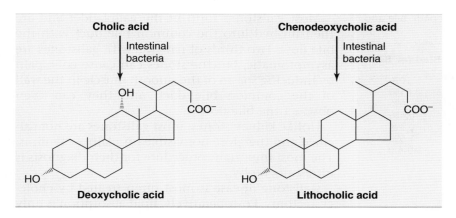

Figure 24.12 Synthesis of the secondary bile acids by intestinal bacteria.

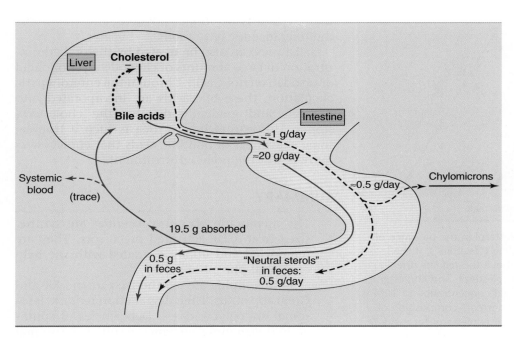

Figure 24.13 Disposition of bile acids and cholesterol in the enterohepatic system.

of bile acids are secreted per day. Each bile acid molecule is recycled five to eight times every day, and it remains in the system for an average of 1 week before it is finally excreted.

Bile acids are synthesized round the clock by the liver, but their release into the intestine from the gallbladder is intermittent, being stimulated by the intestinal hormone cholecystokinin after a fatty meal. The gallbladder concentrates the bile in addition to storing it. Inorganic ions are actively removed across the gallbladder epithelium, followed by passive water flux. Therefore, all solids except inorganic ions are more concentrated in bladder bile than in hepatic bile.

A very small portion of the bile acids that are absorbed from the ileum fail to return to the liver. They escape into the peripheral circulation, in which their presence can be determined in the clinical laboratory. Plasma bile acid levels are elevated

in patients with biliary obstruction because bile backs up, and the bile acids enter the blood from the liver. Plasma bile acid levels are also elevated in liver cirrhosis and portal hypertension when portal blood is shunted around the cirrhotic liver. Although otherwise not very toxic, the bile acids can cause a most distressing itching (pruritus) in these patients.

Most Gallstones Consist of Cholesterol

The bile contains cholesterol, bile acids, phosphatidylcholine (lecithin), and the heme-derived bile pigments. *Cholesterol is the least soluble constituent of bile.* Although less abundant than some of the other components (Table 24.2), *cholesterol can be kept in solution only by being incorporated into mixed bile salt/phospholipid micelles.*

Table 24.2 Approximate Composition of Hepatic Bile and Bladder Bile

Component	Hepatic Bile	Bladder Bile
Total solids	2.5%	10%
Inorganic salt	0.85%	0.85%
Bile acids	1.2%	6%
Cholesterol	0.06%	0.4%
Lecithin	0.04%	0.3%
Bile pigments	0.2%	1.5%
pH	7.4	5.0-6.0

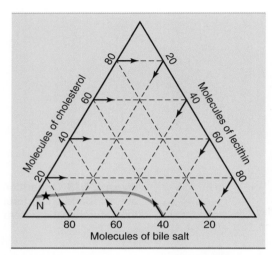

Figure 24.14 Solubility of cholesterol in the presence of bile acids and phosphatidylcholine ("lecithin"). If the relative composition of bile is above the *red line,* the system is supersaturated with cholesterol, and cholesterol is likely to precipitate. A total lipid concentration of 10% is assumed. Point *N* represents a "normal" composition of bladder bile, with 10 molecules of cholesterol for every 5 molecules of lecithin and 85 molecules of bile acid.

When the cholesterol level in the bile is too high, or when the levels of the emulsifying lipids are too low, cholesterol tends to precipitate and form **gallstones.** The "solubility triangle" of Figure 24.14 shows the solubility of cholesterol at different concentrations of bile salts and lecithin. *Most patients with gallstone disease have an elevated cholesterol level in their bile.*

Gallstones afflict about 20% of all people in Western countries at some point in their lives, being most common in fat, fertile females. The risk rises with increasing age. Some gallstones contain both cholesterol and bile pigments, but others are pure cholesterol. Only 10% of all gallstones consist of substances other than cholesterol, usually bilirubin and other bile pigments.

Most gallstones form in the gallbladder and are then flushed into the common bile duct with the bile flow. Two thirds of patients with gallstones are asymptomatic, but the stones can cause colic pain by inducing spasm of the smooth muscle in the wall of the common bile duct, and they can even obstruct the bile flow.

Unlike kidney stones, most gallstones are not calcified and therefore not visible on plain x-ray films. The most important procedure for their diagnosis is ultrasonography.

Gallstone disease is most often treated by cholecystectomy. Postoperatively, lipid absorption is only mildly abnormal because bile acids can still reach the small intestine. Only the accurate timing of their release is no longer possible, and this limits the tolerance for fatty foods.

Gallstones can also be treated by the oral administration of large amounts of chenodeoxycholic acid or ursodeoxycholic acid. Through the enterohepatic circulation, these bile acids are incorporated into the bile and gradually dissolve the cholesterol stones. Unfortunately, diarrhea is such a troublesome side effect of oral bile acids that cholecystectomy is still the preferred treatment.

SUMMARY

The membrane phosphoglycerides are synthesized from CDP-activated precursors. They are remodeled and finally degraded with the help of several phospholipases.

Sphingolipids are synthesized in the ER and Golgi apparatus. Their degradation requires lysosomal endoglycosidases. Deficiencies of sphingolipid-degrading enzymes result in lysosomal storage diseases, with progressive accumulation of the nondegradable lipid, neurological degeneration, and hepatosplenomegaly.

Cholesterol is derived in part from dietary sources and in part from endogenous synthesis in liver and other tissues. Endogenous cholesterol synthesis starts with acetyl-CoA. It is feedback-inhibited at the level of HMG-CoA reductase. Cholesterol is transported as a constituent of plasma lipoproteins, mainly in the form of cholesterol esters.

About one half of the total body cholesterol is eventually converted to bile acids. The bile acids are subject to an extensive enterohepatic circulation. The bile also contains some free cholesterol. This biliary cholesterol can form gallstones, especially in people with an elevated cholesterol level in the bile.

Further Reading

Kosters A, Jirsa M, Groen AK: Genetic background of cholesterol gallstone disease. Biochim Biophys Acta 1637:1-19, 2003.

Merrill AH: De novo sphingolipid biosynthesis: a necessary, but dangerous, pathway. J Biol Chem 277:25843-25846, 2002.

Russell DW: The enzymes, regulation, and genetics of bile acid synthesis. Annu Rev Biochem 72:137-174, 2003.

Sandhoff K, Kolter T: Biosynthesis and degradation of mammalian glycosphingolipids. Phil Trans R Soc Lond B 358:847-861, 2003.

Vance JE, Vance DE: Phospholipid biosynthesis in mammalian cells. Biochem Cell Biol 82:113-128, 2004.

QUESTIONS

1. **The ABO blood group substances are oligosaccharides in plasma membrane glycolipids of erythrocytes and other cells. The biosynthetic enzymes that are encoded by the ABO gene can be characterized as**

   A. Glycosidases.
   B. Glycosyltransferases.
   C. Lipases.
   D. Glycolipases.
   E. Phospholipases.

2. **Gallstones can easily form when the bile contains an increased amount of**

   A. Free (unesterified) fatty acids.
   B. Bile salts.
   C. Phospholipids.
   D. Cholesterol.
   E. Calcium.

3. **An 8-month-old child of Jewish parents is examined for failure to thrive and abnormal neurological development. The child is found to have hepatosplenomegaly and a cherry-red spot on the macula of the eye. Chromatography of lipids from cultured leukocytes shows abnormally high levels of ganglioside G_{M2}. This child has**

   A. Refsum disease.
   B. Tay-Sachs disease.
   C. Gaucher disease.
   D. Metachromatic leukodystrophy.
   E. Hurler disease.

CHAPTER 25

Lipid Transport

The plasma levels of the major lipids are not only higher than the normal blood glucose level of 100 mg/dL (Table 25.1), but they also fluctuate over a wider range, depending on nutrition, lifestyle, and individual constitution. This is possible because none of the major tissues depends on lipids as its only energy source, although there are tissues that depend on glucose.

Unesterified ("free") fatty acids are transported in noncovalent binding to serum albumin, but triglycerides, phospholipids, and cholesterol esters form large noncovalent aggregates with proteins that are collectively called **lipoproteins.** Overall, there are four pathways of lipid transport in the human body:

1. *The transport of fatty acids from adipose tissue to other tissues.*
2. *The transport of dietary lipids from the intestine to other tissues.*
3. *The transport of endogenously synthesized lipids from the liver to other tissues.*
4. *The **reverse transport** of cholesterol from extrahepatic tissues to the liver. This pathway is required because cholesterol cannot be degraded locally and has to be transported to the liver for biliary excretion.*

Most Plasma Lipids Are Components of Lipoproteins

The general structure of a lipoprotein (Fig. 25.1) can be predicted from the solubility properties of the lipids: *the hydrophobic triglycerides and cholesterol esters always avoid contact with water.* They form the core of the lipoprotein. *The amphipathic phospholipids prefer the water-lipid interface.* They form a monolayer covering the surface of the particle. The protein components, or apolipoproteins, are also amphipathic and reside on the surface of the particle. Large lipoprotein particles with a high volume/surface ratio have a high content of nonpolar lipids, and small particles contain more polar lipid and protein.

The composition of lipoproteins keeps changing because most lipids and apolipoproteins can be transferred from one lipoprotein particle to another, and lipids can be acquired from cells, processed by enzymes while in the lipoprotein, and given off to cells. For their final destruction, many lipoproteins are taken up into cells by receptor-mediated endocytosis, which is followed by the lysosomal hydrolysis of their constituents.

The plasma lipoproteins can be separated by **electrophoresis,** along with the other plasma proteins (see Chapter 15). In fasting serum or plasma, the two most prominent lipoprotein bands are in the α_1 and β fractions and are designated, accordingly, as α- and β-**lipoproteins.** A less prominent band, the **pre-β-lipoproteins,** moves slightly ahead of the β-lipoproteins. The **chylomicrons,** found only after a fatty meal, do not move upon electrophoresis.

The behavior of lipoproteins in **density gradient centrifugation** depends on their protein/lipid ratio. Nonpolar lipids have densities near 0.9 g/cm³. With increasing protein content, the densities of the lipoprotein particles increase from 0.9 to 0.96 in the most lipid-rich particles to well above 1.0 g/cm³ in the protein-rich types. In increasing order of density and protein content, we can distinguish chylomicrons, very-low-density lipoprotein (VLDL), low-density lipoprotein (LDL), and high-density lipoprotein (HDL). The correspondence of these density classes to the electrophoretic separation pattern is shown in Figure 25.2.

Lipoproteins Have Characteristic Lipid and Protein Compositions

Table 25.2 shows the approximate compositions of the lipoprotein classes. In the fasting state, *most of the plasma triglyceride is in VLDL, and 70% of the total cholesterol is in LDL.* Therefore, elevations of plasma triglycerides are usually caused by increased

Table 25.1 The "Normal" Concentrations of Plasma Lipids in the Adult, Determined in the Postabsorptive State 8 to 12 Hours after the Last Meal

Lipid	Normal Range (mg/dL)
Total lipid	400–800
Triglycerides	40–280
Total cholesterol	120–280
LDL cholesterol	65–200
HDL cholesterol	30–90
Phospholipids	125–275
Free fatty acids	8–25

HDL, high-density lipoprotein; LDL, low-density lipoprotein.

amounts of VLDL, and elevations of cholesterol are usually caused by increased amounts of LDL.

Each lipoprotein class contains a characteristic combination of apolipoproteins (Table 25.3). With the exception of the B-apolipoproteins, however, which are major structural proteins of LDL, VLDL, and chylomicrons (but not HDL), apolipoproteins can be transferred between different lipoprotein classes. The apolipoproteins

- regulate lipid-metabolizing enzymes in the blood.
- facilitate the transfer of lipids between lipoprotein classes and between lipoproteins and cells.
- mediate the endocytosis of lipoproteins by binding to cell surface receptors.

Lipids of Dietary Origin Are Transported by Chylomicrons

Approximately 100 g of dietary triglycerides have to be transported daily from the small intestine to other tissues. As discussed in Chapter 23, these triglycerides are transported as constituents of

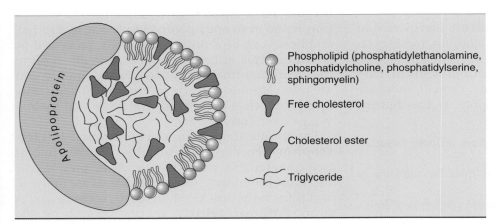

Phospholipid (phosphatidylethanolamine, phosphatidylcholine, phosphatidylserine, sphingomyelin)

Free cholesterol

Cholesterol ester

Triglyceride

Figure 25.1 General structure of a lipoprotein.

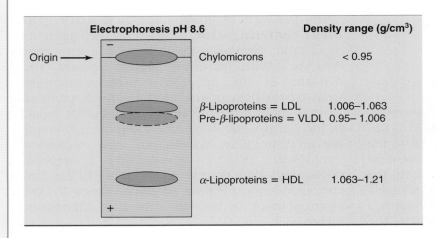

Electrophoresis pH 8.6

Density range (g/cm³)

Origin →

Chylomicrons   < 0.95

β-Lipoproteins = LDL   1.006–1.063
Pre-β-lipoproteins = VLDL 0.95–1.006

α-Lipoproteins = HDL   1.063–1.21

Figure 25.2 Electrophoretic mobilities and density classes of plasma lipoproteins. Intermediate-density lipoprotein (IDL) is included here in low-density lipoprotein (LDL). HDL, high-density lipoprotein; VLDL, very-low-density lipoprotein

Table 25.2 Typical Compositions of Plasma Lipoproteins

Lipoprotein Class	Source	Diameter (nm)	Density (g/cm³)	Protein (%)	Lipid %			
					Triglycerides	Phospholipid	Cholesterol Esters	Cholesterol
Chylomicrons	Intestine	100-1,000	0.95	1-2	86	8	3	2
Very-low-density lipoprotein (VLDL)	Liver	30-80	0.95-1.006	6-10	55	18	13	7
Intermediate-density lipoprotein (IDL)	VLDL	25-30	1.006-1.019	15-20	25	21	28	9
Low-density lipoprotein (LDL)	VLDL, IDL	20-25	1.019-1.063	22	9	20	40	8
High-density lipoprotein	Liver, intestine							
HDL₂		9-12	1.063-1.125	35-45	5	33	17	5
HDL₃		5-9	1.125-1.21	50-55	3	28	12	3

Table 25.3 Characteristics of the Apolipoproteins

Apolipoprotein	Molecular Weight (D)	Plasma Concentration (mg/dL)	Lipoproteins	Source	Function
A-I	29,000	130	HDL, chylomicrons	Liver, intestine	Major structural proteins of HDL, also in chylomicrons; apo A-I activates LCAT
A-II	17,000	40			
B-48	241,000	Variable	Chylomicrons	Intestine	Structural protein of chylomicrons
B-100	513,000	80	VLDL, LDL	Liver	Structural protein of VLDL, IDL, and LDL; only apoprotein of LDL; mediates tissue uptake of LDL
C-I	6,600	6	Most lipoproteins	Liver	Readily transferred between different classes; C-II activates extrahepatic lipoprotein lipase (LPL)
C-II	8,900	3			
C-III	8,800	12			
D	19,000	10	HDL		Unknown
E	34,000	5	VLDL, IDL, chylomicrons	Liver	Mediates the uptake of chylomicron remnants and IDL by the liver

HDL, high-density lipoprotein; IDL, intermediate-density lipoprotein; LCAT, lecithin-cholesterol acyl transferase; LDL, low-density lipoprotein; VLDL, very-low-density lipoprotein.

chylomicrons. *Chylomicrons are present only after a fatty meal.* They are formed with **apoB-48** and the A-apolipoproteins as their only apolipoproteins. ApoE and the C-apolipoproteins are acquired in the blood by transfer from HDL.

The extrahepatic lipoprotein lipase (**LPL**) removes 80% to 90% of the triglycerides. Its activity depends on the presence of **apoC-II** on the surface of the chylomicron. During triglyceride hydrolysis, surface phospholipids and some of the apolipoproteins peel off from the surface of the shrinking particle and are transferred to HDL. Phospholipid transfer requires a specialized **phospholipid transfer protein.** Thus the large chylomicron, with a diameter of about 1 µm, is converted into a far smaller **chylomicron remnant.**

The remnant particles bind to lipoprotein receptors in the liver including the **LDL receptor** and the LDL-receptor-related protein (**LRP**), followed by *receptor-mediated endocytosis into the hepatocytes.* Receptor binding and endocytosis depend on **apoE** on the surface of the remnant particle. In the cell, lipids and apolipoproteins are hydrolyzed by lysosomal enzymes.

The life span of a chylomicron, from its secretion by the intestinal cell to the uptake of the remnant by the liver (Fig. 25.3), is less than 1 hour. Once in the blood stream, the life expectancy of the chylomicron triglycerides is only 5 to 10 minutes.

VLDL Is a Precursor of LDL

The liver synthesizes 25 to 50 g of triglycerides and smaller amounts of other lipids per day. These lipids

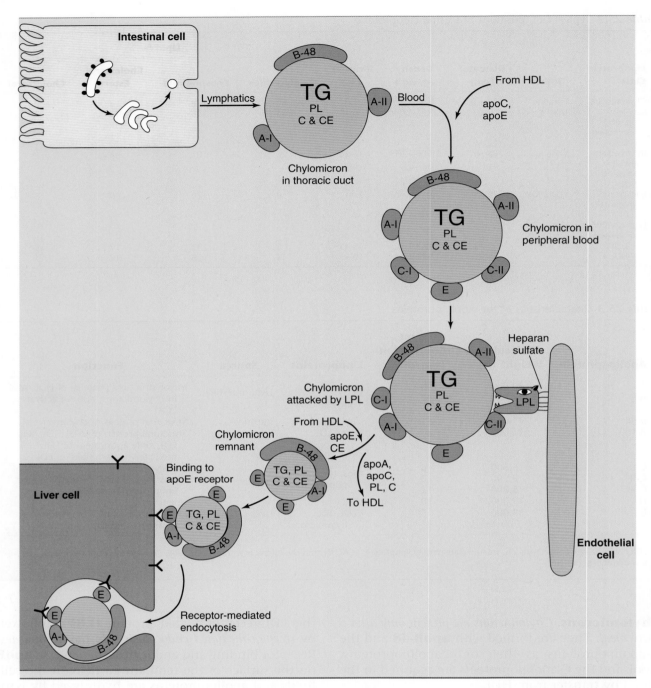

Figure 25.3 Metabolism of chylomicrons. C, free cholesterol; CE, cholesterol ester; HDL, high-density lipoprotein; LPL, lipoprotein lipase; PL, phospholipid; TG, triglyceride.

are released as **VLDL**. Like the chylomicrons, VLDL is synthesized in the endoplasmic reticulum (ER) and Golgi apparatus and is released by exocytosis. Unlike the intestinal capillaries, the liver sinusoids have a fenestrated endothelium that allows the passage of the lipoproteins into the sinusoidal blood.

VLDL is released with **apoB-100** and small amounts of apoE and the C-apolipoproteins. Like the chylomicrons, it acquires more C-apolipoproteins and apoE from HDL. Nascent VLDL contains only a modest quantity of cholesterol esters. Additional cholesterol esters are acquired from circulating HDL. This requires a **cholesterol ester transfer protein** (**CETP**).

The major apolipoprotein of VLDL, apoB-100, is a single polypeptide of 4536 amino acids. It is encoded by the same gene as apoB-48, the major

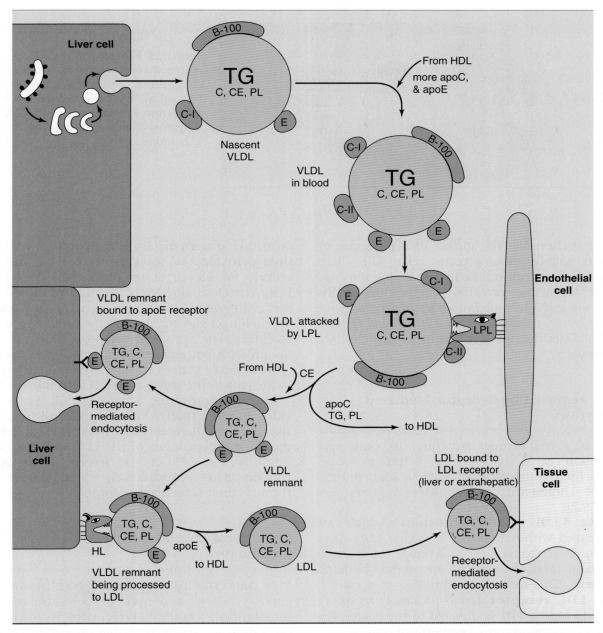

Figure 25.4 Metabolism of very-low-density lipoprotein (VLDL) and low-density lipoprotein (LDL). C, free cholesterol; CE, cholesterol esters; HDL, high-density lipoprotein; HL, hepatic lipase; LPL, Lipoprotein lipase; PL, phospholipid; TG, triglyceride.

apolipoprotein of chylomicrons. Indeed, apoB-48 consists of the first 2152 amino acids of apoB-100, counting from the N-terminus. In the intestine, a CAA codon that codes for glutamine in position 2153 is post-transcriptionally changed into the stop codon UAA. This is an example for the *tissue-specific editing of an RNA transcript.*

Like the chylomicrons, *VLDL is metabolized by LPL,* although VLDL triglycerides are hydrolyzed a bit more slowly than those in chylomicrons. Like chylomicrons, VLDL transfers C-apolipoproteins to HDL during triglyceride hydrolysis but retains most of its apoE.

About one half of the VLDL remnants, especially the larger specimens that contain multiple copies of apoE, are taken up by the liver. Smaller remnant particles appear initially as **intermediate-density lipoprotein** (IDL) and are eventually remodeled to **LDL.** This requires the hydrolysis of excess triglyceride and phospholipid by the **hepatic lipase (HL),** as well as the transfer of excess apolipoproteins to HDL (Fig. 25.4).

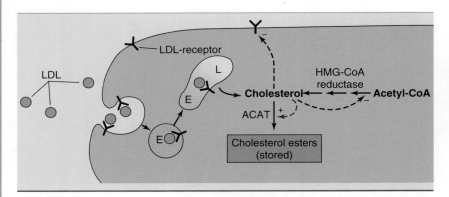

Figure 25.5 Regulation of cholesterol metabolism by low-density lipoprotein (LDL)–derived cholesterol in extrahepatic cells. ACAT, acyl-CoA–cholesterol acyl transferase; E, endosome; HMG-CoA, 3-hydroxy-3-methylglutaryl–CoA; L, lysosome.

HL is anchored to the surface of hepatocytes by heparan sulfate proteoglycans. Like LPL, it is released by heparin; unlike LPL, it is not activated by apoC-II and does not attack triglycerides in chylomicrons and VLDL. *It hydrolyzes triglycerides and, to some extent, phosphoglycerides in IDL and HDL.* It also facilitates the uptake of remnant particles into hepatocytes.

LDL Is Removed by Receptor-Mediated Endocytosis

LDL has a well-defined structure. Its only apolipoprotein is a solitary apo B-100 molecule, and its lipid component includes a high proportion of cholesterol and cholesterol esters (see Table 25.2).

Unlike VLDL and chylomicrons, which are metabolized within minutes to hours, LDL circulates in the plasma for an average of 3 days. Eventually, *LDL is removed by receptor-mediated endocytosis.* This requires the binding of apoB-100 to the **LDL receptor** (apoB-100/apoE receptor). The endocytosed LDL is directed to the lysosomes, and its apolipoproteins, cholesterol esters, and other lipids are hydrolyzed by lysosomal enzymes.

Approximately two thirds of the LDL ends up in the liver. However, for the extrahepatic tissues, *LDL acquired through the LDL receptor is the major external source of cholesterol.*

Not all LDL is cleared by the LDL receptor. Macrophages and some endothelial cells possess alternative lipoprotein receptors, collectively known as **scavenger receptors.** They have a 4 to 7 times higher Michaelis constant (K_m), or lower affinity, for LDL than does the regular LDL receptor. Therefore, their contribution to LDL metabolism is greatest when the plasma LDL concentration is high.

LDL that has been chemically modified by acetylating or oxidizing agents or by exposure to the crosslinking agent malondialdehyde (formed during lipid peroxidation; see Chapter 23) has a higher affinity for scavenger receptors than does virgin LDL. Therefore, one likely function of these receptors is the *removal of aberrant or aged lipoproteins* that are no longer good ligands for the other lipoprotein receptors. The scavenger receptors bind not only lipoproteins but also other particles, even bacteria, with negative surface charges. Therefore, they can participate in the defense against infections.

In the liver, ovaries, adrenal glands, lungs, and kidneys, more than 90% of cholesterol is utilized through the LDL receptor. However, 44% of the LDL uptake is independent of the LDL receptor in the intestine and 72% in the spleen. These organs contain many macrophages, which remove LDL through their scavenger receptors.

Cholesterol Regulates Its Own Metabolism

Most cells can obtain cholesterol both from endogenous synthesis and from LDL. In the cell, free (unesterified) cholesterol regulates its own concentration by acting on three important proteins (Fig. 25.5):

1. *It induces acyl-CoA-cholesterol acyl transferase (ACAT).* This enzyme converts free cholesterol into highly insoluble cholesterol esters that are stored in the cell:

$$\text{Cholesterol} + \text{Acyl-CoA}$$
$$\downarrow$$
$$\text{Cholesterol ester} + \text{CoA-SH}$$

2. *It represses HMG-CoA reductase,* the rate-limiting enzyme of cholesterol biosynthesis.
3. *It reduces the synthesis and/or accelerates the degradation of the LDL receptor.*

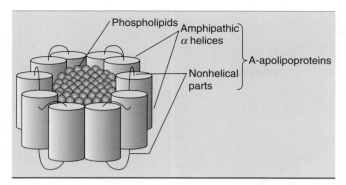

Figure 25.6 Hypothetical structure of nascent high-density lipoprotein (HDL) from liver and intestine. It consists of a little piece of lipid bilayer whose edge is occupied by amphipathic helices of the apolipoproteins. The A-apolipoproteins have amphipathic α-helical portions that are separated by short, nonhelical segments.

Cholesterol regulates gene expression by binding to nuclear transcription factors that act as cholesterol sensors. Macrophages tend to accumulate cholesterol when the LDL level is high because their scavenger receptors, unlike the "regular" LDL receptor, are not down-regulated by excess cellular cholesterol.

HDL Is Needed for Reverse Cholesterol Transport

HDL occurs in several subtypes that represent different stages in its metabolism. **Nascent HDL,** released from liver and intestine, is a small, phospholipid-rich particle, not spherical like the other lipoproteins but resembling a little disk of lipid bilayer with apolipoproteins at the edge (Fig. 25.6).

Nascent HDL from the liver contains apoA-I, apoA-II, apoE, and the C-apolipoproteins, but intestinal HDL is formed with only apoA-I. It acquires the other apolipoproteins later, especially during the processing of chylomicrons and VLDL by LPL.

Once in the circulation, *nascent HDL attracts free, unesterified cholesterol both from other lipoproteins and from cells.* Through apoA-I or apoE, HDL particles can dock to the cell surface. The cellular membrane protein **ABC1** (ATP-binding cassette protein-1) then pumps free cholesterol into the particle. The subsequent fate of this cell-derived cholesterol depends on two proteins that are bound to the surface of the HDL particle:

1. **Lecithin-cholesterol acyl transferase** (**LCAT**) is an otherwise soluble enzyme that binds to the surface of HDL, where it becomes activated by apo A-I. It catalyzes the reaction

Cholesterol + Phosphatidylcholine

↓

Cholesterol ester + 2-Lysophosphatidylcholine

Lysophosphatidylcholine (lysolecithin) is transferred to albumin, and the hydrophobic cholesterol esters sink into the center of the HDL particle. The originally flat HDL bulges into a spherical particle called HDL_3, with a hydrophobic core of cholesterol esters.

2. **Cholesterol ester transfer protein (CETP)** transfers cholesterol esters from HDL to other lipoproteins, either alone or in exchange for triglycerides. During the lipolysis of chylomicrons and VLDL by LPL, cholesterol esters are transferred from HDL to the remnant particles, mostly in exchange for triglycerides; this process is stimulated by the high local concentration of fatty acids. The remnant particles bring the cholesterol esters to the liver.

In the liver, HDL is exposed to the hepatic lipase (HL). The hydrolysis of triglycerides and phospholipids by HL converts larger HDL particles, known as HDL_2, to the smaller HDL_3. Whereas triglycerides and phospholipids are removed by HL, cholesterol esters are transferred selectively to the cells with the help of **SR-BI** (scavenger receptor class B type I). This membrane protein is structurally related to the CD36 protein that mediates the cellular uptake of fatty acids (see Chapter 23).

Thus, there is a fundamental difference between cholesterol delivery to cells by LDL and HDL. *LDL is endocytosed in one piece, but HDL remains intact while giving off cholesterol esters to the cells.* Only a few of the larger HDL particles acquire multiple copies of apoE, and this leads to their endocytosis by hepatocytes (Fig. 25.7). It is now apparent that cholesterol from the extrahepatic tissues can reach the liver by three routes:

- *The apo-E mediated endocytosis of remnant particles,* which have obtained part of their cholesterol esters from HDL.
- *The direct transfer of cholesterol esters from HDL during lipolysis by HL, mediated by SR-BI.*
- *The endocytosis of large apo-E containing HDL particles.*

Of these three mechanisms, the pathway through CETP and remnant particles is quantitatively the most important in humans.

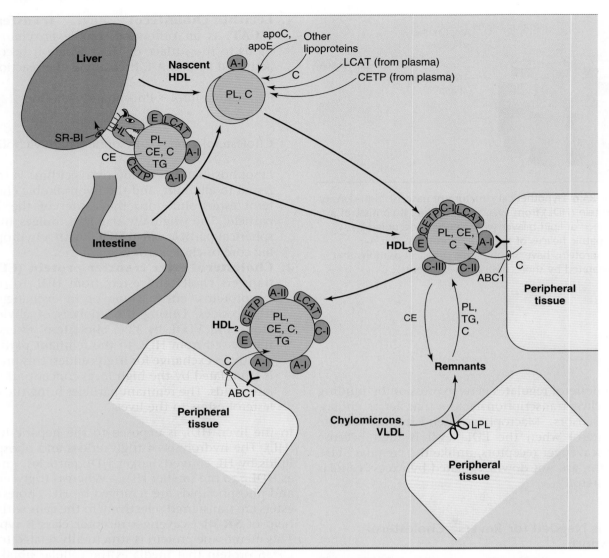

Figure 25.7 Metabolism of high-density lipoprotein (HDL). All HDL apolipoproteins can be exchanged with other lipoprotein classes. A-I, A-II, C-I, C-II, C-III, and E, apoA-I, apoA-II, apoC-I, apoC-II, apoC-III, and apoE; ABC1, ATP-binding cassette protein 1; C, cholesterol; CE, cholesterol esters; CETP, cholesterol ester transfer protein; HL, hepatic lipase; LCAT, lecithin-cholesterol acyl transferase; LPL, lipoprotein lipase; PL, phospholipid; SR-BI, scavenger receptor B-I; TG, triglyceride; VLDL, very-low-density lipoprotein.

Lipoproteins Are Risk Factors for Atherosclerosis

Atherosclerosis is the most common form of arteriosclerosis. Its complications include coronary heart disease (CHD) and acute myocardial infarction, gangrene, strokes, and even some forms of senile dementia. Together, these complications account for between one third and one half of all deaths in affluent societies.

The characteristic lesion of atherosclerosis is the **atheromatous plaque** in the intima of large arteries. Typical plaques contain a core of cholesterol esters surrounded by an area of fibrosis, often with calcification. The plaque impairs blood flow by narrowing the lumen of the artery, and it can lead to further changes and complications, including hemorrhage into the plaque and thrombosis.

The origins of atheromatous plaques are still somewhat obscure, but the deposition of cholesterol esters in the arterial wall is considered an early event. In essence, LDL enters the arterial wall by transcytosis across the endothelium. Macrophages take up the LDL through their scavenger receptors and store the LDL-derived cholesterol as cholesterol ester in cytoplasmic lipid droplets. These lipid-laden macrophages are called **foam cells.** Some of the foam cells die, and their cholesterol esters end up

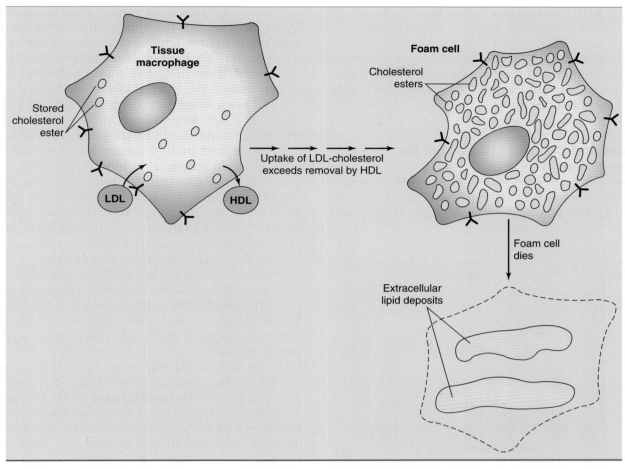

Figure 25.8 Hypothetical model for the formation of a fatty streak. The extracellular lipid deposits of the fatty streak are thought to induce a fibroproliferative response, leading eventually to the formation of an atheromatous plaque. Y indicates a scavenger receptor. HDL, high-density lipoprotein; LDL, low-density lipoprotein.

in the extracellular matrix. This extracellular lipid, damaged by nonenzymatic oxidation, is hard to metabolize. The resulting **fatty streak** is an early, reversible lesion that is common even in children. Most fatty streaks regress spontaneously, but some progress into atheromatous plaques.

The lipid deposits can act as a proinflammatory stimulus on surrounding cells, stimulating the release of soluble cytokines and growth factors. Some of the cytokines attract additional monocytes that become tissue macrophages, and growth factors cause the abnormal proliferation of fibroblasts and smooth muscle cells, leading to the excessive deposition of extracellular matrix.

Lipids and cytokines also help to induce or maintain the expression of cell adhesion molecules on the surface of endothelial cells that attract additional monocytes into the vessel wall. This is most likely at places where the endothelium is otherwise stressed or damaged: for example, by rheological

stress at arterial bifurcations or by hypertension. Platelets that are activated at the site of endothelial damage release platelet-derived growth factor, which attracts smooth muscle cells and fibroblasts.

LDL cholesterol is the "bad cholesterol" that promotes atherosclerosis. HDL cholesterol, in contrast, is the "good cholesterol" that reduces atherosclerosis. Presumably, LDL is bad because it brings cholesterol into the arterial wall, and HDL is good because it removes excess cholesterol. In essence, *a fatty streak develops when the amount of cholesterol supplied by LDL exceeds the amount of cholesterol removed by HDL* (Fig. 25.8).

In the clinical laboratory, the total cholesterol and triglyceride levels are determined directly from fresh plasma or serum. HDL cholesterol is determined after the selective precipitation of LDL and VLDL by phosphotungstate or some other polyanion. LDL cholesterol (in mg/dL) is estimated with the formula

LDL cholesterol = Total cholesterol −
(HDL cholesterol + 0.16 × Triglycerides)

The reagents used for routine cholesterol determination contain a cholesterol esterase, and therefore the measured "cholesterol" is actually free cholesterol + cholesterol esters.

Genes and Diet Are Risk Factors for Atherosclerosis

The most important risk factors of atherosclerosis and CHD are *advanced age, male gender, smoking, dia-* *betes mellitus, hypertension, and hypercholesterolemia.* Figure 25.9 shows the relationship between the total plasma cholesterol level and the incidence of death from CHD. Because two thirds of the plasma cholesterol is in LDL, the total cholesterol level reflects mainly the level of LDL cholesterol.

Some environmental effects on LDL and HDL cholesterol are summarized in Table 25.4. The effects of saturated and unsaturated fatty acids are most likely mediated by nuclear receptors that regulate gene expression after binding the fatty acid, but, overall, disappointingly little is known about the mechanisms by which environmental agents affect blood lipoprotein levels. However, there is evidence that dietary and pharmacological interventions that raise the HDL level or decrease the LDL level actually reduce the risk of CHD.

Other risk factors are less easily manipulated. Premenopausal women have less CHD than do men, possibly because their HDL level is 20% higher. Mother Nature is not politically correct. She discriminates against males and even more against senior citizens.

Lipoprotein(a) [**Lp(a)**] is an important genetic risk factor. This unusual form of LDL contains the glycoprotein **apolipoprotein(a)** disulfide-bonded to apoB-100. *Elevated Lp(a) concentrations are an independent risk factor for atherosclerosis.* The plasma level of Lp(a) can range from less than 5 to more than 100 mg/dL, depending on promoter variations in the *lp(a)* gene. Unlike ordinary LDL, Lp(a) does not seem to respond to dietary manipulations.

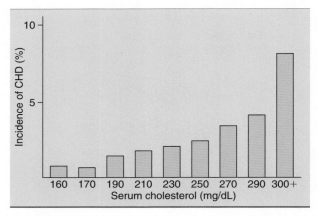

Figure 25.9 Relationship between the plasma cholesterol level and death from coronary heart disease (CHD).

Table 25.4 Effects of Various Manipulations on Plasma Lipid Levels and the Risk of CHD*

Manipulation	LDL Cholesterol	HDL Cholesterol	VLDL Triglycerides	Risk of CHD	Other Effects
Weight gain	(↑)	↓	↑	↑	High CETP
Weight reduction	(↓)	↑	↓	↓	
Saturated fat	↑	(↑)		↑	
Polyunsaturated fat	↓	(↓)		↓	
Dietary cholesterol	↑	(↑)		↑	
Regular alcohol consumption	(↑)	↑	↑	(↓)	Can cause alcoholic cardiomyopathy
Cigarette smoking		↓		↑	Causes oxidative damage of lipoproteins
Regular exercise		↑		↓	High lipoprotein lipase, low hepatic lipase
Diabetes mellitus	(↑)	(↓)	↑	↑	
Hypothyroidism	↑			↑	
Androgen treatment	(↑)	↓			
Estrogen-rich birth control pills	(↑)	↑	↑	(↓)	
Progesterone-rich birth control pills	(↑)	↓	↑	(↑)	
Antioxidant vitamins (C and E)				↓	Prevent oxidative damage of lipoproteins

*↑, increase; ↓, decrease. Weak and/or inconsistent effects are in parentheses.
CETP, cholesterol ester transfer protein; CHD, coronary heart disease; HDL, high-density lipoprotein; LDL, low-density lipoprotein; VLDL, very-low-density lipoprotein.

Deficiencies of Individual Lipoprotein Classes Are Cause of Severe Diseases

The functions of the lipoprotein classes are highlighted by some rare genetic diseases.

Abetalipoproteinemia is caused by the inherited *deficiency of a triglyceride transfer protein in the ER.* This makes the liver and intestine of affected homozygotes unable to assemble and secrete the triglyceride-rich, apoB-containing lipoproteins. LDL, VLDL, and chylomicrons are essentially absent, and plasma cholesterol and triglyceride levels are reduced to 20% or 25% of normal.

This disease leads to severe fat malabsorption and steatorrhea and to the accumulation of triglycerides in the intestinal mucosa and the liver. In the absence of LDL, cholesterol transport to the tissues depends on apoE-rich HDL particles. These particles undergo endocytosis through "LDL" receptors that recognize both apoB and apoE. Deficiencies of fat-soluble vitamins are often severe, and untreated patients develop spinocerebellar ataxia, an atypical form of retinitis pigmentosa, myopathy, and acanthocytosis (star-shaped red blood cells). These clinical signs respond to treatment with megadoses of vitamin E.

Tangier disease is characterized by the virtual absence of HDL in affected homozygotes. It is caused by the *absence of the membrane protein ABC1,* which transfers free cholesterol from cells to HDL particles that are docked at the cell surface. In its absence, the A-apolipoproteins never acquire their lipid component, and HDL particles cannot be formed.

The LDL level is also reduced to about one third of normal, probably because the transfer of cholesterol esters from HDL to VLDL remnants is no longer possible, but the VLDL level is normal or mildly elevated.

Affected patients have deposits of cholesterol esters in reticuloendothelial cells, bone marrow, and Schwann cells, and they develop peripheral neuropathy, hepatosplenomegaly, and lymphadenopathy. A telltale orange discoloration of the tonsils is caused by cholesterol esters that are colored by dietary carotene. Despite the HDL deficiency, there is only a mild tendency for early atherosclerosis, because the decreased LDL level reduces the need for reverse cholesterol transport.

Defects of LDL Receptors Cause Familial Hypercholesterolemia

Familial hypercholesterolemia (**FH**) is caused by a *deficiency of LDL receptors in liver and extrahepatic tissues.* The number of functional LDL receptors is reduced to 50% of normal in heterozygotes, and this is sufficient to double the level of LDL cholesterol. The total plasma cholesterol level is between 250 and 500 mg/dL, with an average of 350 mg/dL. Being impaired in their ability to acquire cholesterol from LDL, the cells respond by increasing the rate of endogenous synthesis (see Fig. 25.5).

Xanthomas, typically in the form of tendon xanthomas, develop in most affected patients after 20 years of age. Xanthomas are visible subcutaneous lipid deposits, usually yellow or brownish in color. Like the fatty streaks in arterial walls, they represent accumulations of lipoprotein-derived lipids, initially within tissue macrophages. Xanthomas occur not only in FH but in many other hyperlipidemic states as well. They are important for the differential diagnosis of lipoprotein disorders.

More serious than the xanthomas is CHD. In a study in England, 5% of male FH heterozygotes suffered their first myocardial infarction by age 30, 51% by age 50, and 85% by age 60. *Approximately 5% of all myocardial infarctions before age 60 occur in patients with FH.* The diagnosis is based on the presence of plasma cholesterol levels in excess of 260 mg/dL, tendon xanthomas, and a positive family history for CHD.

Heterozygous FH has a frequency in the vicinity of 1 per 500 in many populations. Homozygosity is rare, with a frequency of 1 per 1 million. The homozygotes have no functional LDL receptors, and their plasma cholesterol is in the range of 600 to 1200 mg/dL. They develop rampant atherosclerosis, and many die of CHD before age 20. The pathways in normal individuals and in FH are summarized in Figure 25.10.

Many mutations in the LDL receptor gene have been identified as causes of FH. They include complete and partial gene deletions, receptors that are not translocated from their site of synthesis in the ER to the plasma membrane, receptors that cannot bind LDL, and receptors that fail to trigger endocytosis even though they can bind LDL. These mutations are common because in the heterozygous state, they usually kill their victims only after the end of the reproductive age, when the mutation has already been transmitted to their offspring. Thus, there is not much selection against them.

Deficiencies of LCAT and CETP Prevent Reverse Cholesterol Transport

Other inherited diseases impair reverse cholesterol transport. In **familial LCAT deficiency,** the cholesterol acquired by HDL cannot be esterified to cholesterol esters. This inability leads to variable hypercholesterolemia and hypertriglyceridemia, and most of the lipoprotein cholesterol is in the

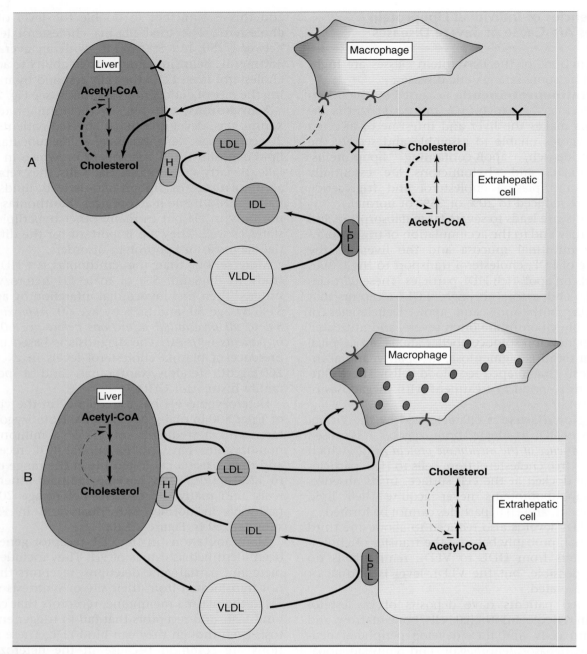

Figure 25.10 Metabolism of LDL in normal individuals and in patients with homozygous familial hypercholesterolemia. **A,** Normal: Both liver and extrahepatic tissues obtain most of their cholesterol from receptor-mediated low-density lipoprotein (LDL) uptake. The LDL-derived cholesterol inhibits endogenous synthesis at the level of HMG-CoA reductase. Y indicates a LDL receptor; Υ, a scavenger receptor. HL, hepatic lipase; IDL, intermediate-density lipoprotein; LPL, lipoprotein lipase; VLDL, very-low-density lipoprotein. **B,** Familial hypercholesterolemia, homozygous. LDL is redirected from parenchymal cells in liver and extrahepatic tissues to tissue macrophages, which become foam cells. These foam cells contribute to the formation of xanthomas, fatty streaks, and atherosclerotic lesions.

form of free cholesterol rather than cholesterol esters. The lipoproteins have abnormal shapes, and both LDL and HDL levels are reduced. Free cholesterol accumulates in many tissues, and clinical findings include severe corneal clouding and kidney disease. There is only a mild tendency for early atherosclerosis.

CETP deficiency is a benign condition in which the cholesterol esters formed by LCAT cannot be transferred from HDL to other lipoproteins.

Table 25.5 Important Determinants for Hyperlipidemia and Atherosclerosis

Risk Factor	Normal Functoin	Relation to Plasma Lipids and Atherosclerosis
Lipoprotein lipase (LPL)	Hydrolysis of triglycerides in chylomicrons and VLDL	Deficiency leads to hyperchylomicronemia but not atherosclerosis
Hepatic lipase (HL)	Hydrolysis of triglycerides and phosphoglycerides in HDL and remnant particles; possibly facilitates hepatic uptake of chylomicron remnants and transfer of cholesterol esters from HDL to the liver	Activity is inversely related to the plasma HDL concentration; lower in females than in males; complete deficiency causes severe hypercholesterolemia, hypertriglyceridemia, and possibly increased atherosclerosis
ApoB-100	Major structural apolipoprotein of VLDL and LDL; ligand of the "LDL receptor"	High in patients with type II or type IV hyperlipoproteinemia; high levels are associated with high atherosclerosis risk
ApoA-I	Major apolipoprotein of HDL; mediates binding of HDL to cells, facilitates transfer of unesterified cholesterol from cells to HDL	High level of apoA-I—(but not apoA-I—*and* apoA-II—) containing HDL is associated with decreased atherosclerosis risk; higher in females than in males; low in patients with CHD and their relatives; high in octogenarians
ApoE	Cellular uptake of remnant particles; stimulation of cholesterol transfer from cells to HDL	Homozygosity for apoE-2 causes dysbetalipoproteinemia; knockout mice lacking apoE have impaired flux of cholesterol from cells to HDL and develop rampant atherosclerosis
LDL receptor (apoB-100/ apoE receptor)	Cellular uptake of LDL, in both liver and extrahepatic tissues	Deficiency leads to high LDL and atherosclerosis
Lecithin-cholesterol acyl transferase (LCAT)	Formation of cholesterol esters in HDL	Homozygous deficiency leads to moderately increased atherosclerosis risk
Cholesterol ester transfer protein (CETP)	Transfer of cholesterol esters from HDL to triglyceride-rich lipoproteins; activated in the presence of LPL	Inversely related to plasma HDL level; induced by hypercholesterolemia
ABC1	Transfer of free cholesterol from cells to HDL	Homozygous deficiency causes Tangier disease
SR-BI	Transport of cholesterol esters from HDL into cells	Unknown

CHD; coronary heart disease; HDL, high-density lipoprotein; LDL, low-density lipoprotein; VLDL, very-low-density lipoprotein.

Affected homozygotes have a fourfold elevation of HDL cholesterol (100 to 250 mg/dL), but LDL cholesterol is normal or low (35 to 150 mg/dL). The HDL particles are oversized, with abundant cholesterol ester and very little triglyceride. Even heterozygotes have mildly elevated HDL cholesterol levels. Reverse cholesterol transport is possible even in homozygotes because cholesterol esters can still reach the liver by direct transfer from HDL through SR-BI and by the endocytosis of apo-E–coated HDL particles.

CETP deficiency is common in Japan, where 1% of the population are heterozygous for an allele that causes a complete lack of cholesterol ester transfer in homozygotes. Another 5% of Japanese are heterozygous for a CETP variant that causes more moderate increases of HDL cholesterol levels. The effect of these traits on the risk of CHD is uncertain.

The roles of various apolipoproteins, lipoprotein receptors, and enzymes of lipoprotein metabolism are summarized in Table 25.5.

Hyperlipoproteinemias Are Grouped into Five Phenotypes

The hyperlipidemias are said to have a combined prevalence of 5% to 20% in affluent populations although, as usual, the cutoff between normal and abnormal is more than a bit arbitrary. Five types are distinguished, depending on the lipoprotein class that is affected (Table 25.6). They are not diseases but phenotypes that occur in a variety of contexts. In rare instances—as in FH—the condition can be blamed on a single faulty gene. More commonly, it is related to a chronic disease, diet and lifestyle, and/or multifactorial genetic predisposition.

TYPE I HYPERLIPOPROTEINEMIA

Type I hyperlipoproteinemia, or **hyperchylomicronemia,** is caused by impaired hydrolysis of chylomicron triglycerides. It is a rare condition

Table 25.6 The Five Hyperlipoproteinemia Phenotypes. Elevations of lipid levels range from minimal (↑) to massive ↑↑↑

| Type | Name | Plasma Lipids | | Fraction Elevated | Incidence | Causes |
		Triglyceride	Cholesterol			
I	Hyperchylomicronemia	↑↑↑	(↑)	Chylomicrons	Rare	Inherited deficiency of LPL or apoC-II, systemic lupus erythematosus, or unknown
II	Hypercholesterolemia	(↑)	↑↑	LDL	Common	Primary: familial hypercholesterolemia; secondary: obesity, poor dietary habits, hypothyroidism, diabetes mellitus, nephrotic syndrome
III	Dysbetalipoproteinemia	↑	↑	Chylomicron remnants, VLDL remnants	Rare	Homozygosity for apoE2 (does not bind to hepatic apoE receptors), combined with poor dietary habits
IV	Hypertriglyceridemia	↑↑	↑	VLDL	Common	Diabetes mellitus, obesity, alcoholism, poor dietary habits
V	—	↑↑	↑	Chylomicrons, VLDL	Rare	Obesity, diabetes mellitus, alcoholism, oral contraceptives

LDL, low-density lipoprotein; LPL, lipoprotein lipase; VLDL, very-low-density lipoprotein.

(prevalence, 1 per 10,000) that can be caused by inherited deficiencies of LPL or its activator, apoC-II. In severe cases, the hypertriglyceridemia can reach a level of 1000 mg/dL. LDL level, however, is decreased to 20% of normal or less, and most of the plasma cholesterol is present in VLDL rather than LDL. This shows the importance of VLDL lipolysis for the formation of LDL. *The type I pattern does not lead to atherosclerosis and CHD.* Affected patients have eruptive cutaneous xanthomas, abdominal pain after fatty meals, and recurrent attacks of pancreatitis. The treatment consists of a low-fat diet.

TYPE II HYPERLIPOPROTEINEMIA

Type II hyperlipoproteinemia, or **hypercholesterolemia,** is an elevation of the LDL level. It includes FH, but multifactorial and secondary forms are at least 10 times more common. In some affected patients, only LDL level is elevated (type IIa). Others have a combined elevation of LDL and VLDL (type IIb). Weight gain and obesity, diabetes mellitus, and a diet high in cholesterol and saturated fat are the main culprits, but genetic factors other than a deficiency of LDL receptors are also involved. *This pattern is a major risk factor for atherosclerosis and CHD.*

TYPE III HYPERLIPOPROTEINEMIA

Type III hyperlipoproteinemia, or **dysbetalipoproteinemia,** is caused by homozygosity for apoE2, a genetic variant of apoE that does not bind to hepatic apoE receptors. This results in the accumulation of chylomicron remnants and IDL-like VLDL remnants in the blood. The presence of *cholesterol-rich β-migrating lipoproteins with VLDL-like density* in a hyperlipidemic patient is diagnostic for type III hyperlipoproteinemia.

The phagocytosis of remnant particles by macrophages leads to palmar xanthomas and tuboeruptive xanthomas on knees, elbows, and buttocks. Atherosclerosis shows a predilection for peripheral arteries, but the CHD risk is increased as well. Although 1% of the population have the offending apoE genotype, only 2% to 10% of these persons actually become hyperlipidemic. Most patients respond well to dietary management.

TYPE IV HYPERLIPOPROTEINEMIA

Type IV hyperlipoproteinemia, or **hypertriglyceridemia,** consists of elevated VLDL. Although triglyceride levels are elevated to a greater extent than is cholesterol, some hypercholesterolemia is usually present and *the atherosclerosis risk is increased.* This is a common type that is

Table 25.7 The Most Commonly Used Antihyperlipidemic Drugs

Drug Type	Mechanism of Action	Uses	Lipoprotein Effects
Statins (e.g., lovastatin)	Inhibition of HMG-CoA reductase	First-line treatment for hypercholesterolemia	↓↓ LDL
Bile acid binding resins (e.g., cholestyramine)	Interruption of enterohepatic circulation of bile acids	Hypercholesterolemia	↓ LDL
Niacin	Reduces lipolysis in adipose tissue and VLDL formation in the liver	Both type II and type IV hyperlipoproteinemia, but many side effects	↓ VLDL ↓ LDL ↑ HDL
Fibrates (e.g., clofibrate, gemfibrozil)	PPAR-α agonists that increase LPL, apoA-I, apoA-II, and decrease apoC-III	Hypertriglyceridemia	↓↓ VLDL ↑ HDL

HDL, high-density lipoprotein; HMG-CoA, 3-hydroxy-3-methylglutaryl–coenzyme A; LDL, low-density lipoprotein; LPL, lipoprotein lipase; PPAR, peroxisome proliferator–activated receptor; VLDL, very-low-density lipoprotein.

related to obesity, type II diabetes mellitus, alcoholism, progesterone-rich contraceptives, and excess dietary carbohydrate (especially sugar).

TYPE V HYPERLIPOPROTEINEMIA

Type V hyperlipoproteinemia consists of combined elevations of chylomicrons and VLDL. Although this pattern often has a familial background, it is also associated with uncontrolled diabetes mellitus, alcoholism, obesity, and kidney disease. Dietary treatment is effective.

Both Diet and Drugs Affect Plasma Lipoproteins

Most hyperlipoproteinemias respond to dietary modification. As a rule, hypertriglyceridemias tend to be more responsive than hypercholesterolemias. The recommendation for hypertriglyceridemic patients is *a reduction of caloric intake, alcohol, and simple carbohydrates.* For hypercholesterolemia, *less cholesterol and saturated fat and more unsaturated fat and dietary fiber* are recommended. In obese patients, a balanced weight-reduction diet is likely to normalize the lipoprotein levels without the need for any further treatment.

Dietary treatment is of little practical use because few patients comply with a physician-imposed diet; pill-popping is far easier. Therefore, hyperlipidemias, and especially hypercholesterolemias, are usually treated with drugs. Two important drug classes reduce the plasma cholesterol level by interfering with critical steps in cholesterol metabolism:

1. The **statins** are inhibitors of HMG-CoA reductase. Endogenous cholesterol synthesis is blocked, and the reduced level of free cholesterol in the cells induces the synthesis of LDL receptors. (Fig. 25.11C; see also Fig. 25.5). By this mechanism, *the statins reduce LDL cholesterol levels with little effect on HDL cholesterol.*

2. **Cholestyramine** is an insoluble, nonabsorbable anion exchanger that binds bile acids in the lumen of the small intestine, preventing their absorption from the ileum. Instead of returning to the liver, the bile acids are excreted in the stools. Because bile acids feedback-inhibit their own synthesis in the liver (see Chapter 24), their diminished supply by the enterohepatic circulation *increases the conversion of cholesterol to bile acids by the liver.* The resulting depletion of the cellular cholesterol pool leads to an *upregulation of hepatic LDL receptors* and a reduction of the LDL (but not HDL) level in the plasma (see Fig. 25.11B). A high-fiber diet lowers LDL cholesterol by the same mechanism as cholestyramine: by impairing the absorption of bile acids from the ileum.

Some other lipid-lowering drugs are included in Table 25.7. **Antioxidant vitamins** do not reduce the LDL level but slow down the oxidation of LDL. Because oxidized LDL is a preferred substrate for macrophage scavenger receptors, these vitamins reduce cholesterol accumulation in macrophages.

SUMMARY

The plasma lipoproteins transport triglycerides, phospholipids and cholesterol in the blood. There are three highways of lipoprotein-based lipid transport:

1. Lipids of dietary origin are transported from the intestine to other tissues as constituents of chylomicrons. Lipolysis by the extrahepatic LPL produces remnant particles that undergo endocytosis by hepatocytes through apoE receptors.

2. Lipids from endogenous synthesis in the liver are released as constituents of VLDL. The

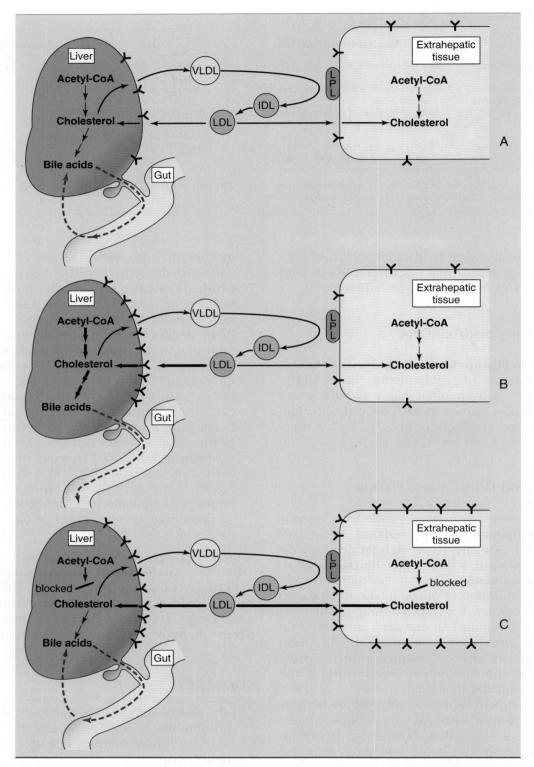

Figure 25.11 Effects of a bile acid binding resin (cholestyramine) and a 3-hydroxy-3-methylglutaryl–coenzyme A (HMG-CoA) reductase inhibitor (lovastatin) on cholesterol metabolism. **A,** Normal or hyperlipidemic. **Y** indicates a low-density lipoprotein (LDL) receptor. LPL, extrahepatic lipoprotein lipase; IDL, intermediate-density lipoprotein; VLDL, very-low-density lipoprotein. **B,** Effect of cholestyramine: Hepatic LDL receptors are up-regulated. The liver removes an increased amount of LDL to obtain cholesterol for bile acid synthesis. **C,** Effect of lovastatin: LDL receptors are up-regulated in all tissues. The cells require an increased amount of LDL cholesterol because they are unable to obtain cholesterol from endogenous synthesis.

VLDL triglycerides are hydrolyzed by LPL, and some of the resulting remnant particles are processed to LDL. Most of the triglyceride in normal fasting serum is present in VLDL, and most of the cholesterol is in LDL. LDL undergoes endocytosis both in the liver and in extrahepatic tissues.

3. In the reverse transport of cholesterol from extrahepatic tissues to the liver, HDL acquires free cholesterol from the cells. This cholesterol is esterified by the HDL-associated enzyme LCAT. The resulting cholesterol esters are transferred either to other lipoproteins or directly to hepatocytes.

The deposition of cholesterol esters in the arterial wall can promote atherosclerosis. A high level of LDL favors lipid deposition and atherosclerosis, and a high level of HDL is protective against those developments.

Some hyperlipidemias are caused by major genetic defects, but most cases result from lipid-elevating lifestyles and polygenic inheritance or are secondary to chronic diseases.

📖 Further Reading

Bruce C, Chuinard RA, Tall AR: Plasma lipid transfer proteins, high-density lipoproteins, and reverse cholesterol transport. Annu Rev Nutr 18:297-330, 1998.

Choy PC, Siow YL, Mymin D, et al: Lipids and atherosclerosis. Biochem Cell Biol 82:212-224, 2004.

Glass CK, Witztum JL: Atherosclerosis: the road ahead. Cell 104:503-516, 2001.

Jin W, Marchadier D, Rader DJ: Lipases and HDL metabolism. Trends Endocrinol Metab 13:174-178, 2002.

Krieger M: Charting the fate of the "good cholesterol": identification and characterization of the high-density lipoprotein receptor SR-BI. Annu Rev Biochem 68:523-558, 1999.

Lippi G, Guidi G: Lipoprotein(a): an emerging cardiovascular risk factor. Crit Rev Clin Lab Sci 40:1-42, 2003.

Mead JR, Irvine SA, Ramji DP: Lipoprotein lipase: structure, function, regulation, and role in disease. J Mol Med 80:753-769, 2002.

Moreno JJ, Mitjavila, MT: The degree of unsaturation of dietary fatty acids and the development of atherosclerosis. J Nutr Biochem 14:182-195, 2003.

Stender S, Dyerberg J: Influence of trans fatty acids on health. Ann Nutr Metab 48:61-66, 2004.

Young SG, Fielding CJ: The ABCs of cholesterol efflux. Nat Genet 22:316-318, 1999.

QUESTIONS

1. **A pharmaceutical company wants to develop a drug for the treatment of type IV hyperlipoproteinemia. The most promising approach would be an agent that**

   A. Increases the synthesis of apoB-100 in the liver.
   B. Prevents the synthesis of apoE.
   C. Stimulates the hormone-sensitive adipose tissue lipase.
   D. Inhibits LPL.
   E. Inhibits triglyceride synthesis in the liver.

2. **Cholestyramine can reduce the level of LDL cholesterol by increasing the activity of the liver enzyme**

   A. HMG-CoA reductase.
   B. LPL.
   C. HL.
   D. 7α-hydroxylase.
   E. LCAT

3. **The statins inhibit the endogenous synthesis of cholesterol, thereby reducing the level of free cholesterol in the cell. The reduced level of cellular cholesterol, in turn, leads to**

   A. Increased activity of ACAT.
   B. Increased synthesis of LDL receptors in most tissues.
   C. Reduced synthesis of LDL receptors in most tissues.
   D. Increased transfer of cholesterol esters from the cell to HDL.
   E. Increased synthesis of bile acids by the liver.

4. **If you are looking for ways to increase the reverse transport of cholesterol from peripheral tissues to the liver, the best bet would be a drug that**

   A. Inhibits the synthesis of LDL receptors.
   B. Inhibits hepatic lipase.
   C. Inhibits lipoprotein lipase.
   D. Stimulates the transcription of the apoB gene.
   E. Stimulates the transcription of the gene for the ABC1 protein.

CHAPTER 26

Amino Acid Metabolism

Amino acids are used for three major purposes:

1. *They are substrates for the generation of metabolic energy.* Most people in affluent countries obtain 15% to 20% of their metabolic energy from protein.
2. *They are substrates for protein synthesis.* Human body proteins are degraded and resynthesized continuously. Therefore, pools of free amino acids have to be maintained in all nucleated cells.
3. *They are substrates for the synthesis of many products,* including heme, purines, pyrimidines, several coenzymes, melanin, and the biogenic amines.

Only 11 of the 20 amino acids can be synthesized in the human body. Those that cannot be synthesized are called **essential amino acids.** They include

- Valine
- Threonine
- Leucine
- Methionine
- Isoleucine
- Lysine
- Phenylalanine
- Histidine
- Tryptophan

The nonessential amino acids are synthesized either from common metabolic intermediates or from other amino acids. This chapter describes the fate of the amino nitrogen during amino acid catabolism, the pathways by which amino acids are degraded to simple nitrogen-free metabolic intermediates, and the biosynthesis of the nonessential amino acids.

Most Amino Acids in the Human Body Are Present as Constituents of Proteins

The adult human body contains approximately 10 kg of protein, but the free amino acids are not abundant in tissues and body fluids. In the blood, the concentrations of the 20 amino acids combined are only 20 to 30 mg/dL, one fourth of the blood glucose level.

Figure 26.1 shows the metabolic fates of amino acids and proteins. The dietary intake is variable, but 100 g/day is typical. Another 250 to 300 g of amino acids comes from protein breakdown, but the same amount is consumed for protein synthesis. The life expectancy of an average protein is 35 to 40 days, but it differs widely from one protein to another. Most metabolic enzymes live for only one or a few days, but most plasma proteins circulate for 1 to 3 weeks. Hemoglobin survives for 120 days, collagen lasts up to several years in some tissues, and the lens proteins last for a lifetime.

Glucogenic amino acids feed into the TCA cycle or glycolysis. They can be used for gluconeogenesis. **Ketogenic amino acids** are degraded to acetyl-CoA. They are substrates for ketogenesis. Only leucine and lysine are purely ketogenic. Some of the larger amino acids, including isoleucine and the three aromatic amino acids phenylalanine, tyrosine, and tryptophan, are both. All other amino acids are glucogenic.

The nitrogen of the amino acids is incorporated in **urea,** a soluble, nontoxic product that is excreted in the urine.

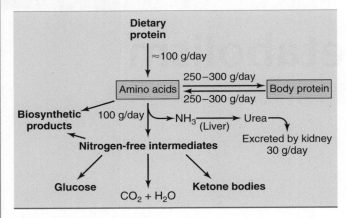

Figure 26.1 Metabolic interrelationships of amino acids.

The Nitrogen Balance Indicates the Net Rate of Protein Synthesis

Approximately 16 g of nitrogen is contained in 100 g of dietary protein. Approximately 83% of this ingested nitrogen eventually leaves the body as urea, 7% as ammonium ion, and 10% as organic waste products, including uric acid and creatinine. Ninety-five percent of the urea and a large majority of the other nitrogenous wastes are excreted in the urine, but 1 to 2 g of nitrogen from undigested protein is excreted in the stools.

The **nitrogen balance** is the difference between the nitrogen entering the body and that leaving it. A normal adult with adequate protein intake should be in **nitrogen equilibrium** (Fig. 26.2). This means that the amount of outgoing nitrogen matches exactly the amount of incoming nitrogen, and the amount of body protein remains constant.

A **positive nitrogen balance** is observed when nitrogen intake exceeds nitrogen excretion. It implies that the amount of body protein increases. Growing children, pregnant women, and bodybuilders have a positive nitrogen balance. Therefore, they have an increased requirement for dietary protein.

A **negative nitrogen balance** is observed in dietary protein deficiency. Even the protein-starved body degrades 30 to 40 g of amino acids every day. This amount defines the dietary requirement. Essential amino acid deficiency has the same effect because protein synthesis is impaired even if only one of the essential amino acids is missing.

Patients with chronic infections, cancer, or other severe diseases have a negative nitrogen balance because *glucocorticoids and other stress hormones favor protein degradation over protein synthesis,* thereby supplying amino acids for gluconeogenesis. Also, some **cytokines**—biologically active proteins released by

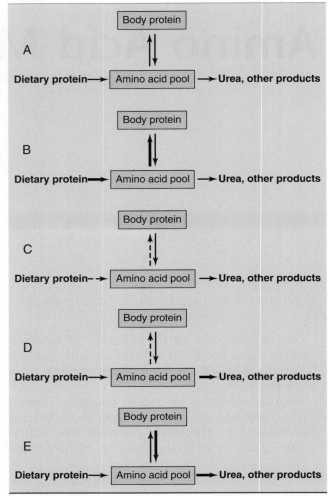

Figure 26.2 Nitrogen balance in different normal and abnormal states. **A,** Normal adult: nitrogen equilibrium. **B,** Growth, pregnancy: positive nitrogen balance. **C,** Protein deficiency: negative nitrogen balance. **D,** Essential amino acid deficiency: negative nitrogen balance. **E,** Wasting diseases, burns, trauma: negative nitrogen balance.

white blood cells in many diseases—have catabolic effects similar to those of the stress hormones.

The Amino Group of the Amino Acids Is Released as Ammonia

During amino acid catabolism, the nitrogen of the amino acids produces urea. Initially, however, it is released as ammonia. The most important ammonia-forming reaction, catalyzed by **glutamate dehydrogenase** in liver and other tissues, is shown in Figure 26.3A.

This oxidative deamination/reductive amination is freely reversible and can function both in the synthesis and the degradation of glutamate. Either

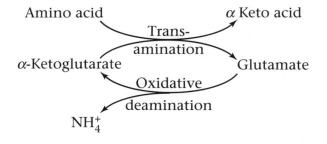

A

Glutamate

$\xrightarrow{\text{Glutamate dehydrogenase}}$ α-Ketoglutarate

with H$_2$O, NAD(P)$^+$ in, NH$_4^+$, NAD(P)H, H$^+$ out

B

Alanine + α-Ketoglutarate $\underset{\text{Alanine transaminase}}{\overset{B_6}{\rightleftharpoons}}$ Pyruvate + Glutamate

Aspartate + α-Ketoglutarate $\underset{\text{Aspartate transaminase}}{\overset{B_6}{\rightleftharpoons}}$ Oxaloacetate + Glutamate

Figure 26.3 The fate of the amino group during amino acid catabolism. **A,** The release of ammonia from glutamate in the glutamate dehydrogenase reaction. Although reversible, this reaction functions in glutamate degradation under most conditions. NAD(P), nicotinamide adenine dinucleotide (phosphate); NAD(P)H, reduced form of NAD(P). **B,** The transamination of alanine and aspartate. These reversible reactions transfer the amino group to α-ketoglutarate, forming glutamate. From glutamate, the nitrogen can be released as ammonia in the glutamate dehydrogenase reaction.

nicotinamide adenine dinucleotide (NAD) or nicotinamide adenine dinucleotide phosphate (NADP) can serve as a cosubstrate, but NAD$^+$ is mainly used for glutamate degradation, and NADPH is used for its synthesis. The glutamate dehydrogenase reaction implies that *glutamate is both nonessential and glucogenic.*

Most other amino acids do not form ammonia directly. *They transfer their α-amino group to α-ketoglutarate to form glutamate.* The enzymes that catalyze these reversible amino group transfers are called **transaminases** or **aminotransferases.** Examples are shown in Figure 26.3B.

At least a dozen different transaminases have been described in mammalian tissues. Most of them use glutamate/α-ketoglutarate as one of their substrates/products. *All amino acids except threonine, lysine, and proline can be transaminated.*

All transaminases contain **pyridoxal phosphate (PLP),** the coenzyme form of vitamin B$_6$, as a prosthetic group. PLP is bound to the active site of the enzyme by electrostatic interactions and by a Schiff base (aldimine) bond with a lysine side chain of the apoprotein. PLP participates directly in the reaction as shown in Figure 26.4.

Thus, the α-amino group is turned into ammonia by successive transamination and oxidative deamination:

Amino acid → α Keto acid (Transamination)

α-Ketoglutarate ← Glutamate (via Transamination)

Glutamate → α-Ketoglutarate + NH$_4^+$ (Oxidative deamination)

Ammonia Is Detoxified into Urea

Ammonia is a hazardous waste. It is neurotoxic even in low concentrations, and therefore it has to be disposed of quickly. Being unable to excrete ammonia fast enough, humans turn it into nontoxic, water-soluble, and therefore easily excretable urea.

Urea is the diamide of carbonic acid. This dry statement implies that *urea can be cleaved into carbonic acid and ammonia.* The reaction is catalyzed by the bacterial enzyme **urease:**

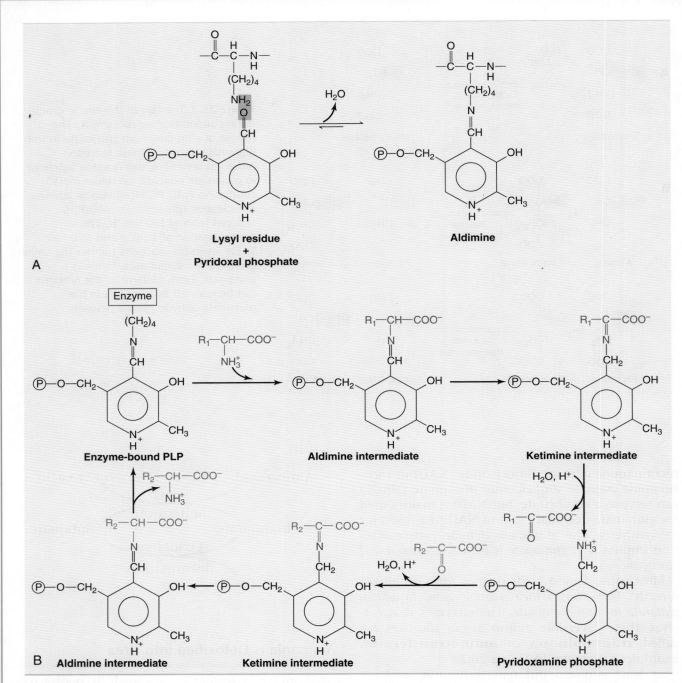

Figure 26.4 Mechanism of transamination reactions. **A,** Pyridoxal phosphate (PLP) is bound to a lysine side chain in the apoprotein by an aldimine ("Schiff base") bond. **B,** The catalytic cycle. The transamination is actually a sequence of two reactions in which the prosthetic group of the enzyme participates as a reactant.

$$H_2N-\overset{\overset{\displaystyle O}{\|}}{C}-NH_2$$

Urea

$$2\,H_2O \searrow \Big|\text{Urease}$$

$$HO-\overset{\overset{\displaystyle O}{\|}}{C}-OH + 2\,NH_3$$

Carbonic acid

This reaction does not normally occur in the human body, but it is important in urinary tract infections by the urease-producing bacterium *Proteus mirabilis*. The ammonia formed by the bacterial urease alkalinizes the urine, causing the precipitation of insoluble magnesium ammonium phosphate and the formation of large kidney stones. The sharp smell of latrines is ammonia formed by urease-producing bacteria.

Because urea contains 48% nitrogen by weight and proteins contain 16%, 1g of urea is formed from 3g of dietary protein—a total of 33g urea on a diet of 100g protein per day.

The blood urea level is measured as **blood urea nitrogen (BUN)**. In health, it is 250 to 700 µmol/liter (8 to 20 mg/dL). *The BUN rises sharply in renal failure.* This condition is called **uremia.** Urea is not responsible for most of the clinical manifestations of uremia, but BUN is a convenient measure for the retention of nitrogenous wastes.

Urea Is Synthesized in the Urea Cycle

Most amino acid catabolism takes place in the liver, and the liver is also the only important site for ammonia detoxification in the **urea cycle.** One of the substrates of the urea cycle is **carbamoyl phosphate,** which is synthesized from ammonia, carbon dioxide, and adenosine triphosphate (ATP):

$$NH_4^+ + CO_2 + 2\,ATP + H_2O$$

Carbamoyl phosphate synthetase (mitochondria) $\searrow$ 2 ADP, P$_i$, 3 H$^+$

$$H_2N-\overset{\overset{\displaystyle O}{\|}}{C}-O-\overset{\overset{\displaystyle O^-}{|}}{\underset{\underset{\displaystyle O}{\|}}{P}}-O^-$$

where ADP = adenosine diphosphate and P$_i$ = inorganic phosphate.

The use of two ATP molecules makes this reaction irreversible. The carbamoyl phosphate synthetase catalyzing this reaction requires **N-acetylglutamate** as an activator. This regulatory metabolite is formed by a separate enzyme from glutamate and acetyl-CoA. Carbamoyl phosphate synthetase is abundant in liver mitochondria, and its Michaelis constant (K_m) for ammonia (250 µmol/liter) is not much higher than the physiological ammonia concentration (30 to 60 µmol/liter). Therefore, it can maintain ammonia at this low level.

The reactions of the urea cycle proper are shown in Figure 26.5. *One of the two nitrogen atoms in urea*

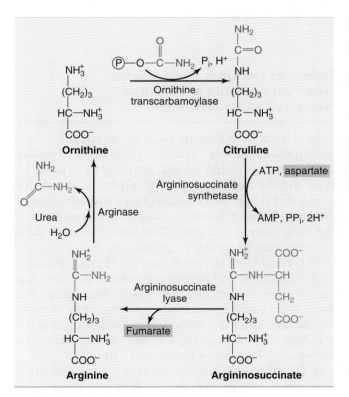

Figure 26.5 The reactions of the urea cycle.

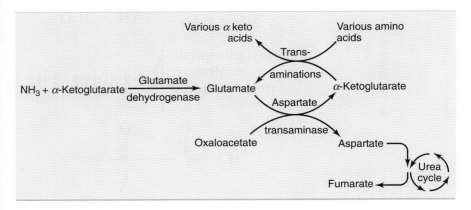

Figure 26.6 The sources of nitrogen for the argininosuccinate synthetase reaction of the urea cycle.

comes from ammonia via carbamoyl phosphate, and the other from aspartate. The aspartate nitrogen is derived either from ammonia, through the glutamate dehydrogenase reaction followed by transamination with oxaloacetate, or directly from transamination reactions (Fig. 26.6).

The synthesis of one urea molecule requires four high-energy phosphate bonds. Two ATP molecules are converted to ADP in the carbamoyl phosphate synthetase reaction, and another two phosphate bonds are consumed for the formation of argininosuccinate when one ATP molecule is hydrolyzed to AMP and inorganic pyrophosphate. *The nitrogen is committed to urea synthesis because the two reactions that introduce it into the cycle are made irreversible by ATP hydrolysis.*

Failure of the Urea Cycle Causes Hyperammonemia and Central Nervous System Dysfunction

Inherited deficiencies of urea cycle enzymes lead to *hyperammonemia and encephalopathy.* Feeding difficulties, vomiting, ataxia, lethargy or irritability, poor intellectual development, and a tendency for coma and death are common in all these disorders. Death in infancy or severe disability is inevitable if the deficiency is complete, but partial enzyme deficiencies lead to milder impairments.

The condition is aggravated by dietary protein, and therefore many patients spontaneously develop an aversion to protein-rich foods. The glutamine level is elevated in addition to ammonia because excess ammonia is diverted into glutamine synthesis. Also, the immediate substrate of the deficient enzyme is elevated in blood and urine.

A far more common cause of hyperammonemia is advanced **liver cirrhosis.** This condition is an end point of many pathological processes, alco-holism being the most common cause. Cirrhosis is characterized by *a progressive loss of hepatocytes, which are replaced by fibrous connective tissue.*

The proliferating connective tissue impairs blood flow through the liver. This leads to portal hypertension and the development of a collateral circulation. Venous channels in the lower esophagus and in the periumbilical, rectal, and retroperitoneal areas dilate, shunting blood from the portal vein to the systemic circulation. Portal hypertension is dangerous because it can result in the rupture of veins and fatal hemorrhage, especially from veins in the lower esophagus.

The biochemical derangements in liver cirrhosis cause **hepatic encephalopathy,** also known as **portal-systemic encephalopathy** because the shunting of blood around the cirrhotic liver is important in its pathogenesis. It is manifested by slurring of speech; blurring of vision; motor incoordination (ataxia); a characteristic coarse, flapping tremor (asterixis); and mental derangements. The condition can progress to **hepatic coma** and death. Although other biochemical abnormalities have been implicated as well, *hyperammonemia is a major cause of the central nervous system disorder.*

Foul-smelling breath is an important diagnostic sign. It is caused by volatile sulfhydryl compounds (mercaptans). These products are formed from dietary cysteine and methionine by intestinal bacteria. Ordinarily, the mercaptans are oxidized to nonvolatile, odorless products in the liver. In liver cirrhosis, however, they can reach the lungs and are exhaled.

For long-term management, *a low-protein, alcohol-free diet is the mainstay of treatment for liver cirrhosis.* The replacement of essential amino acids by their corresponding α-keto acids is an effective (but expensive) way of reducing the total nitrogen intake without precipitating essential amino acid deficiencies. Because of the transamination reac-

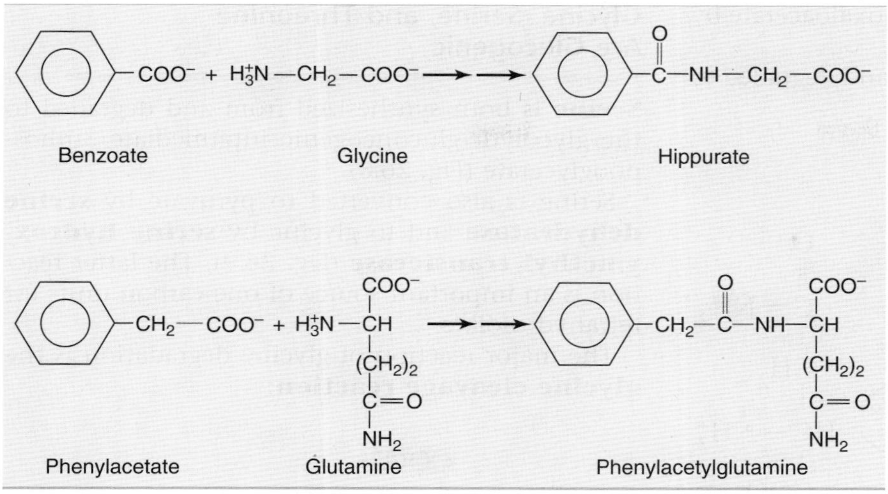

Figure 26.7 The use of benzoate and phenylacetate for the treatment of hyperammonemia in liver cirrhosis and inherited urea cycle enzyme deficiencies. The amino acid conjugates of these organic acids provide alternative routes of nitrogen excretion.

tions, most of the essential amino acids are no longer essential when their corresponding α-keto acids are present in the diet.

Other treatments exploit alternative routes of nitrogen excretion. High oral doses of **benzoic acid** and **phenylacetic acid** are helpful because these organic acids become conjugated with glycine and glutamine, respectively, as shown in Figure 26.7.

The conjugation products are excreted in the urine. Ordinarily, these reactions are not important for nitrogen excretion, but they are used for the disposal of unwanted organic acids from dietary sources.

Intestinal bacteria are an important source of ammonia. Undigested dietary proteins are fermented by bacteria in the ileum and colon, and part of their nitrogen is released as ammonia. Additional ammonia is formed from urea in digestive secretions, which is cleaved to carbonic acid and ammonia by bacterial ureases. Sterilization of the gastrointestinal tract by broad-spectrum antibiotics can therefore be beneficial for patients with hepatic encephalopathy, although there is a danger of overgrowth by drug-resistant bacteria with resulting enterocolitis.

Some Amino Acids Are Closely Related to Common Metabolic Intermediates

Some amino acids are close relatives of metabolic intermediates that were described previously in the major metabolic pathways. **Alanine,** for example, is structurally and metabolically related to pyruvate. These two molecules are interconverted in the reversible **alanine transaminase** reaction:

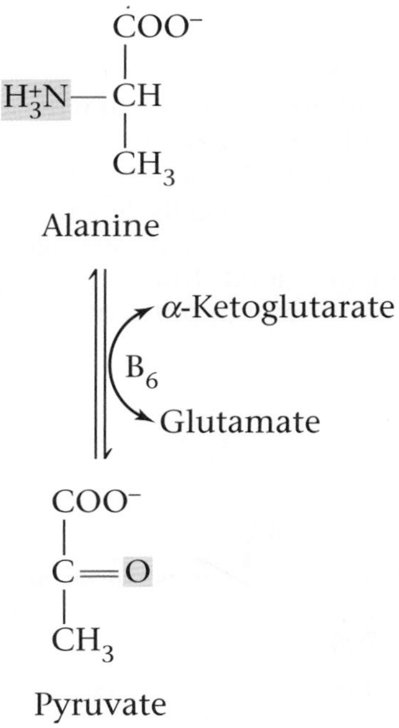

Glutamate is similarly related to α-ketoglutarate, both by transamination reactions and through glutamate dehydrogenase. **Glutamine** is both synthesized from and degraded to glutamate:

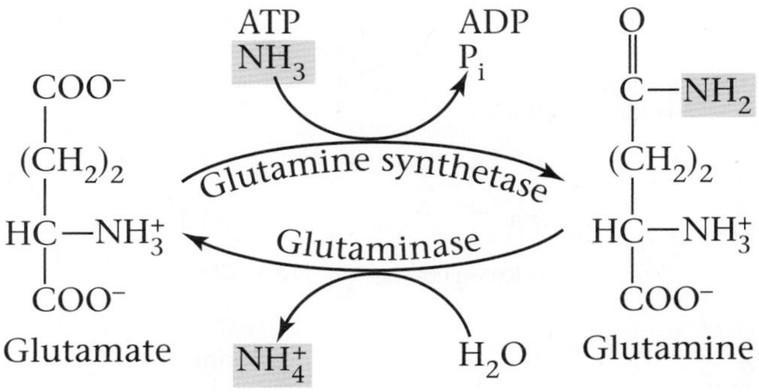

Aspartate is interconvertible with oxaloacetate by transamination.

Asparagine is synthesized from and degraded to aspartate:

Parenterally administered asparaginase has been used in cases of adult leukemia in which the malignant cells have lost the ability to synthesize asparagine. These cancer cells depend on asparagine from the blood. The injected asparaginase destroys asparagine in the blood, thus depriving the malignant cells of an essential nutrient.

Glycine, Serine, and Threonine Are Glucogenic

Serine is both synthesized from and degraded to the glycolytic-gluconeogenic intermediate 3-phosphoglycerate (Fig. 26.8).

Serine is also converted to pyruvate by **serine dehydratase** and to glycine by **serine hydroxymethyl transferase** (Fig. 26.9). The latter reaction is an important source of one-carbon units for tetrahydrofolate.

The major reaction of glycine degradation is the **glycine cleavage reaction:**

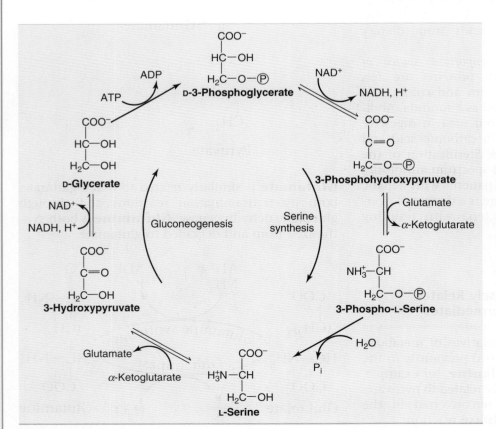

Figure 26.8 Metabolic interconversion of serine and the glycolytic intermediate 3-phosphoglycerate. ADP, adenosine diphosphate; ATP, adenosine triphosphate; NAD$^+$, nicotinamide adenine dinucleotide; NADH, reduced form of NAD; P$_i$, inorganic phosphate.

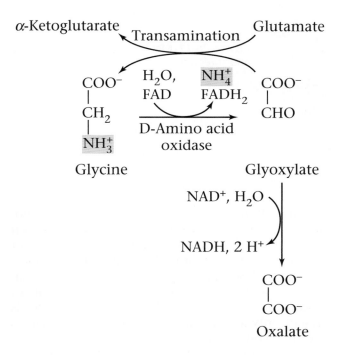

Figure 26.9 The catabolism of serine.

Inherited deficiencies in the glycine-cleaving enzyme cause **nonketotic hyperglycinemia.** This rare, recessively inherited disease (1 per 250,000 liveborn infants) can cause death in infancy and profound mental retardation in the not-so-lucky survivors.

Glycine can also form **glyoxylate,** in a reaction that is catalyzed by the peroxisomal flavoprotein **D–amino acid oxidase.** Glyoxylate is either transaminated back to glycine or oxidized to **oxalate:**

where FAD = flavin adenine dinucleotide, FADH$_2$ = reduced form of FAD, and NADH = reduced form of NAD. *Most kidney stones consist of calcium oxalate.* Some of this oxalate is derived from leafy vegetables in the diet, and some is formed in the body from glycine. Bacteria (but not humans) can convert glycine into **trimethylamine:**

where SAH = *S*-adenosyl homocysteine and SAM = *S*-adenosyl methionine. Trimethylamine is distinguished by its scent, which resembles that of stale fish. It is formed during the bacterial decomposition of many protein-rich substrates. The typical smell is most noticeable under alkaline conditions (for example, in the presence of soap) when the volatile free base is released from the protonated form.

Threonine cannot be synthesized in the human body, but there are several pathways for its degradation, as shown in Figure 26.10. Figure 26.11 summarizes the metabolic relationships of serine, glycine, and threonine.

Proline, Arginine, Ornithine, and Histidine Are Degraded to Glutamate

Proline, arginine, and **ornithine** are degraded to glutamate, as shown in Figure 26.12. Proline can

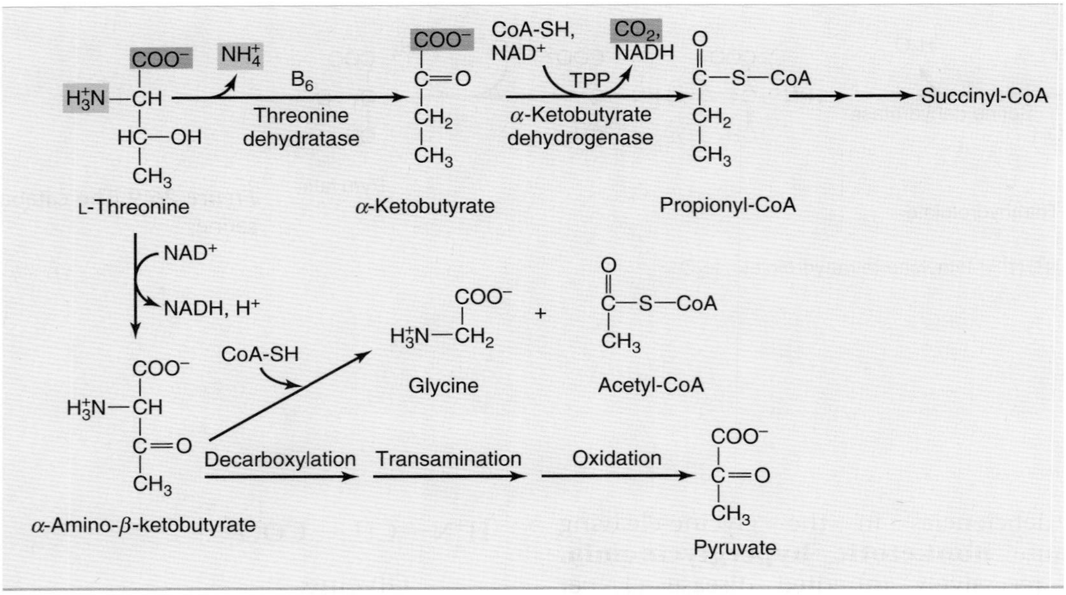

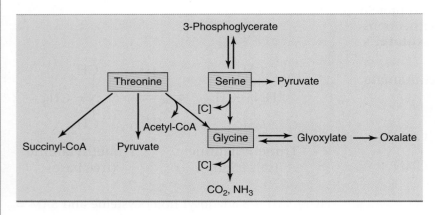

Figure 26.10 The catabolism of threonine. TPP, thiamine pyrophosphate.

Figure 26.11 Metabolism of serine, glycine, and threonine.

be synthesized freely from glutamate and is therefore not nutritionally essential. However, the capacity for arginine synthesis is so limited that arginine is considered a "semiessential" amino acid.

Histidine is degraded to glutamate by an unrelated pathway, as shown in Figure 26.13. Transamination is normally a minor pathway, but it becomes the major reaction in patients with **histidinemia,** a rare (incidence, 1 per 10,000), recessively inherited condition in which histidase is deficient.

Histidinemia first was detected during the screening of newborns for phenylketonuria when urinary imidazole pyruvate produced a false-positive color reaction in the ferric chloride test for urinary phenylpyruvate. The condition is considered benign, despite early reports of mental deficiency

and speech disorders in some affected children. Dietary treatment by histidine restriction, which corrects the biochemical abnormality, is not required. Diagnostic procedures include the determination of serum histidine, enzyme determination in skin biopsy, and the measurement of urocanate concentration in sweat. Histidase is present only in the skin and liver, and urocanate is a normal constituent of sweat.

The last reaction in the pathway of histidine catabolism contributes a formimino group to tetrahydrofolate. The folate requirement of this reaction is exploited in a laboratory test for folate deficiency. After an oral histidine load, the excess is normally degraded without the accumulation of metabolic intermediates. In folate deficiency, however, formiminoglutamate (FIGLU) is no longer

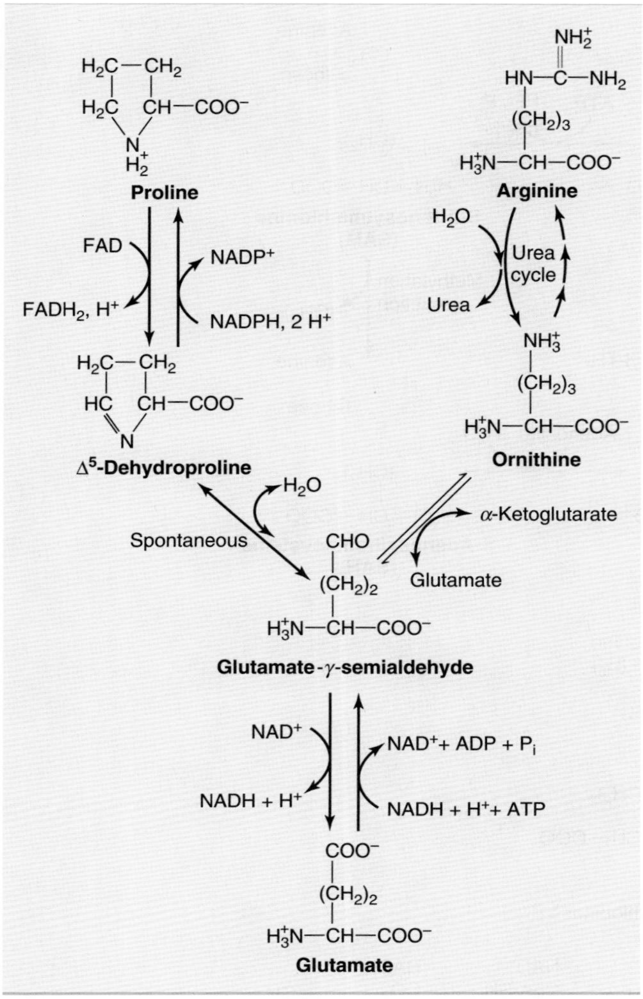

Figure 26.12 Metabolism of proline, arginine, and ornithine.

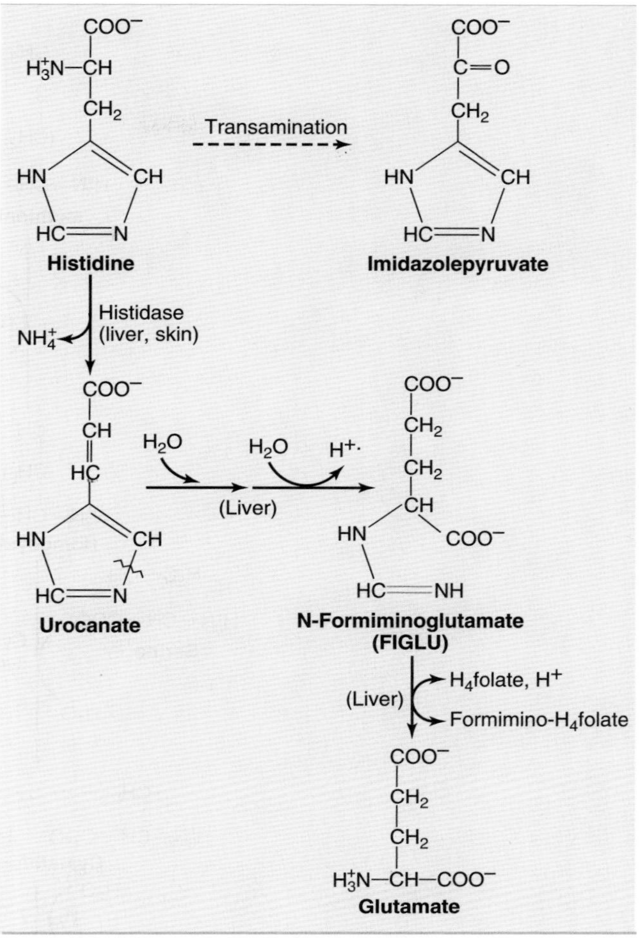

Figure 26.13 The catabolism of histidine.

Carnosine

converted to glutamate and can be demonstrated in the urine.

However, false-positive reactions are not uncommon in this test, because some people lack the formimino transferase and habitually excrete FIGLU as an end product of histidine degradation. This enzyme deficiency is benign.

Although histidine cannot be synthesized in the human body, people can subsist on a histidine-free diet for many weeks without ill effects. The reason is that histidine can be formed from the dipeptide **carnosine** (β-alanyl-histidine), which is present in large quantity in muscle tissue:

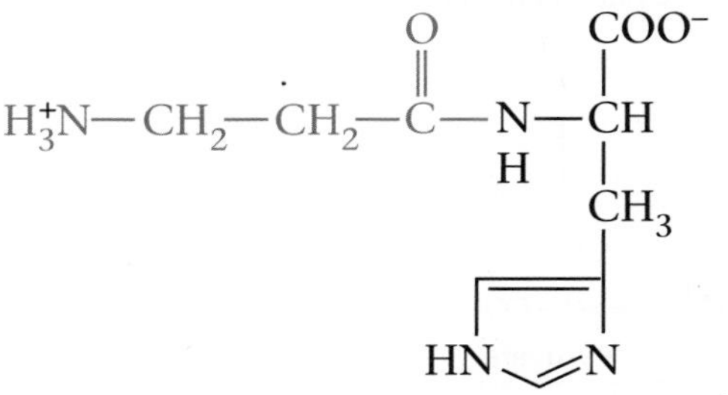

Carnosine is a pH buffer that limits the effect of lactic acid on the tissue pH during anaerobic contraction.

Methionine and Cysteine Are Metabolically Related

The essential amino acid **methionine** is a precursor of the methyl group donor **S-adenosylmethionine (SAM)** (see Chapter 5). SAM is synthesized from

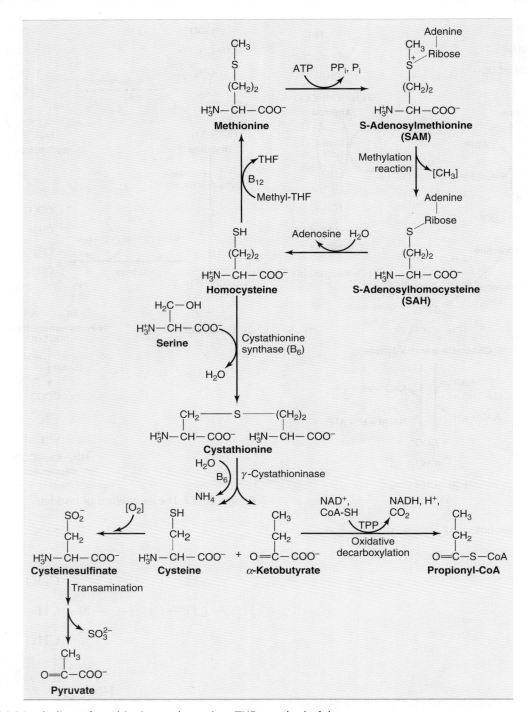

Figure 26.14 Metabolism of methionine and cysteine. THF, tetrahydrofolate.

methionine and ATP in an unusual reaction in which all three phosphates of ATP are released. By donating its methyl group during methylation reactions, SAM becomes S-adenosylhomocysteine (SAH). SAH forms **homocysteine** and finally methionine (Fig. 26.14). The methylation of homocysteine to methionine requires both folate (as methyl-tetrahydrofolate) and vitamin B_{12} (as methylcobalamin).

Figure 26.14 also shows how **cysteine** is made from the carbon skeleton of serine and the sulfur of methionine. Cysteine catabolism releases the sulfur as inorganic sulfite, which is rapidly oxidized and excreted in the urine as sulfate. Humans excrete 20 to 30 mmol of sulfate per day, and most of this is derived from dietary cysteine and methionine.

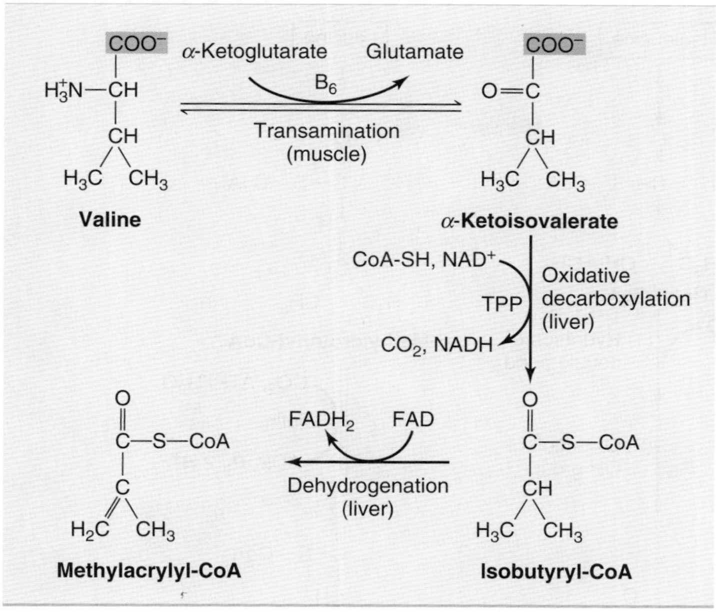

Figure 26.15 The first three reactions in the catabolism of valine. Analogous reactions take place with leucine and isoleucine.

Homocysteine Is a Risk Factor for Vascular Disease

The most important aberration in the metabolism of the sulfur amino acids is **homocystinuria,** caused by a recessively inherited deficiency of cystathionine synthase. Homocysteine, homocystine, and methionine accumulate. Patients with this rare condition (incidence, 1 per 200,000) show thinning and lengthening of the long bones, osteoporosis, lens dislocation, a tendency for vascular thrombosis, and mental deficiency. These symptoms are caused by the accumulation of homocysteine, not methionine.

Homocystinuria can be treated by the restriction of dietary methionine. Some patients have abnormal cystathionine synthase with a reduced affinity for pyridoxal phosphate. They respond to megadoses of vitamin B_6, the dietary precursor of pyridoxal phosphate. Supplements of vitamin B_{12} and folic acid can also be tried in an attempt to boost the homocysteine $\rightarrow$ methionine reaction. Betaine (N,N,N-trimethylglycine), which is a methyl group donor in an alternative reaction for the synthesis of methionine from homocysteine, can be employed with the same reasoning.

The high plasma level of homocysteine predisposes homocystinuric patients to vascular disease, but homocysteine levels are quite variable in normal people also. Indeed, *a high plasma homocysteine level is a risk factor for cardiovascular disease,* even in the "normal" range. A rise of homocysteine from $10\,\mu$mol/liter to $15\,\mu$mol/liter raises the risk of cardiovascular disease to about the same extent as a rise of the cholesterol level from 180 to $200\,$mg/ dL. The mechanism of this effect is unknown.

Homocysteine-lowering treatments are known to reduce the cardiovascular disease risk. The most consistently effective measure is treatment with folic acid supplements. Vitamins B_6 and B_{12} are also sometimes found effective. The coenzyme forms of these vitamins are cofactors for the homocysteine-metabolizing enzymes.

The Degradation of Valine, Leucine, and Isoleucine Begins with Transamination and Oxidative Decarboxylation

The first three steps in the degradation of valine, leucine, and isoleucine are identical for all three amino acids, as shown for valine in Figure 26.15.

These amino acids are transaminated in skeletal muscle and other extrahepatic tissues, but the resulting α keto acids are transported to the liver, in which they are oxidatively decarboxylated by a mitochondrial enzyme complex. This complex resembles the pyruvate dehydrogenase complex (see Chapter 21) in structure, coenzyme requirements, and reaction mechanism. The third reaction in the sequence resembles the first step of β-oxidation (see Chapter 23).

The remaining reactions differ for the three amino acids (Fig. 26.16). Valine is glucogenic, leucine is ketogenic, and isoleucine is both. The final reactions for valine and isoleucine are shared with the pathways of odd-chain fatty acids (see Chapter 23), threonine (threonine dehydratase; see Fig. 26.10) and methionine (see Fig. 26.14).

The most important disorders of branched-chain amino acid degradation affect the first and the last reactions. The deficiency of the branched-chain

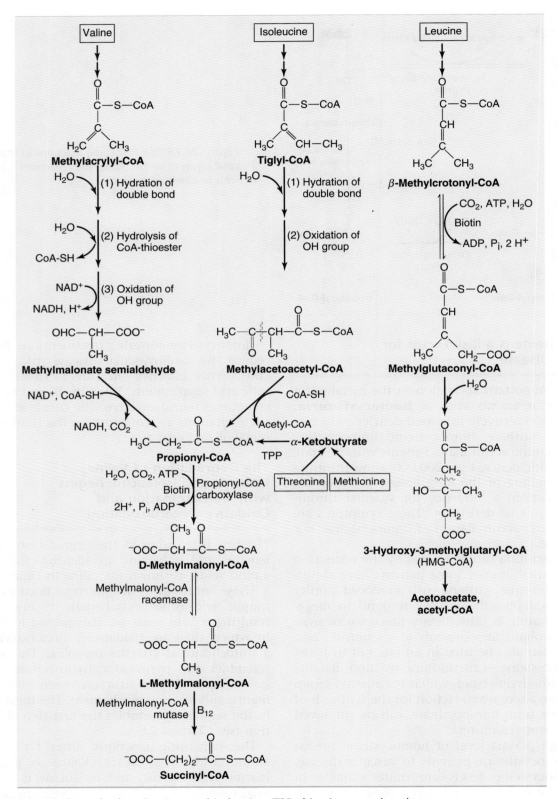

Figure 26.16 Catabolism of valine, leucine, and isoleucine. TPP, thiamine pyrophosphate.

α keto acid dehydrogenase, which oxidatively decarboxylates all three branched-chain α keto acids, causes **maple syrup urine disease.** Complete enzyme deficiency leads to severe mental retardation, acidosis, sweet odor of the urine, and early death. Megadoses of thiamine are effective in only a few patients, and even the restriction of dietary valine, leucine, and isoleucine is not always successful. The prevalence in newborns is approximately 1 per 200,000.

Methylmalonic aciduria is the most common inherited defect in the last reactions of valine and isoleucine degradation (incidence, 1 per 10,000). The vitamin B_{12}-dependent methylmalonyl-CoA mutase reaction is blocked, and methylmalonic acid accumulates in blood and urine. Being an acid, methylmalonic acid causes serious and often fatal acidosis in affected infants. Treatment can be attempted by the cautious restriction of valine, isoleucine, threonine, and methionine. However, substantial restrictions of these essential amino acids will cause signs of protein deficiency.

In some patients, the disease is caused not by a defective enzyme protein but by an inability to convert dietary vitamin B_{12} to the coenzyme form deoxyadenosylcobalamin. They respond to injected adenosylcobalamin. Predictably, a deficiency of dietary vitamin B_{12} raises the methylmalonic acid level in the absence of any genetic defect.

Phenylalanine and Tyrosine Are Both Glucogenic and Ketogenic

The ring systems of the aromatic amino acids cannot be synthesized in the body. Tyrosine is nevertheless considered nonessential because it is synthesized from phenylalanine in the **phenylalanine hydroxylase** reaction:

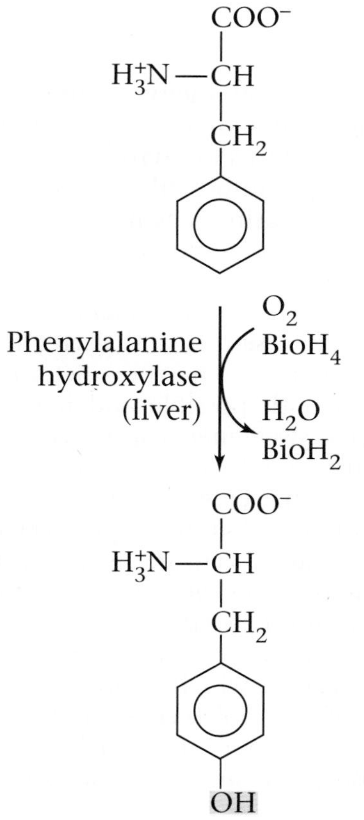

This irreversible reaction takes place only in the liver. It is a monooxygenase reaction requiring molecular oxygen and **tetrahydrobiopterin (BioH₄).** $BioH_4$ becomes oxidized to dihydrobiopterin ($BioH_2$) during the reaction. $BioH_2$ has to be reduced back to $BioH_4$ by an NADH-dependent **dihydropteridine reductase:**

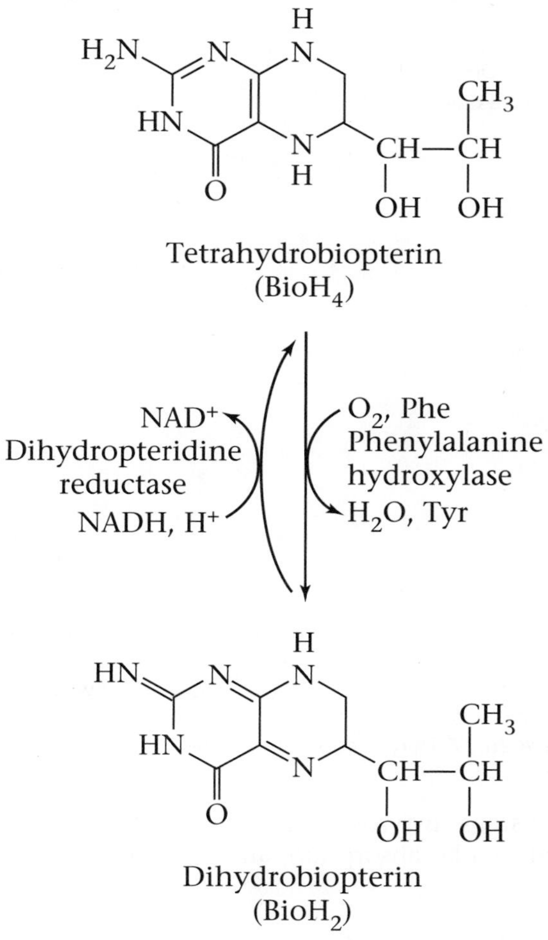

This is the same reaction mechanism as in the tyrosine hydroxylase and tryptophan hydroxylase reactions in Chapter 16.

The catabolism of tyrosine in the liver is shown in Figure 26.17. This pathway is affected in several genetic diseases. The deficiency of homogentisate oxidase causes **alkaptonuria.** Affected patients excrete homogentisate in their urine, which is oxidized to black products on exposure to light and air. Although the ink-colored diapers of affected babies look alarming, the condition is relatively benign. Black pigments gradually accumulate in connective tissues, a condition known as **ochronosis,** and many older patients develop painful arthritis.

In **type I tyrosinemia,** caused by a deficiency of fumarylacetoacetate hydrolase, the accumulation of fumarylacetoacetate and related organic acids causes a cabbage-like smell, an inhibition of the

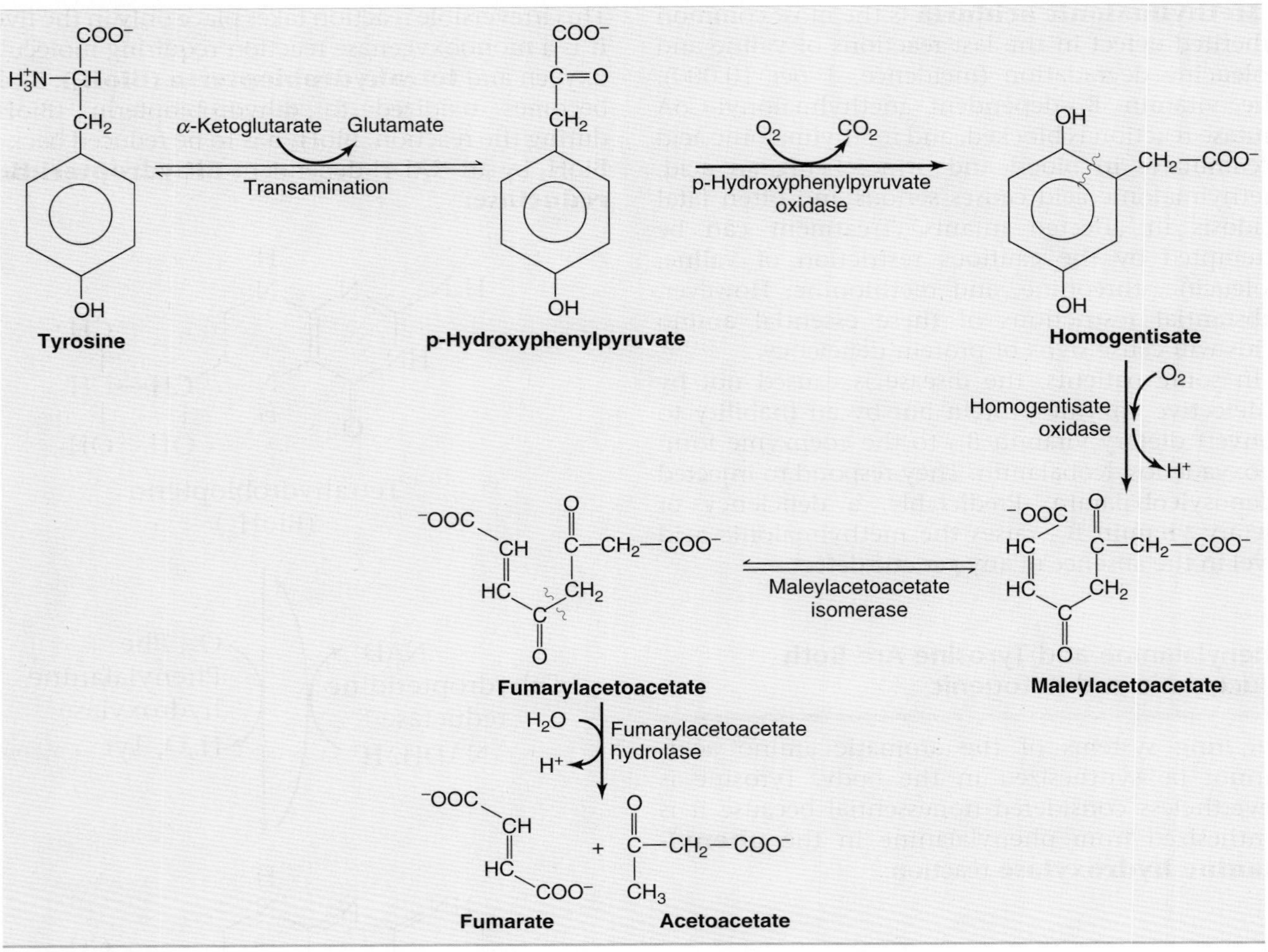

Figure 26.17 Degradation of tyrosine.

early steps in tyrosine degradation, impairment of renal tubular absorption, and liver failure.

Phenylketonuria Causes Mental Deficiency

Classical **phenylketonuria (PKU)** is caused by a complete deficiency of phenylalanine hydroxylase. This enzyme deficiency raises plasma phenylalanine from its normal level of 0.5 to 2.0 mg/dL to more than 20 mg/dL. *Most of the accumulating phenylalanine is transaminated to phenylpyruvate,* although this is otherwise a very minor pathway of phenylalanine metabolism. Phenylpyruvate is then converted to other products that are excreted in the urine along with phenylalanine and phenylpyruvate (Fig. 26.18).

There are no abnormalities at birth because phenylalanine and its metabolites are transferred across the placenta, but serum phenylalanine and urinary phenylpyruvate rise within a few days after birth. *Untreated patients develop mental retardation.*

Some also develop spasticity, seizures, or other neurological signs. In comparison with unaffected siblings, patients with PKU have a light complexion because phenylalanine inhibits the synthesis of melanin from tyrosine. The mechanisms leading to mental retardation are not known.

Mental retardation in PKU can be prevented by the restriction of dietary phenylalanine. Phenylalanine is nutritionally essential and therefore cannot be omitted entirely from the diet, but massive restriction is both possible and required in PKU. The artificial sweetener **aspartame** (*N*-aspartyl-phenylalanine methylester) is hazardous to the patient's health. One quart of Kool-Aid, for example, contains 280 mg of phenylalanine in the form of aspartame. Tyrosine is an essential amino acid for phenylketonuric patients, but dietary supplements are not needed.

Only the developing brain is vulnerable to PKU. Therefore, the diet, which is not very palatable, can be tapered off in adolescence. However, treatment must be started soon after birth to prevent irreversible damage. Thus, early diagnosis is essential.

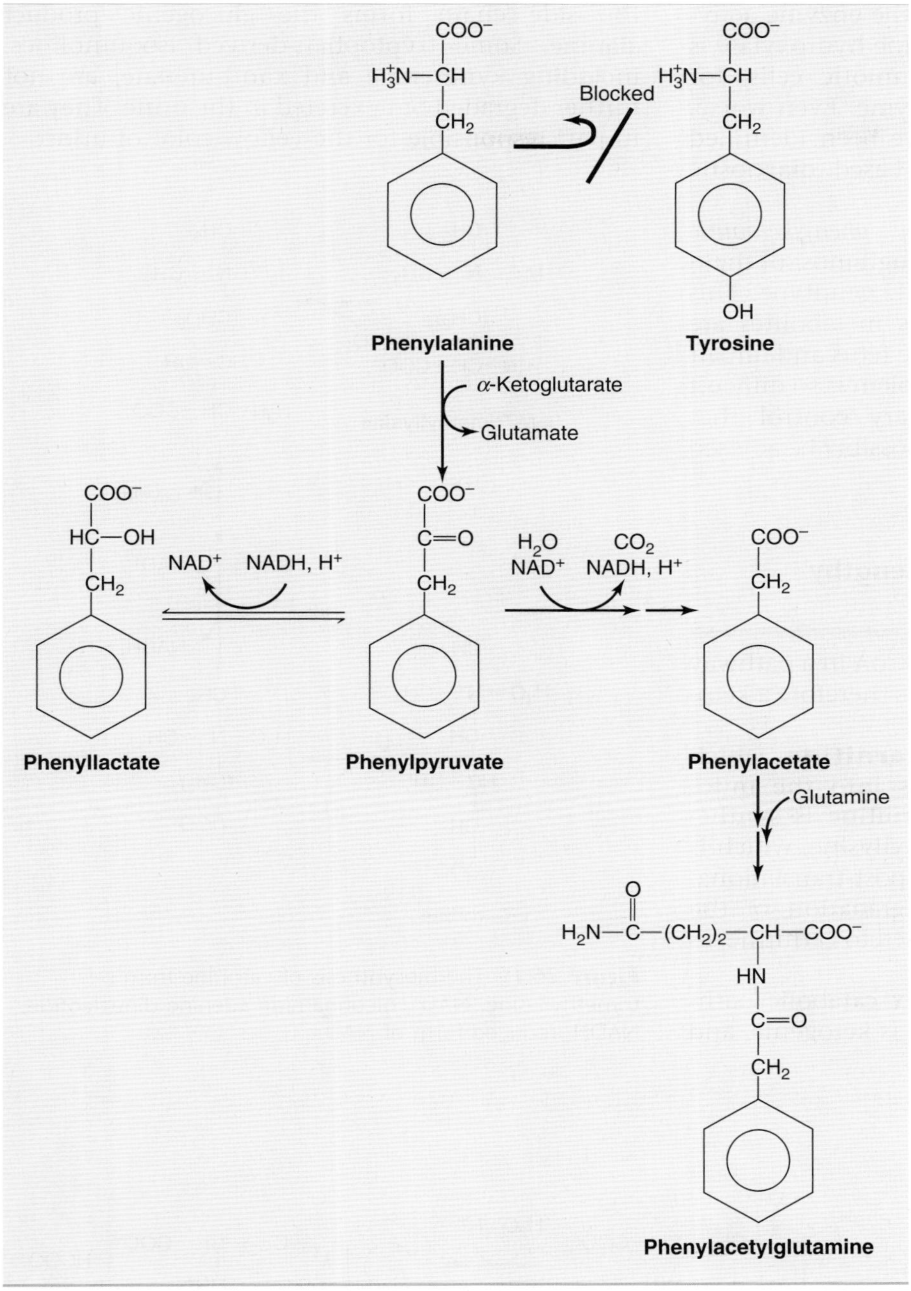

Figure 26.18 Phenylalanine metabolism in phenylketonuria (PKU).

Newborn screening for PKU is mandatory in the United States. PKU can be diagnosed with the **ferric chloride test** for urinary phenylpyruvate or by the determination of blood phenylalanine. The most commonly employed laboratory test is the **Guthrie bacterial inhibition assay** in which phenylketonuric blood, but not the blood of normal individuals, supports the growth of a phenylalanine-dependent bacterial strain. The test should be done no less than 2 days after birth because false-negative results are common during the first 24 or even 48 hours. PKU is most common in people of white European ancestry, with highest frequency (1 per 6000) in Britain and Ireland. It is far less common in other racial groups (e.g., 1 per 200,000 in Japan).

Only a complete deficiency of phenylalanine hydroxylase causes PKU. Therefore, the mode of inheritance is recessive. Heterozygotes have about half of the normal enzyme activity. They can be identified in the **phenylalanine tolerance test** because they have a greater and longer lasting rise in plasma phenylalanine after a standardized oral dose of the amino acid.

Diagnosis by determination of the enzyme activity is difficult because phenylalanine hydroxylase is expressed only in the liver. Amniotic cells, for example, do not express this enzyme. Even worse, so many different mutations have been identified in different patients that DNA-based diagnostic methods are of limited use.

Interestingly, *the children of phenylketonuric mothers are mentally retarded,* although most of them do not have the homozygous PKU genotype. This is because phenylalanine and its metabolites are transferred from the mother to the fetus and impair fetal brain development. This problem is so difficult to manage even by strict dietary control that phenylketonuric women should possibly be advised against pregnancy.

Lysine and Tryptophan Have Lengthy Catabolic Pathways

Lysine is degraded to acetoacetyl-CoA in a pathway with nine enzymatic reactions. It is therefore a ketogenic amino acid.

Lysine is also a precursor of **carnitine,** which transports long-chain fatty acids into the mitochondrion (see Chapter 23). Carnitine is synthesized from protein-bound trimethyllysine, which is formed in some proteins by the post-translational modification of lysine. After degradation of the protein, trimethyllysine is converted to carnitine, as shown in Figure 26.19.

Tryptophan also has complex catabolic pathways (Fig. 26.20). The indole ring is ketogenic, and the side chain forms the glucogenic product alanine. Some tryptophan-derived isoquinolines, including kynurenate and xanthurenate, are not further degraded but excreted in the urine. They are in part responsible for the yellow color of urine:

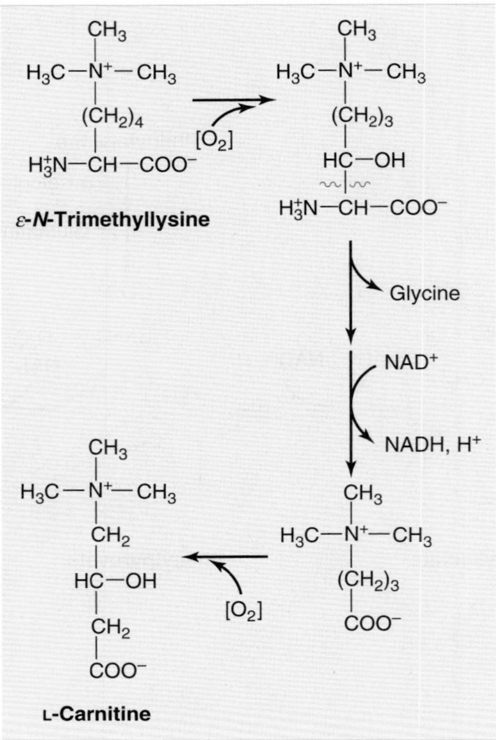

Figure 26.19 The biosynthesis of carnitine from ε-N-trimethyllysine. NAD⁺, nicotinamide adenine dinucleotide; NADH, reduced form of NAD.

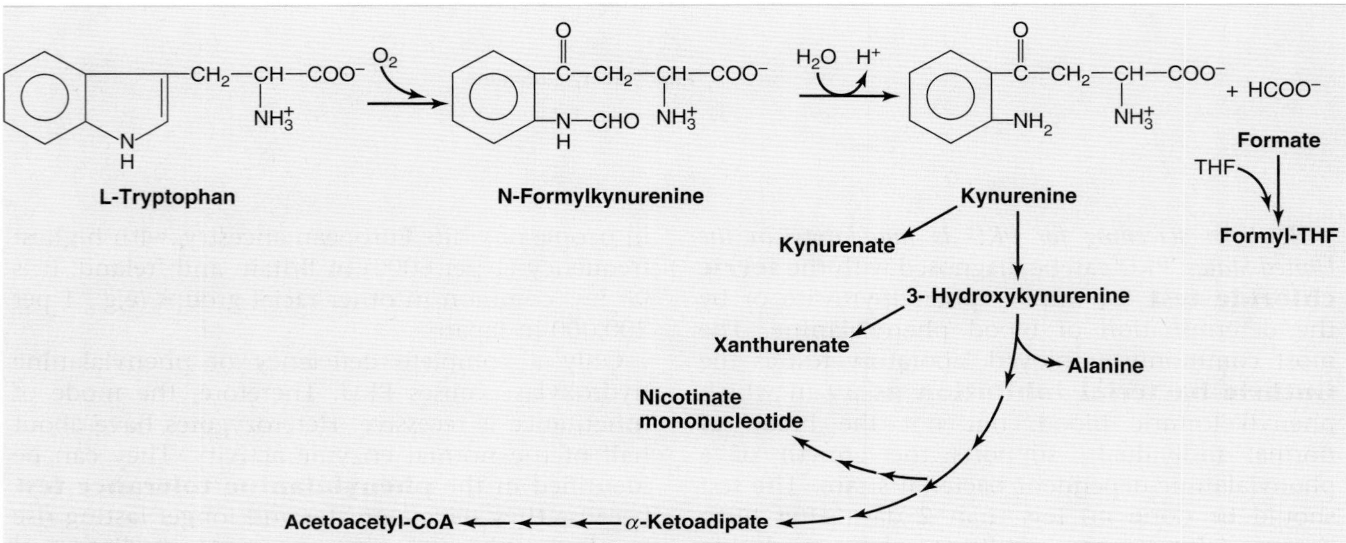

Figure 26.20 Catabolism of tryptophan. THF, tetrahydrofolate.

Kynurenate

Xanthurenate

The Liver Is the Most Important Organ of Amino Acid Metabolism

Although nearly half of human protein is present in muscle tissue, *enzymes of amino acid catabolism are most abundant in the liver.* This makes sense because during fasting, amino acids have to be channeled into the hepatic pathways of gluconeogenesis (glucogenic amino acids) and ketogenesis (ketogenic amino acids).

After a meal (Fig. 26.21A), most of the dietary glutamine and glutamate is metabolized in the intestinal mucosa. Most of the other amino acids go to the liver. Some are used for the synthesis of plasma proteins, but most are catabolized. Only the branched-chain aliphatic amino acids valine, leucine, and isoleucine pass through the liver and go to muscle and other peripheral tissues, in which they are transaminated. The resulting branched-chain α keto acids return to the liver for further catabolism.

Muscle tissue is the major source of plasma amino acids in the fasting state (see Fig. 26.21B). Alanine accounts for 50% and glutamine for 25% of the released amino acids. Most of the alanine goes to the liver for gluconeogenesis, and most of the glutamine goes to kidneys and intestine. In the kidneys, the glutaminase reaction produces ammonia for urinary excretion. For the intestine, glutamine is a major substrate for the generation of metabolic energy besides glucose.

Nitrogen is transported to the liver either as a constituent of amino acids or as free ammonia (Fig. 26.22). Ammonia is produced by glutamate dehydrogenase (most tissues), glutaminase (kidney), histidase (skin), and other enzymes. More important is the

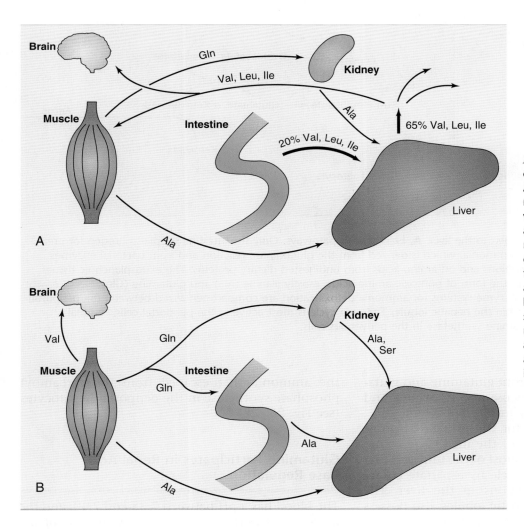

Figure 26.21 Interorgan exchange of amino acids. **A,** After a protein-containing meal: All amino acids except valine (Val), leucine (Leu), and isoleucine (Ile) are metabolized extensively during their first passage through the liver. Ala, alanine; Gln, glutamine. **B,** In the postabsorptive state: Muscle tissue is the main source of plasma amino acids. Alanine and glutamine are quantitatively most important. Ser, serine.

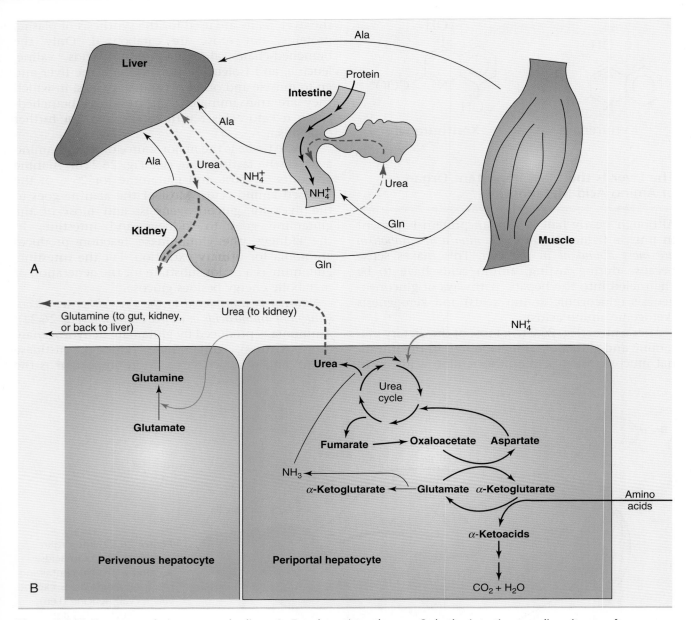

Figure 26.22 Transport of nitrogen to the liver. **A,** Extrahepatic pathways. Only the intestine supplies nitrogen for urea synthesis mostly in the form of ammonia, which is derived from the glutaminase reaction and from bacterial enzymes acting on urea in digestive secretions and on amino acids from undigested dietary proteins. The extrasplanchnic tissues supply most of their nitrogen in the form of nontoxic amino acids, mostly alanine (Ala) and glutamine (Gln). **B,** Intrahepatic pathways. The enzyme systems for ammonia detoxification are compartmentalized between the periportal and perivenous hepatocytes within the hepatic lobule. The urea cycle is most active in the periportal cells; residual ammonia is scavenged by glutamine synthetase in the perivenous cells.

production of ammonia from glutamine and glutamate in the intestinal mucosa and from urea and leftover dietary protein by intestinal bacteria.

Most of the ammonia for the carbamoyl phosphate synthetase reaction of the urea cycle comes from outside the liver, but most of the nitrogen that is brought into the urea cycle by aspartate comes from transamination reactions in the liver. The perivenous cells of the hepatic lobules also possess **glutamine synthetase,** which mops up most of

the ammonia that escaped from the carbamoyl phosphate synthetase in the periportal hepatocytes (see Fig. 26.22B).

Glutamine Participates in Renal Acid-Base Regulation

The blood has a pH between 7.35 and 7.40, and *the long-term maintenance of this pH is the task of the*

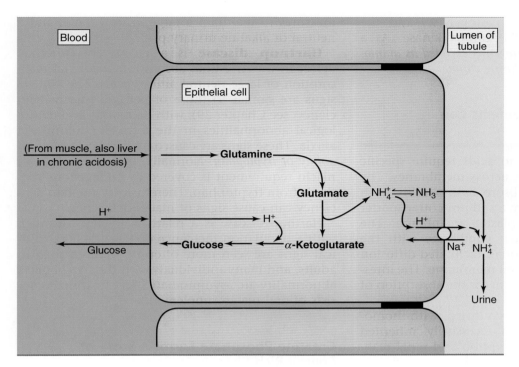

Figure 26.23 Glutamine metabolism and acid-base regulation in the renal tubules. The reactions shown here are most active during chronic acidosis, when a large proportion of the total nitrogen is excreted as the ammonium ion rather than as urea.

kidney. In acidosis, the kidney excretes excess protons; in alkalosis, it retains protons. Therefore, the urinary pH can range anywhere between 4 and 8. Figure 26.23 shows how the kidneys use glutamine-derived ammonia as a vehicle for the excretion of excess protons during chronic acidosis.

In the tubular epithelium, blood-derived glutamine is deaminated first to glutamate and then to α-ketoglutarate. Being small and uncharged, the ammonia (NH_3) formed in these reactions diffuses passively into the urine of the tubular lumen. The urine is more acidic than the cytoplasm because the epithelial cells secrete protons through a sodium-proton antiporter. Therefore, the ammonia in the urine combines with a proton to form the ammonium ion (NH_4^+). Being charged, the ammonium ion cannot diffuse back into the cell and is flushed down the sewage system of the urinary tract. Although NH_3 equilibrates across the membrane, *ammonium ions accumulate in the urine as long as the urine is more acidic than the cytoplasm of the epithelial cells.*

The glutamine-derived α-ketoglutarate is converted to glucose by gluconeogenesis in the kidney. This process absorbs four protons for each molecule of glucose formed according to the following equation:

$$2\ C_5H_4O_5^{2-} + 4\ H_2O + 4\ H^+$$
α-Ketoglutarate

$$\downarrow$$

$$C_6H_{12}O_6 + 4\ CO_2 + 8\ [H]$$
Glucose

The eight hydrogen atoms ([H]) in this equation are exchanged with NAD and FAD in the α-ketoglutarate dehydrogenase, succinate dehydrogenase, malate dehydrogenase, and glyceraldehyde-3-phosphate dehydrogenase reactions.

The excretion of ammonium ions—but not urea—as an end product of amino acid metabolism is accompanied by the removal of protons. Even without the details shown in Figure 26.23, this is apparent from a stoichiometric comparison of the oxidation of a typical amino acid such as alanine:

$$C_3H_7O_2N + 3\ O_2 + H^+$$
Alanine

$$\downarrow$$

$$NH_4^+ + 3\ CO_2 + 2\ H_2O$$
Ammonium ion

and

$$2\ C_3H_7O_2N + 6\ O_2$$
Alanine

$$\downarrow$$

$$CH_4N_2O + 5\ CO_2 + 5\ H_2O$$
Urea

During acidosis, the liver diverts an increasing fraction of the incoming ammonia from urea synthesis in the periportal cells to glutamine synthesis in the perivenous cells (see Fig. 26.22B). The liver becomes a net producer of glutamine, which is forwarded to the kidneys. In the kidney itself, acidosis induces glutaminase, glutamate dehydrogenase, and the gluconeogenic enzyme PEP carboxykinase. As a result, *up to 50% of the nitrogen is excreted as ammonium ion rather than urea during chronic acidosis.*

Amino Acid Transport Defects Can Cause Disease

Being water soluble, amino acids require specific carriers for their transport across membranes. The proximal renal tubules absorb amino acids from the lumen into the cell by a sodium cotransporter in the apical (luminal) plasma membrane. The absorbed amino acids then equilibrate with the blood through a bidirectional, facilitated-diffusion type carrier in the basolateral membrane. The intestine uses the same mechanism for the absorption of dietary amino acids.

Cystinuria (not to be confused with homocystinuria) is caused by a recessively inherited defect in the intestinal absorption and renal reabsorption of the dibasic amino acids lysine, arginine, ornithine, and cystine. Although lysine is nutritionally essential and arginine is semiessential, signs of amino acid deficiency are not common in this condition, probably because amino acids can still be absorbed from the small intestine as dipeptides and tripeptides.

Cystine, however, is problematic. It is poorly soluble under acidic conditions, and, therefore, *it forms kidney stones.* The diagnosis of cystinuria is established by the demonstration of abnormal quantities of dibasic amino acids in the urine. Cystinuria has an incidence of 1 per 7000, and it accounts for a fairly small proportion of kidney stones in the population. The treatment consists of measures to maintain a large urine volume and a neutral or alkaline urinary pH.

Hartnup disease is a recessively inherited defect in the intestinal absorption and renal reabsorption of large neutral amino acids. The clinical signs are similar to those of pellagra (niacin deficiency; see Chapter 29), with dermatitis and neurological abnormalities in the form of intermittent ataxia. These signs are caused by the *decreased availability of tryptophan.* Normally, part of the human niacin requirement is covered by endogenous synthesis from tryptophan. Therefore, tryptophan deficiency can cause signs of niacin deficiency.

Hartnup disease is a relatively benign disorder, with a population incidence of 1 per 24,000. Clinical signs are seen more often in children than in adults, and many individuals with the biochemical abnormality are asymptomatic. The treatment consists of oral niacin supplements.

Creatine Phosphate Forms a Store of Energy-Rich Phosphate Bonds in Muscle Tissue

Creatine and **creatine phosphate** are present in muscle and, to a lesser extent, nervous tissue, in which creatine phosphate provides a store of high-energy phosphate bonds. Creatine phosphate is formed in the reversible **creatine kinase (CK)** reaction (Fig. 26.24). The phosphate bond in creatine phosphate is energy-rich, with a standard free energy of hydrolysis of −10.3 kcal/mol.

In resting muscle, the [ATP]/[ADP] ratio is so high that most of the creatine is present as creatine phosphate. During contraction, when the [ATP]/[ADP] ratio declines, *ATP is rapidly regenerated by the*

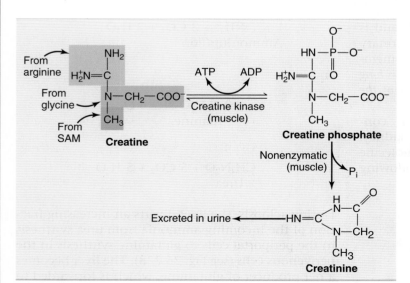

Figure 26.24 Creatine and the creatine kinase reaction. SAM, *S*-adenosyl methionine.

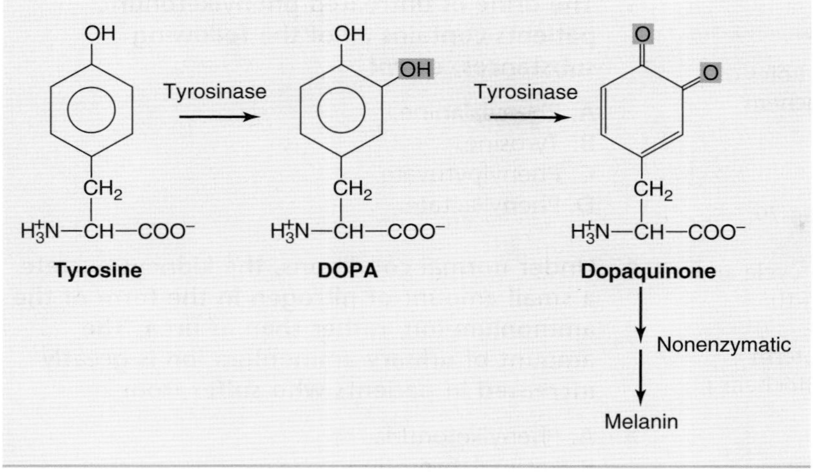

Figure 26.25 The synthesis of melanin from tyrosine.

reversible creatine kinase reaction. This is the most important source of ATP during the first seconds of muscle contraction. For more sustained muscular activity, however, ATP has to be regenerated by glycolysis or oxidative metabolism (see Chapter 30).

Creatine is not degraded enzymatically, but creatine phosphate cyclizes spontaneously to **creatinine.** This product is excreted in the urine.

Melanin Is Synthesized from Tyrosine

Melanin is the dark pigment of skin, hair, the iris, and the retinal pigment epithelium. *Melanin protects the skin* because it absorbs not only visible light but also the ultraviolet component of sunlight. Ultraviolet radiation, especially at wavelengths of 280 to 320 nm, is dangerous because it damages DNA, causing sunburn and skin cancer. In the eye, the melanin of the pigment epithelium underlying the sensory cells of the retina absorbs stray light, thereby enhancing visual acuity and preventing overstimulation of the photoreceptors.

Melanin is a polymeric product with a heterogeneous molecular weight and poorly defined structure. In the first steps of melanin synthesis, tyrosine is oxidized first to **L-dopa** and then to dopaquinone by the copper-containing enzyme **tyrosinase** (Fig. 26.25). Most or all of the subsequent reactions are thought to be nonenzymatic.

Recessively inherited defects of melanin synthesis are the cause of **oculocutaneous albinism.** Some albinos are lacking tyrosinase, whereas others have a defect in the carrier that transports tyrosine across the melanosome membrane.

SUMMARY

Amino acids are degraded to carbon dioxide, water, and urea. The separation of the amino nitrogen from the carbon skeleton is an early event in the catabolism of most amino acids. In most cases, the amino group is initially transferred to α-ketoglutarate in a transamination reaction. The glutamate formed in these reactions is oxidatively deaminated by glutamate dehydrogenase, forming free ammonia.

Because ammonia is toxic, it has to be converted to nontoxic urea in the urea cycle. This pathway is present only in the liver. Therefore, patients with advanced liver cirrhosis suffer from hyperammonemia, with encephalopathy and coma resulting from ammonia toxicity.

The excretion of the ammonium ion rather than urea is accompanied by the elimination of excess protons from the body. The kidneys increase ammonium excretion during acidosis in an attempt to eliminate excess protons.

The carbon skeletons of the amino acids are channeled either into gluconeogenesis (glucogenic amino acids) or into ketogenesis (ketogenic amino acids). Many deficiencies of amino acid–degrading enzymes are known, and some of them are severe diseases. The clinical manifestations of these inborn errors of amino acid metabolism are caused by the abnormal accumulation of the affected amino acid or its metabolites.

Several specialized products, including creatine, carnitine, carnosine, and melanin, are synthesized from amino acids.

📖 Further Reading

Medina MA, Urdiales JL, Amores-Sanchez MI: Roles of homocysteine in cell metabolism. Eur J Biochem 268:3871-3882, 2001.

Moat SJ, Lang D, McDowell IF, et al: Folate, homocysteine, endothelial function and cardiovascular disease. J Nutr Biochem 15:64-79, 2004.

Morris SM: Regulation of enzymes of the urea cycle and arginine metabolism. Annu Rev Nutr 22:87-105, 2002.

Thony B, Auerbach G, Blau N: Tetrahydrobiopterin biosynthesis, regeneration and functions. Biochem J 347:1-16, 2000.

QUESTIONS

1. A 4-month-old child is evaluated for irritability, vomiting after feeding, and delayed motor development. Blood tests show an ammonia level 10 to 20 times higher than the upper limit of normal, as well as marked elevations of ornithine and glutamine. Most likely, this child has a deficiency of the enzyme

   A. Arginase.
   B. Ornithine decarboxylase.
   C. Glutaminase.
   D. Ornithine transcarbamoylase.
   E. Ornithine transglutaminase.

2. A 55-year-old alcoholic is brought to the hospital in a confused state. The emergency room physician notes that the patient's breath has a foul smell, but there is no sign of acute alcohol intoxication. A blood test shows an abnormally high ammonia level. The *worst* treatment for this patient would be

   A. To give him a lot of good, protein-rich food.
   B. To give him benzoic acid or phenylacetic acid.
   C. To give him a diet low in proteins but with plenty of vitamins.
   D. To give him a broad-spectrum antibiotic to eliminate intestinal bacteria.

3. The urine of untreated phenylketonuric patients contains all of the following substances, *except*

   A. Phenylalanine.
   B. Tyrosine.
   C. Phenylpyruvate.
   D. Phenyllactate.

4. Under normal conditions, the kidneys excrete a small amount of nitrogen in the form of the ammonium ion, rather than as urea. The amount of urinary ammonium ion is greatly increased in patients who suffer from

   A. Phenylketonuria.
   B. Fat malabsorption.
   C. Hartnup disease.
   D. Glutaminase deficiency.
   E. Chronic acidosis.

5. All transamination reactions require the coenzyme

   A. Tetrahydrofolate.
   B. Thiamine pyrophosphate.
   C. Pyridoxal phosphate.
   D. Biotin.
   E. SAM.

CHAPTER 27

Heme Metabolism

Heme is a tightly bound prosthetic group of many proteins, including hemoglobin, myoglobin, and the cytochromes. It is bound to its apoproteins either noncovalently, as in hemoglobin and myoglobin, or by a covalent bond, as in cytochrome *c*. Heme consists of a porphyrin, known as **protoporphyrin IX,** with an iron chelated in its center. The porphyrin system consists of four pyrrole rings linked by methine (—CH=) bridges:

Heme
(Fe-protoporphyrin IX)

The conjugated (alternating) double bonds absorb visible light. Therefore, *the heme proteins are colored.* **Porphyrinogens** are important intermediates in heme biosynthesis. Their pyrrole rings are connected by methylene (—CH₂—) bridges, and they do not absorb light because the double bonds are not conjugated over the whole system:

Protoporphyrinogen IX
(a porphyrinogen)

Porphyrinogens are prone to nonenzymatic oxidation to the corresponding porphyrins.

Although a small amount of dietary heme is absorbed in the small intestine, *essentially all the heme in the human body is derived from endogenous synthesis.* This chapter describes the pathways for the biosynthesis and degradation of heme and the diseases in which these pathways are disrupted.

Bone Marrow and the Liver Are the Most Important Sites of Heme Synthesis

The 800 to 900 g of hemoglobin in the adult body contains 30 to 35 g of heme; 250 to 300 mg of heme have to be synthesized in the red bone marrow every day, most of this in the erythroblasts and

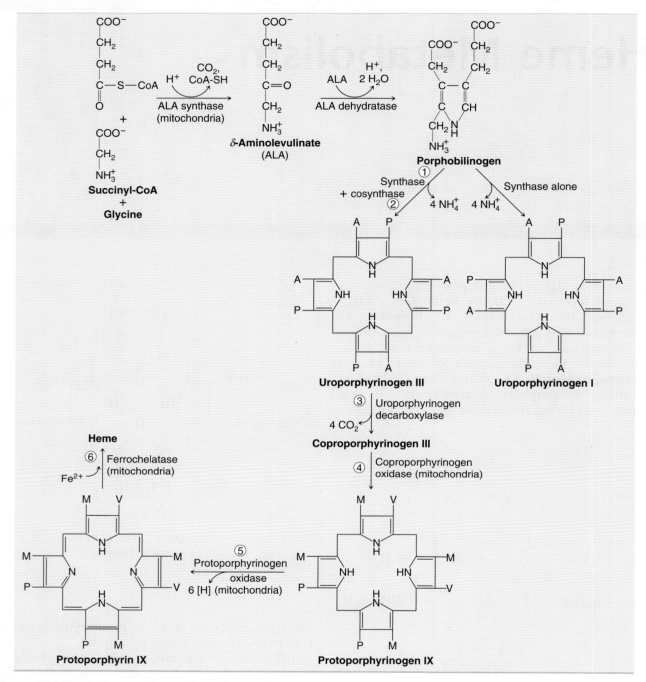

Figure 27.1 The pathway of heme biosynthesis. The numbered reactions refer to Table 27.1. A, acetate (carboxymethyl) group; M, methyl group; P, propionate (carboxyethyl) group; V, vinyl group.

proerythroblasts. *The bone marrow accounts for 70% to 80% of the total heme synthesis in the body.*

The second most important site is the liver because of its high content of cytochrome P-450 and other heme enzymes. These enzymes have far shorter half-lives than does hemoglobin. Therefore, hepatic heme synthesis is quite productive, accounting for approximately 15% of the total.

Heme Is Synthesized from Succinyl-CoA and Glycine

Heme biosynthesis starts with the formation of δ-**aminolevulinate (ALA)** from succinyl-CoA and glycine, catalyzed by the heme-containing, vitamin B$_6$–dependent enzyme δ-**aminolevulinate (ALA) synthase.** This is the committed step of the pathway in Figure 27.1.

The second reaction, catalyzed by **ALA dehydratase,** forms the pyrrole ring of **porphobilinogen.** Lead and other heavy metals can inhibit this enzyme by binding to sulfhydryl groups in the enzyme protein.

The third enzyme, **uroporphyrinogen I synthase (**also called **porphobilinogen deaminase),** links together four molecules of porphobilinogen. Left on its own, this product can spontaneously cyclize to form **uroporphyrinogen I.** In the cell, however, a second protein, **uroporphyrinogen III cosynthase,** channels the reaction into the formation of the isomer **uroporphyrinogen III.** All naturally occurring porphyrins, including heme, belong to the III series. Uroporphyrinogen III is processed to heme by the reactions shown in Figure 27.1.

The first reaction and the last three reactions of the pathway are mitochondrial. The others are cytoplasmic. *Aminolevulinic acid (ALA) synthase is the regulated enzyme.* ALA synthase has an unusually short biological half-life of 1 to 3 hours in the liver, and *its synthesis is very effectively suppressed by heme.* Only free, non–protein-bound heme acts as a feedback inhibitor.

Porphyrias Are Caused by Deficiencies of Heme-Synthesizing Enzymes

The **porphyrias** are caused by a *partial deficiency of one of the heme-synthesizing enzymes other than ALA synthase.* Any one of the numbered enzymes in Figure 27.1 can be affected. A complete deficiency would be fatal, and the offending mutations are generally expressed as autosomal dominant traits; affected heterozygotes have 50% of the normal enzyme activity. Clinically, we can distinguish between *hepatic porphyrias and erythropoietic porphyrias.*

Acute intermittent porphyria (AIP) is caused by a dominantly inherited deficiency of uroporphyrinogen I synthase (porphobilinogen deaminase). The enzyme activity is reduced to 50% of normal in all tissues, but clinical manifestations are caused by impaired heme synthesis in the liver because the activity of this enzyme, in relation to the other heme biosynthetic enzymes, is rather low in this organ.

However, 90% of individuals with the genetic trait never show clinical signs and symptoms. If problems develop, they usually take the form of acute attacks lasting from a few days to several months.

The clinical manifestations of AIP are caused by the accumulation of ALA and porphobilinogen in blood and cerebrospinal fluid. These metabolites act on the central and peripheral nervous systems,

causing abdominal pain, constipation, muscle weakness, and cardiovascular abnormalities. Agitation, seizures, or mental derangement may be present. Undiagnosed AIP appears to be overrepresented among patients of psychiatric institutions in which the condition is worsened by inappropriate drug treatment.

Acute attacks of AIP can be precipitated by barbiturates, phenytoin, griseofulvin, and other drugs that induce the synthesis of **cytochrome P-450.** This family of heme proteins accounts for 65% of the total heme in the liver (see Chapter 30). It is concerned with the metabolic inactivation of drugs and other foreign molecules, and the transcription of their genes is stimulated by many drugs.

As a result of drug exposure and enzyme induction, the small amount of free, unbound heme in the cell rapidly binds to the newly synthesized apoenzymes. This depletes the pool of free, unbound heme, and *heme depletion derepresses ALA synthase.* Large amounts of ALA and porphobilinogen are formed but cannot be processed fast enough by uroporphyrinogen I synthase.

The symptoms of AIP are not accompanied by specific physical findings, and they are therefore often misdiagnosed as "psychosomatic." The patient is treated symptomatically with sedative-hypnotics, tranquilizers or anticonvulsants, and these drugs aggravate the condition by inducing cytochrome P-450 synthesis in the liver. Patients have died of this treatment.

Adequate treatment consists of the withdrawal of any offending drugs and the infusion of **hematin.** Hematin is a stable derivative of heme in which the heme iron is in the ferric form and coordinated with a hydroxyl ion. Like heme, hematin represses the synthesis of ALA synthase. Also, a carbohydrate-rich diet is beneficial by repressing the synthesis of ALA synthase.

Several other porphyrias have been described. Their most important features are summarized in Table 27.1. The most common of them is **porphyria cutanea tarda.** Although some cases are caused by a dominantly inherited defect of uroporphyrinogen decarboxylase, this disease is expressed mainly in people with alcoholism or liver damage. Iron overload is an important factor because the affected enzyme is sensitive to inhibition by iron salts.

The clinical manifestation is very different from that of AIP. Neurological and abdominal symptoms are absent, and *the patient presents with cutaneous photosensitivity.* The condition is most common in older men during the summer months. It is treated by the avoidance of sunlight, abstinence from alcohol, and phlebotomy for the reduction of iron overload.

Table 27.1 The Porphyrias

Enzyme Deficiency*	Disease (and Class)	Inheritance	Signs and Symptoms*			Laboratory Tests
			Visceral	Neurological	Cutaneous	
1	Acute intermittent (hepatic)	AD	++	++	–	Urinary ALA, urinary PBG
2	Congenital erythropoietic (erythropoietic)	AR			+++	Urinary uroporphyrin,† urinary coproporphyrin,† fecal coproporphyrin†
3	Porphyria cutanea tarda (hepatic)	AD‡			++	Urinary uroporphyrin, urinary uroporphyrin, coproporphyrin
4	Hereditary coproporphyria (hepatic)	AD	+	+	(+)	Urinary ALA, urinary PBG, urinary coproporphyrin, urinary uroporphyrin
5	Variegate porphyria (hepatic)	AD	++	++	+	Urinary ALA, urinary PBG, urinary coproporphyrin, fecal protoporphyrin, fecal coproporphyrin
6	Protoporphyria (erythropoietic)	AD			+	Fecal protoporphyrin, RBC protoporphyrin

*Severity ranging from minimal (+) to profound (+++).
† The numbers refer to the numbered reactions in Fig. 22.1.
‡ Type I uroporphyrin and coproporphyrin are elevated.
§ In many cases no specific inheritance can be demonstrated.
AD, autosomal dominant; ALA, δ-aminolevulinate; AR, autosomal recessive; PBG, porphobilinogen; RBC, red blood cell.

Cutaneous photosensitivity occurs in porphyrias in which porphyrins or porphyrinogens accumulate. The porphyrinogens are oxidized nonenzymatically to the corresponding porphyrins. In the skin, the porphyrins become photoexcited by the action of sunlight, which leads to the formation of highly reactive and therefore toxic singlet oxygen. These porphyrias frequently result in unusually dark or colorful urine. The color deepens when the urine is exposed to light and air because of the nonenzymatic oxidation of the porphyrinogens to porphyrins.

For the diagnosis of porphyrias, urinary ALA and porphobilinogen can be quantified by colorimetric tests. Uroporphyrin and coproporphyrin are determined fluorometrically.

Two enzymes of heme synthesis, ALA dehydratase and ferrochelatase, are sensitive to inhibition by lead. This results in increased levels of urinary ALA and an increased concentration of protoporphyrin IX in erythrocytes. Some of the neurological impairments in lead poisoning are attributed to this inhibition of heme biosynthesis and the resulting accumulation of metabolic intermediates.

Heme Is Degraded to Bilirubin

Per day, 300 to 400 mg of heme is degraded in the human body, and close to 80% of this is derived from hemoglobin. The splenic macrophages that dispose of senile erythrocytes convert heme first to the green pigment **biliverdin** and then to yellow **bilirubin.** The heme oxygenase that catalyzes the first of these reactions is the only known CO-forming enzyme in the human body (Fig. 27.2).

The stages of heme degradation can be observed in the color changes of a hematoma; for example, when a punch to the face leaves a so-called black eye. After rupture of the capillaries, red blood cells are stranded in the interstitial spaces, in which their hemoglobin becomes deoxygenated. Deoxyhemoglobin is blue. Within a few days, the erythrocytes are scavenged by tissue macrophages and the heme is degraded first to biliverdin and then to bilirubin. The blue coloration disappears and is replaced by first a greenish and then a yellow coloration.

Bilirubin Is Conjugated and Excreted by the Liver

From the macrophages, bilirubin is *transported to the liver in tight, noncovalent binding to serum albumin.* It enters the hepatocytes on a facilitated-diffusion type carrier of high capacity and is then *conjugated to bilirubin diglucuronide* by two successive reactions with UDP–glucuronic acid. The water-soluble bilirubin diglucuronide is actively secreted into the bile canaliculi against a steep concentration gradient. This is an important rate-limiting step in hepatic bilirubin metabolism.

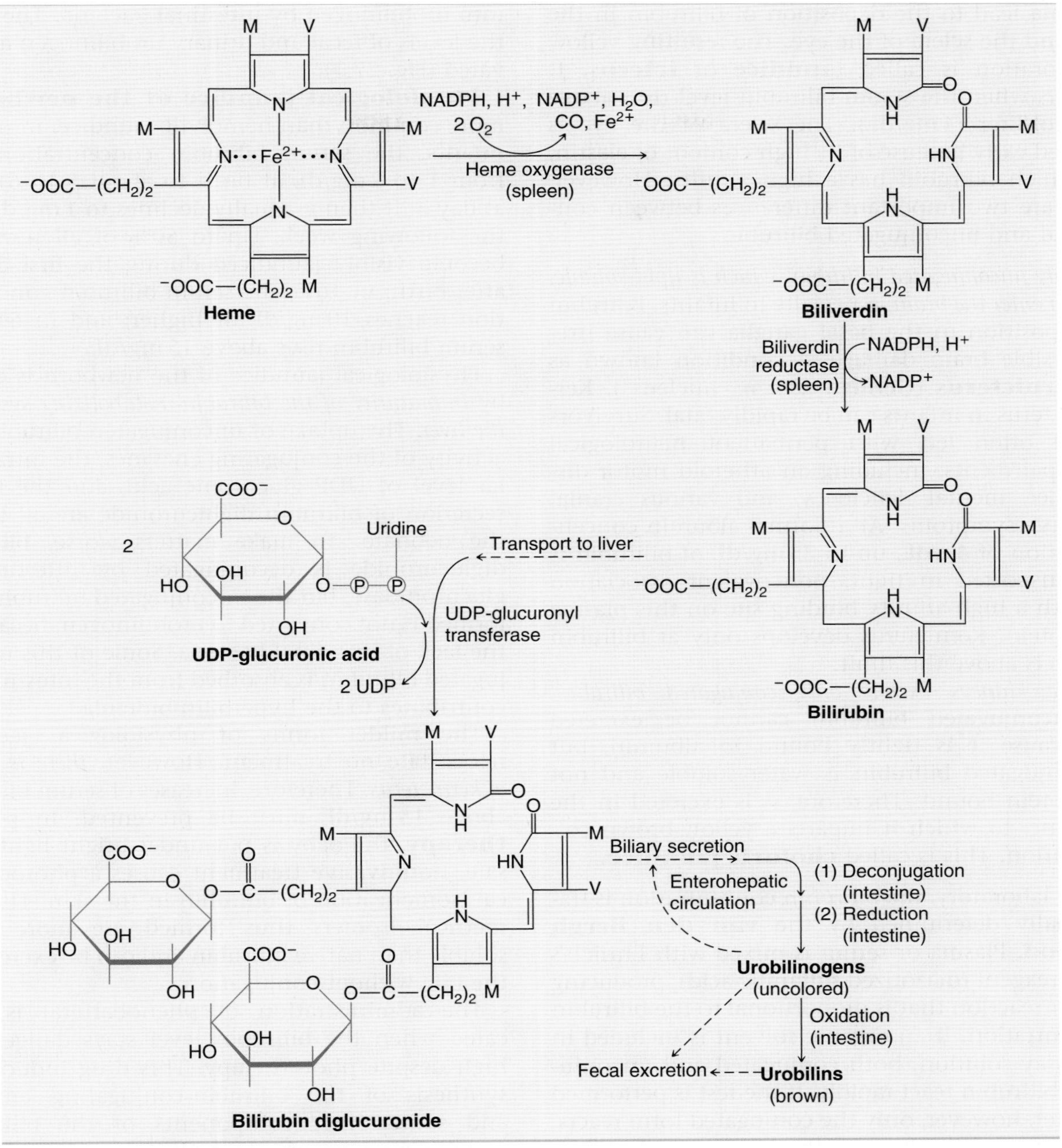

Figure 27.2 Heme degradation and bilirubin metabolism. M, methyl; V, vinyl.

In the intestine, bacteria deconjugate the bilirubin diglucuronide and reduce it to uncolored **urobilinogens.** Some of the urobilinogens are oxidized to urobilins and other colored products, which are responsible for the brown color of the stools. A small amount of urobilinogen is absorbed in the terminal ileum, returned to the liver, and secreted in the bile. Less than 4 mg/day finds its way to the kidneys, to be excreted in the urine.

Elevations of Serum Bilirubin Cause Jaundice

Normal blood contains less than 17 μmol/liter (1 mg/dL) of bilirubin. Most of this is unconjugated, apparently in transit from the spleen to the liver. Both unconjugated and conjugated bilirubin levels can be elevated in diseases. This condition is called **hyperbilirubinemia.** All types of hyperbilirubinemia lead to the deposition of bilirubin in the skin and the sclera of the eye. The resulting yellow discoloration is called **jaundice** or **icterus.** It appears when the serum bilirubin level rises above 70 μmol/liter (4 mg/dL). The sclera of the eye is affected early because of its high content of elastin, for which bilirubin has a high affinity. However, there are two important differences between conjugated and unconjugated bilirubin:

1. *Only unconjugated bilirubin, which is lipid soluble, can enter the brain,* especially in infants. Bilirubin deposition in the basal ganglia can cause irreversible brain damage, a condition known as **kernicterus** (German *kern* = "nucleus"). Kernicterus in infants can be rapidly fatal. Survivors are often left with permanent neurological impairments, including an athetoid motor disorder, mental deficiency, and various cranial nerve symptoms. At a normal albumin concentration of 4 g/dL, up to 25 mg/dL of bilirubin is transported in tight, noncovalent association with a high-affinity binding site on this plasma protein. Kernicterus develops only at bilirubin levels above this limit.

2. *The kidneys excrete only conjugated bilirubin.* Unconjugated bilirubin cannot be excreted because it is tightly bound to albumin, but conjugated bilirubin is water soluble and not protein bound. Therefore, it is excreted in the urine, to which it imparts a yellow-brown coloration. This is called **choluric jaundice.**

In the laboratory, the bilirubin concentration is traditionally determined by the **van den Bergh method.** Plasma or serum is mixed with Ehrlich's diazo reagent (diazotized sulfanilic acid), producing a color reaction that is proportional to the bilirubin concentration. If an organic solvent is included in the assay solution, both conjugated and unconjugated bilirubin react rapidly. If the test is performed in water, however, only the conjugated form reacts. Conjugated bilirubin is therefore called *"direct (reacting)" bilirubin,* and unconjugated bilirubin is called *"indirect (reacting)" bilirubin.*

Unconjugated Hyperbilirubinemia Is Most Common in Newborns

In hemolytic conditions, heme from the destroyed erythrocytes is turned into bilirubin. This can lead to hyperbilirubinemia and **hemolytic jaundice.** Fortunately, the healthy adult liver has a very high capacity for bilirubin metabolism, and the hyperbilirubinemia of hemolytic diseases thus rarely exceeds 3 to 4 mg/dL. The excess bilirubin is conjugated by the liver, secreted in the bile, and turned

into urobilinogen by intestinal bacteria. Therefore, the levels of fecal and urinary urobilinogen are elevated (Fig. 27.3).

Physiological jaundice of the newborn is more common than hemolytic jaundice. In normal infants, the serum bilirubin concentration rises from 1 to 2 mg/dL at birth to about 5 to 6 mg/dL at day 3. It then gradually declines to 1 mg/dL over the following week. Up to 50% of all newborns become visibly jaundiced during the first 5 days after birth; in 16%, the serum bilirubin concentration reaches 10 mg/dL or higher; and in 5%, the serum bilirubin rises above 15 mg/dL.

Physiological jaundice of the newborn is caused by *immaturity of the bilirubin-metabolizing system of the liver.* The uptake of unconjugated bilirubin, the activity of the conjugating enzymes, the intracellular level of UDP–glucuronic acid, and the biliary secretion of bilirubin diglucuronide are all low in the neonate. To make matters worse, bilirubin diglucuronide is deconjugated by intestinal β-glucuronidase, but the unconjugated bilirubin thus formed is not converted to urobilinogen, because of the lack of intestinal bacteria. Some of this unconjugated bilirubin is absorbed from the intestine and contributes to the hyperbilirubinemia.

The milder forms of physiological jaundice necessitate no treatment. However, *there is a risk of kernicterus.* Therefore, increases of serum bilirubin above 15 mg/dL must be prevented. In **phototherapy,** the baby is put under bright light. This safe, noninvasive treatment causes a photochemical isomerization of bilirubin in the skin. The geometrical isomers thus formed are more water soluble than native bilirubin and can be excreted in the bile without conjugation.

The administration of phenobarbital is indicated when the bilirubin level stays dangerously high despite phototherapy. This drug induces the synthesis of the bilirubin-conjugating enzymes and some other components of the bilirubin-metabolizing system. In addition, orally administered agar, which binds intestinal bilirubin and thereby prevents its absorption, is sometimes used.

Hemolytic conditions in the neonatal period are especially dangerous. In **rhesus incompatibility,** a maternal immunoglobulin G (IgG) antibody to a fetal blood group antigen causes severe hemolysis in the newborn. In some cases, exchange transfusion is required immediately after birth or even before birth.

Unconjugated hyperbilirubinemia can also be caused by inherited defects of bilirubin conjugation. A complete deficiency of the conjugating enzyme bilirubin–UDP glucuronyl transferase causes **Crigler-Najjar syndrome type I.** This rare, recessively inherited disease leads to massive

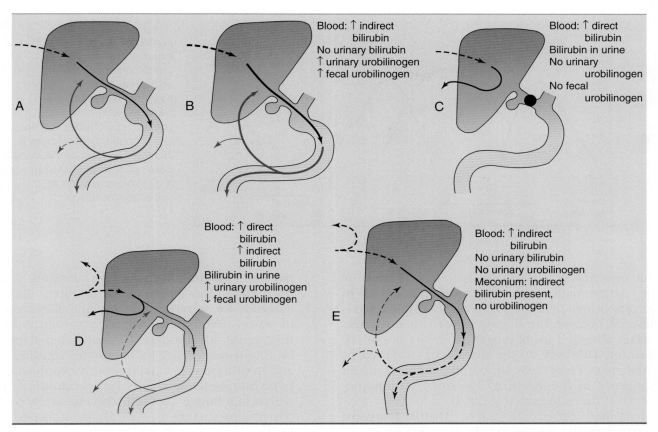

Figure 27.3 Bilirubin and urobilinogen in different types of jaundice. *Dashed black line* represents unconjugated (indirect) bilirubin; *solid line* represents conjugated (direct) bilirubin; *red line* represents urobilinogen. **A,** Normal pattern. **B,** Hemolysis. **C,** Biliary obstruction. **D,** Hepatitis (no cholestasis). **E,** Physiological jaundice of the newborn.

hyperbilirubinemia (>20 mg/dL). Most affected patients die within weeks after birth. **Crigler-Najjar syndrome type II** is a less severe defect of bilirubin conjugation with milder hyperbilirubinemia (5 to 20 mg/dL).

Gilbert syndrome is a benign condition in which mildly elevated unconjugated bilirubin is the only abnormality. It is caused by homozygosity for a mutation in the TATA box of the gene for bilirubin–UDP glucuronyl transferase. These individuals have only 30% of the enzyme. In Europe, 9% of the population are homozygous for the promoter variant, and 50% are heterozygous. However, only some of the homozygotes have hyperbilirubinemia.

Biliary Obstruction Causes Conjugated Hyperbilirubinemia

Conjugated hyperbilirubinemia has to be expected when *the liver still conjugates bilirubin but the flow of bile to the intestine is obstructed.* Having nowhere else to go, bilirubin diglucuronide over-

flows into the blood. The result is called **cholestatic jaundice.**

Urobilinogen, normally formed from bilirubin by intestinal bacteria, disappears from blood, stool, and urine. In complete biliary obstruction, the stools lose their normal brown color, which is caused by urobilins, and appear clay-colored. The urine, however, is colored yellow-brown by bilirubin diglucuronide (choluric jaundice). Liver function is unimpaired in acute biliary obstruction, but long-standing cholestasis causes irreversible liver damage.

Extrahepatic biliary obstruction can be caused by gallstones or, less commonly, by carcinoma of the head of the pancreas. **Intrahepatic biliary obstruction** occurs in many liver diseases in which either the bile canaliculi are blocked or the hepatocytes lose the ability for bile formation. The secretion of bile requires the energy-dependent transport of bile salts and inorganic ions across the intact hepatocyte membrane, and these processes are often impaired in severe liver diseases.

Nonspecific liver diseases typically cause a mixed conjugated and unconjugated hyperbilirubinemia.

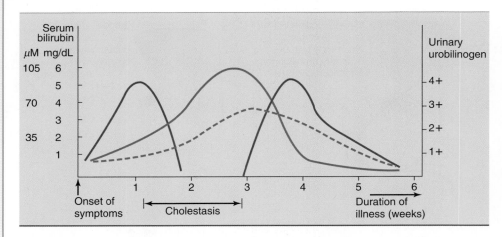

Figure 27.4 Levels of serum bilirubin and urinary urobilinogen in a patient with acute viral hepatitis. Dashed blue line, unconjugated bilirubin; solid blue line, conjugated bilirubin; red line, urobilinogen. Urobilinogen is increased as long as the disease does not lead to cholestasis, but it disappears as soon as cholestasis develops.

The presence of cholestasis can be evaluated by the determination of urinary urobilinogen. In uncomplicated liver disease, urinary urobilinogen is elevated because the diseased liver can no longer extract absorbed urobilinogen from the portal circulation. However, if the disease has resulted in intrahepatic cholestasis, urobilinogen can no longer be formed in the intestine. The urinary urobilinogen level drops to zero (Fig. 27.4).

Two rare genetic disorders, **Dubin-Johnson syndrome** and **Rotor syndrome,** are associated with conjugated hyperbilirubinemia. Dubin-Johnson syndrome is caused by a defect in the membrane carrier that pumps bilirubin diglucuronide into the bile canaliculi, but the molecular defect in Rotor syndrome is unknown.

SUMMARY

Heme is synthesized in bone marrow, the liver, and other tissues that produce heme proteins. The pathway starts with the formation of δ-aminolevulinic acid (ALA) from succinyl-CoA and glycine. This reaction, catalyzed by ALA synthase, is feedback-inhibited by free, non–protein-bound heme. In the porphyrias, one of the biosynthetic enzymes other than ALA synthase is impaired by genetic or environmental insults. Toxic intermediates of heme biosynthesis accumulate as a result, leading to neurological symptoms or cutaneous photosensitivity.

The heme of hemoglobin is degraded to bilirubin by macrophages in the spleen and other organs. The bilirubin is transported to the liver in tight binding to serum albumin. The liver conjugates bilirubin to bilirubin diglucuronide for secretion into the bile. Elevations of serum bilirubin, known as hyperbilirubinemia, result in jaundice. Unconjugated hyperbilirubinemia occurs in hemolytic conditions and in otherwise normal newborns; conjugated hyperbilirubinemia results from conditions in which bile flow is blocked (cholestasis). Mixed hyperbilirubinemia is typical for nonspecific liver diseases, including viral hepatitis and toxic liver damage.

QUESTIONS

1. **Porphyrias can be caused by a reduced activity of any of the following enzymes** *except*

   A. Ferrochelatase.
   B. Uroporphyrinogen decarboxylase.
   C. Uroporphyrinogen synthase.
   D. ALA synthase.
   E. Protoporphyrinogen oxidase.

2. **A combination of elevated conjugated bilirubin, near-normal unconjugated bilirubin, and absence of fecal urobilinogen in a jaundiced patient suggests**

   A. Mild hepatitis.
   B. Cholestasis.
   C. Hemolysis.
   D. Absence of bilirubin–UDP glucuronyl transferase.
   E. Gilbert syndrome.

CHAPTER 28

The Metabolism of Purines and Pyrimidines

The purine and pyrimidine bases (Fig. 28.1) are constituents of nucleotides and nucleic acids. The **ribonucleotides** include adenosine, guanosine, uridine, and cytidine triphosphates (ATP, GTP, UTP, and CTP). They are present in millimolar concentrations in the cell, and they serve important coenzyme functions, in addition to being precursors of RNA synthesis. The **deoxyribonucleotides** deoxyadenosine, deoxyguanosine, deoxycytidine, and deoxythymidine triphosphates (dATP, dGTP, dCTP, and dTTP) are present in micromolar concentrations and are required only for DNA replication and DNA repair. Their cellular concentrations are highest during S phase of the cell cycle.

Although dietary nucleic acids and nucleotides are digested to nucleosides and free bases in the intestine, the products are poorly absorbed. Also, especially in the case of the purines, the absorbed bases are extensively degraded in the intestinal mucosa. Therefore, *humans depend on the endogenous synthesis of purines and pyrimidines*. This chapter is concerned with the pathways for the synthesis and degradation of the nucleotides.

Purine Synthesis Starts with Ribose-5-Phosphate

The de novo synthesis of purines is most active in the liver, which exports the bases and nucleosides to other tissues. Most tissues have a limited capacity for de novo purine synthesis, although they can synthesize the nucleotides from externally supplied bases.

The pathway of purine biosynthesis is shown in Figure 28.2. It starts with ribose-5-phosphate, a product of the pentose phosphate pathway (see Chapter 22). In the reactions of the pathway, all of them cytoplasmic, *the purine ring system is built up step-by-step, with C-1 of ribose-5-phosphate used as a primer.*

The first enzyme, **5-phosphoribosyl-1-pyrophosphate (PRPP) synthetase,** transfers a pyrophosphate group from ATP to C-1 of ribose-5-phosphate, forming **PRPP.** *PRPP is the activated form of ribose for nucleotide synthesis.* In the next reaction, catalyzed by **PRPP amidotransferase,** a nitrogen from the side chain of glutamine replaces the pyrophosphate group at C-1 of PRPP. *This reaction is the committed step of purine biosynthesis.* In the ensuing reaction sequence, the purine ring is constructed from simple building blocks:

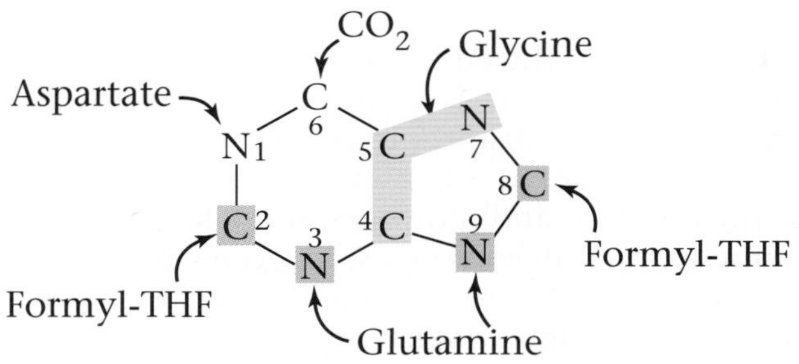

where THF = tetrahydrofolate. The first nucleotide formed in the pathway is **inosine monophosphate (IMP)**, which contains the base **hypoxanthine.** IMP is a branch point in the synthesis of AMP and GMP (Fig. 28.3). These nucleoside monophosphates are in equilibrium with their corresponding diphosphates and triphosphates through kinase reactions.

As expected, purine synthesis is regulated by feedback inhibition (Fig. 28.4). *The first two enzymes of the pathway, PRPP synthetase and PRPP amidotransferase, are inhibited by the purine nucleotides.* Also, the reactions leading from IMP to AMP and GMP are

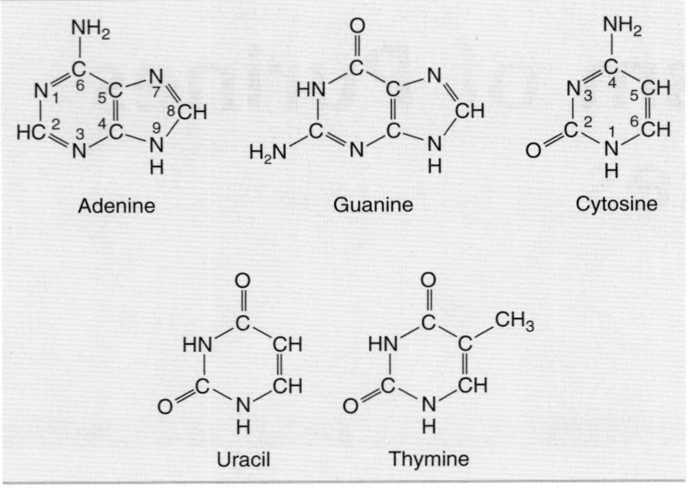

Figure 28.1 The structures of the purine and pyrimidine bases.

feedback-inhibited by the end products, in both cases by competitive inhibition (see Fig. 28.4).

Purines Are Degraded to Uric Acid

The degradation of purine nucleotides starts with the hydrolytic removal of phosphate from the nucleotides. The nucleosides thus formed are then cleaved into ribose-1-phosphate and the free base by the **purine nucleoside phosphorylase.** Adenosine is a poor substrate of the nucleoside phosphorylase. It is therefore catabolized through inosine, as shown in Figure 28.5.

Uric acid is the end product of purine degradation in humans. It is synthesized by **xanthine oxidase** via hypoxanthine and xanthine (reaction (6) in Fig. 28.5). This enzyme contains FAD, nonheme iron, and molybdenum. Like other non-mitochondrial flavoproteins, it regenerates its FAD by transferring hydrogen from $FADH_2$ to molecular oxygen, forming hydrogen peroxide.

Free Purine Bases Can Be Salvaged

As an alternative to degradation, the free bases can be recycled into the nucleotide pool. This requires the PRPP-dependent salvage enzymes **hypoxanthine-guanine phosphoribosyltransferase (HGPRT)** and **adenine phosphoribosyl transferase (APRT):**

$$\text{Hypoxanthine} + \text{PRPP} \xrightarrow{\text{HGPRT}} \text{IMP} + \text{PP}_i$$
$$\text{Guanine} + \text{PRPP} \xrightarrow{\text{HGPRT}} \text{GMP} + \text{PP}_i$$
$$\text{Adenine} + \text{PRPP} \xrightarrow{\text{APRT}} \text{AMP} + \text{PP}_i$$

The salvage reactions are the only source of purine nucleotides for tissues that cannot synthesize the nucleotides de novo. HGPRT is quantitatively by far the more important salvage enzyme. It is competitively inhibited by IMP and GMP, whereas APRT is inhibited by AMP.

Pyrimidines Are Synthesized from Carbamoyl Phosphate and Aspartate

Whereas the purine ring is synthesized on ribose, the pyrimidine ring is synthesized before the ribose is added (Fig. 28.6). The pathway starts with **carbamoyl phosphate** and **aspartate,** and **orotic acid** is formed as the first pyrimidine. Orotic acid is processed to the uridine nucleotides, which are the precursors of the cytidine nucleotides. The enzymes of the pathway are cytosolic except for dihydroorotate dehydrogenase (reaction (4) in Fig. 28.6), which is on the outer surface of the inner mitochondrial membrane.

The carbamoyl phosphate for pyrimidine synthesis is made in the cytoplasm, although the carbamoyl phosphate for the urea cycle is made in the mitochondria (see Chapter 26). Unlike the mitochondrial carbamoyl phosphate synthetase, which obtains its nitrogen from ammonia, the cytoplasmic enzyme uses the nitrogen in the side chain of glutamine. Both the cytoplasmic carbamoyl phosphate synthetase and the CTP synthetase are feedback-inhibited by CTP.

Hereditary orotic aciduria is caused by a deficiency of either orotate phosphoribosyltransferase or orotidylate decarboxylase (reactions (5) and (6) in Fig. 28.6). This rare condition is characterized by megaloblastic anemia, a crystalline sediment of

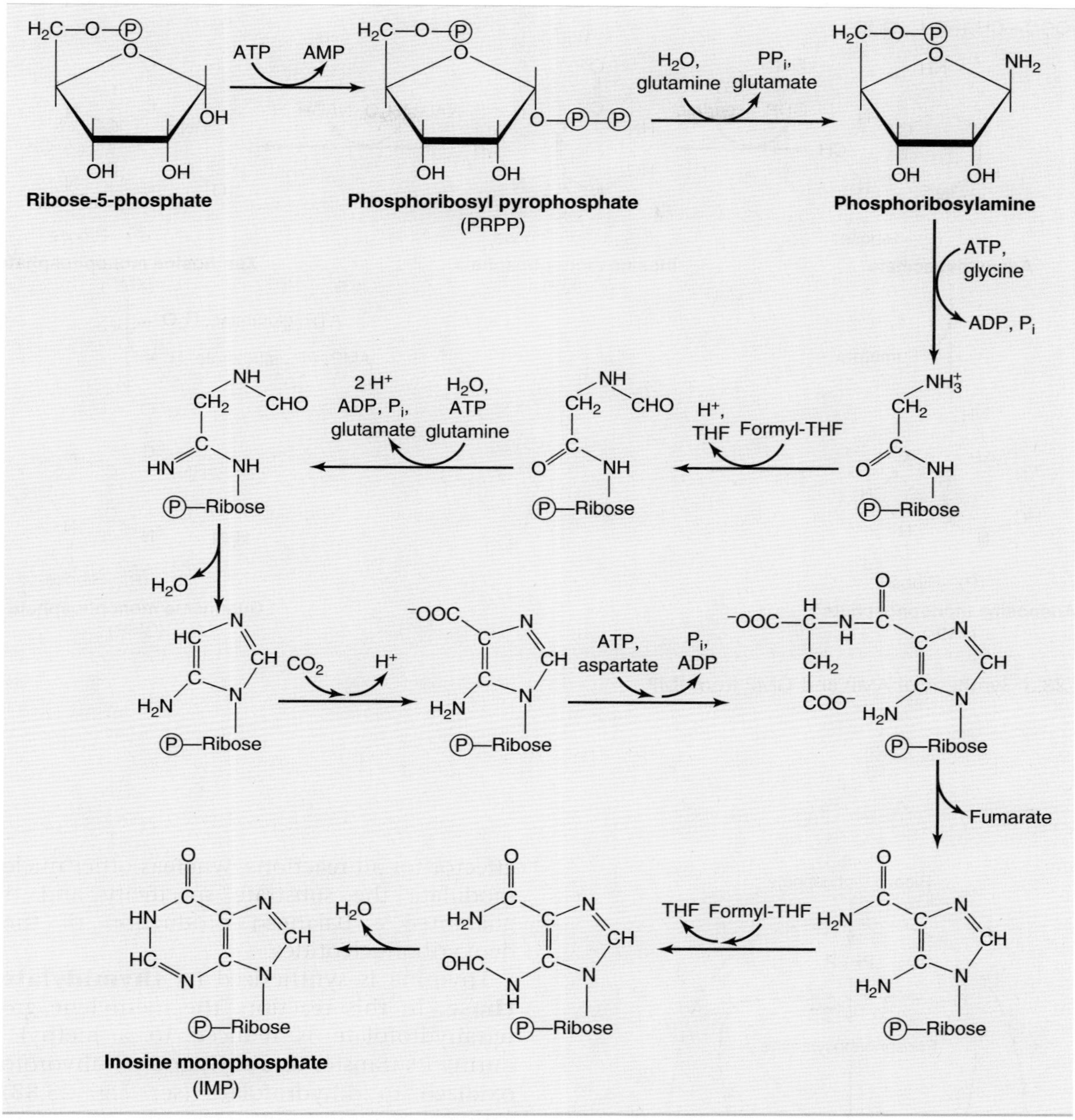

Figure 28.2 The de novo pathway of purine biosynthesis. THF, tetrahydrofolate.

orotic acid in the urine, and poor growth. The important clinical signs are caused not by orotic acid accumulation but by pyrimidine deficiency. The patients are pyrimidine auxotrophs who can be treated quite effectively with large doses of orally administered uridine.

Mild orotic aciduria is also seen in ammonia toxicity and in patients with ornithine transcarbamoylase deficiency. These conditions lead to an accumulation of carbamoyl phosphate in liver mitochondria. Some of this leaks into the cytoplasm, where it is converted to orotic acid.

The pyrimidines are degraded to water-soluble products that are either excreted as such or oxidized to carbon dioxide and water (Fig. 28.7).

DNA Synthesis Requires Deoxyribonucleotides

The synthesis of 2-deoxyribonucleotides from the corresponding ribonucleotides requires two reactions: *the reduction of ribose to 2-deoxyribose* and *the methylation of uracil to thymine*.

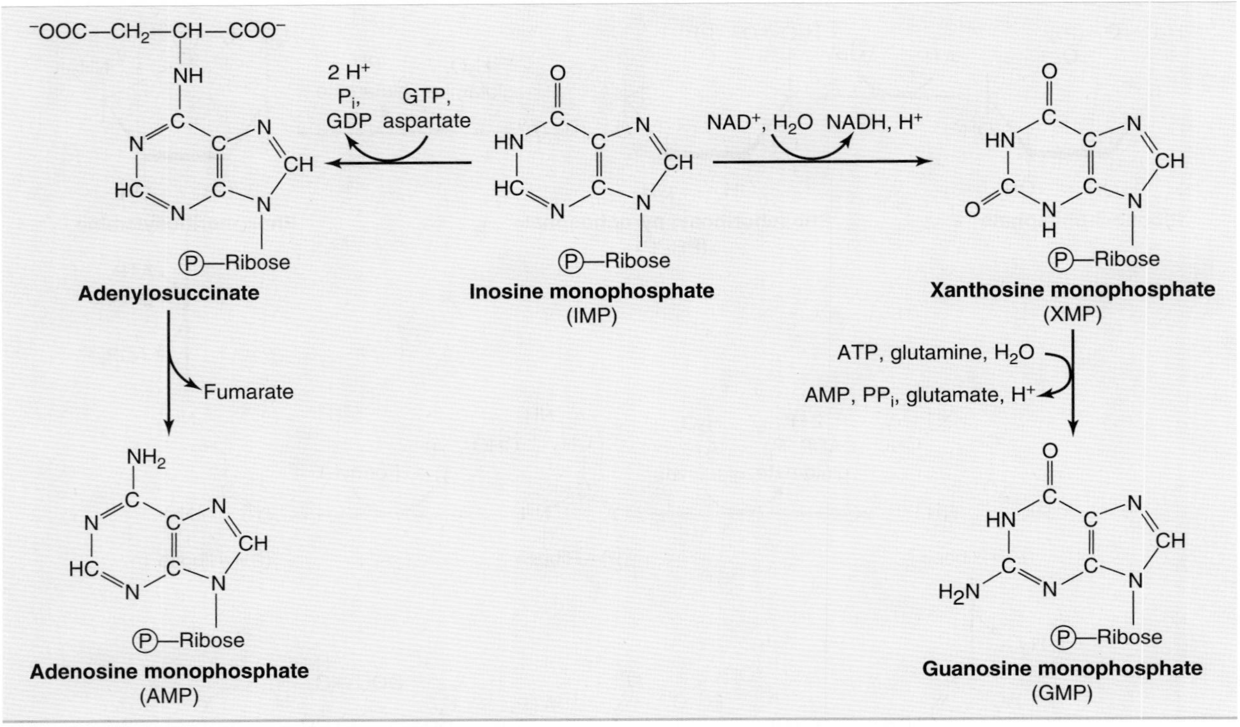

Figure 28.3 Synthesis of AMP and GMP from IMP.

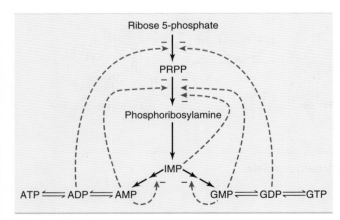

Figure 28.4 Feedback inhibition of de novo purine biosynthesis by nucleotides. IMP, inosine monophosphate; PRPP, 5-phosphoribosyl-1-pyrophosphate.

Ribonucleotide reductase reduces the ribose residues in all four ribonucleoside diphosphates (Fig. 28.8A). Its level rises immediately preceding the S phase of the cell cycle, and it is also subject to intricate allosteric control. dATP is a negative effector for all reactions, whereas other nucleotides modulate the substrate specificity and thereby guarantee a balanced production of the four deoxyribonucleotides.

Thymine is synthesized by **thymidylate synthase.** In this reaction, the methylene group of tetrahydrofolate is reduced to a methyl group during its transfer to dUMP, and tetrahydrofolate is oxidized to dihydrofolate (see Fig. 28.8B). The active coenzyme form, tetrahydrofolate, has to be regenerated by **dihydrofolate reductase** (see Fig. 28.8C).

Many Antineoplastic Drugs Inhibit Nucleotide Metabolism

The development of drugs with selective toxicity for cancer cells is difficult because cancer cells are too similar to normal cells. Therefore, agents that are toxic for cancer cells are toxic also for normal cells. Cancer cells do, however, have a higher mitotic rate than normal cells. Therefore, *they have a higher requirement for DNA synthesis.* With this in mind, drugs have been developed as antagonists of nucleotide synthesis:

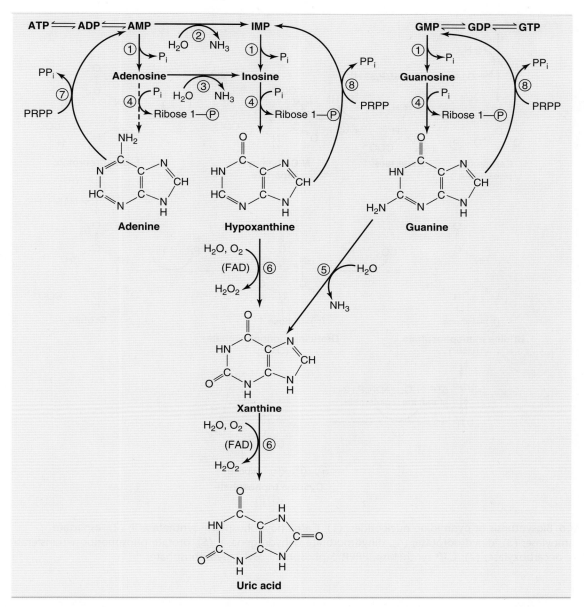

Figure 28.5 Degradation of purine nucleotides to uric acid, and the salvage of purine bases. (1), 5′-Nucleotidase; (2), adenosine monophosphate (AMP) deaminase; (3), adenosine deaminase; (4), purine nucleoside phosphorylase; (5), guanine deaminase; (6), xanthine oxidase; (7), adenine phosphoribosyltransferase; (8), hypoxanthine-guanine phosphoribosyltransferase. IMP, inosine monophosphate; PRPP, 5-phosphoribosyl-1-pyrophosphate.

1. *Glutamine antagonists* inhibit the steps in purine and pyrimidine synthesis in which glutamine donates a nitrogen: the incorporation of N-3 and N-9 into the purine ring, and the IMP→GMP and UTP→CTP reactions. Azaserine is an example:

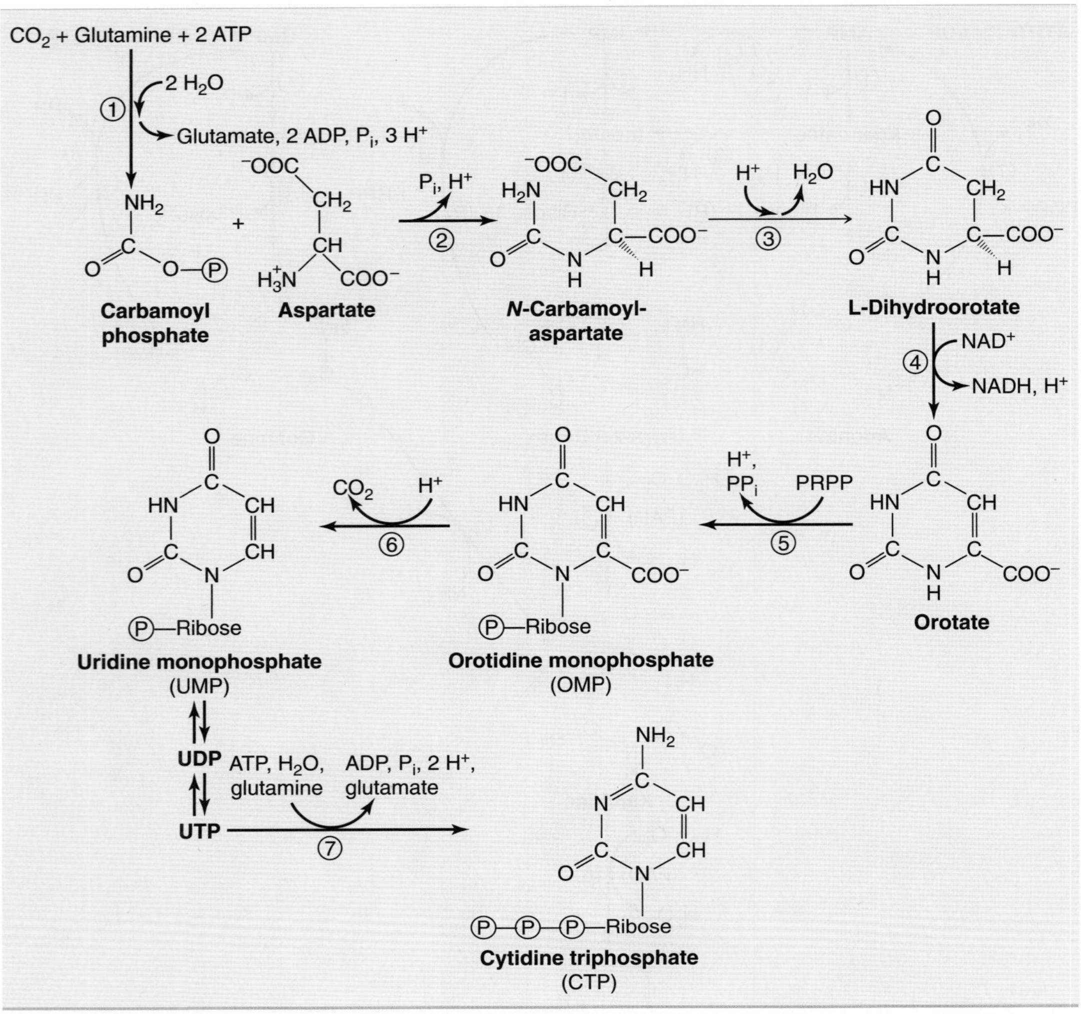

Figure 28.6 Biosynthesis of pyrimidine nucleotides. (1), Carbamoyl phosphate synthetase II; (2), aspartate transcarbamoylase; (3), dihydroorotase; (4), dihydroorotate dehydrogenase; (5), orotate phosphoribosyltransferase; (6), orotidylate decarboxylase; (7), CTP synthetase. PRPP, 5-phosphoribosyl-1-pyrophosphate.

2. Some *structural analogs of bases or nucleosides* are useful as antineoplastic drugs. They act either as inhibitors of nucleotide biosynthesis or through their incorporation into DNA or RNA. A typical example is **5-fluorouracil,** a uracil analog that has been used in the treatment of several solid tumors. 5-Fluorouracil is processed to fluorodeoxyuridine monophosphate in the body:

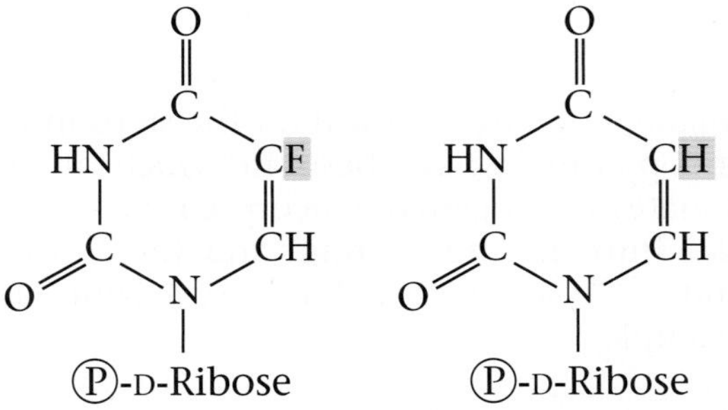

5-Fluorodeoxyuridine monophosphate

Deoxyuridine monophosphate (dUMP)

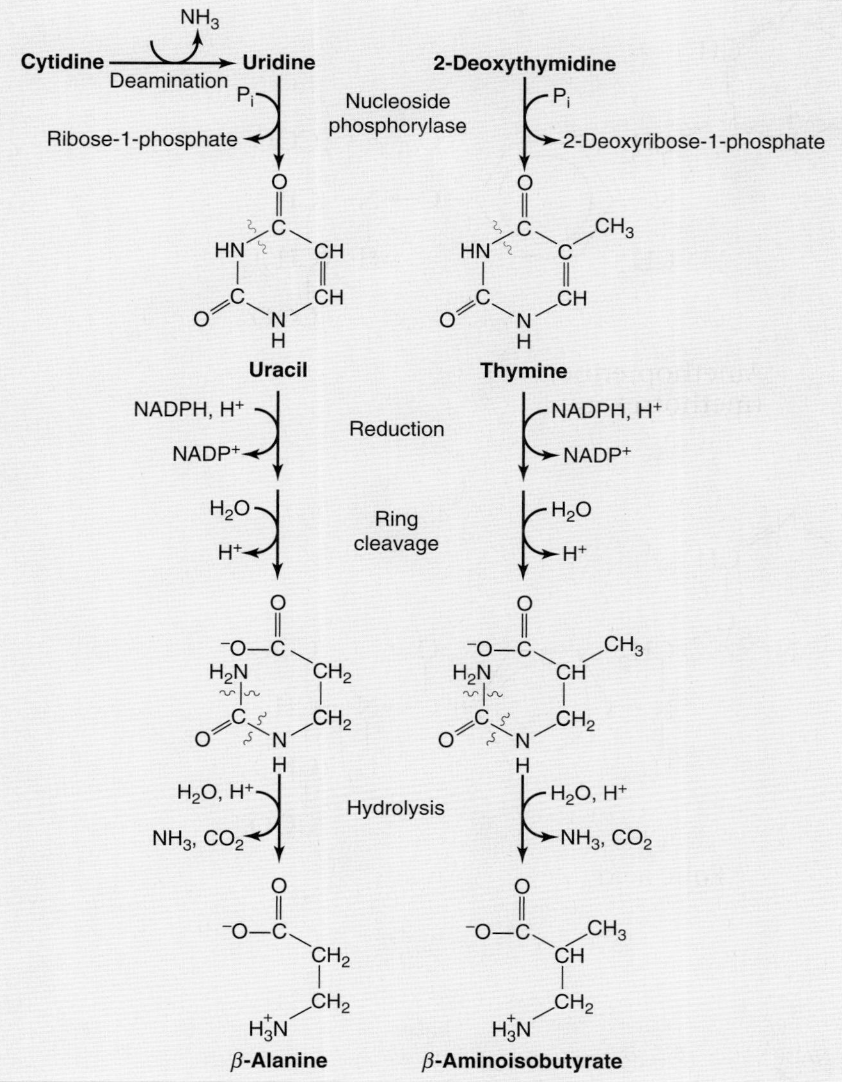

Figure 28.7 Degradation of pyrimidines.

This product binds tightly to thymidylate synthase as a structural analog of its natural substrate dUMP. Eventually, it reacts covalently with the enzyme, resulting in irreversible inhibition. 5-Fluorouracil is also incorporated into RNA in place of uracil, and this contributes to its antineoplastic activity.

3. *Antifolates* are best exemplified by **amethopterine (methotrexate):**

Amethopterine
(methotrexate)

Folic acid

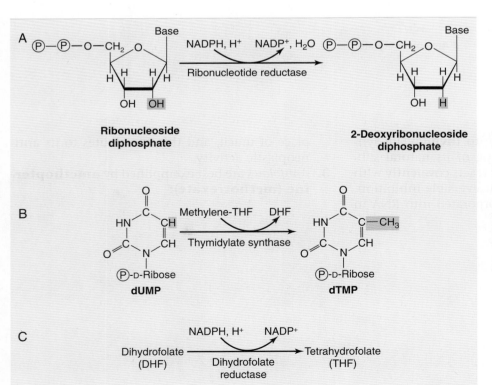

Figure 28.8 The synthesis of 2-deoxyribonucleotides, the precursors for DNA synthesis. DHF, dihydrofolate; dTMP, deoxythymidine monophosphate; dUMP, deoxyuridine monophosphate; NADP+, nicotinamide adenine dinucleotide phosphate; NADPH, reduced form of NADP; THF, tetrahydrofolate.

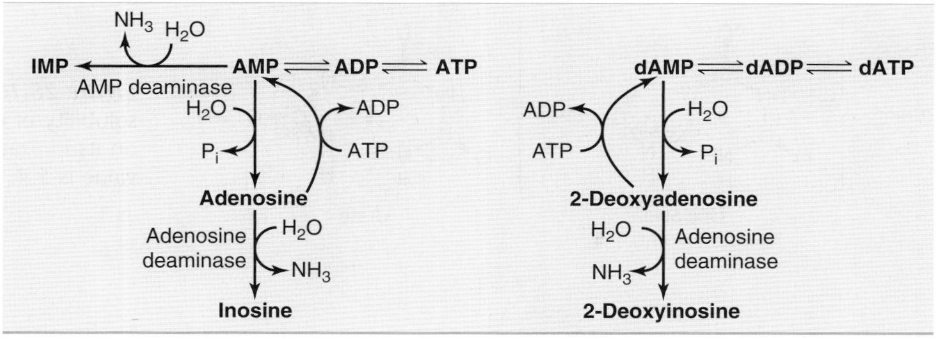

Figure 28.9 The role of adenosine deaminase in the metabolism of adenine nucleotides. The ribonucleotides can be catabolized by adenosine monophosphate (AMP)–deaminase, but the deoxyribonucleotides accumulate in adenosine deaminase deficiency. ADP, adenosine diphosphate; ATP, adenosine triphosphate; dADP, deoxyadenosine diphosphate; dAMP, deoxyadenosine monophosphate; dATP, deoxyadenosine triphosphate; P_i, inorganic phosphate.

Table 28.1 Inherited Disorders of Purine and Pyrimidine Metabolism

Disease	Enzyme Deficiency	Signs and Symptoms
Adenosine deaminase deficiency	Adenosine deaminase	Severe combined immunodeficiency
Purine nucleoside phosphorylase deficiency	Purine nucleoside phosphorylase	Immunodeficiency with T cell defect
Familial orotic aciduria	Orotate phosphoribosyltransferase	Accumulation of orotic acid in blood and urine, failure to thrive
Lesch-Nyhan syndrome	Hypoxanthine-guanine phosphoribosyltransferase	Mental retardation with self-mutilation, hyperuricemia

Methotrexate inhibits dihydrofolate reductase competitively, thereby depleting the cell of tetrahydrofolate. Thymidylate synthase is the only important enzyme that converts a tetrahydrofolate coenzyme to dihydrofolate. Therefore, rapidly dividing cells, with their high activity of this enzyme, are most vulnerable to methotrexate.

All these antineoplastic drugs are toxic not only for cancer cells but for all rapidly dividing cells, including those in bone marrow, intestinal mucosa, and hair bulbs. Therefore, bone marrow depression, diarrhea, and hair loss are common side effects of cancer chemotherapy.

Some Immunodeficiency Diseases Are Caused by Defects in Nucleotide Metabolism

Combined defects of B cells and T cells are known as **severe combined immunodeficiency (SCID)**. Some patients with recessively inherited SCID were found to be deficient in **adenosine deaminase.** This enzyme deaminates adenosine to inosine and deoxyadenosine to deoxyinosine (Fig. 28.9). Both adenosine and deoxyadenosine can also be phosphorylated to the corresponding nucleoside monophosphate.

However, whereas AMP can be deaminated to IMP by AMP deaminase, dAMP has no alternative route of degradation. Therefore, it accumulates, together with its diphosphate and triphosphate derivatives. dATP is thought to cause the immunodeficiency by inhibiting ribonucleotide reductase, thus depriving the cell of the precursors for DNA synthesis. However, the selective impairment of lymphocytes but not other cell types in this condition remains an enigma.

The deficiency of **purine nucleoside phosphorylase** results in a different type of immunodeficiency that affects T cells but not B cells. The mechanism of the selective T cell impairment in this condition is unknown (Table 28.1).

Uric Acid Has Limited Water Solubility

All purines are catabolized to uric acid. Although not very toxic, uric acid has a serious problem: *low water solubility.* It can form damaging crystals in the urine and even in the tissues. Uric acid is a weak acid with a pK of 5.7, and its water solubility depends on its ionization state (Fig. 28.10).

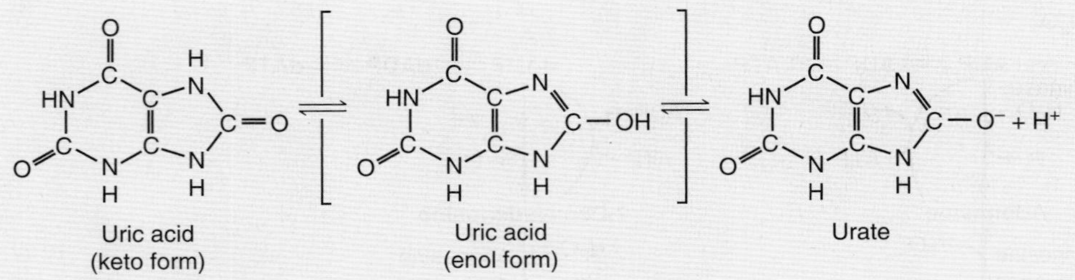

Figure 28.10 The water solubility of uric acid depends on its ionization state. Its pK value is 5.7.

The protonated form is usually less soluble than the deprotonated form. In urine of pH 5.0, uric acid becomes insoluble at concentrations above 0.9 mmol/liter (15 mg/dL). Thus, uric acid stones can form in the collecting ducts, where the urine becomes concentrated and acidified. Between 5% and 10% of all kidney stones consist of uric acid.

In plasma and interstitial fluids, with a pH of 7.3 to 7.4 and a high sodium concentration, sodium urate is the least soluble form. It tends to precipitate at concentrations above 0.4 mmol/liter (7 mg/dL). Most adults have serum urate levels between 3 and 7 mg/dL. Therefore, *even a moderate rise of the serum urate concentration will exceed the limit of solubility.* The average uric acid level is higher in men than in women by about 1 mg/dL and rises with increasing age.

Hyperuricemia Causes Gout

Elevations of the serum uric acid level above the limit of solubility are called **hyperuricemia.** As a result, sodium urate crystals can precipitate in the tissues. Focal deposits of sodium urate in subcutaneous tissues, known as **tophi,** are asymptomatic, but sodium urate crystals in the joints trigger the inflammatory response of **gouty arthritis.** This disease is most common in middle-aged and older men, with a prevalence of 0.4% to 0.8% in this population in the United States.

Gouty arthritis takes the form of acute attacks of severe joint pain and inflammation, separated by long asymptomatic intervals. The disease has a predilection for small peripheral joints, and the metatarsophalangeal joint of the big toe is initially affected in about half of the patients. This is because the solubility of sodium urate is temperature dependent, and crystals form in the coldest parts of the body first.

Any sustained hyperuricemia is likely to cause gouty arthritis, but uric acid levels are somewhat variable over time. On random sampling, between 2% and 18% of healthy people have uric acid levels above the solubility limit of 7 mg/dL, and 10% to 20% of gouty patients have levels below this limit at the time of their first attack.

Synovial fluid analysis from an acutely inflamed joint shows *needle-shaped optically birefringent crystals of sodium urate,* often within polymorphonuclear leukocytes. These cells phagocytize sodium urate crystals, but the razor-sharp, undigestible crystals damage their lysosomes and thereby kill the cell.

The cause of **primary hyperuricemia** is usually unknown, but **secondary hyperuricemia** is caused by an underlying disease. It is seen in psoriasis, chronic hemolytic anemias, pernicious anemia, malignancies, and other conditions with increased cell turnover. Radiation treatment or chemotherapy for neoplastic diseases can cause massive hyperuricemia, with a risk of **uric acid nephropathy** and renal failure.

Uric acid production is also increased in metabolic disorders in which the activity of the pentose phosphate pathway is increased. In type I glycogen storage disease (von Gierke disease; see Chapter 22), for example, accumulating glucose-6-phosphate is converted into ribose-5-phosphate by the pentose phosphate pathway. Ribose-5-phosphate feeds into purine nucleotide biosynthesis, and the excess nucleotides are degraded to uric acid. Purines cannot be stored in the body; therefore, *any increase in the rate of their de novo synthesis has to be matched by an increased rate of degradation to uric acid.*

Primary hyperuricemia is caused either by *overproduction of uric acid, impairment of its renal excretion, or both.* Urinary excretion in excess of 600 mg/day is evidence of uric acid overproduction. Of patients with primary gout, 15% to 25% are overproducers; the other 75% to 85% have impaired renal excretion. The handling of uric acid by the kidneys is complex, inasmuch as it is first reabsorbed and then actively secreted in the tubular system.

Most animals other than the higher primates do not develop gout because they degrade uric acid to water-soluble products. Why do humans use uric acid as the end product of purine metabolism, and why is our uric acid level so high that we are teetering on the brink of gout? One possible reason is that uric acid is an effective antioxidant that scavenges hydroxyl radicals, superoxide radicals, singlet oxygen, and other aggressive oxygen derivatives. It contributes to the body's defenses against oxidative damage.

Some Patients with Gout Have Abnormalities of Purine-Metabolizing Enzymes

Abnormalities of two enzymes have been identified in a minority of patients with uric acid overproduction:

1. *Overactivity of PRPP synthetase* increases de novo purine biosynthesis, and purine breakdown must rise in proportion. Elevated levels of IMP, GMP, and AMP from increased de novo biosynthesis inhibit the salvage enzymes and thereby favor uric acid formation over recycling. The hyperuricemia in individuals with an overactive PRPP synthetase shows that this enzyme is normally rate limiting for de novo purine synthesis. The rate of the amidotransferase reaction depends largely on the concentration of its rate-limiting substrate PRPP.
2. *Reduced activity of the salvage enzyme HGPRT* causes hyperuricemia because the substrates of the deficient enzyme accumulate, whereas the levels of its product are reduced:
   • *The cellular levels of the free bases are increased,* thus providing more substrate for uric acid synthesis.
   • *The cellular PRPP level is increased* because of decreased consumption in the salvage reactions, and more substrate is available for the PRPP amidotransferase of the de novo pathway.
   • *The cellular concentrations of the nucleotides are reduced.* This disinhibits the regulated enzymes of the de novo pathway. The result is an increased rate of de novo synthesis, balanced by an equally increased rate of uric acid formation.

Both PRPP synthetase and HGPRT are encoded by genes on the X chromosome, and the enzyme abnormalities are expressed as X-linked recessive traits.

Partial deficiencies of HGPRT cause only hyperuricemia, but complete deficiency results in **Lesch-Nyhan syndrome.** This rare X-linked recessive disorder is characterized by choreoathetosis, spasticity, mental retardation, and bizarre self-mutilating behavior. If unrestrained, affected patients chew off their lips and fingers or jam their hands in the spokes of their wheelchair. The presence of uric acid crystals in the urine is an early sign of the disease, and most patients eventually die of uric acid nephropathy.

The brain disorder, however, is not caused by uric acid overload but by the deficiency of purine nucleotides. The brain has a very low capacity for de novo purine biosynthesis, and therefore it depends on the salvage enzyme for its purine nucleotides.

Gout Can Be Treated with Drugs

The immediate aim in the treatment of gout is the alleviation of pain and inflammation, but long-term treatment is aimed at reducing the serum uric acid level. The most important drug treatments are as follows:

1. *Anti-inflammatory drugs.* **Colchicine** is the classical treatment for the acute attack. It is not very effective in other forms of arthritis, and therefore it can be used for the differential diagnosis of gout. This approach, in which the response to the treatment confirms (or refutes) a preliminary diagnosis, is called a diagnosis *ex juvantibus.* Because of gastrointestinal side effects, however, colchicine has been largely replaced by indomethacin, ibuprofen, and other nonsteroidal anti-inflammatory drugs.
2. *Uricosuric agents* increase the renal excretion of uric acid. **Probenecid** is an example.
3. *Inhibition of xanthine oxidase* is possible with **allopurinol.** This purine analog is oxidized to alloxanthine by xanthine oxidase, but this product remains bound to the enzyme as a competitive inhibitor. As a result, the patient excretes a mix of uric acid, xanthine, and hypoxanthine. This mix is more soluble than uric acid alone. Hypoxanthine and xanthine are timed into IMP and xanthosine monophosphate (XMP), respectively. These salvage reactions consume PRPP and produce nucleotides that feedback-inhibit the regulated enzymes of the de novo pathway, thereby reducing de novo purine biosynthesis.

Dietary manipulations are less effective. Dietary purines are degraded to uric acid in the intestinal mucosa. Although much of this uric acid ends up in the stools, in which it is degraded by intestinal bacteria, the consumption of 4 g of yeast RNA per day raises the blood urate to levels typical for gout. On the other hand, eliminating all purines from a typical diet would reduce the serum urate level by only 1 mg/dL.

Alcohol should be avoided because of associated dehydration and because the increased lactate level during alcohol intoxication can impair the renal excretion of uric acid. Acute attacks of gouty arthritis are often triggered by an alcoholic binge.

SUMMARY

Humans obtain nearly all their purines and pyrimidines from endogenous synthesis rather than from the diet. The heterocyclic ring systems are assembled from simple precursors, whereas the ribose portion of the nucleotides comes from PRPP, the activated form of ribose-5-phosphate. The first reactions of the biosynthetic pathways are always feedback-inhibited by the nucleotides.

The ribonucleotides are synthesized first, and they are the precursors of the corresponding 2-deoxyribonucleotides. Rapidly dividing cells depend on a high rate of nucleotide biosynthesis, and therefore many inhibitors of nucleotide biosynthesis can be used for cancer chemotherapy.

Purine nucleotides are catabolized to the free bases first, and these are either oxidized to the excretory product uric acid or recycled to the corresponding nucleotides in PRPP-dependent salvage reactions. Uric acid is poorly soluble in water. Therefore, it can cause kidney stones, and it causes gout when it forms crystals of sodium urate in the joints.

QUESTIONS

1. Enzyme abnormalities that can lead to hyperuricemia and gout include

   A. Reduced activity of PRPP synthetase.
   B. Reduced activity of xanthine oxidase.
   C. Reduced activity of hypoxanthine-guanine phosphoribosyltransferase.
   D. Reduced activity of PRPP amidotransferase.
   E. Reduced activity of dihydroorotate dehydrogenase.

2. A coenzyme form of tetrahydrofolate is required for

   A. The de novo synthesis of pyrimidines.
   B. The synthesis of thymine-containing nucleotides from uracil-containing nucleotides.
   C. The synthesis of xanthine from purine nucleotides.
   D. The cleavage of the purine ring in uric acid by an enzyme in the human liver.
   E. The reduction of ribonucleotides to 2-deoxyribonucleotides.

CHAPTER 29

Vitamins and Minerals

Vitamins are organic nutrients that are required in small quantities in the diet and serve specialized functions in the body. Traditionally, scientists distinguish between water-soluble and fat-soluble vitamins. Most of the water-soluble vitamins are nearly always precursors of coenzymes, but the fat-soluble vitamins are more often encountered as physiological regulators or antioxidants.

There are also metabolic differences between these two classes of vitamins. Water-soluble vitamins are readily absorbed in the intestine, but the absorption of fat-soluble vitamins depends on mixed bile salt micelles. Therefore, deficiencies are most likely to be present in patients with fat malabsorption. Also, supplements of these vitamins are most effective when taken with a fatty meal.

Whereas water-soluble vitamins are transported in the blood as such, fat-soluble vitamins are transported either as constituents of lipoproteins or in binding to specific plasma proteins. Finally, the renal excretion of excess water-soluble vitamins is unproblematic, whereas fat-soluble vitamins require prior metabolism to water-soluble products before they can be excreted. Therefore, fat-soluble vitamins are more likely to accumulate in the body and cause toxicity.

Minerals are inorganic nutrients. The **macrominerals,** including sodium, potassium, calcium, magnesium, and phosphate, are required in quantities of more than 100 mg/day. They are components of the body fluids and the inorganic matrix of bone. The **microminerals,** or **trace minerals,** in contrast, are required in only small quantities and serve specialized biochemical functions. Only the vitamins and trace minerals are discussed in this chapter.

The **recommended daily allowances** (**RDAs**) of vitamins and minerals are published by the Food and Nutrition Board of the National Academy of Science in the United States and by similar agencies in other countries. The RDA defines not a minimal requirement but *a dietary intake that is considered optimal under ordinary conditions.*

Experts often disagree about "optimal" levels of intake, and RDAs are therefore frequently revised. Also, the requirement depends on sex, age, body weight, diet, and physiological status. Increases in dietary intake of many nutrients are recommended during pregnancy and lactation. Figure 29.1 summarizes the RDAs of the most important vitamins and minerals for the standard 70-kg textbook man.

Riboflavin Is a Precursor of FMN and FAD

Riboflavin (vitamin B_2) consists of a dimethylisoalloxazine ring that is covalently bound to the sugar alcohol ritbitol. Its only biological function is as a *precursor of flavin adenine dinucleotide (FAD) and flavin mononucleotide (FMN),* the prosthetic groups of the **flavoproteins** (Latin *flavus* = "yellow"). Both free riboflavin and the flavin coenzymes are yellow in their reduced form, with an absorption band at 450 nm. Although riboflavin and its derivatives are heat-stable, they are rapidly degraded to inactive products on exposure to visible light.

Dietary riboflavin is absorbed by an energy-dependent transporter in the upper small intestine and transported to the tissues, in which it is converted to the coenzyme forms FMN and FAD (Fig. 29.2). The excess is excreted in the urine or metabolized by microsomal enzymes in the liver.

The adult male RDA of riboflavin is set at 1.3 mg/day, and most people readily obtain this amount from their diet. Good sources include liver, yeast, eggs, meat, enriched bread and cereals, and milk. Riboflavin deficiency usually occurs along with other vitamin deficiencies and is most common in alcoholics. The symptoms include glossitis (magenta tongue), angular stomatitis, sore throat, and a moist (seborrheic) dermatitis of the scrotum and nose. This deficiency may be accompanied by a normochromic normocytic anemia.

Riboflavin deficiency can occur in infants receiving phototherapy for hyperbilirubinemia (see Chapter 27). Not only bilirubin but also riboflavin is destroyed by light in the skin, and therefore riboflavin supplements are given routinely in this situation.

The dietary status can be assessed by the fluorometric or microbiological determination of urinary riboflavin. Alternatively, the activity of erythrocyte glutathione reductase (see Chapter 22) is determined in freshly lysed red blood cells before and after the addition of its coenzyme FAD. In riboflavin deficiency, the apoenzyme is not completely saturated with its cofactor, and the enzymatic activity is therefore increased by added FAD.

Niacin Is a Precursor of NAD and NADP

The term **niacin,** originally applied to nicotinic acid, is now often used as a generic term for the vitamin-active pyrimidine derivatives **nicotinic acid** and **nicotinamide:**

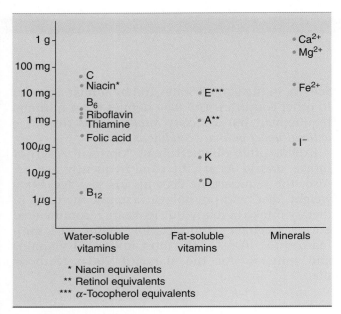

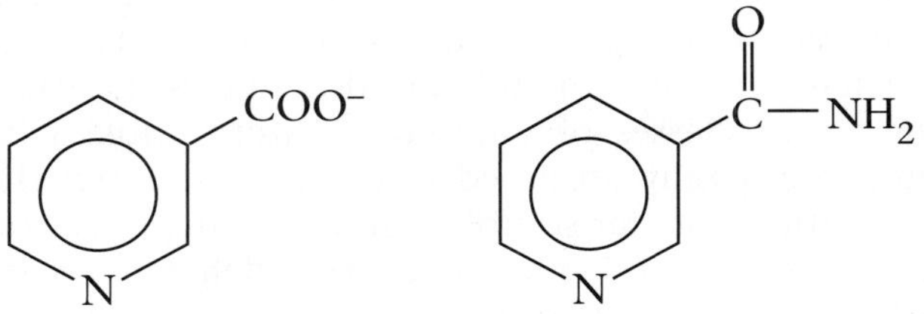

Figure 29.1 Recommended daily allowances of vitamins and minerals for a young, healthy, 70-kg man.

Nicotinic acid (niacin)

Nicotinamide (niacinamide)

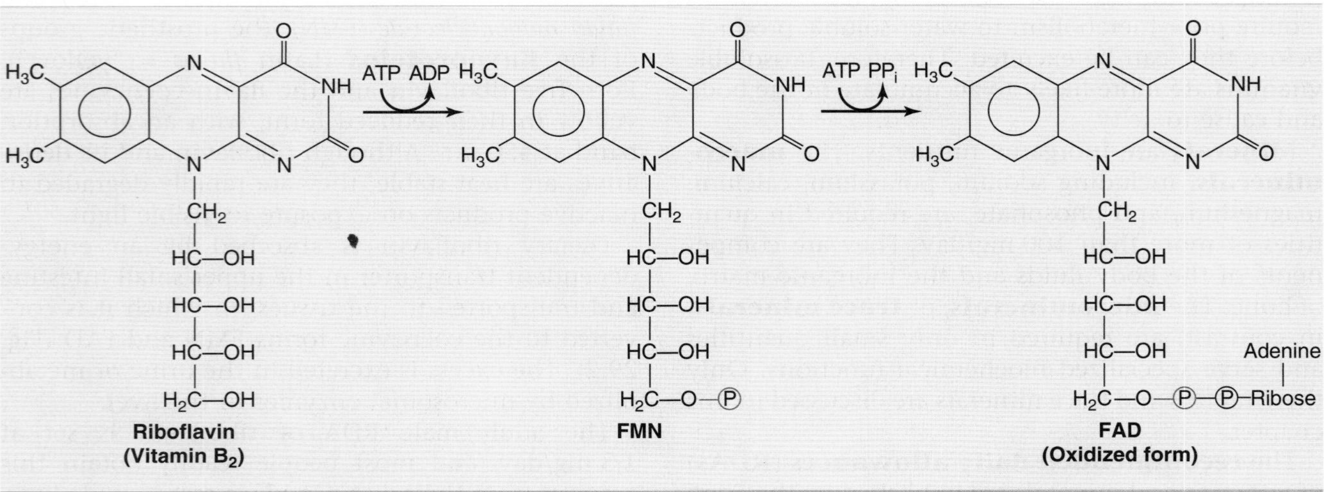

Figure 29.2 Synthesis of flavin mononucleotide (FMN) and flavin adenine dinucleotide (FAD) from dietary riboflavin.

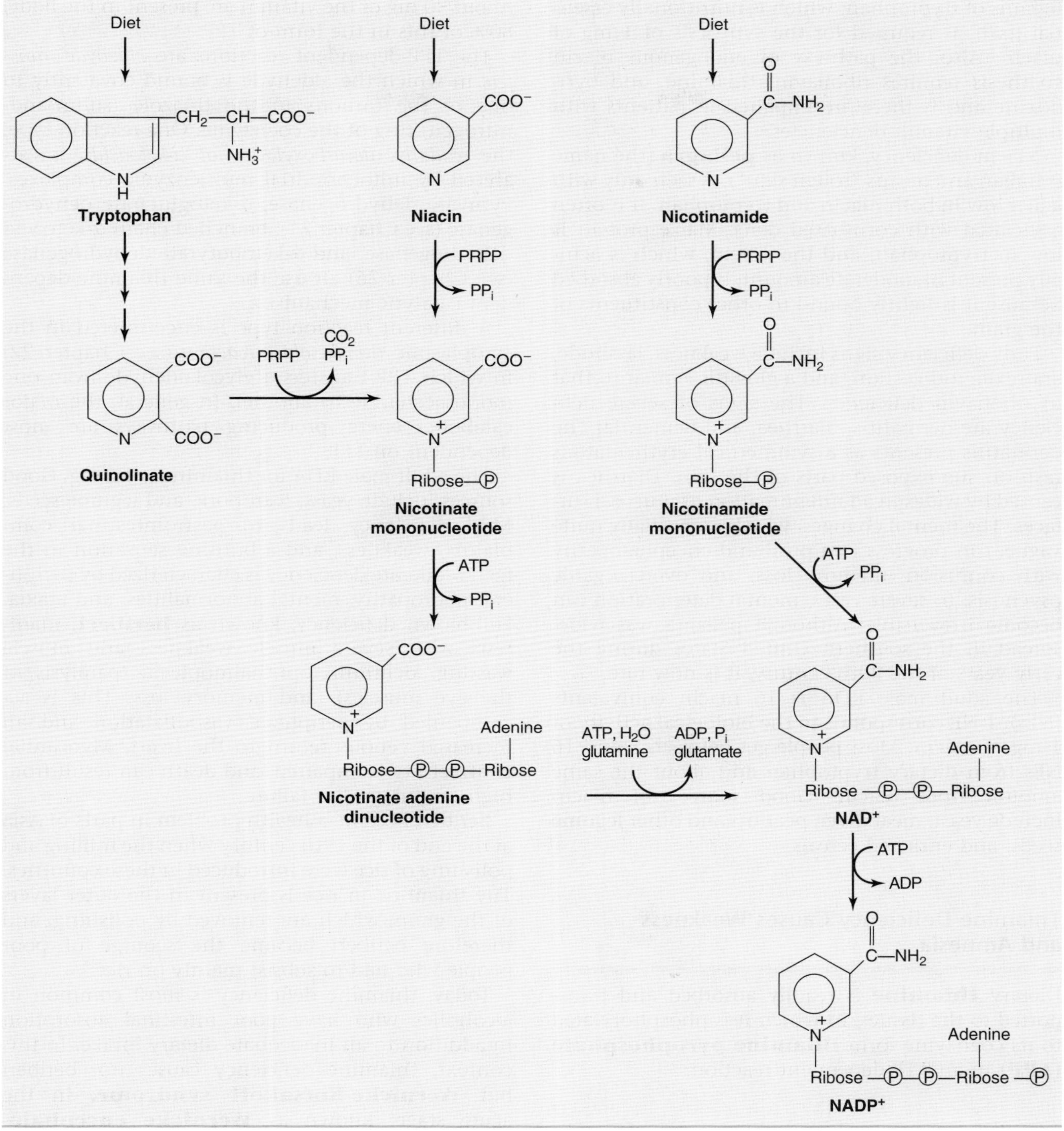

Figure 29.3 Synthesis of nicotinamide adenine dinucleotide (NAD) and nicotinamide adenine dinucleotide phosphate (NADP). PRPP, 5-phosphoribosyl-1-pyrophosphate.

Both in the human body and in dietary sources, *niacin is present as a constituent of nicotinamide adenine dinucleotide (NAD) and nicotinamide adenine dinucleotide phosphate (NADP).* The dietary coenzymes are hydrolyzed in the gastrointestinal tract, and free nicotinic acid and nicotinamide are absorbed in the small intestine. After their transport to the tissues, the vitamin forms are incorporated into the coenzymes (Fig. 29.3). Excess niacin is readily excreted by the kidneys.

NAD and NADP can also be synthesized from dietary tryptophan, but the pathway is inefficient. Sixty milligrams of tryptophan, which is nutritionally essential itself, is required for the synthesis of 1 mg of niacin. Also, the pathway of endogenous niacin synthesis requires riboflavin, thiamine, and pyridoxine and is therefore impaired in patients with multiple vitamin deficiencies.

Niacin deficiency, known as **pellagra** (the name is Italian and means "rough skin"), is seen only with a diet low in both niacin and tryptophan. It is often associated with corn-based diets. Maize protein is low in tryptophan, and the niacin, which is actually present in moderate amount, is poorly absorbed because it is tightly bound to other constituents of the grain.

Early deficiency signs include weakness, lassitude, anorexia, indigestion, and a glossitis similar to that in riboflavin deficiency. The signs of severe deficiency are dermatitis, diarrhea, and dementia. The dermatitis presents as a symmetrical erythematous rash on sun-exposed parts of the skin. Diarrhea is caused by widespread inflammation of mucosal surfaces. The mental changes, which are initially quite vague, can progress to a profound encephalopathy with confusion, memory loss, and overt organic psychosis. In severe cases, mental deterioration can become irreversible. Although pellagra was widespread in the southern United States during the early years of the 20th century, it is now rare.

The adult male RDA is 16 niacin equivalents (NEs); 1 NE corresponds to the biological activity of 1 mg of niacin. Most people get between 8 and 16 NEs from dietary tryptophan and about the same amount from niacin. Good sources of niacin include yeast, meat, liver, peanuts and other legume seeds, and enriched cereals.

Thiamine Deficiency Causes Weakness and Amnesia

Dietary **thiamine** is readily absorbed and transported to the tissues, in which it is phosphorylated to its coenzyme form **thiamine pyrophosphate (TPP)** in an ATP-dependent reaction:

Thiamine pyrophosphate
(TPP)

About 30 mg of the vitamin are present in the body, 80% of this in the form of TPP.

The TPP-dependent reactions are *aldehyde transfers* in which the aldehyde is bound covalently to one of the carbons in the thiazole (sulfur-and-nitrogen) ring of the coenzyme. One reaction type, the *oxidative decarboxylation of α-ketoacids,* is catalyzed by mitochondrial multienzyme complexes. Pyruvate dehydrogenase, α-ketoglutarate dehydrogenase (see Chapter 21), branched-chain α-ketoacid dehydrogenase, and α-ketobutyrate dehydrogenase (see Chapter 26) all use the same thiamine-dependent catalytic mechanism.

A different reaction type is encountered in the cytoplasmic *transketolase reaction* (see Chapter 22) in which TPP transfers a glycolaldehyde from one monosaccharide to another. In general, the major catabolic, energy-producing pathways are most dependent on TPP.

The adult male RDA for thiamine is 1.2 mg. Good sources include yeast, lean pork, and legume seeds. Mild deficiency leads to gastrointestinal complaints, weakness, and a burning sensation in the feet. Moderate deficiency is characterized by peripheral neuropathy, mental abnormalities, and ataxia. Full-blown deficiency, known as **beriberi,** manifests with severe muscle weakness and muscle wasting, delirium, ophthalmoplegia (paralysis of the eye muscles), and memory loss. This is accompanied by peripheral vasodilatation and an increased venous return to the heart. Myocardial contractility is impaired, and death can result from high-output cardiac failure.

Beriberi became a health problem in parts of Asia at the end of the 19th century when the milling and polishing of rice were introduced in these countries. The thiamine in rice is present in the outer layers of the grain, which are removed by polishing, and therefore beriberi became the scourge of poor people who had to subsist mainly on rice.

Today, thiamine deficiency is most common in alcoholics who have poor intestinal absorption in addition to an inadequate dietary intake. In this context, thiamine deficiency causes not beriberi but **Wernicke-Korsakoff syndrome.** In the acute stage, known as **Wernicke encephalopathy,** the patient presents with mental derangements and delirium, ataxia (motor incoordination), and paralysis of the eye muscles. The chronic stage, known as **Korsakoff psychosis,** is a severely debilitating anterograde amnesia. Affected patients can still remember events from the distant past, and short-term memory is intact, but they can no longer transcribe information from short-term to long-term memory.

Korsakoff psychosis is the most common form of amnesia in most countries. The disease is related to a

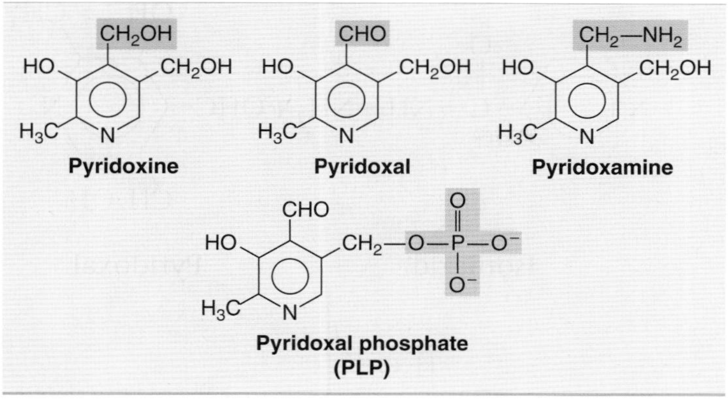

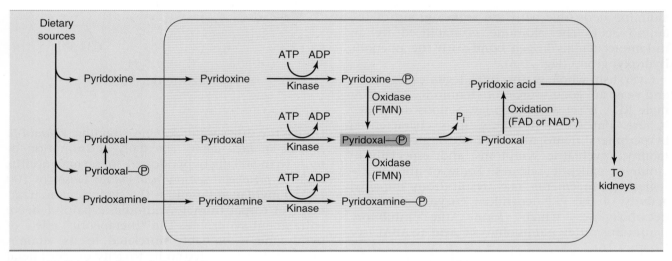

Figure 29.4 The molecular forms of vitamin B_6. All vitamin forms can be converted to the coenzyme form pyridoxal phosphate in the human body.

Figure 29.5 Metabolism of vitamin B_6.

recognizable pattern of brain damage. At autopsy, focal lesions are found in the periventricular areas of the thalamus and hypothalamus, the periaqueductal gray of the midbrain, and the mammillary bodies.

Wernicke encephalopathy can be treated with thiamine injections, but *immediate treatment is essential* because the amnesia, once established, is irreversible.

Thiamine deficiency can be evaluated by the determination of transketolase activity in whole blood or erythrocytes, both before and after the addition of TPP. Alternatively, the plasma levels of lactate and pyruvate can be determined after an oral glucose load. These acids accumulate in persons with thiamine deficiency because pyruvate dehydrogenase requires TPP for its activity.

Vitamin B_6 Plays a Key Role in Amino Acid Metabolism

Vitamin B_6 is the generic name for the dietary precursors of the active coenzyme form, **pyridoxal phosphate** (**PLP**). They include **pyridoxine, pyridoxal,** and **pyridoxamine,** as well as their phosphorylated derivatives (Fig. 29.4).

The phosphate is removed by intestinal alkaline phosphatase, and the dephosphorylated forms are absorbed. The total body content of PLP is only 25 mg in adults, and pyridoxal and PLP are the major circulating forms of the vitamin. The synthesis of the coenzyme form is described in Figure 29.5.

Several dozen enzymes of amino acid metabolism contain PLP as a tightly bound prosthetic group. In these reactions, the aldehyde group of PLP forms an

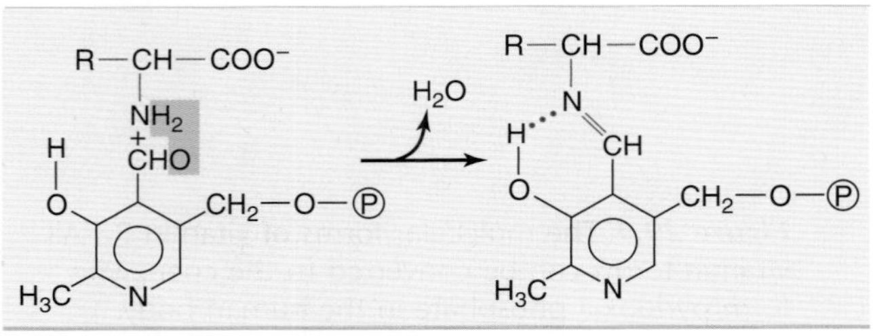

Figure 29.6 In reactions of amino acid metabolism, pyridoxal phosphate forms an aldimine (Schiff base) derivative with the amino group of the amino acid. The further path of the reaction depends on the catalytic specificity of the enzyme.

Isoniazid   Pyridoxal

Hydrazone derivative

aldimine derivative with the amino group of the amino acid. The aldimine is stabilized by an intramolecular hydrogen bond with the phenolic hydroxyl group (Fig. 29.6).

Liver, fish, whole grains, nuts, legumes, egg yolk, and yeast are good sources of vitamin B_6. The adult male RDA is set at 1.3 mg/day. Serious deficiency is rare, but when it occurs, it is characterized by peripheral neuropathy, stomatitis, glossitis, irritability, psychiatric symptoms, and, especially in children, epileptic seizures. Some of the neurological derangements may result from impaired activity of the PLP-dependent enzyme glutamate decarboxylase, which forms the inhibitory neurotransmitter γ-aminobutyric acid (GABA) (see Chapter 16).

Dermatitis, glossitis, and **sideroblastic anemia** are other abnormalities in vitamin B_6 deficiency. Sideroblastic anemia is a microcytic hypochromic anemia, similar to iron deficiency anemia but in the presence of normal serum iron. It is most likely caused by reduced activity of the PLP-dependent aminolevulinic acid (ALA) synthase in the bone marrow and the resulting impairment in heme biosynthesis. Without heme, iron cannot be used for hemoglobin synthesis but accumulates in erythroblasts in the bone marrow. These iron-loaded erythroblasts are called sideroblasts.

Vitamin B_6 deficiency is most common in alcoholics, in whom it contributes to sideroblastic anemia, peripheral neuropathy, and seizures. Some drugs, including the tuberculostatic **isoniazid** and the metal chelator **penicillamine,** can precipitate vitamin B_6 deficiency by reacting nonenzymatically with the aldehyde group of pyridoxal or PLP.

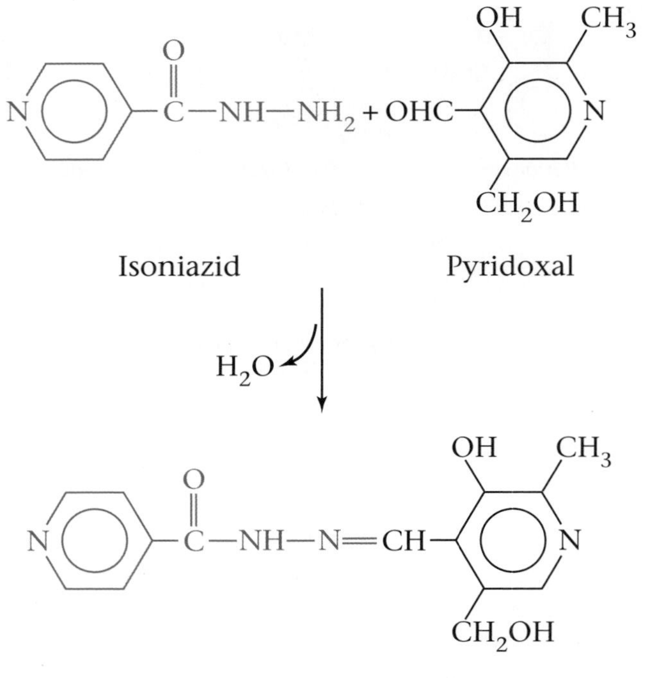

Unlike the other water-soluble vitamins, *vitamin B_6 is toxic in high doses.* The daily consumption of more than 500 mg of pyridoxine for several months leads to *peripheral sensory neuropathy.* Doses of 100 to 150 mg/day are used for the symptomatic treatment of carpal tunnel syndrome, a painful nerve entrapment syndrome. The "therapeutic" effect of pyridoxine is probably unrelated to its vitamin function but is related to its toxicity on peripheral nerves.

The vitamin B_6 status can be evaluated by determining the plasma level of PLP (normal: 5 to 23 ng/mL) or from the urinary excretion of the PLP metabolite 4-pyridoxic acid. Alternatively, the urinary excretion of xanthurenic acid can be determined after an oral load of 2 to 5 g of tryptophan. Vitamin B_6 deficiency blocks the major catabolic pathway of this amino acid by preventing the PLP-dependent cleavage of 3-hydroxykynurenine, thereby diverting tryptophan catabolism to the yellow product xanthurenic acid (see Chapter 26).

Pantothenic Acid Is a Building Block of Coenzyme A

Pantothenic acid consists of pantoic acid and β-alanine:

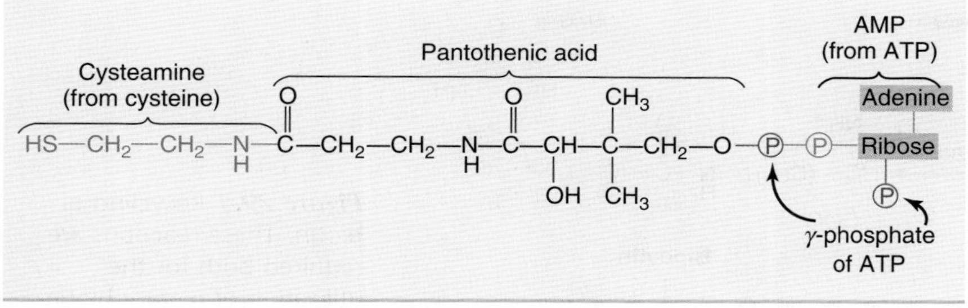

Figure 29.7 The structure of coenzyme A. Pantothenic acid is the only nutritionally essential component of this coenzyme.

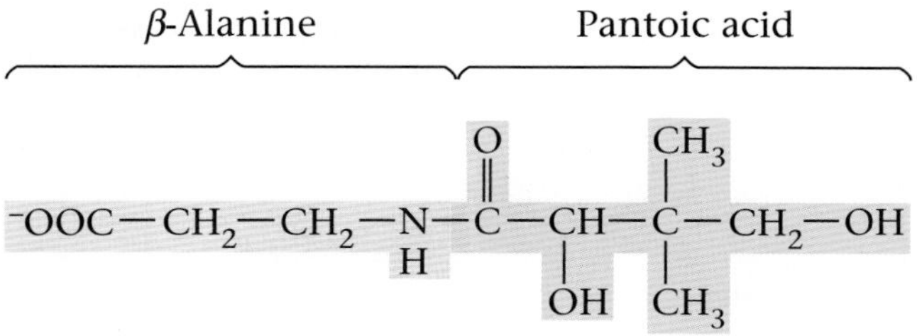

Pantothenic acid

Pantothenic acid functions as *a constituent of coenzyme A (CoA)* and of the phosphopantetheine group in the fatty acid synthase complex (see Chapter 23). The structure and biosynthesis of CoA are summarized in Figure 29.7.

Pantothenic acid deficiency has never been observed under ordinary conditions, and an isolated deficiency in humans could be induced only under rigorously controlled experimental conditions. An amount of 5 mg/day is recommended as a "safe and adequate intake." This amount is readily supplied by most ordinary diets.

Biotin Is a Coenzyme in Carboxylation Reactions

Biotin is a prosthetic group of pyruvate carboxylase, acetyl-CoA carboxylase, propionyl-CoA carboxylase, and other *ATP-dependent carboxylases.* These multisubunit enzymes contain biotin covalently bound to the ε-amino group of a lysine residue:

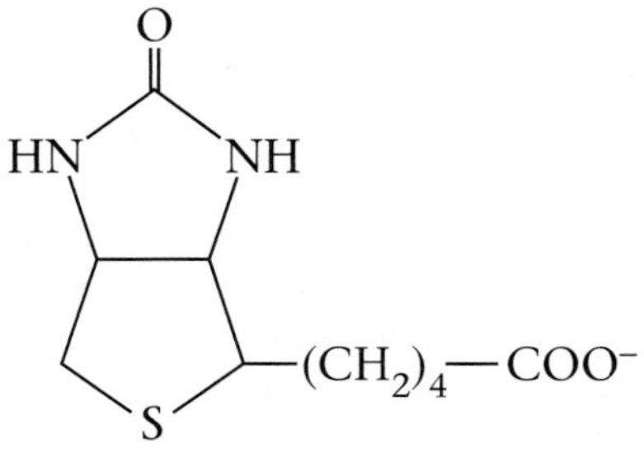

Biotin

In the reaction, biotin functions as a carrier of a bicarbonate-derived carboxyl group:

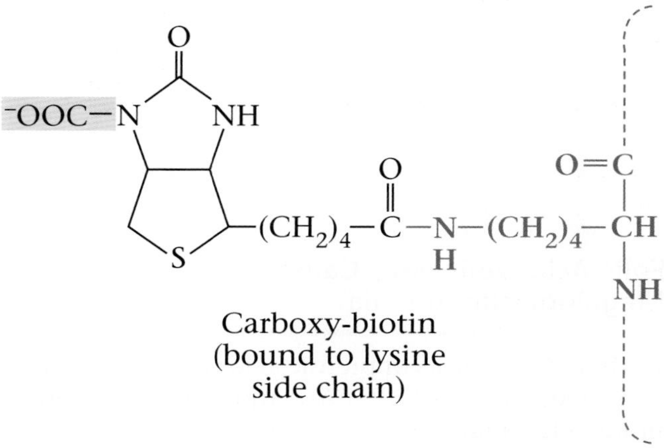

Carboxy-biotin
(bound to lysine
side chain)

Yeast, liver, eggs, peanuts, milk, chocolate, and fish are good sources of biotin, and intestinal bacteria make a sizeable contribution. Humans need only 30 µg of biotin per day, and the only way to induce biotin deficiency is to eat at least 20 raw egg whites per day. Egg white contains the protein **avidin,** so called because it binds biotin avidly, preventing its intestinal absorption.

The proteolytic degradation of biotin-containing enzymes, both in the intestinal lumen and in the tissues, produces the biotin-lysine conjugate **biocytin** (Fig. 29.8). Biotin is released from biocytin by **biotinidase.** *Biotinidase deficiency causes nondietary biotin deficiency.* Affected infants present with hypotonia, seizures, optic atrophy, dermatitis, and conjunctivitis. This condition can be cured easily with biotin supplements. *Biotinidase deficiency is often included in newborn screening programs,* along with other treatable congenital diseases. It can be diagnosed by enzyme assay in fresh serum or, as a screening test, on a strip of blood-soaked filter paper.

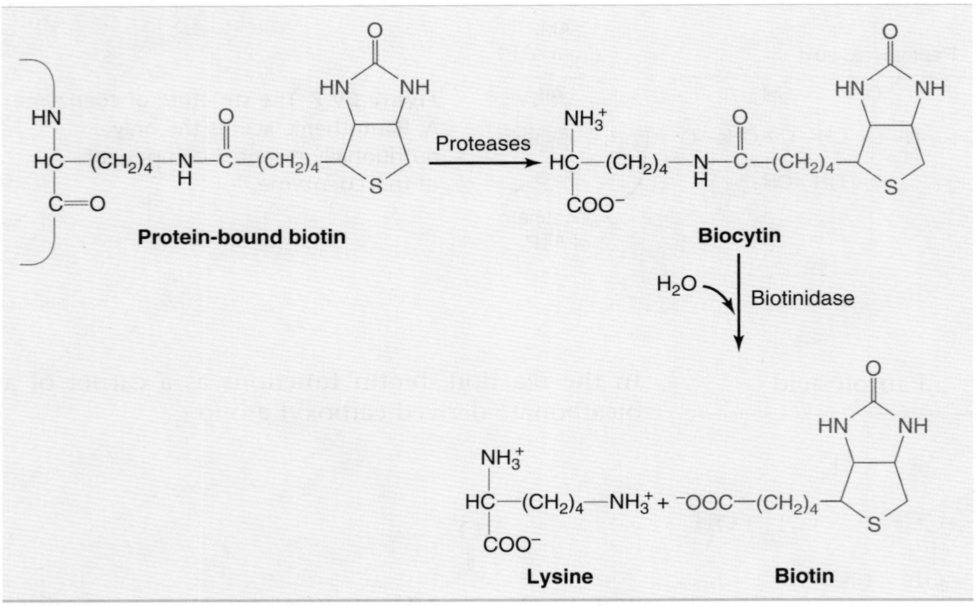

Figure 29.8 Recycling of biotin. These reactions are required both for the utilization of dietary biotin and for the recycling of biotin during the degradation of biotin-containing carboxylase enzymes in the tissues.

Folic Acid Deficiency Causes Megaloblastic Anemia

Folic acid consists of pteroic acid (pteridine + para-aminobenzoic acid [PABA]) and one to seven γ-linked glutamate residues:

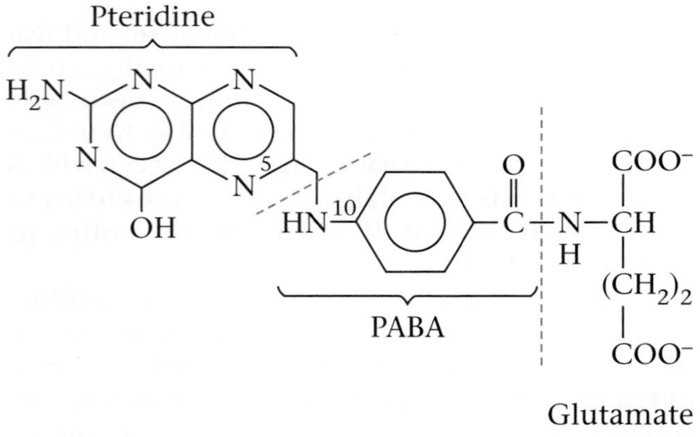

Pteroyl-monoglutamate
(the absorbed form of folic acid)

Dietary polyglutamate forms of folic acid are hydrolyzed to pteroyl monoglutamate in the intestinal lumen. The monoglutamate is absorbed and reduced to the active coenzyme form **tetrahydrofolate (THF)** by **dihydrofolate reductase** in the intestinal mucosa. The monoglutamate conjugate of methyl-THF is the major circulating form of THF, but intracellular THF is present in the form of polyglutamate conjugates.

THF is a carrier of one-carbon units, which are bound to one or both of two nitrogen atoms in the molecule, N-5 and N-10 (Fig. 29.9):

1. *A one-carbon unit is acquired by THF during a catabolic reaction.* The major one-carbon sources are serine in the hydroxymethyl transferase reaction, glycine in the glycine cleavage reaction, and formimino-glutamate in the pathway of histidine degradation (see Chapter 26).
2. *The THF-bound one-carbon unit is oxidized or reduced enzymatically.* Most of these reactions are reversible. They create an assortment of one-carbon units for use by biosynthetic enzymes.
3. *The one-carbon unit is transferred from THF to an acceptor molecule.* THF-dependent biosynthetic processes include the synthesis of purine nucleotides, the thymidylate synthase reaction, and the methylation of homocysteine to methionine.

The clinical signs of folate deficiency are caused by *impairment of DNA replication in dividing cells,* resulting from reduced synthesis of purine nucleotides and thymine. In the bone marrow, hemoglobin is synthesized normally and the cytoplasm grows at a normal rate, but cell division is delayed. Therefore, the production of mature cells slows down, and the cells that are formed are oversized. The result is called **megaloblastic anemia** or **macrocytic anemia.** Megaloblasts are oversized erythrocyte

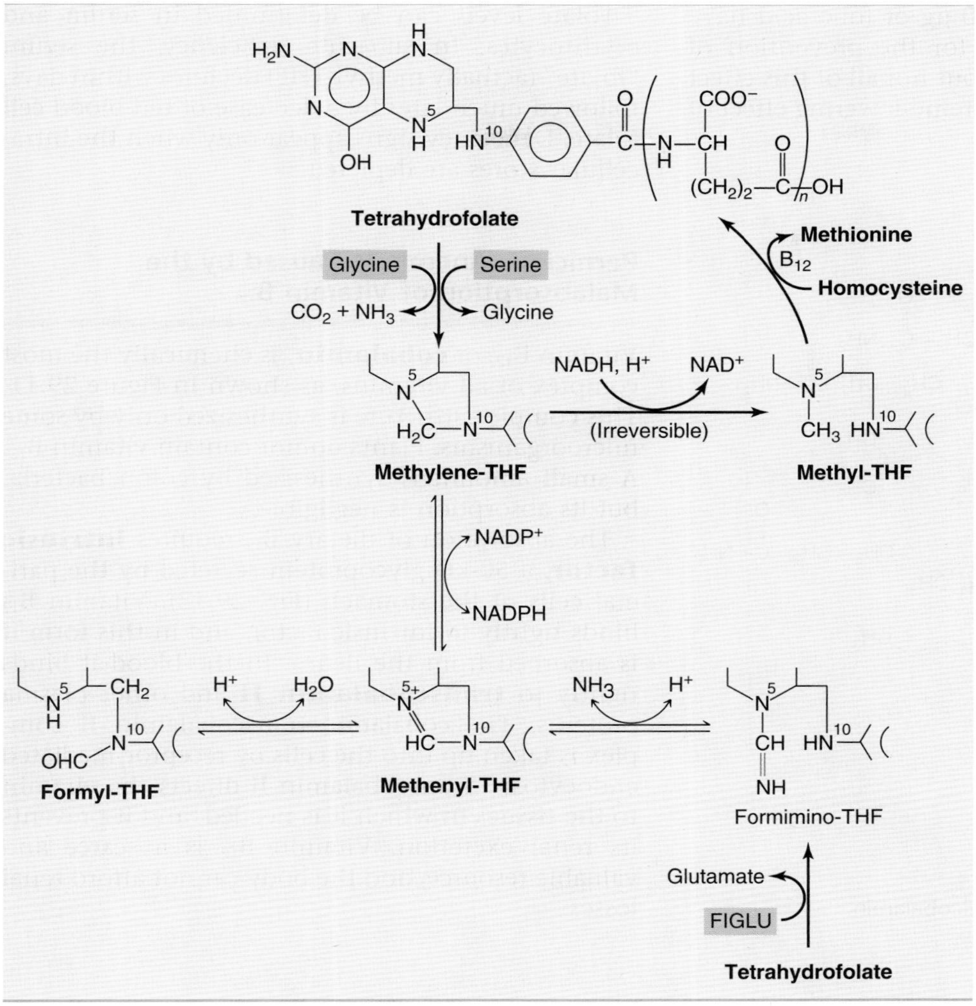

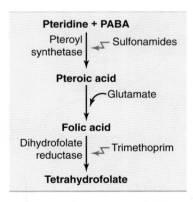

Figure 29.9 Tetrahydrofolate (THF) as a carrier of one-carbon units. FIGLU, formiminoglutamate (formed during histidine degradation).

precursors in the bone marrow, and macrocytes are oversized erythrocytes in the blood.

Unlike humans, most bacteria make their own folate. Their growth can therefore be inhibited with drugs that block folate synthesis. The **sulfonamides** are structural analogs of PABA that inhibit the synthesis of pteroic acid in bacteria, and **trimethoprim** is an inhibitor of bacterial but not human dihydrofolate reductase (Fig. 29.10). These drugs are still used for the treatment of some infections.

Good dietary sources include yeast, liver, some fruits, and green vegetables (Latin *folium* = "leaf"). However, folate is heat-labile, and losses during food processing can be extensive. The RDA is 400 μg, and total body stores are 5 to 10 mg. Low levels of serum folate are often encountered in late pregnancy, and *megaloblastic anemia can be precipitated by pregnancy*. Alcoholism and intestinal malabsorption syndromes can also cause folate deficiency.

Folate supplements are recommended for the *prevention of neural tube defects* (spina bifida and

Figure 29.10 Pharmacological inhibition of tetrahydrofolate synthesis in bacteria. PABA, para-aminobenzoic acid.

anencephaly). These congenital malformations are present in about 1 per 400 births. The current recommendation is that all women who might possibly become pregnant should consume 400 μg of folic acid per day.

Daily doses of at least 500 μg of folic acid have also been found beneficial for the prevention of coronary heart disease. Part but not all of this effect is explained by the homocysteine-lowering effect of this vitamin.

Folate levels can be determined in serum and erythrocytes. In subacute deficiency, the serum "folate" (actually methyl-THF) declines within days, followed much later by a decrease of red blood cell folate. Deficiency signs appear only when the intracellular stores are depleted.

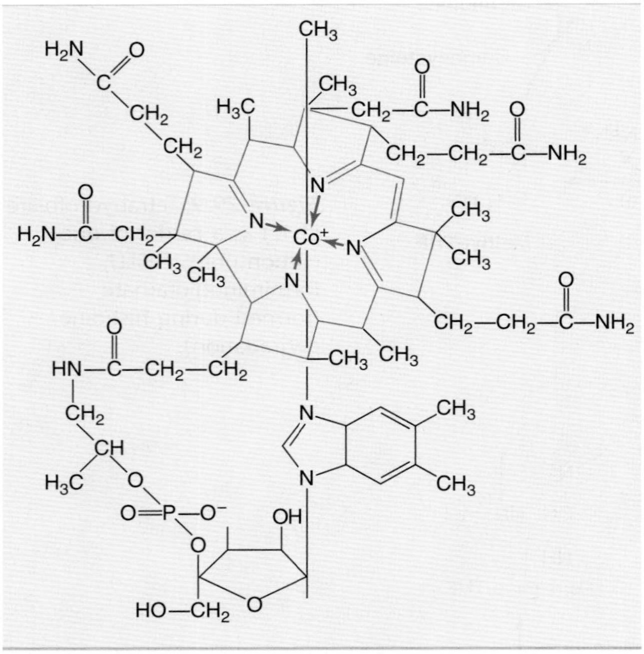

Pernicious Anemia Is Caused by the Malabsorption of Vitamin B_{12}

Vitamin B_{12}, or **cobalamin,** is chemically the most complex of all vitamins, as shown in Figure 29.11. This complex structure is synthesized only by some microorganisms. Plants do not contain vitamin B_{12}. A small amount is synthesized by colon bacteria, but its absorption is negligible.

The absorption of dietary B_{12} requires **intrinsic factor,** a 50-kD glycoprotein secreted by the parietal cells of the stomach (Fig. 29.12). Vitamin B_{12} binds tightly to intrinsic factor, and in this form it is absorbed from the ileum. In the blood it binds tightly to **transcobalamin II** and other plasma proteins. The cobalamin–transcobalamin II complex is taken up into the cells by receptor-mediated endocytosis. Transcobalamin II directs the vitamin to the tissues in which it is needed, and it prevents its renal excretion. Vitamin B_{12} is a scarce and valuable resource, and the body cannot afford renal losses.

Figure 29.11 Structure of methylcobalamin.

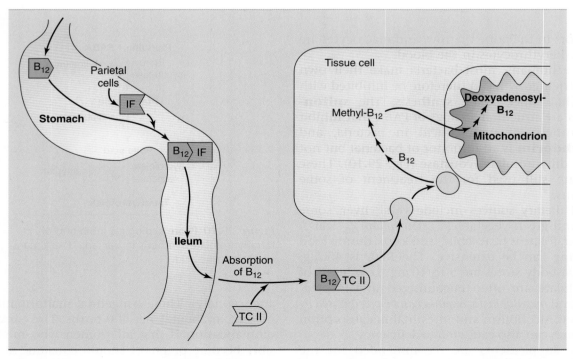

Figure 29.12 Absorption, transport, and tissue utilization of vitamin B_{12}. IF, intrinsic factor; TC II, transcobalamin II.

Only two reactions are known to require cobalamin coenzymes in human tissues. The cytoplasmic *methylation of homocysteine to methionine* (see Chapter 26) requires methylcobalamin, and the mitochondrial *methylmalonyl–CoA mutase reaction* (see Chapter 23) requires deoxyadenosylcobalamin.

The RDA for vitamin B_{12} is 2.4 µg, but as little as 0.1 to 0.2 µg/day are probably sufficient to prevent deficiency. Because essentially all dietary vitamin B_{12} is derived from animal products, *vegans are at risk of vitamin B_{12} deficiency* unless their food is habitually contaminated with bacteria or fecal matter. Between 1 and 10 mg of vitamin B_{12} is stored in the body, most of this in the liver. Therefore, a sudden switch to a vitamin B_{12}–free diet will cause serious deficiency only after a few decades.

Impaired intestinal absorption, however, causes deficiency within 2 to 6 years. Every day, between 1 and 10 µg of vitamin B_{12} is secreted into the bile, and most of this is reabsorbed with the help of intrinsic factor. Indeed, most cases of vitamin B_{12} deficiency are caused by malabsorption.

Pernicious anemia is an autoimmune disease that destroys the parietal cells in the stomach. This deprives the patient of intrinsic factor, and neither dietary nor biliary vitamin B_{12} can be absorbed. This disease was invariably fatal until 1926, when the oral administration of liver extracts was found to be curative. Even in the absence of intrinsic factor, 0.1% to 1% of orally administered vitamin B_{12} is absorbed by nonspecific mechanisms, and the large amount of vitamin B_{12} in the liver extracts was sufficient to correct the deficiency. Pernicious anemia is now treated either with large oral vitamin B_{12} supplements or with monthly injections of more moderate doses.

Pernicious anemia shows two types of abnormalities: *megaloblastic anemia,* similar to that of folate deficiency, and *neurological dysfunction,* caused by demyelination in peripheral nerves and the spinal cord. The demyelination is not seen in patients with folate deficiency.

The megaloblastic anemia is explained by the **methyl folate trap** hypothesis. The problem is this: During the metabolism of one-carbon units, a small amount of methylene-THF is irreversibly reduced to methyl-THF (see Fig. 29.9). Being useless for the synthesis of purines and thymine, methyl-THF has to be converted back to one of the other coenzyme forms. *This can be done only by the vitamin B_{12}–dependent methylation of homocysteine to methionine,* which regenerates free THF. Therefore, methyl-THF accumulates in vitamin B_{12} deficiency, to the detriment of the other coenzyme forms. This mechanism explains the megaloblastic anemia of vitamin B_{12} deficiency, but the cause of the demyelination is unknown.

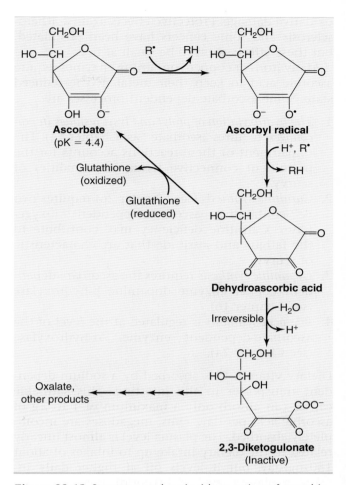

Figure 29.13 Structure and antioxidant action of ascorbic acid (vitamin C). The standard reduction potential of ascorbate/dehydroascorbate is +0.08 V; that of glutathione is –0.23 V. R*, free radical.

Vitamin C Is a Water-Soluble Antioxidant

During recorded history, **scurvy** was one of the most frequently mentioned nutritional deficiencies. The structure of the antiscorbutic agent, now known as **ascorbic acid** or **vitamin C,** was determined in 1932 after its isolation from lemon juice and other natural sources. Its structure is simple, resembling a monosaccharide, and most animals can indeed synthesize ascorbic acid in one of the minor pathways of carbohydrate metabolism (see Chapter 22). Only primates, guinea pigs, and some fruit bats have lost the ascorbate-synthesizing enzyme.

Ascorbic acid is a reducing agent and scavenger of free radicals (Fig. 29.13). As an antioxidant, it suppresses the formation of carcinogenic nitrosamines from dietary nitrite and nitrate in the gastrointestinal tract, and it protects low-density lipoprotein from oxidative damage. Protective effects against atherosclerosis and some cancers have been postulated, but these effects seem to be small at best.

Many iron- or copper-containing enzymes require ascorbic acid to keep their metal in the reduced state. Some ascorbate-dependent processes are:

1. *The hydroxylation of prolyl and lysyl residues in procollagen* requires ascorbate (see Chapter 14). The impairment of these reactions accounts for the prominent connective tissue abnormalities of scurvy.
2. *Carnitine synthesis* (see Chapter 26) requires two Fe^{2+}-containing, ascorbate-dependent ioxygenases. Carnitine deficiency may contribute to the fatigue and lassitude that are characteristic of scurvy.
3. *Dopamine synthesis* requires the ascorbate-dependent copper enzyme dopamine β-hydroxylase (see Chapter 16).
4. *Bile acid synthesis* is regulated at the level of the ascorbate-dependent enzyme 7α-hydroxylase (see Chapter 24).

Dietary vitamin C is absorbed by a sodium-dependent transporter in the intestine. This saturable carrier can absorb only a maximum of 1 to 2 g of ascorbic acid per day. Thus, megadoses are incompletely absorbed. The plasma level is almost linearly related to the dietary intake up to intakes of about 150 mg/day, but it levels off at higher daily intakes. A plasma level of 1.0 mg/dL is typical on a 100-mg/day diet. The total body pool reaches 20 mg per kilogram of body weight on a 150-mg/day diet and is only slightly higher in people consuming megadoses of more than 1 g/day. About 3% of the vitamin C in the body is excreted in the urine every day, some as unchanged ascorbic acid and some after metabolism to water-soluble products, including oxalic acid.

After a sudden switch to a vitamin C–free diet, the first signs of scurvy appear after 2 to 3 months, when the total body pool is reduced to 300 mg. *Cutaneous petechiae and purpura* (small and medium-sized hemorrhages) appear, along with *follicular hyperkeratosis* (gooseflesh). Dry mouth and eyes, decaying peeling gums, and loose teeth are seen in more advanced cases. Wound healing and scar formation are disrupted, and bleeding from old scars can occur. The patient experiences weakness and lethargy, sometimes accompanied by joint pain and aching of the legs.

A daily intake of 20 mg is sufficient to prevent and even cure scurvy. Fresh fruits and vegetables are the major dietary sources. Vitamin C is not very stable under neutral or alkaline conditions, and it is easily oxidized to inactive products by boiling in the presence of oxygen and catalytic amounts of heavy metal ions. The RDA is 60 mg in the United States, but 30 mg/day is considered adequate in the United Kingdom.

The benefits of megadoses of vitamin C were popularized by the late Linus Pauling, whose name is forever linked not only to the structure of the α-helix but also to the claim that high doses of vitamin C can prevent the common cold. A review of 21 placebo-controlled studies with doses of at least 1 g/day concluded that the number of colds is unchanged, but the duration of the episodes and the severity of the symptoms were indeed reduced by an average of 23%. Although the advisability of very large doses is still controversial, Pauling lived to the age of 97 years, consuming several grams of vitamin C per day for his last 40 years.

Retinol, Retinal, and Retinoic Acid Are the Active Forms of Vitamin A

The biologically active forms of vitamin A are the **retinoids:**

All-*trans*-retinol

All-*trans*-retinal

All-*trans*-retinoic acid

Foods of animal origin contain most of their vitamin A in the form of *esters between retinol and a long-chain fatty acid*. The retinol esters are hydrolyzed by a pancreatic enzyme in the small intestine, and free retinol is absorbed with an efficiency of 60% to 90%. The mucosal cells esterify most of the retinol with fatty acids, and the retinol esters thus formed are exported as constituents of

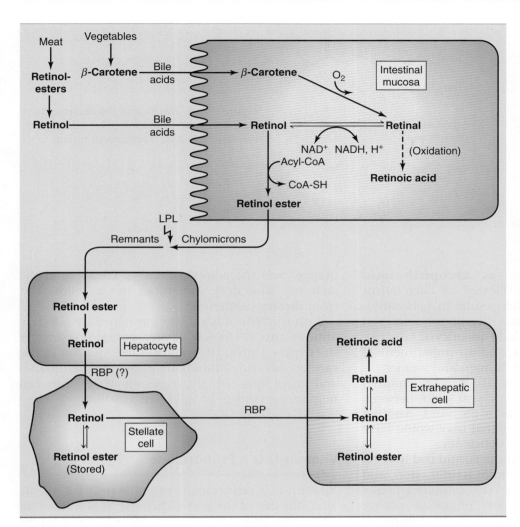

Figure 29.14 Transport and metabolism of retinoids. Retinol is esterified by two different enzymes that use acyl-CoA and lecithin, respectively, as a source of the fatty acid. LPL, lipoprotein lipase; RBP, retinol-binding protein.

chylomicrons. Chylomicron remnants bring the retinol esters to the liver (see Chapter 25), in which up to 100 mg of retinol esters are stored, mainly within the stellate cells (Fig. 29.14).

β-**Carotene,** the orange pigment of carrots and many other vegetables, is the major vitamin A precursor in plants. It is cleaved by β-**carotene dioxygenase** in the cytoplasm of the intestinal mucosal cell (Fig. 29.15). Absorption and cleavage are not very efficient, and 6 mg of β-carotene are needed to produce 1 mg of retinal. Carotenes other than β-carotene can be processed to retinal, but the yield is even lower.

Retinal is in equilibrium with retinol through a reversible, NADH-dependent dehydrogenase reaction. A small amount is irreversibly oxidized to **retinoic acid** (see Fig. 29.14). Retinol is exported from the liver in tight binding to **retinol-binding protein** (**RBP**). Like the intestinal mucosa, the target tissues can oxidize retinol to retinal and

retinal to retinoic acid. Retinal and retinoic acid are the most important biologically active forms:

- **Retinal** is the *prosthetic group of the rhodopsins,* the visual pigments of rods and cones (see Chapter 17).
- **Retinoic acid** is a gene regulator that acts through nuclear receptors, similar to the steroid hormones. Retinoic acid is required for the *maintenance of epithelial tissues.*

In vitamin A deficiency, columnar epithelia are transformed into heavily keratinized squamous epithelia, a process known as **squamous metaplasia.** Follicular hyperkeratosis (gooseflesh) is an early sign, together with night blindness. In the most advanced cases, the conjunctiva of the eye loses its mucus-secreting cells and becomes keratinized, and the glycoprotein content of the tears is reduced as well. These changes disrupt the fluid film that normally bathes the cornea.

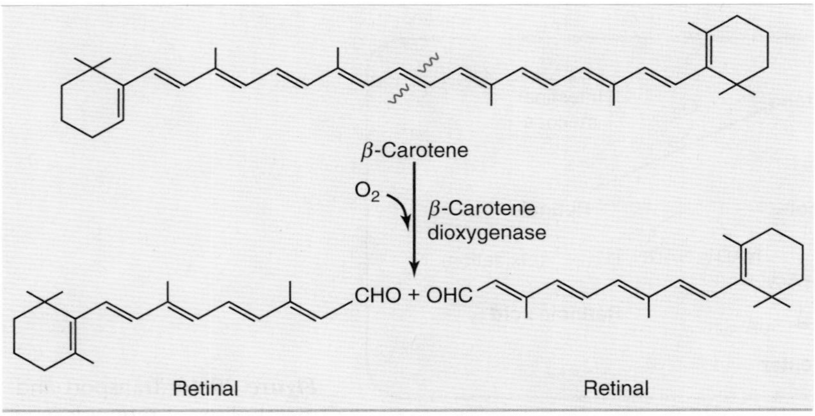

Figure 29.15 The β-carotene dioxygenase reaction cleaves one molecule of dietary β-carotene into two molecules of retinal.

This condition, known as **xerophthalmia** ("dry eyes"), is often complicated by bacterial or chlamydial infection, which results in perforation of the cornea and blindness. Other abnormalities in vitamin A deficiency include microcytic anemia, susceptibility to infections, and an impairment of reproductive function both in men and women.

Worldwide, 3 million to 10 million children become xerophthalmic every year, and between 250,000 and 500,000 of them go blind. Another 1 million die from infections that they would have survived without vitamin A deficiency.

Liver, meat, eggs, dairy products, and cod liver oil provide vitamin A in the form of retinol esters, and vegetables supply carotenes. The carotenes betray their presence by their color. Yellow or orange vegetables and fruits, including carrots, pumpkins, mangoes, and papayas, are excellent sources. Uncolored vegetables have no vitamin A activity. Green leafy vegetables also contain carotenes. The adult male RDA is set at 1000 retinol equivalents (1 mg retinol).

A single dose of more than 200 mg of retinol or retinal, or the chronic consumption of more than 40 mg per day, causes nonspecific signs of toxicity. Of more importance is that retinoic acid is a gene regulator during early fetal development. *Both vitamin A deficiency and vitamin A excess are teratogenic.* Vitamin A preparations are used for the treatment of skin diseases, including common acne, and all it takes for major complications is an acne-plagued teenage girl taking high doses of retinoids and becoming unexpectedly pregnant.

The vitamin A status can be evaluated by the determination of serum retinol. Values between 0.7 and 3.0 μmol/L are considered normal; lower and higher values suggest vitamin A deficiency and toxicity, respectively.

Carotenes are not toxic, but they can accumulate in lipid-rich structures of the body. The skin of babies who are overfed with carrot juice can turn orange, and the adipose tissue of cadavers in the anatomy laboratory sometimes has a yellow tint from dietary carotenes.

Both the retinoids and the carotenes are effective antioxidants at the low oxygen partial pressures in the tissues. Unlike the water-soluble vitamin C, the carotenoids and retinoids are present in membranes and other lipid-rich structures, in which they can help in the control of lipid peroxidation.

Vitamin D Is a Prohormone

Vitamin D is nutritionally essential only for people who stay out of the sun. Otherwise, *it is synthesized photochemically in the skin* (Fig. 29.16), by the action of ultraviolet radiation on the minor membrane steroid **7-dehydrocholesterol.**

The initial product of this reaction, **cholecalciferol** (vitamin D_3), is transferred to a specialized vitamin D–binding plasma protein. Cholecalciferol is not the active form of the vitamin, but it needs to be converted to active **1,25-dihydroxycholecalciferol** (**calcitriol**) by successive hydroxylations in liver and kidney.

25-Hydroxylation in the liver is fast. Its product, 25-hydroxycholecalciferol, is the major circulating form of the vitamin. 1α-Hydroxylation in the kidney is the slow, rate-limiting step, and it is tightly regulated. It is stimulated by parathyroid hormone (PTH), hypocalcemia, and hypophosphatemia. Whereas cholecalciferol and 25-OH-D_3 have biological half-lives of approximately 30 days, calcitriol survives for only 2 to 4 hours.

Calcitriol is a hormone-like substance. Its receptor is a ligand-regulated transcription factor that resembles the receptors for retinoic acid, steroid hormones, and thyroid hormones. Along with PTH, calcitriol regulates the disposition of calcium and phosphate in the body. However, PTH acts through

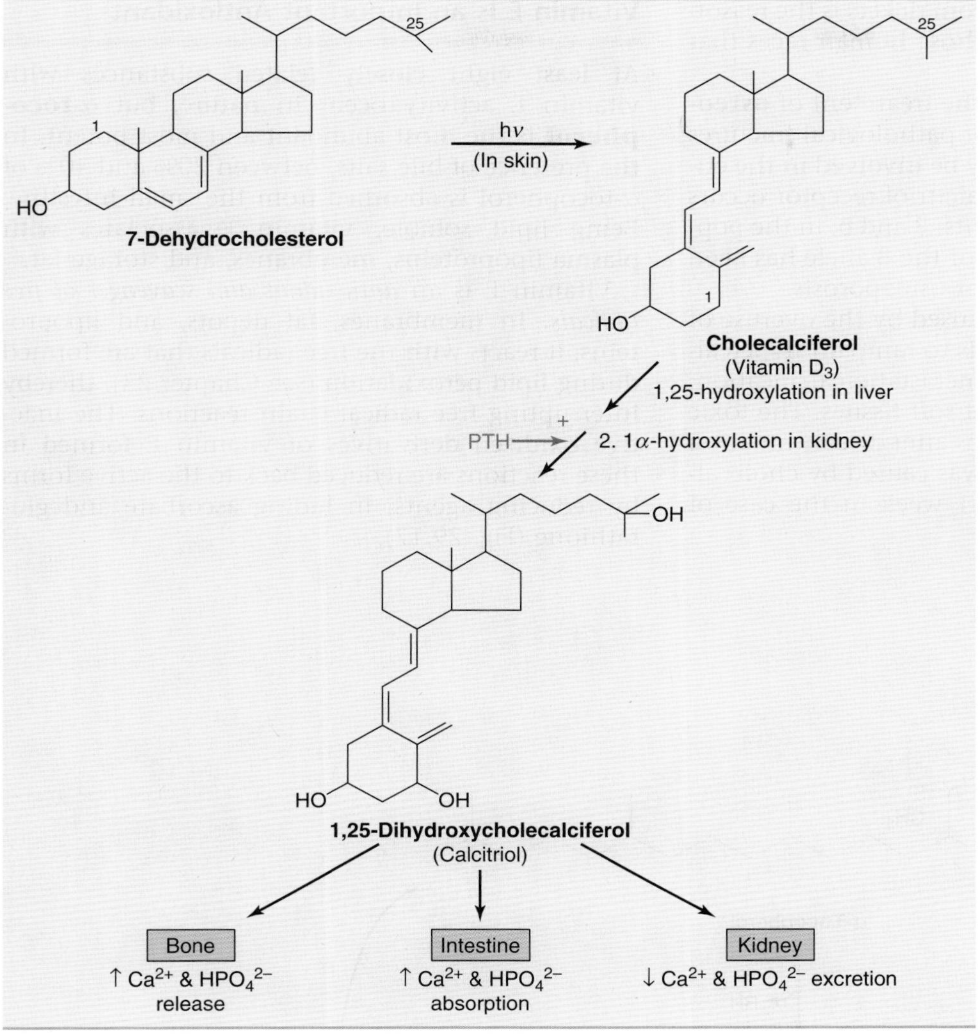

Figure 29.16 Synthesis of calcitriol, the active form of vitamin D, from 7-dehydrocholesterol. PTH, parathyroid hormone.

cyclic AMP and induces its effects within seconds, whereas calcitriol acts through protein synthesis and therefore requires some days for maximal effect. Calcitriol assists PTH in mobilizing calcium and phosphate from the bones and in stimulating calcium reabsorption by the kidneys. Its most important effect, however, is the *stimulation of intestinal calcium and phosphate absorption.*

Extracellular calcium is important for excitable tissues, and therefore its plasma level has to be tightly regulated. In acute hypocalcemia, PTH restores the plasma calcium level within minutes by stimulating osteoclasts, thus inducing the release of calcium and phosphate from the bones. Whereas PTH acts on bone to maintain the plasma calcium level on a minute-to-minute basis, *calcitriol acts on the intestines and kidneys to increase the total amount of calcium and phosphate in the body.*

Vitamin D deficiency is called **rickets** in children and **osteomalacia** in adults. The immediate effect

is reduced intestinal calcium absorption, which tends to reduce the plasma calcium concentration. The maintenance of the blood calcium level has top priority, and therefore PTH is released. Even in long-term vitamin D deficiency, plasma calcium can be maintained at a near-normal level by PTH—at the expense of the bones, which are gradually drained of their mineral content. As a result, affected children have soft, cartilaginous bones that bend easily, and affected adults have brittle bones that break easily.

Rickets used to be common in England and other cloudy countries, but it is now rare. In the absence of sunlight, a daily intake of 5 µg (200 IU) of cholecalciferol is considered adequate. Vitamin D is present in only a few natural foodstuffs, including liver, egg yolk, and saltwater fish (cod liver oil), as well as in fortified foods. The synthesis of cholecalciferol in the skin is affected by skin color. White skin produces about five times more vitamin D than does black skin. Protection from rickets is the reason why white skin evolved in those human races that lived in cloudy climates.

Calcitriol can be used for the treatment of **osteoporosis,** a common cause of pathological fractures in the elderly. It may actually be involved in the etiology of this ailment. The calcitriol receptor occurs in two common allelic variants, B and b, in the population, and homozygosity for the B allele has been claimed to be a risk factor for osteoporosis.

Hypervitaminosis D, caused by the overuse of vitamin D supplements, leads to rampant hypercalcemia, hypercalciuria, and metastatic calcification: the abnormal calcification of soft tissues. The toxic state persists for a few months after discontinuation of the offending agent if it was caused by cholecalciferol, but for only about 1 week in the case of calcitriol.

Vitamin E Is an Important Antioxidant

At least eight closely related substances with vitamin E activity occur in nature, but **α-tocopherol** is the most abundant and most potent. In the presence of bile salts, between 20% and 40% of α-tocopherol is absorbed from the small intestine. Being lipid soluble, vitamin E associates with plasma lipoproteins, membranes, and storage fat.

Vitamin E is an *antioxidant and scavenger of free radicals.* In membranes, fat depots, and lipoproteins, it reacts with the free radicals that are formed during lipid peroxidation (see Chapter 23), thereby interrupting free radical chain reactions. The inactive oxidized derivatives of vitamin E formed in these reactions are reduced back to the active forms by reducing agents, including ascorbate and glutathione (Fig. 29.17).

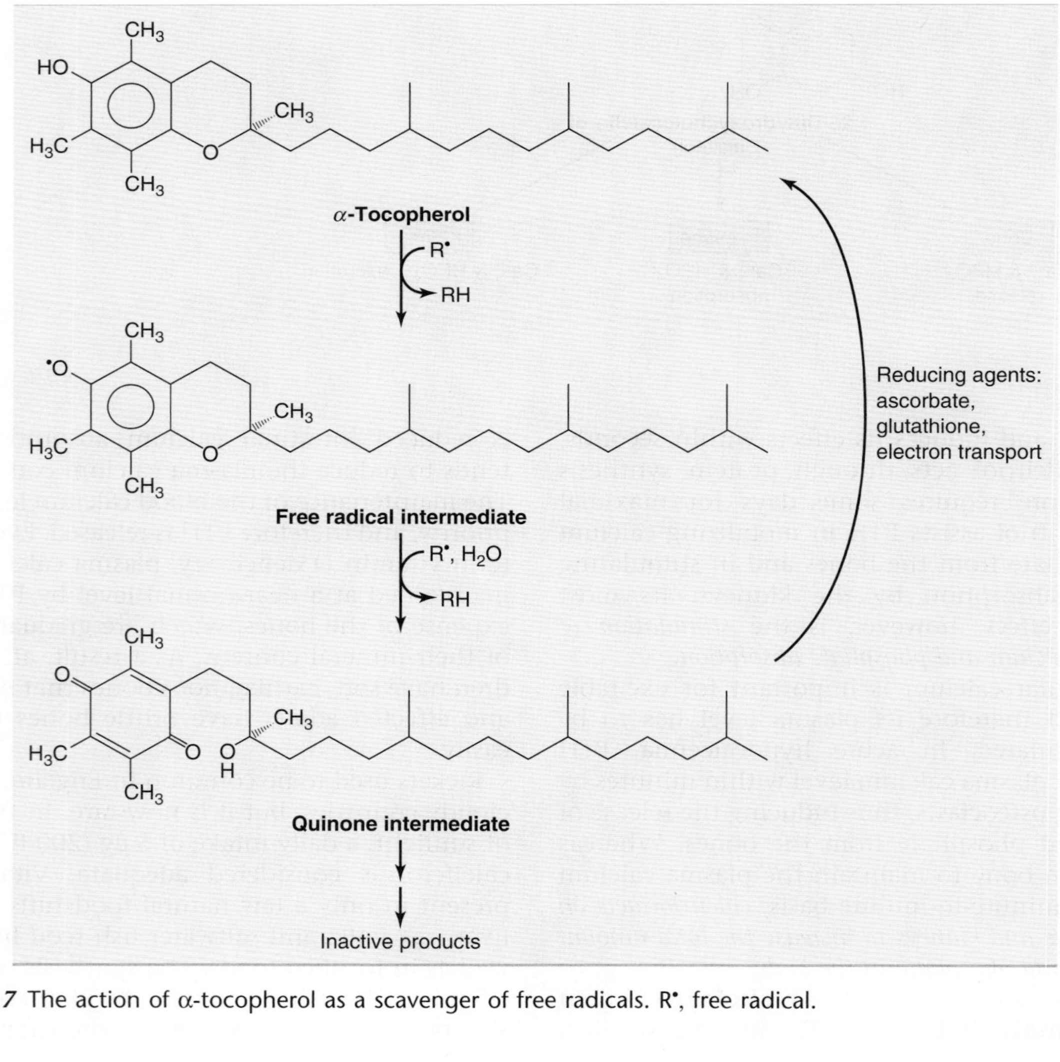

Figure 29.17 The action of α-tocopherol as a scavenger of free radicals. R•, free radical.

Unlike most other vitamins, vitamin E was not discovered by the observation of a deficiency disease in humans but as a result of animal experiments. Although it has been called a "vitamin in search of a disease," human deficiency occasionally does occur, especially in premature infants who are born with low tissue stores and who have poor intestinal absorption for several weeks after birth. Vitamin E deficiency results in a mild hemolytic anemia, both in infants and in children and adults with malabsorption syndromes. The most serious form of vitamin E deficiency occurs in patients with abetalipoproteinemia (see Chapter 25), who develop neuropathic and myopathic changes in addition to hemolysis.

Epidemiological studies suggest an inverse relationship between vitamin E intake and the risk of coronary heart disease. This protective effect tends to be more consistent than similar effects of the other antioxidant vitamins A and C. Intervention studies have shown a reduced risk of coronary heart disease in individuals consuming vitamin E supplements in dosages of approximately 200 mg/day. Like the other antioxidant vitamins, vitamin E is also thought to be protective from some degenerative diseases and some cancers, but in most cases the effects are weak or ambiguous.

A daily intake of 10 mg of α-tocopherol is considered adequate, and this amount is supplied by most diets. Good sources include vegetable oils, various oil seeds, and wheat germ. Although vitamin E is a popular object of abuse by health food enthusiasts, the dangers of overdosage are minimal. Unlike vitamins A and D, vitamin E is nontoxic in doses up to 50 times the recommended intake.

Vitamin K Is Required for Blood Clotting

The name vitamin K is derived from "koagulation," because a clotting disorder is the only abnormality in vitamin K deficiency. The naturally occurring forms of the vitamin are isoprenoids containing a quinoid ring structure. **Phylloquinone** is present in vegetables, and **menaquinone** in bacteria:

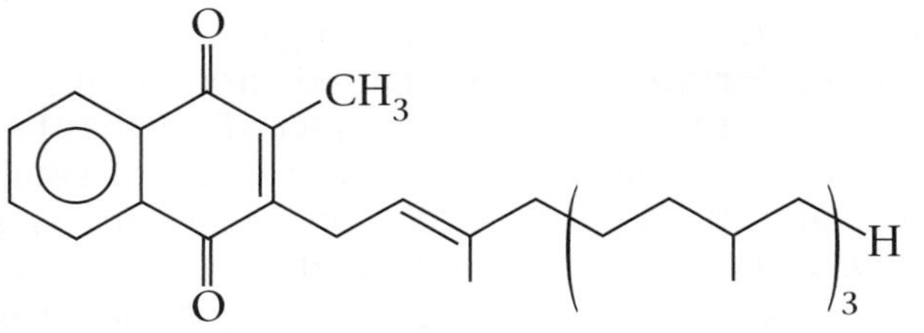

Menadione is a synthetic analog that acts like the natural vitamin forms after its enzymatic alkylation in the human body:

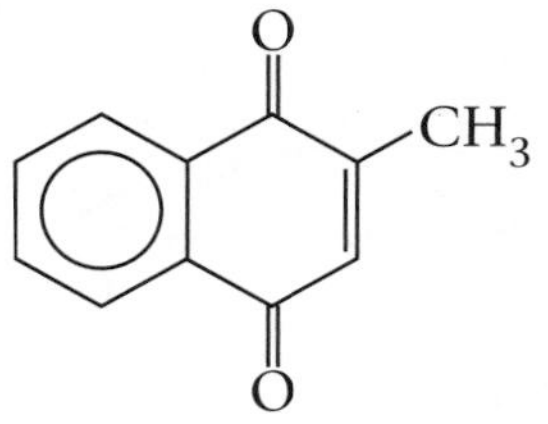

Menadione
(Vitamin K₃)

Unlike the natural forms, menadione is efficiently absorbed even in the absence of bile salts.

Humans get some of their vitamin K as phylloquinone and some as menaquinone produced by intestinal bacteria. Vitamin K has no specific binding protein in the plasma, but is transported from the intestine to the liver in chylomicrons. Unlike the other fat-soluble vitamins, *vitamin K is not stored to any great extent.* Total body stores are as low as 50 to 100 µg, and therefore *vitamin K is the first fat-soluble vitamin to be deficient in acute fat malabsorption.*

Vitamin K participates in the enzymatic carboxylation of glutamyl residues during the synthesis of prothrombin and other clotting factors in the liver (Fig. 29.18). The only important deficiency sign is a clotting disorder, and the determination of the prothrombin time (see Chapter 15) is the most important laboratory test for the evaluation of the vitamin K status.

Vitamin K deficiency is most common in newborns. The tissue stores are low at birth, the intestinal flora is not yet established, and breast milk contains only 1 to 2 µg vitamin K per liter. Because the newborn has a requirement of 5 µg/day (3 liters of breast milk), it is not surprising that, even in normal newborns, the levels of vitamin K dependent clotting factors decline during the first 2 to 3 days after birth. In perhaps 1 per 400 newborns, an abnormal bleeding tendency is evident at this time. This is known as **hemorrhagic disease of the newborn.** *It is the most common nutritional deficiency in newborns.* Most newborns in the United States are now treated with vitamin K either orally or intramuscularly, and vitamin K prophylaxis is mandatory in some states.

Vitamin K deficiency in adults is usually caused by fat malabsorption. It is, for example, common practice to administer vitamin K supplements for a few days before surgery for biliary tract obstruction because these patients have impaired vitamin K absorption, and the resulting impairment of blood

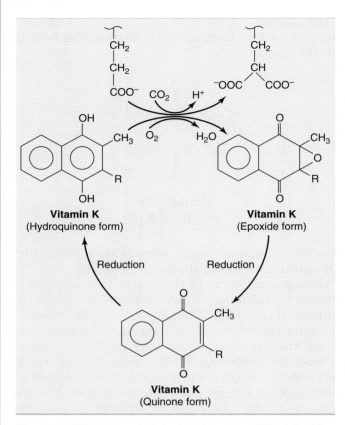

Figure 29.18 Carboxylation of glutamate residues during the post-translational modification of clotting factors in the endoplasmic reticulum of the liver. Unlike other carboxylations, this reaction does not require biotin and ATP; it is driven by the exergonic oxidation of the vitamin K cofactor. R, variable side chain.

clotting makes them vulnerable to surgical complications.

Because of the contribution made by intestinal bacteria, a dietary requirement is hard to define. The RDA is set at 60 to 80 μg but many people consume as much as 300 to 500 μg/day.

Iron Is Conserved Very Efficiently in the Body

Many proteins contain iron, either in the form of a heme group or bound directly to amino acid side chains. In hemoglobin and myoglobin, the ferrous heme iron functions as a binding site for molecular oxygen, and in many enzymes, it participates in redox reactions (electron transfers) by switching back and forth between the ferrous (Fe^{2+}) and ferric (Fe^{3+}) states.

When present in excess or in the wrong place, however, iron is toxic. Like other heavy metals, it binds to many proteins, disrupting their structure

Table 29.1 Distribution of Body Iron in a "Typical" 70-kg *Man* and a 55-kg *Woman*

Protein	Amount (g) in:	
	70-kg Man	**55-kg Woman**
Hemoglobin	2.50	1.70
Myoglobin	0.15	0.10
Enzymes, cytochromes, Fe-S-proteins	0.15	0.10
Storage iron		
Ferritin	0.50	0.30
Hemosiderin	0.50	0.10
Transferrin	0.003	0.002
Total	3.8	2.3

and biological properties. Even worse, it can initiate oxidative damage by forming reactive hydroxyl and peroxide radicals in the presence of molecular oxygen. Ferrous iron is especially dangerous as a catalyst of free radical reactions. Therefore, iron is stored and transported in the ferric state, tightly bound to specialized binding proteins that are not fully saturated under physiological conditions.

The male body contains 3 to 4 g of iron (Table 29.1). Two thirds of this is present in hemoglobin, and much of the rest is storage iron in the liver, spleen, bone marrow, intestinal mucosa, pancreas, myocardium, and other tissues. The amount of stored iron is highly variable. It is near zero in many children and menstruating women but can reach several grams in some older men.

Most iron is stored in the form of **ferritin.** This protein forms a shell of 24 polypeptides, made from two slightly different polypeptide chains (molecular weights, 19 kD and 21 kD). This shell of apoferritin, with an external diameter of 13 nm and an internal cavity 6 nm across, is riddled with pores that allow the entry and exit of ionized iron. The hollow core can accommodate up to 4500 ferric iron atoms in the form of ferric oxide hydroxide (FeOOH) crystals, but, actually, it rarely contains more than 3000.

Hemosiderin is a partially denatured derivative of ferritin. Ferritin is the more abundant storage form when the tissue stores are low, and hemosiderin predominates when tissue stores are high. A small amount of ferritin, consisting mainly of apoferritin with little bound iron, is also present in the blood. This ferritin is released during normal cell turnover in the liver and other organs.

Transferrin is a specialized iron transport protein in the plasma (see Chapter 15). It has two binding sites that bind ferric iron with extremely high affinity. *Almost all the iron in the plasma is bound to transferrin.* In the laboratory, the transferrin concentration is measured as the **total iron**

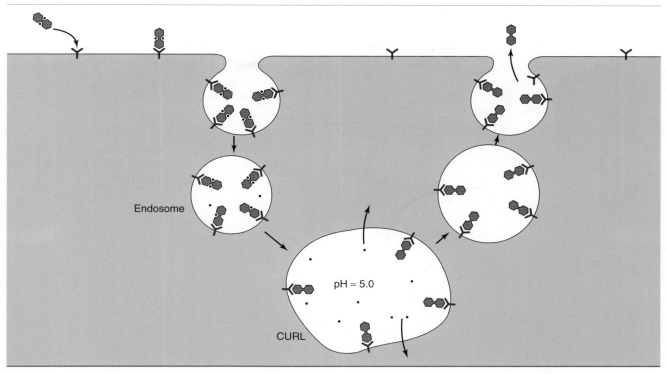

Figure 29.19 Utilization of transferrin-bound iron by receptor-mediated endocytosis. In this variation of the endocytic pathway, the endosome is acidified to a pH of approximately 5.0. In this acidified organelle, known as CURL (compartment of uncoupling of receptor and ligand), iron is released from transferrin. Whereas iron is transported into the cytoplasm, the receptor-bound apotransferrin is returned to the cell surface. ⬡–⬡, Apotransferrin; •, Fe^{3+}; Y, transferrin receptor.

binding capacity (TIBC), and the percentage of high-affinity binding sites that are occupied by iron is expressed as the **iron saturation.** An iron saturation between 10% and 60% is considered normal.

To acquire transferrin-bound iron, the cells use a transferrin receptor in the plasma membrane. This receptor binds iron-loaded transferrin in preference to apotransferrin, and receptor binding is followed by endocytosis. The endocytic vesicle is transformed into an acidified endosome in which the iron dissociates from transferrin and is reduced to the ferrous state for translocation into the cytoplasm. The vesicle itself is recycled to the cell surface, and the apotransferrin can resume its voyage through the circulatory system (Fig. 29.19).

Most people consume between 10 and 20 mg of iron per day. Much of this is derived not from the foodstuffs but from the cooking utensils used for food preparation. The replacement of iron cooking ware by aluminum products and the increasing use of Teflon-coated pots and pans can therefore promote iron deficiency.

Iron is absorbed in the ferrous form, mainly in the duodenum. Although both intracellular storage and transport in the blood are in the ferric form,

only ferrous iron is transported across membranes. The reduction of the ferric iron in food is favored by the low pH in the stomach and the presence of reducing substances, especially ascorbic acid. Therefore, iron absorption is enhanced by vitamin C–rich fruit juices and reduced by achlorhydria (lack of gastric acid) and after gastrectomy (surgical removal of the stomach).

Iron absorption is also reduced by tannins, oxalate, phytate (inositol hexaphosphate), large quantities of inorganic phosphate, and phosphate-containing antacids that form insoluble or nonabsorbable iron complexes. The absorption of nonheme iron varies between 0.8% (rice) and 10% (soybeans), depending on the presence of interfering or facilitating substances in the food. However, the rate of absorption can double in response to iron deficiency. *Any anemic state, regardless of its cause, enhances intestinal iron absorption.* Heme iron, which accounts for a significant portion of iron in meat, is absorbed by separate mechanisms and with an efficiency of 20% to 25%.

Absorbed iron initially binds to ferritin in the intestinal mucosal cell. From intracellular ferritin, it either is transferred to circulating transferrin or

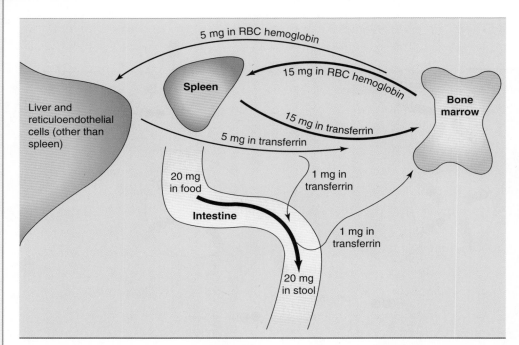

Figure 29.20 Daily transport of iron in the body. RBC, red blood cell.

returns to the intestinal lumen when the mucosal cell is sloughed off from the epithelium at the end of its 2- to 6-day life span. The mucosal cell also accepts iron from transferrin, and this blood-derived iron is again incorporated in ferritin. Total iron absorption is only 1 mg/day in men, and this is balanced by the excretion of 1 mg of blood-borne iron in exfoliated mucosal cells. Because there is virtually no iron in urine, sweat, bile, and digestive secretions, *the intestinal mucosa is the only route for iron excretion.*

Most iron transport in the body is from the spleen and liver, in which aged erythrocytes are destroyed by macrophages, to the bone marrow, in which the iron is used for hemoglobin synthesis (Fig. 29.20).

To adjust their iron uptake to their needs, the cells must regulate the number of transferrin receptors. They achieve this by regulating the stability of the transferrin receptor messenger RNA (mRNA) (Fig. 29.21). The transferrin receptor mRNA has a set of **iron response elements (IREs)** in its 3′-untranslated region: small stem-loop structures that bind **iron regulatory proteins (IRPs)**. The IRPs are active only in the iron-depleted state. When an IRP binds to the IREs, it prolongs the lifespan of the mRNA by protecting it from nucleases. Thus, *the cell makes more transferrin receptors when it needs more iron.*

Ferritin mRNA has an IRE not in the 3′-untranslated region but in the 5′-untranslated region near the cap. When an IRP binds this IRE in the iron-deficient state, it prevents the initiation of transla-tion. Thus, *apoferritin is synthesized only when iron is abundant.*

Iron Deficiency Is the Most Common Micronutrient Deficiency Worldwide

When iron becomes scarce in the body, *storage iron is mobilized first,* without any ill effects. Next, hemoglobin synthesis becomes impaired, with resulting iron deficiency anemia. The iron-containing enzymes that participate in cell respiration become involved in more advanced deficiency states. Iron deficiency is rarely caused by a deficient diet alone. The most important contexts in which it is seen are as follows:

1. **Acute massive hemorrhage.** With a blood loss of 1 liter, approximately 500 mg of iron is drained from the body. Most people have enough storage iron to make up for a loss of this magnitude, and the hematocrit returns to normal within 1 or 2 weeks. Iron supplements are required only if the iron stores of the body are low.

2. **Chronic blood loss.** Most women lose 20 to 40 mL of blood during each menstrual period. This amount contains 10 to 20 mg of iron (0.35 to 0.7 mg/day), which has to be replaced from dietary sources. "Occult" blood loss is caused by chronic hemorrhage into the alimentary canal from esophageal varices, peptic ulcer, hemor-

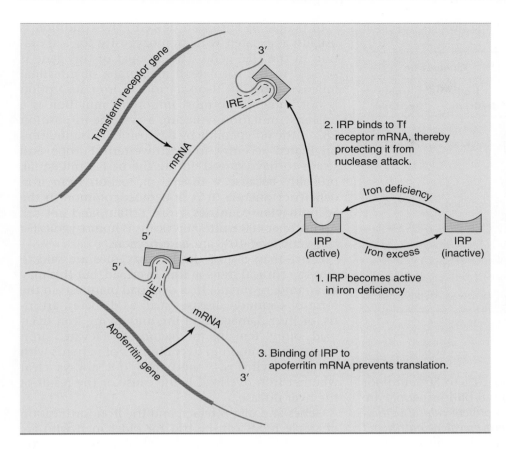

2. IRP binds to Tf receptor mRNA, thereby protecting it from nuclease attack.

Iron deficiency

IRP (active)   Iron excess   IRP (inactive)

1. IRP becomes active in iron deficiency

3. Binding of IRP to apoferritin mRNA prevents translation.

Figure 29.21 Cellular adaptations in the iron-deficient state: more transferrin (Tf) receptors are synthesized to acquire iron from circulating transferrin, and the synthesis of apoferritin is inhibited. The iron response element (IRE) is a regulatory sequence of approximately 30 nucleotides in the messenger RNAs for the transferrin receptor and apoferritin. In iron deficiency, the iron regulatory protein (IRP) is converted to an active form that binds the IREs with high affinity.

rhoids, blood-sucking intestinal parasites, or tumors. Iron deficiency anemia in men should always be evaluated carefully because it may be the first sign of a malignancy.

3. **Growth.** Adults need to absorb iron only to balance iron excretion, but growing children have to maintain a positive iron balance as the blood volume expands. The iron content of the breast milk is low, and therefore the blood hemoglobin concentration normally declines from 18% to 20% at birth to 10% to 14% at 5 months. Oxygen delivery is not much affected by this decline because fetal hemoglobin is replaced by adult hemoglobin during this time period, and adult hemoglobin is the better oxygen carrier after birth. Iron supplements are sometimes given at this time to prevent a decline below 10%, which is arbitrarily considered the lower limit of the "normal" range.

4. **Pregnancy and lactation.** During pregnancy, 250 to 300 mg of iron is transferred to the fetus, and the additional iron loss in the placenta and umbilical cord and in blood loss at birth can range anywhere from 80 to 400 mg. Another 100 to 180 mg is lost during lactation. The drain is minimal during the first months of pregnancy, but up to 5 mg/day are transferred to the fetus during the third trimester. Because many women have negligible iron stores, supplements are routinely given during late pregnancy.

Iron deficiency results in *microcytic hypochromic anemia* (*microcytic* means small red blood cells; *hypochromic* means low hemoglobin content/cell). An important differential diagnosis is the thalassemias, which should be excluded before the initiation of iron therapy because iron supplements are contraindicated in thalassemia (see Chapter 10). Pallor, weakness, and lassitude are typical manifestations of iron deficiency.

Iron deficiency anemia is treated with iron supplements, usually in the form of ferrous sulfate. Some of the commonly used iron supplements also contain ascorbic acid to improve iron absorption. The treatment is given for several months, and it should be continued for some months after hematological improvement to allow for the formation of adequate tissue stores.

Iron deficiency is most prevalent in growing children and in menstruating or pregnant women. Depending on diagnostic criteria, nutritional habits in the population, and the iron fortification of staple foods, the prevalence of iron deficiency anemia in these groups is often reported as 2% to

Table 29.2 Biochemical Indices of Iron Deficiency and Iron Overload

Index	Normal	Changes in: Iron Deficiency	Changes in: Iron Overload
Hematocrit			
Male	43%-49%	Decreased	Normal
Female	41%-46%		
Blood hemoglobin			
Male	14%-18%	Decreased	Normal
Female	12%-16%		
Total plasma iron	50-160 µg/dL	Decreased	Increased
Total iron binding capacity	250-400 µg/dL	Increased	Increased
% Transferrin saturation	20%-55%	Decreased	Increased
Serum ferritin			
Male	5-30 µg/dL	Decreased	Increased
Female	1.2-10 µg/dL		

15% in affluent countries and 10% to 50% in poor countries. Worldwide, 0.5 to 0.6 billion people are affected. *With the exception of protein-calorie malnutrition, iron deficiency is the most prevalent nutritional deficiency worldwide.* Biochemical indices of iron deficiency anemia are summarized in Table 29.2. Serum ferritin and transferrin saturation are the two most important measures in the clinical laboratory.

Iron Overload Can Cause Disease

Apart from the normal turnover of intestinal mucosal cells, which contain iron in the form of ferritin, *there are no effective mechanisms of iron excretion.* If in an adult the amount of absorbed iron exceeds the losses for many years, iron accumulates in the tissues initially as ferritin and later as hemosiderin. This is called **hemosiderosis.** Although initially asymptomatic, excessive iron accumulation is unhealthy because iron catalyzes the formation of destructive free radicals. The longer life span of women may have to do with the fact that they have lower iron stores than do men.

Hemochromatosis is an iron overload syndrome with progressive hemosiderosis and resulting organ damage. It can lead to liver cirrhosis and liver cancer, diabetes mellitus, cardiomyopathy, hyperpigmentation of the skin, endocrine disorders, and joint pain. Accumulating the 10 to 40 g of iron needed to produce symptoms takes some decades, and women are protected by menstruation and childbearing. Therefore, iron overload is seen mainly in older men.

In people of European descent, the condition is usually associated with homozygosity for a mutation in the *HFE* gene. The product of this gene is present in the basolateral membrane of intestinal mucosal cells, but its exact role in iron absorption is not known. The most important mutation is a missense mutation replacing a cysteine in position 282 of the polypeptide by a tyrosine. This mutation originated recently in northwestern Europe and seems to have spread during the past 2 millennia, probably because it offered protection from iron deficiency anemia. It is now most common in the Scandinavian countries, Great Britain, and Ireland. About 1 per 400 white Americans is homozygous for this gene, and 10% are heterozygous.

Fewer than 5% of the homozygotes are said to develop clinical signs of iron overload, but this may be an underestimate. Iron overload manifests in the form of common diseases such as diabetes, arthritis, or liver damage, and the underlying iron overload often remains undiagnosed. Elevated iron levels are common in liver biopsies of patients with "alcoholic cirrhosis," and it is not always clear whether iron overload is the cause or the result of the liver disease.

Genes and diet interact, and the iron fortification of staple foods can be bad for older men who are at risk of iron overload. Also, alcohol increases iron absorption. Many South African Bantus, for example, developed iron overload from the lifelong consumption of iron-rich alcoholic beverages. The excessive iron was derived from the steel vats in which these local brews had been fermented. This "Bantu hemosiderosis" also has a genetic component, but the contributing gene is different from *HFE.*

Hemochromatosis is treated by repeated phlebotomy. Leeches being no longer in fashion, weekly blood donations for up to 1 or 2 years are the best option. The only form of iron overload that cannot be treated with phlebotomy is that of patients with chronic severe anemias who became iron-overloaded by repeated blood transfusions. These cases necessitate **desferrioxamine,** an iron chelator that forms an excretable iron complex.

Because there is only one major hemochromatosis mutation in northern European populations, genetic screening is possible. If the genotype is ascertained early in life, the development of iron overload in genetically predisposed individuals can be prevented by lifestyle adjustments, including regular blood donations.

Zinc Is a Constituent of Many Enzymes

With total body stores of 1.5 to 2.5 g, zinc is the most abundant trace mineral in the body after iron. It is a *constituent of the zinc metalloenzymes,* which include carbonic anhydrase, the cytoplasmic (copper-zinc) superoxide dismutase, alcohol dehydrogenase, carboxypeptidases A and B, DNA and RNA polymerases, and many others. In the *zinc finger proteins,* it serves a structural role by stabilizing small loops in the polypeptide. The human genome is known to code for more than 300 zinc finger proteins.

Some zinc is bound to the storage protein **metallothionein** in the tissues. This protein also binds copper and many other heavy metals, thereby reducing their toxicity. Its synthesis is induced by zinc, cadmium, bismuth, arsenic, and other metals.

Zinc is absorbed incompletely in the small intestine. It is also present in pancreatic juice, and excess zinc is excreted in the stools. Transport in the blood is in association with serum albumin. Only small amounts are lost in urine (0.5 mg/day), sweat (0.2 to 2.0 mg/day), and seminal fluid (up to 1 mg/ejaculate). Meat, nuts, beans, and wheat germ are good dietary sources of zinc. The adult male RDA is set at 15 mg/day.

Zinc deficiency leads to dermatitis and poor wound healing, hair loss, neuropsychiatric impairments, decreased taste acuity, and, in children, poor growth and testicular atrophy. **Acrodermatitis enteropathica** is a rare recessively inherited disease with dermatitis, diarrhea, and alopecia (hair loss), caused by an impairment of intestinal zinc absorption. High doses of orally administered zinc are curative.

Copper Participates in Reactions of Molecular Oxygen

The adult human body contains 80 to 110 mg of copper. Its major function is as a cofactor of enzymes that use either molecular oxygen or an oxygen derivative as one of their substrates. Examples include cytochrome oxidase, dopamine β-hydroxylase, monoamine oxidase, tyrosinase, Δ^9-desaturase, lysyl oxidase, and the cytoplasmic superoxide dismutase.

The dietary requirement is between 1 and 3 mg/day, and the major route of copper excretion is the bile. Of the copper in the serum, 60% is tightly bound in **ceruloplasmin,** and the rest is loosely bound to albumin or complexed with histidine.

Copper deficiency is characterized by a microcytic hypochromic anemia, leukopenia, hemorrhagic vascular changes, bone demineralization, hypercholesterolemia, and neurological problems. It is uncommon and has been seen mainly in patients on total parenteral nutrition and in infants on copper-deficient formulas.

Menkes syndrome is a rare X-linked recessive disorder that is caused by the deficiency of an ATP-dependent membrane transporter for copper. The transfer of copper from the intestinal mucosal cells to the blood is blocked, and its intracellular transport is abnormal as well. This fatal disease is characterized by growth retardation, mental deficiency, seizures, arterial aneurysms, bone demineralization, and brittle hair. It can be treated by the administration of the copper-histidine complex, but affected children nevertheless die during the first years of life.

Wilson disease (**hepatolenticular degeneration**) is a rare recessively inherited deficiency of a different copper transporter. The intestinal absorption of copper is intact, but its biliary excretion is blocked. This leads to copper accumulation in liver and brain, with liver damage, neurological degeneration, or both. This disease can manifest at any time during the life span. It is treated with D-penicillamine, which forms a soluble, excretable copper complex.

Some Trace Elements Serve Very Specific Functions

Some other trace minerals serve highly specialized functions in the body. They include:

- **Manganese:** This metal stimulates the activity of many enzymes but can, in most cases, be replaced by magnesium. An adequate intake is 2 to 5 mg/day. Excess manganese is toxic, causing psychosis and parkinsonism ("manganese madness").
- **Molybdenum:** This metal occurs in a few oxidase enzymes, including xanthine oxidase.
- **Selenium:** In the form of selenocysteine, this element occurs in about 20 human proteins, including the important antioxidant enzyme glutathione peroxidase. Both selenium deficiency and toxicity have been described. **Keshan disease** is an endemic cardiomyopathy in parts of China that is caused by the low selenium content of locally grown foodstuffs. The selenium content of the soil varies widely in different parts of the world, and this is reflected in the selenium content of the food plants grown on these soils.
- **Iodine:** This halogen is needed only for the synthesis of the thyroid hormones.
- **Fluorine:** The fluoride ion can be incorporated in the inorganic substance of bones and teeth. Although not absolutely essential, it strengthens teeth and bones. It may even have some protective effect in osteoporosis.

SUMMARY

Vitamins are essential micronutrients that serve specialized functions in metabolism. Most of the water-soluble vitamins are precursors of coenzymes. Riboflavin, for example, is required for the synthesis of the flavin coenzymes, niacin for NAD and NADP, thiamine for TPP, pantothenic acid for CoA, and folic acid for THF.

Other vitamins, notably vitamins A, D, and E, are antioxidants that scavenge destructive free radicals. They express lipid peroxidation, and they may have antimutagenic properties. They have some use in the prevention of atherosclerosis, cancer, and degenerative diseases.

Other vitamins are precursors of hormone-like products. Vitamin A is converted to retinoic acid, and vitamin D to calcitriol. These vitamin derivatives are gene regulators, with mechanisms of action similar to the steroid hormones.

Macrominerals are bulk constituents of the body fluids that are required in fairly large quantities in the diet. Microminerals serve specialized functions, and they are required only in small quantities. Iron, in particular, is required as a constituent of heme proteins and iron-sulfur proteins.

Nutritional deficiencies of individual vitamins and minerals cause distinctive deficiency states that are related to the metabolic functions of the missing nutrient. Vitamin C deficiency (scurvy), for example, causes connective tissue problems because of impaired collagen synthesis, and iron deficiency causes anemia because of impaired hemoglobin synthesis. Although the incidence of severe nutritional deficiencies has declined in affluent countries, vitamin and mineral nutrition is still a major public health concern for at-risk groups, including infants, pregnant women, alcoholics, and the elderly.

📖 Further Reading

Andrews NC: Iron deficiency and iron overload. Annu Rev Genomics Hum Genet 1:75-98, 2000.
Arrigoni O, De Tullio MC: Ascorbic acid: much more than just an antioxidant. Biochim Biophys Acta 1569:1-9, 2002.
Clagett-Dame M, DeLuca H: The role of vitamin A in mammalian reproduction and embryonic development. Annu Rev Nutr 22:347-381, 2002.
Eisenstein RS: Iron regulatory proteins and the molecular control of mammalian iron metabolism. Annu Rev Nutr 20:627-662, 2000.
Harris ED: Cellular copper transport and metabolism. Annu Rev Nutr 20:291-310, 2000.
Hentze MW, Muckenthaler MU, Andrews NC: Balancing acts: molecular control of mammalian iron metabolism. Cell 117:285-297, 2004.
Kohrle J, Brigelius-Flohe R, Bock A, et al: Selenium in biology: facts and medical perspectives. Biol Chem 381:849-864, 2000.
Leong W-I, Lonnerdal B: Hepcidin, the recently identified peptide that appears to regulate iron absorption. J Nutr 134:1-4, 2004.
McCune CA, Al-Jader LN, May A, et al: Hereditary haemochromatosis: only 1% of adult HFE C282Y homozygotes in South Wales have a clinical diagnosis of iron overload. Hum Genet 111:538-543, 2002.
Reddy MB, Clark L: Iron, oxidative stress and disease risk. Nutr Rev 62:120-124, 2004.
Ricciarelli R, Zingg J-M, Azzi A: The 80th anniversary of vitamin E: beyond its antioxidant properties. Biol Chem 383:457-465, 2002.
Schweizer U, Schomburg L, Savaskan NE: The neurobiology of selenium: lessons from transgenic mice. J Nutr 134:707-710, 2004.
Stahl W, Ale-Agha N, Polidori MC: Non-antioxidant properties of carotenoids. Biol Chem 383:553-558, 2002.
Umeta M, West CE, Haidar J, et al: Zinc supplementation and stunted infants in Ethiopia: a randomised controlled trial. Lancet 355:2021-2026, 2000.
Wessling-Resnick M: Iron transport. Annu Rev Nutr 20:129-151, 2000.

QUESTIONS

1. **A finding that would support a diagnosis of iron deficiency anemia in a 25-year-old woman with a hematocrit of 28% is**

   A. The presence of oversized erythrocytes.
   B. Low iron saturation of transferrin.
   C. A reduced serum transferrin concentration.
   D. An increased level of serum ferritin.
   E. A reduced level of metallothionein in a liver biopsy.

2. **Retinoic acid in high doses is sometimes used for the treatment of skin diseases, including common acne. Retinoic acid can cause many toxic effects at high doses. The *most important* of these toxic effects is**

   A. Bone demineralization, which leads to pathological fractures.
   B. Connective tissue weakness with multiple small subcutaneous hemorrhages.
   C. Teratogenic effects during the first trimester of pregnancy.
   D. Peripheral neuropathy.
   E. Amnesia.

3. Vitamin D can be produced by the action of sunlight on 7-dehydrocholesterol in the skin, but it has to be converted to its biologically active form by hydroxylation reactions in

   A. The lungs and brain.
   B. Endothelium and the intestines.
   C. Skeletal muscle and the adrenal cortex.
   D. Adipose tissue and bone.
   E. The liver and kidneys.

4. Some vitamins have antioxidant properties and are therefore considered promising for the prevention of atherosclerosis, cancer, and age-related degenerative diseases. Antioxidant properties have been demonstrated for all of the following vitamins *except*

   A. Thiamine (vitamin B_1).
   B. α-Tocopherol (vitamin E).
   C. Ascorbic acid (vitamin C).
   D. Retinol (vitamin A).

5. Thiamine deficiency can cause both acute encephalopathy and irreversible memory impairment. These problems are most often seen in thiamine-deficient

   A. Newborns.
   B. Alcoholics.
   C. Diabetics.
   D. Vegetarians.
   E. Medical students.

CHAPTER 30

Integration of Metabolism

For the individual cell, the most immediate challenge is the safeguarding of its own energy supply. Beyond the imperative of self-preservation, however, cells and organs have to cooperate unselfishly for the common good of the body. Together they have to master the everyday challenges of overeating, fasting, and muscular activity and the less routine challenges of infectious illnesses and environmental toxins.

These challenges require the organism-wide coordination of metabolic pathways. This coordination is provided by nervous and hormonal signals that reach every part of the body. This chapter is concerned with the metabolic adaptations to environmental challenges and varying physiological needs. It describes the hormonal mechanisms of metabolic regulation and some clinical conditions in which these regulatory mechanisms are deranged.

Insulin Is a Satiety Hormone

After a hearty meal, the body is flooded with monosaccharides, amino acids, and triglycerides. Not all of this bounty can be oxidized immediately, and *excess nutrients have to be stored as glycogen and fat.*

Insulin is the hormone of the well-fed state. Its synthesis and release are powerfully stimulated by glucose, and this effect is potentiated by amino acids. Therefore, *the plasma level of insulin is highest after a carbohydrate-rich meal.* The list of insulin effects in Table 30.1 shows that insulin stimulates the *utilization of dietary nutrients,* including glucose, amino acids, and triglycerides. It diverts excess nutrients into the synthesis of glycogen, fat, and even protein.

In skeletal muscle and adipose tissue, *glucose uptake into the cell through glucose transporter 4 (GLUT-4) carriers is the rate-limiting step of glucose metabolism.* This step is stimulated 10- to 20-fold by insulin.

The liver has an insulin-independent glucose transporter (GLUT-2) that is not rate-limiting, but *the glucose-metabolizing enzymes are stimulated by insulin.* Insulin induces the synthesis of glycolytic enzymes and represses the synthesis of gluconeogenic enzymes on a time scale of hours to days. Through the dephosphorylation of metabolic and regulatory enzymes, it also stimulates glycolysis and glycogen synthesis and inhibits gluconeogenesis and glycogenolysis on a minute-by-minute time scale (see Chapter 22).

Glucose metabolism in brain and erythrocytes is not insulin dependent. Therefore, these tissues keep consuming glucose even during fasting, when the insulin level is low. They have to because they are inept at metabolizing alternative fuels.

Insulin regulates the metabolism of fat and protein as well as of carbohydrate. It induces the conversion of excess carbohydrate to fat by stimulating glycolysis and fatty acid synthesis. At the same time, it promotes fat synthesis in adipose tissue while preventing fat breakdown. Insulin even stimulates protein synthesis rather nonselectively, in large part by actions at the level of translation. Thus, excess nutrients are used for the synthesis of glycogen, fat, and body protein.

Glucagon Maintains the Blood Glucose Level

The secretion of glucagon from the pancreatic α cells is increased twofold to threefold by hypoglycemia and reduced to half of the basal release by hyperglycemia. Acting through its second messenger, cyclic AMP (cAMP), *glucagon up-regulates the blood glucose level when dietary carbohydrate is in*

Table 30.1 Metabolic Effects of Insulin

Tissue	Affected Pathway	Affected Enzyme
Liver	↑ Glucose phosphorylation	Glucokinase
	↑ Glycolysis	Phosphofructokinase-1,* pyruvate kinase[†]
	↓ Gluconeogenesis	PEP-carboxykinase, fructose-1,6-bisphosphatase,* glucose-6-phosphatase
	↑ Glycogen synthesis	Glycogen synthase[†]
	↓ Glycogenolysis	Glycogen phosphorylase[†]
	↑ Fatty acid synthesis	Acetyl-CoA carboxylase,[†] ATP-citrate lyase, malic enzyme
	↑ Pentose phosphate pathway	Glucose-6-phosphate dehydrogenase
Adipose tissue	↑ Glucose uptake	Glucose carrier
	↑ Glycolysis	Phosphofructokinase-1
	↑ Pentose phosphate pathway	Glucose-6-phosphate dehydrogenase
	↑ Pyruvate oxidation	Pyruvate dehydrogenase[†]
	↑ Triglyceride utilization (from lipoproteins)	Lipoprotein lipase
	↑ Triglyceride synthesis	Glycerol-3-phosphate acyl transferase
	↓ Lipolysis	Hormone-sensitive lipase[†]
Skeletal muscle	↑ Glucose uptake	Glucose carrier
	↑ Glycolysis	Phosphofructokinase-1
	↑ Glycogen synthesis	Glycogen synthase[†]
	↓ Glycogenolysis	Glycogen phosphorylase[†]
	↑ Protein synthesis	Translational initiation complex

*Insulin acts indirectly by promoting the dephosphorylation of phosphofructokinase-2/fructose-2,6-bisphosphatase, thereby increasing the level of fructose-2,6-bisphosphate.
[†]Insulin acts by promoting the dephosphorylation of the enzyme.
Most of the other insulin effects included here are actions on the rate of synthesis or degradation of the affected enzyme.

Table 30.2 Metabolic Effects of Glucagon on the Liver*

Effect on Pathway	Affected Enzyme	Enzyme Affected by		
		Enzyme Induction/Repression	Enzyme Phosphorylation	Other
↓ Glycolysis	Glucokinase	+		
	Phosphofructokinase-1			+[†]
	Pyruvate kinase	+		
↑ Gluconeogenesis	PEP-carboxykinase	+		
	Fructose-1,6-bisphosphatase	+		+[†]
	Glucose-6-phosphatase	+		
↓ Glycogen synthesis	Glycogen synthase		+	
↑ Glycogenolysis	Glycogen phosphorylase		+	
↓ Fatty acid synthesis	Acetyl-CoA carboxylase	+	+	
↑ Fatty acid oxidation	Carnitine-palmitoyl transferase-1	+		

*Both the enzyme phosphorylations and the effects on gene expression are mediated by cAMP.
[†]Mediated by the cAMP-dependent phosphorylation of phosphofructokinase-2/fructose-2,6-bisphosphatase and a decreased cellular concentration of fructose-2,6-bisphosphate.

short supply. Its actions on the pathways of glucose metabolism are opposite to those of insulin (Table 30.2), but, unlike insulin, *glucagon acts almost exclusively on the liver;* it has negligible effects on adipose tissue, muscle, and other extrahepatic tissues.

Catecholamines Mediate the Flight-or-Fight Response

Norepinephrine is the neurotransmitter of postganglionic sympathetic neurons, and both epinephrine and norepinephrine are released from the adrenal medulla in response to nerve stimulation. These two catecholamines are *stress hormones.* They are released during physical exertion and cold exposure and also in response to psychological stress: for example, during a biochemistry examination.

The catecholamines can raise the cellular cAMP level through β-adrenergic receptors, and the calcium level through α_1-adrenergic receptors. Muscle and adipose tissue have mainly β receptors, and the liver has mainly α_1 receptors.

The metabolic actions of the catecholamines are summarized in Table 30.3. These actions, which

Table 30.3 Metabolic Effects of Norepinephrine and Epinephrine

Tissue	Affected Pathway	Affected Enzyme	Second Messenger
Adipose tissue	↑↑↑ Lipolysis	Hormone-sensitive lipase*	cAMP
	↓ Triglyceride utilization (from lipoproteins)	Lipoprotein lipase	?
Liver	↓ Glycolysis	Phosphofructokinase-1†	cAMP
	↑ Gluconeogenesis	Fructose-1,6-bisphosphatase†	
	↓↓ Glycogen synthesis	Glycogen synthase*	Ca²⁺, cAMP
	↑↑↑ Glycogenolysis	Glycogen phosphorylase*	
	↓ Fatty acid synthesis	Acetyl-CoA carboxylase*	cAMP
Skeletal muscle	↑↑↑ Glycolysis	Phosphofructokinase-1†	
	↓↓ Glycogen synthesis	Glycogen synthase*	cAMP
	↑↑↑ Glycogenolysis	Glycogen phosphorylase*	
	↑ Triglyceride utilization (from lipoproteins)	Lipoprotein lipase	?

↑ and ↓, Weak or inconsistent effect; ↑↑ and ↓↓, moderately strong effect; ↑↑↑ and ↓↓↓, strong effect.
*Effects mediated by enzyme phosphorylation.
†Mediated indirectly by phosphorylation of phosphofructokinase-2/fructose-2,6-bisphosphatase.

appear within seconds, are part of the **flight-or-fight response.** Most important is the *mobilization of fat and glycogen reserves for use by the muscles.* In muscle tissue itself, the major effects are the *stimulation of glycogen degradation and glycolysis.*

As in the liver (see Chapter 22), the regulatory metabolite fructose-2,6-bisphosphate activates phosphofructokinase-1 in muscle. However, the phosphofructokinase-2/fructose-2,6-bisphosphatase of skeletal muscle is different from the liver enzyme. Its kinase activity is not inhibited but stimulated by cAMP-induced phosphorylation. Therefore, the catecholamines, acting through β receptors and cAMP, stimulate rather than inhibit glycolysis in skeletal muscle.

The catecholamines are *functional antagonists of insulin* that raise the blood levels of glucose and free fatty acids. They are not very important for blood glucose regulation under ordinary conditions, but *their release is potently stimulated by hypoglycemia.* Therefore, hypoglycemic episodes in metabolic diseases are always accompanied by signs of excessive sympathetic activity, including pallor, sweating, and tachycardia.

Glucocorticoids Are Released in Chronic Stress

Under conditions of *chronic stress,* the hypothalamus of the brain releases corticotropin releasing factor, which stimulates the secretion of adrenocorticotropic hormone (ACTH) from the anterior pituitary gland. ACTH stimulates the secretion of cortisol and other glucocorticoids from the adrenal cortex. The metabolic actions of the glucocorticoids (Table 30.4) can best be understood as adaptations to life in a dangerous world.

By and large, the glucocorticoids are synergistic with epinephrine, but there is an important differ-

Table 30.4 Important Metabolic Actions of Cortisol and Other Glucocorticoids*

Tissue	Affected Pathway	Affected Enzyme
Adipose tissue	↑ Lipolysis	Hormone-sensitive lipase
Muscle tissue	↑ Protein degradation	?
Liver	↑ Gluconeogenesis	Enzymes of amino acid catabolism, PEP-carboxykinase
	↑ Glycogen synthesis	Glycogen synthase

*The glucocorticoid effects are mediated by altered rates of enzyme synthesis.

ence. Epinephrine works through the second messengers cAMP and calcium, whereas the glucocorticoids are gene regulators. Therefore, epinephrine induces its effects in a matter of seconds, but the glucocorticoid effects are cumulative over many hours to days.

The glucocorticoids prepare the body for the action of epinephrine. They stimulate the synthesis of the hormone-sensitive adipose tissue lipase. This is of little consequence under ordinary conditions, but it potentiates the epinephrine effect on lipolysis. They also increase gluconeogenesis from amino acids by causing net protein breakdown in peripheral tissues and inducing PEP carboxykinase in the liver. Excess glucose-6-phosphate produced by gluconeogenesis is diverted into glycogen synthesis, thus providing more substrate for epinephrine-induced glycogenolysis.

It is now apparent how cortisol and epinephrine cooperate in a stressful situation. During an extended hunting expedition by a stone-age caveman, cortisol induced the hormone-sensitive lipase in his adipose tissue and built up the glycogen stores in his liver. As soon as the hunter was attacked

Table 30.5 The Metabolic Rates of Various Organs and Tissues

	Organ Metabolic Rate (kcal/ kg/day)	Tissue or Organ Weight (kg)			% of Body Weight			Metabolic Rate (% of Total)		
		Male	Female	Child (6 Months)	Male	Female	Child (6 Months)	Male	Female	Child (6 Months)
Liver	200	1.8	1.4	0.26	2.57	2.41	3.51	21	21	14
Brain	240	1.4	1.2	0.71	2.00	2.07	9.51	20	21	44
Heart	440	0.33	0.24	0.04	0.47	0.41	0.53	9	8	4
Kidneys	440	0.31	0.28	0.05	0.44	0.47	0.71	8	9	6
Muscle	13	28	17	1.88	40	29.3	25	22	16	6
Adipose tissue	4.5	15	19	1.50	21.4	32.8	20	4	6	2
Others	12	23.2	18.9	3.06	33.1	32.6	40.7	16	19	24
Total		70	58	7.50	100	100	100	100*	100†	100‡

Data from: Kinney JM, Tucker HN: Energy Metabolism. New York: Raven Press, 1992.
*1680 kcal/day. †1340 kcal/day. ‡390 kcal/day.

by a cave bear, epinephrine immediately stimulated the release of fatty acids by the hormone-sensitive lipase in his adipose tissue and of glucose by glycogen phosphorylase in the liver. Thanks to the supply of these fuels to his muscles, the caveman managed to dodge the cave bear's attack, kill the animal with his club, and have a fine dinner.

The stress hormones are still important today. Patients suffering from infections, autoimmune diseases, malignancies, injuries, or any other serious illness have elevated levels of glucocorticoids and catecholamines. Cortisol-induced protein breakdown leads to *negative nitrogen balance and muscle wasting.* Because the stress hormones oppose the metabolic effects of insulin, seriously ill patients also have *insulin resistance and poor glucose tolerance.* The insulin requirement of insulin-dependent diabetic patients rises substantially during otherwise harmless infections or other illnesses.

Some **cytokines,** which are released by white blood cells during infections and some other diseases, also have metabolic effects. **Interleukin-1** stimulates proteolysis in skeletal muscle, and **tumor necrosis factor** promotes lipolysis in adipose tissue. These mediators contribute to the weight loss that is common in patients with malignancies or chronic infections.

Energy Must Be Provided Continuously

The basal metabolic rate (BMR) is the amount of energy that is consumed by a resting subject in the "postabsorptive" state, 8 to 12 hours after the last meal. It is near 24 kcal per kilogram of body weight under ordinary conditions but drops by 15% to 25% during starvation, possibly because of reduced levels of thyroid hormones. The BMR depends on the body composition. Men tend to have a higher BMR

per body weight than do women, because men have relatively more muscle than fat (Table 30.5). Women need more fat as an energy reserve for pregnancy, and men traditionally needed more muscle to fight over the females.

On top of the BMR, humans need some additional energy for **postprandial thermogenesis:** the additional energy expenditure after a meal. It typically amounts to about 10% of the BMR. Postprandial thermogenesis is produced by metabolic interconversions after a meal and by increased futile cycling in metabolic pathways. It depends on the composition of the meal. Thus, the digestion, absorption, and storage of fat require only 2% to 4% of the fat energy, but the conversion of carbohydrate to storage fat requires 24% of the energy content of the carbohydrate.

Thermogenesis also results from other factors, including cold exposure and coffee. **Muscular activity** is the most variable item in the energy budget, but is generally below 1500 kcal/day except in people who engage in very strenuous physical labor all day long.

Unlike ruminants, most people eat not continuously but in well-spaced meals. Humans are flooded with nutrients for only 3 to 4 hours after a meal, and yet they have to expend metabolic energy round the clock. Therefore, they depend on stored energy reserves during fasting.

The fat in adipose tissue contains almost 100 times more energy than the combined glycogen stores of liver and muscle (Table 30.6). Therefore, only fat can keep a human alive during prolonged fasting. It is easy to calculate that with fat stores of 16 kg and a BMR of 1500 kcal/day, people can survive for about 100 days on tap water and vitamin pills alone. The time to death on a hunger strike depends on the fat reserves, but survival times near 100 days are typical.

Table 30.6 Energy Reserves of the "Textbook" 70-kg Man

Stored Nutrient	Tissue	Amount Stored (kg)	Energy Value (kcal)
Triglyceride	Adipose tissue	10-15	90,000-140,000
Glycogen	Muscle	0.3	1200
	Liver	0.08*	320*
Protein	Muscle	6-8	30,000-40,000

*After a meal. Liver glycogen is approximately 20% to 30% of this value after an overnight fast of 12 hours.

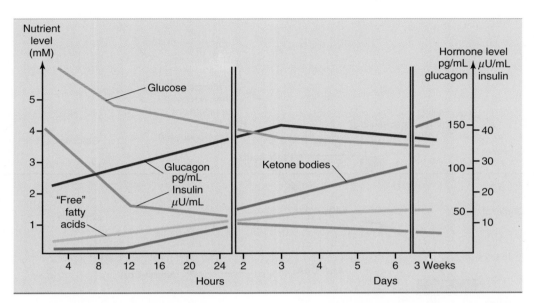

Figure 30.1 Plasma levels of hormones and nutrients at different times after the last meal. mM, mmol/liter.

Glycogen is rapidly depleted. It is a checking account from which withdrawals are made on an hour-by-hour basis, whereas fat is a saving account. Indeed, only liver glycogen supplies energy for the whole body. Muscle glycogen is earmarked strictly for muscular activity.

Unlike fat and glycogen, protein is not a specialized energy storage form. Nevertheless, much of the protein in muscle and other tissues can be mobilized during fasting. Only the protein in brain, liver, kidneys, and other vital organs is taboo, even during prolonged starvation.

During long-term fasting, net protein breakdown is required to supply amino acids for gluconeogenesis. Because even-chain fatty acids are not substrates of gluconeogenesis, only amino acids are available in sufficient quantity to cover the glucose requirement during fasting. Therefore, *the loss of protein from muscle and other tissues is inevitable during prolonged fasting.*

Figure 30.1 shows some of the changes in blood chemistry during the transition from the well-fed state to starvation. The most important hormonal factor is *the balance between insulin and its antagonists,* especially glucagon. During fasting, the plasma level of insulin falls, whereas first epinephrine, then glucagon, and finally cortisol levels rise.

During the first few days on a zero-calories diet of tap water and vitamin pills, between 70 and 150 g of body protein is lost per day. The rate of protein loss then declines in parallel with the rising use of ketone bodies. Nevertheless, 1 kg of protein is lost within the first 15 days of starvation.

Adding 100 g of glucose to the zero-calories diet reduces the need for gluconeogenesis and cuts the protein loss by 40%. Also, the addition of 55 g of protein per day cannot prevent a negative nitrogen balance initially, but many subjects regain nitrogen equilibrium after about 20 days.

Adipose Tissue Is the Most Important Energy Depot

The blood glucose level declines only to a limited extent even during prolonged fasting, but free fatty

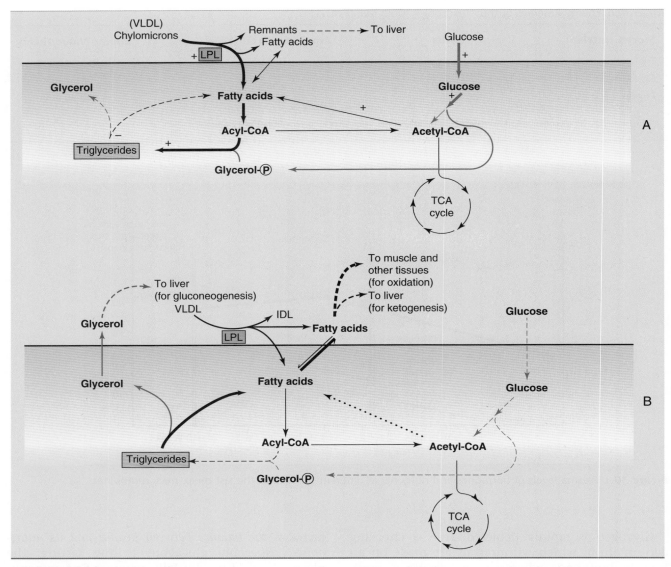

Figure 30.2 Metabolism of adipose tissue after a mixed meal containing all major nutrients and during fasting. **A,** After a meal. Insulin-stimulated or insulin-inhibited steps are marked by + or −, respectively. **B,** During fasting. LPL, lipoprotein lipase; IDL, intermediate-density lipoprotein (VLDL remnant); VLDL, very-low-density lipoprotein.

acid levels rise fourfold to eightfold and the levels of ketone bodies (β-hydroxybutyrate and acetoacetate) rise up to 100-fold.

Plasma free fatty acids are low after a carbohydrate meal because the hormone-sensitive lipase is inhibited by insulin. At the same time, insulin stimulates glucose uptake into adipose cells. This facilitates fat synthesis because glucose is converted into glycerol phosphate, the immediate precursor of the glycerol in stored triglycerides. Insulin also stimulates the lipoprotein lipase in adipose tissue but not in muscle, thus routing chylomicron triglycerides to adipose tissue in the well-fed state (Fig. 30.2).

During fasting, fat synthesis is reduced, while the hormone-sensitive lipase is stimulated by the combination of the low insulin level and the high levels of insulin antagonists. Adipose tissue is very sensitive to insulin, and *lipolysis is inhibited even at moderately high insulin levels* during the early stages of fasting.

The Liver Converts Dietary Carbohydrates to Glycogen and Fat

Being devoid of lipoprotein lipase, *the liver is not a major consumer of triglycerides after a meal.* It obtains only a small amount of dietary triglyceride from chylomicron remnants. However, the liver metabolizes 20% to 30% of the dietary glucose after a carbohydrate-rich meal. Because of the high Michaelis constant (K_m) of glucokinase for glucose, *hepatic glucose utilization is controlled by substrate availability*. Insulin induces the synthesis of glucokinase, but this effect becomes maximal only after 2 or 3 days on a high-carbohydrate diet.

The liver converts a major portion of its glucose allotment into glycogen after a meal. Most of the rest is metabolized by glycolysis, although the liver has only a moderately high capacity for glycolysis. After a mixed meal containing all major nutrients, the liver obtains most of its metabolic energy from amino acids rather than glucose. Therefore, much of the glucose-derived acetyl-CoA is available for fat synthesis. *In the liver, glycolysis is the first step in the conversion of carbohydrate to fat*. Insulin coordinates this process by stimulating both glycolysis and fatty acid biosynthesis.

The Liver Supplies Glucose and Ketone Bodies during Fasting

In the fasting state, *the liver has to feed the glucose-dependent tissues*. The brain is the most demanding customer. It is the most aristocratic organ in the body, and it therefore requires a large share of the communally owned resources. Although it accounts for only 2% of the body weight in the adult, it consumes at least 20% of the total energy in the resting body (see Table 30.5). This large energy demand is covered from glucose under ordinary conditions and from glucose and ketone bodies during prolonged fasting. The brain oxidizes 90 g of glucose per day in the well-fed state and 30 g during long-term fasting.

Three to four hours after a meal, the liver becomes a net producer of glucose. The glucose is initially formed by glycogen breakdown, but *liver glycogen lasts for less than 1 day*. During more extended fasting, humans depend entirely on gluconeogenesis to produce between 80 and 160 g of glucose per day. At least one half of this is consumed by the brain, and the erythrocytes claim another 20 g per day. More than one half of the glucose is produced from amino acids. Other substrates of gluconeogenesis are glycerol from adipose tissue and lactic acid from erythrocytes and other anaerobic cells.

The fasting liver spoon-feeds the other tissues with **ketone bodies** as well as with glucose. In theory, both carbohydrates and fatty acids can be converted into ketone bodies through acetyl-CoA. Actually, however, *the liver forms ketone bodies from fatty acids during fasting but not from carbohydrate after a meal*.

The maximal rate of glycolysis in the liver is only 2 μmol per gram of tissue weight per minute, or 30 g/hour for a 3-pound liver. Much of this is used for lipogenesis, and some is oxidized in the TCA cycle. Therefore, very little is left for ketogenesis. However, the liver has a very high capacity for fatty acid oxidation. Over a wide range of plasma levels, about 30% of the incoming fatty acids are extracted and metabolized. This means that *hepatic fatty acid utilization is controlled by substrate availability*. It rises during fasting, when adipose tissue supplies large amounts of free fatty acids.

The liver has several options for the metabolism of these fatty acids (Fig. 30.3). The first choice is between esterification in the cytoplasm and uptake into the mitochondrion. The liver synthesizes lipids for export in very-low-density lipoprotein (VLDC) at all times. After a meal, the fatty acids for these lipids are made from dietary carbohydrate, but during fasting they come from adipose tissue.

Fatty acid esterification remains at a modest level during fasting, but fatty acid uptake into the mitochondrion is stimulated. Carnitine-palmitoyl transferase-1, which controls the transport of long-chain fatty acids into the mitochondrion, is induced by glucagon through its second messenger cAMP and also by fatty acids through the nuclear fatty acid receptor peroxisome proliferator–activated receptor α (PPAR-α).

In the well-fed state, carnitine-palmitoyl transferase-1 is inhibited by malonyl-CoA. During fasting, however, the production of malonyl-CoA by acetyl-CoA carboxylase is switched off by high levels of acyl-CoA, low levels of citrate, and a high glucagon/insulin ratio. Therefore, the mitochondrial uptake of fatty acids is no longer inhibited by malonyl-CoA.

β-Oxidation is the only major fate of fatty acids in the mitochondrion. Its product acetyl-CoA, however, has to be partitioned between the TCA cycle and ketogenesis.

The activity of the TCA cycle depends on the cell's need for ATP. It is inhibited by ATP and a high [NADH]/[NAD$^+$] ratio (see Chapter 21). β-Oxidation produces NADH and, indirectly, ATP. These products of β-oxidation inhibit the TCA cycle, preventing the oxidation of acetyl-CoA and diverting it into ketogenesis. Enzyme induction is also important. The activity of 3-hydroxy-3-methylglutaryl-CoA lyase, the enzyme that forms acetoacetate from HMG-CoA, is greatly increased during fasting.

Ketogenesis amounts to an incomplete oxidation of fatty acids. Whereas the complete oxidation of one molecule of palmitoyl-CoA produces 131 molecules of ATP (see Chapter 23), its conversion to acetoacetate and β-hydroxybutyrate produces 35 and 23 molecules of ATP, respectively. The conversion of

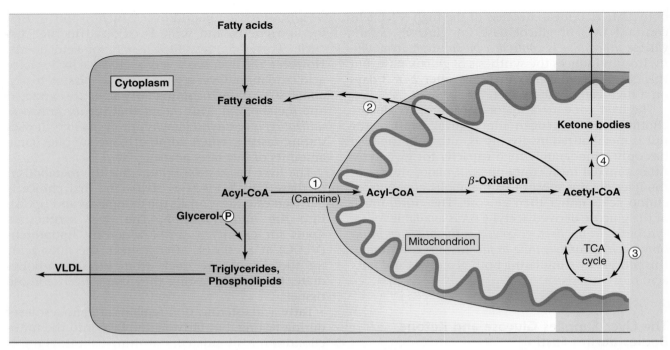

Figure 30.3 Alternative fates of fatty acids in the liver. The regulated steps are as follows: ① Carnitine acyl transferase-1 is induced in the fasting state. It also is acutely inhibited by malonyl-CoA, the product of the acetyl-CoA carboxylase reaction when fatty acid biosynthesis is stimulated after a carbohydrate-rich meal. ② Acetyl-CoA carboxylase is induced in the well-fed state. It is inhibited in the fasting state by high levels of acyl-CoA, low levels of citrate (direct allosteric effects), and a high glucagon/insulin ratio (leading to phosphorylation and inactivation). ③ The TCA cycle is inhibited when alternative sources supply ATP and NADH. Therefore, a high rate of β-oxidation reduces its activity. ④ The ketogenic enzymes are induced during fasting. VLDL, very-low-density lipoprotein.

50 g of fatty acids to acetoacetate during a hungry day supplies enough energy to synthesize 190 g of glucose from lactic acid without any need for the TCA cycle.

Why does the liver convert fatty acids to ketone bodies when carbohydrates are in short supply? The reason is that *ketone bodies are more easily metabolized than are fatty acids by many tissues.* The brain, in particular, which depends almost entirely on glucose under ordinary conditions, is unable to oxidize fatty acids but can cover up to 70% of its energy needs from ketone bodies during prolonged fasting, when ketone body levels are very high. This reduces the need for gluconeogenesis and thereby spares body protein. Liver metabolism in different nutritional states is summarized in Figure 30.4.

Most Tissues Switch from Carbohydrate Oxidation to Fat Oxidation during Fasting

Total body glucose consumption falls precipitously during the transition from the well-fed state to the

fasting state (Fig. 30.5). The place of glucose is taken by fatty acids and ketone bodies. Only tissues that depend on glucose for their energy needs, including brain and red blood cells, continue to consume glucose because their glucose metabolism is insulin independent. The switch from glucose oxidation to fat oxidation is reflected in the **respiratory quotient** (see Chapter 21), which declines from about 0.9 after a mixed meal to slightly above 0.7 in the fasting state.

The nutrient flows in the body change dramatically in different nutritional states. Figure 30.6 shows the flow of nutrients after different kinds of meal, and Figure 30.7 shows the changes during the transition from the well-fed state to prolonged fasting. The intestine provides for all the body's needs after a mixed meal, whereas adipose tissue and liver assume this role during fasting.

The refeeding of severely starved patients is not entirely unproblematic. The levels of glycolytic enzymes in the liver are very low, and the patients show profound carbohydrate intolerance. Therefore, *refeeding should be started slowly,* especially in advanced cases.

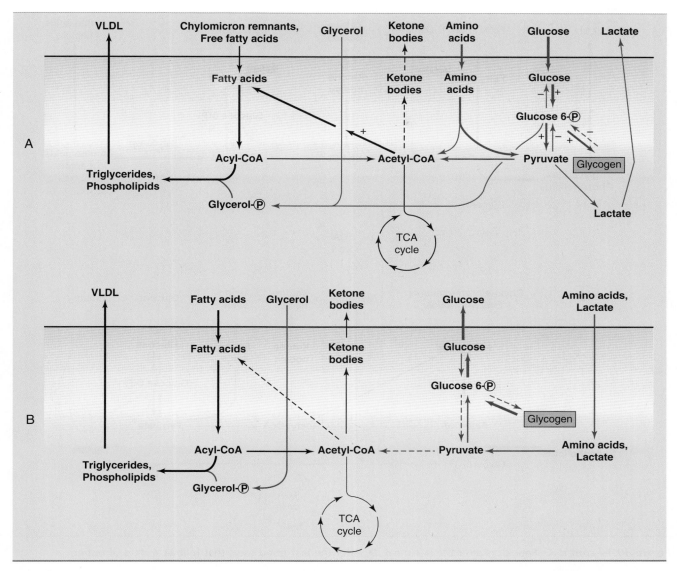

Figure 30.4 Metabolism of the yoyo dieter's liver. **A,** After a meal. Pathways that are stimulated or inhibited by insulin are marked by + or −, respectively. VLDL, very-low-density lipoprotein. **B,** Twelve hours after the last meal.

Obesity Is the Most Common Nutrition-Related Disorder in Affluent Countries

Obesity is the most visible medical problem in modern societies. Its prevalence depends on the definitions used. One convenient measure, the **body mass index (BMI)**, is defined as follows:

$$BMI = weight/height^2$$

A BMI of 20 to 24.9 kg/m^2 is considered normal, a BMI between 25 and 29.9 signifies overweight, and a BMI of 30 and above indicates obesity. The prevalence of overweight and obesity in different popu-lation groups in the United States during the early 1990s is shown in Table 30.7. The problem has worsened since then. Overall, 25% of Americans today are classified as obese, and an additional 35% are overweight but not obese.

Body weight tends to change over the life span. In affluent countries, women tend to gain weight between the ages of 20 and 60. Men tend to gain weight more slowly from age 20 to age 50 and to get thinner again after age 60. However, even with constant weight, the amount of lean body mass declines slowly with advancing age, while fat rises.

Until the early years of the 20th century, body weight was related to social class, rich people being

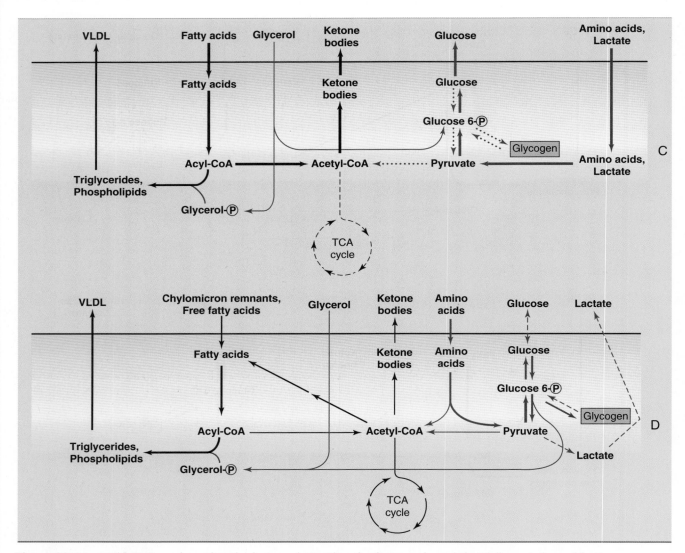

Figure 30.4—cont'd **C,** Four days after the last meal. **D,** After the first good meal that follows 4 days of fasting.

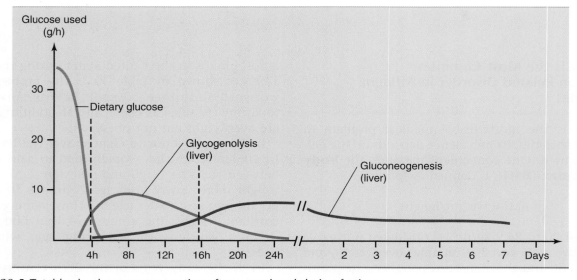

Figure 30.5 Total body glucose consumption after a meal and during fasting.

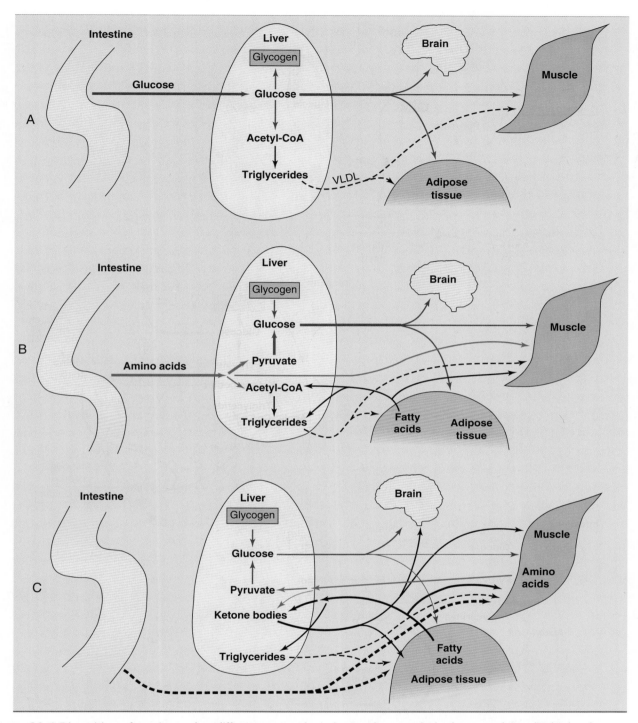

Figure 30.6 Disposition of nutrients after different types of meals. **A,** After a carbohydrate meal (insulin high, glucagon low). CoA, coenzyme A; VLDL, very-low-density lipoprotein. **B,** After a protein meal (insulin moderately high, glucagon high). **C,** After a fat meal (insulin low, glucagon high).

heavier than the poor. Socioeconomic status (SES) is still important today, but now poor people are fatter than the rich. A study in the United States found that 30% of low-SES women, 16% of middle-SES women, but only 5% of upper-SES women were obese. There was a similar but weaker relationship in men.

Another effect of obesity is increased rates of mortality. Actuarial tables of life insurance companies typically show that mortality is lowest in people

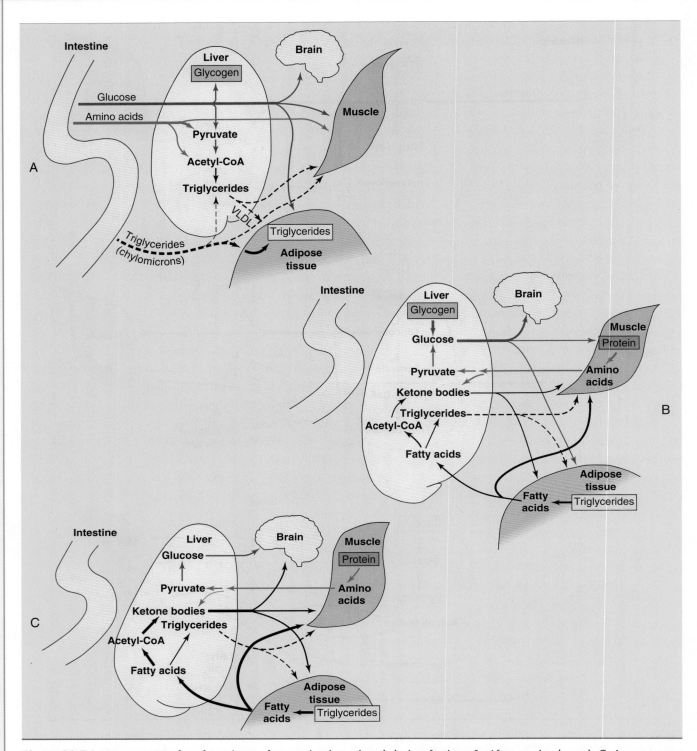

Figure 30.7 Interorgan transfer of nutrients after a mixed meal and during fasting. **A,** After a mixed meal. CoA, coenzyme A; VLDL, very-low-density lipoprotein. **B,** Postabsorptive state, 12 hours after the last meal. **C,** One week after the last meal.

who are considered 10% underweight. Overweight and obese people, but also those who are severely underweight, are more likely to die. Only among the elderly are slightly overweight people less likely to die than are underweight people, probably because weight loss is an effect (rather than a cause) of aging as well as of many chronic diseases.

By and large, however, obesity is unhealthy. For every 10% rise in relative weight, the systolic blood pressure rises by 6.5 mm Hg, cholesterol by

Table 30.7 The Prevalence of Overweight (and Obesity) in Different Population Groups in the United States, Early 1990s

	Male	Female
White	32.0	33.5
Black	31.5	49.6
Mexican	39.5	47.9

Data from Kuczmarski RJ, Flegal KM, Compbell SM, et al.: Increasing prevalence of overweight among US adults. The National Health and Nutrition Surveys, 1960 to 1991. JAMA 272:205–211, 1994.

Table 30.8 Typical Features of the Two Major Types of Diabetes Mellitus

Parameter	Type I	Type II
Age at onset	<20 years	>20 years
Lifetime incidence	0.2%-0.4%	5%-10%
Heritability	≈50%	≈80%
Pancreatic β cells	Destroyed	Normal
Circulating insulin	Absent	Normal, high, or low
Tissue response to insulin	Normal	Reduced (most patients)
Fasting hyperglycemia	Severe	Variable
Metabolic complications	Ketoacidosis	Nonketotic hyperosmolar coma
Treatment	Insulin injections	Diet, oral antidiabetics, or insulin

12 mg/dL and fasting blood glucose by 2 mg/dL in men. These associations are only a bit weaker in women.

Obesity is inevitable when the food intake exceeds the amount that can be oxidized in the body. The BMR can vary by as much as 30% among individuals, even after adjustment for age, sex, weight, and lean body mass versus fat. This means that even the same amount of food intake will cause obesity in some people but not others.

However, food intake is the more important variable. Appetite is normally inhibited by nervous afferents from stretch receptors in the stomach, elevations of blood glucose and other nutrients, intestinal hormones, and the hormone **leptin,** which is released from adipose tissue after a meal. There exist mouse mutants that are morbidly obese because they are deficient in either leptin or the leptin receptor. Similar defects have been observed in some morbidly obese humans.

Overeating initially increases the size of the adipocytes, but once the existing adipocytes are filled, preadipocytes differentiate into additional adipocytes. Normally, the number of adipocytes increases fivefold between the ages of 2 years and 22 years, and a common concern is that overeating, especially at a young age, leads to adipose tissue hyperplasia. Losing excess adipocytes once they have been formed is difficult or impossible.

In general, the metabolic rate of obese people drops by 15% to 20% during weight loss and remains reduced when weight is stabilized at a lower level. Thus the ex-obese have to live permanently with a metabolic rate that is otherwise typical for serious starvation. This is uncomfortable for many such people, and 80% to 85% of weight-reduced obese patients quickly regain until they reach their previous weight.

Diabetes Is Caused by Insulin Deficiency or Insulin Resistance

Diabetes mellitus is caused by a relative or absolute deficiency of insulin action. **Hyperglycemia** (abnormally elevated blood glucose) is the biochemical hallmark of diabetes mellitus, but the pathways of all major nutrients are deranged. There are two primary forms of diabetes: type 1 and type 2 (Table 30.8).

Type 1 diabetes usually starts in childhood or adolescence. It is an autoimmune disease that leads to the *destruction of pancreatic β cells*. Without endogenous insulin production, the patients depend on insulin injections for life. Being a protein, insulin is not orally active because it is destroyed by digestive enzymes. Type 1 diabetes afflicts perhaps 1 per 400 individuals, and its incidence is not strongly related to lifestyle.

Type 2 diabetes is a disease of middle-aged and older individuals. It is far more common than type 1, is less severe, and has more complex origins. The pancreatic β cells are intact, and the plasma level of insulin is normal, reduced, or elevated. The problem is either *reduced insulin secretion* or *insulin resistance* of the target tissues, or a combination of both. Worldwide, 150 million people are affected, and the prevalence rises steeply with rising affluence. Between 4% and 7% of adult Americans are thought to suffer from type 2 diabetes, and the disease costs $100 billion per year in the United States alone.

Most type 1 diabetics are thin, especially if their disease is poorly controlled, but most type 2 diabetics are obese. *Obese patients with type 2 diabetes are invariably insulin-resistant.* Even nondiabetic obese individuals have twofold higher insulin levels than do thin people, and their tissue responsiveness

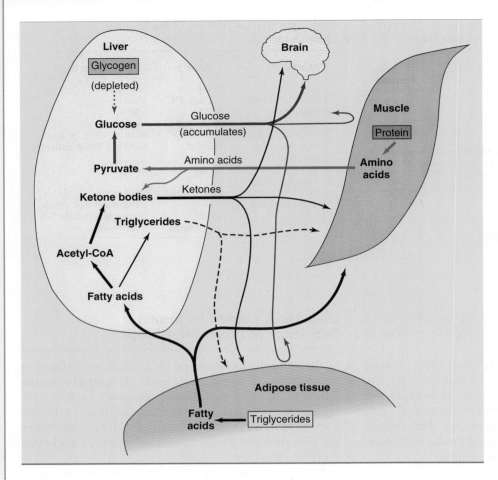

Figure 30.8 Disposition of the major nutrients in diabetes mellitus (postabsorptive state).

is proportionately reduced. Part of their insulin resistance results from a reduced number of insulin receptors, but intracellular insulin signaling is defective as well. The down-regulation of insulin receptors might conceivably be the result of overeating and excessive insulin release (see Chapter 17), but otherwise very little is known about the relationship between insulin resistance and obesity.

Nonetheless, it is known that in most obese persons with diabetes, a balanced weight-reduction diet restores tissue responsiveness and corrects the metabolic derangements. Not all such patients comply with this cruel and unreasonable treatment, and therefore insulin or oral antidiabetic drugs are often required.

In Diabetes, Metabolism Is Regulated as in Starvation

The blood insulin level declines sharply during extended fasting, and this triggers most of the metabolic adaptations to food deprivation. Therefore,

the metabolic changes of diabetes are expected to resemble those of starvation (Fig. 30.8).

The hyperglycemia of diabetes mellitus is caused by *overproduction and underutilization of glucose.* The liver makes rather than consumes glucose, and muscle and adipose tissue fail to take up glucose from the blood. There is also *excessive lipolysis in adipose tissue.* The levels of plasma free fatty acids rise, and the liver turns excess fatty acids into ketone bodies. These are the same changes as in starvation, when liver and adipose tissue have to keep the other organs alive by doling out glucose, fatty acids, and ketone bodies.

VLDL also tends to be elevated because the oversupply of fatty acids promotes triglyceride synthesis in the liver, whereas the activity of lipoprotein lipase in adipose tissue is reduced. The rise in VLDL contributes to the accelerated development of atherosclerosis and coronary heart disease in diabetes.

The complete absence of insulin in type 1 diabetes leads to **diabetic ketoacidosis,** with severe ketonemia, acidosis, and blood glucose levels as high as 1000 mg/dL. Large amounts of glucose and ketone bodies are lost in the urine, and osmotic

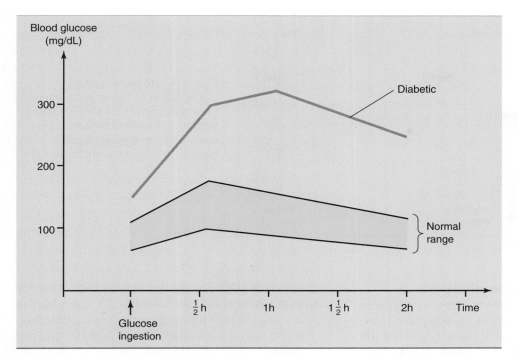

Figure 30.9 The glucose tolerance test. Blood glucose is measured at different time intervals after the oral ingestion of a flavored glucose solution (75 g of glucose). In normal individuals, but not in diabetic patients, the blood glucose returns to the fasting level within 2 hours.

diuresis causes dehydration and electrolyte imbalances. The coma is caused by dehydration, electrolyte disturbances, and acidosis. Hyperglycemia as such is not acutely damaging to the brain. *Untreated ketoacidosis is fatal.* Proper treatment includes fluid replacement, correction of the acidosis, and generous insulin injections.

Patients with type 2 diabetes are not afflicted by ketoacidosis, but elderly patients can develop **non-ketotic hyperosmolar coma.** It is caused by excessive glucosuria with osmotic diuresis. If the patient forgets to drink, the resulting dehydration can become sufficiently severe to affect the central nervous system.

The overtreatment of diabetes with insulin or oral antidiabetic drugs leads to **hypoglycemic shock.** Therefore, affected patients must be educated to time their insulin injections with their meals. In persons without diabetes, hypoglycemic episodes sometimes are caused by an **insulinoma,** a rare insulin-secreting tumor of pancreatic β cells. The diagnosis of insulinoma is established by the measurement of elevated levels of insulin or the C-peptide (see Chapter 16).

Diabetes Is Diagnosed with Laboratory Tests

Urinalysis is a quick screening test for diabetes mellitus. *Whenever the blood glucose level exceeds 9 to 10 mmol/liter (160 to 180 mg/dL), glucose appears in the urine.* Ketone bodies are also excreted in the

urine. There is no true renal threshold for ketone bodies, but ordinarily only trace amounts are excreted. Only in uncontrolled diabetes are ketone bodies excreted in substantial quantity.

Determination of the *fasting blood glucose level* is the most important laboratory test for diabetes. A blood glucose concentration of more than 7.8 mmol/liter (140 mg/dL) on two different occasions is often used as a diagnostic cutoff. Borderline cases can be evaluated with the **glucose tolerance test.** It involves repeated measurements of the blood glucose level both immediately before and at different intervals after the ingestion of a glucose solution (Fig. 30.9). Both the fasting blood glucose concentration and, to a far greater extent, the glucose tolerance test show wide variations among normal individuals. Therefore, the diagnostic cutoff between "normal" and "diabetic" is as arbitrary as that between "pass" and "fail" on a biochemistry examination.

To assess the quality of long-term metabolic control in treated diabetic patients, the blood concentration of **hemoglobin A_{1c}** can be measured. This product is formed by the nonenzymatic glycosylation of the terminal amino groups in the α and β chains as shown in Figure 30.10. *The concentration of glycosylated hemoglobin is proportional to the blood glucose level.* It is 3% to 5% in normal individuals and above 6% in diabetic patients. Because hemoglobin has a life span of 4 months, this test provides information about the average severity of hyperglycemia during the last weeks to months before the test.

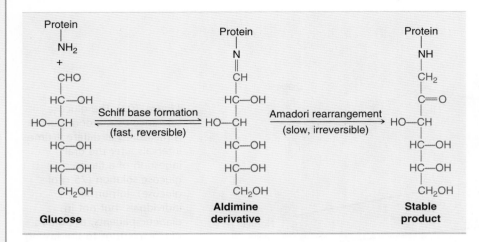

Figure 30.10 Nonenzymatic glycosylation of the terminal amino groups in proteins. A stable fructose derivative is formed in these reactions. Hemoglobin A_{1c} and glycosylated albumin are formed this way.

Diabetes Leads to Late Complications

Diabetic coma can be prevented by adequate treatment, but diabetic patients still have a reduced life expectancy. In the course of many years, they develop accelerated atherosclerosis, nephropathy, retinopathy, cataracts, and peripheral neuropathy. Two biochemical mechanisms have been proposed for these delayed complications:

1. *The nonenzymatic glycosylation of terminal amino groups* (see Fig. 30.10) interferes with the normal function or turnover of proteins. This mechanism has been suggested for the thickening of basement membranes that is observed in the renal glomeruli of diabetic patients.
2. *The increased formation of sorbitol and fructose by the polyol pathway* (see Chapter 22) is favored by hyperglycemia:

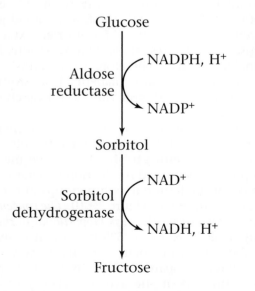

where NADP = nicotinamide adenine dinucleotide phosphate and NADPH = the reduced form of NADP. The K_m of aldose reductase for glucose is near 200 mmol/liter, 40 times higher than the normal blood glucose level. Therefore, the reaction rate depends directly on the glucose concentration. Sorbitol and fructose are not only osmotically active but can also interfere with the metabolism of inositol. Aldose reductase is abundant in Schwann cells of peripheral nerves, the papillae of the kidney and the lens epithelium, sites that are affected in diabetes.

In diabetic patients, the intracellular glucose concentration is not elevated in muscle and adipose tissue, whose glucose uptake is insulin-dependent. However, nerve sheaths, blood vessels, the kidneys, and the retinas have insulin-independent glucose uptake. These tissues are most vulnerable to diabetes.

Contracting Muscle Has Three Energy Sources

Resting muscles consume only a moderate amount of energy. During contraction, however, their energy demand can rise 50-fold above the resting level. The energy is supplied by three metabolic systems:

CREATINE PHOSPHATE

This energy-rich compound is present in skeletal muscle at a concentration of at least 20 mmol/kg (Table 30.9), while the ATP concentration is only 5 to 6 mmol/kg. During vigorous contraction all ATP would be hydrolyzed to ADP and phosphate within 2 to 4 seconds. In this situation, ATP can be regenerated quickly in the reversible **creatine kinase** reaction:

Creatine phosphate + ADP

Creatine
kinase

Creatine + ATP

$$\Delta G^{0\prime} = -3.0 \text{ kcal/mol}$$

where $\Delta G^{0\prime}$ = standard free energy change. The equilibrium of the reaction favors ATP formation. Therefore, creatine phosphate is utilized while the ATP concentration is only slightly reduced from its

Table 30.9 Concentrations of Some Phosphate Compounds in the Quadriceps Femoralis Muscle at Rest

Compound	mmol/kg, Muscle Tissue
Adenosine triphosphate	5.85
Adenosine diphosphate	0.74
Adenosine monophosphate	0.02
Creatine phosphate	24*
Creatine	5*

*Determined in situ, by nuclear magnetic resonance. In biopsy samples, the ratio of phosphocreatine to creatine is approximately 3:2.

resting level. This system requires neither oxygen nor external nutrients, but *it can supply ATP only for 6 to 20 seconds of vigorous exercise.* It is the main energy source for weight lifting and during a 100-meter sprint.

ANAEROBIC GLYCOLYSIS

Stored glycogen $(Glc)_n$, is the major substrate for glycolysis in skeletal muscle:

$$(Glc)_n + 3 \text{ ADP} + 3 \text{ P}_i$$

$$\downarrow$$

$$(Glc)_{n-1} + 2 \text{ Lactate} + 3 \text{ ATP} + 2 \text{ H}_2\text{O}$$

This system requires no oxygen, but it is limited by the *accumulation of lactic acid,* which acidifies the tissue and inhibits phosphofructokinase (Fig. 30.11). Anaerobic glycolysis is the most important energy source between about 20 seconds and 2 minutes after the onset of vigorous exercise.

OXIDATIVE METABOLISM

Oxidative metabolism produces at least 10 times more ATP than does anaerobic glycolysis from glycogen, but *it is limited by the oxygen supply.* Muscle can oxidize glycogen, glucose, fatty acids, ketone bodies, and amino acids. Resting muscle

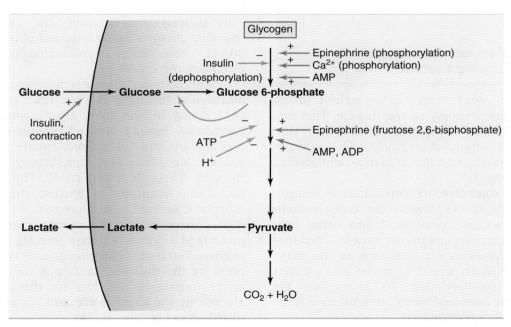

Figure 30.11 Regulation of glycogenolysis and glycolysis in skeletal muscle. The important control points are glycogen phosphorylase, phosphofructokinase, and the glucose carrier in the plasma membrane.

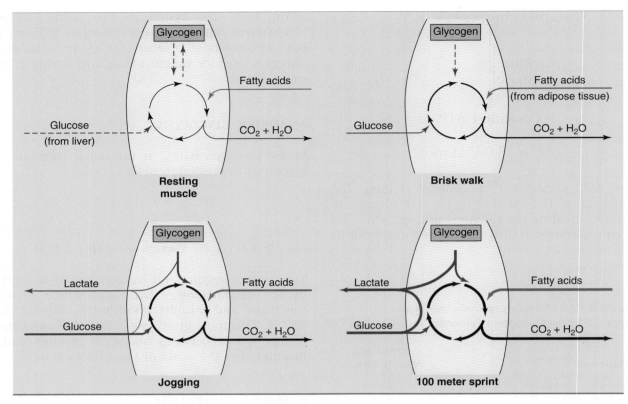

Figure 30.12 Muscle metabolism during exercise.

relies mainly on fatty acid oxidation during the postabsorptive state, although glucose is important after a carbohydrate meal. Fatty acids are still the major fuel during mild to moderate physical activity, but vigorously contracting muscle depends in large part on carbohydrate oxidation (Fig. 30.12).

The Catecholamines Coordinate Metabolism during Exercise

Vigorous tonic contraction, as in weight lifting, impairs the blood supply of the muscle. This type of exercise is called **anaerobic exercise.** It does not require the supply of external fuels; it relies on creatine phosphate and the anaerobic metabolism of stored glycogen.

In **aerobic exercise,** in contrast, as in running and swimming, blood flow to the active muscles is increased because lactic acid and other local mediators relax vascular smooth muscle. Therefore, oxidative metabolism can function as the major energy source. Both stored glycogen and external nutrients are oxidized (Fig. 30.13; see also Fig. 30.12), and *the combined use of all nutrients is necessary for maximum performance.*

The nutrient supply to exercising muscle is under neural and hormonal control. The plasma insulin concentration decreases during strenuous exercise. Glucagon is initially unchanged but tends to rise with prolonged vigorous activity. Most important, however, are norepinephrine and epinephrine. The plasma levels of these two catecholamines rise 10- to 20-fold during strenuous physical activity.

In skeletal muscle itself, the catecholamines *stimulate glycogen degradation and glycolysis* (see Fig. 30.11). These effects are mediated by β-adrenergic receptors and cAMP.

In adipose tissue, the catecholamines *stimulate fat breakdown* through β-adrenergic receptors and cAMP, and in the liver, they *stimulate glycogen degradation* mainly through α_1-adrenergic receptors and inositol-1,4,5-trisphosphate (IP_3). To a far lesser extent, they also stimulate gluconeogenesis through β receptors and cAMP. The liver releases substantial amounts of glucose during exercise, most of it derived from glycogen.

Gluconeogenesis becomes important only during prolonged vigorous exercise (see Fig. 30.13). Most of the substrate for gluconeogenesis is actually supplied by the muscles. Lactate is transported from active muscle to the liver for the resynthesis of glucose in the **Cori cycle** and for alanine in the **alanine cycle** (Fig. 30.14).

The plasma levels of glucose, fatty acids, and ketone bodies are only mildly elevated during phys-

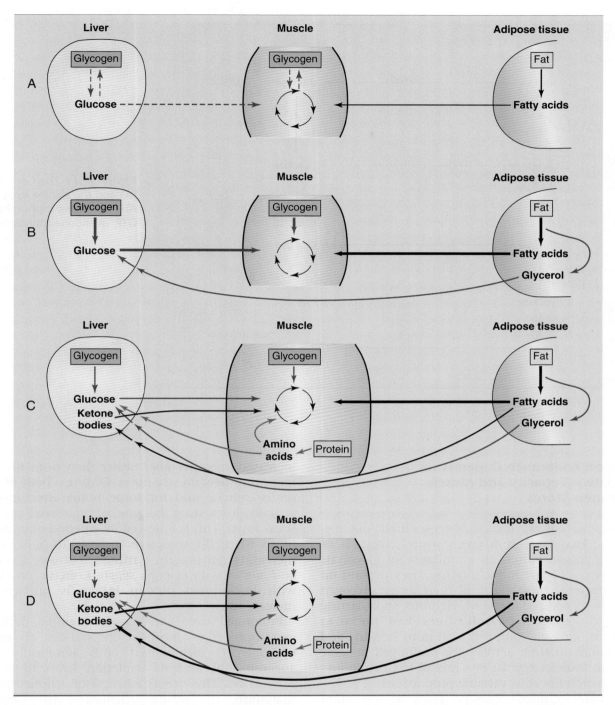

Figure 30.13 The marathoner's plight. **A,** Resting. **B,** After 10 minutes: Muscle glycogen and glucose from liver glycogen are the most important fuels. **C,** After 2 hours: Glycogen reserves in muscle and liver are seriously reduced. Fatty acids become more important. **D,** At the finish line: Both liver and muscle glycogen are depleted. Runner drops from exhaustion.

ical exercise. Although these fuels are produced in quantity by adipose tissue and liver, they are rapidly consumed by the muscles. The uptake of circulating glucose, which is insulin dependent in resting muscle, is stimulated by active contraction without the need for insulin. Ketone bodies (from the liver) and amino acids (from protein breakdown in muscle) are less important except, perhaps, in very extended vigorous exercise, when the glycogen stores are depleted.

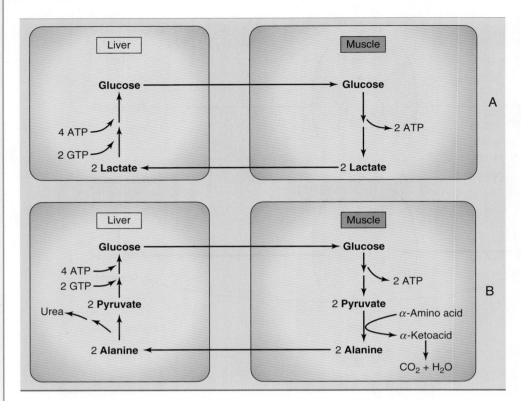

Figure 30.14 The Cori cycle (**A**) and the alanine cycle (**B**). ATP, adenosine triphosphate; GTP, guanosine triphosphate.

Physical Endurance Depends on Oxidative Capacity and Muscle Glycogen Stores

To some extent, the muscle fibers are metabolic specialists. **Fast-twitch fibers** ("white" fibers) have large glycogen stores, an abundance of glycolytic enzymes, and few mitochondria. They depend on the anaerobic metabolism of their stored glycogen and are specialized for rapid, vigorous, short-lasting contractions. **Slow-twitch fibers** ("red" fibers), in contrast, are well equipped with mitochondria and can maintain their activity for prolonged periods. Human muscles consist of a mix of fast-twitch and slow-twitch fibers in variable proportions.

Regular strenuous exercise leads to important adaptive changes. Endurance athletes have an increased capillary density in the trained muscles, and their muscle mitochondria are increased in size and number. The activities of enzymes for fatty acid and ketone body oxidation are increased, and the amounts of both the lactate transporter and GLUT-4 are increased as well. Glucose uptake by GLUT-4 is the rate-limiting step in muscle glucose metabolism.

Muscle mass can also increase in response to physical exercise. This increase results from increased mass per fiber rather than from the formation of new muscle fibers. During a bout of vigorous exercise and for some hours after, muscle actually loses mass because of increased protein breakdown. This is followed by a period of up to 48 hours when the muscle is inclined to bulk up by increasing net protein synthesis, *but only if amino acid substrates are in ample supply.* Exercise combined with low-normal protein intake is unlikely to increase muscle mass.

Prolonged severe exercise—for example, during a marathon race—depends on muscle glycogen. Glycogen is metabolized both aerobically and anaerobically, and its depletion leads to severe exhaustion. This occurs when, 2 or 3 hours into a marathon, the runner encounters the dreaded "wall" (see Fig. 30.13). *The amount of muscle glycogen depends on the carbohydrate content of the diet.* For this reason, methods of **carbohydrate loading** have been devised to build up large glycogen stores before an important athletic contest. Typically, the athlete is placed on a 70% to 80% carbohydrate diet for 3 to 8 days before the event. These regimens are quite effective in endurance athletes, but they are useless in athletic performances of less than 1 or 2 hours' duration, when glycogen depletion is not a problem.

Lipophilic Xenobiotics Are Metabolized to Water-Soluble Products

Along with useful nutrients, humans ingest a great variety of useless chemicals that have to be removed from the body. These **xenobiotics** include a wide variety of plant metabolites, not all of them harmless, and a vast number of synthetic products: drugs, intoxicants, food additives, industrial and agricultural chemicals, and pyrolysis products in cigarette smoke and in fried, roasted, and smoked foods.

Water-soluble products can be excreted in urine or bile, but lipophilic xenobiotics cannot easily be excreted. They tend to accumulate in adipose tissue and other lipid-rich structures. For example, a substantial amount of Δ^1-tetrahydrocannabinol (THC), the active constituent of marijuana, is still present in the body several days after inhalation. *Lipophilic xenobiotics must be metabolized to water-soluble products* before they can be excreted.

The most important organs of xenobiotic metabolism are the liver, intestines, and lungs. The lungs metabolize airborne pollutants, and the liver and intestines guard against food-borne products. Xenobiotics are metabolized in two phases. In **phase 1 reactions,** the substance is oxidized, usually by the attachment of one or more hydroxyl groups. In some cases, these reactions detoxify a toxic substance or terminate the effect of a drug. In other cases, however, an otherwise innocuous substance is converted into a toxin (Fig. 30.15), or an inactive prodrug is processed to a pharmacologically active metabolite.

In **phase 2 reactions,** the foreign substance or its metabolite is conjugated with a hydrophilic molecule, such as glucuronic acid, sulfate, glycine, glutamine, or glutathione (Fig. 30.16). The products of these conjugation reactions not only are water soluble and excretable but also have lost all biological activities of the parent compounds.

Xenobiotic Metabolism Requires Cytochrome P-450

The oxidative reactions in phase 1 metabolism are *monooxygenase reactions* that require **cytochrome P-450** as an electron carrier. This cytochrome is also found in the steroid-producing endocrine glands, in which it participates in hydroxylation and side chain cleavage reactions (see Chapter 16). The balance of these hydroxylation reactions is as follows:

$$Substrate\text{-}H + O_2 + NADPH + H^+$$
$$\downarrow$$
$$Substrate\text{-}OH + H_2O + NADP^+$$

Cytochrome P-450 is not a single protein but a whole superfamily of heme-containing proteins. They are membrane bound in the endoplasmic reticulum ("microsomes") or in the inner mitochondrial membrane. Approximately a dozen of them participate in normal lipid metabolism, including the synthesis of steroid hormones (see Chapter 16) and the ω-oxidation of fatty acids (see Chapter 23). These species of cytochrome P-450 have tight substrate specificities.

The xenobiotic-metabolizing varieties of cytochrome P-450 are found in the smooth endoplasmic reticulum of liver and lungs. The human genome encodes at least 14 families of these enzymes, and about 150 isoforms have been identified from their DNAs and genome sequences. Unlike the steroid-synthesizing varieties of cytochrome P-450, those of xenobiotic metabolism have broad and overlapping substrate specificities. Thus, there is a cytochrome P-450 for nearly every foreign organic molecule that might possibly be encountered.

As a rule, xenobiotic-metabolizing enzymes are inducible either by their own substrates or by other xenobiotics. The antiepileptic drug phenobarbital, for example, induces the synthesis of several cytochrome P-450 species in the smooth endoplasmic reticulum of the liver, including those responsible for its own metabolism. Therefore, tolerance to phenobarbital develops within a week, and this necessitates a threefold to fourfold dosage increase to maintain the original therapeutic effect. Phenobarbital also induces the synthesis of cytochrome P-450 species that metabolize other drugs. Thus, the metabolism of the anticoagulant dicumarol is accelerated when the patient is also treated with phenobarbital. This necessitates an increase in the dose of the anticoagulant and a decrease when the patient stops taking phenobarbital.

The reaction mechanism is shown in Figure 30.17. In essence, an oxygen molecule binds to the heme iron and becomes activated by an electron transfer. This highly reactive oxygen molecule attacks the substrate, depending on the substrate specificity of the enzyme. The activating electron is derived from NADPH and is transmitted to the iron by a flavoprotein.

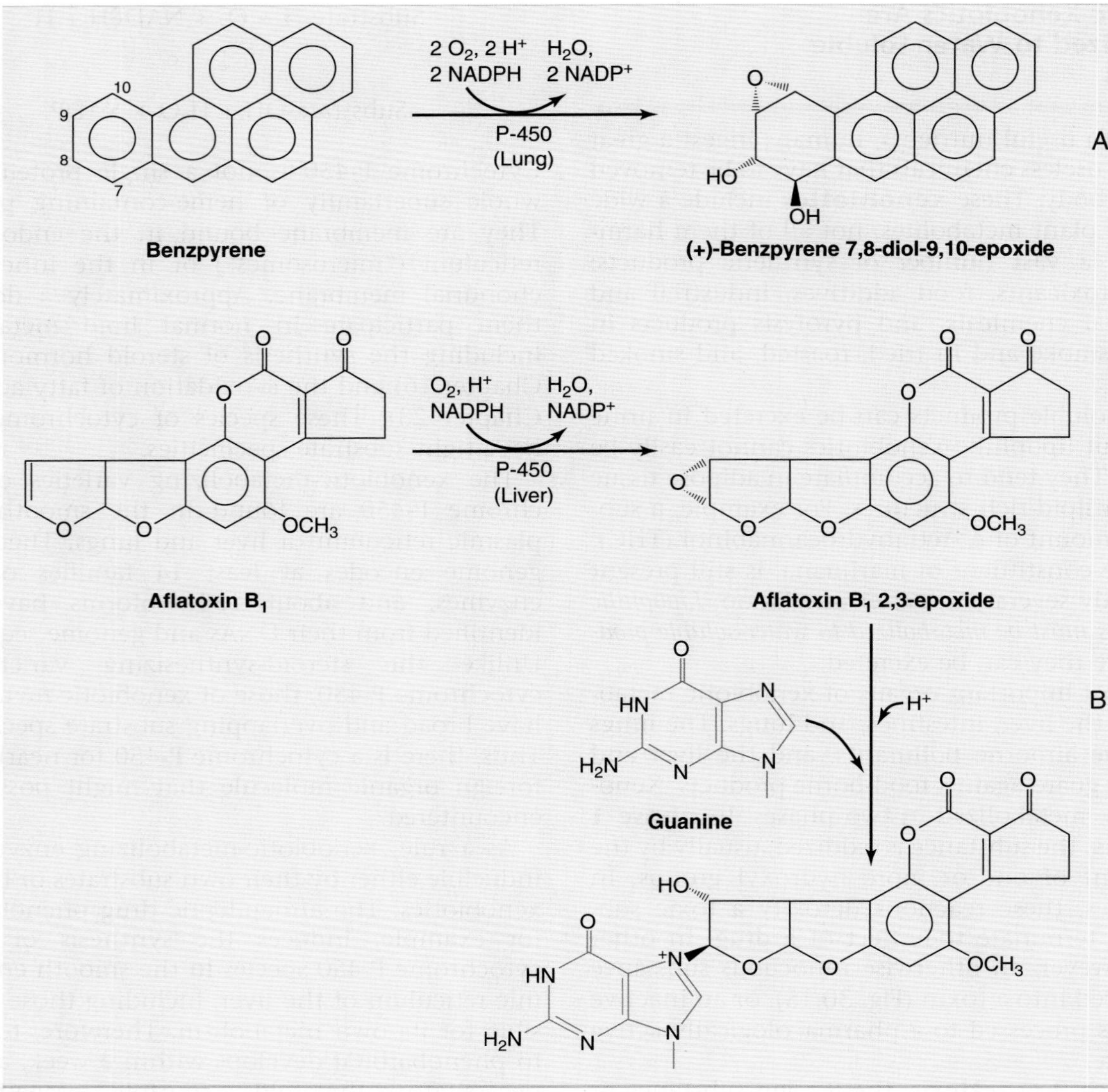

Figure 30.15 Metabolic activation of carcinogens. **A,** Metabolic activation of benzpyrene, a polycyclic hydrocarbon in cigarette smoke. Although benzpyrene itself is innocuous, the epoxide reacts spontaneously with DNA bases, causing point mutations. Individuals with a genetically determined high activity of the activating cytochrome P-450 have an increased risk of lung cancer if they smoke. **B,** Activation of aflatoxin B$_1$, a toxin of the mold *Aspergillus flavus*. The resulting epoxide reacts spontaneously with guanine residues in DNA, causing point mutations. Besides hepatitis B virus, aflatoxins are a major risk factor for liver cancer. The offending mold thrives under hot and humid conditions; thus, liver cancer is common in many tropical countries.

Ethanol Is Metabolized to Acetyl-CoA in the Liver

Ethanol is not only an intoxicant but also a nutrient with an energy value of 7.1 kcal/g. Therefore, a drinker can cover half of his or her BMR from 100 to 120 g of alcohol per day. Distilled alcoholic beverages represent "empty calories," and therefore alcoholics are prone to multiple vitamin and mineral deficiencies.

Being a water-miscible organic solvent, ethanol rapidly distributes through the aqueous compartments of the body, with tissue concentrations similar to the blood alcohol level. It is metabolized by the following reactions:

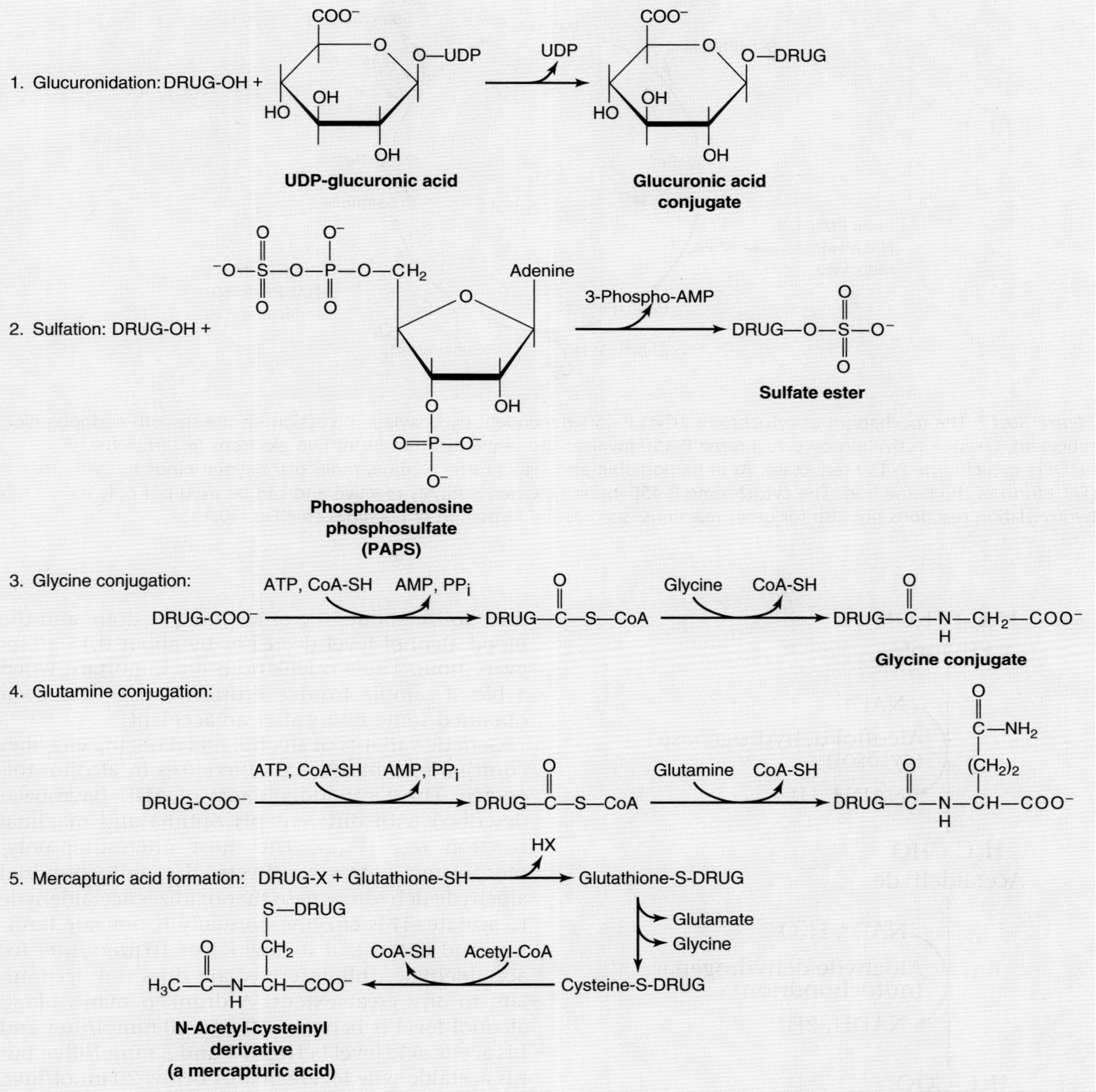

Figure 30.16 Conjugation reactions of drugs (DRUG) and other xenobiotics used in phase 2 of xenobiotic metabolism. Most of these reactions take place in the liver, and the water-soluble products are excreted either in the bile or in the urine.

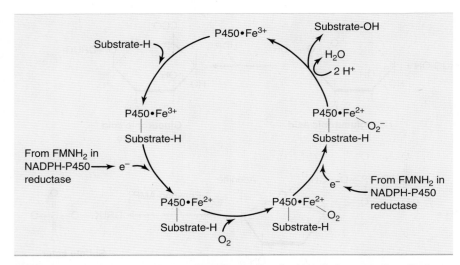

Figure 30.17 The mechanism of cytochrome (Cyt) P-450–dependent hydroxylation reactions in the smooth endoplasmic reticulum. Oxygen activation by cytochrome P-450 involves the sequential transfer of two electrons (e⁻) from the NADPH–cytochrome P-450 reductase. As in hemoglobin and cytochrome oxidase, molecular oxygen binds to the ferrous (Fe²⁺) form of the heme iron. The cytochrome P-450–bound oxygen is highly reactive and can be used not only for hydroxylation reactions but also for other reactions, such as the formation of epoxides (see Fig. 30.15).

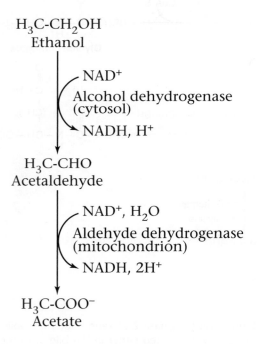

These reactions take place in the liver and, to a lesser extent, in the stomach wall, but most of the acetate is released into the blood and oxidized by other tissues. **Alcohol dehydrogenase (ADH)** catalyzes the rate-limiting step, but the *availability of NAD⁺* is another limiting factor for alcohol metabolism. The K_m of ADH for ethanol is near 1 mmol/liter (46 mg/liter). Therefore, the enzyme is essentially saturated after only one drink, and *alcohol metabolism follows zero-order kinetics*. Most people metabolize about 10 g of alcohol per hour, and the blood alcohol level decreases by about 0.15 g/liter every hour. These calculations are important when a blood sample from a drunken driver has been obtained some hours after an accident.

Genetic variants of alcohol metabolizing enzymes contribute to individual differences in alcohol tolerance. Three genetic variants of ADH have been described with different pH optima and maximal reaction rate (V_{max}). The most interesting polymorphism, however, affects the mitochondrial aldehyde dehydrogenase that oxidizes acetaldehyde to acetate. This enzyme normally is not rate limiting, and because of its low K_m of 10 µmol/liter for acetaldehyde, this intermediate does not accumulate to any great extent. A drunken man's blood alcohol level is between 20 and 50 mmol/liter and his acetic acid level between 1 and 2 mmol/liter, but his acetaldehyde level remains below 20 µmol/liter.

Many East Asian persons, however, have an atypical aldehyde dehydrogenase with a single amino acid substitution (Glu→Lys) in position 487 of the polypeptide. This genetic variant behaves as a "dominant negative" mutation. This means that even heterozygotes, who still produce the normal enzyme in addition to the defective one, have near-zero enzyme activity, possibly because the mutant enzyme forms inactive oligomers with the normal one. In these individuals, acetaldehyde is oxidized by a cytosolic aldehyde dehydrogenase whose K_m for acetaldehyde is close to 1 mmol/liter. Therefore, *toxic acetaldehyde accumulates to high levels after only one or two drinks.*

The result is the **oriental flush** response, with vasodilatation, facial flushing, and tachycardia. These effects are so unpleasant that affected individuals rarely become alcoholics. Thirty to 40 percent of Chinese, Japanese, Mongolians, Koreans, Vietnamese, and Indonesians, and also many South American Indians, have the atypical aldehyde dehydrogenase.

The mitochondrial aldehyde dehydrogenase can be inhibited pharmacologically by **disulfiram** (**Antabuse**). This drug is used for the treatment of alcoholism, but its use requires strict medical supervision. Fatal reactions have occurred when the drug was mixed into an unsuspecting alcoholic's drink.

Alcohol is also metabolized by the cytochrome P-450 system:

$$H_3C\text{-}CH_2OH + O_2 + NADPH + H^+ \text{ (Ethanol)}$$
$$\downarrow$$
$$H_3C\text{-}CHO + NADP^+ + 2\ H_2O \text{ (Acetaldehyde)}$$

This reaction accounts only for a small percentage of total alcohol metabolism in most people, but unlike ADH, cytochrome P-450 synthesis is induced by alcohol. Therefore, an increased proportion of the alcohol is metabolized by this route in alcoholic persons.

The alcohol-induced cytochrome P-450 enzymes metabolize barbiturates and many other drugs in addition to alcohol. Therefore, the sober alcoholic is not very responsive to these drugs, and this can cause problems for the induction of surgical anesthesia. However, alcohol restores responsiveness to the drug because it competes with the drug for the drug-metabolizing enzyme. Fatal reactions have occurred when barbiturates and alcohol were used at the same time.

Liver Metabolism Is Deranged by Alcohol

Unlike carbohydrate and fatty acid oxidation, alcohol metabolism is not subject to negative controls. Therefore, *alcohol oxidation takes precedence over the oxidation of other nutrients.* The reactions of alcohol metabolism evolved presumably for the detoxification of the small amount of alcohol that is normally formed by bacterial fermentation in the colon. Thus, the lack of feedback inhibition was no handicap before the invention of fermented beverages.

Alcohol metabolism produces large quantities of acetyl-CoA, NADH, and ATP. As shown in Figure 30.18, these products inhibit glucose metabolism at the level of phosphofructokinase and pyruvate dehydrogenase. Fatty acid oxidation is impaired by the depletion of NAD^+. The TCA cycle is inhibited by high levels of ATP and NADH and by the depletion of NAD^+. The TCA cycle is dispensable for the drunken liver because the respiratory chain oxidation of the NADH generated in the oxidation of ethanol to acetic acid is more than sufficient to provide for the energy needs of the cell.

Rather than being oxidized, the fatty acids are esterified into triglycerides for export as VLDL. Therefore, VLDL tends to be elevated in alcoholics.

Despite high levels of ATP and NADH, gluconeogenesis from pyruvate and oxaloacetate is inhibited by alcohol because the high [NADH]/[NAD$^+$] ratio drives the reversible lactate dehydrogenase and malate dehydrogenase reactions in the "wrong" direction:

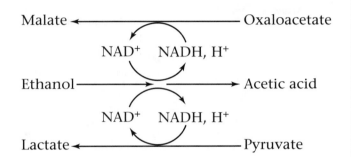

As a result, the gluconeogenic substrates pyruvate and oxaloacetate are depleted, whereas the blood level of lactate is increased. *Alcohol can precipitate hypoglycemia when liver glycogen is depleted.* A marathoner must never consume an alcoholic drink after a race. Alcohol itself is not a substrate for gluconeogenesis. It is ketogenic but not glucogenic.

Alcoholism Leads to Fatty Liver and Liver Cirrhosis

The liver synthesizes triglycerides at all times, not for storage but for export in VLDL. A **fatty liver** develops as a result of *increased triglyceride synthesis* or *reduced VLDL formation* or both (Table 30.10). Fatty liver causes no functional impairment, and it is reversible. Alcohol is the most common cause of fatty liver. It does not prevent VLDL formation but increases fat synthesis. Fatty liver is most likely in alcoholics who also suffer from protein deficiency, because protein deficiency impairs VLDL formation.

In **liver cirrhosis,** hepatocytes degenerate and are replaced by fibrous connective tissue. Cirrhosis is the final outcome of many liver diseases, but in

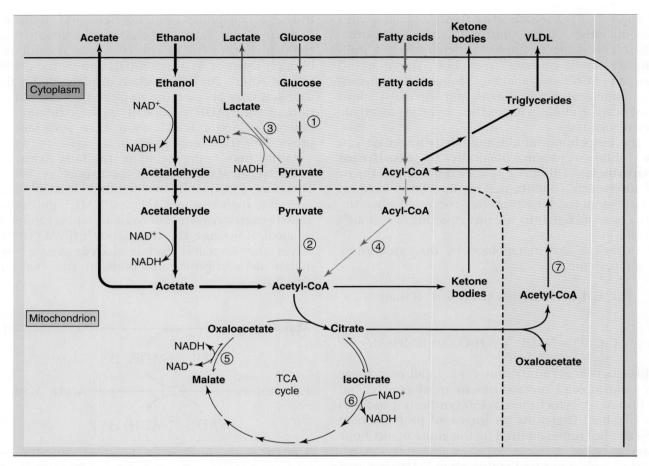

Figure 30.18 Effects of alcohol on liver metabolism. Important control points: ① phosphofructokinase: inhibited by high energy charge; ② pyruvate dehydrogenase: inhibited by high energy charge, high NADH/NAD$^+$ ratio, and high acetyl-CoA; ③ lactate dehydrogenase: high NADH/NAD$^+$ ratio favors lactate formation; ④ β-oxidation: slowed down because of low NAD$^+$; ⑤ malate dehydrogenase: high NADH/NAD$^+$ ratio favors malate formation, oxaloacetate is depleted; ⑥ isocitrate dehydrogenase: inhibited by high energy charge and high NADH/NAD$^+$ ratio; ⑦ acetyl-CoA carboxylase: may be stimulated by high citrate (accumulates because isocitrate dehydrogenase is inhibited). VLDL, very-low-density lipoprotein.

Table 30.10 Conditions Leading to Fat Accumulation in the Liver

Condition	Examples	Mechanism
Increased triglyceride synthesis	Starvation Diabetes mellitus	Increased supply of fatty acids from adipose tissue
	Alcoholism	Decreased fatty acid oxidation; possibly increased intrahepatic fatty acid synthesis
Decreased formation of VLDL	Protein deficiency	Decreased synthesis of VLDL apolipoprotein
	Essential fatty acid deficiency	Decreased phospholipid synthesis
	Toxic liver damage	VLDL formation is impaired to a greater extent than is triglyceride synthesis

VLDL, very-low-density lipoprotein.

Table 30.11 Biochemical Abnormalities in Advanced Liver Cirrhosis

Abnormality	Impaired Function
Fasting hypoglycemia	Glycogenolysis, gluconeogenesis
Prolonged clotting time	Synthesis of clotting factors
Edema	Albumin synthesis*
Hyperammonemia	Urea cycle
"Fetid" breath	Metabolism of sulfhydryl compounds formed by intestinal bacteria
Alcohol intolerance	Alcohol metabolism
Jaundice	Bilirubin metabolism

*Impaired lymph flow is another cause of abdominal edema (ascites).

Table 30.12 The Top 10 Causes of Death in the United States, 1900 and 1998

Rank	Cause of Death	% of All Deaths
	1900	
1	Pneumonia	12
2	Tuberculosis	11
3	Diarrhea and enteritis	8
4	Heart disease	8
5	Chronic nephritis	5
6	Accidents	4
7	Stroke	4
8	Diseases of infancy	4
9	Cancer	4
10	Diphtheria	2
	1998	
1	Heart disease	31
2	Cancer	23
3	Stroke	7
4	Lung diseases	5
5	Pneumonia and influenza	4
6	Accidents	4
7	Diabetes	3
8	Suicide	1
9	Kidney diseases	1
10	Liver diseases	1

industrialized countries, 60% to 70% of cases are associated with alcoholism. Table 30.11 summarizes some of the abnormalities in patients with liver cirrhosis.

Most "Diseases of Civilization" Are Caused by Aberrant Nutrition

The disease patterns in industrialized countries changed dramatically during the 20th century. As shown in Table 30.12, infectious diseases have given way to cardiovascular disease and cancer as the leading causes of death. Even more "ancient" patterns of mortality and morbidity have been described in simple agricultural and preagricultural societies, but *infectious diseases have always been the leading cause of death.*

Thanks to better hygiene and antibiotics, most people now escape the ravages of infectious diseases. In preindustrial societies, infant and childhood mortality hovered near 40%, and the overall life expectancy was in the 25- to 40-year range. Because more people survive to an advanced age today, age-related diseases, including cancer and cardiovascular disease, have become more prevalent.

However, why do nearly half of all people die of cardiovascular disease rather than, say, kidney or brain disease? Why do 5% of all adults in industrialized societies suffer from diabetes mellitus rather than some other endocrine disorder? Why are so many people overweight rather than underweight? And why do 20% of adults suffer from hypertension, whereas hypotension is rare?

"Diseases of civilization" are prevalent today because human beings, like all other creatures, are adapted to their environment by mutation and selection. In essence, only the genetic variants that enabled early humans to reproduce in the environments in which they lived are still with us today.

Ancestral environments were very different from the conditions under which people are living today. Levels of physical activity were high, and food was sometimes scarce. Therefore, humans had to evolve a ravenous appetite and a preference for foods with high caloric density, especially those rich in fat or sugar. They also had to store as much energy as possible in their adipose tissue, to maximize the chance of survival during bad seasons.

The ancient food preferences are still wired into human brains today, and people still store excess energy in adipose tissue. This programming, evolved under conditions of frequent food shortages, is the reason for near-universal obesity in affluent societies.

Until less than 10,000 years ago, all humans lived by hunting and gathering rather than farming. Human metabolic and physiologic systems evolved under these Paleolithic conditions. Table 30.13 compares the typical nutrient intakes under these conditions with the typical modern American diet and the recommended daily allowances set by experts.

Contrary to common prejudice, ancestors of today's humans were not vegetarians; rather, they covered about one third of their energy needs from meat. Meat supplied most of their dietary protein. Whereas modern Americans typically consume 100 g of protein per day, human ancestors consumed closer to 250 g per day. As a result, typical early humans were at least as tall as the tallest

Table 30.13 Nutrient Intake during the Paleolithic Period in Comparison with Current Nutrient Intake in the United States and Recommended Intakes

	Paleolithic Intake	Current U.S. Intake	Recommended Intake
Macronutrients			
% Protein	37	14	12
% Carbohydrate	41	50	
Sugars	3	21	
% Fat	22	36	
Saturated	6	14	<10
Trans-unsaturated	0	3	
Monounsaturated	7.5	13.5	
Polyunsaturated	8.5	5.5	
Cholesterol (mg)	480	450	<300
Vitamins (mg/day)			
Riboflavin	6.5	1.7	1.7
Folic acid	0.4	0.18	0.2
Thiamine	3.9	1.4	1.5
Ascorbic acid	604	100	60
Vitamin A	3.8	1.8	1
Vitamin E	32.8	9	10
Minerals (mg/day)			
Iron	87.4	11	10
Zinc	43.4	13	15
Sodium	768	4000	500-2400
Potassium	10,500	2500	3500
Fiber (g/day)	104	10-20	20-30

populations in modern industrialized countries, muscular, and lean.

Dietary carbohydrate was as abundant in Paleolithic times as in the modern diet. However, modern carbohydrate consists of easily digestible starch and refined sugar. Today, sugars alone contribute 21% of the daily energy intake. Most of the carbohydrate in the Paleolithic diet was in the form of complex carbohydrates with a low **glycemic index.** The glycemic index is a measure for the extent to which the carbohydrate raises the blood glucose after a meal. Even people who are genetically predisposed to type 2 diabetes would rarely ever develop diabetes on a Paleolithic diet.

People who are genetically predisposed to type 2 diabetes are also known to have reduced postprandial thermogenesis. They have a *thrifty genotype* that reduces energy wastage after an ample meal. This genetic predisposition used to be advantageous because it made the conversion of excess food into storage fat more efficient. It became maladaptive only in a world in which people gorge themselves on sugary junk food.

Fat was less abundant in the Paleolithic diet than in modern diets. Wild game animals are always lean. Unlike farm animals, they cannot afford excess fat stores that would compromise running speed. Thus, most of the fat in human ancestral diets was derived from oily seeds and nuts. Saturated fat, which is considered the main dietary risk factor for coronary heart disease, made up only 6% of the energy content in the typical Paleolithic diet, as opposed to 13% or 14% in the modern American diet.

Interestingly, the plasma total cholesterol levels that have been measured in hunter-gatherers average only 125 mg/dL, although the cholesterol content of their diet was quite high. The modern American average is 205 mg/dL. This difference is attributed to the different types of fat consumed and to the deficiency of fiber in modern diets. Modern Americans consume on average less than 20 g of dietary fiber per day, but the "natural" diet of Paleolithic humans contained more than 100 g of fiber per day.

The term **metabolic syndrome** is applied to a constellation of obesity, poor glucose tolerance, and an atherogenic lipid profile. The reason why these abnormalities are often found combined in the same person is that they all have the same underlying cause: overeating foods with high caloric density.

Another reason for the high incidence of cardiovascular disease in modern societies is the aberrant pattern of mineral consumption. As shown in Table 30.13, humans are adapted to a diet that contains almost 14 times more potassium than sodium. Today, the potassium intake has dropped to one third and the sodium intake has risen almost sixfold. Of the sodium consumed today, 75% is bought in processed foods.

A high sodium intake is the principal risk factor for hypertension because it tends to expand the blood volume, at least in people whose kidneys are slow to excrete the excess. In one major study, the average blood pressure of human groups that do not use added salt was 102/62 mm Hg. The average for those groups that did use salt was 119/74. There is a linear relationship between blood pressure and the complications of hypertension even in the "normal" range. The "low" blood pressure typical for no-salt human groups is indeed healthier than the blood pressure that is considered "normal" in modern societies.

Unlike the Paleolithic diet, the diets of traditional farmers often are deficient in protein, vitamins, and minerals. When human groups made the transition from hunting and gathering to agriculture, they typically became shorter, and their skeletal remains show signs of nutritional deficiencies. These nutritional deficiencies are still seen in traditional farmers from the less industrialized parts of the world.

Can humans adapt genetically to the conditions of civilized life? One common observation is that in affluent societies, type 2 diabetes is most common among groups whose ancestors either were nonagricultural or were exposed to frequent famine. For example, type 2 diabetes is twice as common in acculturated Australian aborigines than in white Australians, and in the United States, Pima Indians are at least three times more likely to develop diabetes than are white people. Apparently, populations with a long history of carbohydrate-rich diets in traditional agricultural economies did become genetically less susceptible to type 2 diabetes. Similarly, hypertension seems to be most common in populations whose ancestors had no access to salt.

Aging Is the Greatest Challenge for Medical Research

Aging is not a disease of civilization but an inevitable part of the human condition. Although the *average* life span has increased through advances in medicine, the *maximal* life span has remained the same. But exactly what processes contribute to normal aging? Several mechanisms have been postulated:

1. **Accumulation of somatic mutations.** Somatic mutations are believed to contribute to age-related functional decline, especially in tissues that cannot replace defective cells. However, the extent to which somatic mutations are responsible for the cell loss that occurs in these tissues with advancing age is not known.

2. **Damage by reactive oxygen species.** Reactive oxygen species are incompletely reduced forms of oxygen; they include the superoxide radical, hydrogen peroxide, and hydroxyl radicals. They can cause somatic mutations, lipid peroxidation, and other cellular damage.

3. **Mitochondrial dysfunction.** The mutation rate is higher in mitochondrial DNA than nuclear DNA. This results from the abundance of reactive oxygen species in this organelle and probably also from less efficient DNA repair. Declines in oxidative capacity are commonly observed in aging tissues. Terminally differentiated cells, in particular, tend to accumulate abnormal oversized mitochondria that are inefficient at ATP synthesis but still produce reactive oxygen species.

4. **Telomere shortening.** In most tissues, telomerase is no longer expressed after birth. As a result, telomeres tend to shorten in tissues whose cells keep dividing throughout life. Shortened telomeres can trigger apoptosis.

5. **Accumulation of garbage.** Aged lysosomes of nondividing cells accumulate an undegradable yellow product called **lipofuscin** that is derived from oxidized lipids and crosslinked denatured proteins. Extracellular garbage accumulates in the form of insoluble proteins that are collectively called **amyloid.** Amyloid can be formed from many normal proteins. In the brain, for example, insoluble β-**amyloid** accumulates in patients with Alzheimer disease and, to a lesser extent, in normal aging. β-Amyloid is a fragment of a normal membrane protein.

6. **Collateral damage.** Because infections used to be the leading cause of death until the 20th century, humans evolved a vigilant immune system that responds to the slightest provocation. In allergies, immune responses are mounted against harmless environmental materials; in autoimmune diseases, they are mounted against components of the body. Most age-related diseases have an inflammatory component, and collateral damage can be done by abortive immune responses to such abnormal stimuli as the deposition of cholesterol esters in arterial walls and the deposition of β-amyloid in the brain.

7. **Hormonal mechanisms.** Animal experiments have shown that the signaling system that is represented by insulin and insulin-like growth factor–1 (IGF-1) in humans shortens life, in addition to stimulating growth and metabolism. Mice with reduced numbers of IGF-1 receptors and mice lacking insulin receptors in adipose tissue have a prolonged life span. Whether transgenic humans with similar changes also live longer remains to be seen—in one century, at the earliest.

But why have humans not evolved more effective ways of counteracting these threats to their continued existence? Aging and age-related diseases are explained by the theory of **antagonistic pleiotropy.** In essence, mortality from infections, accidents, and homicide was so high in ancestral populations that few people ever got very old. There would be little selective advantage for a genetic variant that offered better health or continued reproductive capacity at an old age, because most of the potential beneficiaries never reached that age. Worse, any genetic variant that offers a great advantage to the old but at the cost of a slight disadvantage for the young will be selected out of the gene pool. Thus, we must expect that own defenses against aging and age-related diseases are less than optimal. Only genetic engineering can change this sorry state of affairs.

Short of genetic engineering, the only intervention that slows the aging process is caloric restriction. Rats that are kept at 70% of free-feeding weight live 20% longer than those with an unlimited food supply. This life-prolonging effect is accompanied by a reduced metabolic rate and therefore most likely a reduced formation of reactive oxygen derivatives. However, the effect of caloric restriction is not duplicated with antioxidants. Caloric restriction also reduces the level of IGF-1, and this may well be the mechanism of its life-prolonging effect.

We do not know whether humans respond to caloric restriction the way rats do, but slimming down to 70% of free-feeding weight is worth a try. To quit smoking and drinking would not be a bad idea either.

SUMMARY

The major metabolic pathways have to adapt to the nutrient supply. After a meal, insulin stimulates glucose utilization by enhancing glucose uptake in muscle and adipose tissue and by stimulating glucose-metabolizing enzymes in most tissues. It also directs dietary triglycerides to adipose tissue for storage and promotes the conversion of excess carbohydrate into fat.

Fatty acids from adipose tissue are the main energy source during fasting. The fatty acids are oxidized either directly or after their initial conversion to ketone bodies by the liver. A few tissues, including brain and erythrocytes, require glucose even during fasting. The liver supplies these tissues with glucose, initially by glycogen degradation and later by gluconeogenesis from amino acids, lactate, and glycerol. These processes are stimulated by glucagon, the main insulin antagonist in the liver.

During stress and physical exertion, epinephrine and norepinephrine mobilize stored fat and glycogen for use by the muscles. These effects are potentiated by the other important type of stress hormone, the glucocorticoids.

"Diseases of civilization" are caused by the prevalent dietary habits in modern societies. Obesity is caused by overeating; type 2 diabetes, by an overabundance of easily digested carbohydrates; and hypertension, by excessive salt consumption. Alcohol is detoxified in the liver, but this process can lead to liver damage. Other drugs, food additives, and environmental toxins are also handled by detoxifying systems in liver and other organs, but damage by these agents cannot always be prevented.

Further Reading

Brunk UT, Terman A: The mitochondrial-lysosomal theory of aging. Accumulation of damaged mitochondria as a result of imperfect autophagocytosis. Eur J Biochem 269:1996-2002, 2002.

Eaton SB, Eaton SB III, Konner MJ: Paleolithic nutrition revisited: a twelve-year retrospective on its nature and implications. Eur J Clin Nutr 51:207-216, 1997.

Evans RM, Barish GD, Wang Y-X: PPARs and the complex journey to obesity. Nat Med 10:355-360, 2004.

Flier JS: Obesity wars: molecular progress confronts an expanding epidemic. Cell 116:337-350, 2004.

Kenyon C: A conserved regulatory system for aging. Cell 105:165-168, 2001.

Lieber CS: Alcohol: its metabolism and interaction with nutrients. Annu Rev Nutr 20:395-430, 2000.

Ornish D: Was Dr. Atkins right? J Am Diet Assoc 104:537-542, 2004.

Raha S, Robinson BH: Mitochondria, oxygen free radicals, disease and aging. Trends Biochem Sci 25:502-508, 2000.

Saltiel AR: New perspectives into the molecular pathogenesis and treatment of type 2 diabetes. Cell 104:517-529, 2001.

QUESTIONS

1. **How can you best describe the function of cytochrome P-450 in xenobiotic metabolism?**

   A. It transfers an electron to adrenodoxin.
   B. It binds a water molecule, thereby activating it for a nucleophilic attack on the substrate.
   C. It accepts two electrons and a proton from NADPH for transfer to the substrate.
   D. It activates an oxygen molecule.
   E. It acts as an ATPase.

2. **The brain produces most of its energy by the oxidation of glucose; during long-term fasting, however, it can cover more than half of its energy needs from**

   A. Anaerobic glycolysis.
   B. Oxidation of its stored glycogen.
   C. Oxidation of free fatty acids.
   D. Oxidation of amino acids.
   E. Oxidation of ketone bodies.

3. **When an insulin-dependent diabetic patient undergoes surgery (any surgery), you should monitor his or her blood glucose level extra carefully *because***

   A. Stress hormones antagonize insulin, and the patient may therefore require extra insulin.
   B. Stress reduces insulin release from the pancreas, a condition known as insulin shock.
   C. Insulin can inhibit the blood clotting system.
   D. Any physical or psychological stress is likely to cause hypoglycemia.

4. **During long-term fasting, the liver produces acetyl-CoA by the β-oxidation of fatty acids. What is the major metabolic fate of this acetyl-CoA?**

   A. Fatty acid biosynthesis.
   B. Gluconeogenesis.
   C. Amino acid biosynthesis.
   D. Ketogenesis.
   E. Oxidation in the TCA cycle.

5. **The catecholamines epinephrine and norepinephrine adjust metabolic activity throughout the body to satisfy the energy demands of the working muscles. All of the following catecholamine effects are important during physical activity *except***

   A. Stimulation of glycogenolysis in the liver.
   B. Stimulation of glycogenolysis in skeletal muscle.
   C. Inhibition of glycolysis in skeletal muscle.
   D. Inhibition of glycolysis in the liver.
   E. Stimulation of lipolysis in adipose tissue.

6. **When you get up in the morning, 12 hours after dinner, what is the main source of your blood glucose?**

   A. Dietary glucose.
   B. Liver glycogen.
   C. Muscle glycogen.
   D. Gluconeogenesis from lactate.
   E. Gluconeogenesis from amino acids.

Case Studies

The Mafia Boss

Once upon a time there was a Mafia boss in Chicago who had killed a great many people. He used to dispose of his victims' bodies by throwing them into a lake or river. There was one problem, however: even if he tied heavy stones to a victim, the body would be found floating 2 or 3 days later. He finally consulted a physician about this problem.

Questions

1. What is the typical density of the human body? Which tissues are lighter and which are heavier than water? Describe how the content of protein, lipid, and inorganic materials is related to the density of the tissue.
2. Are there gas-filled spaces in the body? What happens to these spaces after death?
3. What advice can you give the Mafia boss?

Viral Gastroenteritis*

Benita was a 6-week-old black girl in a rural district of Alabama who had been born after a normal pregnancy and weighed 3.2 kg at birth. Her parents and two older brothers were reported to be in good health. She had been breast-fed for 4 weeks, and her weight gain had been normal. The composition of human milk is as follows:

Total solids:	13%
Fat:	4%
Lactose:	6.8%
Total protein:	1.5%
Lactalbumin:	0.7%
Casein:	0.5%

*Copyright 1996 Mosby–Year Book.

Minerals:	0.2%
kcal/100 mL:	66

Her stools during this period were described as "loose" but were not considered by her mother to be abnormal. When Benita was 4 weeks of age, breast-feeding had been discontinued and a commercial baby formula was substituted. Within 10 days, the child developed watery diarrhea and vomiting, which was diagnosed as viral gastroenteritis. At the age of 6 weeks she was admitted to a local hospital.

Physical examination at the time of admission revealed only a moderate degree of dehydration (dry mucous membranes, slight depression of the anterior fontanel, and sunken appearance of the eyes). Skin turgor seemed normal, and body weight was 3.4 kg. Urinalysis yielded a 1+ reaction for reducing substance and no reaction for glucose. The infant was hydrated with intravenous (IV) fluids over a period of 24 hours, and then with fluids orally for another 24 hours. During this time, the diarrhea subsided and her weight increased to 3.7 kg. She then was fed the commercial formula (67 kcal/100mL). Within 24 hours her stools became watery and were passed at the time of each feeding.

On the fourth day of hospitalization, a therapeutic formula was substituted for the commercial formula. The number of stools decreased to two or three daily. They contained no reducing substance and became semiformed in character. The infant gained 40 g/day during the next 4 days. However, because of the cost and inconvenience of the therapeutic formula, a single feeding of the commercial formula was given once again as a trial. The infant did not pass a stool, but a second feeding 4 hours later was followed by several explosive, watery stools. The stool pH was 5.0, and it gave a positive reaction for reducing substance.

Table C-1 Formula Compositions. +, present; −, absent

Components	Commercial Formula	Therapeutic Formula
Cow milk protein	+	
Casein hydrolysate		+
Corn oil	+	+
Coconut oil	+	−
Lactose	+	−
Sucrose	−	+
Arrowroot starch	−	+
Protein	1.7%	2.2%
Carbohydrate	6.6%	8.5%
Minerals	0.4%	0.6%

The child was switched back to the therapeutic formula, and the diarrhea subsided within 24 hours. After another 2 days in the hospital, the child was discharged and the mother was given a 1-week supply of the therapeutic formula. There was no recurrence of diarrhea when this formula was gradually replaced by the commercial formula. The compositions of the two formulas are given in Table C-1.

Questions

1. Which tissues are affected in viral gastroenteritis? What functional derangements can you possibly expect?
2. Why did the child show signs of dehydration when admitted to the hospital?
3. Urinalysis showed the presence of small amounts of a reducing substance. What kind of reducing substance was this? Is the presence of reducing substances in the urine normal? Do you know any other diseases in which reducing substances appear in the urine?
4. Which methods are best employed to determine the presence and concentration of glucose in urine, blood, or stool, without interference by other substances?
5. Why was a reducing substance present in the stool after the baby was fed the commercial formula but not after the therapeutic formula?
6. Why was the pH of the stool in the acidic range? Which acids could possibly be present?
7. The bacterial fermentation of undigested carbohydrates in the intestine is accompanied by the formation of gas. Which gases are formed?
8. Do you know of an inherited enzyme deficiency that would cause diarrhea in response to the commercial formula? Is this likely in the present case?
9. Some children and adults have gastrointestinal problems because they are hypersensitive to a dietary component. Which component of the commercial formula could possibly act as an effective antigen that can stimulate B or T lymphocytes?

📖 Suggested Reading

Greenberg HB, Matsui SM, Holodniy M: Small intestine: infections with common bacterial and viral pathogens. In Yamada T, Alpers DH, Laine L, et al (eds): Textbook of Gastroenterology, 4th ed, vol 2. Philadelphia: Lippincott Williams & Wilkins, 2003, pp 2026-2061.

🗂 Death in Installments

A 19-year-old man was admitted to the hospital because of a progressive central nervous system disorder. He had developed disturbances of motor coordination since age 14, had dropped out of college at age 17, and had been evaluated at various hospitals between ages 17 and 19, without clear diagnosis. Repeated lumbar puncture specimens, electroencephalograms (EEGs), pneumoencephalograms, liver function test results, and ceruloplasmin level had been normal.

On admission he showed some insight into his illness but was indifferent about his deficits. He was disoriented in relation to time but could provide information about the previous 10 years. Spasticity and ataxia were present. Verbal IQ was 83, and performance IQ was 67. Pneumoencephalography disclosed ventricular dilatation. A specific diagnosis could not be established at this time.

Over the next years, the patient's condition worsened, and he required total care because of inability to walk and incontinence. At age 34, a computed tomography scan (CT) showed ventricular dilatation, and there was marked peripheral neuropathy, mainly of demyelinative nature. Blood cells, electrolytes, and CO_2 levels were normal; a serological test for syphilis was negative. Lumbar puncture yielded clear, colorless, acellular cerebrospinal fluid (CSF) under normal pressure. The vitamin B_{12} level was normal. Diagnostic procedures included the determination of enzyme activities in cultured leukocytes. Some results were as follows:

Arylsulfatase A (millimoles per milligram of protein per hour):

Patient: 31
Normal: 77 ± 18

Sulfatidase (millimoles per milligram of protein per 2 hours):

Patient: 0.2
Normal: 12.9 ± 3.2

Urine sulfatide excretion (millimoles per milligram of creatinine):

Patient: 0.39
Normal: 0.07 to 0.14

Questions

1. Several diagnostic tests had been performed on the patient before a definitive diagnosis could be established. Give a rationale for each of these tests.
2. What is sulfatide, and where does it occur?
3. Arylsulfatase A and sulfatidase are the same enzyme, assayed either with a synthetic substrate (arylsulfatase A) or with the natural substrate (sulfatidase). What do the discrepancies between the two enzyme activities (each in comparison with normal levels) suggest?
4. Ultrastructural studies were not performed on the patient's leukocytes. If such studies had been performed, what would be the likely observation?
5. Traditionally, leukocytes are cultured in a serum-containing medium. This is done because serum but not plasma stimulates mitosis of leukocytes. Do you know of any mitogen that is present in serum but not in fresh plasma?
6. The patient's enzyme activities were determined only in cultured leukocytes. Do you expect the enzyme deficiency to be present in other cells (cultured skin fibroblasts, for example) as well?
7. Many genetic diseases, including the patient's disease, show subtypes that vary in their severity and age of onset (infantile, juvenile, adult forms). Why?
8. What would abnormally high protein levels or low glucose levels in CSF suggest? Are the patient's values in the normal range?

Suggested Reading

Percy AK: Gangliosidoses and related lipid storage disorders. In Emery AEH, Rimoin DL (eds): Emery and Rimoin's Principles and Practice of Medical Genetics, 4th ed, vol 3. Edinburgh: Churchill Livingstone, 2002, pp 2712-2751.

Sandhoff K, Kolter T: Biosynthesis and degradation of mammalian glycosphingolipids. Phil Trans R Soc Lond B 358:847-861, 2003.

von Figura K, Gieselmann V, Jaeken J: Metachromatic leukodystrophy. In Scriver CR, Beaudet AL, Sly WS, et al (eds): The Metabolic and Molecular Basis of Inherited Disease, 8th ed, vol 3. New York: McGraw-Hill, 2001, pp 3695-3724.

A Mysterious Death*

In the summer of 1989, Patricia Stallings brought her 3-month-old son, Ryan, to the emergency room of Cardinal Glennon Children's Hospital in St. Louis. The child had labored breathing, uncontrolled vomiting, and gastric distress. According to the attending physician, a toxicologist, the child's symptoms indicated that he had been poisoned with the antifreeze ethylene glycol. This suspicion was confirmed by a commercial laboratory. After the child recovered, he was placed in a foster home, and the parents were allowed to see him in supervised visits. However, when the infant became ill and subsequently died after a visit in which Stallings had been left alone briefly with him, she was charged with first-degree murder and held without bail. Both the commercial laboratory and the hospital laboratory personnel found large amounts of ethylene glycol in the boy's blood and traces of it in a bottle of milk that Stallings had fed her son during the visit.

While in custody, Patricia Stallings learned that she was pregnant. In February 1990 she gave birth to another son, David Stallings, Jr. This son was placed immediately in a foster home, but within weeks he started having symptoms similar to Ryan's. Eventually, David was diagnosed with methylmalonic acidemia. Despite this new evidence, Patricia Stallings was convicted of assault with a deadly weapon and sentenced to life in prison.

After hearing about the case from a television broadcast, William Sly, chairman of the Department of Biochemistry and Molecular Biology, and James Shoemaker, head of a metabolic screening laboratory, both at St. Louis University, became interested. Together with Piero Rinaldo, a metabolic-disease expert at Yale University School of Medicine, they analyzed Ryan's blood. Rather than ethylene glycol, they found large amounts of methylmalonic acid. They also found massive amounts of ketone bodies in the boy's blood and urine, another typical finding in methylmalonic acidemia. The bottle could not be tested because it had mysteriously disappeared.

When the previous findings supporting ethylene glycol poisoning were checked, it turned out that workers at one laboratory had claimed the presence of ethylene glycol even though Ryan's blood did not match their own profile for a sample containing ethylene glycol. At the other laboratory, an abnormal substance had been detected in Ryan's blood, and the workers had assumed that it was

---

*Copyright 1991 American Association for the Advancement of Science.

ethylene glycol. Samples from the bottle had produced nothing unusual, but the laboratory had claimed evidence of ethylene glycol in that, too.

After these findings, all charges against Patricia Stallings were dismissed on September 20, 1991.

Questions

1. What causes methylmalonic acidemia, and what signs and symptoms would you expect?
2. How is ethylene glycol metabolized, and why does ethylene glycol poisoning look similar to methylmalonic acidemia?
3. Can you propose a mechanism for the excessive formation of ketone bodies in this disease?
4. What treatments can you suggest for methylmalonic acidemia?
5. Some metabolic diseases can be treated with megadoses of a vitamin or coenzyme. What coenzyme would you try in a patient with methylmalonic acidemia?
6. Is vomiting a sign that is specific for individual diseases? What is the function of the vomiting reflex?

📖 Suggested Reading

Fenton WA, Gravel RA, Rosenblatt DS: Disorders of propionate and methylmalonate metabolism. In Scriver CR, Beaudet AL, Sly WS, et al (eds): The Metabolic and Molecular Basis of Inherited Disease, 8th ed, vol 2. New York: McGraw-Hill, 2001, pp 2165-2193.

🗀 To Treat or Not to Treat?

Becky Brummond was transferred to a specialized metabolic clinic at the age of 14 months. She had first presented with coma at the age of 3 days, and she had developed severe seizures at 4 weeks. Nonketotic hyperglycinemia was diagnosed at 2 months, with a plasma glycine level of 897 µmol/liter (normal, 81 to 436 µmol/liter) and normal urine organic acid levels. She was treated with lorazepam and phenobarbital and with sodium benzoate at 500 mg/kg/day.

At 14 months, she had severe axial hypotonia, spasticity, and frequent myoclonic seizures. She occasionally babbled and had a short attention span. Her plasma glycine level was 917 µmol/liter. The sodium benzoate dosage was increased to 640 mg/kg/day, and the plasma glycine decreased to 352 µmol/liter. Within the next 3 months, she became more awake, her seizures ceased, and she made developmental progress. She learned to roll

from front to back and back to front and to reach for and take objects in her hands. When the benzoate dosage was inadvertently decreased to 64 mg/kg/day at 1 year 8 months of age, she had frequent severe seizures despite increasing doses of anticonvulsants, which made her progressively drowsy. Plasma glycine level was 657 µmol/liter and CSF glycine level was 117 µmol/liter (normal, 3 to 10 µmol/liter). The error soon was noted, and her normal sodium benzoate dosage was reinstated. At the age of 2 years, 6 months, her seizures recurred when her glycine level became elevated. With an increase in the benzoate dosage to 750 mg/kg/day, good control of her plasma glycine level and seizures was achieved.

At the age of 2 years, 8 months, she still had pronounced axial hypotonia with distal spasticity. She had achieved some degree of head control, she could push herself up on her hands, and she could push herself around on the floor. One year later, at the age of 3 years 10 months, no substantial developmental progress was seen. Her adaptive skills were at the 8- to 16-week level, gross motor skills were at the 8- to 12-week level, fine motor skills were at the 4-week level, and personal social skills were at the 4- to 12-week level. Visual inattentiveness was striking. Magnetic resonance imaging showed a static delayed myelinization. When the plasma carnitine level was noted to be in the low-normal range at age 3, L-carnitine therapy (50 mg/kg/day) was started. After the initiation of this treatment, an increased activity level was noted.

Questions

1. Describe the metabolism of glycine and the molecular defect in nonketotic hyperglycinemia.
2. Does glycine serve any specialized functions in the brain that could account for the neurological problems in nonketotic hyperglycinemia?
3. How does benzoic acid lower the plasma glycine level? Which other diseases can be treated with benzoic acid?
4. Benzoic acid treatment induces carnitine deficiency in some patients. How? What are the metabolic consequences of carnitine deficiency?
5. Who makes decisions about the patient's treatment? What would you do if the parents ask you to refrain from any treatment and let the disease take its natural course?

📖 Suggested Reading

Hamosh A, Johnston MV: Nonketotic hyperglycinemia. In Scriver CR Beaudet AL, Sly WS, et al (eds): The

Metabolic and Molecular Basis of Inherited Disease, 8th ed, vol 2. New York: McGraw-Hill, 2001, pp 2065-2078.

van Hove JLK, Kishnani P, Muenzer J, et al: Benzoate therapy and carnitine deficiency in non-ketotic hyperglycinemia. Am J Med Genet 59:444-453, 1995.

Yellow Eyes

Andrew Brown, a 64-year-old civil servant at the Internal Revenue Service, appeared to be in excellent health when he was told at work that the sclerae of his eyes were yellow. He ignored this for 2 weeks and then noted that his stools were pale and his urine was dark. He had slight anorexia and had lost 10 pounds.

Although he did not suffer from abdominal pain and had no fever, he consulted his physician, who noted the jaundice and found a nontender swelling in the right upper abdomen, which appeared to be a dilated gallbladder. Mr. Brown was sent to the local hospital, where some tests were performed on his blood. The results were as follows (normal ranges are in parentheses):

Hematocrit:	48% (40-54)
Platelets:	250,000/μL (150,000 to 450,000)
White blood cells:	17,000/μL (4500 to 11,000)
Prothrombin time:	26 seconds (10 to 13)
Total bilirubin:	14.2 mg/dL (0.1 to 1.2)
Direct bilirubin:	12.0 mg/dL (0.1 to 0.4)
Alanine transaminase (ALT):	12 U/liter (4 to 36)
α-Amylase:	200 U/liter (30 to 220)
Alkaline phosphatase:	650 U/liter (20 to 130)
Lactate dehydrogenase (LDH):	410 U/liter (208 to 378)

The urine was brown and tested positive for bilirubin. Tests for urobilinogen in urine and stool yielded negative results, and the stool was noted to be clay colored. An ultrasound confirmed the presence of a dilated common bile duct, but there was no evidence of gallstones.

Exploratory laparotomy was performed 5 days later. Besides the dilatation of the gallbladder and the common bile duct, the head of the pancreas was found to be swollen, and a small amount of ascitic fluid was noted. Biopsy samples were obtained from the head of the pancreas and from five regional lymph nodes. Routine cytologic studies established a diagnosis of pancreatic adenocarcinoma, and four of the five lymph nodes turned out to be invaded. The patient was offered combination chemotherapy with fluorouracil, methotrexate, and vincristine, but he declined when the likely outcome was

explained to him. He died 4 months later, with morphine as his only medication.

Questions

1. How is bilirubin normally metabolized?
2. What are the possible causes of jaundice in adults? Is the absence of fever significant for the initial diagnosis?
3. Why were the stools clay colored, and why was the urine brown?
4. What is urobilinogen, and why can it be used to distinguish different types of jaundice?
5. Give rationales for the laboratory tests employed.
6. Do you think that an injection of vitamin K would correct the prolonged prothrombin time?
7. Why was no attempt made to treat Mr. Brown's cancer surgically?
8. How do fluorouracil, methotrexate, and vincristine work, and would you expect any side effects?

Suggested Reading

Duffy JP, Reber HA: Nonendocrine tumors of the pancreas. In Yamada T, Alpers DH, Laine L, et al (eds): Textbook of Gastroenterology, 4th ed, vol 2. Philadelphia: Lippincott Williams & Wilkins, 2003, pp 2091-2108.

An Abdominal Emergency

Elma Crawford is a 62-year-old retired housewife, 40 pounds overweight, who was rushed to the emergency room by her husband one Saturday morning after suddenly developing severe pain in the epigastric region. The pain had started suddenly and had become very severe over a period of only 15 minutes, followed shortly by repeated vomiting. On reaching the hospital she was pale and in obvious distress. Her blood pressure was 100/60 in a reclining position and 70/40 in the upright position. The heart rate was 110/minute, and the respiratory rate was 35/minute. Physical examination was unremarkable except for extreme tenderness in the epigastric region.

Two ampules of blood were drawn for blood tests. Because Ms. Crawford was in extreme pain, she was given 75 mg of meperidine intramuscularly, and a history was obtained from her husband. She had been in good health until that morning, but 5 years ago she had had episodes of abdominal pain, which had been due to stones in her gallbladder. She had been treated with chenodiol (chenodeoxycholic acid); after 1 year, the gallstones had disappeared and the treatment was discontinued.

The following results of the blood tests were available 3 hours later (normal ranges are in parentheses):

Hematocrit:	41% (38 to 47)
Na⁺:	146 mmol/liter (136 to 142)
K⁺:	4.6 mmol/liter (3.8 to 5.0)
Ca²⁺:	2.4 mmol/liter (2.30 to 2.74)
Cl⁻:	104 mmol/liter (95 to 103)
Glucose (fasting):	130 mg/dL (70 to 110)
Total bilirubin:	<1 mg/dL (0.1 to 1.2)
Blood urea nitrogen (BUN):	22 mg/dL (8 to 23)
Creatinine:	1.0 mg/dL (0.6 to 1.2)
LDH:	410 U/liter (208 to 378)
ALT:	16 U/liter (4 to 36)
Creatine kinase:	55 U/liter (30 to 135)
Alkaline phosphatase:	120 U/liter (20 to 130)
α-Amylase:	760 U/liter (30 to 220)

She was transferred immediately to the intensive care unit, where she was treated with IV fluids, parenteral nutrition, nasogastric suction, and cimetidine. A blood sample obtained the next morning showed the following laboratory values (again, normal values are in parentheses).

Glucose (fasting):	180 mg/dL (70 to 110)
Na⁺:	135 mmol/liter (136 to 142)
K⁺:	4.0 mmol/liter (3.8 to 5.0)
Ca²⁺:	1.8 mmol/liter (2.30 to 2.74)
Mg²⁺:	0.4 mmol/liter (0.65 to 1.05)
Cl⁻:	92 mmol/liter (95 to 103)
α-Amylase:	850 U/liter (30 to 220)

She was mildly febrile at this time (38.9° C). Ten milliliters of 10% calcium gluconate and 2 mL of 50% magnesium sulfate were added to her IV replacement fluid, and intensive care treatment was continued for another 3 days. After this time, her condition had improved sufficiently to permit her transfer to a regular hospital ward, and she was discharged after another 2 weeks. A cholecystectomy was scheduled for 3 weeks later. Her gallbladder was removed together with four yellow-brown stones that she took home in a glass jar to show to her family and friends.

Questions

1. What possible causes do you know for severe abdominal pain of sudden onset? What procedures can be used to establish a diagnosis?
2. Describe the normal composition of bile and the origin of its constituents.
3. What are the typical constituents of gallstones?
4. Can you think of biochemical and physiological conditions leading to an increased risk of gallstone formation?
5. Most gallstones form not in the bile ducts but in the gallbladder. Why?
6. Is the risk of gallstones affected by the diet, and are there any commonly used drug treatments that either increase or decrease the risk of gallstones?
7. Why can oral chenodeoxycholic acid (chenodiol) be used for the treatment of gallstones? Compare the merits of chenodiol treatment and cholecystectomy.
8. Chenodiol increases the level of low-density lipoprotein cholesterol but not high-density lipoprotein cholesterol in some patients. Can you propose a biochemical mechanism for this?
9. How can gallstones cause pancreatitis?
10. Which pancreatic enzymes are synthesized as zymogens?
11. Can you propose rational treatments for acute pancreatitis?
12. Many patients with severe pancreatitis develop hypocalcemia and hypomagnesemia. Why?
13. Why did the patient have mild hyperglycemia 1 day after the onset of pain?

📖 Suggested Reading

Kosters A, Jirsa M, Groen AK: Genetic background of cholesterol gallstone disease. Biochim Biophys Acta 1637:1-19, 2003.

Lee SP, Co CW: Gallstones. In Yamada T, Alpers DH, Laine L, et al (eds): Textbook of Gastroenterology, 4th ed, vol 2. Philadelphia: Lippincott Williams & Wilkins, 2003, pp 2177-2200.

Paigen B, Carey MC: Gallstones. In King RA, Rotter JI, Motulsky AG (eds): The Genetic Basis of Common Diseases, 2nd ed. Oxford, UK: Oxford University Press, 2002, pp 298-335.

Topazian M, Gorelick FS: Acute pancreatitis. In Yamada T, Alpers DH, Laine L, et al (eds): Textbook of Gastroenterology, 4th ed, vol 2. Philadelphia: Lippincott Williams & Wilkins, 2003, pp 2026-2061.

🗂 Shortness of Breath

Oscar Schnorr, a high school teacher, was 53 years old when he consulted his physician with the first complaints of shortness of breath. He also mentioned several occasions when he felt tightness or pain in the middle of the chest that radiated to the inner side of the left arm. These episodes were always precipitated by physical activity, in several instances by climbing the stairs to his fifth-floor apartment.

Mr. Schnorr's body mass index was found to be 32. He had been a one-pack-a-day smoker since age 18 but had quit smoking 3 years before this visit. Physical examination findings were unremarkable. His blood pressure was 155/100, and his heart sounds were normal. His breath sounds were near normal, with only mild evidence of chronic bronchitis. Laboratory tests for fasting blood glucose and lipids showed the following results (normal values in parentheses):

Glucose: 105 mg/dL (70 to 110 mg/dL)
Total cholesterol: 240 mg/dL (140 to 250 mg/dL)
Triglycerides: 310 mg/dL (10 to 190 mg/dL)

The level of lipoprotein (a) was in the normal range. The electrocardiogram showed evidence of mild myocardial damage in the wall of the left ventricle, consistent with an old infarction in the area of the descending branch of the left coronary artery. A coronary arteriogram showed a moderately severe stenotic lesion near the origin of the main left coronary artery that narrowed the arterial lumen by approximately 50%.

Mr. Schnorr agreed with his physician that conventional treatment should be tried first. On the doctor's advice, he adopted a diet with a reduced amount of animal fat and cholesterol, to normalize his blood lipids. However, a blood test taken 4 weeks later showed no improvement of his hyperlipidemia. After a telephone conversation with the dietitian at the local hospital, the physician placed Mr. Schnorr on a low-carbohydrate, high-fiber diet. Much to everyone's surprise, Mr. Schnorr found this diet quite acceptable. He lost 10 pounds during the following year, and repeated laboratory tests showed cholesterol and triglyceride levels in the normal or near-normal range. He also bought a blood pressure monitor and managed to keep his blood pressure in the normal range with dietary adjustments and mild medication.

Although his condition was stable over the following years, he was scheduled for bypass surgery at age 56. In the years after the surgery, he no longer suffered any chest pain after exertion, and he said that he felt 20 years younger.

Six weeks after surgery, he was enrolled in a double-blind, placebo-controlled clinical trial of the effects of antioxidant vitamins on late complications and survival of coronary bypass patients. He is now taking one daily capsule with 200 mg of vitamin E plus 1 g of vitamin C, and he must go to the hospital once every 2 months to have his blood lipids and plasma ascorbic acid checked and to receive his supply of vitamin (or placebo?) capsules. He is still doing well 5 years after surgery.

Questions

1. What are the possible causes for "shortness of breath"? Which features in Mr. Schnorr's initial clinical presentation suggest that he had a cardiac problem?
2. How would you classify the pattern of hyperlipidemia in this patient? Which type of lipoprotein is elevated?
3. What is lipoprotein (a)? Is it a risk factor for atherosclerosis?
4. Why was the patient's hyperlipidemia ameliorated on a low-carbohydrate diet but not on a low-fat diet?
5. Polyunsaturated fats tend to normalize blood lipid levels in hyperlipidemic patients. By what mechanisms can these fatty acids possibly influence lipid metabolism?
6. Is smoking a risk factor for coronary heart disease? By what mechanism can smoking affect the underlying disease process and its clinical expression?
7. How does nitroglycerin work (in medicine, not terrorism)?
8. What is "stenosis," and what is the likely nature of the "stenotic lesion" in the patient's coronary artery?
9. Describe the role of lipoproteins in the formation of atherosclerotic lesions.
10. Besides lipoproteins, what other blood metabolites have been linked to atherosclerotic disease?
11. What abnormal processes, possibly triggered by lipid deposition, take place during the development of atheromatous lesions?
12. Why is hypertension so common among people in industrialized countries, and what kind of dietary measures would you recommend to normalize an elevated blood pressure?
13. There was evidence for an old infarction in one of the terminal branches of the patient's left coronary artery. Could the lesion at the root of the left coronary artery be responsible for this infarction, and if so, how?
14. When you detect a myocardial lesion in the electrocardiogram, how can you find out whether this is a fresh infarction or the scar of an old infarction?
15. How long can myocardial tissue survive under ischemic conditions, and what is the immediate mechanism of cell death during ischemia?
16. ATP is required for all major energy-dependent processes in the cell. What are these energy-dependent processes in the myocardium? Failure of which of them is most likely to kill the cells during an ischemic attack?

17. Cell death during ischemia could be caused, in theory, either directly by the lack of oxygen or indirectly by the accumulation of metabolic end products. Can you design an animal experiment that distinguishes between these two possibilities?
18. Would anticoagulant therapy make sense for this patient, and what are the risks?
19. What is coronary bypass surgery?
20. How are placebo-controlled, double-blind clinical trials designed?
21. Does anything in the patient's history suggest that he is particularly suitable for participation in a clinical trial?
22. During the clinical trial, the laboratory checks not only the patient's blood lipid levels but also his ascorbate level. Why?
23. Antioxidant vitamins have been proposed as prophylactic agents for coronary heart disease. What is their proposed mechanism of action?
24. Compare the effects of lipid-lowering drugs (lovastatin, colestipol, fibrates, niacin) on blood lipid levels with the effects of dietary manipulations. In which situations would you rely on diet, and in which situations do you use drugs?
25. What are the pros and cons of heart surgery, as opposed to conventional management of coronary heart disease?

Suggested Reading

Choy PC, Siow YL, Mymin D, et al: Lipids and atherosclerosis. Biochem Cell Biol 82:212-224, 2004.
Foody J (ed): Preventive Cardiology: Strategies for the Prevention and Treatment of Coronary Artery Disease. Totowa, NJ: Humana Press, 2001.
Lippi G, Guidi G: Lipoprotein(a): an emerging cardiovascular risk factor. Crit Rev Clin Lab Sci 40:1-42, 2003.
Moreno JJ, Mitjavila MT: The degree of unsaturation of dietary fatty acids and the development of atherosclerosis. J Nutr Biochem 14:182-195, 2003.
Motulsky AG, Brunzell JD: Genetics of coronary atherosclerosis. In King RA, Rotter JI, Motulsky AG (eds): The Genetic Basis of Common Diseases, 2nd ed. Oxford, UK: Oxford University Press, 2002, pp 105-126.
Sainani GS, Bhatia MS, Sainani R: Endothelial cell dysfunction—a key factor in atherogenesis and its reversal. In Pierce GN, Nanago M, Dhallia NS, et al (eds): Atherosclerosis, Hypertension and Diabetes. Boston: Kluwer, 2003, pp 27-51.
Wilson PWF (ed): Atlas of Atherosclerosis: Risk Factors and Treatment, 3rd ed. Philadelphia: Current Medicine, 2002.
World Health Organization: Prevention of Recurrent Heart Attacks and Strokes in Low- and Middle-Income Populations: Evidence-Based Recommendations for Policy-Makers and Health Professionals. New York: World Health Organization, 2003.

Itching

Margaret Mallon was a 55-year-old librarian at the public library when she saw her doctor with a complaint of diffuse itching at night, which had troubled her for the past 3 months. Physical examination was unremarkable except for slight liver enlargement. There was no urticaria. The patient was prescribed chlorpheniramine maleate, 4 mg four to five times daily. When she returned 3 weeks later, commenting that the medication made her drowsy but was otherwise useless, a series of laboratory tests was performed on her blood, with the following results (normal ranges are in parentheses):

Hematocrit:	41% (38 to 47)
Red blood cells:	$4.5 \times 10^6/\mu L$ (4.2 to 5.4)
White blood cells:	$22 \times 10^3/\mu L$ (4.5 to 11)
Platelets:	250,000/μL (150,000 to 450,000)
Total protein:	6.9 g/dL (6.0 to 7.8)
Albumin:	2.7 g/dL (3.2 to 4.5)
Globulin:	4.2 g/dL (2.3 to 3.5)
Prothrombin time:	12 seconds (10 to 13)
Glucose:	80 mg/dL (70 to 110)
Cholesterol:	330 mg/dL (150 to 250)
Triglyceride:	75 mg/dL (10 to 190)
Bilirubin (total):	3.5 mg/dL (<1)
LDH:	280 U/liter (90 to 310)
ALT:	55 U/liter (4 to 36)
Creatine kinase:	45 U/liter (30 to 135)
Alkaline phosphatase:	680 U/liter (20 to 130)
γ-Glutamyltransferase:	220 U/liter (5 to 40)
BUN:	15 mg/dL (8 to 23)

After these test results were received, Ms. Mallon was referred to the gastroenterology department of the local hospital for cholangiography, a transcutaneous needle biopsy of the liver, and some additional laboratory tests. The cholangiogram showed normal structure of the extrahepatic biliary system. The biopsy showed degeneration of intrahepatic bile ducts. There was inflammation with an infiltrate of mononuclear cells, and the ductular epithelial cells were in disarray. The bile canaliculi between the hepatocytes were dilated, and the hepatocytes adjacent to the portal tract had a swollen and foamy appearance. Excess copper was shown with a rhodamine stain. Blood tests revealed a serum copper level of 85 μmol/dL (normal, 13 to 24) and a fasting bile acid level of 12.5 mg/dL (normal, 0.3 to 3.0). Immunoelectrophoresis showed mildly elevated IgG and strongly elevated IgM levels, and antimitochondrial antibodies could be detected.

Treatment with cholestyramine, 10 g/day, was initiated, and this improved the itching. She also was treated intermittently with cortisol and with penicillamine. She remained in reasonably good health during the next 3 years, although she retired from her job at the public library because the work was too strenuous and she felt that she needed more rest.

Four years after the initial diagnosis, she was brought to the emergency room by her husband. She was in a mildly confused state, had a coarse tremor, and was unable to walk without support. In the emergency room, she was unable to complete a number-connection test in the allotted time of 60 seconds. The EEG showed a bilateral synchronous decrease in wave frequency and increase in wave amplitude with disappearance of the normal α rhythm. A series of blood tests was performed, with the following results (normal ranges are in parentheses):

Hematocrit:	37% (38 to 47)
Total protein:	6.5 g/dL (6.0 to 7.8)
Albumin:	1.9 g/dL (3.2 to 4.5)
Globulin:	4.6 g/dL (2.3 to 3.5)
Prothrombin time:	25 seconds (10 to 13)
Glucose:	100 mg/dL (70 to 110)
Cholesterol:	210 mg/dL (150 to 250)
Triglyceride:	40 mg/dL (10 to 190)
Bilirubin:	8.6 mg/dL (<1.0)
ALT:	115 U/liter (4 to 36)
Alkaline phosphatase:	450 U/liter (20 to 130)
Ammonia:	450 μg/dL (40 to 80)
BUN:	16 mg/dL (8 to 23)

She was treated initially with mannitol enemas, followed on the next day by neomycin. Sodium phenylbutyrate and sodium benzoate, 10 g/day each, were given, and she was kept on a diet with 40 to 50 g of protein per day. With this treatment, she regained her previous state of health within a few days, and she was discharged on a regimen of cholestyramine, vitamin K, and phenylacetate and on a diet that provided 40 to 50 g of high-quality protein per day.

Six months later she was rushed to the hospital after throwing up copious amounts of blood. She died in the hospital a few hours later.

Questions

1. What illness did the doctor suspect on Mrs. Mallon's first visit, before the laboratory and biopsy tests established the diagnosis of a hepatobiliary disease?

2. Which of the initial laboratory test results suggested a biliary problem?
3. Why was cholangiography performed?
4. What is the significance of elevated levels of immunoglobulin M and the antimitochondrial antibodies?
5. Why were levels of serum bile acids, cholesterol, and copper elevated?
6. What was the rationale for the use of mannitol and neomycin?
7. Do you expect that vitamin K treatment was effective in this patient?
8. Why was the patient treated with a low-protein diet?
9. How do sodium phenylbutyrate and sodium benzoate work?
10. What caused Ms. Mallon's sudden death?

Suggested Reading

Heathcote EJ: Primary biliary cirrhosis. In Schiff ER, Sorrell MF, Maddrey WC (eds): Schiff's Diseases of the Liver, 9th ed, vol 1. Philadelphia: Lippincott Williams & Wilkins, 2003, pp 701-712.

Mayo MJ, Thiele DL: Primary biliary cirrhosis. In Yamada T, Alpers DH, Laine L, et al (eds): Textbook of Gastroenterology, 4th ed, vol 2. Philadelphia: Lippincott Williams & Wilkins, 2003, pp 2374-2387.

Weinman SA, Kemmer N: Bile secretion and cholestasis. In Yamada T, Alpers DH, Laine L, et al (eds): Textbook of Gastroenterology, 4th ed, vol 1. Philadelphia: Lippincott Williams & Wilkins, 2003, pp 366-388.

Abdominal Pain

Betty Belmaker was a 29-year-old woman who had been a secret but heavy drinker for a few years, ever since she married a physician who neglected her in favor of his patients and his secretary. One day she developed acute pain in the lumbar region and abdomen. On the following day, she entered a hospital and was treated initially with ampicillin for a suspected urinary tract infection. Shortly after admission, she had two grand mal seizures. Her serum sodium was 119 mmol/liter at that time (normal, 136 to 142), and the EEG was mildly abnormal.

She was treated with hypertonic saline and phenytoin. This resulted in initial improvement, and she was discharged on the ninth hospital day. However, the pain persisted, and muscle weakness developed.

The patient was readmitted 4 days later. Temperature, pulse rate, and blood pressure were normal, and no rash or lymphadenopathy was found. Lungs, heart, breasts, abdomen, and extremities were normal. Pelvic and rectal examinations yielded negative findings. There was, however, considerable muscle tenderness and weakness. On the neurological examination, the patient was alert but irritable and mildly confused. There were no signs of aphasia or apraxia.

Urine: Amber, with specific gravity of 1.022 and pH of 5.0; few white blood cells and bacteria

Stool: No occult blood

One day after admission, several laboratory tests were performed on the patient's blood with the following results (normal ranges are in parentheses):

Hematocrit:	38.9% (38 to 47)
White blood cells:	6300/μL (4,500 to 11,000)
58% Neutrophils (56%)	
40% Lymphocytes (34%)	
2% Monocytes (4%)	
Platelets:	291,000/μL (150,000 to 450,000)
Protein:	6.4 g/dL (6 to 7.8)
Albumin:	3.7 g/dL (3.2 to 4.5)
Globulin:	2.7 g/dL (2.3 to 3.5)
Urea nitrogen:	23 mg/dL (8 to 23)
Glucose (fasting):	123 mg/dL (70 to 110)
Uric acid:	3.0 mg/dL (2.7 to 7.3)
Bilirubin:	0.3 mg/dL (0.1 to 1.2)
Na^+:	138 mmol/liter (136 to 142)
K^+:	4.1 mmol/liter (3.8 to 5.0)
Ca^{2+}:	2.3 mmol/liter (2.30 to 2.74)
Phosphate:	1.2 mmol/liter (0.74 to 1.52)
Cl^-:	92 mmol/liter (95 to 103)
CO_2:	28 mmol/liter (22 to 26)
Aspartate transaminase:	31 U/liter (8 to 33)
LDH:	235 U/liter (208 to 378)
Creatine kinase:	13 U/liter (30 to 135)
α-Amylase:	10 U/liter (30 to 220)
Alkaline phosphate:	54 U/liter (20 to 130)
γ-Glutamyltransferase:	115 U/liter (5 to 40)
Heart rate:	126/min (70 to 95)
Chest radiograph:	normal

Lumbar puncture produced clear, colorless CSF with two red blood cells, one lymphocyte, and one mononuclear cell per microliter, and no bacteria:

Glucose:	80 mg/dL (40 to 80)
Protein:	21 mg/dL (12 to 60)
Plasma electrophoresis:	Mild increase in the γ-globulin fraction

Immunoelectrophoresis:	Mild increase of immunoglobulin G, mild decrease of immunoglobulin A

The patient remained afebrile. A urine sample obtained 3 days after readmission showed an orange discoloration. The sediment had few white blood cells and bacteria.

After a tentative diagnosis was made, phenytoin was withdrawn and the patient was treated with IV glucose and hemin (hematin). This resulted in gradual improvement over the following days.

Questions

1. Give rationales for the blood tests that were performed on this patient. On the basis of the normal results of most of these tests, which diseases can be ruled out?
2. Why was the γ-glutamyltransferase level elevated?
3. Are alcoholics prone to seizures? Under what circumstances are they most likely to have seizures?
4. Do you know of diseases that cause an abnormal color of the urine?
5. Why was a lumbar puncture performed?
6. What was the tentative diagnosis that was confirmed by the effectiveness of the treatment? Can you think of a laboratory test that would establish a definitive diagnosis?
7. Were the symptoms caused by the deficiency of a metabolic product or by the accumulation of toxic metabolites?
8. What is hemin, and why was it effective?
9. Could the phenytoin treatment have worsened the patient's condition?

📖 Suggested Reading

Desnick RJ, Astrin KH, Anderson KE: Alcoholism. In King RA, Rotter JI, Motulsky AG (eds): The Genetic Basis of Common Diseases, 2nd ed. Oxford, UK: Oxford University Press, 2002, pp 876-913.

Sassa S, Shibahara S: Disorders of heme production and catabolism. In Handin RI, Lux SE, Stossel TP (eds): Blood: Principles and Practice of Hematology, 2nd ed. Philadelphia: Lippincott Williams & Wilkins, 2002, pp 1435-1501.

🗀 Rheumatism

Charles Fillmore is a 62-year-old racetrack bookie who saw his doctor with complaints of stiffness and pain in his hands and wrists, which troubled him during his work. A radiograph showed joint space narrowing of the metacarpophalangeal joints and chondrocalcinosis in the area of the wrist joint. A tentative diagnosis of rheumatoid arthritis was made, and aspirin was prescribed. Eight weeks later, Mr. Fillmore was in his doctor's office again with complaints of serious stomach pain that could be relieved only by eating. The radiograph showed evidence of a gastric ulcer. Aspirin was discontinued, and with treatment with cimetidine (Tagamet), a histamine H_2 receptor blocker, the ulcer healed within 2 months.

Subsequently Mr. Fillmore occasionally used phenacetin or acetaminophen for his "rheumatism," but with little success. After another year he noticed that he felt increasingly weak and lethargic, and the last of his libido was gone. He underwent a complete medical checkup. At this time he was noted to have a brown discoloration of the skin. Echocardiography showed moderately severe ventricular enlargement, and his blood pressure was 140/95. Physical examination was normal except for a mild swelling and tenderness of the metacarpophalangeal joints, restricted mobility of the wrist joint, and some tenderness of the medial aspect of the left knee joint. A series of blood tests were performed, with the following results (normal ranges are in parentheses):

Hematocrit:	44% (40 to 54)
Red blood cells:	$5.1 \times 10^6/\mu L$ (4.6 to 6.2)
White blood cells:	8,000/μL (4,500 to 11,000)
Platelets:	380,000/μL (150,000 to 450,000)
Hemoglobin:	14.8% (13.5 to 18.0)
Total protein:	7.3% (6.0 to 7.8)
Albumin:	2.9% (3.2 to 4.5)
Globulin:	4.4% (2.3 to 3.5)
Prothrombin time:	11 seconds (10 to 13)
Glucose:	240 mg/dL (70 to 110)
BUN:	20 mg/dL (8 to 23)
Bilirubin:	1.5 mg/dL (0.1 to 1.2)
Total iron-binding capacity:	330 μg/dL (250 to 400)
Transferrin saturation:	92% (20 to 55)
Serum ferritin:	680 ng/mL (15 to 200)
Creatine kinase:	75 U/liter (55 to 170)
ALT:	65 U/liter (4 to 36)
Alkaline phosphatase:	160 U/liter (20 to 130)

Mr. Fillmore was referred to the gastroenterology unit for a liver biopsy. Histological examination revealed fibrous degeneration of moderate severity. A Prussian blue stain showed extensive iron accumulation in hepatocytes, with less intense staining of Kupffer cells. The iron concentration was determined, by atomic absorption spectroscopy, to be 320 μmol/g dry weight (normal, 5 to 40).

Questions

1. What disease does Mr. Fillmore have, and what is the most likely cause?
2. Although the propensity for iron overload is based on genetics, environmental factors contribute to iron overload. What lifestyle factors are likely to contribute to iron overload?
3. The major hemochromatosis mutation originally occurred in a single individual sometime between 2000 and 4000 years ago. How can you estimate the age of the mutation?
4. Today more than 10% of the population in Ireland, Great Britain, and the Scandinavian countries carry at least one copy of the hemochromatosis mutation. How could this mutation have become so common so fast?
5. Is genetic screening of children or adults for the disease predisposition possible? Would screening make sense?
6. Which blood tests are most important for the diagnosis?
7. What treatment would you use?
8. In which tissues is iron normally stored, and why does this require specialized iron storage proteins?
9. The patient presented initially with symptoms of arthritis. What types of arthritis do you know?
10. The patient developed a gastric ulcer after using aspirin for several weeks. Can aspirin be absorbed into the cells of the gastric mucosa? Can it accumulate in these cells? The structure of aspirin is shown in Figure C-1:

11. Aspirin inhibits cyclooxygenase (COX). Do you know stomach-friendly COX inhibitors that do not cause gastritis and stomach ulcers and that can be used instead of aspirin?
12. How is gastric acid formed, and which components of this process can be used as drug targets?
13. The patient had a dark discoloration of the skin. Do you know of other diseases in which the color of the skin is abnormal?
14. A loss of libido in men can be caused by insufficient testosterone secretion. Malfunction of which other endocrine gland (besides the testis) can cause this? Which laboratory tests can you use to distinguish among the different possibilities?

Suggested Reading

Adams PC: Hemochromatosis. In Yamada T, Alpers DH, Laine L, et al (eds): Textbook of Gastroenterology, 4th ed, vol 2. Philadelphia: Lippincott Williams & Wilkins, 2003, pp 2388-2396.

Andrews NC: Disorders of iron metabolism. In Handin RI, Lux SE, Stossel TP (eds): Blood: Principles and Practice of Hematology, 2nd ed. Philadelphia: Lippincott Williams & Wilkins, 2002, pp 1399-1433.

Busfield F, Anderson GJ, Powell LW: Hereditary hemochromatosis. In King RA, Rotter JI, Motulsky AG (eds): The Genetic Basis of Common Diseases, 2nd ed. Oxford, UK: Oxford University Press, 2002, pp 366-381.

Chu TW, Bowlus C, Gruen JR: Iron metabolism and related disorders. In Emery AEH, Rimoin DL (eds): Emery and Rimoin's Principles and Practice of Medical Genetics, 4th ed, vol 3. Edinburgh: Churchill Livingstone, 2002, pp 2638-2665.

Hentze MW, Muckenthaler MU, Andrews NC: Balancing acts: molecular control of mammalian iron metabolism. Cell 117:285-297, 2004.

Reddy MB, Clark L: Iron, oxidative stress, and disease risk. Nutr Rev 62:120-124, 2004.

Rouault TA, Klausner RD: Molecular basis of iron metabolism. In Stamatoyannopoulos G, Majerus PW, Perlmutter RM, et al (eds): The Molecular Basis of Blood Diseases, 3rd ed. Philadelphia: WB Saunders, 2001, pp 363-387.

A Bank Manager in Trouble

J.C. Penny, a bank manager in a small town in the Midwest, was 46 years old when he was admitted to the hospital after collapsing at a business meeting. Results of some blood tests performed immediately after admission are shown in Table C-2.

At 4:00 the following morning, he woke up with excruciating pain in the left big toe. On questioning, Mr. Penny reported that he had had spasmodic pain in that toe on a few occasions during the past few months and admitted that he had been a heavy drinker for some time. Nodules could be seen and felt in his earlobes, and the joint of the toe was swollen and exquisitely tender. The serum urate level was determined on the same day. It was

Table C-2 Blood Test Results

| Substance | Concentration | |
	mmol/liter*	mg/dL*
Alcohol	55	250
Glucose	3.0 (3.9–6.1)	54 (70–110)
Lactate	3.2 (0.6–2.2)	29 (5–20)

*Normal values in parentheses.

0.6 mmol/liter, or 10.1 mg/dL (normal, 0.24 to 0.51 mmol/liter, or 4.0 to 8.5 mg/dL).

Mr. Penny was given indomethacin and allopurinol. His urate level was in the normal range when he was discharged 3 days later.

Questions

1. How is alcohol metabolized, and how is alcohol metabolism regulated?
2. How can alcohol affect the blood levels of glucose and lactate?
3. Which diseases can result in joint pain? Are there typical differences in the clinical manifestation of gout versus other forms of arthritis?
4. Is an elevated serum urate level diagnostic for gout? Which laboratory test would establish a definitive diagnosis?
5. Why does gout affect small peripheral joints first? Why are nodules often found in the earlobes?
6. Outline the rationales of pharmacological treatments for the acute attack of gouty arthritis and for the long-term maintenance of the patient.
7. What recommendations can you make to Mr. Penny concerning his diet and lifestyle?

Suggested Reading

Becker MA: Hyperuricemia and gout. In King RA, Rotter JI, Motulsky AG (eds): The Genetic Basis of Common Diseases, 2nd ed. Oxford, UK: Oxford University Press, 2002, pp 518-536.

Emmerson BT: Hyperuricemia, gout, and the kidney. In Schrier RW (ed): Diseases of the Kidney and Urinary Tract, 7th ed, vol 3. Philadelphia: Lippincott Williams & Wilkins, 2001, pp 2255-2279.

Lieber CS: Alcohol: its metabolism and interaction with nutrients. Annu Rev Nutr 20:395-430, 2000.

Wortmann RL, Kelley WN: Gout and hyperuricemia. In Ruddy S, Harris ED, Sledge CB, et al (eds): Kelley's Textbook of Rheumatology, 6th ed. Philadelphia: WB Saunders, 2001, pp 1339-1376.

Kidney Problems

Cathy Stout is a 33-year-old typist who has been diabetic since the age of 14. She controls her disease with daily insulin injections, measures her blood glucose daily, and must see her physician once a month. Regular laboratory tests have shown fasting blood glucose levels anywhere between 100 and 400 mg/dL, and her insulin medication has been adjusted repeatedly for optimal blood glucose control. During this month's visit, she complained about lassitude, nausea, and appetite loss, and she also mentioned a distressing itching that typically appears in the late evening and interferes with sleep. She had tried unsuccessfully to self-medicate for this problem with phenacetin and sleeping pills. Her blood pressure at this time was 175/120. She was sent to the laboratory for some tests. Results of urinalysis were as follows:

Dipstick tests:

Glucose:	2+
Ketones:	Trace
Protein:	4+
Blood:	2+

Sediment:

Red blood cells:	260/µL (normal, 3 to 20)
White blood cells:	210/µL (normal, 5 to 30)
Some casts	

The 24-hour urine sample contained 3.7 g of protein. A series of blood tests was performed, with the following results (normal ranges are in parentheses):

Hematocrit:	29% (38 to 47)
Red blood cells:	3.1×10^6/µL (4.2-5.4×10^6)
White blood cells:	12.6×10^3/µL (4.5 to 11.0×10^3)
Platelets:	240,000/µL (150,000 to 450,000)
Total protein:	6.3 g/dL (6.0 to 7.8)
Albumin:	2.5 g/dL (3.2 to 4.5)
Globulin:	3.8 g/dL (2.3 to 3.5)
Na^+:	148 mEq/liter (136 to 142)
K^+:	6.2 mEq/liter (3.8 to 5.0)
Ca^{2+}:	4.0 mEq/liter (4.6 to 5.5)
Mg^{2+}:	3.9 mEq/liter (1.3 to 2.1)
Phosphorus:	8.5 mg/dL (2.3 to 4.7)
Total CO_2:	18 mmol/liter (24 to 30)
pH:	7.35 (7.35 to 7.45)
Glucose:	220 mg/dL (70 to 110)
Total bilirubin:	<1.0 mg/dL (<1.0)
BUN:	185 mg/dL (8 to 23)
Uric acid:	8.3 mg/dL (2.7 to 7.3)
Creatinine:	4.5 mg/dL (0.6 to 1.2)
ALT:	8 U/liter (4 to 36)
Alkaline phosphatase:	325 U/liter (20 to 130)
Creatine kinase:	48 U/liter (30 to 135)
Ferritin:	175 µg/liter (15 to 150)

The creatinine clearance was 12 mL/minute (normal 87 to 107). Ophthalmoscopy showed vascular changes with numerous microaneurysms. At this point, extra attention was given to the control of her blood glucose, including regular determination of hemoglobin A_{1C}. She also was placed on a diet with restricted protein, potassium, and sodium, and she was given sodium bicarbonate, 1.2 g/day,

and calcium carbonate, 500 mg with each meal. Her hypertension was treated with captopril. After initial improvement, her condition worsened again and she was placed on hemodialysis 8 months later. She now is receiving hemodialysis three times a week while waiting for a kidney transplant.

Questions

1. Which type of diabetes does Cathy Stout have? What histologic abnormalities do you expect in her pancreas?
2. Why does the patient depend on insulin injections? Do you know of alternative methods for treating diabetes?
3. The patient complains about itching. Do you know of any other diseases that cause itching?
4. Should the patient ask her doctor before she self-medicates for such problems as itching and indigestion?
5. Explain the electrolyte abnormalities in this patient.
6. Why is the level of alkaline phosphatase high?
7. The parathyroid hormone (PTH) level was not determined. How would you determine PTH, and what results can you expect in this patient?
8. Why is the total CO_2 low?
9. How do the kidneys participate in acid-base regulation?
10. What is BUN, and in which disease is it elevated?
11. Why is the hematocrit low? What would be the best treatment for the patient's anemia?
12. The blood pressure is elevated in many kidney diseases. Why?
13. Is there any reason to examine the eyes in patients with chronic diabetes?
14. Give rationales for the initial treatment.
15. What is hemodialysis?

📖 Suggested Reading

Bailey JL, Mitch WE: Pathophysiology of uremia. In Brenner BM (ed): Brenner & Rector's The Kidney, 6th ed, vol 2. Philadelphia: WB Saunders, 2000, pp 2059-2078.

Brownlee M, Aiello LP, Friedman E, et al: Complications of diabetes mellitus. In Larsen PR, Kronenberg HM, Melmed S, et al (eds): Williams Textbook of Endocrinology, 10th ed. Philadelphia: WB Saunders, 2003, pp 1509-1583.

Mauer M, et al: Diabetic nephropathy. In Schrier RW (ed): Diseases of the Kidney and Urinary Tract, 7th ed, vol 3. Philadelphia: Lippincott Williams & Wilkins, 2001, pp 2083-2127.

Parving HH, Osterby R, Ritz E: Diabetic nephropathy. In Brenner BM (ed): Brenner & Rector's The Kidney, 6th ed, vol 2. Philadelphia: WB Saunders, 2000, pp 1731-1773.

A Sickly Child*

PART I: HISTORY

David was 5 months old when he was brought by his mother to the emergency room at Children's Hospital at 8:00 A.M. after 12 hours of fever with increasing wheezing and coughing. On admission he was found to be in acute respiratory distress, with a temperature of 40.5° C (105° F). He was also somewhat underweight for his age.

David's mother reported that he had experienced several episodes of fever, congestion, and noisy breathing over the last month, which had improved with ampicillin until the day of admission. David was the product of a normal full-term pregnancy, labor, and delivery. His mother described him as a sickly child. She was concerned about his feeding behavior, because he would vomit frequently, particularly during the first hour after feeding. She also commented that during these times his skin became clammy and tasted salty.

Questions

1. Is vomiting after feeding a common problem in infants? Name some possible causes.
2. On the basis of the history, what is the most likely acute problem that brought David to the emergency room?
3. The boy's condition seems to require immediate intervention. What treatment can you propose at this point?

PART II: PHYSICAL EXAMINATION AND LABORATORY TESTS

On physical examination David was found to be a pale, somewhat thin, extremely weak, lethargic child who was slightly cyanotic. His respiratory rate was 80/minute (normal, 40) and his heart rate was 220/minute (normal, 90 to 100). He was clammy and was in extreme respiratory distress. His liver was palpable 10 cm below the right costal margin, and the spleen was felt 3 cm below the left costal margin. Both organs were firm and nontender. A liver scan showed profound liver enlargement without focal lesions.

Some laboratory data were obtained (normal ranges are in parentheses):

Urinalysis: Glucose negative
              Ketones present in moderate amounts

*Copyright 1990 President and Fellows of Harvard College.

Exhaled gases in face mask oxygen:
Partial pressure of oxygen (pO_2) = 189 torr (150 in room air)
Partial pressure of carbon dioxide (pCO_2) = 14 torr (36 to 40)

Blood tests:

White blood cells:	17,150/mm³ (6000 to 12,000)
Hematocrit:	29% (33 to 40)
Total CO_2:	5 mEq/liter (25 to 28)
pH:	7.08 (7.35 to 7.45)
Blood glucose:	<25 mg/dL (80 to 110)
ALT:	86 U/liter (5 to 30)
LDH:	587 U/liter (208 to 378)
Total protein:	9.4 g/dL (6.4 to 8.1)
Total cholesterol:	270 mg/dL (110 to 200)
Triglycerides:	480 mg/dL (10 to 150)
Bilirubin:	0.5 mg/dL total, 0.1 direct (0 to 1.0, direct)
Uric acid:	8.5 mg/dL (3.5 to 7.2)
Lactate:	15 mmol/liter (0.6 to 1.5)

Questions

1. David's respiratory rate was too high. On the basis of the history (presence of fever, slightly cyanotic, previous response to ampicillin), what seems to be the most obvious mechanism for this? Is this mechanism confirmed by the laboratory results?
2. Why was the patient treated with oxygen? Do you think this treatment was continued once the laboratory results were in?
3. The patient had tachycardia, and his skin felt "clammy." What physiological mechanism mediates these effects? Could the same mechanism explain the slight cyanosis?
4. Why was a liver scan performed?
5. Which were the most immediately life-threatening abnormalities revealed by the laboratory tests? Is there anything you can do to help this patient immediately?
6. Why were LDH, ALT, and bilirubin levels determined, and what do the results tell you?
7. A hematocrit of 33% to 40% is indicated as normal for a 5-month-old, although 40% to 50% is considered normal for adults. How does the hematocrit normally change during the first months after birth? What are the evolutionary reason and physiological significance for this?

PART III: HOSPITAL COURSE

David was treated with IV antibiotics, and he became afebrile within 24 hours. The rest of his hospital course was devoted to a diagnostic workup of his hypoglycemia. He underwent an oral glucose tolerance test. With glucose given in a single 2.5-g/kg dose via a nasogastric tube, his blood glucose level rose to within normal limits (90 mg/dL), but within 4 hours it fell to 14 mg/dL. Glucagon administered intramuscularly had no effect on the blood glucose level, but it caused a marked increase in the blood levels of lactate and uric acid.

When David was given a constant glucose infusion at 0.5 g/kg/hour via a nasogastric tube, a normal blood glucose level of 90 to 100 mg/dL was maintained.

While in the hospital, David was maintained on feedings of 150 mL of 10% glucose (IV) every 4 hours in addition to his other food. Before one of the 8:00 A.M. feedings, he was noted to have twitching and jerking movements, which resolved rapidly when he was fed additional glucose.

Questions

1. How is the blood glucose level normally maintained during fasting?
2. How does glucagon affect blood glucose, and what does the atypical response to glucagon suggest?
3. Can "twitching and jerking movements" be caused by hypoglycemia?

PART IV: DIAGNOSIS

A gastrointestinal consultation was sought, and a liver biopsy was performed. A histological examination revealed the presence of abnormal amounts of fat and glycogen within the hepatocytes. Biochemical tests included the determination of glucose-6-phosphatase activity in liver microsomes. Enzyme activity was absent both from fresh microsomes and from microsomes that had been subjected to repeated freezing and thawing.

Questions

1. Give examples of enzyme deficiencies that result in glycogen accumulation.
2. Does the liver normally produce triglycerides? What is the normal fate of liver-derived triglycerides, and under what conditions can fat accumulate in the liver?
3. What are microsomes, and how are they prepared?
4. The enzyme activity was determined both in fresh microsomes and in microsomes that had been frozen and thawed repeatedly. Can you give a rationale for this approach?

5. What diagnosis can you give for this patient?
6. David had increased amounts of glycogen and fat in his liver. Do you expect elevations of other metabolic intermediates as well?
7. Knowing the molecular defect in the patient, how can you explain his abnormal blood chemistry, including the hypoglycemia, lactic acidemia, hyperuricemia, hyperlipidemia, and the presence of ketone bodies? Do hormones play a role in these abnormalities?

PART V: FOLLOW-UP

David was discharged from the hospital after 2 weeks. At home, he was maintained on a regimen of lactose-free milk preparation with added glucose, approximately 2 g/kg every 4 hours. This formula was given around the clock, with a baby soft diet as tolerated. He did well on this therapy, although periodically he had hypoglycemic spells between 3 and 4 hours after feeding.

When David was 3 years old, his glucose formula gradually was tapered off, and he received cornstarch several times daily. He did well on this schedule, although nightly feeding remained a major inconvenience. It was necessary to wake him up once every night for his cornstarch porridge. Periodic blood tests showed near-normal blood lipid levels, although lactate and uric acid levels remained elevated. Starting at age 5, he was treated with allopurinol.

Questions

1. Why was David given lactose-free milk? Compare the metabolism of glucose and galactose. Would sucrose be better than lactose?
2. Why was he given cornstarch?
3. How does allopurinol work?

PART VI: PRENATAL DIAGNOSIS

David's parents had been told by his physician that his condition was inherited and that there was a considerable risk of the disease in future children. For this reason, they refrained from having more children until, quite by accident, his mother became pregnant, again by her husband, when David was 4 years old. Frozen blood samples from David and his parents were sent to a laboratory that could perform molecular studies on David's DNA. The DNA was extracted, and the coding regions and intron-exon junctions of the gene were amplified by the polymerase chain reaction (PCR). The five exons of the gene were amplified to yield products of 306 base pairs (exon 1), 192 base pairs (exon 2), 209 base pairs (exon 3), 259 base pairs (exon 4), 292 base pairs (exon 5, 5′-terminal part) and 389 base pairs (exon 5, 3′-terminal part).

Amplification products of the expected size were obtained. Sequencing of the PCR products showed two known mutations. One was a C → T transition in exon 3 in which Arg-83 was replaced in the polypeptide by cysteine, and the other was a C → T transition in exon 5 in which the codon for Gln-347 was converted to a strop codon. Also, a copy of the unmutated exon was present in both cases. David's mother had only the mutation in exon 3, and his father had only the mutation in exon 5. Amniocentesis was performed as soon as these results were available, and after a 6-day culturing period, the cells were sent to the laboratory for analysis. The fetus turned out to have the exon 5 mutation but not the exon 3 mutation. Five months later, David had a healthy sister.

Questions

1. Describe in general terms the situations in which prenatal diagnosis is indicated.
2. What is the mode of inheritance for David's disease, and how high exactly is the risk that a next child of his parents is affected?
3. Why is a DNA-based method used for prenatal diagnosis in this case, rather than determination of the enzyme activity?
4. PCR-based methods are preferred to Southern blotting for the prenatal diagnosis of genetic diseases. Why?
5. The two mutations found in David account for most cases of glucose-6-phosphatase deficiency in people of European ancestry. Try to design a routine diagnostic test for the detection of these two mutations in which PCR and allele-specific probes are used. Do you expect that this test can be used for the diagnosis of glucose-6-phosphatase deficiency in patients from other ethnic backgrounds?
6. Prenatal diagnosis with the selective termination of affected pregnancies is used increasingly for the prevention of genetic diseases. Is this practice likely to reduce the incidence of recessive disease genes in the population?

Suggested Reading

Chen Y-T: Glycogen storage diseases. In Scriver CR, Beaudet AL, Sly WS, et al (eds): The Metabolic and Molecular Basis of Inherited Disease, 8th ed, vol 1. New York: McGraw-Hill, 2001, pp 1521-1551.

Lei KJ, Shelly LL, Lin B, et al: Mutations in the glucose-6-phosphatase gene are associated with glycogen storage disease types Ia and IaSP and not Ib and Ic. J Clin Invest 95:234-240, 1995.

Van de Werve G, Lange A, Newgard C, et al: New lessons in the regulation of glucose metabolism taught by the glucose 6-phosphatase system. Eur J Biochem 267:1533-1549, 2000.

The Missed Examination

Annemarie is a 22-year-old medical student who has been diabetic since the age of 4. She controls her diabetes with daily insulin injections, 20 U/day, and she has been free from complications so far. One Monday morning, however, she is rushed to the emergency room unconscious.

In the ambulance, Annemarie has the following vital signs: blood pressure, 80/40; pulse rate, 124; and respiratory rate, 35. The paramedics draw several tubes of blood and then administer 50 mL of 50% dextrose solution and 2 mg of naloxone.

Annemarie's parents, who arrive at the emergency room only a few minutes after the ambulance in their own car, report that their daughter spent the night in her room studying for a biochemistry examination. She had been extremely apprehensive about this examination for a number of days. Her mother was not able to wake her up in the morning for this examination, which was scheduled for 8 A.M. Although the paramedics in the ambulance had noticed a suspect smell on her breath, the parents insist that their daughter has not touched any alcohol recently.

On physical examination, the patient is thin and nonjaundiced. She is in no obvious distress but is breathing deeply and rapidly. Her blood pressure is 100/80 when she is lying down, but the systolic pressure falls to 40 in a sitting position. Examination of her chest reveals normal heart and breath sounds. The abdomen is normal. The only abnormal finding is inflammation of the vulva and deposits in the folds of the labia, suggestive of a yeast infection. The laboratory reports the following results:

Urinalysis:
4+ glucose
4+ Ketones
0+ Blood
1+ Protein

Blood tests (normal ranges are in parentheses):

Na^+:	130 mEq/liter	(136 to 142)
Cl^-:	95 mEq/liter	(95 to 103)
K^+:	5.5 mEq/liter	(3.8 to 5.0)
Bicarbonate:	10.8 mEq/liter	(21 to 30)
Glucose:	720 mg/dL	(70 to 110)

Creatinine: 1.7 mg/dL (0.6 to 1.2)
BUN: 35 mg/dL (8 to 23)
Osmolality: 340 mOsm/kg (275 to 295)
pH: 7.22 (7.35 to 7.45)

Complete blood cell count: Mildly elevated white blood cell count

Arterial blood gases:
pO_2:   102 mm Hg (95 to 100)
pCO_2:   22 mm Hg (35 to 40)

Treatment is started with regular insulin, 8 U/hour, and with isotonic saline. Annemarie receives 1.5 liters of saline during the first hour and another 1.0 liter during the second hour, all IV. A blood sample taken at this time yields the following values:

Glucose: 540 mg/dL
Na^+:   142 mmol/liter
K^+:   2.2 mmol/liter
pH: 7.25

Treatment is continued with the infusion of insulin, hypotonic saline (1 liter/hour for another 2 hours), and potassium. Annemarie is fully conscious by this time and gradually regains her previous state of health. She is released the next day, with an increase in her insulin dose to 30 U/day and with keto-conazole for the infection.

Three days later she is brought into the emergency room unconscious. After blood samples are drawn, she is given 50 mL of 50% dextrose and wakes up in less than one minute. She reports that over the 30 minutes before losing consciousness, she had felt increasingly confused, cold, and sweaty.

The blood glucose level at the time of the second admission is 15 mg/dL. A concerned emergency room physician immediately suspects an insulinoma and requests a serum C-peptide level.

Questions

1. What causes of unconsciousness do you know?
2. Can you propose physiological mechanisms for the patient's hypotension, tachycardia, and hyperventilation?
3. What biochemical and physiological abnormalities account for the patient's loss of consciousness at the times of the first and second admissions?
4. Why did the paramedics in the ambulance give Annemarie dextrose and naloxone?
5. A suspect smell on Annemarie's breath was noted in the ambulance. What caused this smell? Are there any other situations in which an abnormal smell on the breath can point to the cause of unconsciousness?
6. Patients with diabetic coma suffer from dehydration. Why?
7. What metabolic aberrations account for Annemarie's markedly elevated serum glucose level at the time of the first admission, although she had consumed no food for several hours?
8. The initial presentation of this patient included a reduced blood pH. Discuss the factors contributing to this and the metabolic pathways responsible for the acidosis.
9. Is ketoacidosis the only type of "diabetic coma"?
10. Why did the potassium level decrease within 2 hours after the treatment was started?
11. At the time of the patient's second visit, an insulin-secreting tumor was suspected, and this was investigated by measuring the levels of circulating C-peptide. How is this peptide formed, and what controls its secretion? In which clinical situations might its measurement be a useful test?
12. Diabetic ketoacidosis often is precipitated by an infection or some other stressful condition. What counter-regulatory hormones might be involved in this process? Do you know of other physiological situations that increase the insulin requirement of diabetic patients?
13. Some patients with type 2 diabetes have elevated levels of circulating insulin, despite displaying many classic signs of the disease. In some cases, cells taken from such a patient display normal binding of insulin, but the hormone does not induce an appropriate biological response. What biochemical defects might be the cause of such a problem?
14. Which genetic and environmental risk factors contribute to the risk of type 1 diabetes? Are these the same that contribute to the risk of type 2 diabetes?
15. What evolutionary reason could account for the relatively high incidence of type 1 diabetes in the population, although in the absence of modern medical care affected individuals used to die before they could produce children? What about type 2 diabetes?

📖 Suggested Reading

Eisenbarth GS, Polonsky KS, Buse JB: Type 1 diabetes mellitus. In Larsen PR, Kronenberg HM, Melmed S, et al (eds): Williams Textbook of Endocrinology, 10th ed. Philadelphia: WB Saunders, 2003, pp 1485-1508.

Elbein SC, Chiu KC, Permutt MA: Type 2 diabetes mellitus. In King RA, Rotter JI, Motulsky AG (eds): The Genetic Basis of Common Diseases, 2nd ed. Oxford, UK: Oxford University Press, 2002, pp 457-480.

Gardner DG, Greenspan FS: Endocrine emergencies. In Greenspan FS, Gardner DG (eds): Basic & Clinical

Endocrinology, 7th ed. New York: Lange/McGraw-Hill, 2004, pp 867-892.

LeRoith D, Taylor SI, Olefsky JM: Diabetes Mellitus: A Fundamental and Clinical Text, 3rd ed. Philadelphia: Lippincott Williams & Wilkins, 2004.

Masharani U, Karam JH, German MS: Pancreatic hormones and diabetes mellitus. In Greenspan FS, Gardner DG (eds): Basic & Clinical Endocrinology, 7th ed. New York: Lange/McGraw-Hill, 2004, pp 658-746.

Raffel LJ: Type 1 diabetes mellitus. In King RA, Rotter JI, Motulsky AG (eds): The Genetic Basis of Common Diseases, 2nd ed. Oxford, UK: Oxford University Press, 2002, pp 431-456.

Gender Blender

An otherwise healthy baby is born with unusual genitalia: There is a small penis, or possibly an enlarged clitoris, and the labioscrotal folds are partially fused, with no palpable testis present. To test for the possibility of a chromosomal abnormality, a buccal smear is made, and a Barr body is identified. Karyotype analysis shows a normal 46,XX karyotype. A urine sample shows elevated levels of 17-ketosteroids, and the 17-hydroxyprogesterone level is found elevated in the plasma. Next, blood electrolytes are determined with the following results (normal range in parentheses):

Na^+:	125 mmol/liter (135 to 148)
K^+:	6.8 mmol/liter (4.0 to 5.9)
Ca^{2+}:	2.3 mmol/liter (2.12 to 2.60)
Mg^{2+}:	1.8 mmol/liter (1.3 to 2.1)
Cl^-:	100 mmol/liter (98 to 106)
HCO_3^-:	18 mmol/liter (22 to 29)

An ultrasound scan of the abdomen shows enlargement of the adrenal glands.

On seeing the results, the chief resident mumbles that they better start hormone treatment soon. However, a medical student accompanying him on his rounds questions whether this should be done. She had learned in medical ethics class that doctors should respect the patient's autonomy and never start treatment without the patient's consent. For this reason, and to prevent gender discrimination, she proposes to wait until the child is 18 and then let the child decide what sex he or she wants to be.

Questions

1. What is a Barr body?
2. What is a karyotype, and which procedures are used for karyotype analysis?
3. Describe the synthesis of steroid hormones in the adrenal cortex. How is the production of these hormones regulated?
4. How do the steroid hormones act on their target tissues? Are their effects short term (seconds to minutes) or long term (days to years)?
5. What enzyme is most likely deficient in this child, and how does this affect the blood levels of the different types of steroid hormone?
6. Blood electrolytes were determined in this patient. Do the levels of inorganic ions fluctuate over a wide range, or are they kept fairly constant in the healthy body?
7. Why does this child have abnormal electrolyte levels?
8. What kind of hormone treatment does the chief resident have in mind?
9. The student's proposal certainly has its merits, but can you expect gender identity problems if treatment is delayed? Could there be gender identity problems even if treatment is started immediately after birth?
10. Without treatment, is there a risk of abnormal physical development during childhood and adolescence?
11. When the parents ask you about whether this condition is heritable and whether a next child will be at risk, what do you tell them?
12. This patient has a serious developmental problem. However, are there also normal or near-normal variations in adrenal steroid synthesis that cause mild virilization of girls and women without an intersex phenotype?

Suggested Reading

Coate FA, Grumbach MM: Abnormalities of sexual determination and differentiation. In Greenspan FS, Gardner DG (eds): Basic & Clinical Endocrinology, 7th ed. New York: Lange/McGraw-Hill, 2004, pp 564-607.

Miller WL, New MI: Genetics of adrenal steroid disorders. In Baxter JD, Melmed S, New MI (eds): Genetics in Endocrinology. Philadelphia: Lippincott Williams & Wilkins, 2002, pp 331-363.

New MI, Wilson RC: Genetic disorders of the adrenal gland. In Emery AEH, Rimoin DL (eds): Emery and Rimoin's Principles and Practice of Medical Genetics, 4th ed, vol 3. Edinburgh: Churchill Livingstone, 2002, pp 2277-2314.

Man Overboard!

Crispin Darroux is an Afro-Caribbean who was born on a small Caribbean island. He had spent his youth without major health problems, and by the age of 20 he was earning his living with temporary jobs in addition to small-scale farming.

One day he went to sea with some fishermen from his village. Far off the coast, they located a shoal of fish. It was close to midday. The sun was bright and the weather was hot, but a fresh breeze kept the men cool when they were finally ready to throw their net. While throwing the net, Mr. Darroux suddenly fainted and fell overboard.

The next thing he remembered was lying in the ambulance, in which somebody told the driver to drive as fast as possible because otherwise they would have a dead man. However, he passed out again and did not regain full consciousness until 2 days later in the local hospital, with saline solution from a bag above his head gently dripping toward his vein.

The doctor then told him that he had sickle cell disease. Mr. Darroux had already heard about sickle cell disease because one of his uncles, whom he had never met, was said to have died of it. However, he was surprised that he had the disease, since he had not had attacks of pain or fainting before. Physical examination findings at that time were inconspicuous except for a scar on the leg. Mr. Darroux said this scar was from a sore that he had had for more than a year before it finally healed.

Thirty years later, the patient reports that since this first episode, he has had recurrent attacks of joint pain. These attacks typically started with pin-prick-like pain in one or a few joints, which then intensified and spread more widely to other joints and bones. Self-medication with Tylenol or other mild analgesics was sometimes effective, but at other times he had to go to the hospital, where he was treated with intravenous fluids. On several occasions, when the pain was especially bad, he was given an injection that put him to sleep for about 6 hours, but the pain always returned after he woke up. The doctor had told him that he must not get this injection too often, because it would lose its effectiveness. Blood tests were done in the hospital on two occasions. The results are shown in Table C-3.

The patient reports that the attacks are unpredictable and occur without relation to food, weather, or time of day. However, he noticed that he did not take well to vigorous physical activity. Once he had to stop digging a septic tank when he noticed the first signs of joint pain while feeling cold and dizzy. For the past 15 years, he has been working as a security guard for a local hotel.

Over the years, his attacks decreased in frequency and severity. Lately he has had serious attacks only once or twice a year on average. He ascribes this improvement to his religious faith and to better adherence to his doctor's advice to drink plenty of water.

Mr. Darroux is married and has three children. His daughter is healthy, but both his sons have sickle cell disease. One of them has recurrent attacks of joint pain, like his father, and the other has pain mainly in the abdomen. One of Mr. Darroux's nieces died of sickle cell disease a few years ago, at the age of 10. After a cold, the girl became severely ill. She was flown to a neighboring island where better treatment facilities were available. She improved initially and returned home but died suddenly a few days later. According to the autopsy report, her death was caused by a problem with her spleen.

Mr. Darroux understands the heritable nature of his disease, although he did not know about it when he was young. He says he does not want others to suffer the way he is suffering. Therefore, he told his children that before marrying, they should have their partners tested and should marry only if a partner is not a carrier.

Questions

1. What is the normal hemoglobin concentration in erythrocytes? What is the normal hemoglobin concentration in whole blood, and how does this relate to hematocrit and intracorpuscular hemoglobin concentration?
2. Describe the normal life cycle of erythrocytes, from the cradle to the grave. How does the sickle cell mutation affect this life cycle?
3. What kind of mutation causes sickle cell disease, and how does this mutation lead to sickling?

Table C-3 Results of Blood Tests, Determined During Two Different Admissions for Sickling Crisis (Patients 1 and 2, respectively)

	Patient (1)	Patient (2)	Normal
Red blood cells/μL × 10^6	4.83	4.88	4.2–5.8
Hemoglobin (% w/v)	10.8	10.6	14–18
Hematocrit (%)	34.8	34.7	42–52
Mean corpuscular volume (μm³)	72.1	71.2	80–94
Mean corpuscular hemoglobin (pg)	22.5	21.8	27–31
Mean corpuscular hemoglobin concentration (% w/v),	31.2	30.6	33–37
Platelets/μL × 10^3	183.0	176.0	130–400
White blood cells/μL × 10^3	8.9	5.0	4.8–10.8

4. Can you estimate (or even calculate) the frequency of sickle cell disease in a population in which 10% are carriers?

5. What causes the recurrent pain episodes of sickle cell disease?

6. Can frequent sickling lead to lasting organ damage?

7. What external circumstances triggered the patient's near-fatal attack on the fishing boat?

8. During this first attack, the patient lost consciousness. What sequence of physiological events is likely to have caused this?

9. Why does strenuous physical activity precipitate pain attacks in some patients?

10. Even if they do not develop a pain attack, patients with sickle cell disease tire easily during strenuous physical activity. Why?

11. By what mechanisms can dehydration precipitate an attack, and why are intravenous fluids used for treatment?

12. What kind of injection was used to put Mr. Darroux to sleep when he suffered severe pain? Other than the loss of effectiveness, could there be another reason for using these injections sparingly?

13. Patients with sickle cell disease are sometimes treated with blood transfusions. What are the benefits and risks of this treatment, and under what circumstances do the benefits outweigh the risks?

14. Oxygen treatment is not very effective during sickling crisis and is therefore rarely used. Why?

15. In addition to religious faith and plenty of water, what else can be tried to reduce the frequency of pain attacks?

16. Would gene therapy be a promising treatment option?

17. In principle, could new drugs that manipulate erythrocyte pH or 2,3-bisphosphoglycerate concentration be effective in sickle cell disease?

18. In one case, a dramatic spontaneous improvement of a patient with sickle cell disease was reported, with complete cessation of pain attacks and hemoglobin concentration rising to the normal range. This improvement could finally be attributed to a leak in his gas stove. How can a leak in the gas stove cure sickle cell disease?

19. What kinds of complications could Mr. Darroux possibly develop as he gets older?

20. The spleen is not essential for life, inasmuch as its functions are duplicated by reticuloendothelial cells in other parts of the body. How could a splenic problem cause the death of Mr. Darroux's niece?

21. Mr. Darroux advised his sons not to marry someone with the sickle cell trait. Is this a sensible attitude? Should he give the same advice to his unaffected daughter?

22. Is it appropriate for a physician in Europe or the United States to tell an affected patient not to marry someone with the sickle cell trait? What about in China?

23. Mr. Darroux was healthy before age 20, and has only infrequent attacks today. Looking at his laboratory values, what could be responsible for the relatively benign course of his disease?

24. Is HbS the only hemoglobin mutation that can cause sickling?

25. In which parts of the world is the sickle cell mutation found, and why is it common only in certain human populations but not others?

26. Does the sickle cell mutation arise frequently in human populations? Or are all sickle cell patients the descendants of one person with an original mutation?

27. How can you determine whether a mutation occurred only once or more than once, and can you use molecular methods to determine the geographic area in which a new mutation first occurred?

28. Does the severity of sickle cell disease vary with the geographic origin of the mutation? Are there any other genetic traits that modulate the severity of sickle cell disease?

📖 Suggested Reading

Bunn HF: Human hemoglobins: sickle hemoglobin and other mutants. In Stamatoyannopoulos G, Majerus PW, Perlmutter RM, et al (eds): The Molecular Basis of Blood Diseases, 3rd ed. Philadelphia: WB Saunders, 2001, pp 227-273.

Hesketh T: Getting married in China: pass the medical first. BMJ 326:277-279, 2003.

Michie S, Bron F, Bobrow M, et al: Nondirectiveness in genetic counseling: an empirical study. Am J Hum Genet 60:40-47, 1997.

Old J: Hemoglobinopathies and thalassemias. In Emery AEH, Rimoin DL (eds): Emery and Rimoin's Principles and Practice of Medical Genetics, 4th ed, vol 3. Edinburgh: Churchill Livingstone, 2002, pp 1861-1898.

Platt OS: Sickle syndromes. In Handin RI, Lux SE, Stossel TP (eds): Blood: Principles and Practice of Hematology, 2nd ed. Philadelphia: Lippincott Williams & Wilkins, 2002, pp 1655-1708.

🗂 Spongy Bones

Fred Knickerbocker is a 72-year-old man who has been living alone since the death of his wife 5 years ago. Long retired, he spends his days mainly at home housekeeping, reading, and watching TV.

One day in March, while changing a bulb in the ceiling light of his living room, he lost balance and fell from the stool he was standing on. Immediately he felt a sharp pain in his right hip joint. Although every movement of the hip caused him severe pain, he finally managed to reach for the telephone and call the ambulance.

In the hospital, the hip joint was found to be broken, and a cast was applied. He asked the doctor, "How could this happen? Just a little fall. I never had a broken bone in my life." However, on questioning he mentions that he had had occasional bone pain during the past years and that this was perhaps one reason why he was not as physically active as he should be.

Physical examination findings were unremarkable. The sclera of the eye had a normal color. One day after admission, blood was taken for laboratory tests. Some of the results were as follows:

Na^+:	144 mmol/liter (136 to 145)
K^+:	3.6 mmol/liter (3.5 to 4.5)
Ca^{2+}:	1.55 mmol/liter (2.20 to 2.55)
Mg^{2+}:	0.80 mmol/liter (0.66 to 1.07)
Cl^-:	105 mmol/liter (98 to 107)
HCO_3^-:	24 mmol/liter (22 to 29)
HPO_4^{2-}:	0.52 mmol/liter (0.74 to 1.20)

Several blood enzymes were also measured. The only abnormality was an elevation of alkaline phosphatase to 480 U/liter, five times the upper limit of normal. When questioned about his lifestyle, the patient says that he rarely leaves the house during the day. He likes to sleep long and is most active in the evenings, when he also does most of his shopping. He spends one or two evenings every week with friends in the pub playing cards. He gave up smoking 40 years ago and does not drink alcohol except for "two or three drinks" with his friends in the pub. He lives mainly on canned food, soft drinks, and supper from the fast food place round the corner. He does not drink any milk, nor does he like milk products such as cheese and yogurt. A radioimmunoassay for vitamin D showed that the blood level of 25-OH-vitamin D_3 was 2 ng/mL (normal, 14 to 60 ng/mL).

Questions

1. What protein is most abundant in bone, and how is it synthesized? Does this require any vitamins or trace minerals?
2. What is the inorganic component of bone? How is its formation in the bones regulated? Does alkaline phosphatase play a role in this process?
3. How can age-related hormonal changes influence bone structure?
4. The patient's sclera was found to have a normal color. Do you know a bone disease that is accompanied by an unusual color of the sclera? What feature in the patient's history suggests that he does not have this disease?
5. How is 25-OH-vitamin D_3 formed? Is this the biologically active form of vitamin D?
6. Could the low vitamin D level be related to the season?
7. What are the biological functions of vitamin D, and how do they relate to the bone problems that are typical for vitamin D deficiency?
8. Is a milk-free diet bad for this patient?
9. How do abnormal plasma levels of calcium or phosphate affect bone mineralization?
10. How do vitamin D and PTH interact in the regulation of calcium and phosphate metabolism? Would you expect a high or a low PTH level in this patient?
11. Is hormone replacement recommended as a treatment strategy for bone problems in old people?

Suggested Reading

Delaney MF, LeBoff MS: Metabolic bone disease. In Ruddy S, Harris ED, Sledge CB, et al (eds): Kelley's Textbook of Rheumatology, 6th ed. Philadelphia: WB Saunders, 2001, pp 1635-1652.

Foroud T, Econs MJ, Johnston CC: Genetics of osteoporosis. In King RA, Rotter JI, Motulsky AG (eds): The Genetic Basis of Common Diseases, 2nd ed. Oxford, UK: Oxford University Press, 2002, pp 510-517.

Raisz LG, Kream BE, Lorenzo JA: Metabolic bone disease. In Larsen PR, Kronenberg HM, Melmed S, et al (eds): Williams Textbook of Endocrinology, 10th ed. Philadelphia: WB Saunders, 2003, pp 1373-1410.

Shoback D, Marcus R, Bikle D: Metabolic bone disease. In Greenspan FS, Gardner DG (eds): Basic & Clinical Endocrinology, 7th ed. New York: Lange/McGraw-Hill, 2004, pp 295-361.

Blisters

The patient is an 18-year-old woman with a chronic skin disease. She presented at birth with multiple blisters of the arms and legs. Mechanically induced and spontaneous blisters continued to appear, the extremities, head, and face being most often affected. The blisters healed without scars but with some atrophy and hyperpigmentation. Periungual blistering and paronychia led to dystrophy of all nails. Beginning at the age of 6 years, patchy alopecia of the scalp developed, leading to loss of all parietal hair. The oral mucosa and the tongue were regularly involved with erosions. Electron microscopy showed junctional blistering and

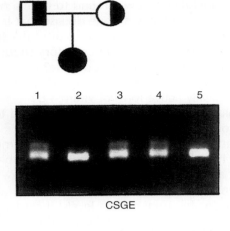

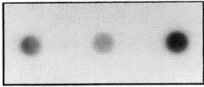

ASO: Wildtype sequence

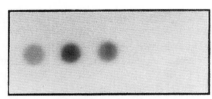

ASO: Mutated sequence

hypoplastic hemidesmosomes. The patient is the only child of healthy parents. There is no family history of related skin diseases or similar genetic disorders. There was no known history of consanguinity, but both parents were from the same region in the Swiss Alps.

The condition was diagnosed as a form of junctional epidermolysis bullosa, a disease that is known to be caused by mutations in the gene for collagen 17 in many affected patients. The sequence of this gene is known. To identify the mutation responsible for her disease, several exons of the patient's *COL17A1* gene were amplified with PCR. Amplification products were subjected to a mutation scan, with the use of conformation-sensitive gel electrophoresis. In this procedure, gel electrophoresis is performed with a heteroduplex formed between the patient's DNA and normal DNA. Exon 45 showed a mismatch, and the PCR product was sequenced. The patient was found to be homozygous for a C → T transition in exon 45 that converted a glutamine-coding codon into a stop codon.

Figure C-2 above shows the appearance of the stained gel on conformation-sensitive gel elec-

trophoresis for the amplified patient DNA (lane 2), the DNA of the patient's parents (lanes 1 and 3), an unrelated normal person (lane 5), and the patient's DNA mixed with the normal person's DNA (lane 4). It also shows dot-blots with allele-specific oligonucleotides for the normal (wild-type) sequence and the mutation.

Questions

1. Skin blistering diseases are caused by abnormalities in the dermal-epidermal junction. Describe the normal structure of this junction and the more important structural proteins.
2. What types of blistering diseases are commonly distinguished, and what proteins are involved?
3. Some skin blistering diseases are caused not by abnormalities of proteins in hemidesmosomes or the extracellular matrix but by defects in cytoskeletal proteins. What cytoskeletal proteins are present in the epidermis, what is their structure, and how do they interact with the cell-cell junctions that hold the epidermal cells together?
4. In this case, one of the collagen genes is mutated. Describe the general structure of the collagens and their biosynthesis.
5. What types of collagen occur in the skin, and what are their functions?
6. The DNA was amplified by PCR. Describe this procedure.
7. For conformation-sensitive gel electrophoresis, you have to adjust the conditions in such a way that annealing is complete in a homoduplex (no base mismatch) but incomplete in a heteroduplex (mismatch present), so that only the mismatched DNA smears over the gel. How can you manipulate the strength of base-pairing by adjustments of temperature, ionic strength, and pH?
8. Could DNA microarrays (DNA chips) be used for mutation scanning?

📖 Suggested Reading

Anton-Lamprecht I, Gedde-Dahl T: Epidermolysis bullosa. In Emery AEH, Rimoin DL (eds): Emery and Rimoin's Principles and Practice of Medical Genetics, 4th ed, vol 3. Edinburgh: Churchill Livingstone, 2002, pp 3810-3897.

Schumann H, Hammami-Hauasli N, Pulkkinen L, et al: Three novel homozygous point mutations and a new polymorphism in the COL17A1 gene: relation to biological and clinical phenotypes of junctional epidermolysis bullosa. Am J Hum Genet 60:1344-1353, 1997.

Uitto J, Pulkkinen L: Epidermolysis bullosa: the disease of the cutaneous basement membrane zone. In

Scriver CR, Beaudet AL, Sly WS, et al (eds): The Metabolic and Molecular Basis of Inherited Disease, 8th ed, vol 4. New York: McGraw-Hill, 2001, pp 5655-5674.

📁 The Sunburned Child

A Hispanic girl developed freckles on sun-exposed areas of the skin at the age of 10 months. Squamous and basal cell carcinomas, as well as premalignant lesions (keratoacanthomas and actinic keratoses) began to develop in these damaged areas at 17 months of age. The condition was diagnosed as xeroderma pigmentosum, and strict avoidance of sunlight was prescribed. Over the next 3 years, several malignant tumors had to be surgically removed from various parts of her face. When she was 4 years, 8 months old, a full-face dermabrasion was performed. In this procedure, performed with the patient under general anesthesia, the epidermis is abraded along with the topmost part of the dermis. A small (2 × 2 cm) squamous cell carcinoma was also removed from near her left ear on this occasion.

Healing proceeded well during the months after the procedure, and the child avoided sun exposure altogether. However, several malignancies appeared again in the course of the following 5 years, and these were promptly excised. She is again developing disfiguring skin lesions but has led a relatively normal life except for strict sun avoidance.

Questions

1. Describe the DNA repair system that is defective in this patient. What proteins are involved, and what type of sunlight-induced damage does this system repair in the skin?
2. What other DNA repair systems do you know? Can defects in these other systems also lead to diseases?
3. The malignant skin tumors that this patient develops are otherwise seen mainly in older people. Why is this the case, although young people are as much exposed to the sun as are older people?
4. Exposure to sunlight is the most important risk factor for skin cancer, and the formation of melanin is an important protective mechanism. How is melanin formed? What cell types are involved, and from which precursor is melanin made?
5. What is the rationale for dermabrasion, and how can the abraded epidermis regenerate?
6. The exact molecular defect in this patient has not been determined, but all forms of xeroderma pigmentosum are known to be inherited as autosomal recessive traits. How high is the risk of the disease in a younger sibling? Can you think of a method for prenatal diagnosis that can be used even if it is not known which gene is involved?
7. What methods for prenatal diagnosis could be used if scientists knew which gene is mutated but not the mutation itself? What could be done if the exact mutations in the parents were known?

📖 Suggested Reading

Bootsma D, et al: Nucleotide excision repair syndromes: xeroderma pigmentosum, Cockayne syndrome, and trichothiodystrophy. In Scriver CR, Beaudet AL, Sly WS, et al (eds): The Metabolic and Molecular Basis of Inherited Disease, 8th ed, vol 1. New York: McGraw-Hill, 2001, pp 677-703.

Moses RE: DNA damage processing defects and disease. Annu Rev Genomics Hum Genet 2:41-68, 2001.

Ocampo-Candiani J, Silva-Siwady G, Fernandez-Gutierrez L, et al: Dermabrasion in xeroderma pigmentosum. Dermatol Surg 22:575-577, 1996.

📁 Too Much Ammonia

The patient is a boy, now 2 years old, who was the product of an uncomplicated pregnancy. There was no family history of problems during the neonatal period. Two days after birth, while still in the hospital nursery, he was noted to have feeding difficulties. In essence, he refused to drink at all. The next morning, he was found in an agitated state, breathing heavily and in obvious distress.

An infection was suspected, and he was treated with intravenous antibiotics, although there was no fever. Actually, the body temperature was below normal. However, the child's condition worsened, and the antibiotics were soon discontinued when blood and sputum cultures failed to produce evidence of bacterial pathogens.

The blood tests showed a blood pH of 7.5 (normal, 7.35 to 7.45), and the blood pCO_2 level was 8 mEq/liter (normal, 25 to 28). Otherwise, blood electrolyte levels were in the normal range. Blood glucose, ketone bodies, and bilirubin levels were normal. The levels of transaminases, creatine kinase, and BUN also showed no abnormality. However, the blood ammonia level was 1800 μmol/liter (normal, 10 to 40).

When this result was in, treatment with intravenous sodium benzoate and sodium phenylacetate was started immediately, and the patient's condition stabilized over the next days. Additional blood samples had been taken before the initiation of treatment and sent to a metabolic screening laboratory. The metabolic screen showed the following abnormalities (normal ranges in parentheses):

Ammonia: 2100 µmol/liter (15 to 40)
Glutamine: 3200 µmol/liter (470 to 750)
Citrulline: <2 µmol/liter (11 to 21)

Amino acid analysis of the urine showed the presence of a large amount of ornithine. The presence of orotic acid was also demonstrated in the urine. A liver biopsy was taken for enzymatic tests, and ornithine transcarbamoylase was found to be completely absent. The child was treated with a combination of sodium phenylacetate and sodium benzoate. The dose had to be readjusted repeatedly and was varied between 100 mg/kg and 200 mg/kg of benzoate and 250 mg/kg and 500 mg/kg of phenylacetate. At 18 months, phenylbutyrate was substituted for phenylacetate. The child had to be kept in the hospital throughout because of feeding difficulties that necessitated the use of a nasogastric tube. Ammonia determinations were done frequently, and values between 250 and 1000 µmol/liter were obtained.

Seizures developed at age 14 months, and these were controlled with clonazepam. At 2 years of age, neurological development was severely impaired. The child had spastic quadriparesis and still had difficulty sitting without support. Although he babbled or showed distress vocalizations at times, he was unable to form intelligible words. Social responses were limited mainly to simple orienting responses.

Questions

1. Describe the reactions of the urea cycle. Where in the cell do these reactions occur?
2. Levels of which urea cycle intermediates are likely to be elevated in this patient, and which ones are likely to be reduced? What about carbamoyl phosphate?
3. All urea cycle enzyme deficiencies lead to the accumulation of glutamine. Describe the reactions that are responsible for this. What are the normal functions of these reactions?
4. Ammonia damages the nervous system. Can you speculate about possible mechanisms for this neurotoxicity?
5. The presence of orotic acid was noted in the patient's urine. From which pathway is orotic acid derived, and why does it accumulate?

6. Why was the patient treated with phenylacetate, phenylbutyrate, and benzoate? Do you know any other disease in which this treatment can be used?
7. Dietary manipulations are not mentioned in the treatment regimen. If you were in charge of this patient, what kind of special diet would you design?
8. Patients with ornithine transcarbamoylase deficiency are sometimes given supplementary citrulline or arginine. Why?
9. The patient had alkalosis during the first attack of hyperammonemia shortly after birth. Was this respiratory or metabolic alkalosis?
10. Would patients with inherited urea cycle enzyme deficiencies be candidates for liver transplantation? Do you know any other metabolic diseases in which liver transplantation could be tried?
11. Most patients with ornithine transcarbamoylase deficiency have a "guarded" prognosis, but some are less seriously affected and do fairly well with adequate treatment. Why do some patients have a better prognosis than others?
12. What diagnostic tests can you consult to find out which patients are likely to do well and which ones are going to die or end up with profound neurological defects?
13. Once the diagnosis is made, how would you go about explaining the situation to the parents? Can the parents elect to withhold treatment from the child?
14. Ornithine transcarbamoylase deficiency is inherited as an X-linked recessive disease. Do you expect that a sizable fraction of the patients have a new mutation? How would you go about genetic counseling, and what strategies can be used for prenatal diagnosis?

📖 Suggested Reading

Brusilow SW, Horwich AL: Urea cycle enzymes. In Scriver CR, Beaudet AL, Sly WS, et al (eds): The Metabolic and Molecular Basis of Inherited Disease, 8th ed, vol 2. New York: McGraw-Hill, 2001, pp 1909-1963.

Wilcox WR, Cederbaum SD: Amino acid metabolism. In Emery AEH, Rimoin DL (eds): Emery and Rimoin's Principles and Practice of Medical Genetics, 4th ed, vol 3. Edinburgh: Churchill Livingstone, 2002, pp 2405-2440.

Answers to Case Studies

The Mafia Boss

Sixty percent of the adult human body is water. Therefore, the density of the body is close to 1.0 g/cm^3. The bones have densities exceeding 1.0 g/cm^3, as do protein-rich tissues. The fat in adipose tissue (typically 10 to 15 kg) has a density close to 0.9 g/cm^3. Gas-filled spaces are present in lungs and intestine. Shortly after death, a body will sink in water as much of the air is forced out of the lungs. However, within 1 to 3 days after death, intestinal bacteria form large quantities of gas (carbon dioxide, methane, and hydrogen) as they start invading the surrounding tissues. The body floats to the surface at this time. According to the source of this case study (a popular book about organized crime in America), the doctor advised the Mafia boss to make a hole in the abdomen with an ice pick, so that the trapped gas could escape.

Viral Gastroenteritis

Gastroenteritis is a common viral infection, especially in children. Vomiting and diarrhea can lead to serious dehydration and general weakness, but most cases are mild and self-limited. Breast-feeding provides some protection through maternal immunoglobulin A antibodies. The infection tends to compromise the digestive and absorptive functions of the intestinal mucosa. In this case, small amounts of a "reducing substance" were demonstrated in the urine. This was probably undigested lactose, which entered the blood stream through the damaged intestinal mucosa. Like other disaccharides, lactose is not metabolized in the tissues once it has entered the blood but is excreted in the urine.

Monosaccharides and disaccharides with at least one free anomeric carbon, including all monosaccharides and most disaccharides (but not sucrose), have reducing properties. The nature of a reducing substance in the urine can be determined by enzymatic tests, such as the glucose oxidase test for free glucose.

This patient seems to have an impaired ability of lactose digestion. The lactose intolerance is secondary, caused by the infection. Primary lactose intolerance, caused by functional polymorphisms in the regulator regions of the lactase gene, is uncommon in infants although it is very common in older children and adults.

Undigested lactose is readily fermented by intestinal bacteria (e.g., the *lac* operon of *Escherichia coli*). Bacterial fermentation produces acetic, propionic, and lactic acids, as well as the gases methane, hydrogen, and carbon dioxide. Diarrhea is caused by the osmotic effect of lactose and by the irritant effects of the acids on the intestine.

The beneficial effects of the therapeutic milk formula probably arose from the absence of lactose. Also, the use of casein hydrolysate instead of intact milk proteins may have contributed to the effect. The hydrolysate is more easily digested and, unlike some of the milk proteins, the small peptides in the hydrolysate are unlikely to trigger immune responses.

Death in Installments

This patient suffers from metachromatic leukodystrophy, a lipid storage disease caused by a recessively inherited deficiency of sulfatidase. Undegraded sulfatide (sulfated galactocerebroside) accumulates in the lysosomes. Because lysosomal enzymes as a rule are not tissue specific, the deficiency is expressed in all tissues. However, because the turnover of sulfatide tends to be highest in nervous tissue (especially myelin), the dominant feature of the disease is neurological deterioration.

A complete deficiency of the enzyme causes death in infancy or early childhood, but incomplete deficiencies result in a milder and more protracted course. This patient seems to have an abnormal enzyme that acts poorly on its natural substrate, although it works quite well on arylsulfates, phenolic sulfate esters that can be used for the assay of sulfatidase ("arylsulfatase A") in the laboratory.

Lipid storage diseases are rare, and therefore the diagnosis is often missed. Histological examinations can be helpful because they show the abnormal accumulation of lipids in lysosomes. Definitive diagnosis requires either enzyme determinations or the electrophoretic separation of lipids from biopsy samples or cultured cells. These tests are often done with cultured leukocytes or fibroblasts. The cultured cells grow better on serum than on plasma because blood clotting is induced when serum is prepared from fresh blood. When platelets are activated during blood clotting, they release platelet-derived growth factor (PDGF). PDGF is an excellent stimulus for the growth of cultured cells.

Many diseases can cause neurological degeneration. Therefore the differential diagnosis requires a broad range of diagnostic tests. This patient had been tested specifically for pernicious anemia (vitamin B_{12} level), Wilson disease (ceruloplasmin level, liver function tests), and syphilis. Pneumoencephalography is an obsolete method for the diagnosis of ventricular dilatation and cerebral atrophy; it was replaced long ago by computed tomography and other imaging techniques.

Lumbar puncture is most commonly performed for the diagnosis of central nervous system (CNS) infections. An elevated cerebrospinal fluid (CSF) protein concentration and reduced CSF glucose are typical for bacterial infections. CSF protein levels are normally very low in comparison with protein levels in the plasma (20 mg/dL versus 7000 mg/dL), and the CSF glucose concentration is about two thirds of the blood glucose concentration. Glucose is transported into the brain by facilitated diffusion, which is a passive process that can transport glucose only down a concentration gradient. Because glucose is consumed but not produced in the brain, its CSF level must be less than the plasma level.

A Mysterious Death

Methylmalonic acidemia (also called methylmalonic aciduria) is caused by a recessively inherited deficiency of the vitamin B_{12}–dependent enzyme methylmalonyl-CoA mutase, which converts methylmalonyl-CoA to succinyl-CoA. This reaction participates in the catabolism of valine, isoleucine, methionine, threonine, and odd-chain fatty acids. Methylmalonic acid accumulates and

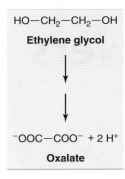

causes life-threatening acidosis. Methylmalonic acidemia can be mistaken for ethylene glycol poisoning because ethylene glycol is metabolized to oxalic acid, which also causes severe acidosis, as shown in Figure C-3 above.

Acidosis results in peripheral vasodilation and circulatory shock. Through baroreceptors, the drop in blood pressure triggers a massive release of epinephrine from the adrenal medulla and norepinephrine from sympathetic nerve terminals. Epinephrine and norepinephrine not only upregulate the blood pressure but also induce fat breakdown in adipose tissue. Fatty acids are transported from adipose tissue to the liver, in which they are converted to ketone bodies. This amounts to a vicious cycle because the ketone bodies, being acidic, aggravate the acidosis.

In a substantial minority of patients, the disease is caused not by a deficiency of methylmalonyl-CoA mutase but by an inability to convert dietary vitamin B_{12} to the active coenzyme form adenosyl-cobalamin. These patients can be treated with adenosyl-cobalamin. The possibilities for dietary treatment by the restriction of valine, isoleucine, methionine, and threonine are limited because these amino acids are nutritionally essential and cannot be excluded from the diet.

To Treat or Not to Treat?

Nonketotic hyperglycinemia is caused by a recessively inherited deficiency of the glycine cleavage enzyme, the major enzyme of glycine degradation. Glycine serves important functions in the central nervous system. It is an inhibitory neurotransmitter in the spinal cord and brain stem, and it acts as coligand for the N-methyl-D-aspartate (NMDA) receptor, an important excitatory amino acid receptor in the brain. Therefore the abnormal accumulation of glycine in patients with nonketotic hyperglycinemia induces both CNS depression and CNS excitation. Untreated patients die of sudden apnea or status epilepticus within a few months after birth, and survivors develop severe CNS dysfunction and mental deficiency.

Dietary treatment is not effective because glycine is formed endogenously from serine, which in turn is synthesized from a glycolytic intermediate. Benzoic acid can be used for treatment because it becomes conjugated with glycine. The hippuric acid thus formed is excreted in the urine. However, the doses of benzoic acid necessary to reduce the blood and CSF levels of glycine are enormous, and the treatment does not prevent brain damage, although it makes survival possible. Because the conjugation reaction takes place in the liver and other peripheral tissues, benzoic acid lowers the glycine level mainly in the periphery but less so in the CNS.

Carnitine deficiency can develop because carnitine reacts enzymatically with many organic acids, including benzoic acid. The resulting conjugation product is excreted in the urine.

Ethical problems arise because the patient would not be viable without heroic treatment; her capacity for suffering is uncertain because there is no possibility of communication; and the patient cannot give informed consent to her treatment. Some parents may request the discontinuation of life-prolonging treatment. In addition, insurance companies are reluctant to pay for prolonged treatment, although the treating physician can derive substantial income from the patient's continued existence.

Yellow Eyes

Jaundice in an adult can be caused by hemolytic conditions, liver disease, or obstructive biliary disease. In this patient, biliary obstruction is suggested by the abnormal color of stool and urine. In normal individuals, the brown color of the stool is caused by colored stercobilin and other urobilins that are generated from bilirubin diglucuronide by intestinal bacteria. Biliary obstruction prevents bilirubin diglucuronide from reaching the intestine. Therefore, the urobilins cannot be formed. The bilirubin diglucuronide that cannot reach the intestine "overflows" into the blood and is eventually excreted in the urine, to which it imparts a brownish color. Unlike the unconjugated variety, conjugated bilirubin is water soluble and not protein-bound. Therefore, it is excreted by the kidneys.

The substantially elevated level of alkaline phosphatase in the presence of only mildly elevated alanine transaminase suggests that the jaundice is caused by acute biliary obstruction rather than liver disease. The same is suggested by the preponderance of "direct" (conjugated) bilirubin over "indirect" (unconjugated) bilirubin.

The absence of urobilinogen in stool and urine also suggests cholestasis. Urobilinogen is formed from bilirubin diglucuronide by intestinal bacteria. Its urinary level would be increased in hemolysis because of increased formation of bilirubin diglucuronide and in liver disease because of impaired enterohepatic circulation of urobilinogen. The normal hematocrit in this case argues against hemolysis.

The patient's prolonged prothrombin time is caused by impaired vitamin K absorption. Like the other fat-soluble vitamins, vitamin K requires bile salts for efficient intestinal absorption. The clotting problem would therefore respond to vitamin K injection or to large doses of oral vitamin K.

Biliary obstruction can result from a number of diseases, including malignancies. This patient has cancer of the head of the pancreas. About two thirds of pancreatic cancers originate in the head of the pancreas. They compress the common bile duct and often manifest with obstructive jaundice before other signs of malignant disease (weight loss, pain) are evident. Most pancreatic cancers are highly aggressive, and surgical resection is rarely possible.

Cancer chemotherapy is based on the use of agents with selective toxicity for rapidly dividing cells. Some antineoplastic drugs, including methotrexate (a folate antagonist) and fluorouracil (a base analog), inhibit nucleotide metabolism and DNA synthesis. Others, including vincristine, bind to tubulin and interfere with the formation of the mitotic spindle.

An Abdominal Emergency

Abdominal pain with acute onset can be caused by many diseases, including food poisoning, peptic ulcer, biliary disease, intestinal infarction, hernia, renal disease, malignancies, and pancreatitis. Blood tests are essential for the diagnosis. This patient shows no evidence of liver or biliary disease (normal alanine transaminase, alkaline phosphatase, and bilirubin levels) or renal disease (normal urea and creatinine levels). The α-amylase level, however, is elevated to a degree typical for patients with acute pancreatitis.

Acute pancreatitis is a disease in which pancreatic zymogens, including proteases and phospholipases, become activated in the pancreas rather than the duodenum. The activated enzymes destroy pancreatic tissue and spill over into the abdominal cavity and the blood stream. The action of pancreatic lipase on intra-abdominal adipose tissue produces free fatty acids. The binding of calcium by these fatty acids can lead to hypocalcemia. Hypomagnesemia is the result of excessive vomiting, and hyperglycemia can develop when the endocrine pancreas is damaged by the out-of-control enzymes.

The treatment of acute pancreatitis is based on the complete avoidance of food because food constituents, particularly fat and protein, stimulate pancreatic enzyme production and fluid secretion. These effects are mediated by the hormones cholecystokinin (pancreozymin) and secretin.

The immediate cause for an attack of acute pancreatitis is rarely known with certainty, but a dislodged gallstone is the culprit in some cases. A gallstone lodged in the ampulla of Vater can impair the patency of the pancreatic duct and even, in patients with joint pancreatic and common bile ducts, lead to a reflux of bile into the pancreatic duct system.

Normal bile contains a substantial amount of bile salts (deprotonated bile acids) along with smaller amounts of phospholipid, free (unesterified) cholesterol, inorganic ions, and "bile pigments" (bilirubin diglucuronide and its derivatives). Cholesterol is insoluble in water and must be kept in solution as a constituent of mixed bile salt–phospholipid micelles. Most gallstones consist of cholesterol. They form when the cholesterol concentration of the bile is increased or the concentration of bile salts and phospholipid is reduced ("lithogenic" bile). Gallstones usually form in the gallbladder, where the bile becomes concentrated by the absorption of water and electrolytes across the gallbladder epithelium.

High-calorie diets and obesity favor the formation of gallstones by raising the cholesterol level in the bile. Bile acid–binding resins such as cholestyramine, which are sometimes used for the treatment of hypercholesterolemia, can trigger gallstone formation in susceptible individuals by reducing the supply of bile salts through the enterohepatic circulation. Conversely, orally administered bile acids, such as chenodeoxycholic acid (chenodiol) and ursodeoxycholic acid, can be helpful because they enter the bile through the enterohepatic circulation, in which they help dissolve the stones. However, these bile acids can raise LDL cholesterol by inhibiting the conversion of cholesterol to bile salts by 7α-hydroxylase in the liver. The accumulating cholesterol inhibits the synthesis of LDL receptors in the liver.

Shortness of Breath

Death rates from coronary heart disease have been declining since the mid-1970s, not because of improved lifestyle but because of more aggressive treatment. However, coronary heart disease is still the most important cause of death in the United States and in most other Western countries as well. It is caused by atheromatous lesions in the coronary arteries that encroach on the arterial lumen and impair blood flow to the myocardium.

High levels of LDL are known to promote atherosclerosis, whereas high levels of high-density lipoprotein (HDL) are protective. Also, elevated very-low-density lipoprotein (VLDL) levels in patients with type IV hyperlipoproteinemia increase the risk of coronary heart disease. These lipid abnormalities promote the accumulation of cholesterol esters in the walls of large arteries to form fatty streaks. Fatty streaks are reversible lesions, but some appear to progress to full-blown atheromatous plaques.

Additional risk factors include smoking, hypertension, and diabetes mellitus. Smoking probably promotes atherosclerosis because cigarette smoke contains oxidants that damage LDL. Oxidized LDL is a preferred substrate for macrophage scavenger receptors and is more readily taken up by macrophages than is virgin LDL. This is an important first step in the formation of a fatty streak. Hypertension exposes the arteries to physical stress, and diabetes mellitus is injurious to arterial walls as well.

Coronary heart disease can result in acute myocardial infarction, typically after the formation of a thrombus (intravascular blood clot) on the surface of the lesion. The thrombus either blocks the artery at the site of the lesion or it causes infarction after being carried into one of the terminal branches of the coronary system. The myocardium can survive acute ischemia for 30 to 60 minutes. After this time, the cells die because of the failure of ATP-dependent ion pumps and the excessive formation of lactic acid from stored glycogen. New infarctions can be distinguished from old scars by the determination of plasma enzymes that leak out of damaged myocardium, including creatine kinase MB, LDH 1, and aspartate transaminase.

Other patients have chronic impairments, including exercise intolerance, shortness of breath, and chest pain on exertion. The last condition is called angina pectoris. This patient has angina pectoris associated with obesity, a sedentary lifestyle, smoking, and type IV hyperlipoproteinemia.

Type IV hyperlipoproteinemia is more likely to respond to dietary carbohydrate restriction rather than lipid restriction. This is because VLDL triglycerides are synthesized from excess carbohydrate in the well-fed liver. The reaction sequence involves glycolysis, fatty acid biosynthesis, and esterification of the fatty acids. Otherwise, polyunsaturated fatty acids rather than saturated fatty acids are recommended because they promote fatty acid oxidation over lipogenesis and reduce the plasma levels of

VLDL and LDL. This effect of polyunsaturated fatty acids is most likely mediated by actions on nuclear receptors.

Nitroglycerin is used for the treatment of angina pectoris because it is a potent vasodilator. It is metabolized to nitric oxide, a short-lived product that activates the cytoplasmic guanylate cyclase in vascular smooth muscle cells. Nitric oxide is otherwise formed by endothelial cells in response to agents that raise the cytoplasmic calcium concentration in the endothelial cells, including histamine, bradykinin, and acetylcholine. Being small and lipid soluble, it diffuses readily from the endothelium into the vascular smooth muscle, in which it acts as an endothelium-derived relaxing factor.

For long-term management of coronary heart disease, smoking should be discouraged. Dietary recommendations for hyperlipidemic patients include a low-cholesterol diet with a high ratio of polyunsaturated to saturated fatty acids, a lot of dietary fiber, and reduced carbohydrate for patients with elevated VLDL. Antioxidant vitamins, particularly vitamins C and E, are recommended because they protect LDL from oxidation. Nonvitamin phytochemicals in tea, red wine, broccoli, and other fruits and vegetables seem to be beneficial, perhaps because of their antioxidant properties.

Coumarin-type anticoagulants can be used in patients with coronary heart disease to prevent acute myocardial infarction, but they are dangerous. Patients receiving long-term anticoagulant treatment have died of cerebral hemorrhages and other complications. Fibrinolytic treatments, either streptokinase or tissue-type plasminogen activator, can be used within 1 hour after acute myocardial infarction in an attempt to dissolve the existing clot and thereby limit the extent of tissue damage.

Several lipid-lowering drugs are available. The statins (e.g., lovastatin) inhibit 3-hydroxy-3-methylglutaryl (HMG)–CoA reductase, the rate-limiting enzyme of cholesterol biosynthesis. They lead initially to a reduced level of free cholesterol in the cells, both in the liver and in many other tissues. The cells respond by increasing the synthesis of LDL receptors. They try to obtain more cholesterol from the blood in an attempt to make up for the shortfall of newly synthesized cholesterol.

Cholestyramine is a nonabsorbable ion exchange resin that binds bile salts and prevents their intestinal absorption. Their reduced supply through the enterohepatic circulation activates 7α-hydroxylase, thereby increasing the conversion of cholesterol to bile salts in the liver. The resulting decrease of the intracellular cholesterol pool stimulates the synthesis of LDL receptors in the liver. Fibrate drugs (e.g., bezafibrate) and niacin reduce the formation of VLDL. The fibrates induce their effects by actions on nuclear receptors of the PPAR-α type.

Coronary bypass surgery has become an increasingly important source of income for the medical profession. It consists of an autograft from the patient's own saphenous vein that bypasses the affected portion of the coronary artery. Bypass surgery can be highly effective, but it carries a nontrivial risk of surgical mortality, and restenosis of the graft in the course of some years is not uncommon.

This patient was enrolled in a double-blind, placebo-controlled clinical study of the protective effects of antioxidant vitamins. A double-blind study is a study in which neither the patient nor the physician knows whether the patient is getting the active treatment or the placebo. A placebo—an inactive substance such as lactose or starch administered in the same form as the active treatment—is essential in clinical trials because the psychological effects of receiving treatment can cause a beneficial therapeutic outcome in the absence of any active ingredient at all.

This patient appears suitable for participation in the clinical trial because he had quit smoking and complied with dietary changes in the past. Noncompliance is a major problem in long-term clinical trials as it is in general medical practice. His blood level of vitamin C was determined because the plasma ascorbic acid level depends on the dietary intake. Noncompliance with the active treatment would be revealed by a low plasma level.

Itching

This patient has primary biliary cirrhosis, an autoimmune disease that leads to inflammation and degeneration of intrahepatic bile ducts. The diagnosis is established by the results of the liver biopsy and the presence of antimitochondrial antibodies. The biochemical abnormalities are those of biliary obstruction, with elevated serum levels of bilirubin, bile acids, alkaline phosphatase, and γ-glutamyltransferase. The serum cholesterol level is elevated because the biliary excretion of cholesterol and bile acids is impaired. The backlog of bile acids inhibits 7α-hydroxylase, the rate-limiting enzyme of bile acid synthesis. Bile acid synthesis is the major metabolic fate of cholesterol in the liver (besides incorporation in VLDL), and the inhibition of bile acid synthesis therefore results in an elevated cholesterol level in the liver. Free cholesterol downregulates the hepatic LDL receptors, and this leads to elevated levels of LDL cholesterol.

Copper accumulates in patients with cholestasis because the bile is the normal vehicle for copper excretion. Like other heavy metals, copper is toxic if it accumulates in the tissues. The copper accumulation in patients with chronic cholestasis resembles that in Wilson disease, an inherited deficiency of a copper transporter in which copper accumulates because it cannot be excreted into the bile.

The initial symptom of itching in this patient is probably the result of elevated blood levels of bile acids, which irritate free nerve endings in the skin. Unlike the itching of allergic reactions, itching in patients with biliary disease is not accompanied by pustular or erythematous changes ("hives"), and it does not respond to antihistamines. Itching also occurs in patients with uremia and in those with polycythemia vera, a neoplastic disease with excessive formation of erythrocytes. However, renal failure and uremia can be ruled out in this patient because of the normal blood urea nitrogen (BUN) level, and polycythemia vera can be ruled out because of her low-normal hematocrit.

There are several treatment strategies for primary biliary cirrhosis, none of them entirely satisfactory. The inflammatory process can be suppressed by anti-inflammatory steroids. The accumulation of copper, which contributes to liver damage, can be treated with penicillamine. This copper chelator forms a soluble copper complex that is excreted in the urine. Cholestyramine is a nonabsorbable ion exchange resin that binds bile acids in the intestine, preventing their absorption and thereby preventing the excessive accumulation of bile acids in liver and blood, at least as long as the bile flow is not interrupted entirely. By removing excess bile acids, it also permits an increased metabolism of cholesterol to bile acids.

Chronic cholestasis leads to liver cirrhosis, a condition in which normal hepatocytes gradually die out and are replaced by fibrous connective tissue. The proliferation of fibrous connective tissue in the liver is a typical response to injury, similar to scar formation in other tissues. Liver cirrhosis is also accompanied by capillary metaplasia of the sinusoids, which essentially replaces the wide sinusoids by narrow capillaries with a far greater resistance to blood flow. This leads to portal hypertension.

Biochemical abnormalities in liver cirrhosis include an increased globulin/albumin ratio and reduced levels of prothrombin and other clotting factors. The liver is the principal source of most plasma proteins, including albumin and the clotting factors. The clotting disorder in cirrhotic patients is not likely to respond to vitamin K because it is caused by a reduced capacity for clotting factor synthesis, not by vitamin K malabsorption. The deficiency of clotting factors is important because cirrhotic patients are prone to hemorrhages from peptic ulcer disease and from dilated lower esophageal veins, which form part of a collateral circulation around the diseased liver.

Besides hemorrhage, hepatic encephalopathy is a major complication of liver cirrhosis. Although its etiology is complex, hyperammonemia is an important factor. Ammonia accumulates in cirrhotic patients because it can no longer be detoxified in the urea cycle. The liver is the only major organ with a complete urea cycle. Patients with hepatic encephalopathy must be kept on a low-protein diet because ammonia is produced from dietary protein.

Intestinal bacteria are an important source of ammonia. They degrade leftover dietary protein, and they cleave the urea in digestive secretions to carbon dioxide and ammonia. In acute episodes of hepatic encephalopathy, a mannitol enema can be helpful immediately because mannitol (a sugar alcohol) stimulates the growth of intestinal bacteria by providing them with a carbon source. It does not provide any nitrogen, and the growing bacteria therefore must assimilate nitrogen from ambient ammonia. The eradication of intestinal bacteria by broad-spectrum antibiotics is an alternative strategy.

The removal of excess nitrogen from the body can also be achieved by the liberal use of benzoic acid or phenylacetic acid. These organic acids are conjugated with glycine and glutamine, respectively, and the conjugation products are excreted by the kidneys. These reactions are actually detoxification reactions that are designed to remove unwanted foreign organic acids, but in cirrhotic patients they can be exploited as an alternative route of nitrogen excretion. This reduces the need for urea synthesis.

Abdominal Pain

The most remarkable feature of this patient is the lack of gross abnormalities, both on physical examination and in blood chemistry. There was evidence of neurological dysfunction, including seizures, but no evidence of a physical disorder. There is no indication of an infection (normal white blood cell and globulin counts), infectious or inflammatory CNS disease (normal lumbar CSF findings), focal brain damage (no aphasia or apraxia), kidney disease (normal BUN, normal appearance of the urine), liver disease (normal aspartate transaminase and bilirubin levels), pancreatitis (normal/low amylase level), muscle disease (normal/low creatine kinase level), and anemia (normal hematocrit). The seizures can possibly be related to alcohol withdrawal. Patients like this are usually diagnosed as psychiatric cases, but some do indeed have an identifiable physical disorder.

The final diagnosis was a porphyria, probably acute intermittent porphyria. Porphyrias can be caused by a partial deficiency of any of the heme-synthesizing enzymes other than aminolevulinic acid (ALA) synthase. Such deficiencies can be genetic, but in many cases, they are also related to environmental agents such as lead or excess iron. ALA synthase catalyzes the committed and rate-limiting step in heme biosynthesis. It is feedback-inhibited by free heme.

The symptoms of porphyria are caused not by a deficiency of heme but by the accumulation of biosynthetic intermediates. In the hepatic porphyrias, the accumulating intermediates are formed in the liver, but the symptoms are caused by actions of these intermediates on the nervous system. Autonomic dysfunctions are caused by actions on the sympathetic, parasympathetic, and enteric nervous systems; pain is caused by a stimulation of visceral pain fibers; and weakness, irritability, and seizures result from toxic effects on the central nervous system.

Patients with neuropsychiatric disorders are usually treated symptomatically with tranquilizers, sedative-hypnotics, or anticonvulsants. Many of these drugs are contraindicated in patients with hepatic porphyrias because they induce drug-metabolizing microsomal enzymes in the liver. One component of these enzyme systems is a family of heme-containing enzymes collectively known as cytochrome P-450. The drugs induce the synthesis of the P-450 apoproteins. The apoproteins bind heme, thereby depleting the pool of free, unbound heme in the cell. Free heme but not protein-bound heme represses ALA synthase, the first enzyme of the heme biosynthetic pathway. By this mechanism, drugs can induce ALA synthase and cause the accumulation of biosynthetic intermediates.

Porphyrias are rare diseases, and therefore they often go undiagnosed. An abnormal color of the urine, caused by the accumulated biosynthetic intermediates, is a clue to the diagnosis. In many cases, the urine assumes an abnormal color only after exposure to light and air. These conditions favor polymerization reactions and the conversion of uncolored porphyrinogens to colored porphyrins. Other disorders with abnormally colored urine include conjugated hyperbilirubinemia ("choluric jaundice"), hemoglobinuria in massive hemolysis, and myoglobinuria in some muscle diseases. The levels of porphobilinogen and other intermediates of the heme biosynthetic pathway should be determined in the urine whenever a porphyria is suspected.

The treatment of porphyria consists of measures to reduce the activity of ALA synthase and thereby curtail the supply of the offending biosynthetic intermediates. Drugs that induce hepatic enzyme synthesis have to be withdrawn. Hematin (a chemically stable oxidized form of heme) can be given intravenously to repress ALA synthase. Intravenous glucose and a high-carbohydrate diet also repress ALA synthase by unknown mechanisms.

Rheumatism

Most patients with joint pain are given one of two diagnostic labels: rheumatoid arthritis, if autoimmune/inflammatory reactions predominate, or osteoarthritis, if degenerative changes predominate. The treatment of these major forms of arthritis is symptomatic and not always satisfactory. Aspirin is still a mainstay of treatment for the painful inflammatory process of rheumatoid arthritis, but it can cause gastritis and gastric ulcers.

The patient in this case study does not have one of the common forms of arthritis; instead, he suffers from hemochromatosis. The most important laboratory findings are the elevated level of serum ferritin and the abnormally high transferrin saturation. The transferrin concentration (total iron-binding capacity) is not a very useful diagnostic parameter because it can be either normal or elevated in hemochromatosis.

Ferritin is the principal intracellular iron storage protein. It is present in the intestinal mucosa, spleen, liver, pancreas, heart, bone marrow, and other tissues. Its synthesis is induced by the presence of free iron in the cells. Free iron is toxic because it binds to proteins and, in particular, because it catalyzes the formation of highly reactive free radicals from molecular oxygen. Therefore, the tissue levels of ferritin are low in iron deficiency and high in iron overload. Small amounts of ferritin normally enter the blood during cell turnover in the liver and other ferritin-rich tissues. Its level can be determined in the serum by sensitive radioimmunoassays. Transferrin is the principal iron transport protein of the blood. It has two binding sites for ferric iron. In most people, about 30% of these sites are occupied by iron. This percentage is reduced in iron deficiency and increased in iron overload.

Hemochromatosis develops only when iron absorption exceeds iron excretion for a very long time. Therefore, it causes problems only in middle-aged and older people. Essentially all affected patients are men; women are protected by menstruation and childbearing. Iron overload (hemosiderosis) can develop as a result of unusual dietary habits: for example, in alcoholics drinking large amounts of iron-rich wines. Most affected patients, however, are homozygous for a recessive gene that increases intestinal iron absorption. This gene originated only recently (perhaps 2000 years ago) in northern Europe and is now present in more than 10% of people of Irish, British, or Scandinavian origin. Its spread is most likely related to a high prevalence of iron deficiency in prehistoric and early historic farming communities.

The first signs of hemochromatosis can include liver dysfunction, heart failure, diabetes mellitus, reduced pituitary and testicular function, joint pain, and abnormal skin pigmentation. Unsatisfactory testicular androgen production in hemochromatosis is caused by pituitary dysfunction. Hormone determinations in these patients would show low levels of pituitary gonadotropins in addition to reduced androgen levels. Testicular failure, in contrast, would cause low levels of androgens but elevated levels of gonadotropins because the androgens normally inhibit gonadotropin secretion. The signs of hemochromatosis are so nonspecific that the diagnosis is often missed. A correct diagnosis requires biochemical determinations.

Specific treatment of hemochromatosis is aimed at the removal of the excess iron. Dietary restrictions are ineffective. Daily iron excretion amounts to about 1 mg/day, and more than 20 g of iron may be stored in the patient's tissues. Therefore, the removal of the excess iron stores by eliminating all dietary sources of iron (which would be hard to achieve) would take almost a century. Treatment with the iron chelator desferrioxamine is possible, but it is too cumbersome (the drug must be administered with a subcutaneous infusion pump) and removes excess iron too slowly. Therefore, desferrioxamine is reserved for patients who have developed iron overload in the course of severe anemia or after repeated blood transfusions, such as those with thalassemia.

Repeated phlebotomy is a far better option. The removal of blood increases erythropoiesis via erythropoietin, and the iron for the increased hemoglobin synthesis is mobilized from stored ferritin and hemosiderin. Treatment must be continued for a long time—for example, removing 0.5 to 1.0 liter of blood per week for half a year or more—until the excess iron stores are nearly depleted. Early clinical signs of hemochromatosis improve with treatment, but more advanced lesions, such as liver cirrhosis, advanced diabetes mellitus, or cardiac damage, are irreversible. Therefore, early diagnosis and prompt treatment are essential.

🗀 A Bank Manager in Trouble

This patient has an attack of gouty arthritis that was precipitated by alcohol abuse. Alcohol is metabolized in the liver. It is oxidized to acetaldehyde by the cytosolic alcohol dehydrogenase, and the acetaldehyde is oxidized to acetic acid by a mitochondrial aldehyde dehydrogenase. The acetic acid either is activated to acetyl-CoA in the liver mitochondria or is transported to other parts of the body for oxidation.

Alcohol metabolism is not feedback-inhibited. Therefore, large amounts of the products acetyl-CoA, ATP, and NADH are formed in the drinker's liver. Drunken individuals can develop hypoglycemia because the high [NADH]/[NAD$^+$] ratio favors the formation of lactate from pyruvate and of malate from oxaloacetate, thereby depleting the liver of gluconeogenic precursors. The lactate level is elevated because of the high [NADH]/[NAD$^+$] ratio and because pyruvate dehydrogenase in the liver is inhibited by high energy charge and by high levels of acetyl-CoA and NADH.

Alcohol abuse can precipitate attacks of gouty arthritis by causing dehydration and possibly because the elevated lactic acid level during alcohol intoxication interferes with the renal excretion of uric acid. Gout develops when crystals of sodium urate precipitate in the joints, where they cause an inflammatory response. Unlike rheumatoid arthritis and osteoarthritis, gouty arthritis typically manifests with acute attacks of severe pain that are separated by asymptomatic intervals.

Most, but not all, patients have an elevated serum uric acid level at the time of the acute attack. Therefore, a definitive diagnosis requires synovial fluid analysis from the inflamed joint. An acute attack develops when phagocytic cells engulf the needle-sharp sodium urate crystals. This results in lysosomal damage and death of the cell, with the release of lysosomal enzymes. Gout has a predilection for the small joints of the toes and fingers because the low temperature in these peripheral joints reduces the solubility of sodium urate.

Dietary treatments are not very effective, and most patients require drugs. The acute attack is treated with nonsteroidal anti-inflammatory drugs. Colchicine is useful but is rarely used because of gastrointestinal side effects. Long-term treatment is aimed at reducing the hyperuricemia. Allopurinol inhibits the formation of uric acid from xanthine and hypoxanthine by xanthine oxidase. Alternatively, uricosuric agents such as probenecid can be used to increase the renal excretion of uric acid.

🗀 Kidney Problems

This patient has type 1 diabetes, a severe chronic disease caused by the autoimmune destruction of pancreatic β cells. This disease can be controlled only by regular insulin injections. Insulin is not active orally because it is destroyed by proteases in the stomach and intestines. Neither dietary management nor oral antidiabetic drugs are effective.

Acute complications of type 1 diabetes, including ketoacidosis, can be prevented by insulin treatment, but late complications are likely to develop in the course of many years. These late complications include microangiopathy, early atherosclerosis, peripheral neuropathy, retinopathy, and nephropathy. Diabetes is an important cause of cardiovascular disease, blindness, and renal failure.

The patient is suffering from diabetic nephropathy. The most important diagnostic test for this condition is the determination of urinary protein. Healthy urine is essentially protein free. Patients with diabetic nephropathy gradually develop proteinuria, and the amount of protein in the 24-hour urine sample is proportional to the extent of renal damage.

Renal failure leads to the accumulation of all substances that are normally excreted in the urine, including nitrogenous wastes (urea, uric acid, creatinine) and inorganic ions (sodium, potassium, magnesium, phosphate). There is also a mild chronic acidosis because the normal kidney participates in acid-base regulation by excreting excess protons, mainly in the form of the ammonium ion (ammonia + proton). The urinary pH usually is below 7. In most patients, renal acidosis is compensated by hyperventilation. The result is a normal or near-normal blood pH with reduced serum carbon dioxide and bicarbonate concentrations.

Patients with kidney disease are also prone to hypertension because reduced diuresis increases the blood volume. Abnormal activation of the renin-angiotensin system contributes to hypertension in some patients. Anemia is caused by the inability of the diseased kidneys to produce adequate amounts of erythropoietin, a growth factor that stimulates erythropoiesis in the bone marrow. Recombinant erythropoietin is available for treatment.

Another common problem in patients with kidney disease is bone demineralization (renal osteodystrophy). One reason is the chronic acidosis, which increases the solubility of the calcium phosphates in bone. Even a slight reduction of the pH causes a large increase in the solubility of the "bone salt." Another reason for renal osteodystrophy is the inability to convert 25-hydroxyvitamin D to the active form 1,25-dihydroxyvitamin D (calcitriol). Calcitriol is required for the intestinal absorption of dietary calcium. In its absence, the plasma calcium level must be maintained by parathyroid hormone (PTH), which mobilizes calcium from the bones. Over time, the bones become depleted of calcium and phosphate. PTH can be measured by radioimmunoassay in the clinical laboratory. Its plasma level is high in patients with renal failure, whereas the calcium level is either normal or low. The level of the bone isoenzyme of alkaline phosphatase is elevated in the serum of many patients.

The kidneys are responsible for the excretion of many drugs. Drugs that are normally excreted in the urine should be used with caution in order to avoid toxicity. Also, some drugs are significantly nephrotoxic and can therefore aggravate the condition. Some antacids contain magnesium. This ion tends to accumulate in patients with renal failure.

The best way of treating incipient diabetic nephropathy is improved metabolic control of the disease. Supportive measures include the restriction of dietary constituents that must be excreted by the kidneys. Excess electrolytes, in particular, should be avoided. Also, dietary protein should be low. One gram of urea is formed from every 3 g of protein, and urea must be excreted by the kidneys. Advanced renal failure necessitates the use of hemodialysis. This treatment is based on the diffusion of small molecules and ions through a system of semipermeable membranes. Low-molecular weight waste products are removed, whereas plasma proteins and blood cells are retained.

A Sickly Child

The presenting problem of this patient is a respiratory infection with high fever and coughing. Although isolated respiratory infections are not unusual in infants, this patient had repeated bouts of infection that suggest a "special reason" for his susceptibility.

The most remarkable finding of the physical examination was the presence of profound liver enlargement. The liver scan was performed to investigate the possibility of a tumor. Malignant liver tumors, known as hepatoblastoma, do occasionally occur in this age group. The abnormally high heart rate suggests overactivity of the sympathetic nervous system. Also the mother's remark that "his skin becomes clammy and it tastes salty" suggests excessive sympathetic activity with peripheral vasoconstriction and sweating.

Slight cyanosis can be caused by poor tissue oxygenation in the wake of a respiratory infection. This patient was apparently given oxygen because his hyperventilation and cyanosis suggested an impairment of gas exchange in the lungs. However, the low blood CO_2 shows that gas exchange is unimpaired and the slight cyanosis is most likely caused by peripheral vasoconstriction. Oxygen treatment is therefore not indicated.

The laboratory tests reveal severe acidosis. The low level of carbon dioxide in the blood proves that the acidosis is metabolic, not respiratory. The low level of carbon dioxide in the exhaled air is simply the result of hyperventilation. The hyperventilation is caused not by impaired gas exchange but by a direct effect of the acidosis on the respiratory center in the brainstem. The high blood lactate concentration and the presence of ketone bodies in the urine show that the patient has a mixed lactic acidosis and ketoacidosis.

The other major finding is an abysmally low blood glucose level, suggesting a defect of the glucose-producing pathways in the liver. Both the hypoglycemia and the acidosis are so severe as to be immediately life-threatening. There is no indication of acute liver failure, however, because the bilirubin concentration is normal and alanine transaminase is only mildly elevated. The not very abnormal hematocrit suggests that the patient does not suffer from a severe hemolytic condition, either.

The hematocrit of infants normally declines from 50% to 55% at birth to 30% to 40% at 6 months. This decline does not reduce the efficiency of oxygen delivery because fetal hemoglobin (HbF) is replaced by adult hemoglobin at the same time, and adult hemoglobin is the more effective oxygen transporter after birth. The declining hematocrit is related to the low iron content of breast milk. The supply of maternal iron to the fetus before birth is more efficient than the supply of iron in milk because less than 30% of the iron in milk is absorbed by the infant. Because iron is valuable for the mother as well as for the infant, transfer before birth is the better option.

Further investigations showed that the hypoglycemia was relieved by oral glucose, but the patient was unable to maintain a normal blood glucose level during fasting. The "twitching and jerking movements" that were noted were a seizure. Hypoglycemia can cause seizures both in infants and in adults. At one time, insulin shock treatment has been used in psychiatry in place of electroconvulsive therapy.

Normally, glucagon stimulates both glycogen breakdown and gluconeogenesis in the liver. The complete failure of glucagon to raise the blood glucose suggests that both pathways are blocked in the patient. The rise in lactate and uric acid further suggests that intermediates of these two pathways cannot be converted into glucose but are diverted into alternative metabolic channels. The only reaction that is common to gluconeogenesis and glycogen degradation in the liver is the glucose-6-phosphatase reaction. Therefore, there is a first indication that this reaction might be blocked.

The biochemical determinations on the liver biopsy confirmed the absence of glucose-6-phosphatase and established a diagnosis of type I glycogen storage disease, also known as von Gierke disease. Microsomes are obtained by mechanical disruption of the cells followed by centrifugation. The microsomal fraction is enriched in small membranous vesicles that are derived from the endoplasmic reticulum. Glucose-6-phosphatase is in the endoplasmic reticulum, although the other enzymes of glycogen degradation and gluconeogenesis are cytoplasmic.

Repeated freezing and thawing was performed to disrupt the endoplasmic reticulum membrane. In intact microsomes, the glucose-6-phosphatase is locked in the vesicles. A carrier in the membrane is needed to bring glucose-6-phosphate to the enzyme, and another carrier is needed to release free glucose from the vesicle. Some patients with type I glycogen storage disease possess glucose-6-phosphatase but are lacking one of the carriers. These patients cannot form glucose because either glucose-6-phosphate cannot reach the enzyme or glucose cannot leave the endoplasmic reticulum.

The hypoglycemia of type I glycogen storage disease is more severe than that seen in other enzyme deficiencies (for example, fructose-1,6-bisphosphatase or glycogen phosphorylase) because glucose can be formed neither by glycogen breakdown nor by gluconeogenesis.

The hypoglycemia inhibits insulin release and stimulates the release of glucagon, epinephrine, norepinephrine, and cortisol. Low insulin and high epinephrine or norepinephrine levels stimulate the hormone-sensitive adipose tissue lipase. Large amounts of fatty acids are released into the blood, and some of them are converted into ketone bodies by the liver. As in normal fasting, the products of β-oxidation (acetyl-CoA, NADH, and ATP) inhibit the pyruvate dehydrogenase complex, thereby preventing the mitochondrial oxidation of glycolytic intermediates.

Without glucose-6-phosphatase, these intermediates cannot be converted into glucose, either. They accumulate and are diverted into the formation of lactic acid and glycogen. Glycogen accumulates because the excessive level of glucose-6-phosphate in the patient's liver stimulates glycogen synthase, in addition to providing ample substrate for glycogen synthesis. Hyperuricemia is present because some of the accumulating glucose-6-phosphate is diverted into the pentose phosphate pathway to form ribose-5-phosphate, a precursor for purine biosynthesis. This increases the rate of de novo purine biosynthesis, which must be matched by an equally increased rate of purine degradation to uric acid.

The fat accumulation in the liver and the elevated level of plasma triglycerides suggest a high level of lipogenesis (fat synthesis) in the liver. The excess fat is synthesized from adipose tissue–derived fatty acids. Although most of these fatty acids are used for ketogenesis, some are esterified into triglycerides by the liver.

Patients with von Gierke disease can be kept alive and well only by continuous glucose feeding day and night. Not only hypoglycemia but also the excessive accumulation of glycolytic intermediates in the liver must be avoided. The accumulation of glucose-6-phosphate and other phosphorylated intermediates not only leads to lactic acidosis, hyperuricemia, and abnormal glycogen deposition but also can deplete the cells of inorganic phosphate. This damages the cells by interfering with ATP synthesis.

Why was the patient given lactose-free milk with extra glucose? In normal adults, only 20% or 25% of the dietary glucose is metabolized in the liver after a carbohydrate-rich meal. This proportion is even lower in infants because of the relatively greater size of the brain in infants than in adults. The brain accounts for 60% of the basal metabolic rate in infants, as opposed to 20% in adults, and it subsists almost entirely on glucose. Moreover, in patients with von Gierke disease, the insulin level is so low that the phosphorylation of glucose by glucokinase in the liver is reduced to perhaps 10% of normal.

On the other hand, about one half of the dietary galactose is metabolized by the liver. Unlike glucose phosphorylation, galactose metabolism is not tightly controlled. Therefore, large amounts of glucose-6-phosphate and other glycolytic intermediates can be formed from galactose. This depletes the cells of inorganic phosphate and aggravates lactic acidosis, hyperuricemia, and glycogen formation. Like galactose, fructose is rapidly converted to glycolytic intermediates in the liver and should therefore be avoided.

Glucose is absorbed rapidly from the intestine. Therefore, it must be fed frequently to maintain an adequate blood glucose level. Some forms of starch are digested as rapidly as glucose. Some starchy foods, however, are retained in the stomach for up to 3 or 4 hours, and some forms of starch are digested more slowly than others. Slowly digested forms of starch are most suitable for the management of patients with von Gierke disease because they maintain the blood glucose level for many hours.

Von Gierke disease is inherited as an autosomal recessive trait. This implies that the patient has inherited mutations both from the father and the mother. When both parents carry the disease gene in the heterozygous state, the risk of the disease in a future child is 25%. Although the conception of an affected child cannot be prevented, the parents can be offered prenatal diagnosis. Fetal cells are obtained by chorionic villus sampling at week 9 or 10 or by amniocentesis at weeks 14 to 16. The fetal cells are cultured, and the disease is diagnosed from the cultured cells. This procedure makes sense only if the parents plan to terminate the pregnancy in case the fetus is affected.

Von Gierke disease cannot be diagnosed by enzyme determination from cultured fetal cells because the enzyme is not present in these cells. Glucose-6-phosphatase is expressed only in liver, kidney, intestine, and pancreatic β cells.

Allele-specific probes require exact knowledge of the mutation. Most genetic diseases, however, including von Gierke disease, can be caused by a large number of different mutations in the affected gene. These low-frequency mutations usually are of recent origin and represent "mutational load" (i.e., "genetic garbage") that is continuously being removed by natural selection.

In prenatal diagnosis, these disease genes can be tracked by linkage with genetic markers that are located close to the gene. Alternatively, a scanning method can be used to identify the exact mutation in the patient. More commonly, the brute-force approach of amplifying and sequencing all exons of the gene is used. Once the mutations in the patient and his or her parents are known, allele-specific probes can be used in a next pregnancy.

Prenatal diagnosis is always done on a tight schedule because late pregnancy termination should be avoided. Therefore, methods that do not require exceedingly long periods for cell culturing and testing are preferred. Polymerase chain reaction (PCR) is ideal because it requires only a minute amount of DNA that can be obtained without cell culturing, and the amplification can be done in a single day. The mutated section of the fetal DNA is amplified, the denatured amplification product applied to a nitrocellulose filter, and an allele-specific probe applied. This PCR/dot-blotting procedure obviates the need for gel electrophoresis, and it can be used for the detection of single-base substitutions that do not change the length of the PCR product.

The Missed Examination

This patient has ketoacidosis, a life-threatening complication of type 1 diabetes. Ketoacidosis manifests with coma, and it must be differentiated from other causes of unconsciousness. The emergency measures used in this case were the administration of dextrose (glucose) and naloxone. Dextrose is effective only when the loss of consciousness is caused by hypoglycemia, and naloxone is an opiate antagonist that revives patients after an opiate overdose (and induces withdrawal in addicts). Neither dextrose nor naloxone can do much harm. Even in patients with ketoacidosis, the injected glucose adds little to the hyperglycemia.

Ketoacidosis is suggested by a typical acetone odor that resembles the smell of alcohol. Acetone is produced by the nonenzymatic decarboxylation of acetoacetate. Hyperventilation is a response to the metabolic acidosis.

Signs of circulatory shock, with an inability to maintain a normal blood pressure, appear for two reasons. First, massive glucosuria causes dehydration and hypovolemia through osmotic diuresis. Everything else being equal, reduced blood volume means lower blood pressure. A second reason is acidosis. Low pH dilates peripheral resistance vessels (arterioles, precapillary sphincters). This is a normal physiological mechanism that increases the blood supply to hypoxic tissues in which lactic acid is produced, such as contracting muscles. In generalized acidosis, however, vasodilatation is generalized. The blood pressure drops, and this is a powerful stimulus for the sympathetic nervous system. Increased sympathetic activity up-regulates the blood pressure and also causes sweating and tachycardia.

Patients with diabetic ketoacidosis have severe hyperglycemia. This is caused both by the overproduction of glucose in the liver and its underutilization in peripheral tissues. In the liver, insulin stimulates glycolysis and glycogen synthesis while inhibiting gluconeogenesis and glycogen degradation. Therefore, patients with uncontrolled diabetes have rampant gluconeogenesis and glycogen degradation. Gluconeogenesis is more important than glycogen degradation for the hyperglycemia because liver glycogen is depleted rapidly in severe diabetes.

Glucose utilization is impaired in diabetic patients. Muscle and adipose tissue have insulin-dependent glucose transporters of the GLUT-4 type and are therefore unable to take up glucose in severe diabetes. In other tissues, the glucose-metabolizing pathways are stimulated by insulin, although glucose uptake is insulin independent. Only the brain and erythrocytes still consume normal amounts of glucose in diabetic patients, because their glucose metabolism is insulin independent.

Hyperglycemia by itself is innocuous to the brain. It contributes to the development of "diabetic coma" by causing dehydration. As an osmotic diuretic, it impairs the reabsorption of water in the tubular system. The acidosis also contributes to the coma.

The accumulation of ketone bodies is caused by uncontrolled fat breakdown in adipose tissue. Although the free fatty acids thus formed are a major fuel for most tissues, a substantial portion is converted to ketone bodies in the liver. Ketoacidosis develops when ketogenesis in the liver exceeds the capacity for ketone body oxidation in the peripheral tissues. Ketone bodies cause acidosis simply because they are acidic products (acetoacetic acid, β-hydroxybutyric acid) that are formed from a nonacidic substrate (fat). Ketoacidosis is not the only type of "diabetic coma." In nonketotic hyperosmolar coma, massive hyperglycemia causes coma by inducing osmotic diuresis and dehydration. This type is seen also in type 2 diabetes, although ketoacidosis is limited to type 1 diabetes.

Diabetic ketoacidosis is treated with intravenous fluids and insulin injections. Some patients have elevated plasma levels of potassium, which is derived from intracellular sources. Some of this potassium is lost in the urine. When the patient recovers, however, potassium is pumped back into the cells, and hypokalemia can develop.

Ketoacidosis is the result of insufficient insulin treatment of an insulin-dependent diabetic patient. It can also be precipitated by psychological stress and physical illness because the "stress hormones," including epinephrine and the glucocorticoids, stimulate gluconeogenesis in the liver and lipolysis in adipose tissue. They are functional antagonists of insulin. Some cytokines, hormone-like proteins that are released by white blood cells during infections and other illnesses, also have insulin-antagonistic metabolic effects. Therefore, the insulin requirement of diabetic patients is always increased during even minor illnesses and psychological stress. Once the metabolic derangements of ketoacidosis develop, the patient is in a vicious cycle that can be broken only by vigorous treatment.

Whereas patients with type 1 diabetes are unable to produce insulin, those with type 2 diabetes have a reduced capacity for glucose-stimulated insulin release, a reduced insulin responsiveness of the target tissues ("insulin resistance"), or both. Many insulin-resistant patients have a reduced number of insulin receptors, whereas others seem to have feeble insulin-triggered signaling cascades. The insulin receptor is a tyrosine kinase that triggers intracellular phosphorylation cascades.

A few days after the first episode, this patient was admitted to the emergency room with hypoglycemia. Hypoglycemic spells can be caused by a combination of insulin overuse and fasting, and they respond immediately to intravenous dextrose. Hypoglycemia is also seen in patients with insulinoma, an insulin-secreting tumor of pancreatic β cells. Clinical laboratories routinely determine C-peptide rather than insulin levels for the investigation of pancreatic function and the diagnosis of insulinoma because C-peptide is released from the pancreas along with insulin. Unlike insulin, which may be derived from insulin injection, C-peptide is definitely derived from the patient's own pancreas. In this case, C-peptide determination was not justified because the patient's history (ketoacidosis only a few days ago) was incompatible with the presence of an insulinoma.

Gender Blender

In the absence of androgens, the external genitalia develop in the female direction before birth. This developmental path does not depend on female hormones. However, normal male genital development depends on the presence of androgens, irrespective of karyotypic and gonadal sex.

Congenital adrenal hyperplasia (CAH) is a virilizing disorder that is caused by a defect in adrenal steroid synthesis. The deficient enzyme is 21-hydroxylase in 90% of affected patients and 11β-hydroxylase in most of the remaining 10%. The gene for 21-hydroxylase is prone to deletions and gene conversions because it is located in a duplicated DNA segment next to a nonfunctional pseudogene. This accounts for the relatively high incidence of 21-hydroxylase deficiency in newborns (up to 1 per 10,000).

These enzymes are required for the synthesis of corticosteroids but not the synthesis of adrenal androgens. This patient has an elevated plasma level of 17-hydroxyprogesterone, an immediate substrate of 21-hydroxylase in the pathway of glucocorticoid synthesis. Thus, the deficient enzyme is in all likelihood the 21-hydroxylase.

The diagnosis depends on the measurement of 17-hydroxyprogesterone and adrenal androgens in the blood and of 17-ketosteroids in the urine. A sex chromatin determination from a buccal smear, or karyotype analysis from cultured leukocytes, is done routinely to verify the chromosomal sex, because intersex phenotypes can also be caused by insufficient prenatal androgen action in karyotypic male patients. Karyotype analysis has traditionally been done with mitotic cells but can now be done with fluorescent probes applied to interphase cells.

Adrenal steroid synthesis is stimulated by the adrenocorticotropic hormone (ACTH) from the pituitary gland, whose secretion is feedback-inhibited by glucocorticoids. In CAH, lack of glucocorticoids leads to insufficient inhibition of ACTH release. ACTH stimulates the rate-limiting desmolase reaction of steroid synthesis (choles-

terol→pregnenolone), with resulting overproduction of progestins. Because their conversion to corticosteroids is blocked, the accumulating progestins are diverted into androgen synthesis. If the enzyme deficiency is complete, the lack of mineralocorticoids leads to dangerous electrolyte abnormalities that necessitate immediate treatment. In partial enzyme deficiencies, electrolyte imbalances are mild or absent, and virilization of the female infant is the only abnormality at birth.

Untreated, both boys and girls with CAH develop precocious puberty, with pubic hair starting to grow between the ages of 6 months and 2 years. Skeletal and even mental development is accelerated initially, but skeletal growth ceases early, and adult height is below average.

Treatment consists of the chronic administration of cortisol or some other glucocorticoid (prednisone or prednisolone), with mineralocorticoids as required. This treatment suppresses ACTH secretion and androgen synthesis, and normalizes any electrolyte imbalances. To ensure normal growth and sexual development, cortisol treatment should be continued for life in female patients and at least to puberty in male patients. However, gender identity disorder and homosexuality seem to be frequent even in successfully treated female patients. These outcomes are attributed to a virilizing effect of prenatal androgens on the brain.

All forms of CAH are inherited as autosomal recessive disorders, with a 25% recurrence risk in families with an affected child. Prenatal diagnosis is possible, and prenatal treatment is possible with the synthetic glucocorticoid dexamethasone administered to the mother. Cortisol cannot be used because of poor placental transfer.

Man Overboard!

Sickle cell disease is caused by a point mutation that replaces a glutamate in the hemoglobin β chain by valine. This subtle change reduces the water solubility of deoxygenated (but not oxygenated) hemoglobin S (HbS) to a point at which an insoluble precipitate of HbS forms in erythrocytes. This insoluble precipitate distorts the shape of the cell ("sickling"); damages the erythrocyte membrane; causes both intravascular and extravascular hemolysis; and entails a risk of capillary blockage.

Recurrent pain attacks are the hallmark of this disease. The attacks are part of a vicious cycle in which sickled cells block capillary flow, resulting in further deoxygenation and even more sickling. Sickling is favored by dehydration because dehydration increases the concentration of everything, including HbS in the erythrocytes. The higher the intracorpuscular concentration of HbS, the greater is the risk of sickling. This patient's first attack was precipitated by dehydration, and drinking plenty of water is standard advice for sickle cell patients.

Intravenous fluids are the mainstay of treatment for the acute attack. They rehydrate the red blood cells, and they raise blood volume and blood pressure. The latter effect helps flushing sickled cells out of blocked capillaries. Minor analgesics are also used routinely. Morphine and other opiates should be used sparingly because higher doses depress the respiratory center in the medulla oblongata. This can lead to suboptimal oxygenation in the lungs.

Oxygen treatment is not very effective because normally the blood in the lung capillaries is about 96% oxygenated; thus, further increases in oxygenation have little effect. Repeated blood transfusions can be used but entail risks of infectious disease transmission, immunological reactions, and iron overload. This treatment is therefore reserved for patients with severe anemia, such as those with splenic sequestration crisis. Drugs that increase the oxygen binding affinity of HbS (e.g., cyanate), or stimulate the synthesis of hemoglobin γ chains (butyrate derivatives, hydroxyurea, azacytidine) can be tried but usually prove too toxic for long-term use. In theory, drugs that inhibit the synthesis of 2,3-BPG or raise the intracorpuscular pH would be beneficial because they would increase the oxygen affinity of HbS. However, such drugs are not currently available.

A leak in the gas stove can prevent sickling because carbon monoxide (CO) converts HbS into a nonsickling conformation resembling oxygenated hemoglobin. With a fraction of the HbS tied up as CO hemoglobin, the concentration of the sickling-prone deoxy-HbS in the cell is reduced. With this kind of treatment, the size of the leak needs to be controlled very carefully.

Patients with sickle cell disease have reduced exercise tolerance because of their moderately severe anemia (typical hemoglobin concentration, 7% to 11%). Superficial ulcers ("sores"), especially on the legs, heal poorly because sickling impedes blood flow to the poorly oxygenated margins of the ulcer. As they get older, these patients are prone to developing small infarctions in many tissues. Multiple kidney infarctions can lead to end-stage renal disease, and the spleen is destroyed in many middle-aged and older patients.

In affected children, however, the spleen is still intact and actually enlarged. Splenic sequestration crisis is an acute complication of sickle cell disease in which large numbers of erythrocytes get trapped in the enlarged spleen. The hematocrit drops precipitously, and death can occur within a few days. This patient's niece died of a splenic sequestration crisis.

Loss of consciousness, as in this patient's first attack, can occur when massive sickling leads to capillary blockage in widespread peripheral tissues. Poor oxygenation of the involved tissues causes a metabolic switch to anaerobic glycolysis, resulting in generalized lactic acidosis. The acidosis dilates peripheral resistance vessels and causes a severe drop in blood pressure, in addition to reducing the oxygen affinity of HbS and thereby promoting further sickling.

Only patients homozygous for the HbS allele have sickle cell disease. Heterozygotes have 30% HbS in addition to 70% adult hemoglobin but are healthy. Because the heterozygotes have improved malaria resistance, the HbS mutation is common in many malaria-infested tropical regions but rare or absent in people whose ancestors lived in colder climates.

Today's patients are the descendants of about five original mutants. One mutation occurred in Arabia or India or somewhere in between, and the other four occurred in Africa. The number of original mutations can be deduced from the number of haplogroups (groups of related haplotypes) that are linked to the sickle cell mutation, inasmuch as each mutation presumably originated on a unique haplotype (combination of closely linked genetic polymorphisms). The diversity within each haplogroup, which has been created by mutations occurring after the sickle cell mutation, is a rough measure for the age of the sickle cell mutation. The geographic origin of a mutation is most likely in the geographic area with the greatest haplotype diversity.

An elevated production of HbF during adulthood produces a milder course of sickle cell disease because HbF dilutes HbS and suppresses its crystallization. Patients with either the Indo-Arabian or one of the African mutations (the Senegalese mutation) have somewhat better prospects than do those with the more common Benin and Bantu mutations. This is because the two former mutations occurred on haplotypes with increased HbF expression. The β and γ chain genes are closely linked on chromosome 11.

This patient has low corpuscular volume and a low intracorpuscular hemoglobin concentration. These signs of microcytic, hypochromic anemia are not typical for sickle cell disease but for thalassemia. Patients with sickle cell disease who also have α-thalassemia minor have a milder course of the disease because the reduced intracorpuscular concentration of HbS makes sickling less likely. This can account for the relatively benign course of this patient's disease.

The patient's wife must be a carrier inasmuch as she produced two affected sons with her affected husband. This constellation implies a 50% risk of an affected child. The more common matings between two carriers entail a 25% risk. Population screening is useful for alerting couples of the risk of an affected child. Most physicians in modern industrialized societies would reject Mr. Darroux's method of genetic counseling as too directive and paternalistic. However, this emphasis is of recent origin and is not shared by all physicians, nor is it prevalent in all societies. In China, for example, more directive approaches are generally preferred.

Spongy Bones

Fractures are a major cause of disability in geriatric patients. The underlying bone disease, known as osteoporosis, is so common that it can almost be considered part of the normal aging process. Sex steroids stimulate the synthesis of type 1 collagen in the bones, and sagging levels of these hormones in postmenopausal women and elderly men impair the proper formation of the organic bone matrix. Hormone replacement therapy can delay or prevent osteoporosis. Insufficient collagen deposition leads to poor mineralization, and radiological determinations of bone mineral density can be used for diagnosis.

In this patient, osteoporosis is confounded by vitamin D deficiency. Vitamin D is present in few foods (liver, egg yolk, cod liver oil). Therefore, most of the time, humans depend on its endogenous synthesis from 7-dehydrocholesterol in the skin. Cholecalciferol is formed by the photolytic cleavage of 7-dehydrocholesterol. This product needs to be activated by successive hydroxylations in liver and kidney to form biologically active calcitriol. Calcitriol is a hormone-like substance that regulates the disposition of calcium and phosphate by actions on bones, the kidneys, and the intestines. Its most important effect is the stimulation of calcium absorption in the duodenum.

In vitamin D deficiency, which is known as rickets in children and osteomalacia in adults, impaired intestinal calcium absorption results in an initial drop of the plasma calcium level that triggers the release of PTH. PTH restores the plasma calcium level to near normal by mobilizing calcium from the bones. Thus, the shortage of calcitriol is compensated by the elevated PTH level, and the calcium that would otherwise come from the food is extracted from the bones instead. In time, the bones are deprived of their mineral content.

Predictably, the plasma levels of vitamin D tend to fall during the winter, when sunlight intensity is reduced. The aggravation of osteomalacia by dietary calcium deficiency is equally predictable. Milk and milk products are the most concentrated sources of calcium in common diets, and they are often recommended for people at risk of combined osteoporosis and osteomalacia.

Also, deficiencies of other vitamins and minerals should be avoided. For example, the synthesis of type 1 collagen requires both ascorbic acid for amino acid hydroxylations and copper for the lysyl oxidase reaction. Lysyl oxidase is the key enzyme for the covalent crosslinking of collagen.

Blisters

A blister forms when the epidermis separates from the dermis, resulting in a fluid-filled space in between. Any damage to the "glue" that holds the two layers together is bound to cause a blister. Such damage can result from autoantibodies, toxins (e.g., some insect venoms), and mutations in the glue-encoding genes.

The epidermal side of the junctional region is formed by the cells of the stratum germinativum. The most prominent structural protein of these cells is a form of keratin that consists of subunits K5 and K14. Mutations in the genes for these two keratin polypeptides cause epidermolysis bullosa simplex.

The keratin cytoskeleton of the germinal cells is connected to the basal lamina by hemidesmosomes. Hemidesmosomal proteins are frequent targets of autoantibodies but can also be affected in inherited blistering diseases. Inherited defects in the laminins of the basal lamina leave the cells of the stratum germinativum intact but lead to separation at the level of the basal lamina. This type is called junctional epidermolysis bullosa.

The basal lamina is attached to the extracellular matrix of the underlying dermis by anchoring fibrils that consist of collagen VII. This collagen is encoded by an unusually large gene with 118 exons. As is true of other large genes, mutations in the COL7A1 gene are not extremely rare. These mutations cause the dystrophic form of epidermolysis bullosa. The severity of the disease and the inheritance pattern depend on the specific mutation. Severe mutations are expressed clinically in the heterozygous state and cause dominantly inherited disease, whereas milder mutations are expressed only in the homozygous state and cause recessively inherited disease.

This patient has a recessive form of epidermolysis bullosa dystrophica. Because both the patient's parents carry the same mutation and come from the same geographic region, they probably inherited this mutation from a long-forgotten shared ancestor. Sometimes a mutation that originated in a single individual not too long ago becomes common in a restricted geographic area simply by chance. This occurrence is called genetic drift.

In this case, the exact mutation was identified by PCR amplification of exons in the *COL7A*1 gene, followed by a scanning method (conformation-sensitive gel electrophoresis). With wider availability of user-friendly DNA sequencers, scanning methods now tend to be replaced by the direct sequencing of all PCR-amplified exons.

The ability to scan the whole gene with oligonucleotide microarrays is on the horizon. Ideally, a DNA chip would scan all genes that are known to be involved in skin blistering diseases. This would simplify definitive diagnosis in affected individuals. It would also permit the genetic testing and screening of potential carriers for recessive mutations.

The Sunburned Child

Genome maintenance requires multiple DNA repair systems with overlapping specificities. This patient has xeroderma pigmentosum (XP), caused by a recessively inherited defect in genome-wide nucleotide excision repair. This system repairs bulky DNA lesions throughout the genome. Such lesions occur in all cells of the body at a low rate, but the clinical picture is dominated by cutaneous photosensitivity and skin cancer. The skin is by far the most exposed tissue because it suffers extensive damage from the ultraviolet (UV) component of sunlight. Also, many other tissues, including the brain, depend not on genome-wide nucleotide excision repair but on a transcription-coupled system that is specific for the transcribed strand of expressed genes. Defects in this transcription-coupled system cause not XP but Cockayne syndrome.

At least seven different polypeptides are required for genome-wide nucleotide excision repair. They serve different functions in the repair system, including damage recognition, helicase activity, and nuclease activities. Any one of these seven polypeptides can be absent or defective in a patient. Thus, there are seven biochemically distinct types, or "complementation groups," of this disease. Matters are even more complex because some of the XP proteins also play roles in transcription-coupled repair or in basal transcription. Mutations in these proteins can cause combined XP/Cockayne syndrome or involve hair abnormalities in addition to photosensitivity and Cockayne-like signs. These patients are diagnosed with trichothiodystrophy.

The type of XP is determined by complementation tests in which cells from a new patient are fused with cells from patients with known molecular defects. If the hybrid cells are homozygous (or compound heterozygous) for mutations in the same gene, they are abnormally sensitive to UV radiation.

Nucleotide excision repair in the skin is essential, although some of the UV radiation in sunlight is absorbed by melanin. This dark pigment is synthesized from tyrosine in melanocytes. Ordinarily, the combination of light skin and excessive sun exposure is the most important risk factor of skin cancers, including basal cell carcinoma, squamous cell carcinoma, and, to a lesser extent, malignant melanoma.

The treatment of XP is based on strict sun avoidance and the excision of any premalignant or malignant lesions. Dermabrasion is an unpleasant procedure in which the stratum germinativum is abraded along with the rest of the epidermis. Regeneration takes place from the epithelium of the deep adnexa: hair follicles, sweat glands and sebaceous glands. The hope is that the genomes of cells in these more sheltered locations are less corrupted by sun exposure than are those of the superficial epidermis.

Prenatal diagnosis from cultured amniotic cells is possible. Even without knowledge of the complementation group and the exact mutation, the diagnosis of the homozygous state can be made from the unusual sensitivity of the cells to UV radiation. The heterozygous state is asymptomatic except for a tendency in some light-skinned carriers to develop freckles on sun-exposed skin.

Too Much Ammonia

Inherited deficiencies have been described for each of the urea cycle enzymes. They all cause hyperammonemia and lead to neurological derangements. Multiple mechanisms probably contribute to the neurotoxicity of ammonia. As a substrate of the reversible glutamate dehydrogenase reaction, ammonia drives this reaction toward glutamate synthesis. The conversion of α-ketoglutarate to glutamate depletes TCA cycle intermediates and thereby impairs mitochondrial oxidation.

Glutamate is also an important excitatory neurotransmitter in the brain, and it is the precursor of the inhibitory neurotransmitter γ-aminobutyric acid (GABA). Excessive levels of these neurotransmitters can contribute to CNS dysfunction. Another mechanism is the accumulation of glutamine in astrocytes, resulting in cerebral edema. These cells have high activity of glutamine synthetase. Ordinarily, glutamine synthesis functions as a short-term buffer for ammonia in the brain.

Complete deficiency of any urea cycle enzyme leads to a severe disease that manifests with neurological derangements shortly after birth: poor feeding, hyperventilation leading to respiratory alkalosis, seizures, coma, and speedy death in untreated cases. Partial enzyme deficiencies lead to milder disease, with variable time of onset and severity of symptoms, depending on the severity of the enzyme deficiency. The affected enzyme and its residual activity (if any) can be determined in a liver biopsy.

The patient in this case study has a deficiency of ornithine transcarbamoylase, inherited as an X-linked recessive trait. The substrates of this enzyme, ornithine and carbamoyl phosphate, accumulate, whereas the citrulline product is depleted. Accumulating ornithine is released from the liver into the blood and eventually is excreted by the kidneys. Like other phosphorylated intermediates, carbamoyl phosphate cannot pass the plasma membrane. However, some of it leaks out of the mitochondria where it is formed, and that amount is used for pyrimidine biosynthesis in the cytoplasm. This leads to enhanced pyrimidine synthesis and elevated levels of the pyrimidine biosynthetic intermediate orotic acid.

Also, the downstream intermediates argininosuccinate and arginine are depleted. Arginine becomes a fully essential amino acid because it continues to be degraded by arginase without being resynthesized from ornithine. Therefore, arginine or citrulline is given to prevent arginine deficiency. Citrulline is preferable to arginine because it picks up a nitrogen atom during its conversion to arginine.

Otherwise, treatment is based on the use of benzoate, phenylacetate, and/or phenylbutyrate. Phenylbutyrate is converted to phenylacetate through the reactions of β-oxidation. Benzoic acid is conjugated with glycine, and phenylacetic acid with glutamine. The water-soluble conjugation products are excreted in the urine, thereby eliminating excess nitrogen from the body.

In theory, ammonia formation can be minimized by a low-protein diet. However, major reductions of dietary protein are not possible without compromising the growth and general health of the infant. A better, although expensive, option is to reduce the nonessential amino acids and replace essential amino acids by their α-keto analogs. The α-keto analogs are converted to the corresponding amino acids by transamination.

Answers to Questions

Chapter 1
1. D
2. C
3. A

Chapter 2
1. C
2. D
3. D
4. D

Chapter 3
1. B
2. B
3. A

Chapter 4
1. E
2. C
3. E
4. A
5. D
6. B

Chapter 5
1. E
2. D
3. A

Chapter 6
1. B
2. D
3. C
4. E
5. B

Chapter 7
1. A
2. C
3. E

Chapter 8
1. B
2. C
3. E
4. D
5. E

Chapter 9
1. A
2. D

Chapter 10
1. E
2. B
3. D
4. C
5. B

Chapter 11
1. E
2. E
3. C
4. D
5. D
6. A
7. C
8. C
9. A
10. E
11. D

Chapter 12
1. D
2. D
3. D
4. A

Chapter 13
1. E
2. B
3. C
4. A

Chapter 14
1. A
2. E
3. B
4. D
5. A

Chapter 15
1. A
2. D
3. D
4. A
5. C

Chapter 16
1. E
2. B
3. C
4. E

Chapter 17
1. D
2. C
3. A
4. E
5. D

Chapter 18
1. C
2. B
3. D
4. C
5. C
6. B
7. E
8. A
9. D

Chapter 19
1. C
2. D

Chapter 20
1. D
2. B

Chapter 21
1. A
2. E
3. C
4. B
5. C
6. D
7. E

Chapter 22
1. B
2. E
3. A
4. E
5. C

Chapter 23
1. D
2. C
3. B
4. A

Chapter 24
1. B
2. D
3. B

Chapter 25
1. E
2. D
3. B
4. E

Chapter 26
1. D
2. A
3. B
4. E
5. C

Chapter 27
1. D
2. B

Chapter 28
1. C
2. B

Chapter 29
1. B
2. C
3. E
4. A
5. B

Chapter 30
1. D
2. E
3. A
4. D
5. C
6. B

Glossary

ABC1 A protein that transfers cholesterol from cell membranes to high-density lipoprotein (HDL).

Abetalipoproteinemia An inherited inability to form chylomicrons and very-low-density lipoprotein (VLDL).

Abl An oncogene or proto-oncogene coding for a nuclear tyrosine protein kinase.

Acetyl-CoA carboxylase The rate-limiting enzyme of fatty acid biosynthesis.

Acetylcholinesterase An extracellular acetylcholine-degrading enzyme in cholinergic synapses.

Acid A proton donor.

Acid phosphatase A marker for prostatic cancer.

Acidosis Abnormally low blood pH.

Acrodermatitis enteropathica A disease caused by an inherited defect of intestinal zinc absorption.

Actin A globular protein that polymerizes into microfilaments.

Actinomycin D An inhibitor of transcription that binds to double-stranded DNA.

Active site The place on the enzyme protein to which the substrate binds and where catalysis takes place.

Acute intermittent porphyria A hepatic porphyria, with abdominal pain and neurological symptoms.

Acute-phase reactants Plasma proteins whose levels are elevated or reduced within 1 to 2 days of an acute stress.

Acyl-CoA The activated form of a fatty acid.

Acyl-CoA dehydrogenase The first enzyme of β-oxidation.

Adenomatous polyposis coli (APC) An inherited cancer susceptibility syndrome.

Adenosine deaminase deficiency A cause of severe combined immunodeficiency.

S-Adenosylmethionine (SAM) A cosubstrate that supplies an activated methyl group.

Adenylate cyclase The cyclic adenosine monophosphate (cAMP)–synthesizing enzyme, located in the plasma membrane.

Adrenergic receptors Receptors for epinephrine and norepinephrine.

β-Adrenergic receptor kinase (BARK) Desensitizes the β-adrenergic receptor.

Adrenodoxin A mitochondrial iron-sulfur protein that participates in hydroxylation reactions of steroids.

Adrenogenital syndrome An inherited defect of corticosteroid synthesis that leads to overproduction of adrenal androgens.

Aggrecan A large, aggregating proteoglycan in cartilage.

Agonist A stimulatory ligand for a receptor.

Aminolevulinic acid (ALA) synthase The regulated enzyme of heme biosynthesis.

Alanine transaminase A liver enzyme; the serum level is elevated in liver diseases.

Albinism A condition that is caused by recessively inherited defects of melanin synthesis.

Albumin A plasma protein; it accounts for approximately 60% of the total plasma protein.

Alcohol dehydrogenase A cytosolic liver enzyme that oxidizes ethanol to acetaldehyde.

Aldose Monosaccharide with an aldehyde group.

Alkalosis Abnormally high blood pH.

Alkaptonuria A rare inborn error of tyrosine metabolism, with accumulation of homogentisate.

Allele-specific oligonucleotide probes Probes that can distinguish between two different alleles (variants) of a gene.

Allelic heterogeneity Different disease causing mutations in the same gene.

Allopurinol An inhibitor of xanthine oxidase, used to treat gout.

Allosteric effector A ligand that affects the equilibrium between the alternative conformations of an allosteric protein.

Allosteric protein A protein that can exist in alternative conformations.

Alu sequences A large family of short interspersed elements.

α-Amanitine A mushroom poison that inhibits RNA polymerase II.

Aminoacyl-tRNA A transfer RNA (tRNA) with an amino acid covalently bound to its 3′ terminus.

Aminoacyl-tRNA synthetases Cytoplasmic enzymes that attach an amino acid to a tRNA.

γ-Aminobutyric acid (GABA) An inhibitory neurotransmitter in the central nervous system that is synthesized from glutamate.

Ammonotelic Ammonia excreting.

Amphipathic Containing hydrophilic and hydrophobic portions in the same molecule.

α-Amylase A starch-degrading endoglycosidase in saliva and pancreatic juice.

Anabolic pathway Biosynthetic pathway.

Anaerobic Oxygen deficient.

Anaplerotic reactions Reactions that result in the net production of a TCA cycle intermediate.

Anchorage dependence The inability of cultured cells to grow in the absence of a solid support.

Androgens 19-Carbon steroids derived from progestins by a side chain cleavage reaction.

Anemia Abnormal decrease of the blood hemoglobin concentration.

Aneuploidy Deficiency or excess of a chromosome.

Angiotensin II The active form of angiotensin, synthesized from angiotensinogen by the successive action of renin and converting enzyme.

Anhydride bond Bond between two acids.

Anion Negatively charged ion.

Annealing Formation of a double strand from two complementary nucleic acid strands.

Anomers Monosaccharides that differ only in the orientation of substituents around their carbonyl carbons.

Antagonist An inhibitory ligand for a receptor.

Anticodon The base triplet of the tRNA that base-pairs with the codon during protein synthesis.

Antigen-antibody complex A noncovalent aggregate between antigen and antibody.

Antimycin A An inhibitor of electron flow through the QH_2-cytochrome c reductase complex.

Antiport The coupled membrane transport of two substrates in opposite directions.

α₁-Antiprotease A circulating protease inhibitor, deficiency of which causes lung emphysema.

Antisense gene A gene whose transcript is complementary to a functional RNA.

Antisense technology The use of synthetic nucleic acid analogs in an attempt to block the translation of a specific mRNA.

Antithrombin III A circulating inhibitor of thrombin and some other activated clotting factors.

AP endonuclease An endonuclease that cleaves a phosphodiester bond formed by a baseless ("apurinic") nucleotide in DNA.

ApoA-I, apoA-II The major apolipoproteins of high-density lipoprotein (HDL).

ApoB-100 The major apolipoprotein of very-low-density lipoprotein (VLDL) and low-density lipoprotein (LDL).

ApoB-48 The major apolipoprotein of chylomicrons.

ApoC-II An apolipoprotein that activates lipoprotein lipase.

ApoE An apolipoprotein that mediates the endocytosis of remnant particles by binding to hepatic apo-E receptors.

Apoprotein The polypeptide component of a conjugated protein.

Apoptosis Programmed cell death.

Apoptosome A cytoplasmic protein complex that activates caspases, causing apoptosis.

Arachidonic acid A 20-carbon polyunsaturated fatty acid, precursor of prostaglandins and leukotrienes.

Arginase The urea-forming enzyme of the urea cycle.

Aromatase The enzyme that converts androgens to estrogens.

Arrestin A cytoplasmic protein that binds to activated hormone receptors, inactivating them and marking them for endocytosis.

Arsenate A poison that competes with phosphate in many phosphate-dependent reactions.

Arsenite An inhibitor of pyruvate dehydrogenase that binds to dihydrolipoic acid.

Ascorbic acid Vitamin C, a water-soluble antioxidant.

Asialoglycoprotein Glycoprotein that has lost the terminal sialic acid residues from its oligosaccharides; undergoes endocytosis by the liver.

Aspartate transaminase Serum enzyme, levels of which are elevated in liver diseases, muscle diseases, and acute myocardial infarction.

Ataxia-telangiectasia A syndrome that is caused by impaired repair of DNA double-strand breaks.

Atheromatous plaque The typical lesion of atherosclerosis.

Adenosine triphosphate (ATP) The "energetic currency" of the cell.

Atrial natriuretic factor A hormone from the heart that stimulates a membrane-bound guanylate cyclase.

Autosome Non–sex chromosome.

Avidin A biotin-binding protein in egg white.

Azaserine An antineoplastic drug that inhibits the use of glutamine for nucleotide biosynthesis.

B lymphocyte A type of lymphocyte that produces membrane-bound immunoglobulin.

Bacteriophages "Phages"; bacteria-infecting viruses.

Basal metabolic rate The energy consumed in the absence of physical activity.

Basal mutation rate The mutation rate in the absence of mutagens.

Base A proton acceptor.

Base excision repair Removal of an abnormal base by a DNA glycosylase.

Base pairing The specific interaction between two bases in opposite strands of a double-stranded nucleic acid.

Base stacking The noncovalent interaction between successive bases within a nucleic acid strand.

Basement membrane An extracellular matrix structure beneath single-layered epithelia.

Bence Jones protein Immunoglobulin light chains overproduced by some patients with multiple myeloma (a malignant plasma cell dyscrasia).

Beriberi Thiamine deficiency, with severe neuromuscular weakness.

Bile acids Emulsifiers in bile; required for lipid absorption.

Bilirubin A yellow pigment formed from biliverdin.

Biliverdin A green pigment formed from heme.

Biotin The prosthetic group of carboxylase enzymes.

2,3-Bisphosphoglycerate (BPG) An allosteric effector that reduces the oxygen affinity of hemoglobin.

Blood group substances Polymorphic constituents of the erythrocyte membrane.

Body mass index Weight/height^2.

Bohr effect Decrease in the oxygen-binding affinity of hemoglobin at low pH.

BRCA1, BRCA2 Two tumor suppressor genes associated with inherited susceptibility to breast and ovarian cancers.

Bromouracil An analog of thymine that causes mutations after being incorporated in DNA.

Brush border enzymes Enzymes on the luminal surface of intestinal mucosal cells.

Buffer A solution whose pH value is stabilized by the presence of ionizable groups.

Burkitt lymphoma A B cell malignancy in which the *myc* proto-oncogene has been translocated to an immunoglobulin locus.

C-peptide A biologically inactive fragment of proinsulin that is released together with insulin (C = connecting).

C-reactive protein The most sensitive acute-phase reactant.

Cadherins Membrane-spanning cell adhesion proteins in the zonula adherens.

Calcitriol 1,25-Dihydroxycholecalciferol, the active form of vitamin D.

Calcium channel blockers Drugs that block voltage-gated calcium channels in excitable cells.

Calmodulin A calcium-dependent enzyme activator.

Cap A methylguanosine-containing structure at the 5′ end of eukaryotic messenger RNA.

Capsid The protein coat of the virus particle.

Carbamino hemoglobin Hemoglobin with carbon dioxide covalently bound to its terminal amino groups.

Carbamoyl phosphate An intermediate in the synthesis of urea and pyrimidines.

Carbohydrate loading A procedure aimed at the buildup of large muscle glycogen stores in endurance athletes.

α-Carbon The carbon next to the carboxyl carbon.

Carbon monoxide A competitive inhibitor of oxygen binding to hemoglobin and myoglobin.

Carbonic anhydrase An enzyme that establishes equilibrium among carbon dioxide, water, and carbonic acid.

γ-Carboxyglutamate A post-translationally formed amino acid in prothrombin and factors VII, IX, and X.

Carboxypeptidases A and B Two pancreatic carboxypeptidases.

Carcinoma Cancer of epithelial tissues.

Cardiolipin A phosphoglyceride in the inner mitochondrial membrane.

Cardiotonic steroids A class of drugs that inhibit the sodium-potassium ATPase.

Carnitine A coenzyme that carries long-chain fatty acids into the mitochondrion.

Carnosine The dipeptide β-alanyl-histidine; used as a pH buffer in muscle tissue.

Carotenes Dietary precursors of vitamin A in vegetables.

Caspases Proteases whose activation triggers apoptosis.

Catabolic pathway Degradative pathway.

Catabolite repression Repression of catabolic operons in the presence of glucose.

Catalase A hydrogen peroxide-degrading enzyme.

Catalytic rate constant The rate constant k_{cat} that describes the rate of product formation from the enzyme-substrate complex.

Catecholamines Biogenic amines derived from tyrosine: dopamine, norepinephrine, and epinephrine.

Cation Positively charged ion.

cDNA library A collection of complementary DNA (cDNA)–containing bacterial clones.

Centromere The region of the chromosome that interacts with microtubules during mitosis.

Ceramide A lipid consisting of sphingosine and a fatty acid.

Cerebrosides Sphingolipids containing a monosaccharide.

Ceruloplasmin A copper-containing plasma protein.

Chaperone A protein that assists in the folding of other proteins.

Chirality Optical isomerism, created by alternative configurations of substituents around an asymmetrical carbon.

Cholera toxin The enterotoxin of *Vibrio cholerae*. Causes cAMP accumulation in the intestinal mucosa by covalent modification of the G_s protein.

Cholestasis Lack of bile flow.

Cholesterol The only important membrane steroid in humans.

Cholesterol ester transfer protein A protein that transfers cholesterol esters from high-density lipoprotein (HDL) to other lipoproteins.

Cholesterol esters Esters of cholesterol with a fatty acid.

Cholestyramine A bile acid–binding resin that is used as a cholesterol-lowering agent.

Choline-acetyltransferase The acetylcholine-synthesizing enzyme in nerve terminals.

Cholinesterase A serum enzyme that participates in the metabolism of some drugs.

Choluric jaundice Jaundice accompanied by the urinary excretion of bilirubin diglucuronide.

Chondrodysplasias A group of skeletal deformity syndromes, often caused by abnormal cartilage collagens.

Chondroitin sulfate The most abundant glycosaminoglycan (GAG) in many connective tissues.

Chromatin DNA complexed with histones.

Chromosome A large, double-stranded DNA molecule with associated proteins.

Chylomicrons Lipoproteins that carry dietary lipids from the intestine to other tissues.

Chymotrypsin A serine protease from the pancreas.

Cirrhosis Fibrous degeneration of the liver.

Class switching A change in the class of the immunoglobulin expressed by a B lymphocyte.

Clathrin The protein that forms the coat of coated vesicles.

Clonal selection Selective growth stimulation by an antigen of a B cell clone carrying a matching surface antibody.

Clone A population of genetically identical cells that are all descended from the same ancestral cell.

Cloning vector A plasmid or bacteriophage into which cloned DNA is integrated.

Cobalamin Vitamin B_{12}.

Cockayne syndrome Inherited defects of transcription-coupled nucleotide excision repair, with neurological degeneration and early senility.

Coding strand The strand of a gene whose base sequence corresponds to the base sequence of the RNA transcript.

Codon A base triplet on messenger RNA that specifies an amino acid.

Coenzyme A (CoA) A cosubstrate that forms energy-rich thioester bonds with many organic acids.

Coiled coil Two or three α helices coiled around each other.

Colchicine An alkaloid that inhibits the formation of microtubules.

Collagen A family of fibrous proteins in the extracellular matrix, with a characteristic triple-helical structure.

Colloid-osmotic pressure The osmotic pressure of macromolecules.

Committed step The first irreversible reaction unique to a pathway.

Competitive inhibition Inhibition by an agent that binds noncovalently to the active site of the enzyme.

Complementary DNA (cDNA) The double-stranded DNA copy of a single-stranded RNA.

Compound heterozygote Person who carries two different mutations in different copies of the same gene.

Catechol-*O*-methyltransferase (COMT) A catecholamine-inactivating enzyme.

Condensation reaction Bond formation with release of a water molecule.

Conformation The noncovalent higher order structure of a protein.

Conjugation Transfer of a self-transmissible plasmid from one cell to another.

Conjugation reactions Reactions in which a hydrophilic molecule becomes covalently linked to a chemical.

Connexin A channel-forming transmembrane protein in gap junctions.

Consensus sequence The sequence of the most commonly encountered bases in a functionally defined nucleic acid sequence.

Constitutive proteins Proteins that are synthesized at all times.

Contact inhibition Inhibition of cell proliferation by contact with neighboring cells.

Contact-phase activation The very first reactions in the intrinsic pathway of blood clotting.

Cooperativity Interactions between multiple binding sites for the same ligand in an allosteric protein.

Copper A trace mineral; present in many enzymes that use molecular oxygen as a substrate.

Cori cycle The shuttling of glucose and lactate between muscle and liver during physical exercise.

Corticosteroids Glucocorticoids and mineralocorticoids; C-21 steroids that are derived from progestins by hydroxylation reactions.

Cortisol The most important glucocorticoid; a stress hormone.

Coumarin-type anticoagulants Vitamin K antagonists, which inhibit the post-translational formation of γ-carboxyglutamate in some clotting factors.

Covalent bond Strong chemical bond formed by a binding electron pair.

Covalent catalysis A catalytic mechanism that involves the formation of a covalent bond between enzyme and substrate.

Creatine A metabolite in muscle that forms the energy-rich compound creatine phosphate.

Creatine kinase An enzyme whose level is elevated in the serum of patients with muscle diseases and acute myocardial infarction.

cAMP response element–binding protein (CREB) Protein that mediates effects of cyclic cAMP on gene transcription.

Cretinism The result of untreated congenital hypothyroidism; characterized by mental deficiency and growth retardation.

Crigler-Najjar syndrome Inherited defect of bilirubin conjugation.

Crossing-over The exchange of DNA between homologous chromosomes during meiosis and (rarely) mitosis.

Cryoprecipitate A plasma protein preparation enriched in some clotting factors.

Curare An arrow poison that blocks acetylcholine receptors in the neuromuscular junction.

Cyanide A poison that prevents the reduction of molecular oxygen by cytochrome oxidase.

Cyanosis Blue discoloration of mucous membranes in patients with hypoxia.

Cyclic adenosine monophosphate (cAMP) A second messenger of many hormones.

Cyclic guanosine monophosphate (cGMP) Another second messenger in many cells.

Cyclin-dependent kinases (CDKs) Important as positive regulators of cell cycle progression.

Cyclins Activators of nuclear protein kinases; regulate cell cycle progression.

Cyclooxygenase The key enzyme for the synthesis of prostaglandins, prostacyclin, and thromboxane.

Cystine A dimer of two cysteines.

Cystinuria An inherited defect in the transport of dibasic amino acids in kidney and intestine; causes kidney stones.

Cytidine diphosphate (CDP)–diacylglycerol An activated form of phosphatidic acid for the synthesis of phosphoglycerides.

Cytochrome P-450 A large family of heme-containing proteins that participate in monooxygenase reactions.

Cytochromes Heme proteins that function as electron carriers.

Cytokines Biologically active protein products released by activated lymphocytes and monocytes/macrophages.

Death receptors Receptors for extracellular ligands; their activation triggers apoptosis.

7-Dehydrocholesterol A steroid that is photochemically cleaved to cholecalciferol (vitamin D_3) in the skin.

Dehydrogenase reactions Hydrogen transfer reactions.

Delayed-response genes Genes whose expression is indirectly stimulated by growth factors.

Denaturation Destruction of a protein's higher order structure.

Desaturases Enzymes that introduce double bonds into fatty acids.

Desferrioxamine An iron chelator; used to treat iron overload in anemic patients.

Desmolase A mitochondrial enzyme system that cleaves the side chain of cholesterol, producing pregnenolone.

Desmosine A covalent crosslink in elastin.

Desmosomes Spot welds that hold neighboring cells together.

1,2-Diacylglycerol A second messenger formed by phospholipase C.

Dialysis Removal of small molecules and inorganic ions through a semipermeable membrane.

Diastereomers Geometric isomers.

Dideoxyribonucleotides Nucleotide analogs that are used for chain termination in DNA sequencing and other applications.

Diglyceride Structure formed from glycerol and two fatty acids.

Dihydrofolate reductase An enzyme that reduces dihydrofolate to tetrahydrofolate.

Dihydrotestosterone A potent androgen formed from testosterone by 5α-reductase in androgen target tissues.

Diphtheria toxin A bacterial toxin that inactivates an elongation factor of eukaryotic protein synthesis.

Diploid Containing two copies of each chromosome.

Dipole A structure with asymmetrical distribution of electric charges.

Dipole-dipole interaction Attraction force between the components of two polarized bonds.

Dissociation constant (K_D) A measure for the affinity between a protein and its ligand.

Disulfide bond A covalent bond formed by an oxidative reaction between two sulfhydryl groups.

Disulfiram Antabuse; an aldehyde dehydrogenase inhibitor used for the treatment of alcoholism.

DNA fingerprinting DNA-based methods for the identification of persons in criminal cases.

DNA glycosylases Enzymes that remove abnormal bases from DNA.

DNA ligase An enzyme linking two DNA strands.

DNA methylation A covalent modification of DNA that suppresses transcription.

DNA polymerases DNA-synthesizing enzymes.

Dolichol phosphate A lipid that participates in the synthesis of N-linked oligosaccharides in glycoproteins.

Dominant Determining the phenotype in the heterozygous (as well as the homozygous) state.

Dot blotting A rapid screening method for mutations and DNA polymorphisms.

Down-regulation A long-term type of desensitization that can be overcome only by the synthesis of new protein.

Duchenne muscular dystrophy A severe inherited muscle disease caused by defects of the structural protein dystrophin.

Dynein An ATP-hydrolyzing molecular motor in cilia and flagella.

E2F A transcription factor that is negatively regulated by the retinoblastoma protein.

E6, E7 The oncogenes of the human papillomavirus; they bind and inactivate p53 and pRB, respectively.

Early-response genes Genes whose transcription is induced within approximately 15 minutes after mitogen treatment.

Edema Abnormal fluid accumulation in the interstitial tissue spaces.

Epidermal growth factor (EGF) A growth factor that is mitogenic for many cell types.

Ehlers-Danlos syndrome A type of connective tissue disease characterized by stretchy skin and loose joints; some types are caused by abnormalities of collagen structure or biosynthesis.

Elastase An endopeptidase from pancreas and other sources.

Elastin The major component of elastic fibers.

Electrogenic transport Net transport of electrical charges across a membrane.

Electronegativity The tendency of an atom to attract electrons.

Electrophoresis Separation of molecules in an electrical field.

Electrostatic interaction "Salt bond"; the attraction force between oppositely charged ions.

Emphysema A lung disease, characterized by degeneration of the alveolar walls.

Enantiomers Isomers that are mirror images.

Endergonic reaction Reaction with positive ΔG.

Endocytosis Cellular uptake of soluble macromolecules through an endocytic vesicle.

Endoglycosidases Enzymes that cleave internal glycosidic bonds in complex carbohydrates.

Endonucleases Enzymes cleaving internal phosphodiester bonds in a nucleic acid.

Endopeptidases Enzymes that cleave internal peptide bonds in polypeptides.

Endorphins Peptides with agonist effects on opiate receptors.

Endosome An organelle derived from endocytotic vesicles.

Endosymbiont hypothesis The hypothesis that mitochondria (and chloroplasts) are derived from symbiotic prokaryotes.

Endothermic reaction Reaction with positive ΔH.

Energy charge A measure for the energy status of a cell.

Energy-rich bonds Bonds whose hydrolysis releases an unusually large amount of energy.

Enhancement engineering Attempts to improve the genetic constitution of healthy people by DNA manipulations.

Enhancers DNA sequences that increase the rate of transcription by binding regulatory proteins.

Enterohepatic circulation The cycling of bile acids (and other compounds) through liver and intestine.

Enteropeptidase An enzyme that activates trypsinogen in the duodenum.

Enthalpy The energy content of a molecule.

Entropy The randomness of a thermodynamic system.

Envelope A membrane, acquired from the host cell, that surrounds many animal viruses.

Enzyme-substrate complex Enzyme with a noncovalently bound substrate.

Epidermolysis bullosa Inherited skin-blistering diseases caused by abnormalities of proteins in the dermal-epidermal junction.

Epimers Monosaccharides differing in the configuration of substituents around one of their asymmetrical carbons.

Epinephrine Synonym for adrenaline, a stress hormone from the adrenal medulla.

Equilibrium constant A thermodynamic constant that is defined as product concentration(s) divided by substrate concentration(s) at equilibrium.

Erythropoietin A kidney-derived growth factor that stimulates erythropoiesis in the bone marrow.

Escherichia coli (E. coli) An intestinal bacterium.

Estrogens 18-Carbon steroids, synthesized from androgens by the aromatization of ring A.

Euchromatin A dispersed, transcriptionally active form of chromatin.

Eukaryotes Cells with a membrane-bounded nucleus.

Exergonic reaction Reaction with negative ΔG.

Exocytosis Secretion of water-soluble substances by fusion of an exocytic vesicle with the plasma membrane.

Exons The parts of the gene that are represented in the mature RNA.

Exonucleases Enzymes cleaving terminal phosphodiester bonds in a nucleic acid.

Exothermic reaction Reaction with negative ΔH.

Expressed sequence tags Expressed sections of DNA; identified by the reverse transcription of their RNA transcripts.

Expression cloning Cloning of cDNA for the synthesis of the encoded protein.

Extracellular signal regulated kinases (ERKs) Serine/threonine kinases of the mitogen-activated protein (MAP) kinase family.

F factor A self-transmissible plasmid in *Escherichia coli*.

Fab The antigen-binding fragment of immunoglobulins.

Facilitated diffusion A passive type of carrier-mediated transport.

Familial combined hyperlipoproteinemia A genetic predisposition to type II and type IV hyperlipoproteinemia.

Familial hypercholesterolemia Inherited deficiency of low-density lipoprotein (LDL) receptors.

Fatty streak Accumulation of cholesterol esters in arterial walls.

Fc The crystallizable fragment of immunoglobulins, formed from the carboxyl-terminal halves of the heavy chains.

Feedback inhibition Inhibition of a metabolic pathway by its end product.

Feedforward stimulation Stimulation of a metabolic pathway by its substrate.

Ferritin The principal intracellular iron storage protein; trace amounts also are present in the plasma.

α-Fetoprotein A fetal plasma protein, levels of which are elevated in serum of patients with liver cancer and in amniotic fluid if the fetus has an open neural tube defect.

Fibrate drugs Pharmacological activators of peroxisome proliferator–activated receptor α (PPAR-α), used as lipid-lowering drugs.

Fibrinogen The circulating precursor of fibrin.

Fibronectin A multiadhesive glycoprotein with binding affinities for cell surfaces and extracellular matrix constituents.

First-order reaction Reaction whose velocity is proportional to the concentration of one substrate.

Flavin adenine dinucleotide (FAD) A hydrogen-transferring prosthetic group of flavoproteins.

Flavoproteins Proteins containing flavin adenine dinucleotide (FAD) or flavin mononucleotide (FMN) as a prosthetic group; participate in hydrogen transfer reactions.

Fluid-mosaic model A model of membrane structure that assumes globular proteins embedded in a lipid bilayer.

Fluorouracil A base analog used in cancer chemotherapy.

Foam cell A macrophage filled with droplets of cholesterol esters.

Follicular hyperkeratosis Gooseflesh; occurs in deficiency of vitamin C and vitamin A.

fos An oncogene or proto-oncogene coding for a nuclear transcription factor.

Frameshift mutation Insertion or deletion that changes the reading frame of the messenger RNA.

Free energy The "useful" energy in chemical reactions.

Fructokinase The enzyme that phosphorylates fructose to fructose-1-phosphate.

Fructose-1,6-bisphosphatase An important regulated enzyme of gluconeogenesis.

Fructose-2,6-bisphosphate A regulatory metabolite that mediates hormonal effects on phosphofructokinase and fructose-1,6-bisphosphatase.

Fructose intolerance Hereditary disorders caused by the deficiency of one of the fructose-metabolizing enzymes.

Furanose ring Five-member ring in monosaccharides.

Futile cycle The simultaneous activity of two opposing metabolic reactions, leading to ATP hydrolysis.

G proteins GTP-binding signal transducing proteins that mediate most hormone effects.

G_0 phase The nondividing state of a cell.

G_1 phase The time between mitosis and S phase.

G_2 phase The time between S phase and mitosis.

Galactokinase The enzyme that phosphorylates galactose to galactose-1-phosphate.

Galactosemia A hereditary disease caused by the deficiency of a galactose-metabolizing enzyme.

β-Galactosidase A lactose-hydrolyzing enzyme.

Gallstones Calculi formed from cholesterol or other poorly soluble substances in the biliary system.

Gangliosides Sphingolipids containing an acidic oligosaccharide.

Gap junction A small aqueous channel connecting the cytoplasm of neighboring cells.

Gas gangrene A severe type of wound infection caused by collagenase-producing anaerobic bacteria.

Gelatin Denatured collagen.

Gene A length of DNA directing the synthesis of a polypeptide.

Gene families Structurally related genes with a common evolutionary origin.

Gene therapy The introduction of a functional gene into the patient's cells.

General transcription factors Promoter-binding proteins that are required for the transcription of all genes by a specified DNA polymerase.

Genomic library A collection of bacterial clones containing fragments of genomic DNA.

Germline The cell lineage that gives rise to gametes.

Gilbert syndrome Benign hyperbilirubinemia caused by a promoter mutation in the gene for bilirubin–UDP–glucuronyl transferase.

Glitazone drugs Pharmacological activators of peroxisome proliferator–activated receptor γ (PPAR-γ) that sensitize cells to insulin.

Globular proteins Proteins with a compact shape.

Glucagon A pancreatic hormone that stimulates the glucose-producing pathways of the liver.

Glucogenic Glucose forming.

Glucokinase The liver isoenzyme of hexokinase.

Gluconeogenesis Synthesis of glucose from noncarbohydrates.

Glucose oxidase test An enzymatic method for the selective determination of glucose in the clinical laboratory.

Glucose-6-phosphatase The glucose-producing enzyme in gluconeogenic tissues and glucose-transporting epithelia.

Glucose-6-phosphate dehydrogenase The first enzyme in the oxidative branch of the pentose phosphate pathway.

Glucose-6-phosphate dehydrogenase deficiency A common enzyme deficiency that leads to hemolytic complications after exposure to certain drugs.

Glucose tolerance test A laboratory test that determines the effect of glucose ingestion on the blood glucose level.

Glucose transporter 4 (GLUT-4) An insulin-dependent glucose carrier in muscle and adipose tissue.

Glutamate dehydrogenase An enzyme that catalyzes the oxidative deamination of glutamate and the reductive amination of α-ketoglutarate.

Glutaminase A hydrolytic enzyme that releases ammonia from glutamine.

Glutathione A tripeptide with reducing properties.

Glutathione reductase An NADPH-dependent enzyme that keeps glutathione in the reduced state.

Glycemic index A measure for the extent to which a food raises the blood glucose level.

Glycerol phosphate shuttle The transfer of electrons from cytoplasmic reduced form of nicotinamide adenine dinucleotide (NADH) to the respiratory chain.

Glycocalyx A carbohydrate coat formed by glycolipids and glycoproteins on the cell surface.

Glycogen phosphorylase The enzyme that cleaves glycogen to glucose-1-phosphate.

Glycogen synthase The enzyme that synthesizes glycogen from UDP-glucose.

Glycolipid A lipid whose hydrophilic head group contains carbohydrate.

Glycoprotein A protein that contains covalently bound carbohydrate.

Glycosaminoglycans (GAGs) Polysaccharides containing an amino sugar in every other position.

Glycosidic bond Bond formed by the anomeric carbon of a monosaccharide.

Glycosyl transferases Biosynthetic enzymes that use activated monosaccharides.

Goiter Hypertrophy and/or hyperplasia of the thyroid gland; seen in some forms of hypothyroidism and hyperthyroidism.

Gouty arthritis Arthritis caused by sodium urate deposits in the joints.

Graves disease An autoimmune disease leading to hyperthyroidism.

Growth factors Soluble extracellular messengers, usually proteins, that stimulate the proliferation or differentiation of cultured cells.

Guanylate cyclases Cyclic GMP-synthesizing enzymes.

Half-life The time that it takes for half of the substrate molecules to react in a first-order reaction.

Haploid Containing one copy of each chromosome.

Haptoglobin A hemoglobin-binding protein in serum.

Hartnup disease An inherited defect in the renal and intestinal transport of large neutral amino acids, with pellagra-like symptoms.

Heinz bodies Abnormal protein aggregates in erythrocytes.

Helicases Enzymes separating the strands of double-stranded DNA.

α Helix A compact secondary structure in proteins that is stabilized by intrachain hydrogen bonds between peptide bonds.

Hematin An oxidized derivative of heme containing a ferric iron.

Hematocrit The percentage of the blood volume that is occupied by blood cells.

Hemochromatosis An iron overload syndrome.

Hemoglobin A_{1c} Hemoglobin A modified by a reaction between terminal amino groups and glucose.

Hemoglobin Bart A γ_4 tetramer, in patients with α-thalassemia.

Hemoglobin H A β_4 tetramer, in patients with α-thalassemia.

Hemoglobin S Sickle cell hemoglobin.

Hemoglobinopathies Genetic diseases caused by abnormalities of hemoglobin structure or synthesis.

Hemolysis Destruction of erythrocytes.

Hemopexin A heme-binding protein in serum.

Hemophilia A group of inherited clotting disorders; the most common is factor VIII deficiency.

Hemorrhagic disease of the newborn A neonatal bleeding disorder caused by vitamin K deficiency.

Hemosiderin A partially denatured form of ferritin.

Hemosiderosis Abnormal accumulation of hemosiderin.

Heparan sulfate A glycosaminoglycan (GAG) in many cell surface and connective tissue proteoglycans.

Heparin A sulfated glycosaminoglycan (GAG) made by mast cells and basophils.

Hepatic coma The result of hyperammonemia in patients with advanced liver cirrhosis.

Hepatic lipase An extracellular enzyme in the liver that hydrolyzes triglycerides and phospholipids in remnant particles and high-density lipoprotein (HDL).

Hereditary nonpolyposis colon cancer (HNPCC) An inherited cancer susceptibility syndrome caused by defects of postreplication mismatch repair.

Hereditary persistence of fetal hemoglobin γ-Chain production in an adult.

Heterochromatin A condensed, transcriptionally inactive form of chromatin.

Heterotropic effects Interactions between different ligands of an allosteric protein.

Heterozygous Carrying two different variants of a gene.

Hexokinase The enzyme that phosphorylates glucose to glucose-6-phosphate.

Hexose Six-carbon sugar.

Hinge region The portion of the immunoglobulin heavy chain between the first and second constant domains.

Histidinemia A relatively benign inborn error of histidine metabolism.

Histones Small, basic proteins that are tightly associated with DNA in chromatin.

Holliday intermediate A cross-shaped intermediate in homologous recombination.

Homocysteine An amino acid derived from methionine; elevated serum level is a risk factor for atherosclerosis.

Homocystinuria An inborn error in the metabolism of the sulfur amino acids; it causes skeletal deformities and mental deficiency.

Homologous recombination A reciprocal exchange of DNA between two DNA molecules of related sequence.

Homotropic effects Interactions between identical ligands of an allosteric protein.

Homozygous Carrying two identical variants of a gene.

Hormone-sensitive lipase An enzyme in adipose cells that hydrolyzes stored triglycerides.

Human artificial chromosomes Vectors for germline genetic engineering.

Huntington disease An inherited neurodegenerative disease caused by the expansion of a trinucleotide repeat.

Hyaluronic acid A large, unsulfated glycosaminoglycan (GAG), not bound to a core protein.

Hydrogen bond Dipole-dipole interaction involving a hydrogen atom.

Hydrogen peroxide A toxic product of some oxidative reactions.

Hydrolase Enzyme catalyzing hydrolytic cleavage reactions.

Hydrolysis Cleavage of a bond by the addition of water.

Hydrophobic interactions Interactions between hydrophobic groups, resulting from reduction of the aqueous-nonpolar interface.

3-Hydroxy-3-methylglutaryl–coenzyme A (HMG-CoA) reductase The regulated enzyme of cholesterol synthesis.

Hydroxyapatite The major inorganic component of bone.

Hydroxyl radical An extremely reactive and highly toxic byproduct of oxidative metabolism.

Hydroxylase Enzyme that introduces a hydroxyl group in its substrate.

7α-Hydroxylase The regulated enzyme of bile acid synthesis.

Hyperammonemia Too much ammonia in the blood.

Hyperbilirubinemia Too much bilirubin in the blood.

Hyperlipidemia Too much lipid in the blood.

Hyperuricemia Too much uric acid in the blood.

Hypervariable regions The most variable parts of the variable domains in the immunoglobulins; sites of contact with the antigen.

Hypoglycemic shock Brain dysfunction resulting from lack of blood glucose.

Hypoxanthine A deamination product of adenine.

Hypoxanthine-guanine phosphoribosyltransferase (HGPRT) The most important salvage enzyme for purine bases.

Hypoxia Partial oxygen deficiency.

I-cell disease A lysosomal storage disease caused by the misrouting of lysosomal enzymes.

Immotile cilia syndrome A type of inherited disease caused by abnormalities of structural proteins in cilia and flagella.

Imprinting The silencing of specific genes in the germline, usually by DNA methylation.

Induced-fit model A model that assumes a flexible substrate-binding site in the enzyme.

Inducible proteins Proteins whose synthesis is regulated.

Inosine A nucleoside containing hypoxanthine and ribose.

Insertion sequence A mobile element in prokaryotes that contains a gene for transposase.

In situ hybridization Applying a fluorescent-labeled probe to intact chromosomes.

Insulinoma An insulin-secreting tumor of pancreatic β cells.

Integral membrane proteins Proteins that are embedded in the lipid bilayer.

Integrases Enzymes that catalyze site-specific recombination.

Integrins Integral membrane proteins that function as receptors for components of the extracellular matrix.

Intermediate filament A type of cytoskeletal fiber formed from proteins in a coiled coil conformation.

International unit (IU) The enzyme activity that converts 1 μmol of substrate to product per minute.

Interspersed elements Repetitive, mobile DNA sequences in eukaryotic genomes.

Intrinsic factor A glycoprotein from parietal cells in the stomach, required for efficient vitamin B_{12} absorption.

Introns The parts of a gene that do not appear in the mature, functional RNA product.

Ion channel A pore in the membrane that is selectively permeable for specific ions.

Ion-dipole interaction Attraction force between an ion and a component of a polarized bond.

Inositol 1,4,5-trisphosphate (IP₃) A second messenger formed by phospholipase C; releases calcium from the endoplasmic reticulum.

Iron-sulfur proteins Nonheme iron proteins that participate in electron transfer reactions.

Irreversible inhibition Inhibition by the formation of a covalent bond with the enzyme.

Irreversible reaction A reaction that proceeds in only one direction under physiological conditions.

Ischemia Interruption of the blood supply.

Isoelectric point The pH value at which the number of positive charges on the molecule equals the number of negative charges.

Isoenzymes Enzymes catalyzing the same reaction but composed of different polypeptides.

Isomerase Enzyme that interconverts isomers.

Isomers Alternative molecular forms with identical composition.

Isoniazid A tuberculostatic that can induce vitamin B_6 deficiency.

Isoprenoids Lipids synthesized from branched-chain five-carbon units.

J chain A polypeptide in polymeric immunoglobulins.

J gene A small gene that participates in the assembly of an immunoglobulin gene in developing B lymphocytes.

Janus kinase (JAK) A type of tyrosine kinase that associates with activated receptors for cytokines, growth hormone, prolactin, and erythropoietin.

Jaundice Yellow discoloration of skin and sclera in patients with hyperbilirubinemia.

jun An oncogene or proto-oncogene coding for a nuclear transcription factor.

Junk DNA Noncoding DNA of unknown function.

Keratin A type of intermediate filament protein in epithelial cells.

Kernicterus Brain damage caused by the deposition of bilirubin in the basal ganglia.

Ketoacidosis A metabolic emergency in patients with insulin-dependent diabetes, involving hyperglycemia, acidosis, dehydration, and electrolyte imbalances.

Ketogenesis Synthesis of ketone bodies.

Ketogenic Ketone body forming.

Ketone bodies Acetoacetate, β-hydroxybutyrate, and acetone.

Ketose Monosaccharide with a keto group.

Kinase An enzyme that transfers a phosphate group from a nucleotide.

Kinetics The description of reaction rates.

Knockout mouse A mouse in which a gene has been disrupted by genetic manipulations.

β-Lactamase Penicillinase; an enzyme that inactivates penicillin and related antibiotics.

Lactate dehydrogenase The enzyme that interconverts pyruvate and lactate.

Lactic acidosis Decrease of the blood pH resulting from lactic acid accumulation.

Lactose intolerance Digestive disturbances after the ingestion of milk or milk products, caused by low activity of intestinal lactase.

Lactose operon An operon in *Escherichia coli* that codes for enzymes of lactose metabolism.

Lagging strand The strand that is synthesized piecemeal during DNA replication.

Laminin The most abundant multiadhesive glycoprotein in basement membranes.

LDL receptor A lipoprotein receptor that mediates the endocytosis of low-density lipoprotein (LDL).

Leading strand The strand that is synthesized continuously during DNA replication.

Leber hereditary optic neuropathy Adult-onset blindness caused by mutations in mitochondrial DNA.

Lecithin Synonym for phosphatidylcholine, a phosphoglyceride.

Lecithin-cholesterol acyltransferase (LCAT) An enzyme in high-density lipoprotein (HDL) that converts free cholesterol into cholesterol esters.

Leptin A hormone-like polypeptide from overfed adipose cells that reduces appetite.

Lesch-Nyhan syndrome A neurological disorder caused by a complete deficiency of hypoxanthine-guanine phosphoribosyltransferase.

Leucine zipper proteins A type of DNA-binding protein.

Leukotrienes Biologically active products formed in the lipoxygenase pathway.

Li-Fraumeni syndrome A cancer susceptibility syndrome caused by germline mutations of the *p53* gene.

Ligand A small molecule that binds noncovalently to a protein.

Ligand-gated ion channels Ion channels that are regulated by the binding of a neurotransmitter.

Ligase A type of enzyme that forms a bond while hydrolyzing a high-energy phosphate.

Lineweaver-Burk plot A double-reciprocal plot that describes the relationship between substrate concentration and reaction rate.

Linoleic acid An ω_6-polyunsaturated fatty acid.

Linolenic acid An ω_3-polyunsaturated fatty acid.

Lipase Triglyceride-degrading enzyme.

Lipofuscin "Age pigment," formed from partially oxidized lipids and partially denatured proteins.

Lipoic acid A prosthetic group of pyruvate dehydrogenase.

Lipolysis Triglyceride hydrolysis.

Lipoprotein A noncovalent aggregate of protein and lipid.

α-Lipoprotein High-density lipoprotein (HDL).

β-Lipoprotein Low-density lipoprotein (LDL).

Lipoprotein(a) A form of low-density lipoprotein (LDL) that promotes atherosclerosis.

Lipoprotein lipase An endothelial enzyme that hydrolyzes triglycerides in chylomicrons and very-low-density lipoprotein (VLDL).

Liposome A bilayer-surrounded vesicle.

Lipoxygenase The key enzyme for the synthesis of leukotrienes and hydroxyeicosatetraenoic acids (HETEs).

Lock-and-key model A model that assumes a rigid substrate-binding site in the enzyme.

Long interspersed elements (LINEs) A type of mobile DNA element in the human genome.

Long terminal repeats The terminal repeat sequences of retroviral cDNAs.

LoxP site Recognition site for the DNA-splicing enzyme Cre recombinase, used for genetic engineering.

Lung surfactant A lipid secretion that reduces the surface tension in the lung alveoli.

Lyase An enzyme that removes a group nonhydrolytically from its substrate.

Lysogenic bacterium A bacterium that harbors a prophage.

Lysogenic pathway A reproductive strategy of some bacteriophages that involves the integration of the viral DNA into the host-cell chromosome.

Lysophosphoglyceride A phosphoglyceride with one fatty acid missing.

Lysozyme An enzyme that cleaves a bacterial cell wall polysaccharide.

Lysyl oxidase An enzyme that produces allysyl residues in collagen; required for crosslinking.

Lytic pathway The reproductive strategy of bacteriophages that destroy their host cell.

α₂-Macroglobulin A circulating protease inhibitor, with a very high molecular weight (725,000 D).

Malate-aspartate shuttle The reversible shuttling of hydrogen, in the form of malate, across the inner mitochondrial membrane.

Malondialdehyde A chemically reactive product formed during lipid peroxidation.

Mitogen-activated protein (MAP) kinases A family of protein kinases that are activated in response to growth factors or stress.

Maple syrup urine disease An inborn error of branched-chain amino acid metabolism, causing mental and neurological problems.

Marfan syndrome Dominantly inherited disorder caused by abnormalities of the connective tissue protein fibrillin.

McArdle disease Deficiency of glycogen phosphorylase in muscle, causing muscle weakness.

Mdm2 A protein that inactivates the p53 protein.

Megaloblastic anemia A type of anemia characterized by oversized red blood cells, caused by impaired DNA synthesis.

MEK A protein kinase that activates mitogen-activated protein (MAP) kinases by dual phosphorylation on threonine and tyrosine residues.

Melanin The dark pigment of skin and hair.

Melatonin A pineal hormone derived from serotonin.

Mendelian diseases Single-gene disorders.

Menkes disease An inherited defect of copper absorption.

Metallothionein A protein that binds heavy metals.

Metastable Stable kinetically but not thermodynamically.

Metastatic calcification Abnormal calcification of soft tissues.

Methemoglobin A nonfunctional hemoglobin in which the heme iron is oxidized to the ferric state.

Methotrexate An anticancer drug that inhibits dihydrofolate reductase.

Methylation reaction Transfer of a methyl group from one molecule (often *S*-adenosyl methionine [SAM]) to another.

Methylmalonic aciduria Excretion of methylmalonic acid in the urine, caused by an inherited enzyme deficiency or by vitamin B_{12} deficiency.

Micelle Small globule or sheet formed from amphipathic lipids.

Michaelis constant (K_m) The substrate concentration at which the rate of an enzymatic reaction is half maximal.

Microfilaments Cytoskeletal fibers formed by the polymerization of actin.

Microsatellites Very small tandem repeats.

Microsomes Fragments of the endoplasmic reticulum obtained by cell fractionation.

Microtubules Cytoskeletal fibers formed by the polymerization of tubulin.

Minisatellites Small tandem repeats.

Missense mutation Mutation leading to a single amino acid substitution.

Mitogen Mitosis-inducing agent.

Monoamine oxidase An enzyme that inactivates catecholamines and serotonin.

Monoclonal gammopathy Overproduction of a single immunoglobulin by a plasma cell clone.

Monoglyceride Structure formed from glycerol and one fatty acid.

Monooxygenases Enzymes that incorporate a single oxygen atom from molecular oxygen in their substrate.

Monosaccharide Polyalcohol containing a carbonyl group.

Monounsaturated fatty acid Fatty acid with one carbon-carbon double bond.

Messenger RNA (mRNA) Specifies the amino acid sequence during protein synthesis.

Mucopolysaccharidoses Lysosomal storage diseases caused by deficiencies of glycosaminoglycan (GAG)–degrading enzymes.

Muscarinic receptors G protein–linked receptors for acetylcholine.

Mutagen Mutation-inducing agent.

Mutarotation Spontaneous interconversion of anomeric forms in a monosaccharide.

Mutation Heritable change in DNA structure.

Mutational load "Genetic garbage" that accumulates from generation to generation.

myc An oncogene or proto-oncogene coding for a nuclear transcription factor, amplified in many spontaneous cancers.

Myoglobin An oxygen-binding protein in muscle tissue.

Myosin The protein of the thick filaments in muscle.

Myosin light-chain kinase A calcium-calmodulin activated protein kinase that induces contraction in smooth muscle.

Myxedema Hypothyroidism in adults.

N-Acetylglutamate An activator of mitochondrial carbamoyl phosphate synthetase.

N-Acetylneuraminic acid Sialic acid; an acidic sugar derivative in glycolipids and glycoproteins.

N-Linked oligosaccharides Oligosaccharides bound to asparagine side chains in glycoproteins.

Nicotinamide adenine dinucleotide (NAD), nicotinamide adenine dinucleotide phosphate (NADP) Two cosubstrates that accept or donate electrons (+ proton) in many dehydrogenase reactions.

Natural selection The process that removes pathogenic mutations from the gene pool.

Negative control Inhibition of transcription by the binding of a regulatory protein to DNA.

Neoplasia Abnormal growth of either a benign or a malignant nature.

Nephrotic syndrome A type of kidney disease with massive proteinuria.

Niacin Nicotinic acid; also used as a generic name for nicotinic acid and nicotinamide.

Nicotinic receptors Acetylcholine-operated cation channels.

Nitric oxide (NO) An unstable, diffusible messenger molecule produced in endothelial cells and some other tissues.

Nitrogen balance The difference between ingested nitrogen and excreted nitrogen.

Nitroglycerin A vasodilator drug that is metabolized to nitric oxide.

Noncompetitive inhibition Inhibition by an agent that binds the enzyme noncovalently outside its active site.

Nonketotic hyperosmolar coma A metabolic emergency in patients with non–insulin-dependent diabetes, with hyperglycemia and dehydration but no acidosis.

Nonsense mutation A mutation that creates a stop codon.

Nonsteroidal anti-inflammatory drugs (NSAIDs) A class of drugs that inhibit cyclooxygenase.

Nonviral retroposons DNA sequences produced by the reverse transcription of a cellular RNA.

Northern blotting A method for the identification of RNA after gel electrophoresis, through the use of a probe.

Nucleocapsid The particle formed from viral nucleic acid and protein coat.

Nucleoside A structure formed from a pentose sugar and a base.

Nucleosome The structural unit of chromatin, formed from DNA and histones.

Nucleotide A structure formed from pentose sugar, base, and a variable number of phosphate groups.

Nucleotide excision repair A DNA repair system for bulky lesions.

O-Linked oligosaccharides Oligosaccharides bound to hydroxyl groups in proteins.

Okazaki fragments Pieces of DNA synthesized in the lagging strand during DNA replication.

Oleic acid A C-18 monounsaturated fatty acid.

Oligomycin An inhibitor of the mitochondrial ATP synthase.

Oncogene A growth-promoting gene in cancer cells.

Operator A repressor-binding regulatory DNA sequence in bacterial operons.

Operon The unit of promoter, operator, and structural genes in bacteria.

Opsonization The stimulation of phagocytosis by an antibody or other protein bound to the surface of a particle.

Organophosphates Irreversible inhibitors of acetylcholinesterase, used as pesticides and as nerve gases.

Oriental flush Hypersensitivity to alcohol, caused by the deficiency of a mitochondrial aldehyde dehydrogenase in many Asians.

Orotic acid An intermediate of pyrimidine biosynthesis.

Osteogenesis imperfecta Disorder characterized by brittle bones, caused by inherited defects of type I collagen.

Osteomalacia Rickets in adults.

Osteoporosis Disorder in which bones become brittle and fracture easily, common in elderly people.

Oxalic acid A component of kidney stones that can be formed from glycine.

α-Oxidation A minor catabolic pathway that shortens fatty acids by one carbon.

β-Oxidation The major pathway of fatty acid oxidation.

ω-Oxidation Oxidation of the last carbon in a medium-chain fatty acid.

Oxidoreductase Enzyme catalyzing oxidation-reduction reactions.

Oxygenase Enzyme using molecular oxygen as a substrate.

Oxygenation Reversible binding of oxygen.

_p53_ A tumor suppressor gene (and its encoded protein) that is mutated in at least half of all spontaneous cancers.

Palindrome A type of symmetrical DNA sequence.

Palmitic acid A saturated C-16 fatty acid.

Pancreatic lipase The major enzyme of fat digestion.

Pantothenic acid A nutritionally essential constituent of coenzyme A.

Papillomavirus A DNA virus associated with cervical cancer.

Phosphoadenosine phosphosulfate (PAPS) The "activated sulfate" used for sulfation reactions.

Para-aminobenzoic acid (PABA) A constituent of folic acid.

Paracrine signaling The action of an extracellular messenger on neighboring cells within its tissue of origin.

Passive diffusion Diffusion across the lipid bilayer.

Pasteur effect The stimulation of glycolysis under anaerobic conditions.

λ Phage A temperate bacteriophage of *Escherichia coli*.

Proliferating cell nuclear antigen (PCNA) A clamp protein that holds the DNA template during eukaryotic DNA replication.

Polymerase chain reaction (PCR) A method for amplifying selected DNA sequences.

Platelet-derived growth factor (PDGF) Released from activated platelets during blood clotting.

Pellagra Niacin deficiency; symptoms include dermatitis, diarrhea, and dementia.

Penicillamine A metal chelator used to treat Wilson disease and rheumatoid arthritis.

Pentachlorophenol A wood preservative that uncouples oxidative phosphorylation.

Pentose Five-carbon sugar.

Pepsin An endopeptidase in gastric juice.

Peptide bond Amide bond between two amino acids.

Peptidoglycan The major bacterial cell wall polysaccharide.

Peptidyl transferase The enzymatic activity of the large ribosomal subunit that forms the peptide bond.

Peripheral membrane proteins Proteins that are attached to the surface of the membrane.

Pernicious anemia Megaloblastic anemia and neuropathy caused by vitamin B_{12} malabsorption.

Peroxidases Enzymes that consume hydrogen peroxide or organic peroxides.

Peroxidation The nonenzymatic, free radical–mediated oxidation of polyunsaturated fatty acids.

Peroxisomes Catalase-rich organelles that contain oxidative enzymes.

Pertussis toxin A toxin produced by *Bordetella pertussis;* causes cyclic AMP accumulation by covalent modification of the G_i protein.

pH Value The negative logarithm of the hydrogen ion concentration.

Phagocytosis "Cell eating"; the cellular uptake of a solid particle.

Phenylalanine tolerance test A diagnostic test for phenylketonuria (PKU) heterozygosity.

Phenylketonuria (PKU) An inherited deficiency of phenylalanine hydroxylase, causing mental retardation.

Phenylpyruvate A phenylalanine-derived metabolite in phenylketonuria (PKU).

Phorbol esters Tumor promoters from croton oil; stimulate protein kinase C.

Phosphatase-1 The enzyme that dephosphorylates glycogen synthase, glycogen phosphorylase, and phosphorylase kinase.

Phosphatidic acid Glycerol + two fatty acids + phosphate.

Phosphatidylinositol 3–kinase A lipid kinase that mediates effects of growth factors and insulin.

Phosphodiester bond Bond between phosphate and two hydroxyl groups.

Phosphodiesterases Enzymes that hydrolyze cyclic AMP, cyclic GMP, or both.

Phosphoenolpyruvate (PEP) An energy-rich intermediate of glycolysis and gluconeogenesis.

Phosphoenolpyruvate (PEP)–carboxykinase A gluconeogenic enzyme that is induced by glucagon and glucocorticoids.

Phosphofructokinase The enzyme that catalyzes the committed step of glycolysis

Phosphoglycerides Lipids structurally related to phosphatidic acid.

Phospholipase C A type of enzyme that cleaves phosphoglycerides between glycerol and phosphate.

Phospholipase Cγ (PLCγ) An isoenzyme of phospholipase C that is tyrosine-phosphorylated and activated by growth factor receptors.

Phospholipases Phosphoglyceride-hydrolyzing enzymes.

Phospholipids Lipids with phosphate in their hydrophilic head group.

Phosphopantetheine A prosthetic group of fatty acid synthase.

Phosphoprotein A protein containing covalently bound phosphate.

Phosphoribosyl pyrophosphate (PRPP) The precursor of the ribose in purine and pyrimidine nucleotides.

Phosphorylase A type of enzyme that cleaves a bond by the addition of phosphate.

Phosphorylase kinase A protein kinase that phosphorylates glycogen phosphorylase.

Phosphorylation reactions Reactions in which a phosphate group becomes covalently attached to an acceptor molecule.

Physiological jaundice The common jaundice of newborns.

Phytosterols Steroids from plants.

Pinocytosis Nonselective uptake of fluid droplets into the cell.

pK value The negative logarithm of the dissociation constant for an acid.

Plasmids Circular, double-stranded DNAs that function as "accessory chromosomes" in bacteria.

Plasmin The principal fibrin-degrading enzyme.

Platelet activation A change in shape and membrane structure of platelets, accompanied by the release of various mediators.

Platelet-activating factor (PAF) A soluble, biologically active phosphoglyceride released from white blood cells.

β-Pleated sheet An extended higher order structure in proteins stabilized by hydrogen bonds between polypeptides.

Point mutation Change in a single base pair.

Poly-A tail A structure at the 3′ end of eukaryotic messenger RNA.

Polyacrylamide A type of gel used for the electrophoretic separation of molecules by molecular size.

Polyadenylation signal A conserved sequence at the 3′ end of eukaryotic genes.

Polycistronic mRNA A messenger RNA (mRNA) that has been transcribed from more than one gene.

Polyclonal gammopathy Nonspecific overproduction of immunoglobulins; seen in many diseases.

Polymer A macromolecule consisting of many covalently bonded units (monomers).

Polymerase chain reaction A method used to amplify short segments of DNA.

Polymorphism Sequence variation in DNA.

Polyol pathway A pathway that synthesizes fructose from glucose.

Polyp A benign tumor of mucous membranes.

Polypeptide Polymer of amino acids.

Polysaccharide Polymer of monosaccharides.

Polyunsaturated fatty acids Fatty acids with more than one C=C double bond.

Porphyria cutanea tarda A porphyria characterized by cutaneous photosensitivity.

Porphyrias Diseases caused by an impairment of heme biosynthesis, with the accumulation of biosynthetic intermediates.

Positive control Stimulation of transcription by the binding of a regulatory protein to DNA.

Postprandial thermogenesis Metabolic heat production in response to food intake.

Postreplication mismatch repair A repair system that corrects replication errors.

Post-transcriptional processing Chemical modification of RNA.

Post-translational processing Chemical modification of proteins.

Peroxisome proliferator activated receptors (PPARs) A family of lipid-regulated nuclear receptors.

Preimplantation genetic diagnosis Diagnosis of genetic diseases in the early embryo after in vitro fertilization.

Prenatal diagnosis The diagnosis of diseases in the fetus during early pregnancy.

Pre-procollagen The earliest precursor of collagen.

Primary bile acids Bile acids that are synthesized by the liver.

Primary structure The covalent structure of a protein.

Primase A specialized RNA polymerase that synthesizes a primer during DNA replication.

Probe A labeled oligonucleotide or polynucleotide that is used to identify a specific base sequence in DNA.

Processed pseudogenes Nonviral retroposons derived by the reverse transcription of a messenger RNA.

Processivity The ability of a DNA or RNA polymerase to synthesize long strands without interruption.

Procollagen Pre-procollagen minus the signal sequence.

Progestins 21-Carbon steroids derived from cholesterol, used as precursors for the other steroid hormones.

Prohormone The inactive or less active biosynthetic precursor of an active hormone.

Prokaryote A cell without a nucleus.

Promoter A regulatory DNA sequence at the upstream end of a gene or an operon.

Proopiomelanocortin A prohormone in the anterior pituitary gland.

Propeptides The N- and C-terminal extensions in procollagen.

Prophage The DNA of a temperate bacteriophage after its integration into the host-cell chromosome.

Prostanoids The products of the cyclooxygenase pathway: prostaglandins, prostacyclin, and thromboxane.

Prosthetic group A nonpolypeptide component in a protein.

Proteasome A particle that destroys worn-out cellular proteins.

Protein kinase A The cyclic AMP activated protein kinase.

Protein kinase B (Akt) A protein kinase that mediates effects of growth factors and insulin.

Protein kinase C The diacylglycerol-activated protein kinase.

Protein kinase G The cyclic GMP activated protein kinase.

Proteoglycans Products consisting of core protein and covalently bound sulfated glycosaminoglycans (GAGs).

Proteome The sum total of proteins made by the organism.

Protonation/deprotonation The reversible binding and release of a proton by an ionizable (acidic or basic) group.

Protoporphyrin IX The organic portion of the heme group.

Proximal histidine A histidine residue in hemoglobin and myoglobin that is bound to the heme iron.

Pseudogenes Degenerate, nonfunctional genes that are related to functional genes.

Pseudohypoparathyroidism Reduced responsiveness to parathyroid hormone.

PTEN A lipid phosphatase that hydrolyzes 3-phosphorylated phosphoinositides; the product of an important tumor suppressor gene.

Pyranose ring Six-member ring in monosaccharides.

Pyridoxal phosphate The coenzyme form of vitamin B_6, used as a prosthetic group in many enzymes of amino acid metabolism.

Pyrimidine dimer A DNA lesion caused by ultraviolet radiation.

Pyruvate carboxylase The mitochondrial enzyme that turns pyruvate into oxaloacetate.

Pyruvate dehydrogenase The mitochondrial enzyme complex that turns pyruvate into acetyl-CoA.

Pyruvate kinase The glycolytic enzyme that turns phosphoenolpyruvate (PEP) into pyruvate.

Q_{10} value The factor by which the reaction rate increases in response to a 10° C rise in the temperature.

Quaternary structure The subunit interactions of an oligomeric protein.

R factor A plasmid that carries genes for antibiotic resistance.

Radioimmunoassay A highly sensitive analytical method used for the determination of hormone levels.

raf An oncogene or proto-oncogene coding for a serine/threonine protein kinase.

ras An oncogene or proto-oncogene coding for the Ras protein, a membrane-associated, mitogen-activated G protein.

Rate constant The change in substrate or product concentration per second.

Reading frame The frame in which the codons on the messenger RNA are translated.

Receptor A cellular protein to which an extracellular agent binds and that mediates the physiological effects of this agent.

Recessive Determining the phenotype in the homozygous but not the heterozygous state.

Recommended daily allowances Dietary intakes considered optimal under ordinary conditions.

Reduction potential A measure for the tendency of a redox couple to donate electrons in a redox reaction.

Refsum disease Inherited defect in α-oxidation, causing neurological degeneration.

Remnant particles Lipoproteins that are produced by the action of lipoprotein lipase on very-low-density lipoprotein (VLDL) or chylomicrons.

Repressor A DNA-binding protein that prevents transcription.

Respiratory chain A system of electron carriers (and electron + proton = hydrogen carriers) in the inner mitochondrial membrane.

Respiratory distress syndrome Dyspnea with cyanosis, resulting from insufficient lung surfactant in newborns.

Respiratory quotient The ratio of respiratory CO_2 produced to O_2 consumed.

Response element A regulatory DNA sequence that mediates the effects of a hormone, second messenger, or metabolite on gene transcription.

Restriction endonucleases Bacterial enzymes that cleave specific palindromic sequences in double-stranded DNA.

Restriction fragment DNA fragment produced by a restriction endonuclease.

Restriction site polymorphism A polymorphic cleavage site for a restriction endonuclease.

Retinoblastoma A rare tumor of immature retinal cells in children, occurring in spontaneous and heritable forms.

Retinoblastoma protein (pRB) The "guardian of the G_1 checkpoint," encoded by the retinoblastoma (*Rb*) tumor suppressor gene.

Retinoids The active forms of vitamin A: retinol, retinal, and retinoic acid.

Retinol-binding protein A plasma protein that brings retinol from the liver to other tissues.

Retroposon DNA sequence derived from reverse transcription of an RNA.

Retrovirus A type of virus that inserts a double-stranded DNA copy of its RNA genome into the host cell genome.

Reverse cholesterol transport The transport of cholesterol from extrahepatic tissues to the liver.

Reverse transcriptase A retroviral enzyme that transcribes RNA into a double-stranded DNA.

Restriction fragment length polymorphism (RFLP) DNA sequence variations that can be identified by Southern blotting.

Rhodopsin The light-sensing protein in retinal rod cells.

Radioimmunoassay (RIA) A highly sensitive method for the quantitation of hormones and other substances.

Riboflavin Vitamin B_2, a constituent of flavin adenine dinucleotide (FAD) and flavin mononucleotide (FMN).

Ribonucleotide reductase The enzyme that reduces ribose to 2-deoxyribose in the nucleoside diphosphates.

Ribozyme Catalytic RNA.

Rickets Bone demineralization caused by vitamin D deficiency in children.

Rifampicin An inhibitor of bacterial RNA polymerase.

RNA editing Enzymatic modification of a base in messenger RNA.

RNA interference Selective destruction of a messenger RNA after exposure to the corresponding double-stranded RNA.

RNA polymerases RNA-synthesizing enzymes.

RNA replicase A viral enzyme that synthesizes RNA on an RNA template.

7SL RNA A component of the signal recognition particle and the grandfather of the Alu sequences.

RNase H An enzyme that degrades the RNA strand in a DNA-RNA hybrid.

Rotenone A fish poison that inhibits electron flow through NADH–Q reductase.

Rous sarcoma virus A retrovirus that causes sarcomas in chickens.

Ribosomal RNA (rRNA) A major constituent of the ribosome.

S phase The phase of DNA replication.

Salvage reactions Reactions that convert free bases to nucleotides.

Sarcoma Malignant connective-tissue tumor.

Sarcomere A functional compartment of the muscle fiber.

Sarcoplasmic reticulum The endoplasmic reticulum of muscle cells, specialized as a calcium-storage organelle.

Saturated fatty acids Fatty acids without C=C double bond.

Scanning methods Methods for the detection of unspecified mutations.

Scavenger receptors Lipoprotein receptors with broad substrate specificity that mediate the uptake of low-density lipoprotein (LDL) by macrophages.

Scurvy Disease caused by vitamin C deficiency, with impaired collagen synthesis and connective tissue abnormalities.

Second messengers Small, diffusible molecules that mediate the intracellular effects of hormones.

Secondary active transport Transport that dissipates an ATP-dependent ion gradient.

Secondary bile acids Bile acids that are synthesized from the primary bile acids by intestinal bacteria.

Secondary structure The repetitive folding pattern of a polypeptide.

Secretory pathway The organelles through which secreted proteins are processed: endoplasmic reticulum, Golgi apparatus, and secretory vesicles.

Selectable marker A gene that permits the selective survival of genetically modified cells.

Semiconservative replication The mechanism of DNA replication that leads to a daughter molecule with one old strand and one new strand.

Serotonin 5-Hydroxytryptamine (5-HT), the major indolamine.

Serum Blood plasma from which clotting factors have been removed.

Severe combined immunodeficiency Inherited diseases with combined B cell and T cell defects.

SH2 domain A regulatory domain of many signal-transducing proteins that binds to specific phosphotyrosine-containing proteins.

Shine-Dalgarno sequence A ribosome-binding sequence in the 5′-untranslated region of bacterial messenger RNAs.

Short interspersed elements (SINEs) A form of moderately repetitive DNA.

Sickle cell trait Heterozygosity for hemoglobin S.

Sideroblastic anemia A microcytic anemia in the presence of high iron stores; seen in vitamin B_6 deficiency.

Signal peptidase An enzyme in the endoplasmic reticulum that cleaves off the signal sequence.

Signal recognition particle A cytoplasmic ribonucleoprotein that binds the signal sequence.

Signal sequence An amino acid sequence at the amino end of secreted proteins that directs them to the endoplasmic reticulum.

Sildenafil (Viagra) A phosphodiesterase inhibitor that prevents the degradation of cyclic GMP in the corpora cavernosa.

Silencers DNA sequences that reduce the rate of transcription by binding regulatory proteins.

Single-nucleotide polymorphism (SNP) The most common type of polymorphism in the human genome.

Site-directed mutagenesis The production of specific mutations in the test tube.

Slow-reacting substance of anaphylaxis A mixture of leukotrienes that causes bronchoconstriction in asthmatic patients.

Small nuclear ribonucleoproteins (snRNPs, pronounced "snurps") Components of the spliceosome.

Sodium cotransport A symport system that brings a substrate into the cell together with a sodium ion.

Sodium-potassium ATPase The sodium-potassium pump in the plasma membrane of all cells.

Sodium urate The poorly soluble uric acid salt that deposits in the joints of patients with gout.

Sorbitol A sugar alcohol formed by aldose reductase, intermediate in fructose biosynthesis.

Southern blotting A method for the identification of DNA fragments after gel electrophoresis, with the use of a probe.

Spectrin A membrane-associated cytoskeletal protein in erythrocytes.

Spectrin repeat A three-stranded coiled-coil module in spectrin and dystrophin.

Spherocytosis A group of inherited diseases characterized by sphere-shaped erythrocytes; caused by defects in the membrane skeleton.

Sphingolipidosis Lipid storage disease, a type of disease caused by the deficiency of a sphingolipid-degrading lysosomal enzyme.

Sphingomyelin A phosphosphingolipid.

Sphingosine A long-chain, hydrophobic amino alcohol.

Spike proteins Viral proteins associated with the viral envelope.

Spliceosomes Nuclear ribonucleoproteins that remove introns from primary transcripts.

Spot desmosome A spotlike cell-cell adhesion that is linked to intermediate filaments.

src An oncogene or proto-oncogene coding for a nonreceptor tyrosine protein kinase.

Standard conditions Conditions with 1 mol/liter concentrations of all reactants at a pH of 7.

Statins Lipid-lowering drugs that inhibit 3-hydroxy-3-methylglutaryl–coenzyme A (HMG-CoA) reductase.

Stearic acid A saturated C-18 fatty acid.

Steroids Lipids containing a cyclopentanoperhydrophenanthrene ring system.

Storage disease A type of inborn error of metabolism in which a nonmetabolizable macromolecule accumulates.

Streptokinase A plasmin-activating bacterial protein.

Stress fibers Actin microfilaments underlying the plasma membrane.

Structural gene Gene coding for a functional, nonregulatory protein product.

Substrate The starting material for an enzymatic reaction.

Substrate-level phosphorylation The use of an energy-rich metabolic intermediate for the synthesis of ATP or GTP.

σ Subunit A subunit of bacterial RNA polymerase required for promoter recognition.

Sulfonamides Bacteriostatic agents that inhibit bacterial folate synthesis.

Superoxide dismutase An enzyme that turns superoxide into oxygen and hydrogen peroxide.

Superoxide radical A highly reactive product of oxidative reactions, made by the transfer of a single electron to molecular oxygen.

Supertwisting Overwinding or underwinding of double-helical DNA.

Symport Coupled transport of two substrates in the same direction.

T lymphocytes Lymphocytes possessing no surface antibody but an antigen-recognizing T cell receptor.

Tandem repeats Head-to-tail repeat sequences in eukaryotic genomes.

Tangier disease An inherited disease with near absence of high-density lipoprotein (HDL).

Taq polymerase A heat-stable DNA polymerase used for polymerase chain reaction (PCR).

TATA box A sequence motif in most eukaryotic promoters.

Tay-Sachs disease A lipid storage disease caused by the deficiency of a ganglioside-degrading lysosomal enzyme.

Telomerase An enzyme that extends the telomeres.

Telomere The end piece of the eukaryotic chromosome.

Telopeptides The non–triple-helical end pieces of mature collagen.

Template strand The DNA strand complementary to a newly synthesized DNA or RNA.

Tertiary structure The overall folding of a polypeptide.

Testicular feminization Sex reversal caused by the absence of functional androgen receptor in a genotypic male.

Tetrahydrobiopterin A coenzyme for the hydroxylation of aromatic amino acids.

Tetrahydrofolate The coenzyme form of folic acid. Acts as a carrier of one-carbon units.

Thalassemia Underproduction of hemoglobin α chains (α-thalassemia) or β chains (β-thalassemia).

Thermodynamics The description of reaction equilibria and free energy changes.

Thiamine The dietary precursor of thiamine pyrophosphate.

Thiamine pyrophosphate A prosthetic group that transfers carbonyl compounds.

Thioester bond An energy-rich bond between a sulfhydryl group and a carboxyl group.

Thrombin An activated serine protease in the blood clotting system that acts on fibrinogen and on factors V, VII, VIII, XI, and XIII.

Thromboxane A prostanoid containing a six-member ring structure, produced by platelets and macrophages.

Thrombus A clot formed in an intact blood vessel.

Thymidylate synthase The folate-dependent enzyme that methylates uracil to thymine in deoxyuridine monophosphate.

Thyroglobulin A glycoprotein secreted into the thyroid follicle; precursor of the thyroid hormones.

Thyroperoxidase An enzyme that is required for the iodination and coupling reactions of thyroid hormone synthesis.

Tight junction Belt-like cell-cell adhesion in epithelial tissues that impairs the diffusion of extracellular solutes and of membrane constituents.

Tissue factor A glycoprotein in the plasma membrane of nonendothelial cells, required for the action of factor VII_a.

Titration Treatment of a weak acid or base with a strong base or acid, respectively.

α-Tocopherol The most important form of vitamin E; an important lipid-soluble antioxidant.

Tophi Subcutaneous deposits of sodium urate in gouty patients.

Topoisomerases Enzymes that regulate the supertwisting of double-helical DNA.

Transaminases Enzymes catalyzing the reversible, vitamin B_6–dependent transfer of an amino group from an amino acid to an α keto acid.

Transcription Synthesis of RNA on a DNA template.

Transcription factors DNA-binding proteins that are required for transcription or that increase the rate of transcription.

Transducin A G protein in retinal rod cells that mediates the effects of light exposure on a cyclic GMP-specific phosphodiesterase.

Transduction The cell-to-cell transfer of DNA by a bacteriophage.

Transfection Virus-mediated gene transfer for gene therapy.

Transferase Enzyme that transfers a group between substrates.

Transferrin The iron transport protein in the blood.

Transformation Nonselective uptake of foreign DNA by a cell.

Transgenic mouse Mouse with an artificially inserted gene.

Transglutaminase Clotting factor XIII_a, a fibrin-crosslinking enzyme.

Transition state The most unstable intermediate in a chemical reaction.

Translation Ribosomal protein synthesis.

Translocation (1) Movement of the ribosome along the messenger RNA. (2) Transfer of DNA from one chromosome to another.

Transmembrane helix A membrane-spanning, hydrophobic α helix in integral membrane proteins.

Transposase An enzyme that catalyzes the movement of an insertion sequence or transposon.

Transposon A mobile element in prokaryotes that contains a gene for transposase and other genes.

Transthyretin ("Prealbumin") A plasma protein with binding affinities for thyroxine and retinol binding protein.

Triglyceride Triacylglycerol, a structure formed from glycerol and three fatty acids.

Trimethylamine A fish-smelling product of bacterial glycine degradation.

Triose Three-carbon sugar.

Transfer RNA (tRNA) Brings amino acids to the ribosome.

Tropocollagen The collagen molecule.

Tropomyosin A long, thin, fibrous protein associated with actin microfilaments.

Troponin A calcium-sensing regulatory protein on the thin filaments of striated muscle.

Trypsin A serine protease from the pancreas.

Tryptophan operon An operon in *Escherichia coli* that codes for enzymes of tryptophan biosynthesis.

Tubulin A globular protein that polymerizes into microtubules.

Tumor necrosis factor An apoptosis-inducing cytokine.

Tumor progression The progressive accumulation of oncogenic mutations in neoplastic cells.

Tumor suppressor gene A growth-inhibiting gene in normal cells, whose inactivation contributes to neoplasia.

Turnover number The number of substrate molecules converted to a product by one enzyme molecule per second.

Tyrosinase An enzyme in melanocytes that is required for melanin synthesis.

Tyrosine hydroxylase The enzyme catalyzing the committed step of catecholamine synthesis.

Ubiquinone Coenzyme Q, a lipid that acts as a hydrogen carrier in the inner mitochondrial membrane.

Ubiquitin A ubiquitous protein that marks worn-out cellular proteins for destruction by the proteasome.

Ubiquitin ligases Enzymes that transfer ubiquitin to cellular proteins.

Urea The major nitrogen-containing waste product in urine.

Urease An enzyme in some bacteria and plants that cleaves urea to carbonic acid and ammonia.

Uremia Retention of nitrogenous wastes in patients with kidney failure.

Ureotelic Urea excreting.

Uric acid The end product of purine (but not pyrimidine) degradation.

Uric acid nephropathy Kidney damage caused by urate deposits.

Uricotelic Uric acid excreting.

Urinalysis Semiquantitative determination of urinary metabolites.

Urobilinogens Uncolored products formed from bilirubin by intestinal bacteria.

Urobilins Colored products formed from bilirubin by intestinal bacteria.

Uronic acid pathway The pathway of glucuronic acid metabolism.

Valinomycin A potassium ionophore.

van den Bergh method A colorimetric method for the determination of serum bilirubin.

van der Waals forces Nonspecific attractive and repulsive forces between molecules.

Variable number of tandem repeats (VNTR) Polymorphic microsatellites and minisatellites in eukaryotic genomes.

Very-low-density lipoprotein (VLDL) The lipoprotein that carries triglycerides from the liver to other tissues.

Viral retroposons The remnants of retroviral genomes.

Virion The virus particle.

Vitamin K A fat-soluble vitamin that is required for the synthesis of blood clotting factors.

Voltage-gated ion channels Ion channels that open in response to membrane depolarization.

von Gierke disease Deficiency of glucose-6-phosphatase, causing hepatomegaly and severe fasting hypoglycemia.

von Willebrand factor A plasma protein that mediates the binding of platelets to collagen.

Watson-Crick double helix The principal higher order structure of double-stranded DNA.

Wernicke-Korsakoff syndrome Encephalopathy and amnesia caused by thiamine deficiency in alcoholic persons.

Western blotting A method for the identification of separated proteins, with the use of antibodies.

Wild-type allele The normal form of a gene.

Wilson disease An inherited copper transport defect, with abnormal copper accumulation in liver and brain.

Wobble Freedom of base-pairing between the third codon base and the first anticodon base.

Xanthine oxidase A flavoprotein enzyme that produces uric acid.

Xanthoma Visible subcutaneous lipid deposit.

Xenobiotics Foreign substances without nutritive value.

Xeroderma pigmentosum An inherited defect of nucleotide excision repair, characterized by cutaneous photosensitivity.

Xerophthalmia Dry eyes, in vitamin A deficiency.

Zero-order reaction Reaction whose velocity is independent of the substrate concentration.

Zeta-associated protein 70 (ZAP-70) A protein kinase in T lymphocytes, activated by antigen binding to the T cell receptor.

Zinc A trace mineral in the body; a constituent of many enzymes.

Zinc finger protein A type of DNA-binding protein.

Zonula adherens "Belt desmosome" that holds the cells of single-layered epithelia together.

Zwitterion A molecule that contains at least one positive and at least one negative charge.

Zymogen The catalytically inactive precursor of an enzyme.

Credits

Figure 2.6 Based on illustration © Irving Geis from Dickerson RE, Geis I: The Structure and Action of Proteins. New York: WA Benjamin & Co., 1969. Permission from the estate of Irving Geis.

Figure 2.7 Redrawn from Pauling L: The Nature of the Chemical Bond, 3rd ed. Ithaca, NY: Cornell University Press, 1960. Used with permission of the publisher, Cornell University Press.

Figure 2.9 Redrawn from Richardson JS: The anatomy and taxonomy of protein structure. Adv Protein Chem 34:264-265, 1981.

Figure 3.2 Redrawn from Dickerson RE: The Proteins, 2nd ed. New York: Academic Press, 1964.

Figure 6.8 Redrawn from Devlin TM: Textbook of Biochemistry with Clinical Correlations, 4th ed. © 1997 Wiley-Liss. Redrawn with permission of Wiley-Liss, Inc., a subsidiary of John Wiley & Sons, Inc.

Figure 6.26 Redrawn with permission from Quigley GJ, Rich A: Structural domains of transfer RNA molecules. Science 194:797, 1976. ©1976 American Association for the Advancement of Science.

Figure 8.1 A, Adapted from Kornberg A: DNA Replication. © 1980 WH Freeman and Company. Used with permission. **B,** Adapted from Devlin TM: Textbook of Biochemistry, 4th ed. © 1997 Wiley-Liss. Reprinted with permission of Wiley-Liss, Inc., a subsidiary of John Wiley & Sons, Inc.

Figure 8.12 © Elsevier Trends Journals, 1991. **C,** Modified from Lamb P, McKnight SL: Diversity and specificity in transcriptional regulation: the benefits of heterotypic dimerization. Trends Biochem Sci 16(11):421, 1991.

Figure 10.1 From Behrman RE: Nelson Textbook of Pediatrics, 17th ed. © 2004 Elsevier, p. 385.

Figure 11.16 From Khan J, Simon R, Bittner ML, et al: Gene expression profiling of alveolar rhabdomyosarcoma with cDNA microarrays. Cancer Res 58:5009, 1998.

Figure 13.13 Modified from Stryer L: Biochemistry, 4th ed. New York: WH Freeman, 1995, p 406.

Figure 14.13 From Bowman W: Philos Trans R Soc London Biol Sci 130:457, 1840.

Figure 15.9 Redrawn from Stites PP, Terr AI, Parslow TG: Basic and Clinical Immunology, 8th ed. New York: Appleton & Lange, 1994.

Figure 15.10 A, Modified from Branden C, Tooze J: Introduction to Protein Structure. New York: Garland Publishing, 1991, p 185. **B,** Modified from Silverton EW, Navia MA, Davies DR: Three-dimensional structure of an intact human immunoglobulin. Proc Natl Acad Sci U S A 74:5142, 1977.

Figure 15.12 Redrawn from Stites PP, Terr AI, Parslow TG: Basic and Clinical Immunology, 8th ed. New York: Appleton & Lange, 1994.

Figure 15.13 Redrawn from Stites PP, Terr AI, Parslow TG: Basic and Clinical Immunology, 8th ed. New York: Appleton & Lange, 1994.

Figure 17.3 Redrawn from Unwin N: Neurotransmitter action: opening of ligand-gated ion channels. Cell 72(suppl):31-41, 1993. © 1993 Cell Press.

Case Study: Viral Gastroenteritis Adapted from Montgomery R, Conway T, Spector A, et al: Biochemistry: A Case-Oriented Approach, 16th ed. St. Louis: Mosby–Year Book, 1996.

Case Study: A Mysterious Death Adapted with permission from Hoffman M: Science 254:931, 1991. © 1991 American Association for the Advancement of Science.

Case Studies: A Sickly Child; The Missed Examination Adapted from Folkman J, D'Amore P, Karnovsky M: MAF case 3.91-1: Matthew's feeding difficulties; Birnbaum M: MAF case 8.91-1: Mr. Minkowski's lack of response. Boston: President and Fellows of Harvard College, 1990.

Index

Note: Page numbers followed by the letter f refer to figures and those followed by t refer to tables.